The McGraw-Hill Radiology Series

Series Editor: Robert J. Ward, MD

This innovative series offers indispensable workstation reference material for the practicing radiologist. Within this series is a full range of practical, clinically relevant works divided into three categories:

- **Patterns:** Organized by modality, these books provide a pattern-based approach to constructing practical differential diagnoses.
- **Variants:** Structured by modality as well as anatomy, these graphic volumes aid the radiologist in reducing false positive rates.
- **Cases:** Classic case presentations with an emphasis on differential diagnoses and clinical context.

GENITOURINARY IMAGING CASES

David D. Casalino, MD
Associate Professor of Radiology
Chief, Genitourinary Radiology
Northwestern University Feinberg School of Medicine

Frank H. Miller, MD
Professor of Radiology
Chief, Body Imaging Section and Fellowship
Medical Director, MR Imaging and GI Radiology
Northwestern Memorial Hospital
Northwestern University Feinberg School of Medicine

Paul Nikolaidis, MD
Associate Professor of Radiology
Northwestern University Feinberg School of Medicine

Nancy A. Hammond, MD
Assistant Professor of Radiology
Northwestern University Feinberg School of Medicine

McGraw Hill Medical

New York Chicago San Francisco Lisbon London Madrid Mexico City
Milan New Delhi San Juan Seoul Singapore Sydney Toronto

Genitourinary Imaging Cases

2 3 4 5 6 7 8 9 0 CTP/CTP 14 13 12 11 10

ISBN 978-0-07-147912-7
MHID 0-07-147912-0

Notice

Medicine is an ever-changing science. As new research and clinical experience broaden our knowledge, changes in treatment and drug therapy are required. The authors and the publisher of this work have checked with sources believed to be reliable in their efforts to provide information that is complete and generally in accord with the standards accepted at the time of publication. However, in view of the possibility of human error or changes in medical sciences, neither the authors nor the publisher nor any other party who has been involved in the preparation or publication of this work warrants that the information contained herein is in every respect accurate or complete, and they disclaim all responsibility for any errors or omissions or for the results obtained from use of the information contained in this work. Readers are encouraged to confirm the information contained herein with other sources. For example and in particular, readers are advised to check the product information sheet included in the package of each drug they plan to administer to be certain that changes have not been made in the recommended dose or in the contraindications for administration. This recommendation is of particular importance in connection with new or infrequently used drugs.

This book was set in TradeGothic Light by Glyph International.
The editors were Michael Weitz and Regina Brown.
Project Management was provided by Rajni Pisharody, Glyph International.
The production supervisor was Catherine Sagesse.
The designer was Eve Siegel; the cover designer was the Gazillion Group.
China Translation & Printing Service, Ltd., was the printer and binder.

Library of Congress Cataloging-in-Publication Data

Genitourinary imaging cases / by David Casalino ... [et al.].
p. ; cm.
ISBN-13: 978-0-07-147912-7 (hardcover : alk. paper)
ISBN-10: 0-07-147912-0
1. Genitourinary organs—Imaging—Case studies. 2. Genitourinary organs—Imaging—Atlases. I. Casalino, David.
[DNLM: 1. Female Urogenital Diseases—diagnosis—Atlases. 2. Female Urogenital Diseases—diagnosis—Case Reports. 3. Male Urogenital Diseases—diagnosis—Atlases. 4. Male Urogenital Diseases—diagnosis—Case Reports. 5. Diagnostic Imaging—Atlases. 6. Diagnostic Imaging—Case Reports. 7. Urography—methods—Atlases. 8. Urography—methods—Case Reports. WJ 17 G3305 2010]
RC874.G45 2010
616.6'0754—dc22

2009016002

To my wife, Devora, and our daughter, Kaila.
Thank you for your love, encouragement and patience.

DDC

To my wife, Michelle, children, Scott and Mark, and mother, Relli,
and in memory of my father, Dr. Sheldon Miller.

FHM

To my father, Dr. Demetrios Nikolaidis, who inspired me to pursue a career in academic radiology, and to my mother, Aliki. I thank them both for their love, sacrifices, and endless encouragement and support.

PN

To my husband, Dave, and our children, Brady, Colin, and Bennett.
Thank you for your love, patience, and support.

NAH

CONTENTS

FOREWORD

The depth and breadth of radiology is unlike most other specialties; virtually all human disorders can now be imaged in some way and therefore are under the purview of radiology. In addition, there are few specialties in medicine that are undergoing as much change as radiology. The amount of knowledge that radiologists-in-training must now grasp is greater than ever before. The demands on the practitioner to maintain competency and assimilate new knowledge and advances are extremely challenging and a life-long responsibility.

The subspecialty of genitourinary radiology is a "microcosm" of what is occurring in general radiology. Technological advances in CT, MRI, and ultrasound are replacing older exams, such as intravenous urography. Genitourinary disorders such as prostate cancer, renal cell carcinoma, and gynecologic and testicular cancers, to name a few, simply cannot be managed today without some form of imaging.

Academicians are challenged with the responsibility of educating and training future generations of radiologists, some of whom may become generalists, and others specialists. In either case, learning is a daunting task. To meet the enormous educational demands and time constraints of the radiologist-in-training and the practicing radiologist, many authors are choosing a case-based format when writing textbooks. Indeed, a cursory review of the educational offerings available today will demonstrate that case-based learning is rapidly becoming the norm in textbook writing. The ability to view a large number of cases allows the reader to learn new knowledge rapidly, and in a way that simulates clinical practice.

Drs. Casalino, Miller, Nikolaidis, and Hammond are leading authorities in genitourinary radiology who have assembled a vast and comprehensive array of cases that are a testament to their clinical experience. They have provided a relatively comprehensive treatise that includes both genital and urinary radiology; I doubt many textbooks of this kind include as many illustrative cases across both factions of genitourinary radiology. Their textbook is provided in a readable format that provides key findings, a short, relevant differential diagnosis, and a pithy discussion on each entity. In addition, "pearls" of wisdom are imparted at the end of each discussion in list form and serve as take-home messages. The cases are depicted well with superb images using state-of-the-art US, CT, and MRI examinations; a nice blend of the more 'traditional' techniques such as intravenous urography, retrograde pyelography, and hysterosalpingography are included also. Many cases include images from multiple modalities. In addition, a novel legend is provided with each image that helps readers understand the frequency of the findings. Chapters include common as well as uncommon diseases, and each case is accompanied by related entities. This feature will be particularly helpful to the practicing radiologist, both in forming a differential diagnosis, and selecting which diagnoses are more likely, and why. The authors are to be congratulated for compiling an impressive array of genitourinary radiology cases that will help teach this and future generations of radiologists wishing to learn the burgeoning subspecialty of genitourinary radiology.

Stuart G. Silverman, MD, FACR
Professor of Radiology
Harvard Medical School
Director, Abdominal Imaging and Intervention
Director, CT Scan
Director, Cross-Sectional Interventional Radiology
Department of Radiology
Brigham and Women's Hospital
Boston, Massachusetts

SERIES EDITOR'S FOREWORD

It is with great pride and excitement that we introduce our Genitourinary Cases volume. David Casalino, Frank Miller, Paul Nikolaidis, and Nancy Hammond are recognized experts in genitourinary imaging and have labored hard to bring an astounding breadth and depth of case materials that encompass GU imaging's most essential entities. A veritable feast of GU pathology awaits the reader interested in delving deeper into the common and not-so-common entities encountered in everyday practice.

The text is organized as per the organ system for easy navigation and accessibility. Each case explores common presentations of the entity followed by typical imaging findings, differential diagnoses, a comments section, and useful pearls. The images are strategically formatted with the "index image" (the entity's most representative example) on the left and additional images on the right followed by a useful and practical differential diagnosis section.

The innovative grading system along the right margin indicates the degree to which the images are representative of a case's typical appearance. The scale ranges from "typical" (five squares) to "rare" (one square). Similarly, the differential diagnoses images are graded "common" (five circles) to "unusual" (one circle). The aim is to provide the reader with a sense of appropriateness regarding the practical use of differential diagnoses.

Our ultimate aim for the series is to create a practical resource for radiologists at the workstation for reference on a regular basis. Please look forward to future Cases editions as well as the corresponding Genitourinary Patterns volume featuring extensive differential diagnoses and the Genitourinary Variants volume with its exhaustive cross-modality lists of GU pitfalls and variants.

Congratulations to Drs. Casalino, Miller, Nikolaidis, and Hammond along with their contributors. They have done an exemplary job in creating a practical and comprehensive work.

Robert J. Ward, MD, CCD
Chief, Division of Musculoskeletal Radiology
Department of Radiology
Tufts Medical Center
Director, Medical Student Education
Assistant Professor of Radiology and Orthopaedics
Tufts University School of Medicine
Boston, Massachusetts

Consultant
Sullivan's Island Imaging, LLC
Sullivan's Island, South Carolina

PREFACE

Case-based teaching has long been a tradition in medical education and has enjoyed increasing popularity in radiology as a format for textbooks, web-based education sites, and CME courses. The growing popularity of case-based teaching is not surprising given the practicality of the method. Indeed, radiologists analyze a patient's imaging and clinical information on a case-by-case basis every day in practice, and residents and fellows are required to perform this type of analysis on board examinations. This book is organized in a case-based format with over 1500 images and essential information regarding a wide range of genitourinary tract pathologies and normal variants. The book provides a compilation of the best of the authors' genitourinary tract teaching files with the generous contributions of images from our friends at other academic institutions and from our residents, fellows, and colleagues at Northwestern University.

Genitourinary Imaging Cases consists of 295 cases. Each case features (1) a specific disease process or normal variant, (2) primary and additional images of the entity, (3) common presenting symptoms, (4) concise discussion of the entity's clinical features and common imaging findings, (5) practical differential diagnosis with an emphasis upon distinguishing imaging and clinical features, (6) images of entities in the differential, and (7) a few pearls of wisdom.

While this text is not intended to be a comprehensive radiologic review of all GU tract pathologies and normal variants, those that are most commonly encountered are included in addition to many less common entities. An effort has been made to present the various entities in multiple modalities, including state-of-the-art MR and CT, ultrasonography, and more traditional studies, such as intravenous urography, cystography, and retrograde urography.

We hope you will find *Genitourinary Imaging Cases* an indispensable, efficient reference to be used by radiologists at the workstation or residents as a primer for GU rotations or in preparation for board examinations.

David D. Casalino, MD

ACKNOWLEDGMENTS

We are indebted to many people for helping us complete this book. First and foremost, we would like to thank Laura Merrick for the tremendous work she did in organizing and preparing the manuscript and coordinating communications. David Botos was critical in skillfully preparing images.

We gratefully acknowledge Drs. Earl Nudelman and Suresh Patel and the other members of the Body Imaging Section of the Northwestern University Department of Radiology for contributing many interesting cases to this book and thank them for their encouragement and dedication to teaching.

We thank our residents and fellows throughout the years for contributing to our teaching files, motivating us to strive for excellence in our teaching efforts, and making academic radiology enjoyable.

Finally, we acknowledge the support of the McGraw-Hill team, particularly Michael Weitz, and the efforts of Rajni Pisharody of Glyph International.

DDC, FHM, PN, and NH

I would also like to thank my parents, Connie and Donald, for their support and encouragement; my mentors and former colleagues at the University of Chicago and University of North Carolina at Chapel Hill; my friends and role models in GU radiology and urology; and WJP for his insights and guidance.

DDC

This project would not have been possible without the understanding and support of my wife, Dr. Michelle Naidich Miller, and my sons, Scott and Mark. I would also like to thank my many mentors at Northwestern University, Brigham and Women's Hospital, and Hospital of University of Pennsylvania and colleagues over the years.

FHM

I would like to thank Dr. Nicholas Papanicolaou from the Hospital of University of Pennsylvania for almost two decades of advice and guidance. I would also like to thank my many teachers, mentors and sources, of inspiration at Boston University Medical Center, the MD Anderson Cancer Center, the University of Texas Medical School at Houston, Brigham and Women's Hospital, and Harvard Medical School in Boston. Finally, I would like to thank Amber Mercier for her support and encouragement throughout the process of creating this book.

PN

This book would not have been possible without the help and encouragement from my colleagues and mentors at Northwestern University. I would also like to thank my husband, Dave DuRoss, and three beautiful children, Brady, Colin, and Bennett, for their never-ending support and love.

NAH

CHAPTER 1

SOLID RENAL MASSES

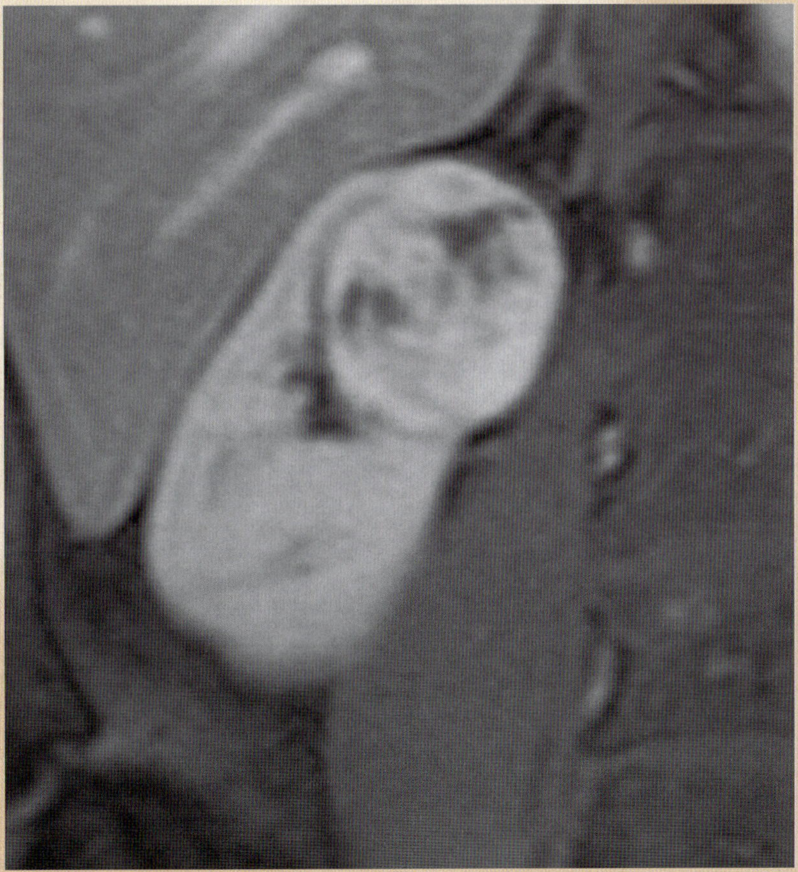

1–1 Clear Cell Renal Cell Carcinoma

David D. Casalino

PRESENTATION

Hematuria and right flank pain.

FINDINGS

MR images demonstrate a right renal round, heterogeneously enhancing mass that is also hyperintense on the T2-weighted image (T2-WI).

DIFFERENTIAL DIAGNOSES

- *Renal cell carcinoma (RCC)*: Papillary and chromophobe RCCs tend to have hypovascularity and intermediate vascularity, respectively, compared to the hypervascularity of most clear cell RCCs, yet there is substantial overlap.
- *Lymphoma*: Usually multiple and bilateral and associated with lymphadenopathy.
- *Metastasis*: Usually multiple and bilateral in patients with a known primary malignancy.
- *Oncocytoma and other benign tumors without detectable fat*: These tumors cannot be reliably differentiated from RCCs based on imaging.
- *Pyelonephritis or abscess*: Findings of pyelonephritis and symptoms of infection are common.

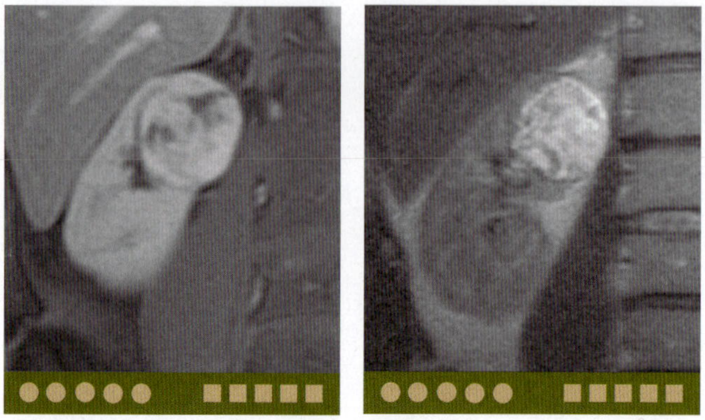

A. Coronal contrast-enhanced T1-WI shows a 3-cm, round, heterogeneously enhancing mass arising from the upper pole of the right kidney.
B. Coronal T2-WI shows the mass to be hyperintense and heterogeneous.

COMMENTS

Approximately 54,000 Americans are diagnosed with kidney cancer and 13,000 die of the disease each year. Renal cell carcinoma comprises approximately 2% of all malignancies, with a median age of 65 years at diagnosis and a slight male predominance. Renal cell carcinoma arises from the renal epithelium and accounts for 85% of renal cancers. Clear cell, or conventional, RCC accounts for 85% of renal cell carcinomas. While the classic presentation of RCC includes flank, pain, hematuria, and a palpable abdominal mass, few patients present with this triad. Renal cell carcinoma is an incidental finding on imaging in approximately 50% of patients. Risk factors for RCC include smoking, obesity, acquired cystic kidney disease, and certain hereditary syndromes, such as von Hippel-Lindau (VHL) disease. For patients with RCC, prognosis is closely related to the tumor grade and stage of disease. Clear cell RCC has a 5-year survival rate of 50% to 60%.

Renal cell carcinoma typically grows by expansion, resulting in a ball-shaped, often exophytic mass. Of the various types of RCC, clear cell tends to enhance most intensely on computed tomography (CT) and MR, yet the degree of enhancement of the tumor subtypes overlaps substantially. Clear cell RCC often enhances heterogeneously because of hemorrhage, necrosis, and/or cystic components. Multilocular cystic RCC accounts for 3% of all cases of RCC and is typically low-grade, clear cell type. Calcifications occur in 20% to 30% of RCC. On ultrasound, RCC may be hypo-, hyper-, or isoechoic. Hyperechoic RCC must be differentiated from angiomyolipomas. On MR, clear cell RCC is typically hypointense on unenhanced T1-weighted images (T1-WI), iso- or hyperintense on T2-WI, and enhances intensely. Some tumors may have sufficient intracellular lipid to result in significant signal loss on opposed phase images.

The treatment of organ confined RCC is usually surgical excision; however, energy ablative therapies are increasingly used in treating small renal cell carcinomas.

PEARLS

- **Clear cell RCC accounts for 85% of renal cell carcinomas and has a 5-year survival rate of 50% to 60%.**
- **Clear cell RCC is typically highly vascular and often heterogeneous.**
- **Multilocular cystic RCC is typically low-grade, clear cell type and cannot reliably be differentiated from multilocular cystic nephroma on imaging.**
- **A hyperechoic renal mass warrants further imaging to determine if it contains macroscopic fat, suggestive of an angiomyolipoma.**

ADDITIONAL IMAGES (C-E)

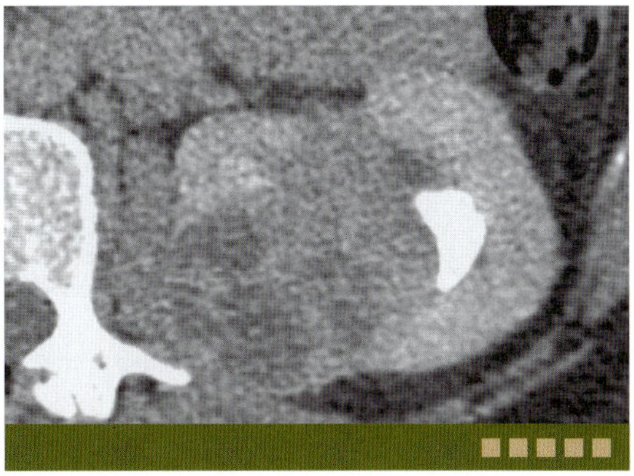

C. Axial CECT, during the excretory phase, from a different patient shows a large, heterogeneous enhancing mass arising from the upper pole of the left kidney.

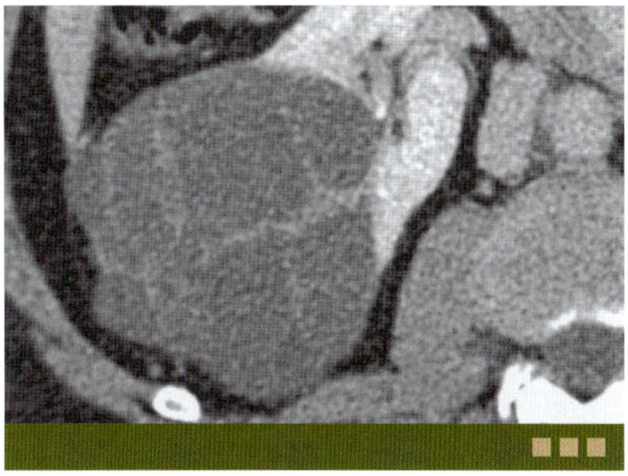

D. Axial CECT shows a large, multiloculated cystic mass with enhancing septations arising from the lateral cortex of the right kidney.

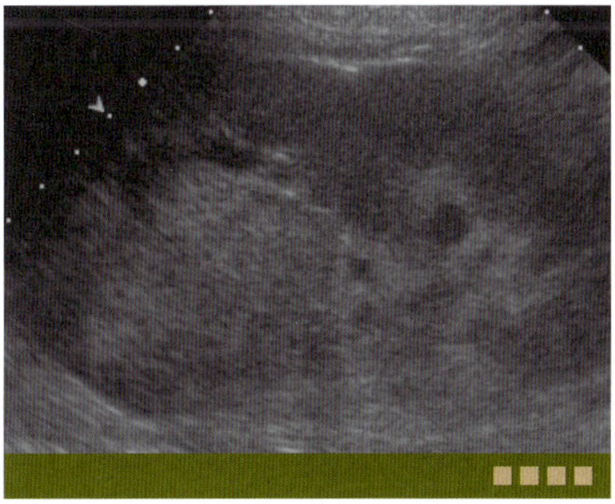

E. Longitudinal sonogram shows a large, heterogeneous, hyperechoic mass arising from the upper pole of the left kidney. Follow-up CT did not show fat within the mass.

DIFFERENTIAL DIAGNOSES IMAGES (F-H)

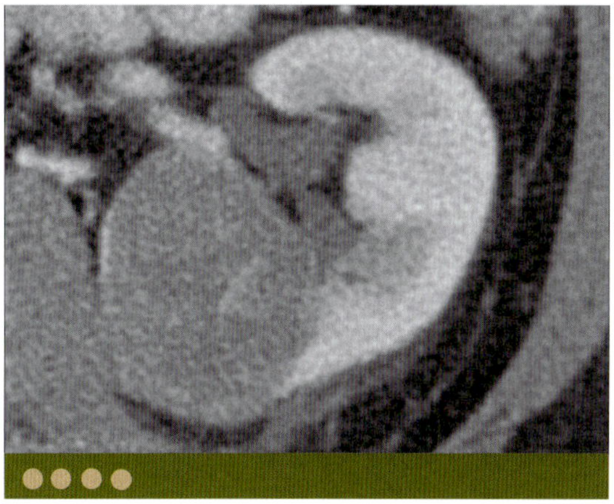

F. Papillary RCC: Axial CECT shows a hypovascular, slightly heterogeneous mass arising from the medial cortex of the left kidney.

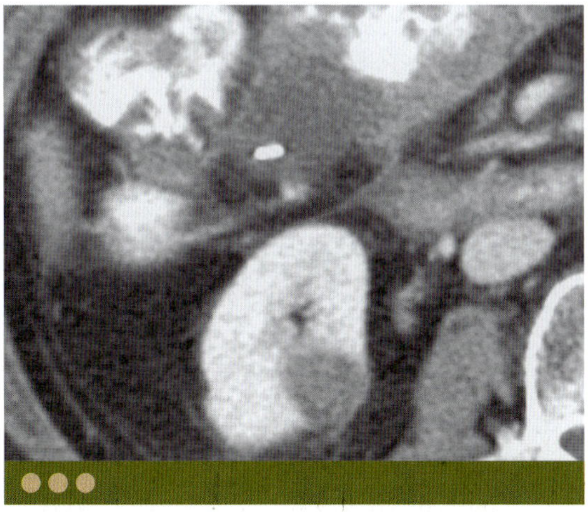

G. Lymphoma: Axial CECT shows an enhancing mass in the medial cortex of the right kidney and adjacent small bowel with gross mural thickening because of lymphoma.

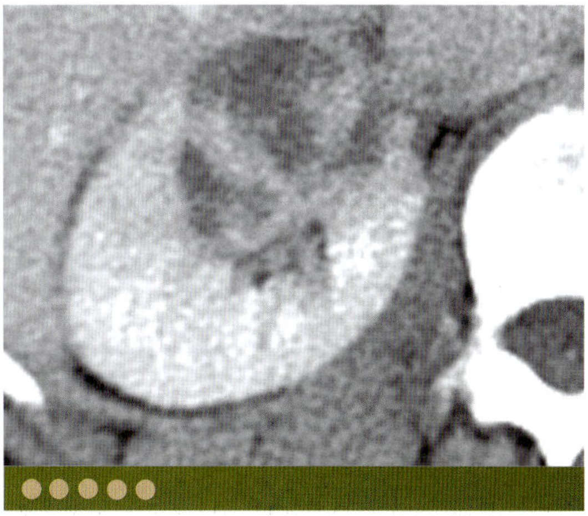

H. Pyelonephritis: Axial CECT shows a round, heterogeneous right renal abnormality in a patient with symptoms of infection and other sites of pyelonephritis in the kidney.

IMAGE KEY

Common

Rare

Typical

Unusual

1–2 Clear Cell Renal Cell Carcinoma with Fat on MR

Frank H. Miller

PRESENTATION

Hematuria, asymptomatic.

FINDINGS

Renal mass which contains microscopic fat and drops in signal on opposed-phase images.

DIFFERENTIAL DIAGNOSES

- *Angiomyolipoma (AML)*: would generally have macroscopic fat and drop in signal on frequency-selective fat-suppressed images.

COMMENTS

Renal cell carcinoma consists of various histopathologic subtypes of which the clear cell subtype is the most common. The intracytoplasmic glycogen and lipid get dissolved during histologic processing, making the cells "clear." Clear cell subtype often appears heterogeneous on imaging resulting from associated hemorrhage, necrosis, and cysts. They show greater enhancement than the other subtypes. They contain intracellular lipid and can be confused with (AML). The amount of lipid is not enough to cause low attenuation fat on CT or show fat-suppression on T1 fat-suppressed images.

Clear cell carcinomas can have microscopic fat and drop in signal intensity on the opposed phase images, as seen in this case. As a result, clear cell cancer can mimic angiomyolipoma. It is important to recognize that the loss of signal on opposed-phase images should not be considered pathognomonic of angiomyolipomas. Unlike angiomyolipomas, clear cell carcinomas do not have macroscopic fat; therefore, they are not high signal intensity on T1-weighted images (unless they bled) and do not drop in signal on the frequency-selective fat-suppressed images. They are typically not hyperintense on T1 in phase images unless they have blood, which would not lose signal on the opposed-phase images. In addition, they do not have macroscopic fat seen as low attenuation on CT scans. Other features to suggest macroscopic fat of an angiomyolipoma includes the presence of India ink or chemical shift artifact on opposed-phase images between the mass and the kidney. If it is unclear if a renal mass is an angiomyolipoma or renal cell carcinoma as it drops in signal on the opposed-phase image, then an unenhanced CT may be helpful.

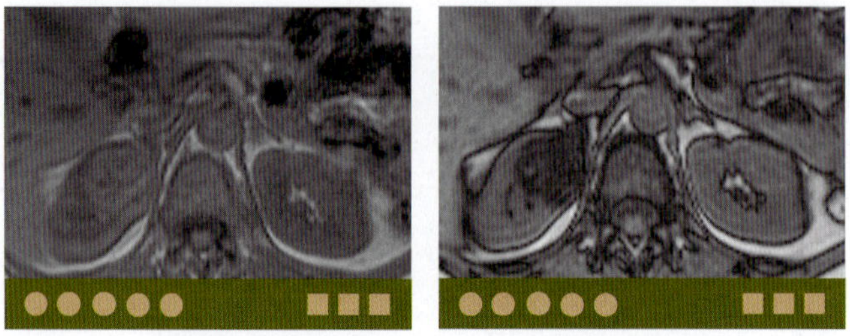

A. Axial in phase T1-WI shows right renal mass (arrow).
B. Axial opposed phase image shows signal loss because of the presence of microscopic lipid in clear cell carcinoma.

Clear cell carcinomas are enhancing masses on MR that are generally iso or hyperintense on T2-weighted images unlike papillary cell carcinomas, which are generally hypointense on T2-weighted images. In addition, microscopic fat may be seen in clear cell carcinomas but generally not papillary renal cell carcinomas.

PEARLS

- **A mass that drops in signal on opposed-phase images is not diagnostic of only angiomyolipoma.**
- **Clear cell carcinomas may contain microscopic fat and drop in signal intensity on the opposed-phase images like angiomyolipomas.**
- **Clear cell carcinomas do not have macroscopic fat and therefore do not drop in signal on frequency-selective fat-suppressed images unlike angiomyolipomas.**
- **CT scans, if necessary, can be helpful in showing that the signal drop associated with clear cell carcinomas is not caused by macroscopic fat.**
- **The use of frequency selective fat suppression is important to distinguish AML, which is high SI on T1 and drops in signal, from clear cell carcinoma, which does not drop in signal on frequency-selective fat suppression.**

ADDITIONAL IMAGES (C-E)

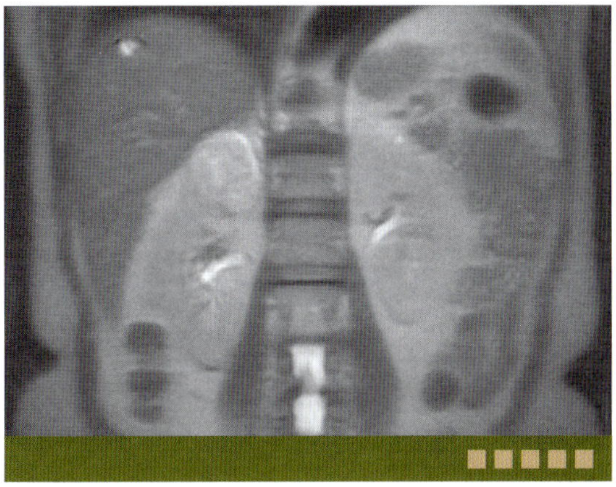

C. Coronal T2-WI shows the lesion is of increased signal. Papillary renal cell carcinomas would generally not be high signal nor contain fat.

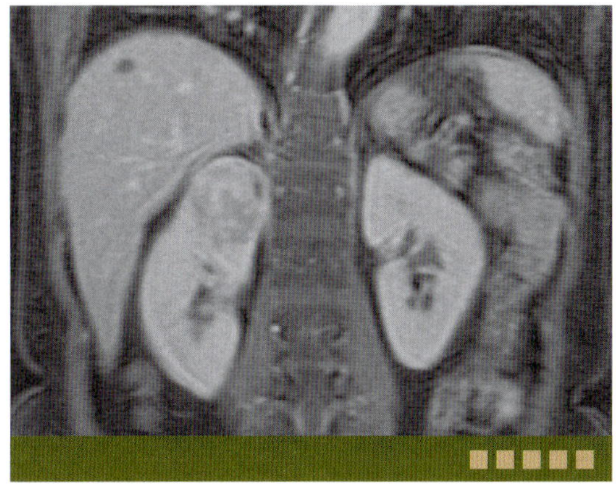

D. Coronal contrast-enhanced T1-WI shows the right upper pole lesion enhances consistent with solid mass because of renal cell carcinoma.

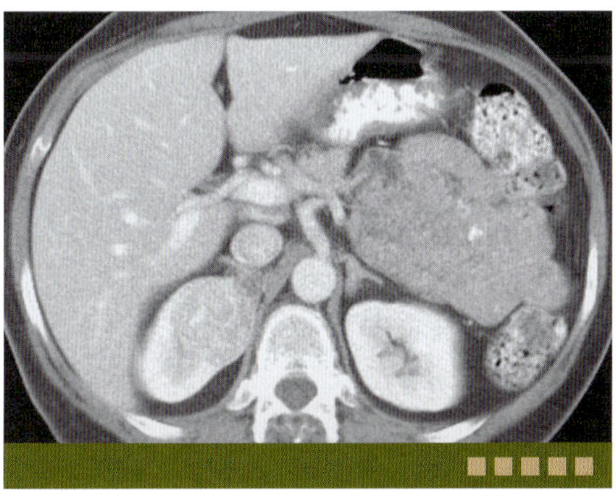

E. Axial CECT shows solid mass which does not contain macroscopic fat to suggest angiomyolipoma.

DIFFERENTIAL DIAGNOSES IMAGES (F-H)

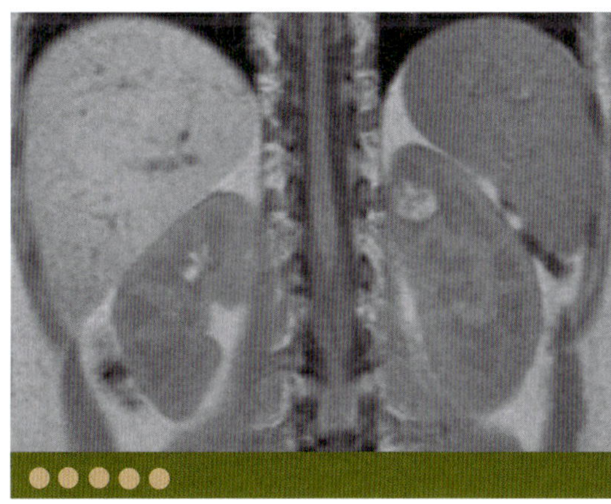

F. Angiomyolipoma: Coronal T1-WI shows left upper pole lesion that is high signal intensity because of fat.

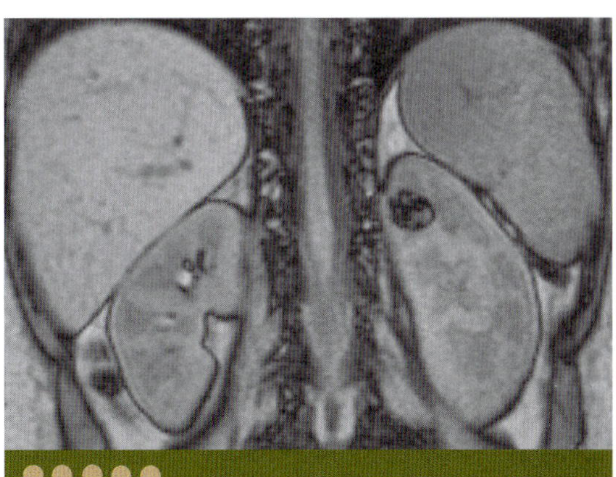

G. Angiomyolipoma: Coronal opposed-phase T1-WI in the same patient shows loss of signal in the lesion from fat in lesion. Based on the loss of signal on opposed-phase images, the lesion could be an angiomyolipoma or a clear cell renal cell carcinoma. The chemical shift artifact between the lesion and the kidney, however,suggests macroscopic fat from an angiomyolipoma.

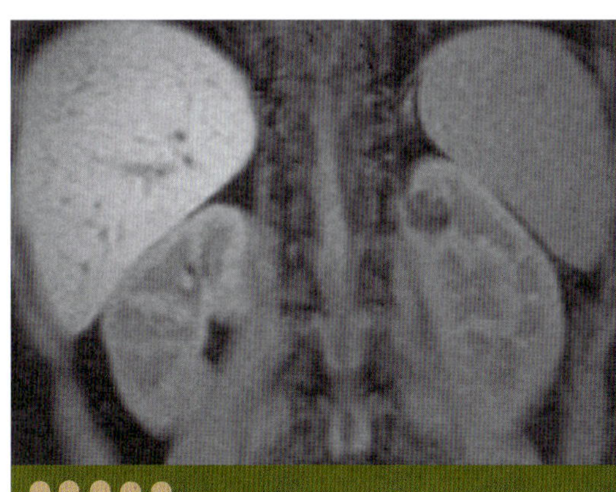

H. Angiomyolipoma: Coronal T1-WI frequency selective fat-suppressed image in same patient shows drop in signal in left upper pole mass confirming macroscopic fat diagnostic of AML.

A-E are the same patient.
F-H are the same patient.

IMAGE KEY

Common

Rare

Typical

Unusual

1–3 Renal Cell Carcinoma in Dialysis Patients

Frank H. Miller

PRESENTATION

Generally asymptomatic. May present with hematuria, flank pain, or mass.

FINDINGS

Atrophic kidneys with enhancing mass caused by renal cell carcinoma.

DIFFERENTIAL DIAGNOSES

- Renal cysts associated with acquired cystic kidney disease appear similar to cysts on imaging studies.
- Hemorrhagic or proteinaceous cysts do not enhance.

COMMENTS

Acquired renal cystic disease, or acquired cystic kidney disease, typically occurs in patients who are on long-term dialysis or have end-stage renal disease. Multiple cysts develop within the native kidneys which tend to be atrophic in the vast majority of patients on dialysis over 5 years. The cysts are generally cortical and bilateral. Patients with acquired cystic disease are at increased risk of renal cell carcinoma. The renal cell carcinomas associated with acquired cystic disease tend to be lower grade neoplasms and do not tend to metastasize as often as typical renal cell carcinomas. The tumors are bilateral in approximately 10%. The appearance of the kidneys and prevalence of multiple cysts and complex hemorrhagic cysts makes the diagnosis of renal cell carcinoma more difficult. Contrast-enhanced studies are generally required to assess if the lesion is malignant. In the past, MR was the ideal imaging modality in this patient population. The association of gadolinium with nephrogenic systemic fibrosis (NSF) makes the use of MR in this patient population with chronic renal insufficiency on dialysis problematic. Contrast-enhanced computed tomography (CECT) may be used in dialysis patients, but because of concerns of nephrotoxicity in the nondialysis population, it is also not ideal. Ultrasound has limitations in visualizing and characterizing renal lesions especially since the kidneys may be difficult to evaluate.

Annual imaging surveillance is generally not required as it has not affected patient outcome. The lesions tend to be lower grade, and the yield of detection of renal cell carcinoma using imaging surveillance is low. Many of these patients have decreased life expectancy and are not ideal surgical candidates.

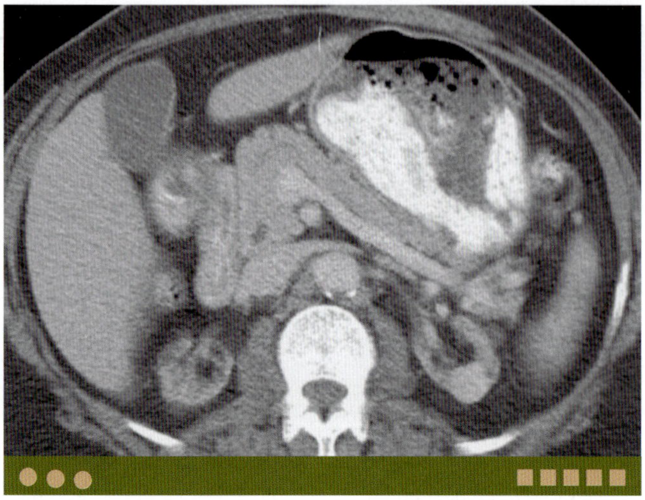

A. Axial CECT shows left renal lesion which is hyperdense to the kidney. With a single phase after contrast, it is difficult to determine if lesion is an enhancing lesion caused by renal cell carcinoma or a hemorrhagic cyst.

PEARLS

- **Acquired cystic kidney disease is generally seen in patients with end-stage renal disease on long-term hemodialysis.**
- **Patients with acquired cystic kidney disease are at increased risk of renal cell carcinoma.**
- **Most of the renal cell carcinomas seen with acquired cystic kidney disease are low grade.**
- **Contrast-enhanced studies are generally required to diagnose renal cell carcinoma in this population.**
- **Association of gadolinium with NSF makes the use of MR in patients on dialysis problematic.**
- **CECT may be used in dialysis patients, but because of concerns of nephrotoxicity in the nondialysis population, it is also problematic.**

ADDITIONAL IMAGES (B-D)

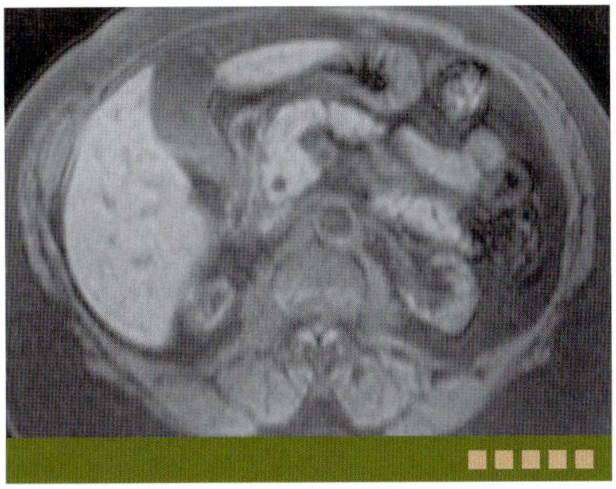

B. Axial unenhanced T1-WI shows lesion in left kidney which is isointense to the kidney. The kidneys are atrophic from chronic renal insufficiency.

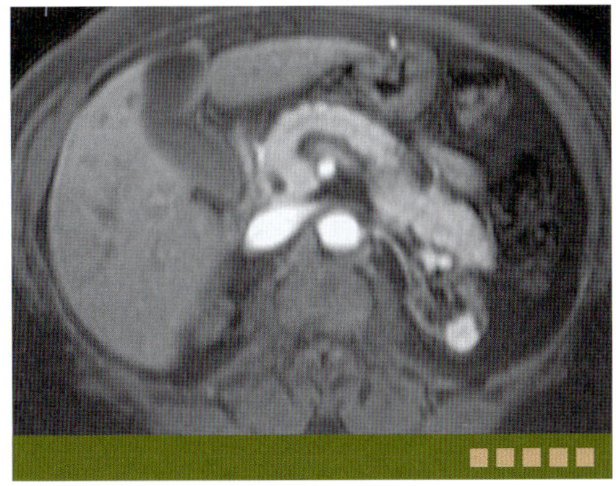

C. Axial early contrast-enhanced T1-WI shows marked enhancement of the left renal lesion consistent with renal cell carcinoma.

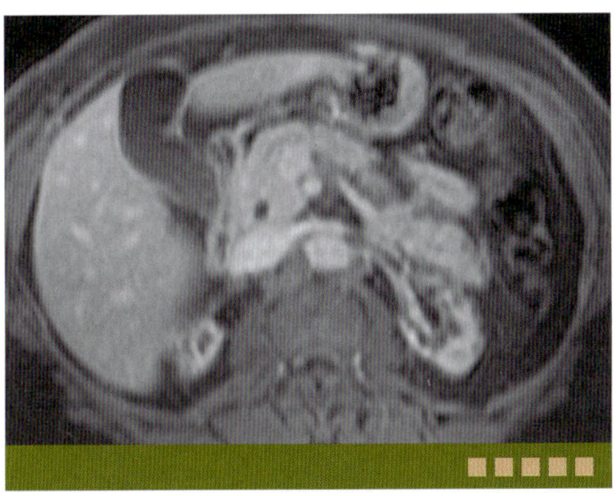

D. Axial more delayed contrast-enhanced T1-WI shows the lesion is less intense.

DIFFERENTIAL DIAGNOSES IMAGES (E-G)

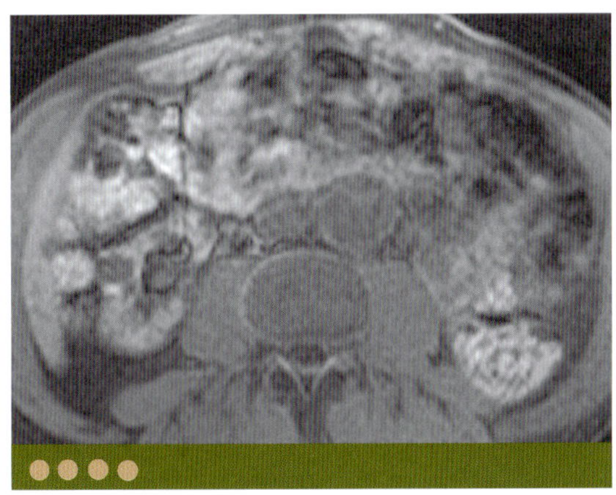

E. Acquired cystic disease: Multiple cystic lesions in acquired cystic disease without renal cell carcinoma. Axial T1-WI image shows atrophic kidneys with mildly complex renal lesions.

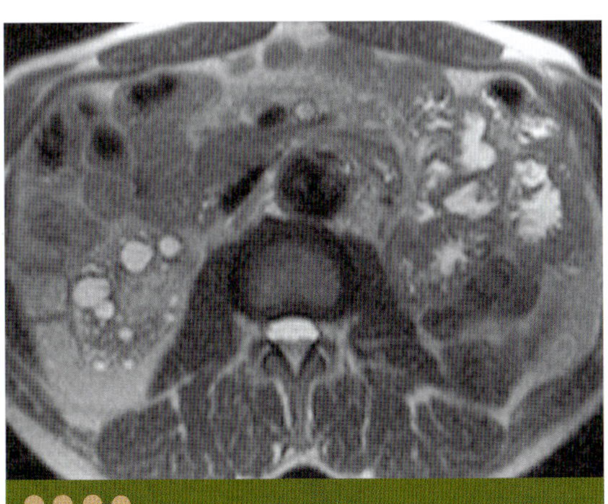

F. Acquired cystic disease: Axial T1-WI shows multiple cystic lesions without renal cell carcinoma. Multiple renal cysts often develop in patients on long-term dialysis.

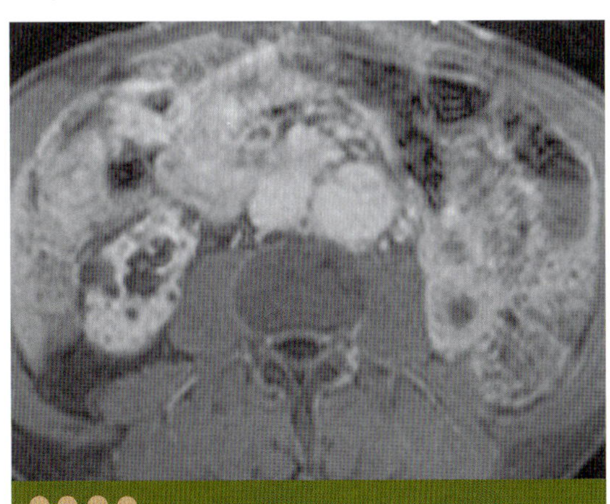

G. Acquired cystic disease: Axial contrast-enhanced T1-WI image shows multiple renal cystic lesions. They did not enhance to suggest cancer. The distinction may be difficult.

IMAGE KEY

Common

Rare

Typical

Unusual

1–4 Chromophobe Renal Cell Carcinoma

David D. Casalino

PRESENTATION

Hematuria.

FINDINGS

CT demonstrates a large hyperdense mass arising from the upper pole of the left kidney.

DIFFERENTIAL DIAGNOSES

- *Renal cell carcinoma (RCC)*: Clear cell and papillary tend to be hypervascular and hypovascular, respectively, compared to the chromophobe type, yet there is substantial overlap.
- *Oncocytoma and other benign tumors without detectable fat*: These tumors cannot be reliably differentiated from RCC based on imaging.
- *Metastasis*: Usually multiple and bilateral in patients with a known primary malignancy.
- *Lymphoma*: Usually multiple and bilateral and associated with lymphadenopathy.
- *Hemorrhagic cyst*: Absence of enhancement may be the only differentiating feature.

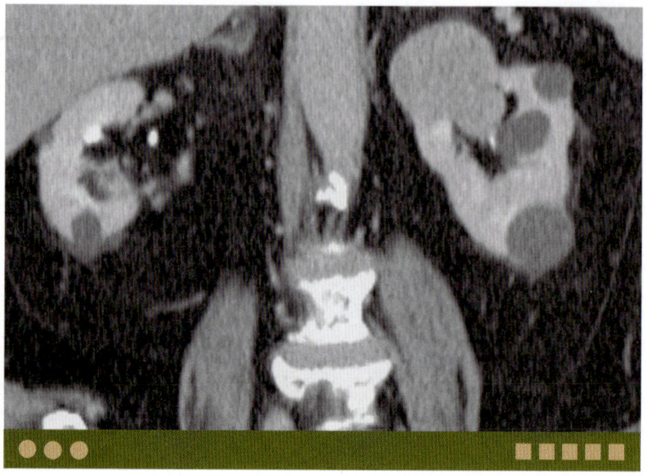

A. Coronal CECT shows a large, homogeneous, enhancing mass arising from the upper pole of the left kidney. There are also bilateral renal cysts.

COMMENTS

Renal cell carcinomas (RCCs) arise from the renal epithelium and account for 85% of renal cancers. Chromophobe RCC accounts for 4% of renal cell carcinomas.

While the classic presentation of RCC includes flank, pain, hematuria, and a palpable abdominal mass, few patients present with this triad. RCC is an incidental finding based on imaging in approximately 50% of the patients. Chromophobe RCC has a higher 5-year survival rate, 80% to 90%, than clear cell RCC, 50% to 60%. Chromophobe RCC is the predominant tumor type in patients with Birt-Hogg-Dubé syndrome, a rare autosomal dominant disorder characterized by hair-follicle hamartomas, pulmonary cysts, and renal tumors

For patients with renal cell carcinoma of any subtype, prognosis is closely related to the stage of disease. Based on the 1997 TMN staging guidelines, stage I disease (tumor <7 cm in greatest dimension and confined to the kidney) has a 90% to 95% 5-year survival; stage II disease (tumor >7 cm in greatest dimension and confined to the kidney) has a 75% to 85% 5-year survival; stage III disease (tumor in major vein, adrenal gland, Gerota's fascia, or one regional lymph node) has a 60% to 70% 5-year survival; and stage IV disease (tumor beyond Gerota's fascia or involving multiple regional lymph nodes) has a 20% to 30% 5-year survival.

Chromophobe RCC tends to enhance moderately, while clear cell and papillary RCCs are usually hypervascular and hypovascular, respectively. The degree of enhancement of the tumor subtypes overlaps substantially. Chromophobe RCC is often homogeneous or shows peripheral enhancement. The treatment is usually surgical excision.

PEARLS

- **Chromophobe RCC accounts for 4% of renal cell carcinomas and has a higher 5-year survival rate.**
- **Prognosis is closely related to the stage of disease.**
- **Imaging features cannot reliably differentiate chromophobe RCC from the other types of RCCs.**
- **Pre- and post-contrast imaging may be necessary to differentiate a hemorrhagic cyst from a solid mass, such as a chromophobe RCC, that is homogeneous.**

ADDITIONAL IMAGES (B-D)

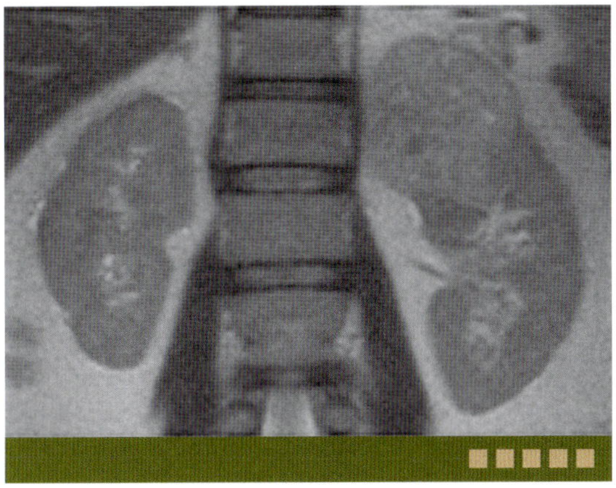

B. Coronal T2-WI from a different patient shows a large, slightly heterogeneous and hyperintense mass arising from the upper pole of the left kidney.

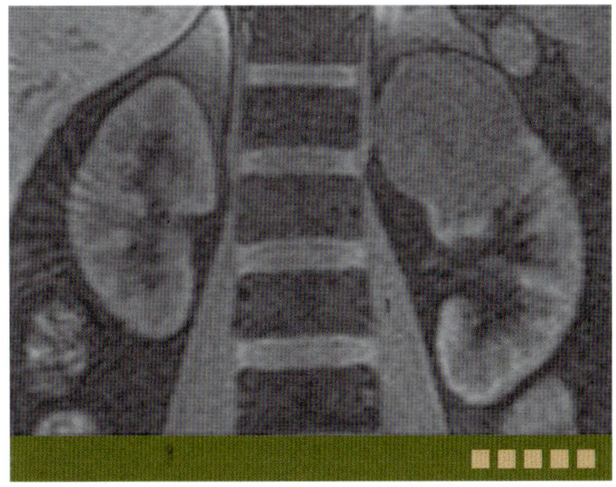

C. Coronal T1-WI shows the mass to be homogeneously hypointense.

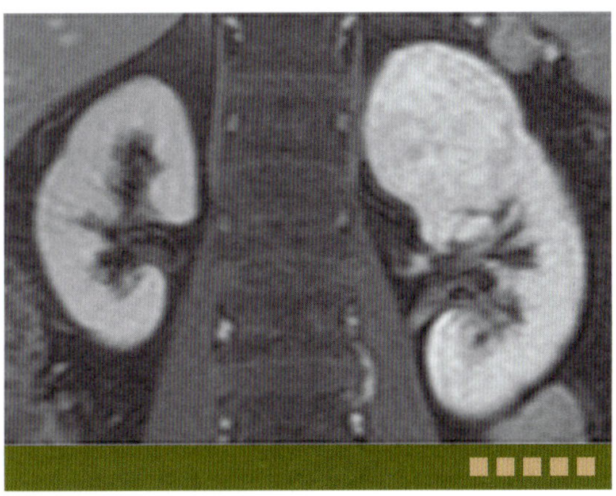

D. Coronal, contrast-enhanced, T1-WI shows marked homogeneous enhancement of the mass.

DIFFERENTIAL DIAGNOSES IMAGES (E-G)

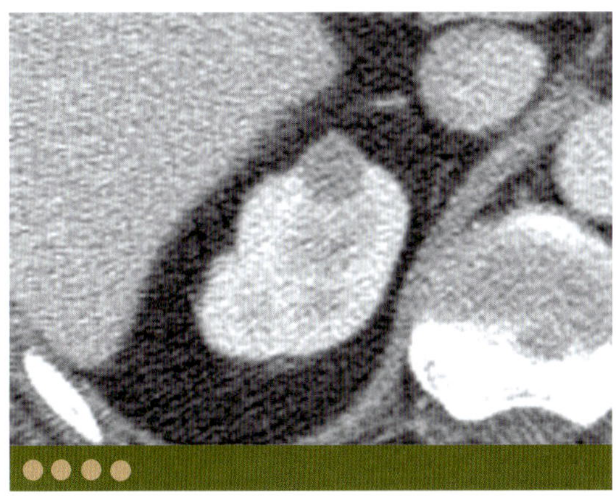

E. Papillary RCC: Axial CECT shows a moderately enhancing, homogeneous mass in the upper pole of the right kidney.

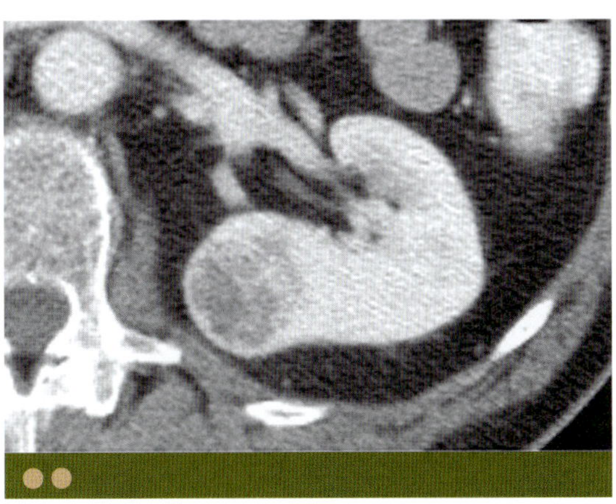

F. Oncocytoma: Axial CECT shows a moderately enhancing, slightly heterogeneous mass in the medial cortex of the left kidney.

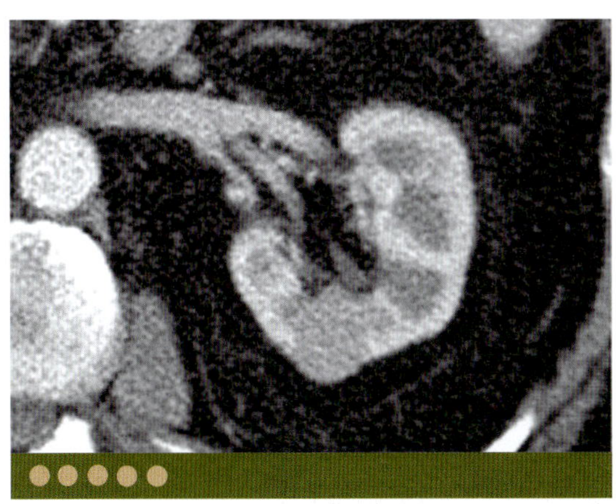

G. Hemorrhagic cyst: Axial CECT shows a homogeneous, hyperdense mass in the posterior cortex of the left kidney. It does not enhance, measuring 70 HU on pre-contrast (not shown) and post-contrast images.

IMAGE KEY

Common

Rare

Typical

Unusual

1–5 Papillary Renal Cell Carcinoma

David D. Casalino

PRESENTATION

Hematuria.

FINDINGS

Pre- and post contrast CT images show a 2.5-cm right renal mass with equivocal enhancement.

DIFFERENTIAL DIAGNOSES

- *Renal cell carcinoma (RCC)*: Clear cell and chromophobe RCCs tend to be more vascular than the papillary type.
- *Hyperdense cyst or hematoma*: Both are nonenhancing and may appear cystic on ultrasound. Hematoma may be caused by trauma or intervention.
- *Abscess*: Nonenhancing and may have a rim of less enhancement than the adjacent cortex. Findings of pyelonephritis and symptoms of infection are common.
- *AML with minimal fat and metanephric adenoma*: Both may be indistinguishable from a papillary RCC. Metanephric adenomas are rare, and only 5% of angiomyolipomas have minimal fat, which is not detectable on imaging.

COMMENT

Renal cell carcinomas arise from the renal epithelium and account for 85% of renal cancers. Papillary RCC accounts for 12% of renal cell carcinomas. While the classic presentation of RCC includes flank, pain, hematuria, and a palpable abdominal mass, few patients present with this triad. RCC is an incidental finding on imaging in approximately 50% of patients. Papillary RCC has a higher 5-year survival rate, 80% to 90%, than clear cell RCC, 50% to 60%. Male predominance is also higher with a 5:1 male-female ratio. Risk factors for RCC include smoking, hypertension, obesity, and acquired cystic kidney disease.

Papillary RCC occurs in several familial syndromes, including hereditary papillary renal carcinoma, an autosomal dominant disorder associated with multifocal papillary RCC, and hereditary leiomyoma RCC, an autosomal dominant disorder associated with cutaneous and uterine leiomyomas and solitary papillary RCC.

Papillary RCC is typically the least vascular type of RCC and shows only mild enhancement after contrast administration. The enhancement is usually homogeneous or peripheral. On T2-weighted MR imaging, papillary RCC is typically hypointense, perhaps because of the iron-containing hemosiderin that may be found in the cytoplasm. On gradient-echo imaging the susceptibility artifact from the hemosiderin will be accentuated.

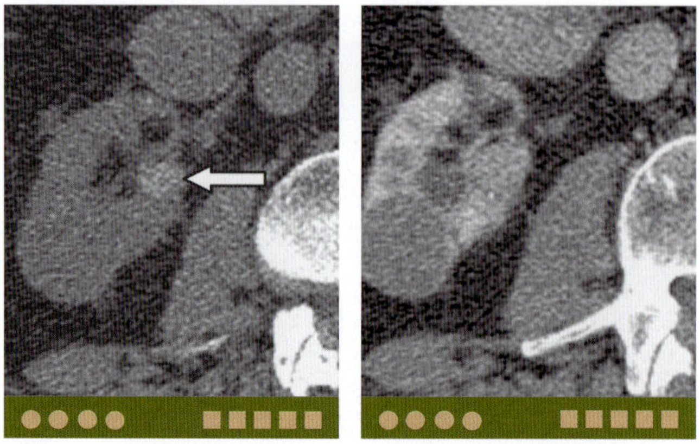

A. and B. Axial NECT and CECT show a 2.5-cm right renal mass with equivocal enhancement, measuring 40 HU precontrast and 50 HU postcontrast. There is also a 7-mm hemorrhagic cyst (arrow).

Some authors advocate biopsy of renal lesions that show enhancement and hyperattenuation on CT, hypointensity on T2-weighted MR imaging, and do not show signal loss on fat-suppressed or opposed-phased gradient-echo imaging. The differential diagnosis for such a lesion would include papillary RCC, AML with minimal fat, and metanephric adenoma. Also occasionally, it may be difficult to differentiate a papillary RCC with minimal enhancement from a hyperdense cyst or hematoma. In such cases, ultrasound may be helpful in differentiating the solid from the cystic lesion.

PEARLS

- **Papillary RCC accounts for 12% of renal cell carcinomas and has a higher 5-year survival rate.**
- **Papillary RCC is typically hypovascular compared to the other types of RCC.**
- **Papillary RCC enhancement may be very mild, making it difficult to differentiate from a hyperdense cyst.**
- **Hypointensity on T2-weighted MR is a common finding.**

ADDITIONAL IMAGES (C-E)

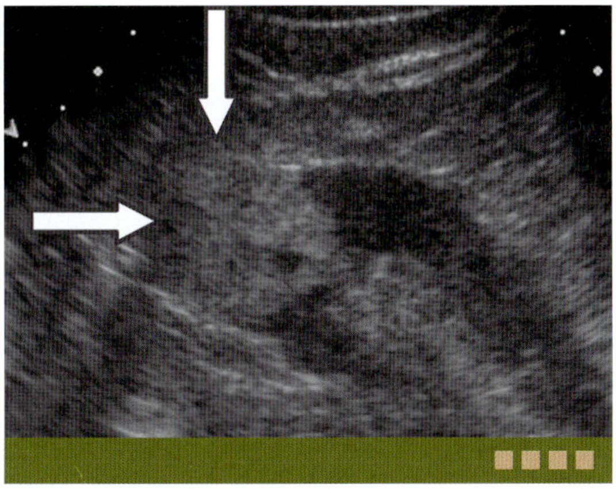

C. Transverse sonogram shows the mass (arrows) to be predominantly hyperechoic.

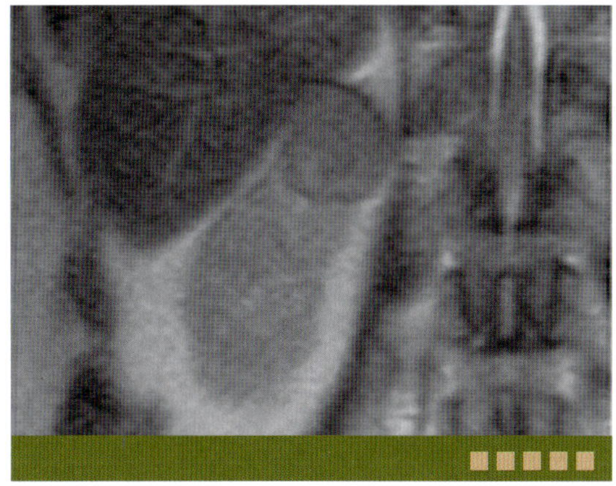

D. Coronal T2-WI shows a hypointense mass arising from the upper pole of the right kidney in a different patient.

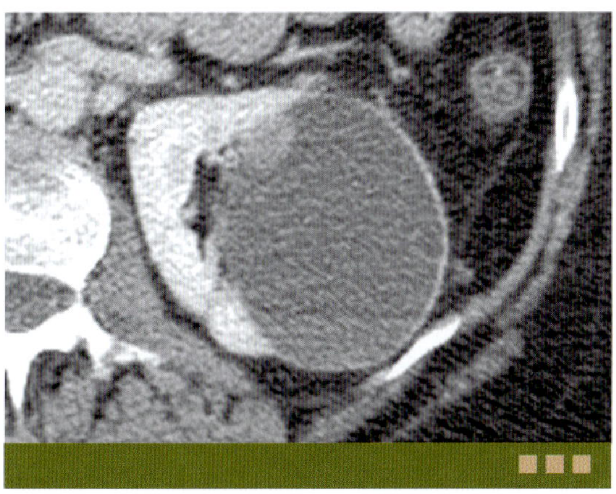

E. Axial CECT shows a papillary RCC that is predominantly cystic with an enhancing mural nodule.

DIFFERENTIAL DIAGNOSES IMAGES (F-H)

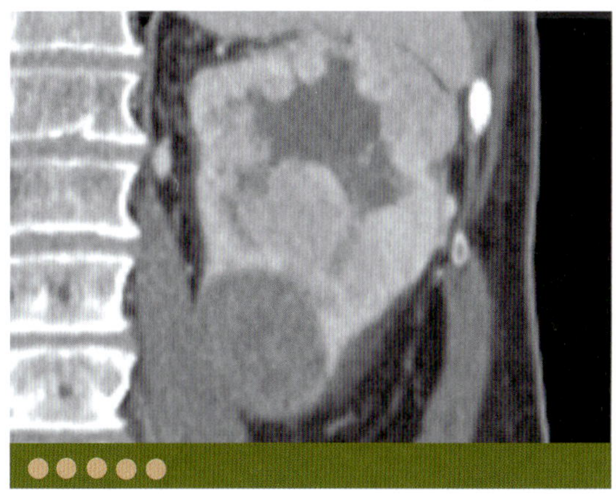

F. Clear cell RCC: Coronal CECT shows a large, upper pole hypervascular clear cell RCC with central necrosis and lower pole hypovascular papillary RCC.

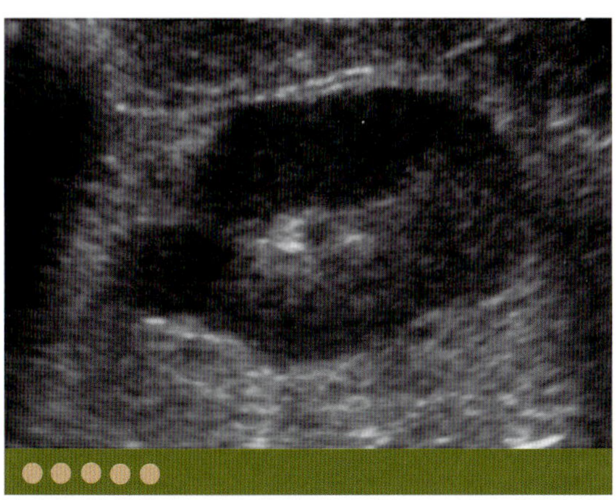

G. Hyperdense cyst: Transverse sonogram from a patient with a 40 HU renal mass on CECT shows the lesion to be anechoic.

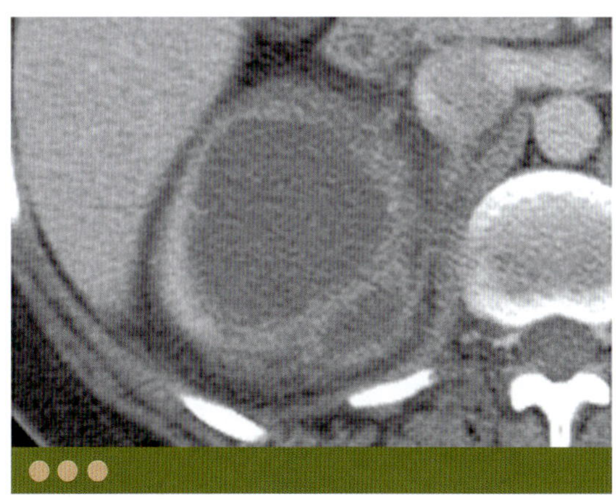

H. Abscess: CECT shows a cystic mass with a rim of hypodensity relative to normal cortex and mild perinephric fatty stranding.

IMAGE KEY

Common

Rare

Typical

Unusual

1–6 Renal Cell Carcinoma Staging

Frank H. Miller

PRESENTATION

Hematuria, flank pain, weight loss, and asymptomatic.

FINDINGS

Renal cell carcinoma

DIFFERENTIAL DIAGNOSIS

None

COMMENTS

Renal cell carcinoma (RCC) is being detected more frequently as an incidental finding because of the frequent use of ultrasonography, CT, and MRI. Following detection of a mass, it is important to characterize the mass as renal cell carcinoma. Following characterization, it is important to stage the tumors with CT or MR, which helps determine the prognosis and guides surgery and therapy. Tumor size can be accurately assessed by all imaging modalities. The most common sites of metastases are lung, bone, skin, liver, and brain.

The Robson classification, first described in 1969, is simpler but less widely used as it does not correlate stage with patient prognosis as well as with the American Joint Committee on Cancer (AJCC) staging method based on the Tumor Node Metastases (TNM) classification. The Robson classification has limitations as lymph node metastases and venous invasion are in the same stage.

Tumor invasion of the renal vein and inferior vena cava (IVC) is important to identify. However, with proper surgical treatment, patients with T3b or T3c disease may have survival similar to stages 1 and 2, as the tumor thrombus can often be removed because it is not attached to the wall. The extent of renal vein and IVC thrombus is important for presurgical planning. It determines whether an abdominal or thoraco-abdominal approach is used and whether cardiac bypass is needed when involving the atrium.

For imaging lymphadenopathy, CT and MR are similar and better than ultrasound. Assessment of tumor involvement of lymph nodes can be difficult as traditional size measurements may not be effective because tumor involvement seen in normal-sized nodes; however, involvement is less critical as the nodes are sampled at the time of surgery. Identification by imaging of bulky lymphadenopathy, which may complicate surgery, especially when encasing the renal artery, would be helpful.

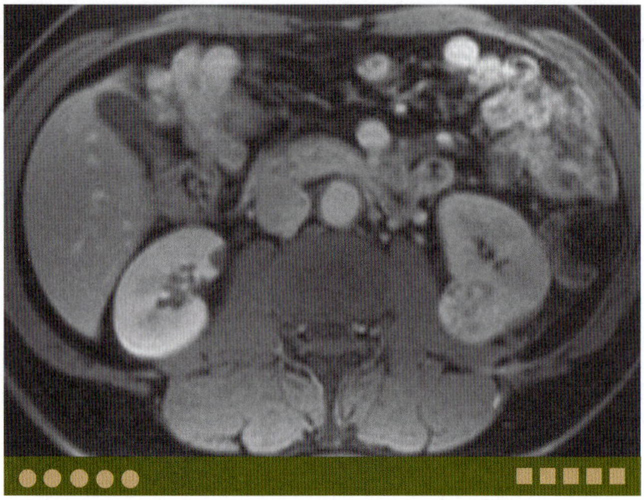

A. Stage 1 renal cell carcinoma: Axial contrast-enhanced T1-WI shows enhancing mass in the left lower pole caused by renal cell carcinoma. There were neither lymph node metastases nor vascular invasion. No perinephric spread was seen.

T4MO disease or contiguous invasion is important for the surgeons to identify. It includes invasion of the liver, diaphragm, psoas muscles, pancreas, and bowel. Multiplanar imaging is helpful, but it can be difficult at times to distinguish invasion from contiguity of the tumor and organ.

Stage 4B or T4M1 disease or distant metastases mainly involves the lungs, bone, liver, and brain. A chest radiograph is considered necessary chest CT although more sensitive is nonspecific in small metastases. Routine bone surveys or bone scans do not appear to be necessary unless abnormal blood tests or bone pain occurs. Metastases can occur to multiple organs including years after nephrectomy.

PEARLS

- **It is important to stage patients with imaging, which helps guide patient treatment and prognosis.**
- **The two most commonly used staging systems are the Robson's staging system and the TNM classification.**
- **Distant metastases mainly involve the lungs, bone, liver, and brain.**

ADDITIONAL IMAGES (B-M)

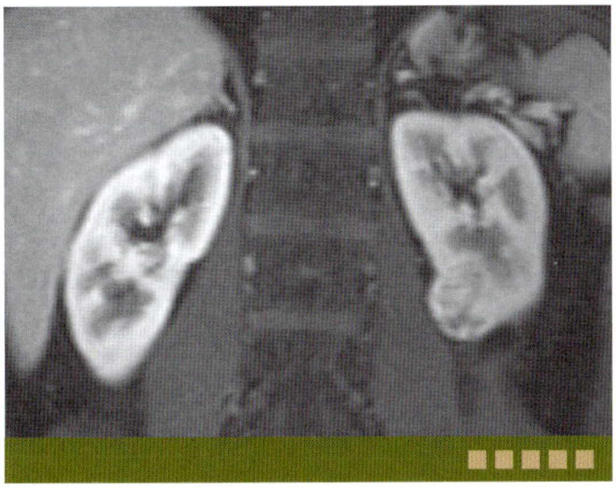

B. Stage 1 renal cell carcinoma: Coronal contrast-enhanced T1-WI shows heterogeneous enhancing renal cell carcinoma. No tumor spread is seen.

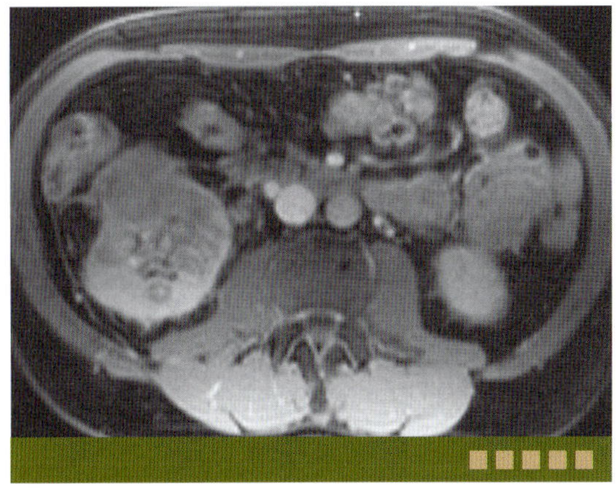

C. Renal cell carcinoma extending into perinephric fat. Axial contrast-enhanced T1-WI shows right renal cell carcinoma with extension into the perirenal fat.

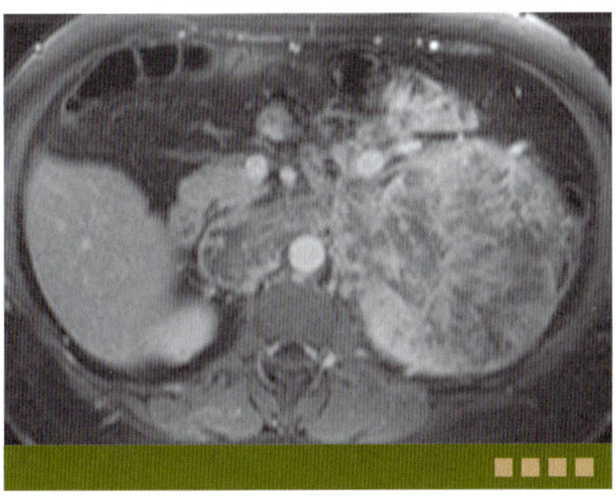

D. Axial contrast-enhanced T1-WI shows tumor larger than 7 cm, which extends into the left renal vein and inferior vena cava.

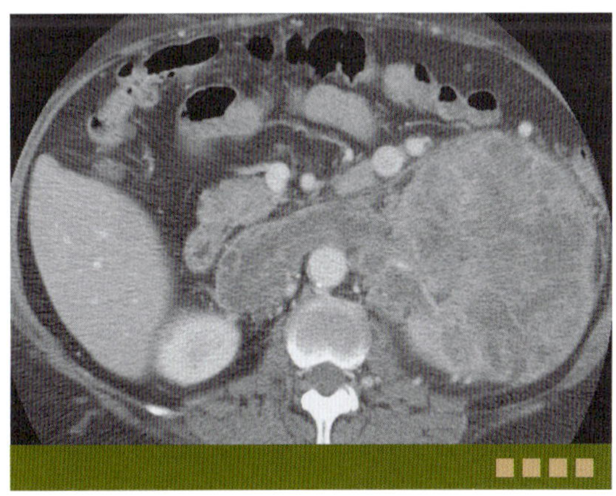

E. Axial CECT scan shows tumor larger than 7 cm, which extends into the left renal vein and inferior vena cava.

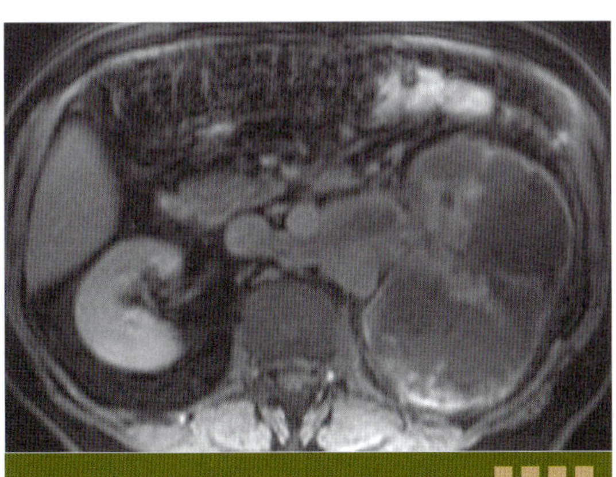

F. Axial contrast-enhanced T1-WI shows left renal cell carcinoma, which extends into the retroaortic left renal vein. Posterior to the left renal vein is metastatic para-aortic lymph node.

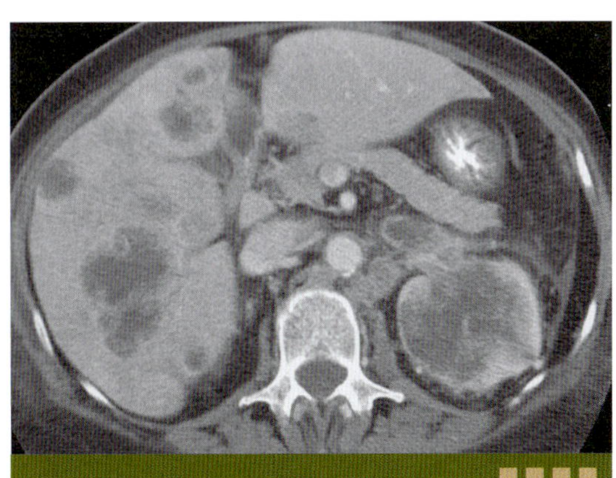

G. Axial CECT shows left renal cell carcinoma with extension into the left renal vein, para-aortic lymphadenopathy, and liver metastases.

IMAGE KEY

Common

Rare

Typical

Unusual

Table 1 Robson Staging System for Renal Cell Carcinoma.

Robson Stage	Disease Extent
I	Confined to renal capsule
II	Spreads to perinephric fat or ipsilateral adrenal gland
IIIA	Extension to renal vein or IVC
IIIB	Involves regional lymph node
IVA	Direct extension of adjacent organs through Gerota fascia
IVB	Distant metastases

Table 2 2002 Version of AJCC TNM Classification for staging Renal Cancer.

Stage	Classification
T1	Tumor <7 cm limited to kidney
T1a	Tumor <4 cm in greatest diameter
T1b	Tumor 4-7 cm
T2	Tumor >7 cm confined to kidney
T3	Tumor extends into major veins or invades the ipsilateral adrenal orperinephric tissue but not beyond Gerota fascia
T3a	Perinephric or adrenal gland
T3b	Grossly extends into renal vein or IVC below the diaphragm
T3c	Grossly extends into IVC above the diaphragm or invades wall of the IVC
T4	Tumor invades beyond Gerota's fascia
N0	No nodes
N1	Metastasis to single regional node
N2	More than one regional lymph node
M0	No distant metastases
M1	Distant metastases

Table 3 Staging Based on TNM Stage.

Stage	Grouping
Stage 1	T1, N0, M0
Stage 2	T2, N0, M0
Stage 3	T1 N1, M0; T2 N1, M0; T3 N1, M0
Stage 4	T2 N1, M0; Any T N2, M0; Any N, M1

ADDITIONAL IMAGES (B-M)

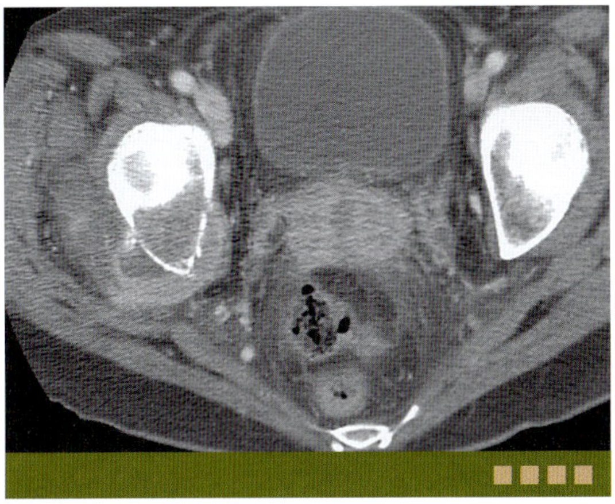

H. Axial CECT shows renal cell carcinoma with bone metastases to the right acetabulum.

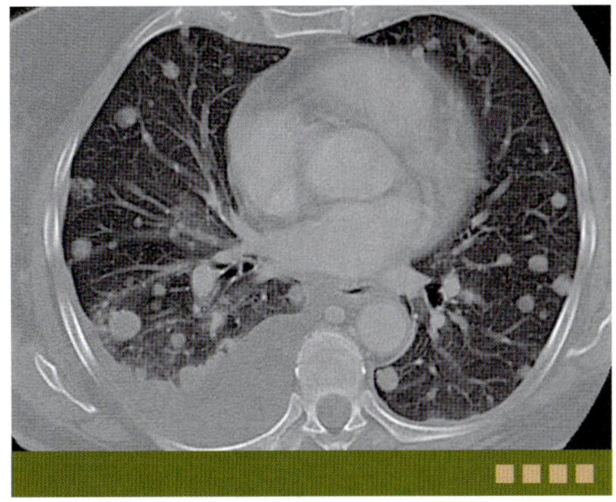

I. Stage 4 renal cell carcinoma. Lung windows from axial CECT show numerous pulmonary metastases resulting from hematogenous spread.

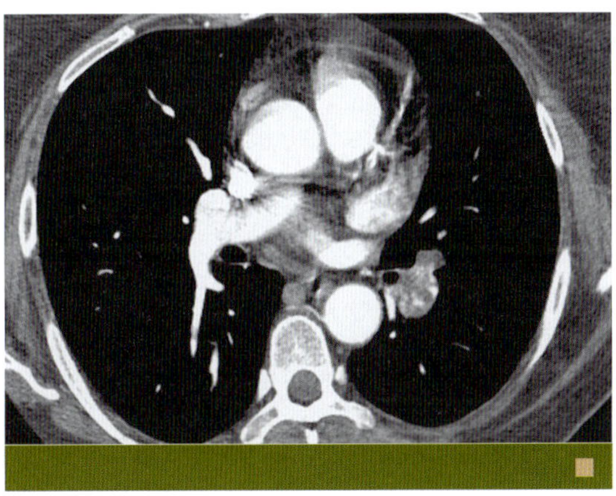

J. Patient with renal cell carcinoma, who had tumor thombus in the IVC. Axial CECT shows pulmonary embolus in left pulmonary artery from tumor thrombus.

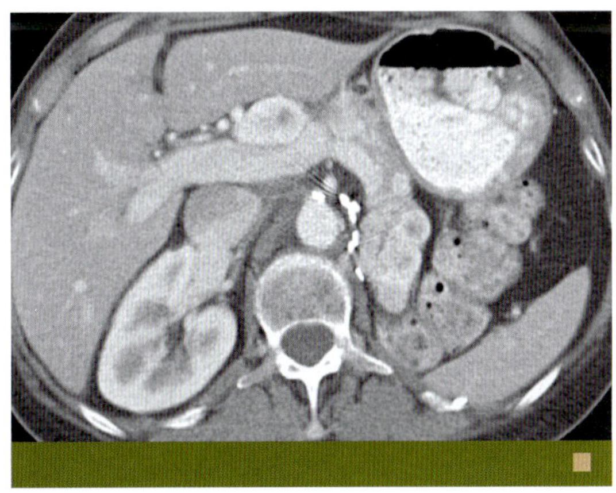

K. Renal cell carcinoma with pancreatic metastases. Axial CECT shows numerous hypervascular pancreatic body and tail metastases in patients with history of renal cell carcinoma and prior left nephrectomy.

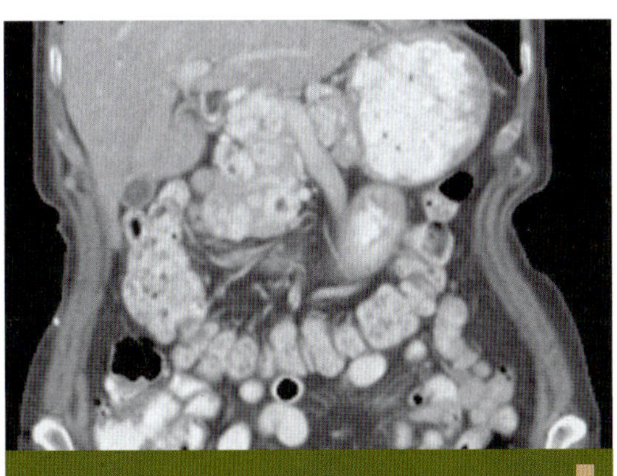

L. Coronal CECT in the same patient shows numerous metastases to the pancreatic head.

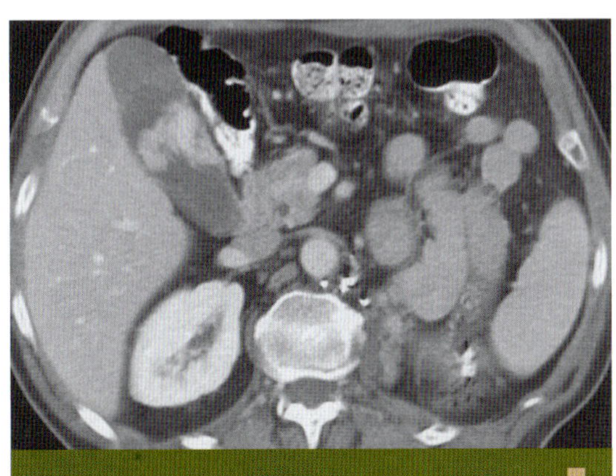

M. Axial CECT in patients with left nephrectomy for renal cell carcinoma shows hypervascular gall bladder mass that is renal cell carcinoma metastasis.

IMAGE KEY

Common

Rare

Typical

Unusual

1–7 Birt-Hogg-Dubé Syndrome

David D. Casalino

PRESENTATION

Acute shortness of breath and history of skin lesions.

FINDINGS

CT shows multiple, bilateral solid renal masses, left lung cysts, and right-side pneumothorax.

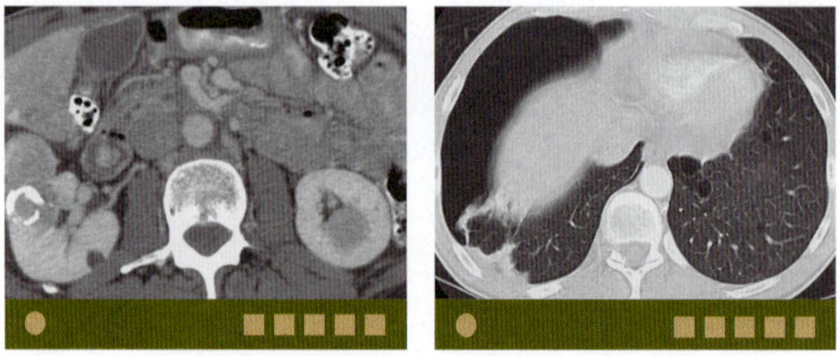

A. Axial CECT shows multiple, bilateral solid renal masses that proved to be chromophobe renal cell carcinomas. In the right kidney, one lesion shows peripheral course calcification, while another lesion is fat density, characteristic of an AML. **B.** Axial CECT shows a large right-side pneumothorax and several cysts in the left lung base.

DIFFERENTIAL DIAGNOSES

- *Multiple metastases*: Usually known primary malignancy with lung, breast, melanoma, and colon cancer being most common.
- *Lymphoma*: Typically associated with lymphadenopathy in retroperitoneum and elsewhere.
- *Tuberous sclerosis*: Angiomyolipomas and cysts are much more frequently seen than renal cell carcinoma. TS may be associated with lymphangiomyomatosis and pneumothorax.
- *Multifocal RCC or benign solid tumors, sporadic or associated with other inherited syndromes*: Extrarenal manifestations and family history may be helpful.

COMMENTS

The Birt-Hogg-Dubé (BHD) syndrome is a rare autosomal dominant disorder. The *BHG* gene, which encodes the protein folliculin, is implicated in the syndrome. Folliculin is a suspected tumor suppressor.

The syndrome is characterized by hair-follicle hamartomas, or fibrofolliculomas, of the neck and face, pulmonary cysts, and renal tumors. The renal tumors occur in 15% to 30% of patients and are usually chromophobe RCC or mixed chromophobe-oncocytomas. Occasionally, patients with BHD may develop papillary or clear cell RCC.

Imaging shows solid renal masses that typically enhance markedly. Cysts may be present but are unrelated to the solid tumors. Pulmonary cysts may be seen on CT in up to 70% of BHD patients and are associated with a history of spontaneous pneumothorax in 25%. Pulmonary cysts are not seen in VHL but can be seen in lymphangiomyomatosis associated with TS.

Approximately 2% of renal cancer cases are associated with inherited syndromes. One should consider the possibility of a hereditary RCC in a patient with multiple enhancing renal masses or in a patient with an enhancing renal mass and family history of RCC, particularly if the patient is less than 50 years old. Some of these syndromes, such as BHD, VHL, TS, and hereditary leiomyoma renal cell carcinoma have extrarenal manifestations, which are often helpful in differentiating these disorders. Others, such as familial clear cell renal cancer and hereditary papillary renal carcinoma, do not have extrarenal manifestations.

Screening guidelines for patients with hereditary renal cancer syndromes vary depending, in part, on the aggressiveness of the phenotype and size of renal lesions. In BHD, tumors less than 3 cm in diameter have a very low risk of metastasis. Once a lesion reaches 3 cm, patients usually undergo nephron-sparing surgery, cryotherapy, or radiofrequency ablation.

PEARLS

- **BHD is characterized by solid renal tumors, pulmonary cysts, and hair-follicle hamartomas.**
- **Chromophobe RCC is the renal malignancy most often associated with BHD.**
- **Twenty-five percent of BHD patients have a history of spontaneous pneumothorax.**
- **Hereditary RCC should be considered in a patient with multiple solid renal masses, particularly if there is a family history of RCC or the patient is younger than 50 years of age.**

ADDITIONAL IMAGES (C-E)

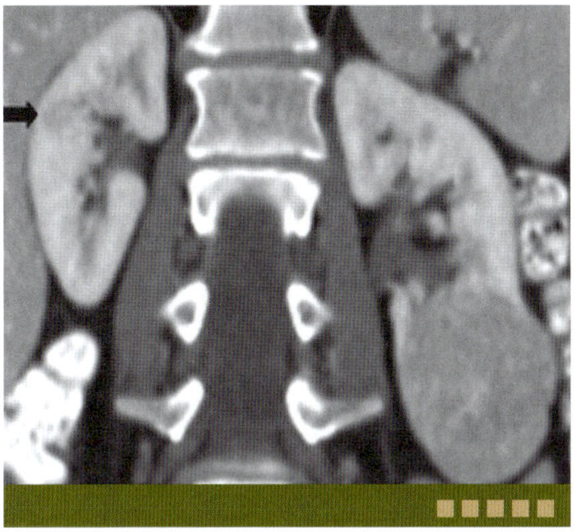

C. Coronal CECT from a different patient with BHD shows a large chromophobe RCC arising from the left lower pole and a smaller carcinoma (arrow) in the right kidney.

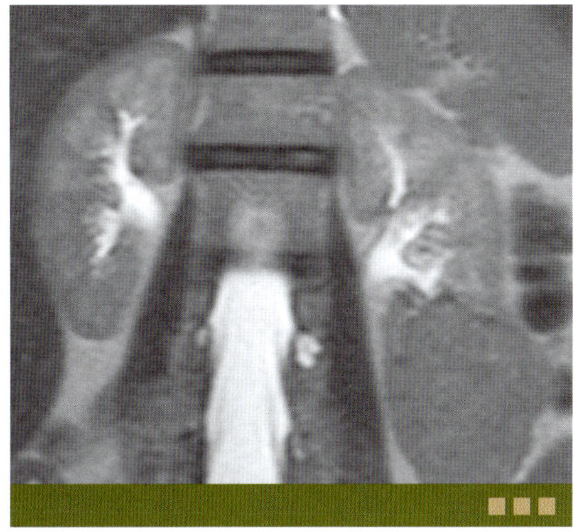

D. Coronal T2-WI shows the left renal lesion to be homogeneously hypointense.

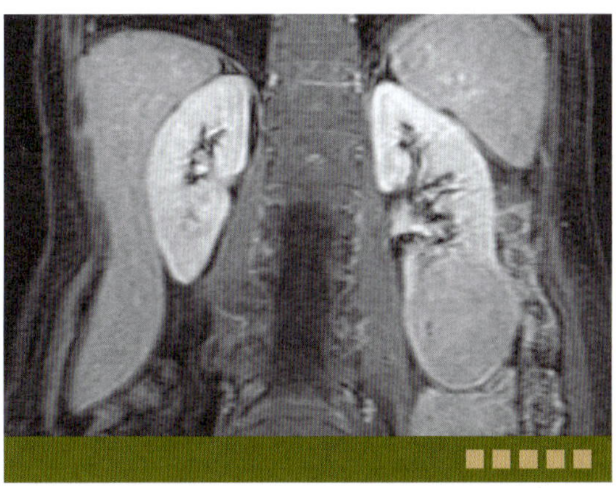

E. Coronal, contrast-enhanced, T1-WI shows the tumor to enhance moderately and with minimal heterogeneity.

DIFFERENTIAL DIAGNOSES IMAGES (F-H)

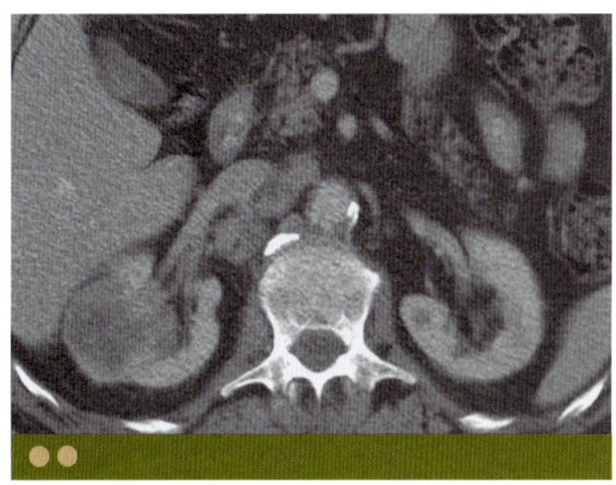

F. Multifocal metastases: Axial CECT shows bilateral solid renal masses and retroperitoneal adenopathy in a patient with known lung carcinoma.

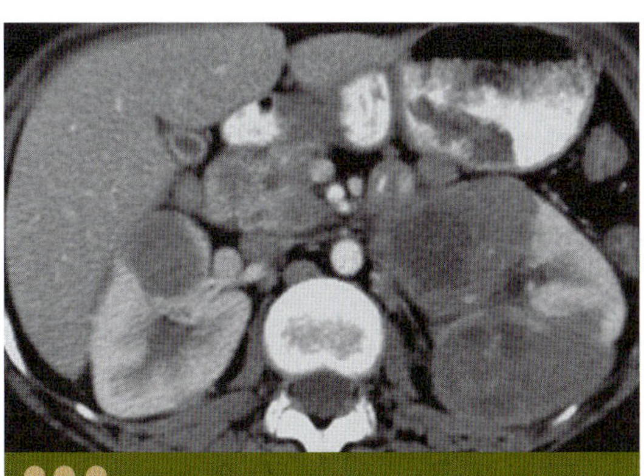

G. Lymphoma: Axial CECT shows bilateral solid renal masses and retroperitoneal adenopathy. NHL was confirmed by biopsy.

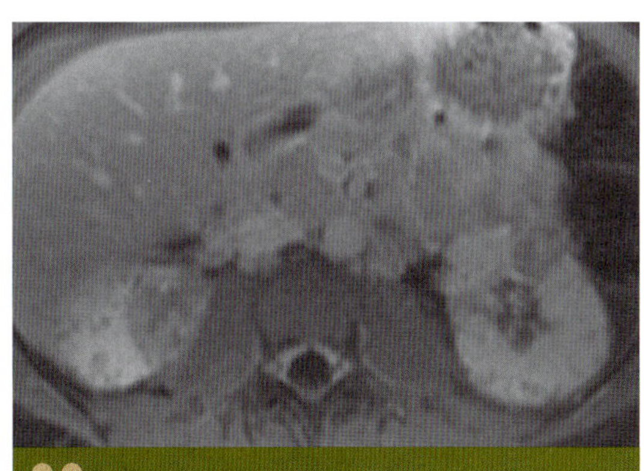

H. Tuberous sclerosis: Axial, contrast-enhanced T1-WI shows numerous, bilateral renal masses. Fat could be confirmed in most of the solid lesions.

IMAGE KEY

Common

Rare

Typical

Unusual

1–8 Renal Medullary Carcinoma

Frank H. Miller

PRESENTATION

Hematuria, abdominal pain, fever, weight loss in patients with sickle cell trait.

FINDINGS

Infiltrative mass in the medullary portion of the right kidney.

DIFFERENTIAL DIAGNOSES

- *Lymphoma*: Generally known history of lymphoma and often multiple or bilateral with associated lymphadenopathy.
- *Renal metastases*: Generally known primary, can be infiltrative in appearance.
- *Renal cell carcinoma (RCC)*: Usually cortical location but can less commonly be medullary and mimic medullary carcinoma.
- *Angiomyolipoma*: Often intratumoral fat.
- *Transitional cell carcinoma (TCC)*: Can have similar infiltrative appearance and arise from collecting system.

COMMENTS

Renal medullary cancer is an extremely aggressive tumor seen typically in young black patients (median age approximately 20 years) with sickle cell trait. It is rare with relatively few reports. Patients most often present with gross painless hematuria as seen in our patient. Patients with sickle cell trait may have microscopic hematuria making the diagnosis more difficult. A high index of suspicion is needed to make an early diagnosis. The tumor is thought to arise from the collecting duct, accounting for its central location in the kidney. The tumor may have hemorrhagic areas and necrosis.

Imaging features include generally large central masses in the medulla and have an infiltrative appearance extending into the renal pelvis. There may be satellite lesions in the renal cortex or adjacent peripelvic tissue. Perinephric spread may also be seen. There is often associated lymphadenopathy and distant metastases to the lung. The lesions need to be detected early as they have lymphatic or vascular invasion and metastasize early. Systemic chemotherapy is often administered, but the prognosis is poor.

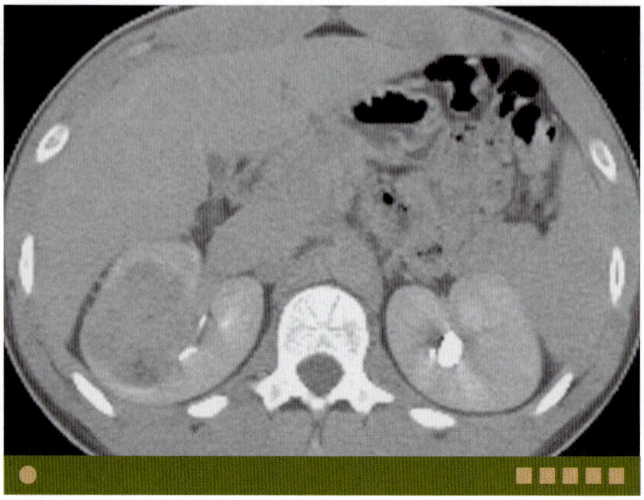

A. Axial CECT in African American male with sickle cell trait shows infiltrative mass involving the medullary portion of right kidney.

The imaging appearance can be similar to other renal masses including renal cell carcinoma and lymphoma. The diagnosis can be suggested, however, based on the relatively young age of the patients, the association with sickle cell trait, and the medullary location of the masses, which helps differentiate it from other malignancies. Biopsy is often required for the diagnosis.

PEARLS

- **Consider medullary carcinoma in patients with sickle cell trait and large central masses.**
- **Medullary cancer has an infiltrative appearance with masses located centrally in the medullary portion of the kidney.**
- **Medullary cancers frequently have associated lymphadenopathy and distant metastases and poor prognosis.**

ADDITIONAL IMAGES (B-C)

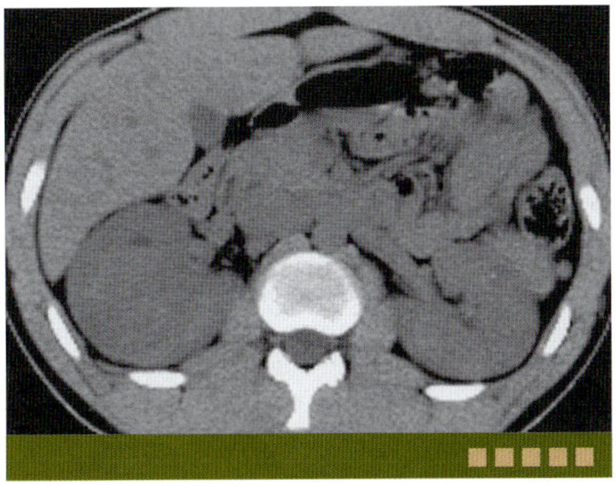

B. On Axial NECT, the mass is more difficult to see than on the CECT.

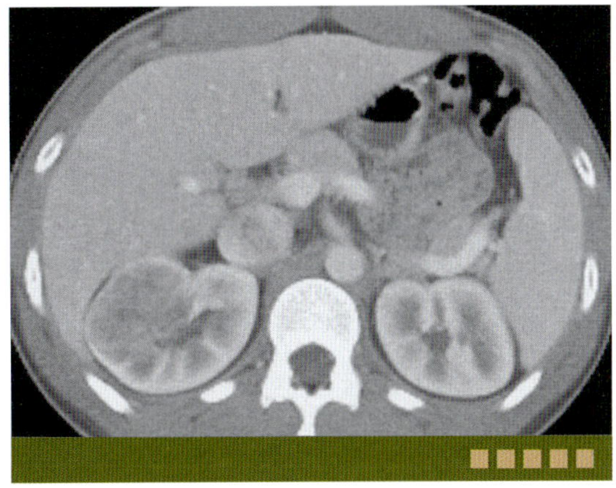

C. On axial cortico-medullary phase CECT image, mass is more difficult to see than on the later contrast-enhanced phase (Figure. A).

IMAGE KEY

Common

Rare

Typical

Unusual

DIFFERENTIAL DIAGNOSES IMAGES (D-E)

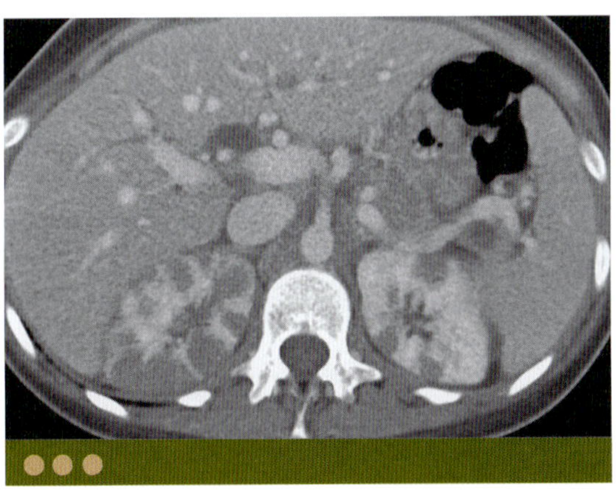

D. Lymphoma: Axial CECT shows multiple solid masses in both kidneys (predominately peripherally) and pancreas with retroperitoneal lymphadenopathy in patients with known non-Hodgkin lymphoma.

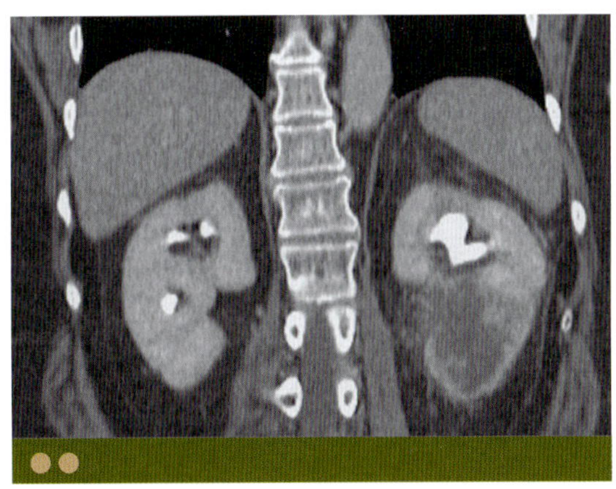

E. Metastasis to the kidney from lung cancer: Coronal CECT shows infiltrative mass in the lower pole of the left kidney. These lesions can usually be distinguished on the basis of the history of primary malignancy.

1–9 Collecting Duct Carcinoma

Paul Nikolaidis

PRESENTATION

Hematuria, abdominal pain, and abdominal mass.

FINDINGS

CT shows an infiltrative mass involving the left kidney, which is globally enlarged. The left renal vein is expanded.

DIFFERENTIAL DIAGNOSES

- *Renal cell carcinoma (RCC)*: May be indistinguishable. Although only about 6% of cortical renal cell carcinomas are infiltrative, RCC represents a large proportion of infiltrative renal tumors, given its higher prevalence.
- *Renal medullary carcinoma*: A rare tumor that may also have an infiltrative appearance associated with sickle cell hemoglobinopathies.
- *Transitional cell carcinoma (TCC)*: A centrally located collecting duct carcinoma with invasion into the renal pelvis may be indistinguishable from an invasive transitional cell carcinoma of the renal pelvis.

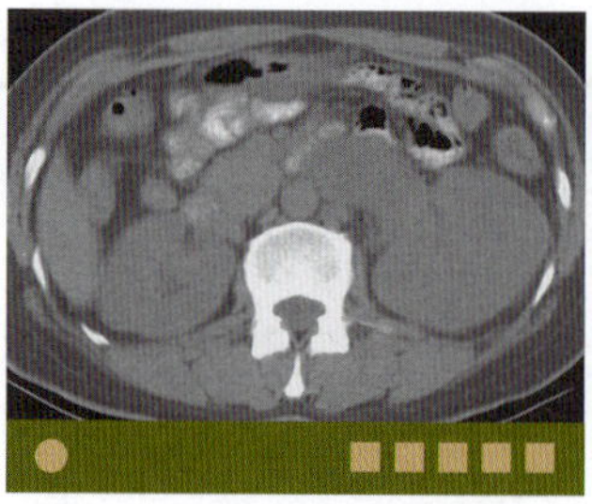

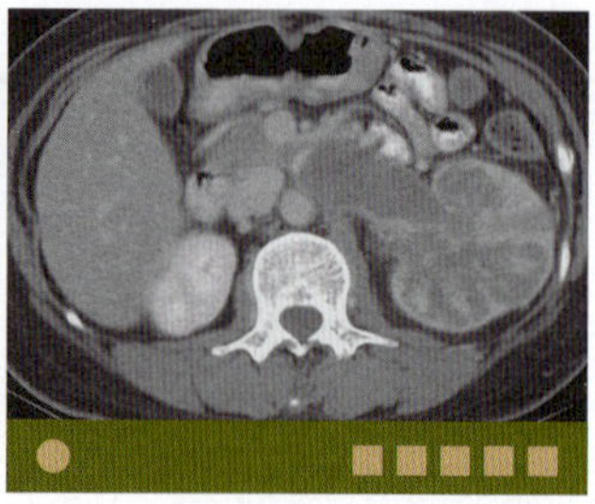

A. Axial NECT shows enlargement of the left kidney, without an obvious renal mass. The renal contour is not distorted. There is no hydronephrosis.
B. Corresponding axial CECT obtained during the nephrographic phase shows a markedly abnormal pattern of enhancement of the left renal parenchyma. There is an infiltrative mass that extends into the left renal vein. *(Images courtesy Dr. Bohyun Kim, Mayo Clinic, Rochester, Minnesota)*

COMMENTS

Collecting duct carcinoma is a rare, aggressive, malignant renal tumor. It accounts for approximately 1% or less of renal neoplasms. It is derived from the epithelium of the collecting ducts in the medulla, whereas most renal cell carcinomas arise from the convoluted tubules of the cortex.

The average age at diagnosis is 53 years, and it predominantly affects men (by a 2:1 ratio). The tumor is metastatic in at least 40% of the cases at the time of diagnosis. Patients typically present with hematuria, often associated with fever, pain, weight loss, and an abdominal mass.

Grossly, collecting duct carcinoma tends to be quite large at the time of presentation. Despite its medullary origin, almost all tumors exhibit extension into the cortex or perinephric space. Histologically, the tumor cells form glands, tubules, solid nests, or cords embedded in a loose desmoplastic stroma.

CT is helpful in identifying the extent of tumor spread. Tumors may metastasize to the lymph nodes, bones, adrenals, lung, skin, and subcutaneous tissues. Medullary location, decreased heterogeneous enhancement, renal sinus involvement, infiltrative pattern of growth, preservation of the renal contour, and cystic components are features frequently seen in patients with collecting duct carcinoma of the kidney.

On MR, the solid portion of the tumor is often hypointense on T2-WI. Areas of necrosis are hyperintense on T2-WI and hypointense on postgadolinium, fat-suppressed T1-WI.

Surgery is the treatment of choice in most patients. The 5-year survival rate is approximately 34%. The use of various adjuvant therapies is controversial.

PEARLS

- **Rare, aggressive tumor arising from the epithelium of the collecting ducts in the medulla.**
- **Frequently metastatic at the time of diagnosis.**
- **On CT, they appear as large infiltrative solid tumors; they may have a significant cystic component.**
- **On T2-WI, hyperintense cystic areas may be seen; the solid components of the tumor are typically hypointense.**

ADDITIONAL IMAGES (C-E)

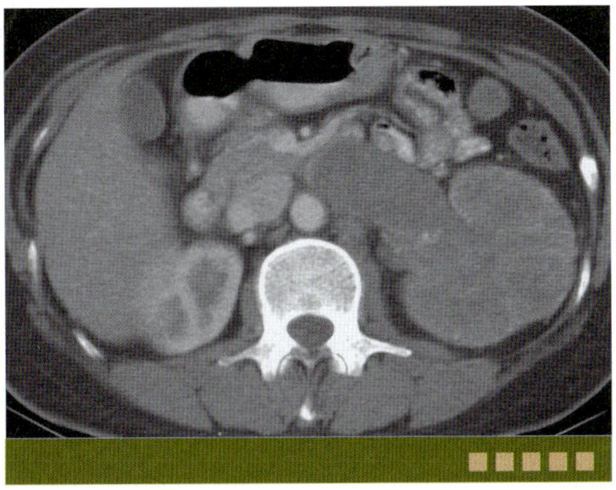

C. Corresponding axial CECT obtained during the excretory shows a markedly hypoenhancing left renal mass involving almost the entire kidney. *(Image courtesy Dr. Bohyun Kim, Mayo Clinic, Rochester, Minnesota)*

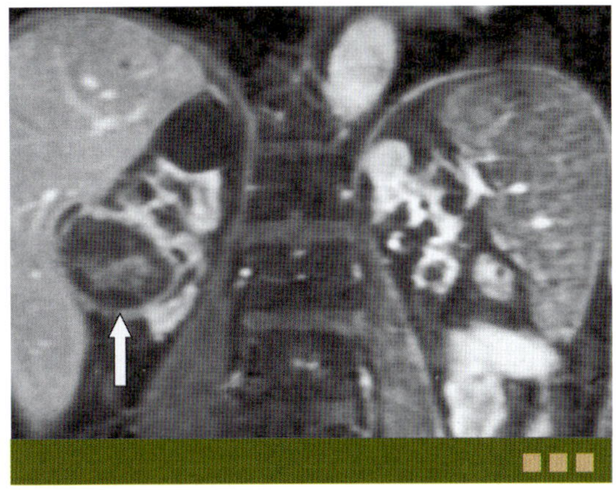

D. Coronal contrast-enhanced T1-WI shows a centrally enhancing mass involving the right kidney (arrow). *(Images D-E courtesy Dr. Christine Menias, Mallinckrodt Institute of Radiology, Washington University, St. Louis, Missouri)*

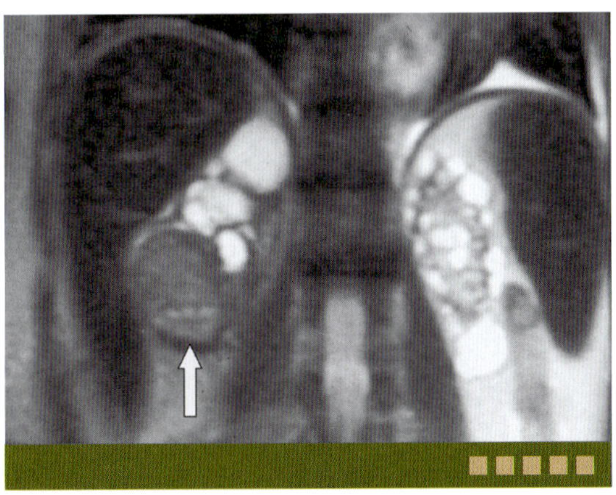

E. Coronal T2-WI on the same patient shows the mass to be hypointense, one of the classic MR features of collecting duct carcinoma. The medullary origin of the tumor is difficult to discern.

DIFFERENTIAL DIAGNOSES IMAGES (F-H)

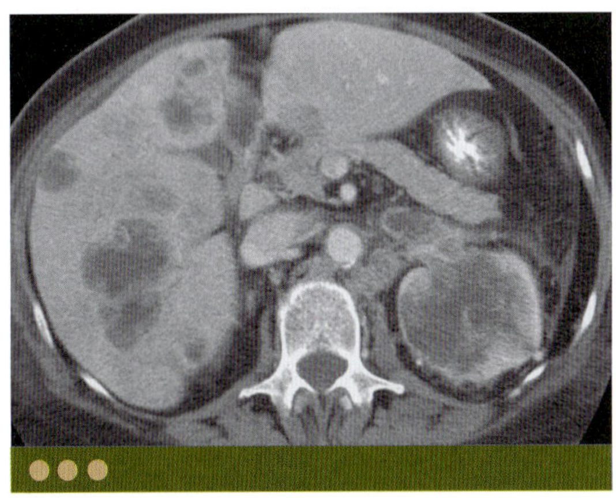

F. Renal cell carcinoma: Axial CECT shows a large infiltrative mass involving the left kidney and extending into the left renal vein. It has also metastasized to the liver.

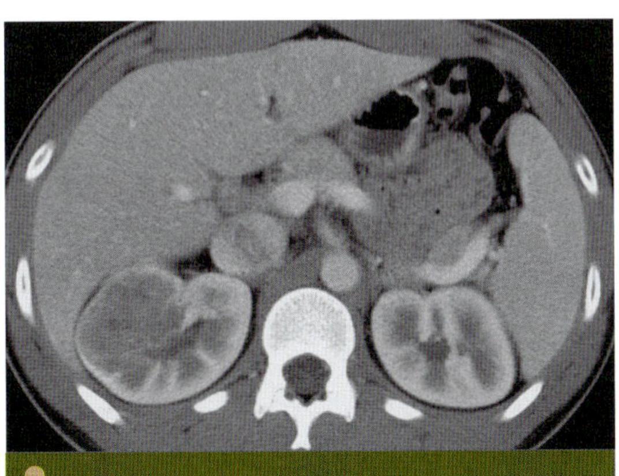

G. Renal medullary carcinoma: Axial CECT shows a large, mildly heterogeneous right renal mass involving the medulla and extending into the cortex. The patient had known sickle cell disease.

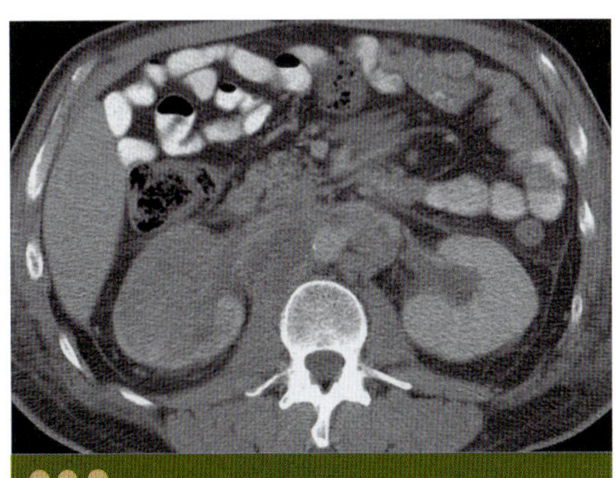

H. Renal lymphoma: Axial CECT shows a large infiltrating mass involving the majority of the right kidney extending medially through the renal sinus, with associated retroperitoneal adenopathy.

IMAGE KEY

Common

Rare

Typical

Unusual

1–10 Renal Lymphoma

Frank H. Miller

PRESENTATION

Asymptomatic, history of non-Hodgkin lymphoma; rare symptoms are flank pain and hematuria.

FINDINGS

Bilateral solid renal masses and hepatic mass.

DIFFERENTIAL DIAGNOSES

- *Renal metastases*: May have similar appearance, can differentiate on the basis of history of malignancy, and often, of metastases in other organs, such as liver and adrenal glands.
- *Renal cell carcinomas (RCC)*: Tends to be hypervascular, unlike lymphoma, and more often solitary, although can be multiple.
- *Angiomyolipomas*: Typically has fat.
- *Renal infarcts*: Typically wedge-shaped hypoenhancement; different clinical presentation.
- *Pyelonephritis*: Associated with striated nephrograms and urinary tract infections.
- *Renal medullary cancer*: Medullary masses and associated with sickle cell trait.

COMMENTS

Primary renal involvement by lymphoma is rare because the kidney does not have lymphoid tissue. Secondary renal lymphoma is common, and most commonly, is the result of non-Hodgkin lymphoma. It can also be seen in immunocompromised patients such as patients with AIDS. There are a number of presentations of non-Hodgkin lymphoma. The most common presentation is that of bilateral renal masses that are homogeneous and of soft tissue-attenuation on CT. Other patterns of involvement include a solitary mass, diffuse infiltrative masses, and extension from retroperitoneal lymph nodes to the renal sinus and perinephric spaces. When perinephric, they often do not invade the kidney. The masses may surround vessels but generally do not occlude them. The least common involvement is diffuse infiltrative masses of the kidneys. Renal failure is not commonly seen.

Features that suggest lymphoma include the lack of hemorrhage, calcifications, or necrosis despite the large size of the masses.

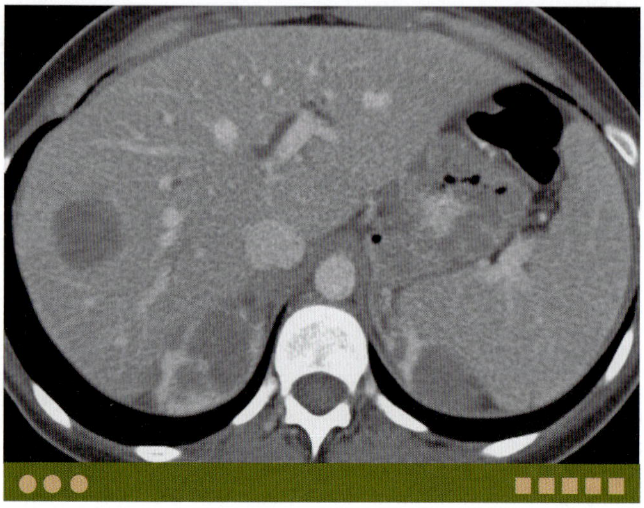

A. Axial CECT shows bilateral solid renal masses with hepatic mass.

CT tends to be the best imaging modality to identify and characterize lymphoma. The masses tend to be hypoenhancing and hypodense relative to the kidney. This differs from renal cell carcinoma which tends to be hypervascular. On ultrasound, masses from lymphoma are often homogenous, hypoechoic in appearance without significant acoustic enhancement which helps differentiate the masses from cysts. On MR, the masses are often hypointense on T1-weighted images (T1-WI) relative to the kidney and variable signal intensity on T2-weighted images (T2-WI) and generally show minimal enhancement.

Patients with renal lymphoma often do not have symptoms related to the urinary tract. Renal involvement is often detected on imaging studies performed for disease staging. Percutaneous biopsy may be required for the diagnosis as the treatment is not surgical and generally involves chemotherapy.

PEARLS

- **Renal lymphoma tends to be hypovascular unlike renal cell carcinoma which tends to be hypervascular.**
- **Masses from lymphoma are often homogenous soft tissue density in density on CT unless large, when they may show necrosis.**
- **Distinguishing renal lymphoma from primary malignancy may require biopsy as the treatment is different (chemotherapy for lymphoma vs. surgery for RCC).**

ADDITIONAL IMAGES (B-D)

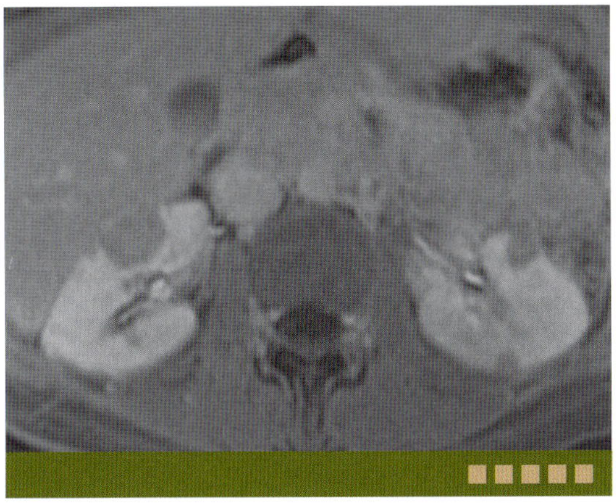

B. Axial CE T1-WI shows solid bilateral hypoenhancing renal masses.

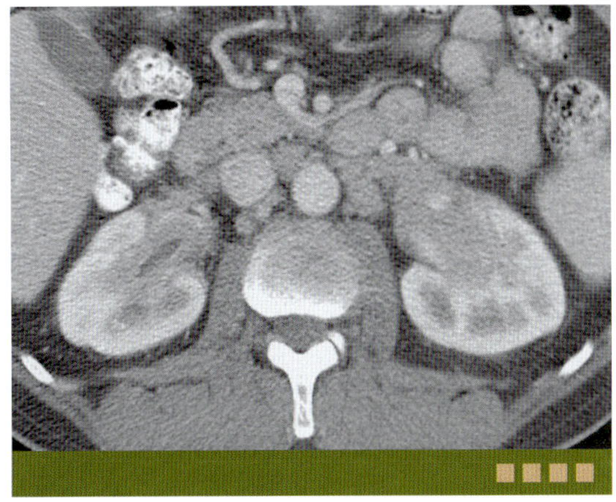

C. Axial CECT in different patient shows bilateral infiltrative masses extending to the renal hilum from adjacent adenopathy, with extension into the kidney. In addition, there was extensive retroperitoneal lymphadenopathy seen at other levels.

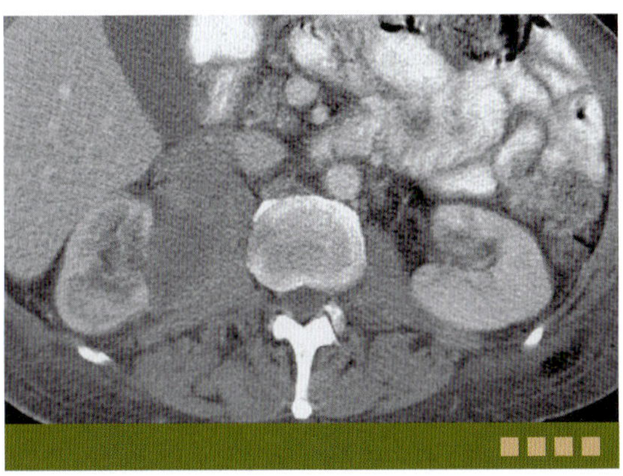

D. Axial CECT in different patient shows large retroperitoneal lymph node invading the right kidney because of non-Hodgkin lymphoma.

DIFFERENTIAL DIAGNOSES IMAGES (E-G)

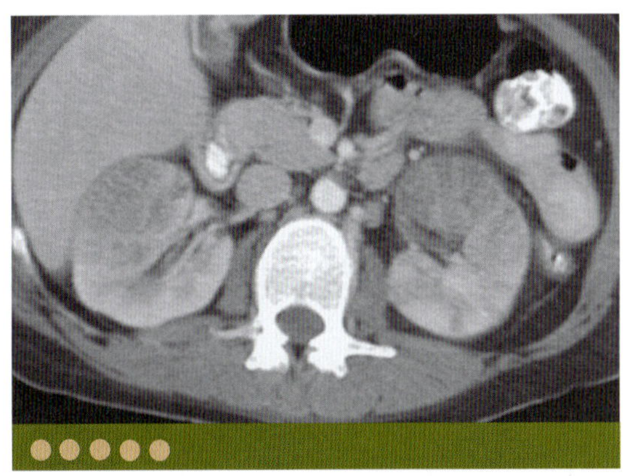

E. Acute pyelonephritis: Axial CECT shows bilateral predominately striated nephrogram in patients with fevers and urinary tract infection caused by pyelonephritis. Following antibiotics, the kidneys returned to normal.

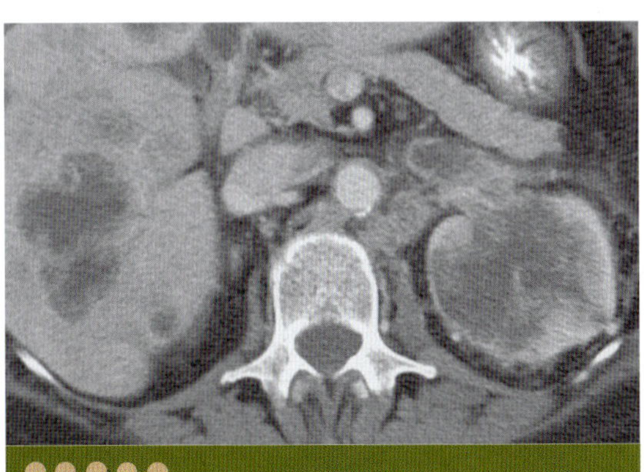

F. Renal cell carcinoma: Axial CECT shows infiltrative mass which invades the left renal vein. There are liver metastases and lymphadenopathy. Lymphoma tends not to invade or obstruct vessels.

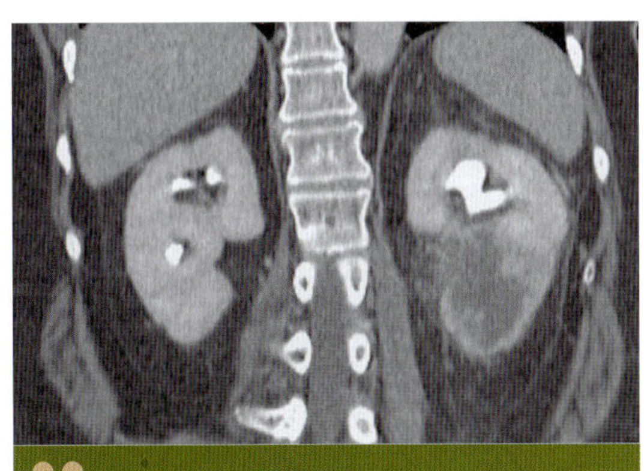

G. Renal cell carcinoma: Axial CECT shows infiltrative mass which invades the left renal vein. There are liver metastases and lymphadenopathy. Lymphoma tends not to invade or obstruct vessels.

Figures A and B are the same patient.

IMAGE KEY

Common

Rare

Typical

Unusual

1–11 Perirenal Lymphoma

Frank H. Miller

PRESENTATION

Generally asymptomatic; generally history of lymphoma or immunocompromised as in this patient with AIDS; may present with abdominal pain.

FINDINGS

Extensive perirenal soft tissue masses.

DIFFERENTIAL DIAGNOSES

- *Perinephric infection*: Distinguish based on history, fevers, chills, elevated white blood count, pyuria.
- *Perinephric metastases*: Typically history of metastases.
- *Perinephric hematoma*: Generally history of trauma or underlying mass that bled.

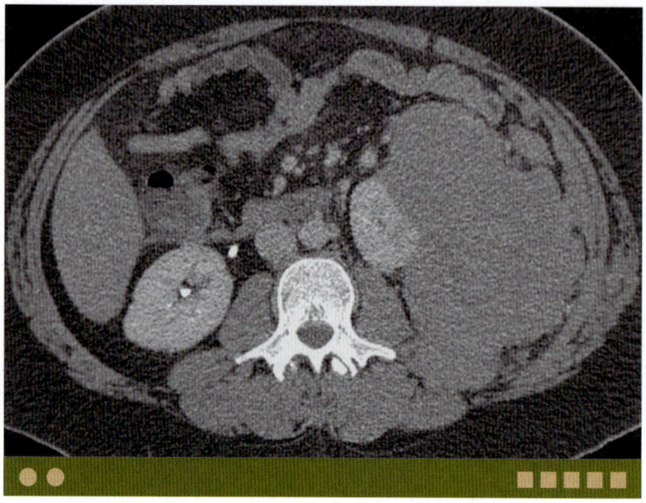

A. Axial CECT in patients with AIDS shows perinephric soft tissue mass from non-Hodgkin lymphoma. The mass enhances less than the kidney.

COMMENTS

Lymphoma involving the kidney is generally secondary involvement as the kidney does not have lymphoid tissue. It is generally associated with systemic non-Hodgkin lymphoma. It can also be seen in patients that are immunocompromised as in this patient with AIDS. The routine use of CT has led to increase in the detection of this disease. The kidney is one of the most common organs involved by extranodal lymphoma.

Renal involvement by lymphoma can be manifested in a number of different ways. The most common appearance is generally multiple solid homogeneous renal masses. Lymphoma may also be seen as a solitary mass. Perirenal involvement may be seen and is generally caused by extension of retroperitoneal lymphadenopathy or transcapsular tumor spread from the kidney. Isolated perirenal involvement may be seen as in this example. Abnormal soft tissue needs to be differentiated from perinephric fluid, inflammation, or blood. When perirenal soft tissue is seen, especially in elderly patients, without an explanation, lymphoma must be considered.

CT is the best method to make the diagnosis. Perirenal lymphoma is often associated with para-aortic or renal hilar lymphadenopathy. It is seen as perirenal soft tissue density masses. The density on unenhanced scans is similar to slightly higher than that of renal parenchyma. Enhancement tends to be homogeneous but less than the kidney itself. Calcifications are uncommon unless lymphoma has been treated.

Biopsy may be required for the diagnosis. Chemotherapy is generally the method of treatment with follow-up imaging with CT. PET scans can be helpful to show the extent of involvement, stage the disease, and assess therapy.

PEARLS

- **Lymphoma may be seen in patients who are immunocompromised by AIDS.**
- **Lymphoma most commonly presents with bilateral solid renal masses.**
- **Lymphoma may be seen as perirenal masses.**
- **CT is the best test to make the diagnosis of perirenal lymphoma.**
- **Biopsy may be required for diagnosis of perirenal lymphoma.**

ADDITIONAL IMAGES (B-D)

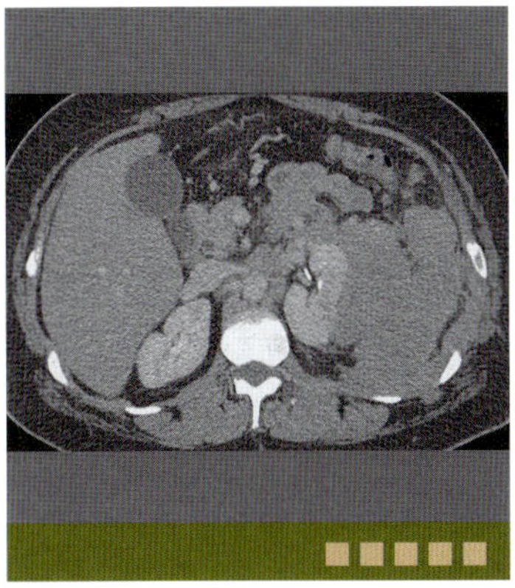

B. Axial CECT shows extensive perinephric soft tissue mass and also lymphadenopathy.

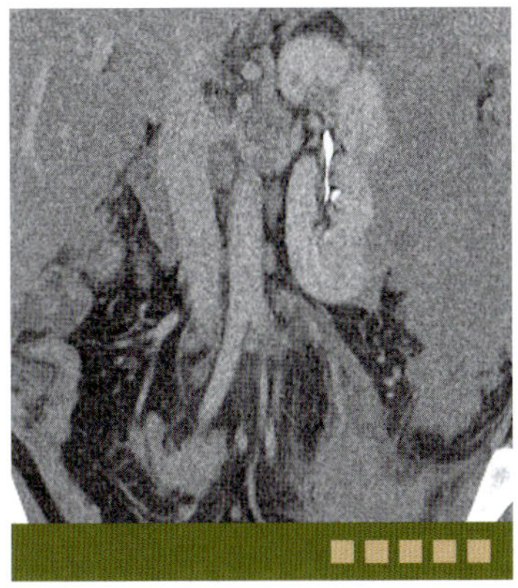

C. Coronal CECT in same patient shows perinephric soft tissue mass with extension to the spleen and into the pelvis.

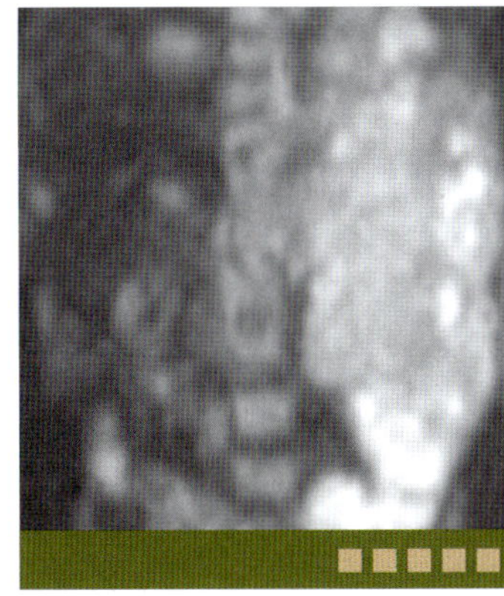

D. PET scan in the same patient shows the extensive involvement of lymphoma.

IMAGE KEY

Common

Rare

Typical

Unusual

DIFFERENTIAL DIAGNOSES IMAGES (E-G)

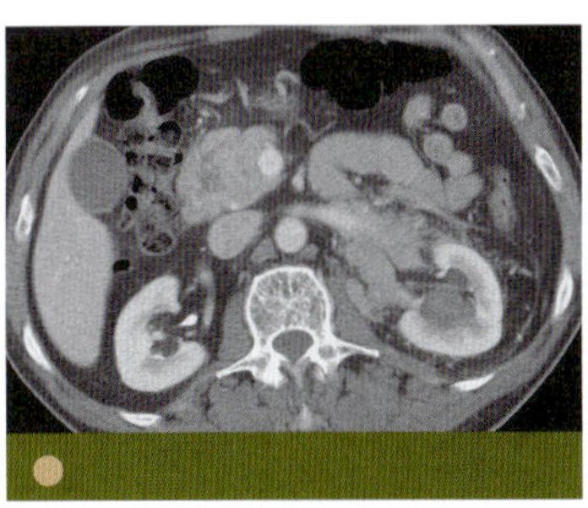

E. Perinephric plasmacytoma: Axial CECT shows perirenal soft tissue mass extending to the renal hilum with associated lymphadenopathy mimicking lymphoma. The distinction is based on clinical history or biopsy as the imaging appearance is similar

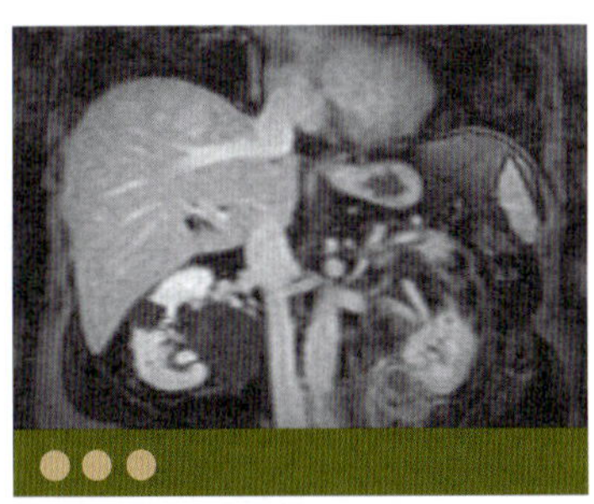

F. Perinephric infection from acute pyelonephritis: Coronal contrast-enhanced T1-WI shows perinephric inflammation from acute pyelonephritis. The clinical history of fevers and chills helps distinguish it from other entities.

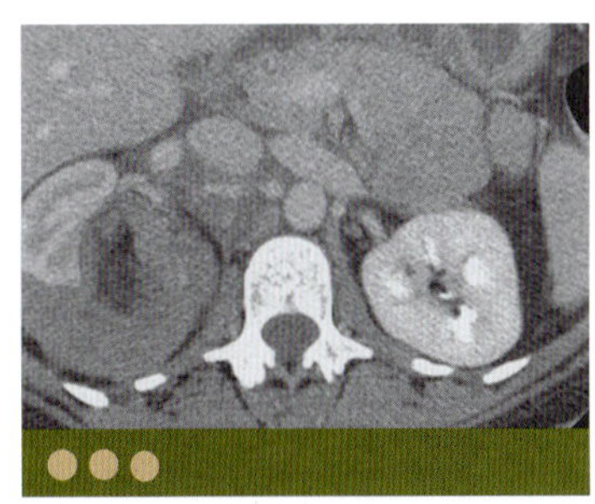

G. Perirenal hemorrhage from angiomyolipoma: Axial CECT shows high-density fluid because of blood in patient with fat-containing mass caused by 5-cm angiomyolipoma in the right kidney.

1–12 Extranodal Lymphoid Hyperplasia Involving the Kidney

Paul Nikolaidis

PRESENTATION

Nonspecific, may be incidental finding on imaging.

FINDINGS

CT shows a relatively ill-defined enhancing lesion in the medullary region of the right kidney.

DIFFERENTIAL DIAGNOSES

- *Renal neoplasms*: In many instances, lymphoid hyperplasia may be indistinguishable from a variety of renal neoplasms. Lymphoid hyperplasia typically presents as a relatively irregularly marginated lesion with features that are suspicious for a neoplasm.
- *Antopol Goldman lesion (subepithelial or renal sinus hemorrhage)*: Similarly ill-defined, always relatively hyperdense on precontrast images; will not enhance.

COMMENTS

Lymphoid hyperplasia, also known as pseudolymphoma, is due to the rapid growth of normal cells that resemble lymphatic tissue. It is an inflammatory response to certain stimuli that results in a lymphomatous-appearing but benign accumulation of inflammatory cells. There is some resemblance to lymphoma histologically, but a definitive distinction can typically be made. The presence of highly reactive germinal centers, numerous cell types, and prominent vascularity are the most important features differentiating this process from lymphoma.

Extranodal lymphoid hyperplasia will very rarely involve the kidney. It is reported to occur throughout the body including the gastrointestinal tract, skin, lung, thyroid, orbit, and pancreas.

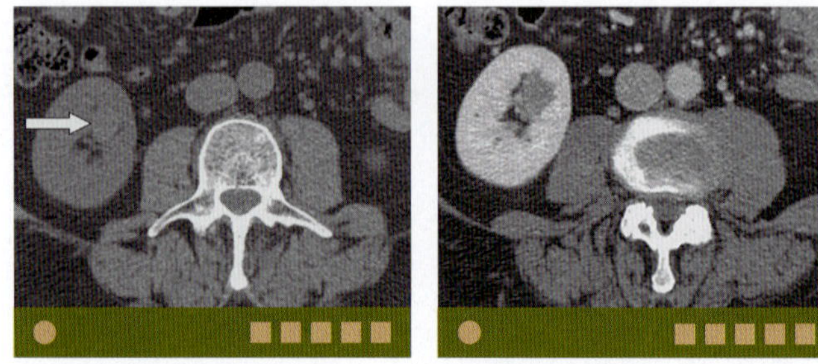

A. Axial NECT shows a subtle rounded area of slightly increased density in the lower pole of the right kidney (arrow).
B. Axial CECT shows mild enhancement of the central right renal lesion.

On cross-sectional imaging, nonspecific enhancing soft tissue lesions are seen and may be located in the renal medulla or sinus. On CT, they appear as space-occupying lesions that are relatively irregularly marginated. They enhance following contrast administration. Their appearance is entirely nonspecific, and many lesions will be managed surgically prior to definitive histologic diagnosis.

PEARLS

- **Rare lesions of the renal medulla and sinus.**
- **May mimic lymphoma histologically, clinically, and on imaging; also known as pseudolymphoma.**
- **Entirely nonspecific appearing on all imaging modalities.**
- **On CT enhancing soft tissue lesions are seen; usually irregularly marginated.**

ADDITIONAL IMAGES (C-E)

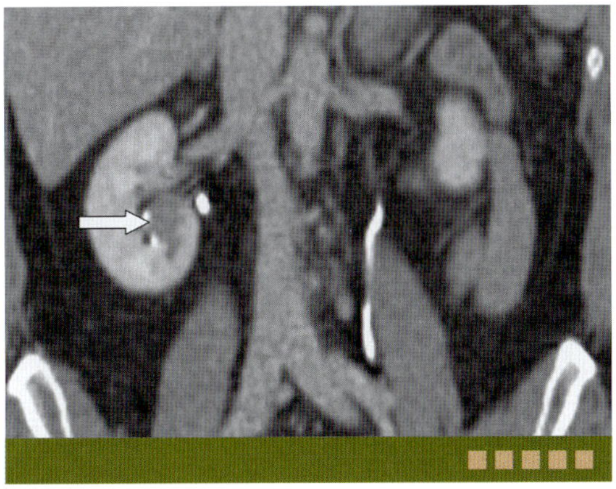

C. Coronal CECT on the same patient again shows the central enhancing right renal mass (arrow).

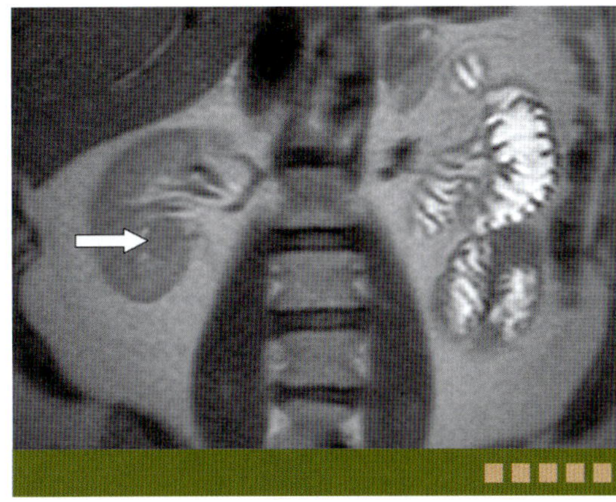

D. Coronal T2-WI on the same patient shows the central lower pole renal mass (arrow) is approximately isointense to the renal parenchyma.

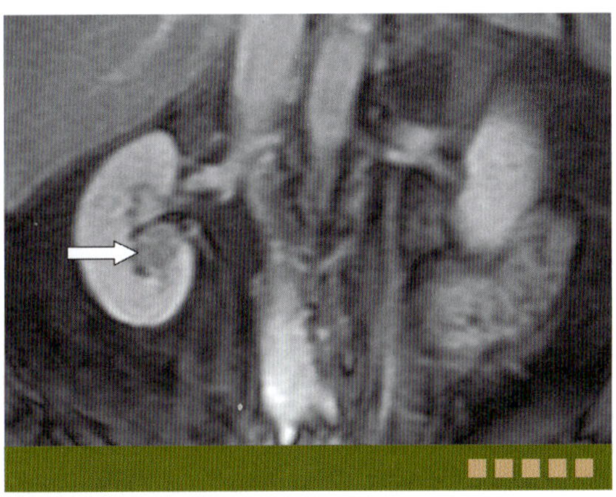

E. Coronal contrast-enhanced T1-WI on the same patient better shows the central enhancing right renal mass (arrow).

DIFFERENTIAL DIAGNOSES IMAGES (F-H)

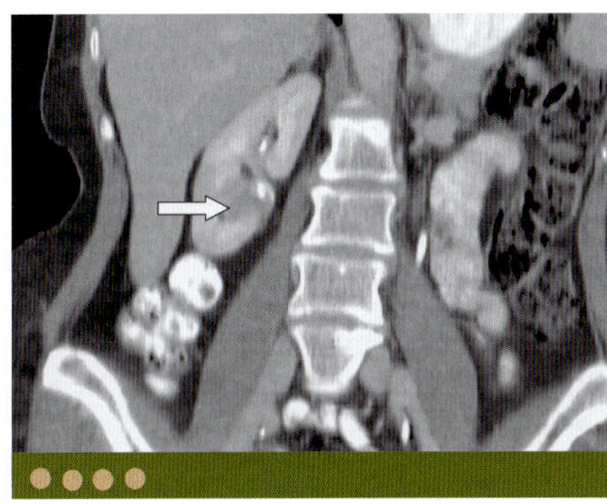

F. Transitional cell carcinoma: Coronal CECT shows a slightly hypoenhancing mass (arrow) centered in the right renal pelvis, invading the medulla.

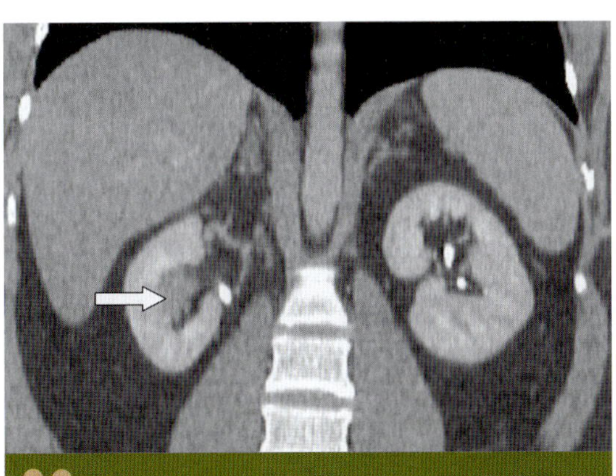

G. Antopol Goldman lesion (subepithelial renal hemorrhage): Coronal CECT shows a right renal mass (arrow) which is more centered in the renal sinus.

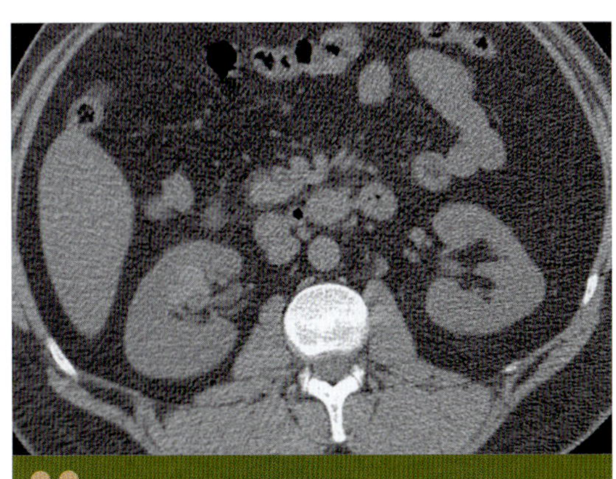

H. Antopol Goldman lesion (subepithelial renal hemorrhage): Corresponding axial NECT on the same patient shows the mass to be slightly ill-defined and hyperdense.

IMAGE KEY

Common

Rare

Typical

Unusual

1–13 Renal Liposarcoma

Frank H. Miller

PRESENTATION

Asymptomatic seen on CT scan for abdominal pain.

FINDINGS

MR shows fat-containing mass of the left renal sinus.

DIFFERENTIAL DIAGNOSES

- *Exophytic angiomyolipomas*: Can be difficult to distinguish from liposarcoma, see comment section.
- *Chronic inflammation*: Inflammation extending into the retroperitoneal fat may mimic liposarcoma.
- *Angiomyolipomas in tuberous sclerosis*: Presence of associated findings of tuberous sclerosis and multiple angiomyolipomas favors diagnosis.

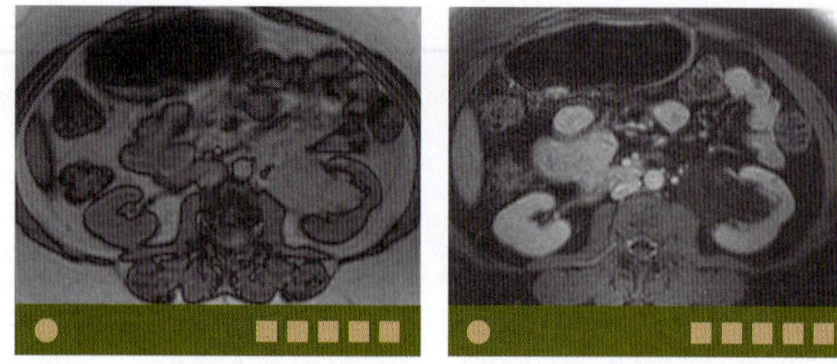

A. Axial, opposed-phase T1-WI shows fat-containing mass of left renal sinus. The lesion does not arise from the kidney and does not show defect with renal parenchyma or significant vascularity. **B.** Axial contrast-enhanced T1-WI shows the mass better and surrounding capsule without large vessels or renal parenchymal defect to suggest angiomyolipoma.

COMMENTS

Renal liposarcomas of the renal sinus are very rare tumors that usually develop in the fourth and sixth decades of life. The exact prevalence is not known because of difficulty in distinguishing retroperitoneal liposarcomas from primary renal liposarcomas. Patients with renal liposarcomas often are clinically asymptomatic for a long period until the mass becomes large. Renal liposarcomas are generally located peripherally between the renal capsule and kidney. They tend to be large at presentation as patients are relatively asymptomatic. They extend into the perirenal space. They are often invasive and should be surgically resected.

Perirenal liposarcomas may be difficult to distinguish from angiomyolipomas. Angiomyolipomas are far more common than liposarcomas. Features that suggest angiomyolipomas include a defect or "claw" sign with the renal parenchyma to suggest that it arises from the kidney. In contrast, liposarcomas do not cause a defect in the kidney parenchyma and have a smooth interface with the kidney. In addition, angiomyolipomas tend to be more vascular with enlarged vessels in the lesion. Liposarcoma tends to be relatively avascular on imaging studies and angiography and tends to be supplied by capsular arteries. The presence of additional angiomyolipomas favors angiomyolipoma, as does intralesional hemorrhage and a smaller overall size.

Based on different treatments and prognoses, it is important to distinguish liposarcomas from angiomyolipomas.

PEARLS

- **Renal liposarcomas are rare, and often, patients are asymptomatic until tumors become large.**
- **Renal liposarcomas often arise from the renal capsule and are seen between the kidney and capsule.**
- **Renal liposarcomas may be difficult to distinguish from angiomyolipomas.**
- **Features that favor angiomyolipoma include a defect in renal parenchyma, greater vascularity, large vessel(s) in lesion, intralesional hemorrhage, and smaller size.**

ADDITIONAL IMAGES (C-E)

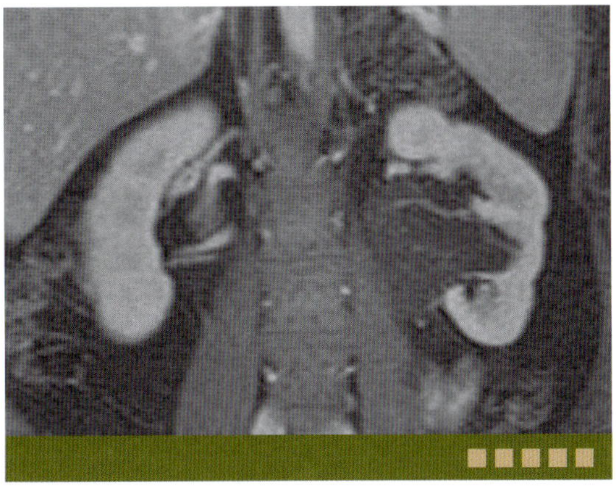

C. Coronal contrast-enhanced T1-WI in the same patient shows relationship to the renal hilum and shows the mass is discrete from the fat surrounding the kidney.

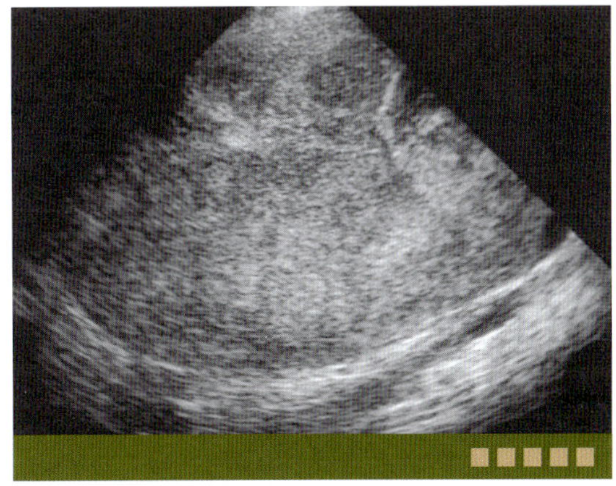

D. In a different patient, longitudinal sonogram shows large complex echogenic mass involving left kidney.

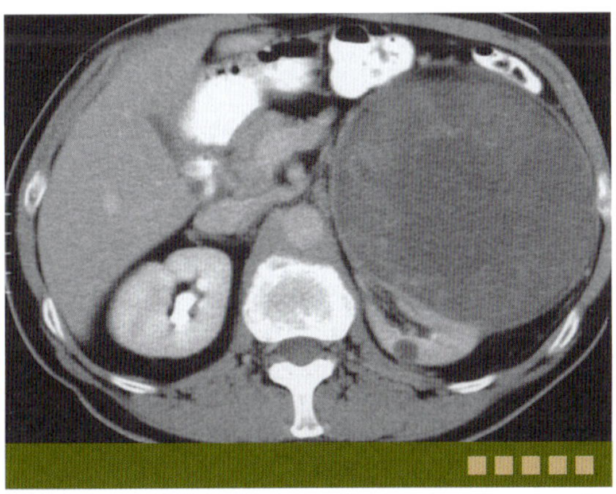

E. Axial CECT shows large hypodense mass displaces the left kidney. It is difficult to tell if it is arising from the kidney or the renal capsule. Smooth compression of kidney favors liposarcoma which was confirmed on biopsy.

DIFFERENTIAL DIAGNOSES IMAGES (F-H)

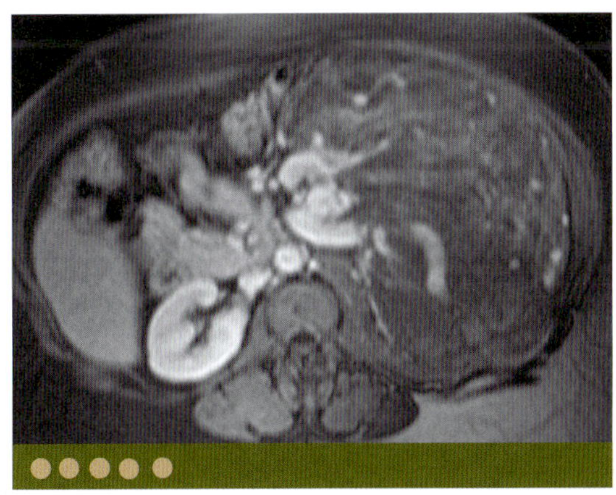

F. Angiomyolipoma: Axial, contrast-enhanced T1-WI shows large, fat-containing mass which shows renal parenchymal defect as it arises from the kidney. There are large vessels in the lesion. These findings are suggestive of angiomyolipoma.

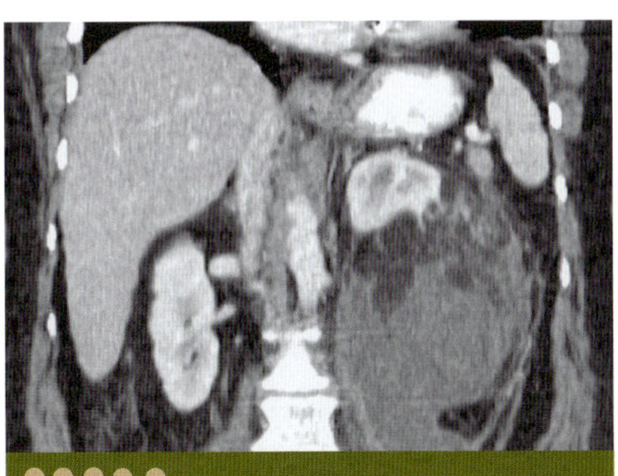

G. Angiomyolipoma: Coronal CECT in the same patient as in Figure F shows large left exophytic fat-containing renal mass with defect in renal parenchyma ("claw" sign) associated with hemorrhage. The presence of the renal parenchyma defect and hemorrhage is generally not seen in patients with liposarcomas.

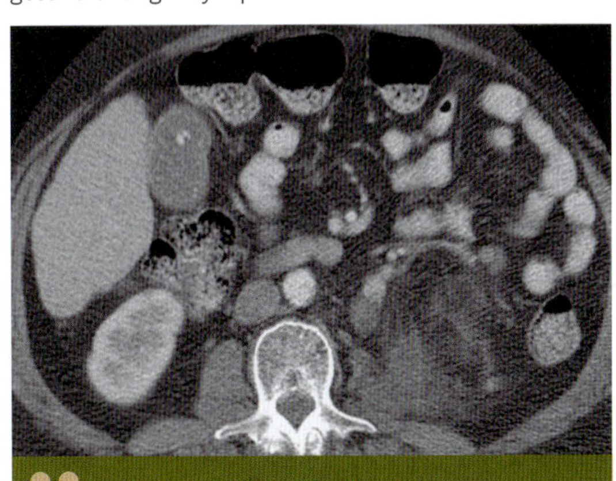

H. Chronic inflammation mimicking fat-containing neoplasm: Axial CECT shows fat-containing mass because of inflammation mimicking liposarcoma and angiomyolipoma.

IMAGE KEY

Common

Rare

Typical

Unusual

1–14 Renal Leiomyosarcoma

Paul Nikolaidis

PRESENTATION

Flank pain, palpable flank, or abdominal mass.

FINDINGS

MR shows a large right renal mass with significant areas of nonenhancement; the mass is predominantly hypointense on T2-WI with central areas of increased signal.

DIFFERENTIAL DIAGNOSES

- *Renal neoplasms*: May be difficult to distinguish from a wide variety of renal neoplasms including renal cell carcinoma (RCC) and other renal sarcomas. Not as likely to invade the renal vein as a large renal cell carcinoma. Areas of low T2 signal are often seen in leiomyosarcoma; T2 hypointensity is typically seen only in the papillary subtype of renal cell carcinoma.

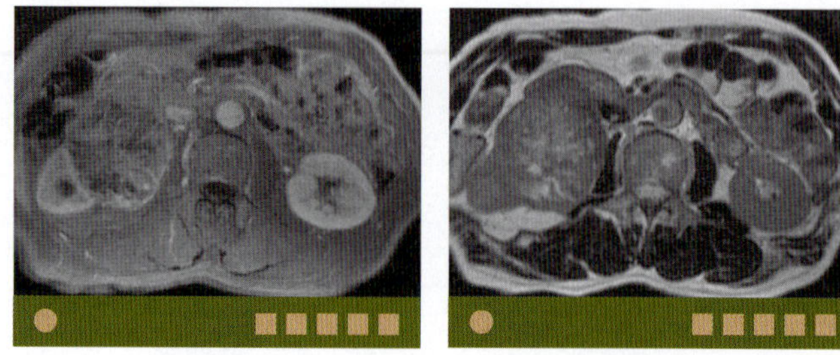

A. Axial, contrast-enhanced T1-WI shows a large mass involving the anterior aspect of the right kidney. It enhances heterogeneously, with large areas of necrosis and degeneration.
B. Axial T2-WI on the same patient shows the mass to be predominantly hypointense with central hyperintense foci. *(Images courtesy Dr. Naoki Takahashi, Mayo Clinic, Rochester, Minnesota)*

COMMENTS

Primary renal sarcomas are rare. They include leiomyosarcoma, angiosarcoma, fibrosarcoma, rhabdomyosarcoma, and osteosarcoma. Leiomyosarcoma is the most common histologic subtype, accounting for 50% to 60% of renal sarcomas.

Renal leiomyosarcoma may arise from the renal capsule, the smooth muscle fibers of the renal pelvis, the sphincteric ring around renal papilla, or the muscle fibers of intrarenal blood vessels. The majority of cases occur between the fourth and eighth decades, and the right kidney is reported to be more frequently involved. Common presenting symptoms include abdominal or flank pain and hematuria. Less frequently, patients may present with anorexia and weight loss. Tumors are typically aggressive, and patients frequently develop systemic metastases prior to initial diagnosis, resulting in poor prognosis.

The imaging findings of renal leiomyosarcoma are variable but usually nonspecific. On ultrasound, a mass that distorts the renal outline is typically seen. Contrast-enhanced CT or MR is necessary to provide more information regarding tumor size, extent of invasion of surrounding structures, and the exact relationship to adjacent vessels and bowel loops.

Renal leiomyosarcoma may appear as a well-defined, heterogeneously enhancing or multinodular mass on CT. In many cases, the mass will displace rather than invade the renal parenchyma. It is not as likely to invade the renal vein as a large renal cell carcinoma. Tumors are characterized by a rapid growth rate and a propensity to metastasize early.

MR will show a heterogeneously enhancing mass. Areas of low signal intensity on T2-WI are classically present, thought to be because of its smooth muscle composition. Areas of degeneration and necrosis will appear hyperintense on T2-WI.

Diagnosis is usually made at the time of biopsy or surgery. Although radical nephrectomy has been suggested as the treatment of choice, partial nephrectomy is an acceptable alternative in patients with a single, 4 to 5 cm or smaller mass with a normal contralateral kidney. Prognosis is poor and the roles of chemotherapy and radiation therapy remain controversial.

PEARLS

- **Tumors usually arise from the renal capsule or the smooth muscle of the renal pelvis or intrarenal vessels.**
- **Rapid growth and a propensity to metastasize early are characteristic features.**
- **Imaging features are typically nonspecific and a preoperative diagnosis is unlikely.**
- **Tumors enhance heterogeneously on CT and MR, and are low-signal on T2-WI.**

ADDITIONAL IMAGES (C-E)

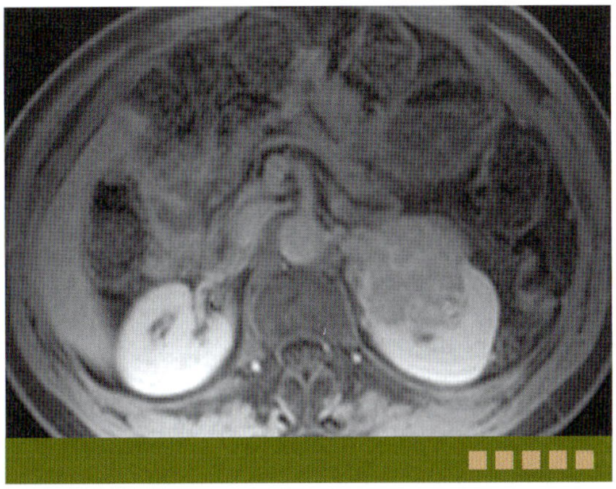

C. Axial contrast-enhanced T1-WI in another patient shows a large centrally located mass extending anteriorly in the mid left kidney. It enhances less than the normal renal parenchyma.

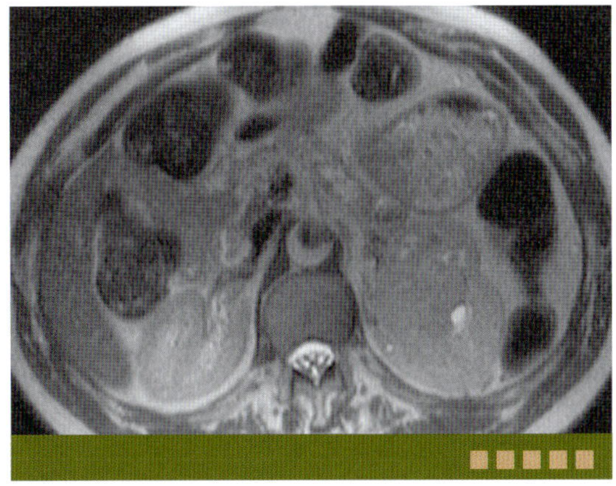

D. Axial T2-WI shows the mass to be slightly hypointense to renal parenchyma. There are a few internal foci of increased signal.

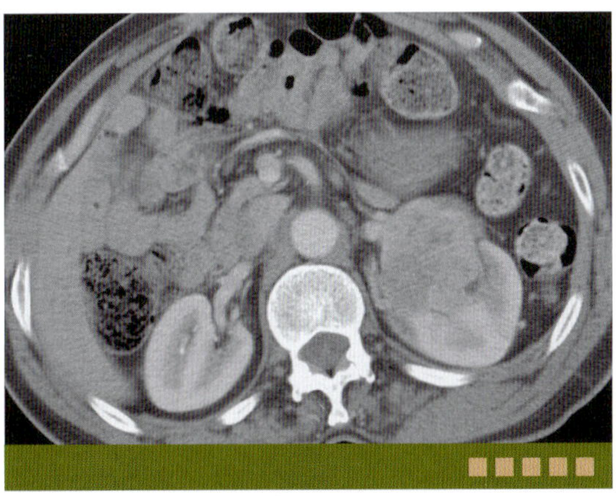

E. Corresponding axial CECT shows that the mass enhances heterogeneously and less than the normal renal parenchyma.

DIFFERENTIAL DIAGNOSES IMAGES (F-H)

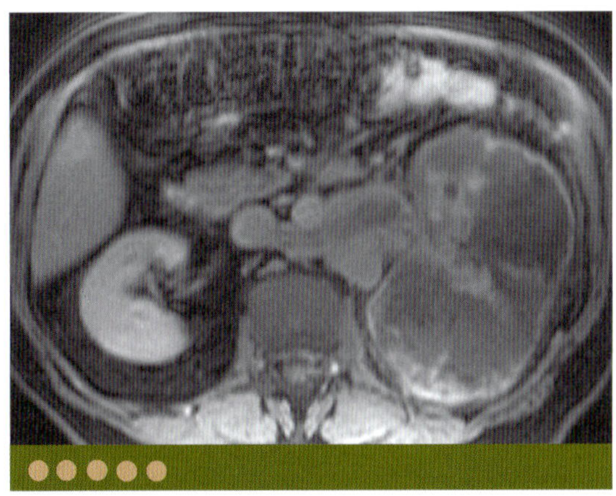

F. Renal cell carcinoma: Axial contrast-enhanced T1-WI shows a large necrotic left renal cell carcinoma with tumor thrombus that extends into the retroaortic left renal vein.

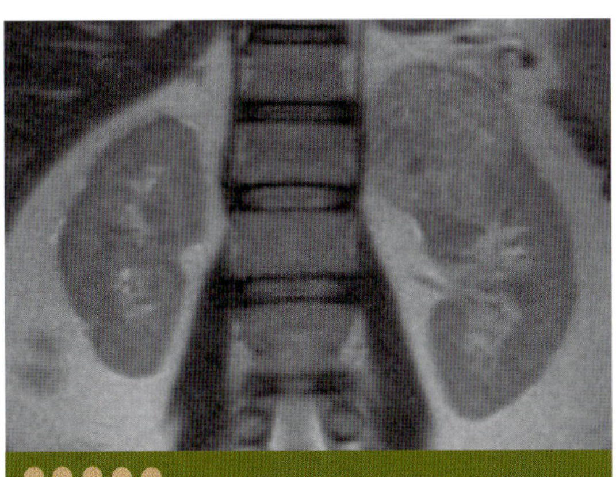

G. Renal cell carcinoma: Coronal T2-WI on another patient shows a large renal cell carcinoma arising from the upper pole of the left kidney. It is predominantly hyperintense comparing to normal renal parenchyma.

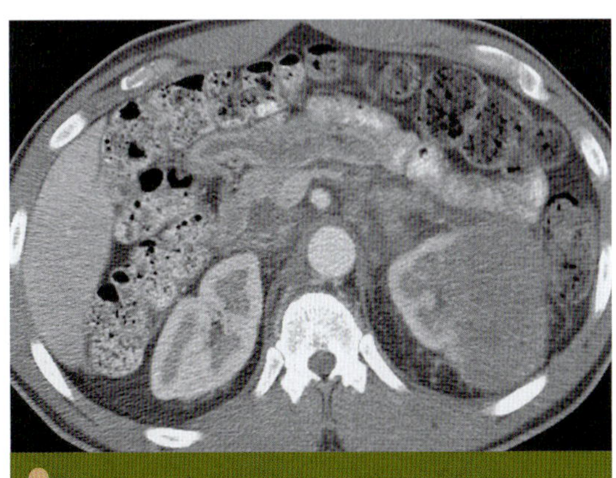

H. Renal malignant fibrous histiocytoma: Axial CECT shows a large mass occupying the lateral portion of the left kidney. It enhances significantly less than the normal renal parenchyma.

IMAGE KEY

Common

Rare

Typical

Unusual

1–15 Renal Malignant Fibrous Histiocytoma

Paul Nikolaidis

PRESENTATION

Flank pain, palpable flank, or abdominal mass.

FINDINGS

CT shows a large mass occupying the lateral portion of the left kidney which enhances significantly less than the normal portions of the kidney.

DIFFERENTIAL DIAGNOSIS

- *Renal neoplasms*: Malignant fibrous histiocytoma (MFH) is almost always indistinguishable from a wide variety of renal neoplasms, including renal cell carcinoma and other renal sarcomas.

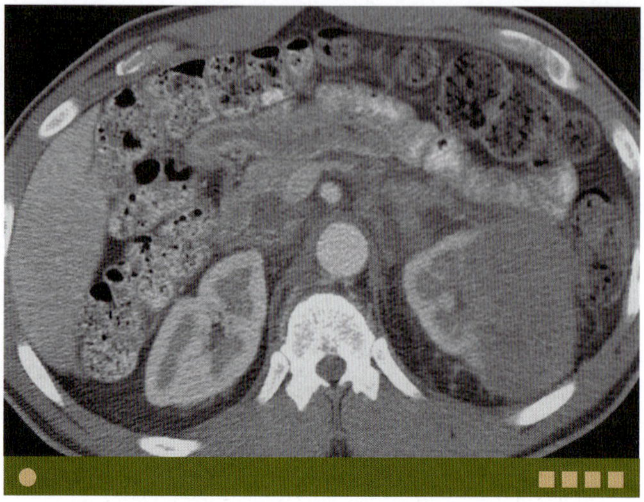

A. Axial CECT shows a large mass occupying the lateral portion of the left kidney. It enhances significantly less than the normal renal parenchyma. While imaging features are nonspecific, areas of decreased attenuation occur in MFH which correspond to areas of myxomatous tissue, cystic degeneration, and necrosis.

COMMENTS

Primary renal sarcomas are rare. Malignant fibrous histiocytoma (MFH) represents less than 6% of primary renal sarcomas. MFH is thought to arise from primitive mesenchymal cells which demonstrate both histiocytic and fibroblastic differentiation. It is the most common soft tissue sarcoma in adults but only rarely arises from the kidney. Approximately 60 cases of MFH have been reported to arise from the kidney or renal capsule.

The majority of cases occur between the fourth and eighth decades, and the left kidney is reported to be more frequently involved. Tumors typically present late with abdominal or flank pain and hematuria. Less frequently, patients may present with anorexia and weight loss. Tumors are aggressive, and patients will frequently develop systemic metastases prior to initial diagnosis, resulting in poor prognosis.

The imaging findings of renal MFH are variable but nonspecific. On ultrasound, a mass that distorts the renal outline is typically seen. CECT or MR is necessary to provide more information regarding tumor size, the presence of any invasion of surrounding structures, as well as the relationship between the mass and adjacent vessels and bowel loops.

By the time of diagnosis, renal MFH usually appears as a large solid, heterogeneously enhancing mass on CT. Central areas of decreased attenuation corresponding to areas of myxomatous tissue, cystic degeneration, and necrosis are often present. Calcifications are unusual. The degree of enhancement varies depending on the amount of fibrosis, tumor vascularity and cellularity, as well as necrosis. Tumors are characterized by a rapid growth rate and a propensity to metastasize early.

On MR, a heterogeneously enhancing mass is seen; tumors show variable signal intensity on T2-WI and low signal on T1-WI. Areas of low signal on T2-WI are thought to represent fibroblast rich regions, whereas high-signal areas are thought to be secondary to necrosis and cystic degeneration.

Diagnosis is usually made at the time of biopsy or surgery. Early radical nephrectomy with postoperative polychemotherapy is the treatment of choice. Prognosis is poor. The role of radiation therapy remains controversial.

PEARLS

- **These rare tumors may arise from the renal capsule or in the renal parenchyma.**
- **Rapid growth and a propensity to metastasize early are characteristic features.**
- **Imaging features are typically nonspecific and a preoperative diagnosis is unlikely.**
- **Tumors enhance heterogeneously on CT and MR, and large areas of necrosis may be present.**

ADDITIONAL IMAGES (B-C)

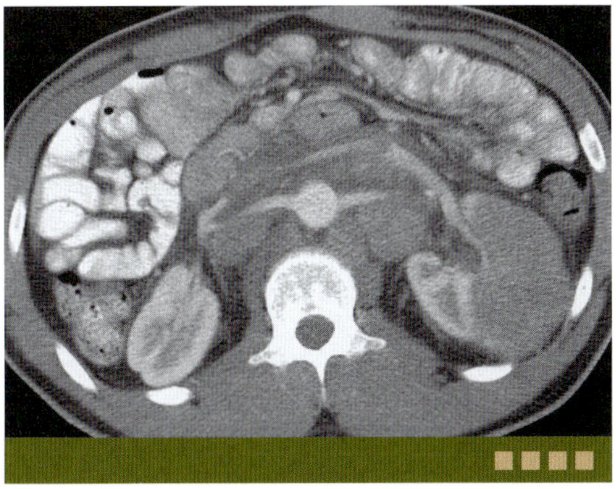

B. Axial CECT on the same patient again shows the large left renal mass along with extensive retroperitoneal adenopathy. Renal sarcomas are characterized by a rapid growth rate and a propensity to metastasize early.

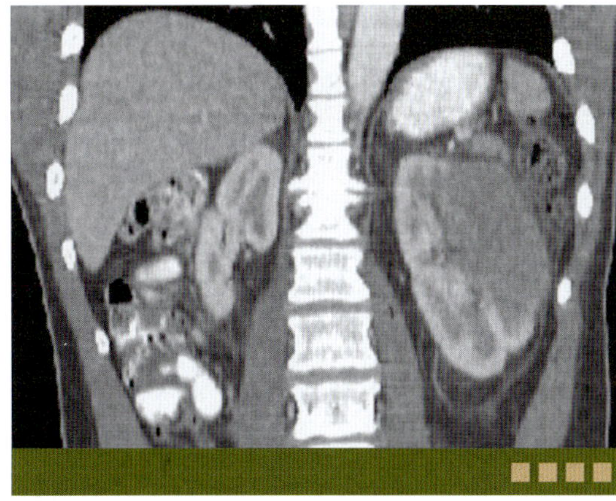

C. Corresponding coronal CECT better shows the extent of renal involvement. It is not certain whether the tumor arose from the renal capsule or the renal parenchyma.

DIFFERENTIAL DIAGNOSES IMAGES (D-F)

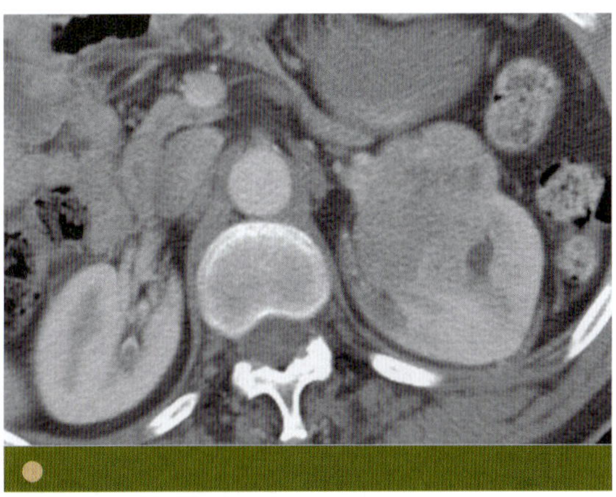

D. Renal leiomyosarcoma: Axial contrast-enhanced T1-WI on another patient shows a large centrally located mass extending anteriorly in the mid-left kidney. It enhances less than the normal renal parenchyma.

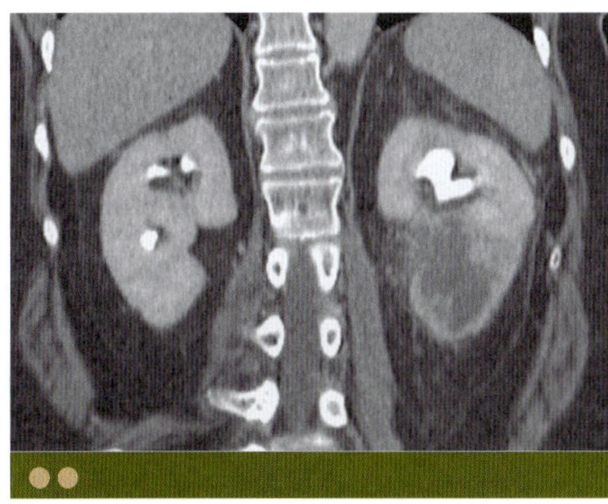

E. Renal metastasis: Coronal CECT shows a large hypoenhancing left lower pole mass. This represented a metastasis in a patient with squamous cell carcinoma.

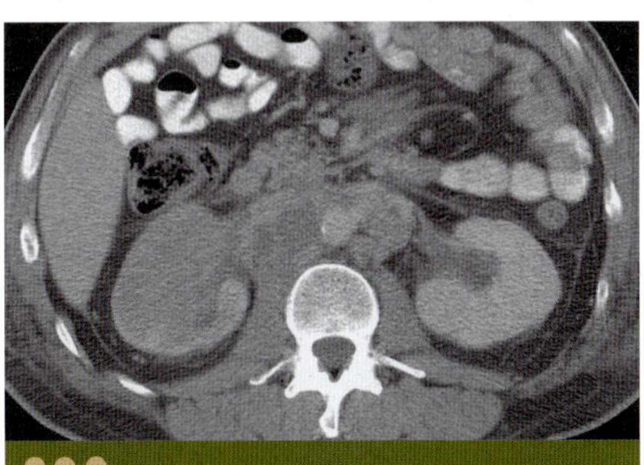

F. Renal lymphoma: Axial CECT shows a large infiltrating mass involving majority of the right kidney. It enhances less than the normal renal parenchyma. It also extends medially through the renal sinus, and there is associated retroperitoneal adenopathy.

IMAGE KEY

Common

Rare

Typical

Unusual

1–16 Perirenal Extramedullary Plasmacytoma

Paul Nikolaidis

PRESENTATION

Abdominal and back pain, may be incidentally discovered, usually in a patient with bone lesions and known multiple myeloma.

FINDINGS

CT shows a large, enhancing soft tissue mass in the retroperitoneum. It encases the left renal artery and vein and extends into the renal sinus. The patient had a known history of multiple myeloma.

DIFFERENTIAL DIAGNOSES

- *Lymphoma*: More common. Similar ill-defined perirenal soft tissue density may be seen; coexisting lymphadenopathy may be extensive.
- *Perirenal hemorrhage*: Similar ill-defined perirenal soft tissue density may be seen; should be hyperdense on precontrast images and should not enhance (unless there is active bleeding).

COMMENTS

Multiple myeloma is a malignant disease affecting primarily the osseous structures, characterized by a proliferation of malignant plasma cells that originate in the bone marrow. Extraosseous myeloma is an uncommon and aggressive form of multiple myeloma. Solitary plasmacytoma of the bone, extramedullary plasmacytoma (EMP), and multiple myeloma are generally considered to be different manifestations of the same basic process. Extramedullary involvement occurs in less than 5% of all patients, with most cases involving the mucous membranes of the upper respiratory tract. Involvement of the gastrointestinal (GI) tract, lymph nodes, breast, spleen, vagina, pancreas, and thyroid has been described. In the genitourinary (GU) tract, involvement of the kidneys and testicles is been reported. Incidence is increased fourfold in males, most often patients in their fifties and sixties.

Extramedullary multiple myeloma arising in the region of the kidney is very rare. Renal disease occurs frequently in patients with myeloma, but is usually from amyloidosis rather than actual plasma cell infiltration of the kidneys. Perinephric soft tissue masses are the most common manifestation of myeloma in the region of the kidneys and retroperitoneum. On imaging studies, renal plasmacytomas may appear as discrete perirenal soft tissue nodules or masses; they may be infiltrative. Both heterogeneous and homogeneous enhancement has been described. They may mimic other perirenal neoplasms and particularly lymphoma (both clinically and radiographically). Rarely, if situated near the renal pelvis, they may mimic neoplasms of the renal pelvis, most notably transitional cell carcinoma. It may be difficult for CT, excretory urography, or arteriography to preoperatively distinguish between perirenal myeloma and malignancy of the renal pelvis. However, this diagnosis should be considered when paraproteins are detected in the blood and urine and the patient has a history of plasma cell dyscrasia.

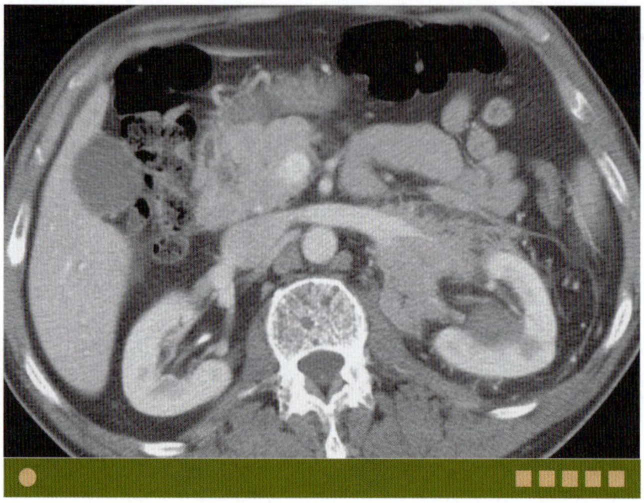

A. Axial CECT shows a large enhancing soft tissue mass in the retroperitoneum. It encases the left renal artery and vein and extends into the renal sinus. The patient had a known history of multiple myeloma.

PEARLS

- **Extraosseous myeloma is an uncommon (occuring approximately in 5%) and aggressive disease.**
- **Most common sites are the upper respiratory tract but the involvement of several other sites throughout the body has been reported.**
- **Renal involvement is usually in the form of perirenal soft tissue masses that may be infiltrative.**
- **In rare instances, more focal involvement of the area of the renal pelvis may occur, suggestive of urothelial neoplasm.**

ADDITIONAL IMAGE

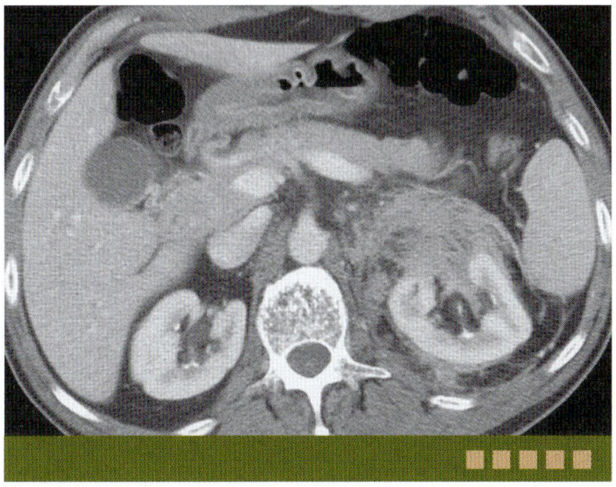

B. Axial CECT on the same patient shows abnormal perirenal enhancing soft tissue both anterior and posterior to the left kidney.

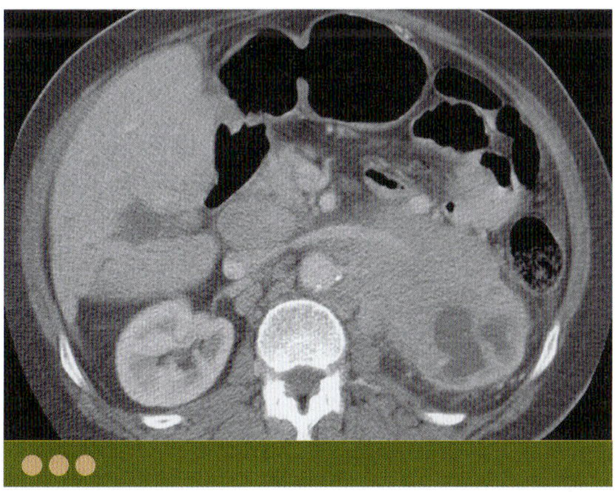

D. Lymphoma: Axial CECT on a different patient shows an infiltrative soft tissue lesion occupying the entire renal sinus and extending medially, surrounding the renal artery and left renal vein.

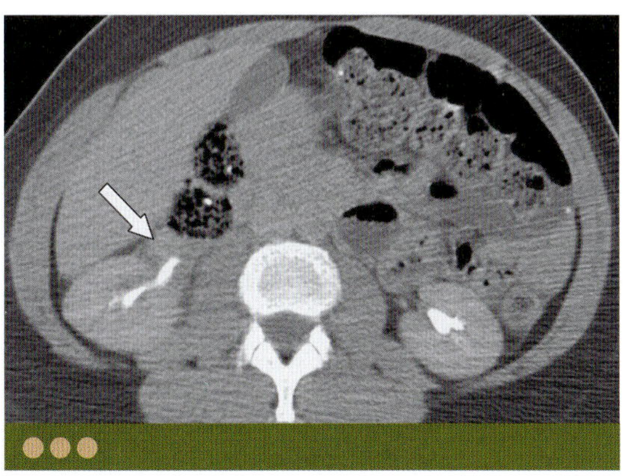

F. Perirenal hemorrhage: Axial CECT on the same patient shows that the lesion does not enhance (arrow). This is compatible with a hematoma. Note excretion of contrast into the proximal right ureter, surrounded by the lesion.

DIFFERENTIAL DIAGNOSES IMAGES (C-F)

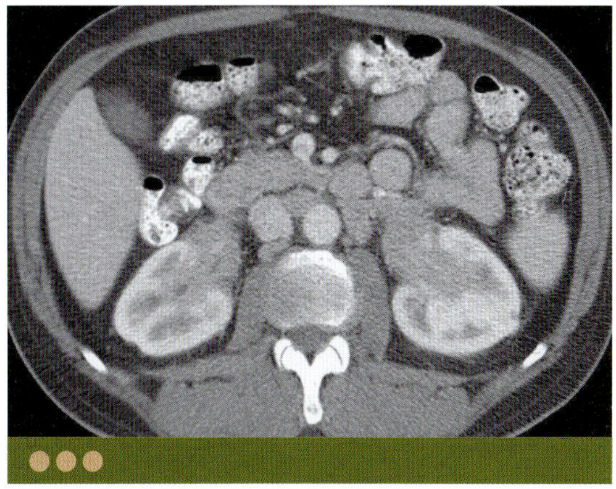

C. Lymphoma: Axial CECT shows enhancing, ill-defined soft tissue lesions infiltrating both renal sinuses. There is retroperitoneal lymphadenopathy.

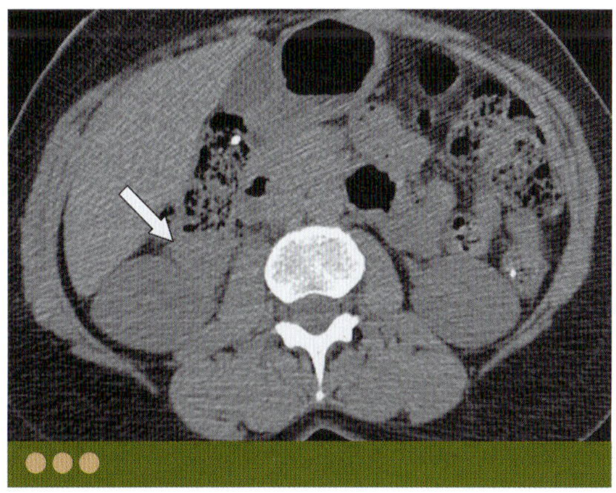

E. Perirenal hemorrhage: Axial NECT shows a small ill-defined hyperdense lesion anterior to the right kidney (arrow).

IMAGE KEY

Common

Rare

Typical

Unusual

1–17 Metastatic Lesion to the Kidney from Squamous Lung Cancer

Frank H. Miller

PRESENTATION

Often asymptomatic, history of malignancy elsewhere.

FINDINGS

CT shows ill-defined infiltrative mass of kidney with metastases elsewhere.

DIFFERENTIAL DIAGNOSES

- *Renal cell carcinoma (RCC)*: Can look similar and may require biopsy to distinguish.
- *Angiomyolipoma (AML)*: Generally contains fat.
- *Renal infection (pyelonephritis or abscess)*: Clinical history and urinalysis are important; follow-up imaging following antibiotics will show whether the mass improves or resolves.
- *Lymphoma*: Biopsy or history helps distinguish.

COMMENTS

Metastases to the kidney are common in patients with advanced stage cancers. At autopsy, approximately 10% of cancer patients have metastases to the kidney, although they may not be seen on imaging studies when the patient is alive. These metastases, however, are often small. They may not be detected prior to autopsy but are being detected more frequently as patients are living longer and are being treated for their primary malignancy and undergo frequent cross-sectional imaging. The more common sources of metastases to the kidneys include cancers from the lung, breast, gastrointestinal (GI) tract, and melanoma.

Renal metastases can have an expansile or infiltrative growth pattern. Most frequently, metastases are seen as multiple bilateral masses that are generally hypodense to the kidney. The lesions often have ill-defined infiltrative margins as seen in this case. Features of cystic necrosis, hemorrhage, or calcifications at imaging studies depend on the primary malignancy.

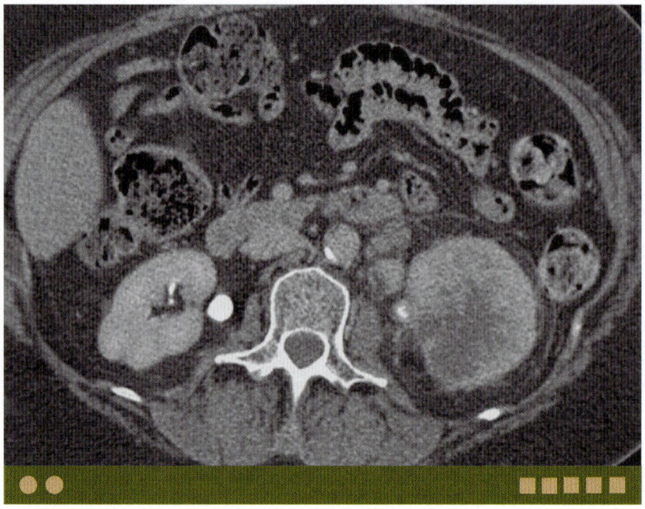

A. Axial CECT in excretory phase shows ill-defined mass in the left kidney.

When solitary lesions are seen in the kidney on imaging studie in patients with a known malignancy biopsy may be required to distinguish primary renal cell carcinoma or lymphoma from metastases to the kidney if it affects treatment. Hypovascular metastases can look similar to papillary renal cell carcinoma or lymphoma.

PEARLS

- **Consider metastases to the kidney when multiple solid masses appear in both kidneys, especially if there is a history of primary malignancy or other metastatic sites.**
- **Metastases are often hypovascular and infiltrative in appearance unless from hypervascular primary malignancy.**
- **Biopsy may be required in patients with primary malignancy if solitary to distinguish from renal cell carcinoma it affects treatment.**

ADDITIONAL IMAGES (B-C)

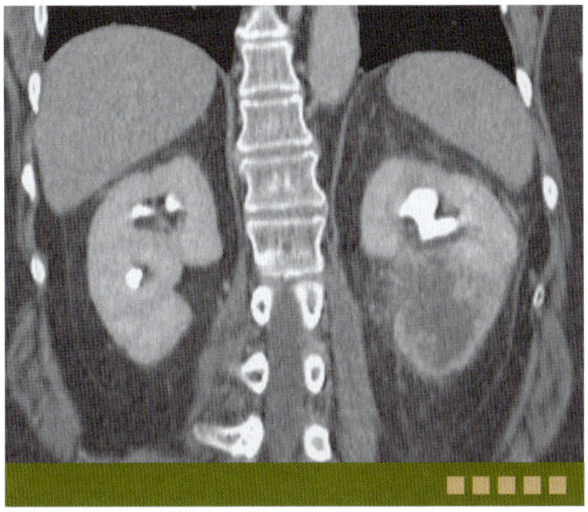

B. Coronal CECT in the patient in Figure A shows the mass is infiltrative and replaces the left lower pole of the kidney.

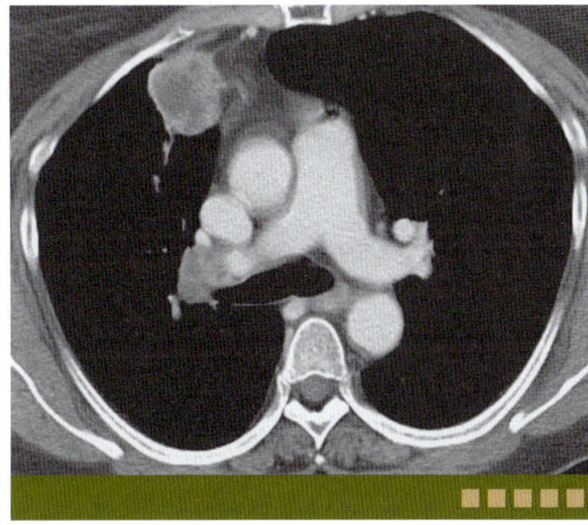

C. Axial CECT in the same patient shows mass in the right lung with lymphadenopathy from squamous cell carcinoma that is the primary source for the kidney metastasis.

DIFFERENTIAL DIAGNOSES IMAGES (D-E)

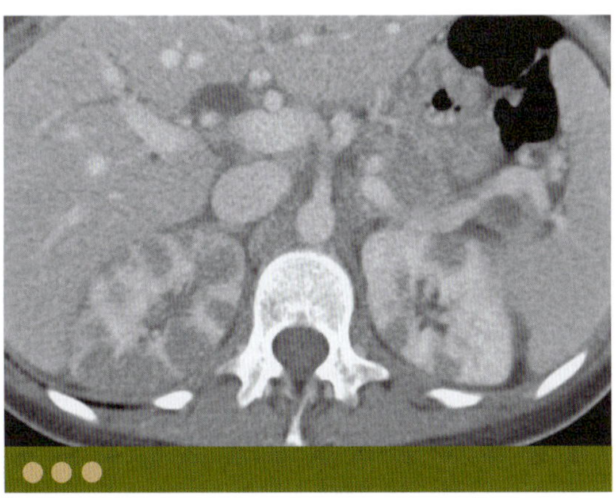

D. Non-Hodgkin lymphoma of kidney: Axial CECT shows bilateral hypodense renal masses from non-Hodgkin lymphoma and pancreatic tail lesion. Diagnosis may require biopsy.

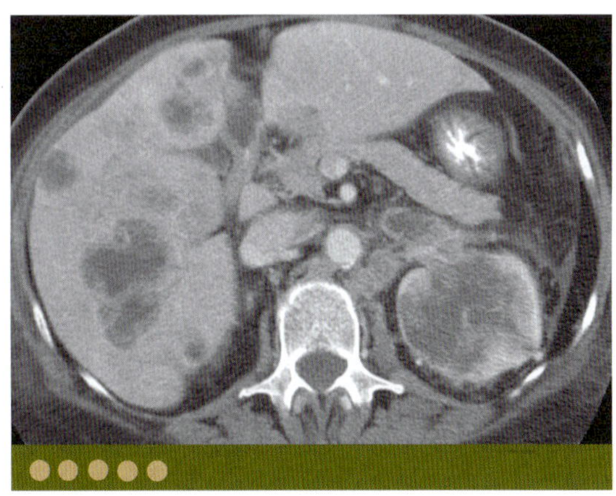

E. Renal cell carcinoma of kidney: Axial CECT shows an infiltrative mass from renal cell carcinoma with liver metastases. Invasion of the renal vein is seen and is generally not present in metastases to the kidneys.

IMAGE KEY

Common

Rare

Typical

Unusual

1–18 Juxtaglomerular Cell Tumor

Paul Nikolaidis

PRESENTATION

Unexplained hypertension, headaches, polyuria.

FINDINGS

CT demonstrates a large well-circumscribed mass arising from the upper pole of the left kidney. It enhances but to a lesser degree than the renal parenchyma.

DIFFERENTIAL DIAGNOSES

- *Renal cell carcinoma (RCC)*: More commonly, markedly hypervascular on arterial phase images; patients have normal renin levels.
- *Medullary carcinoma*: These rare tumors are also hypovascular, but typically less well defined, more heterogenous, and infiltrative in appearance. Patients often have a history of sickle cell disease; renin levels are normal.
- *Pseudomass from focal pyelonephritis*: Usually not confused with a renal neoplasm (clinical history also helps). May be similarly hypoenhancing in relation to the surrounding renal parenchyma.

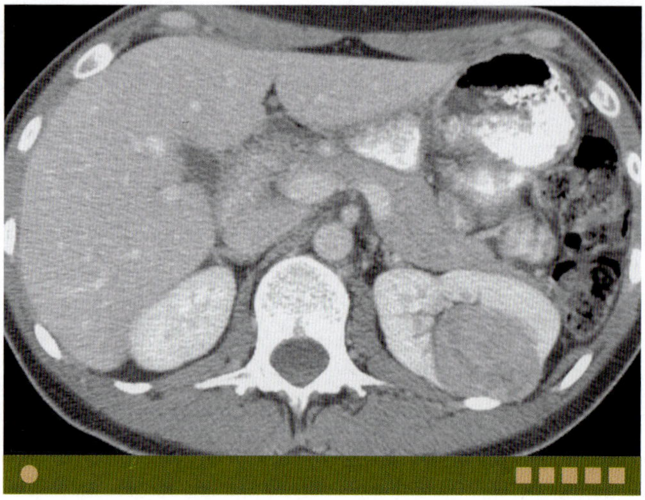

A. Axial CECT obtained during the nephrographic phase shows a large, well-circumscribed left renal mass. It enhances significantly less than the surrounding renal parenchyma. Other than its relative hypovascularity, it is a nonspecific lesion.

COMMENTS

Juxtaglomerular cell tumors, also known as juxtaglomerular apparatus (JGA) tumors are benign tumors of the renal cortex that arise from cells of the juxtaglomerular apparatus. They typically measure 2 to 4 cm. They are a rare cause of hypertension, usually in young adults. Women are more commonly affected. They can be associated with elevated plasma renin levels, two to seven times greater than normal values. In addition to presenting with severe hypertension, clinical manifestations included headaches and polyuria. There may be laboratory evidence of hyperaldosteronism and hypokalemia.

On cross-sectional imaging, JGA tumors are solid, sharply marginated masses. They tend to be isodense with normal renal parenchyma on NECT and, therefore, may not be well seen until administration of IV contrast. They become more conspicuous on postcontrast imaging, particularly on the more delayed phases. Juxtaglomerular apparatus tumors are relatively hypovascular, caused by intimal hyperplasia in the tumor vessel lumina, possibly from the effect of renin. They may demonstrate homogeneous delayed enhancement. CT and MR may also be helpful in identifying the extent of tumor spread and detecting intratumoral hemorrhage or necrosis. The combination of a hypovascular solid renal mass in a patient with elevated renin without any coexisting renal artery lesions should suggest the diagnosis of a juxtaglomerular cell tumor.

Although JGA tumors are benign, they are potentially lethal if left untreated. Preoperative pharmacologic treatment should be undertaken with antihypertensive medications, preferably angiotensin converting enzyme (ACE) inhibitors. Surgery, usually partial nephrectomy, is curative.

PEARLS

- **Rare benign neoplasms of the kidney that arise from the cells of the juxtaglomerular apparatus.**
- **An unusual cause of hypertension, associated with markedly elevated plasma renin levels.**
- **May be difficult to detect on noncontrast CT.**
- **On CECT, they are hypovascular masses, but may demonstrate increased delayed enhancement.**

ADDITIONAL IMAGES (B-C)

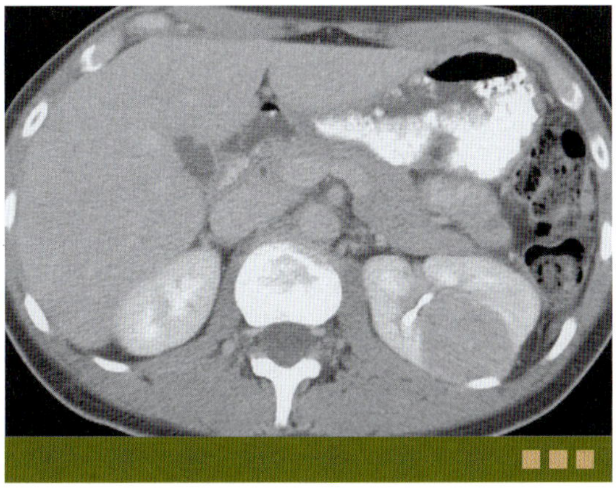

B. Corresponding axial CECT obtained during the excretory phase shows only minimal increased delayed enhancement of the left renal mass.

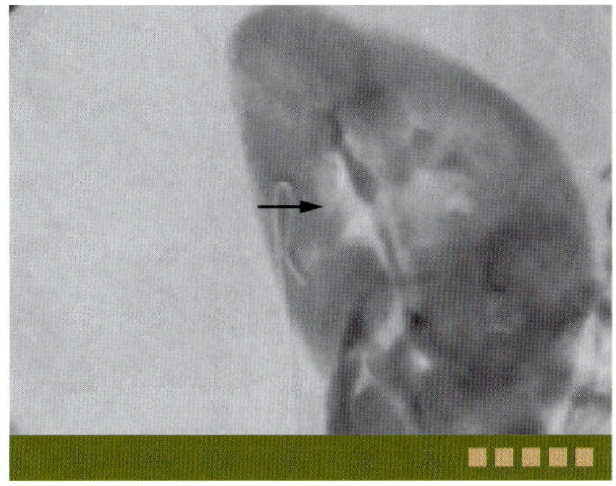

C. Conventional angiogram in another patient with a juxtaglomerular cell tumor shows a hypovascular round mass in the upper pole of the left kidney (arrow).

DIFFERENTIAL DIAGNOSES IMAGES (D-F)

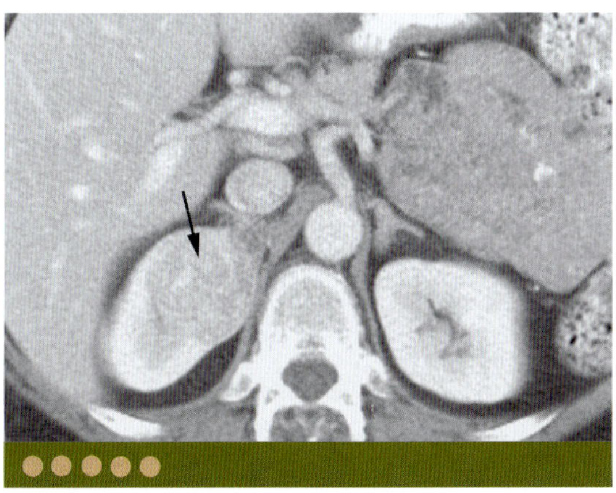

D. Renal cell carcinoma: Axial CECT obtained during the nephrographic phase shows a heterogeneously enhancing right renal mass shown to represent a renal cell carcinoma.

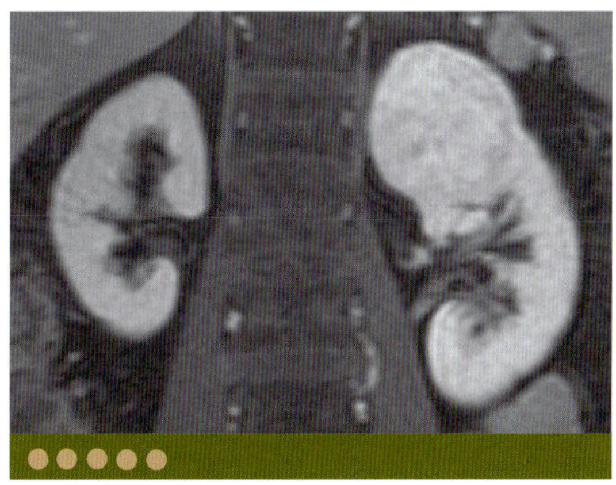

E. Renal cell carcinoma: Coronal contrast-enhanced T1-WI shows an avidly enhancing exophytic mass arising from the upper pole of the left kidney.

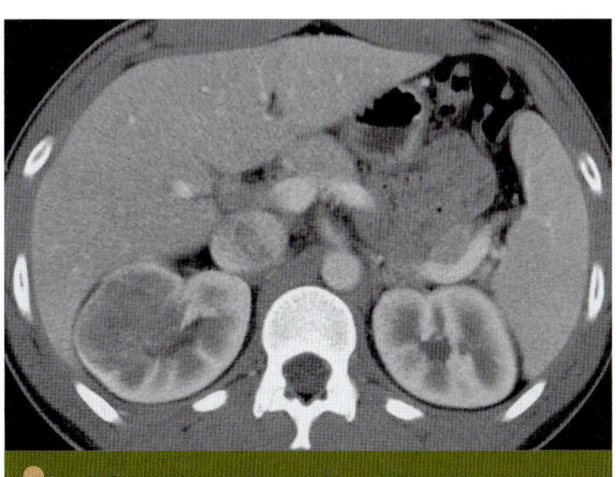

F. Medullary carcinoma of the kidney: Axial CECT shows a large, infiltrative hypovascular right renal mass involving the medulla and extending into the cortex. The patient had sickle cell disease.

IMAGE KEY

Common

Rare

Typical

Unusual

1–19 Renal Oncocytoma

Frank H. Miller

PRESENTATION

Generally asymptomatic; less commonly pain or hematuria.

FINDINGS

Solid enhancing renal lesion with central area of nonenhancement.

DIFFERENTIAL DIAGNOSES

- *Renal cell carcinoma (RCC)*: Can look identical with surgery required to distinguish.
- *Renal metastases*: Generally known malignancy.
- *Angiomyolipoma*: Generally contain fat.

COMMENTS

Oncocytomas are benign renal lesions. Renal oncocytomas are characterized by marked eosinophilic epithelial cells (oncocytes) with cytoplasm rich in mitochondria and arranged in solid trabecular or tubular pattern. The reported prevalence is 4% of renal masses. Oncocytomas generally are seen in the cortex of the kidney. They are generally well-circumscribed, often encapsulated masses lacking necrosis and hemorrhage on imaging studies and pathologic examination. Oncocytoma cannot be distinguished from renal cell carcinoma on the basis of imaging studies. Characteristic imaging findings of oncocytoma include the "spoke-wheel" appearance on angiography and solid mass with central hypodense stellate scar on imaging studies, but these findings are nonspecific as they can be seen in renal cell carcinomas. On MR, the lesions often are hypointense to isointense to renal parenchyma on T1-weighted images (T1-WI) and have variable signal intensity on T2-weighted images (T2-WI). MR is more sensitive to identify a central scar, but this finding is nonspecific.

Imaging studies are helpful to suggest oncocytoma, but removal is generally required for confirmation as the imaging appearance is nonspecific. Solid enhancing masses should generally be considered renal cell carcinoma until proven otherwise. Renal lesions that do not change size especially over a period of years may suggest oncocytoma. Biopsies are not generally performed as the oncocytic type of renal cell carcinoma can show similar results. As a result, most oncocytomas that on imaging studies are solid enhancing renal masses generally are not distinguishable from renal cell carcinoma and are surgically removed with the diagnosis made pathologically. These lesions may be considered more favorably, for partial nephrectomy. Some favorable results have been seen with fine needle aspiration in patients with suspected oncocytomas who are poor surgical candidates.

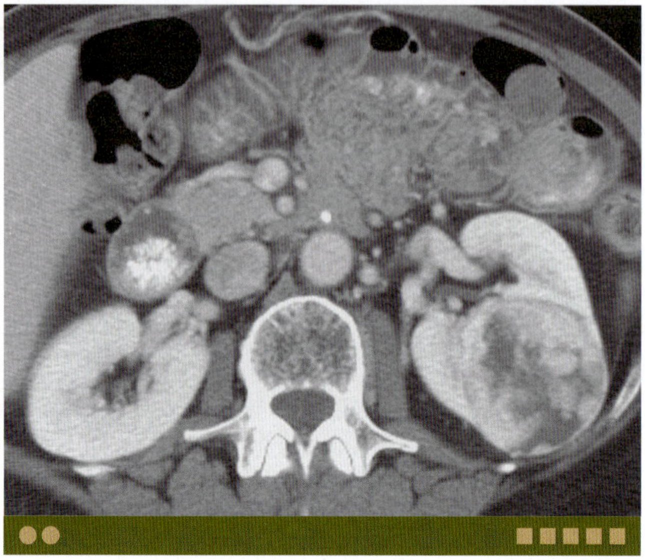

A. Axial CECT shows solid enhancing left renal mass with central area of hypoenhancement.

Bilateral and multifocal oncocytomas and development of metachronic tumors have been reported in 4% to 10% of cases. Oncocytomas may occur in Birt-Hogg-Dubé syndrome and may be genetically inherited. Oncocytoma may coexist with RCC in up to 32% of cases.

PEARLS

- **Oncocytomas are benign renal lesions.**
- **Oncocytomas are generally homogeneously enhancing solid masses with the exception of the scar.**
- **Oncocytoma cannot be distinguished from renal cell carcinoma based on imaging studies.**
- **Oncocytomas may coexist with renal cell carcinoma.**

ADDITIONAL IMAGES (B-D)

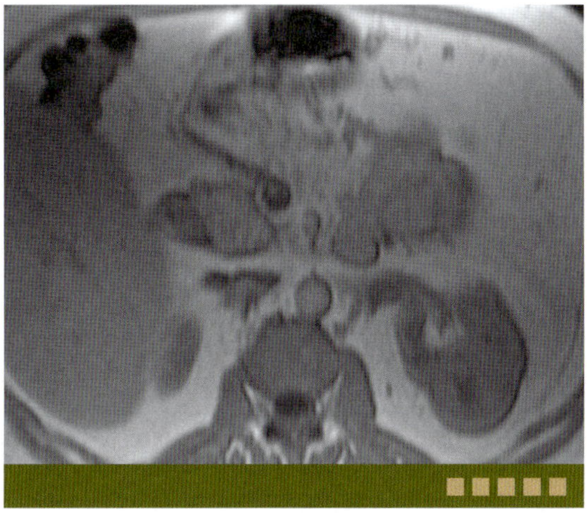

B. Axial T1-WI in different patient shows mass with similar signal intensity to the kidney with central hypointense area.

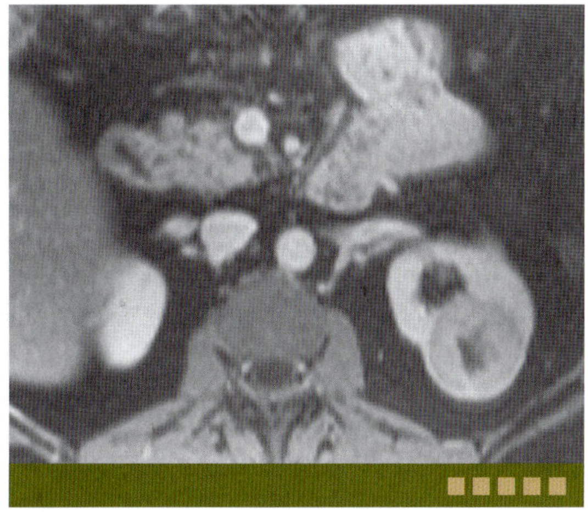

C. Axial contrast-enhanced T1-WI shows the mass enhances less than the kidney with the central scar hypoenhancing.

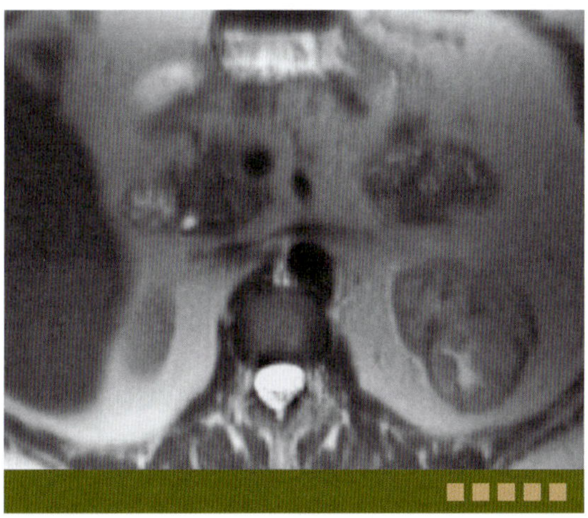

D. Axial T2-WI shows the mass has a central scar which is hyperintense. The oncocytoma was surgically removed as it cannot be distinguished from renal cell carcinoma.

DIFFERENTIAL DIAGNOSES IMAGES (E-F)

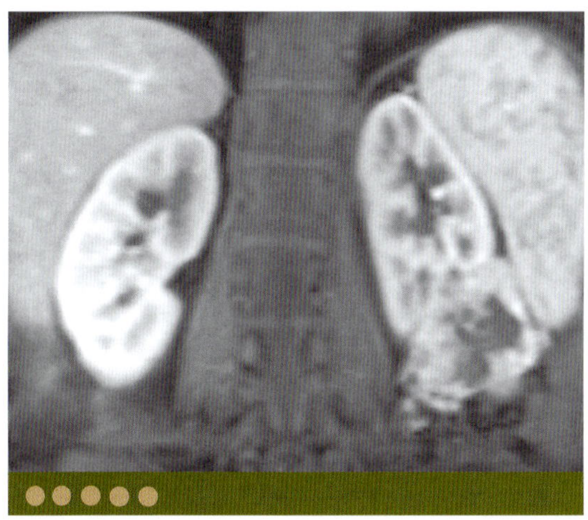

E. Renal cell carcinoma: Coronal contrast-enhanced T1-WI shows lesion in the lower pole of the left kidney with hypoenhancing area because of The appearance of renal cell carcinoma is identical to oncocytoma.

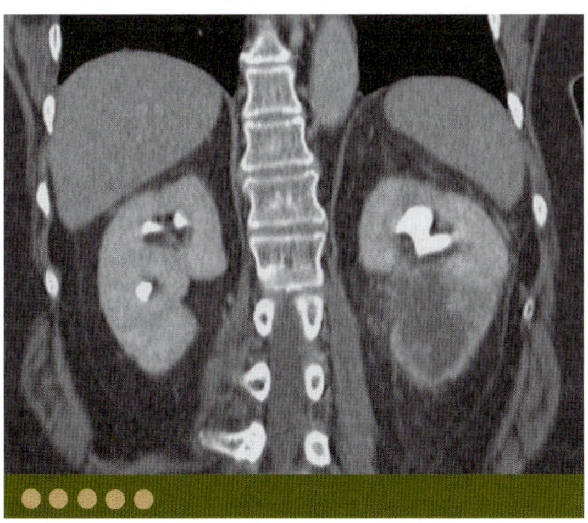

F. Renal cell metastasis from lung cancer: Coronal CECT shows infiltrative mass in left lower pole of kidney. Clinical history of lung cancer helps suggest metastatic lesion and distinguish from oncocytoma or renal cell carcinoma, but biopsy may be required.

IMAGE KEY

Common

Rare

Typical

Unusual

Figures B, C, D are the same patient.

1–20 Angiomyolipoma on CT and Its Complications

Frank H. Miller

PRESENTATION

Generally asymptomatic; rarely acute abdominal pain or hematuria when bleed.

FINDINGS

Fat-containing renal mass on CT caused by angiomyolipoma (AML).

DIFFERENTIAL DIAGNOSIS

Diagnostic of angiomyolipoma (AML) as has macrosopic fat and arises from kidney.

COMMENTS

Angiomyolipomas are benign neoplasms that contain fat, smooth muscle, and vessels. Tuberous sclerosis is associated with AMLs, often multiple. Patients with AMLs are generally asymptomatic; however, patients can present with pain when associated with renal or perirenal hemorrhage. This may require emergent embolization or nephrectomy.

The easiest imaging modality to diagnose AML is CT. The presence of fat (attenuation < –10) in a renal mass is nearly diagnostic of AML. Thin slice CT without contrast may be helpful to detect the relatively smaller foci of fat. Although there are case reports of renal cell carcinoma (RCC) having macroscopic fat, these are rare and are generally associated with osteoid metaplasia, seen as calcifications, or tumor engulfment of perinephric fat. Lipomas and liposarcomas may also have fatty density that can be indistinguishable from AML, but these tumors are extremely rare and often arise from the renal capsule. They tend not to have a renal parenchymal defect with the kidney nor associated prominent vessels as seen with angiomyolipomas. Approximately 5% of AMLs will not have detectable fat on imaging. The absence of fat therefore does not exclude AML, but makes the diagnosis difficult. The diagnosis of AML with minimal fat is generally made at surgical removal or rarely biopsy as these are not easily distinguished from renal cell carcinoma.

Complications of angiomyolipomas include hemorrhage as AMLs have abnormal thin-walled vessels and are predisposed to pseudoaneurysms which may rupture. As a result, AMLs that are large may be embolized. If ruptured, angiography and embolization should be performed. An extremely rare complication of angiomyolipoma is tumor extension into the renal vein or inferior vena cava (IVC), resulting in fat density tumor thrombus similar to the AML.

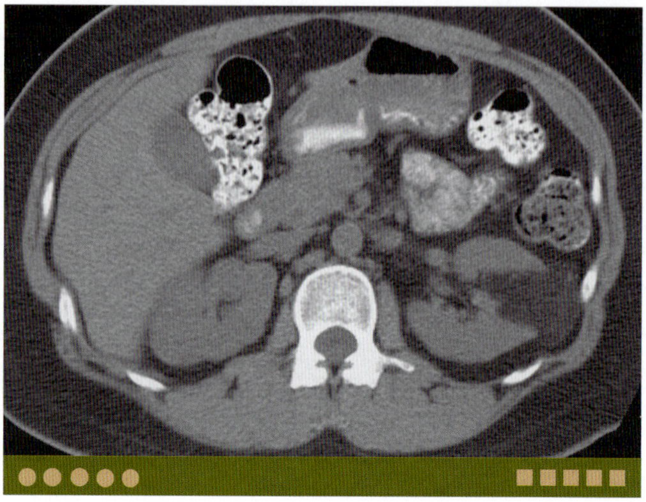

A. Axial NECT shows large left renal mass that is fat density, diagnostic of angiomyolipoma.

PEARLS

- **Angiomyolipomas are benign tumors that contain fat, smooth muscle, and vessels.**
- **Detection of fat on CT is diagnostic for angiomyolipoma.**
- **AMLs are predisposed to pseudoaneurysms, which may hemorrhage.**
- **AMLs that contain minimal or no fat are difficult to distinguish from renal cell carcinoma.**
- **An extremely rare complication of AML is tumor extension into veins.**

ADDITIONAL IMAGES (B-J)

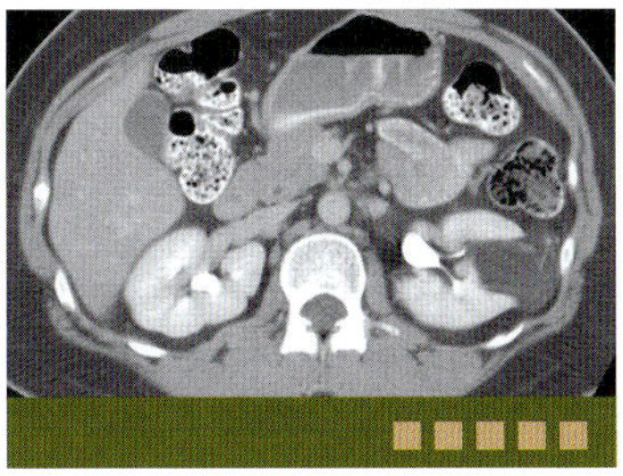

B. Axial CECT scan in the patient in Figure A shows areas of enhancement in the AML.

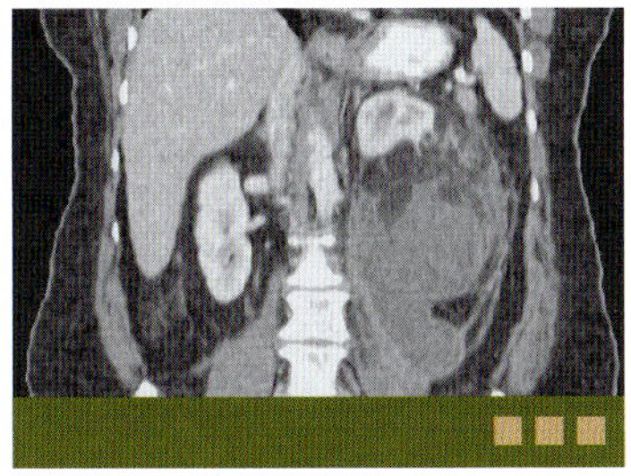

C. AML with perinephric hemorrhage. Coronal CECT in the same patient as in Figure C shows the extent of the hematoma and shows the "claw-sign" from a fat-containing AML of the lower pole of the left kidney.

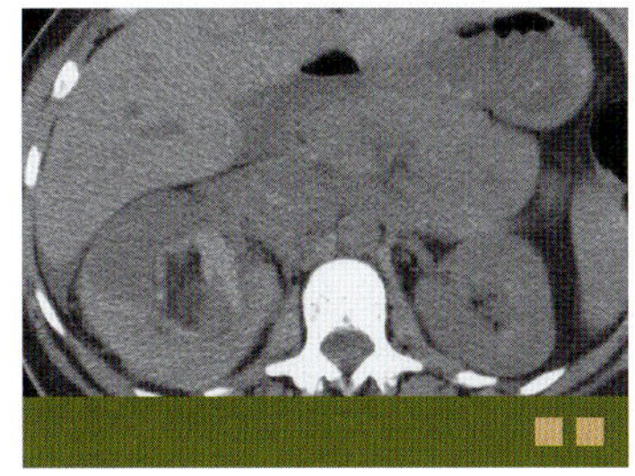

D. AML with perinephric hematoma and pseudoaneurym. Axial NECT shows high-density perinephric fluid from blood adjacent to renal fat-containing mass because of AML.

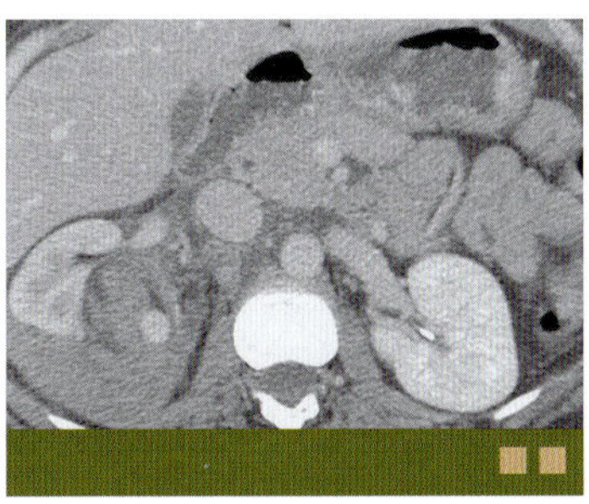

E. Axial CECT shows the cause of the perinephric hematoma is caused by pseudoaneurysm associated with AML.

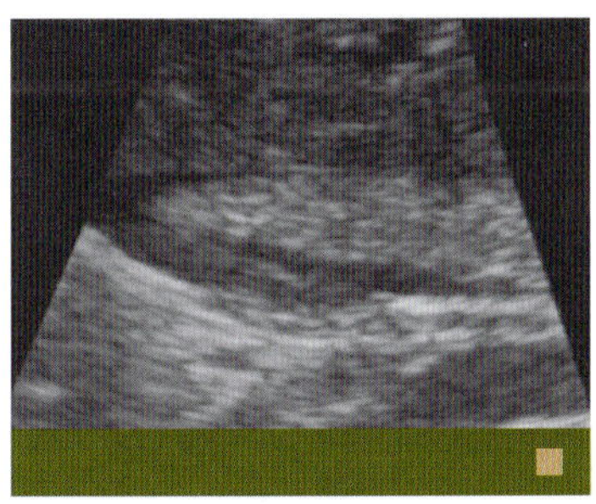

F. AML with tumor thrombus in IVC. Longitudinal sonogram shows echogenic thrombus because of AML invading the inferior vena cava. The thrombus is echogenic caused by the presence of fat.

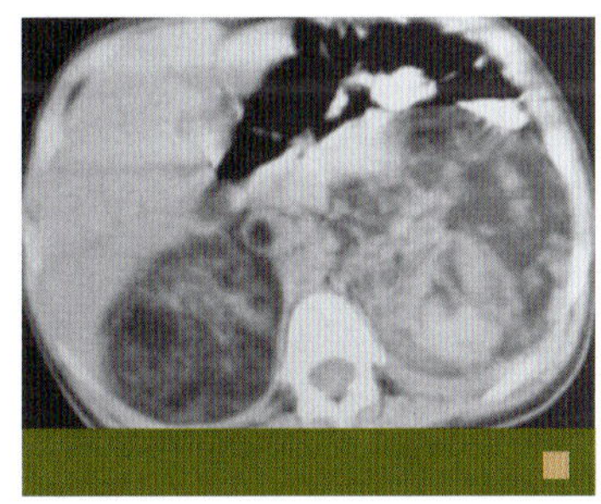

G. AML with tumor thrombus in IVC. Axial NECT in the same patient shows AMLs replacing the kidneys with fat-containing tumor thrombus in the IVC.

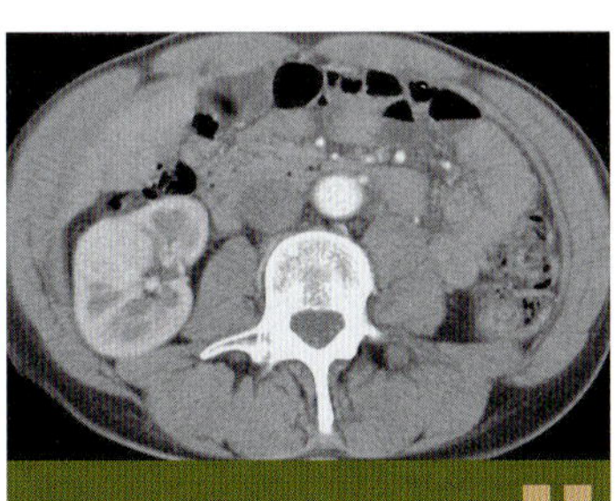

H. AML without fat. Axial CECT in a patient shows tuberous sclerosis shows hypervascular renal lesion caused by AML, which does not have detectable fat. AML with minimal or no fat may be difficult to distinguish from renal cell carcinoma.

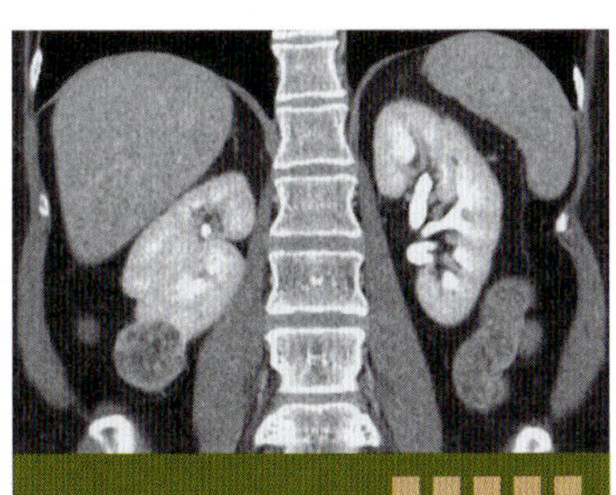

I. Angiomyolipoma: Coronal CECT scan shows right lower pole AML which contained fat.

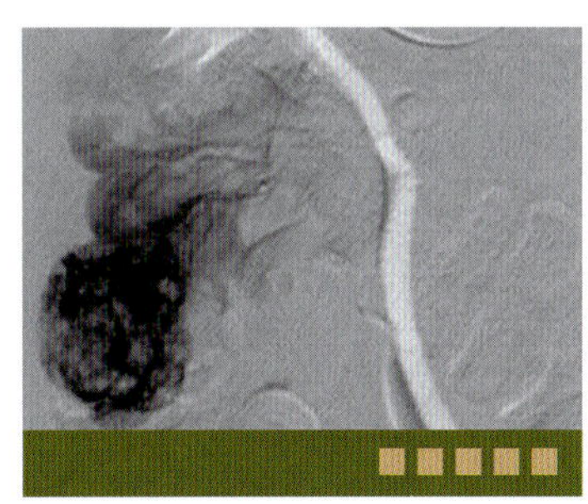

J. Angiogram in the same patient shows hypervascular mass because of angiomyoliopoma. The lesion was embolized.

IMAGE KEY

Common

Rare

Typical

Unusual

1–21 Echogenic Renal Mass Caused by Angiomyolipoma

Frank H. Miller

PRESENTATION

Incidental mass on ultrasound.

FINDINGS

Echogenic mass on ultrasound examination.

DIFFERENTIAL DIAGNOSES

- *Renal cell carcinoma (RCC)*: Can be indistinguishable from AML on ultrasound. CT helps confirm lack of fat unlike AML.
- *Oncocytoma*: Can be indistinguishable from AML and renal cell. Does not have fat on CT.

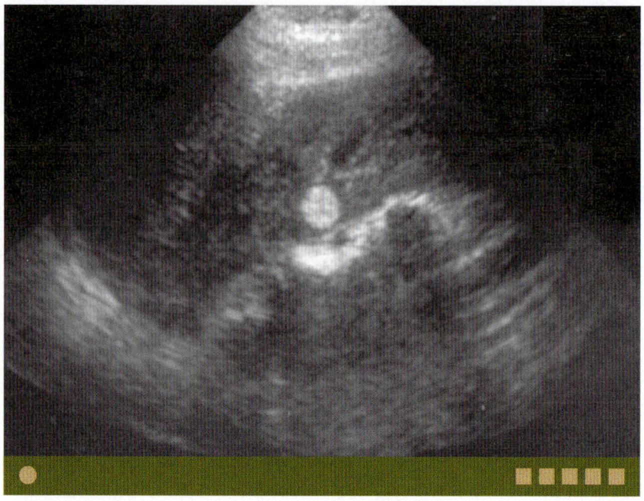

A. Longitudinal sonogram shows very echogenic lesion because of angiomyolipoma.

COMMENTS

Angiomyolipomas are benign, hamartomatous renal tumors. They consist of varying amounts of vascular, fat, and smooth muscle components. When multiple, angiomyolipomas may be associated with tuberous sclerosis. Detection of AMLs has increased considerably as the spatial resolution of ultrasound, CT, and MR has improved. On sonography, AMLs are typically seen as highly echogenic masses on the basis of the fat content of the lesions. If there is a relatively small amount of fat, the lesions are less echogenic. In addition, AMLs on ultrasound may demonstrate less echogenic areas from hemorrhage and necrosis. An echogenic mass, especially in middle-aged women, is often caused by angiomyolipoma; however, the finding is not pathognomonic as it can also be seen in adenocarcinoma of the kidney. Acoustic shadowing may be seen in angiomyolipoma and is not typically seen in renal cell carcinoma.

The distinction between renal cell carcinoma and angiomyolipoma may require CT scans, especially when the lesion is larger than 1 cm. CT shows the mass is of low density (< −10 HU) resulting from fat, confirming the diagnosis of an angiomyolipoma. Unenhanced thin slice MDCT may be best in this distinction instead of contrast-enhanced CT, especially if the amount of fat in the lesion is minimal. MR can diagnose AML by showing fat within the lesions.

The distinction between angiomyolipomas and renal cell carcinoma is critical as renal cell carcinoma is generally a surgical lesion. Angiomyolipomas generally do not require surgery unless large or not able to be diagnosed preoperatively.

PEARLS

- **Angiomyolipomas are benign, hamartomatous renal tumors that contain fat.**
- **Angiomyolipomas are common in middle-aged women.**
- **Echogenic mass may be a result of angiomyolipomas and also of renal cell carcinoma.**
- **The use of CT or MR may be required to show the presence of fat in angiomyolipomas.**

ADDITIONAL IMAGES (B-C)

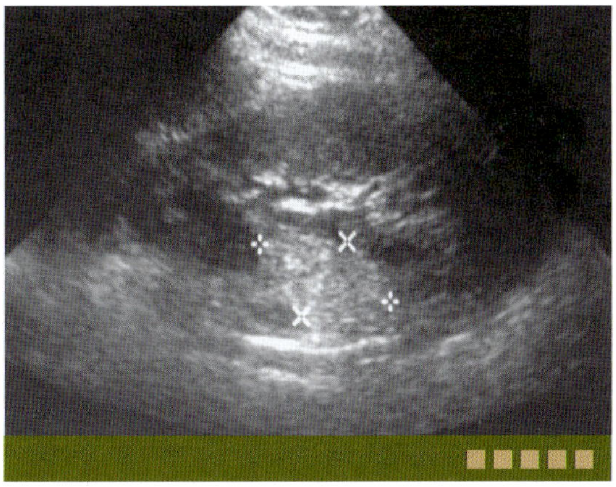

B. Longitudinal sonogram in the same patient shows a larger echogenic lesion.

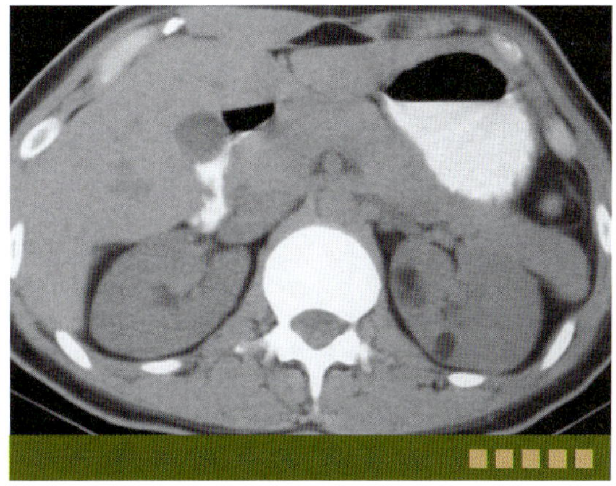

C. Axial NECT shows both lesions are composed of fat consistent with angiomyolipomas.

DIFFERENTIAL DIAGNOSES IMAGES (D-F)

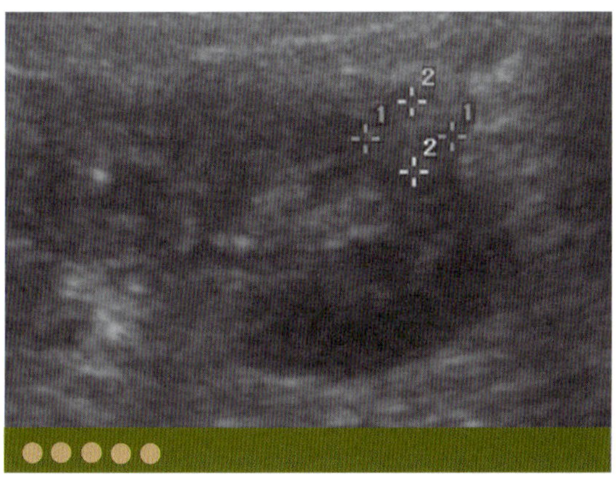

D. Renal cell carcinoma: Longitudinal sonogram shows echogenic right renal lesion.

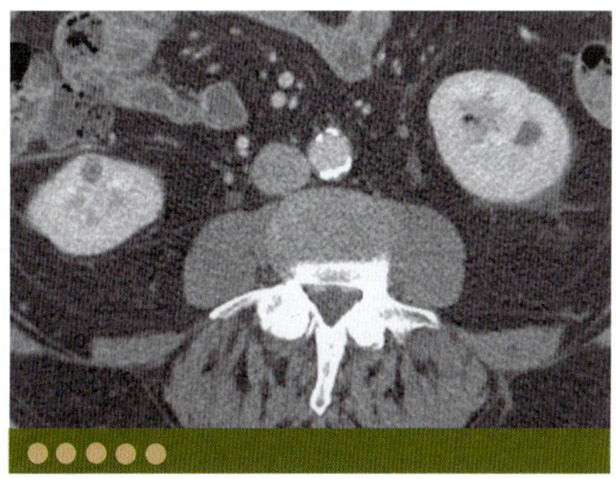

E. Renal cell carcinoma: Axial CECT does not show fat in the lesion in the right kidney. At surgery, lesion was a renal cell carcinoma.

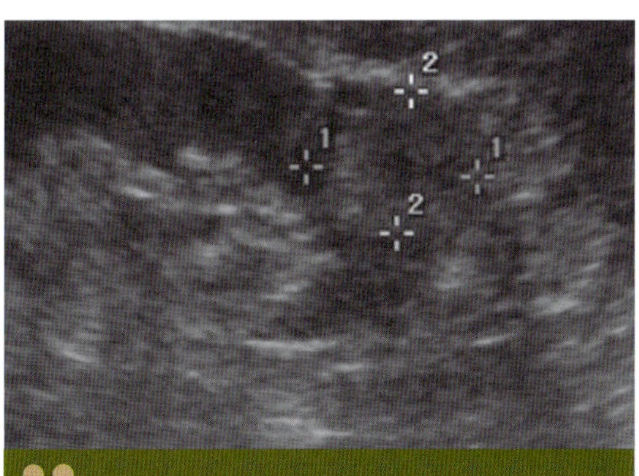

F. Oncocytoma: Longitudinal sonogram shows echogenic renal lesion because of oncocytoma, confirmed at surgery.

IMAGE KEY

Common

Rare

Typical

Unusual

Figures A, B, and C are the same patient.
Figures D and E are the same patient.

1–22 Angiomyolipoma on MR

Frank H. Miller

PRESENTATION

Asymptomatic mass of kidney.

FINDINGS

Renal lesion shows drops in signal on opposed phase images.

DIFFERENTIAL DIAGNOSIS

Clear cell renal cell carcinoma: Would not suppress on the frequency selective T1 fat-suppressed images. Lacks macroscopic fat.

COMMENTS

Angiomyolipomas (AMLs) are benign, hamartomatous renal tumors. They consist of varying amounts of vascular, fat, and smooth muscle components. Most solitary AMLs are seen sporadically (80%), but they are also associated with tuberous sclerosis. MR can diagnose AML by showing fat within the lesions. These masses are seen as high signal intensity similar to subcutaneous fat on T1- and T2-weighted images. Opposed phase images are more sensitive to detect fat especially when there is fat and water in the same voxel. Some AMLs consist predominately of fat and do not have other components and therefore do not drop in signal on opposed phase images. Other features to identify AMLs include the chemical shift or India ink artifact between the mass and the remainder of the kidney or between fatty and nonfatty portions of the angiomyolipoma. When exophytic, fat-containing AMLs lack chemical shift artifact between the angiomyolipoma and the perinephric fat. Unlike hemorrhagic cysts, which also can be bright on T1-weighted images, AMLs show suppression on frequency selective fat-suppressed images because of the presence of fat.

It is important to not identify renal lesions that lose signal intensity on opposed phase imaging as definitive for AML. Other lesions including clear cell subtype of renal cell carcinoma (RCC) can have microscopic fat and mimic angiomyolipomas in this regard. These clear cell RCC can be distinguished from AML on CT and MR as they do not have macroscopic fat. In addition, unlike AMLs, clear cell renal cell carcinomas are not hyperintense on T1-weighted images with associated signal loss on frequency selective T1 fat-suppressed MR images.

When AMLs are small, no treatment is generally required. When large, the lesions may require close follow-up, embolization or surgery because of the risk of bleeding.

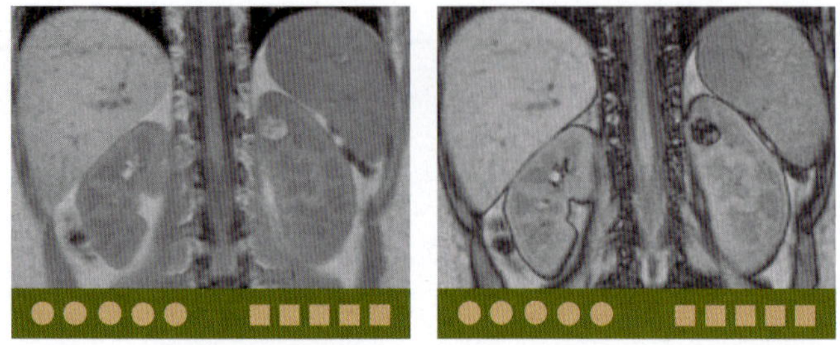

A. Coronal T1-WI shows left upper pole lesion that is high signal intensity because of fat.
B. Coronal opposed-phase T1-WI shows loss of signal in the lesion from fat. On the basis of the loss of signal on opposed phase images the lesion could be an angiomyolipoma or possibly a clear cell renal cell carcinoma. The chemical shift artifact between the lesion and the kidney, however, suggests macroscopic fat from an angiomyolipoma.

PEARLS

- **AMLs are diagnosed based on the presence of macroscopic fat.**
- **Angiomyolipomas with macroscopic fat may not suppress on out of phase images.**
- **T1 frequency selective fat-suppressed images are needed to show fat suppression of macroscopic fat in AML.**
- **AMLs with fat show chemical shift artifact with the kidney but no chemical shift artifact with the retroperitoneal fat.**

ADDITIONAL IMAGES (C-H)

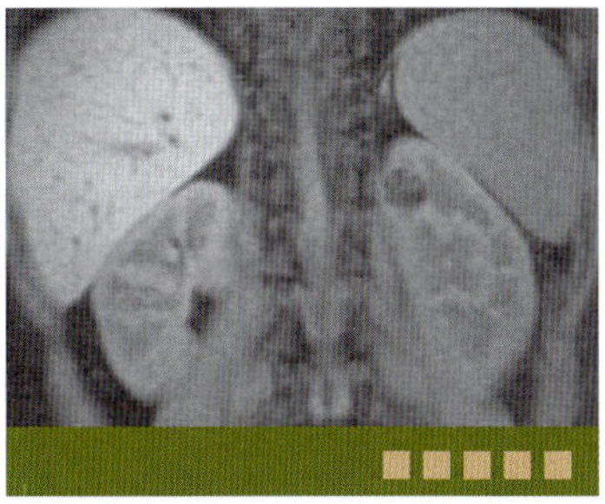

C. Coronal frequency selective fat-suppressed T1-WI shows drop in signal in the mass confirming macroscopic fat diagnostic of AML.

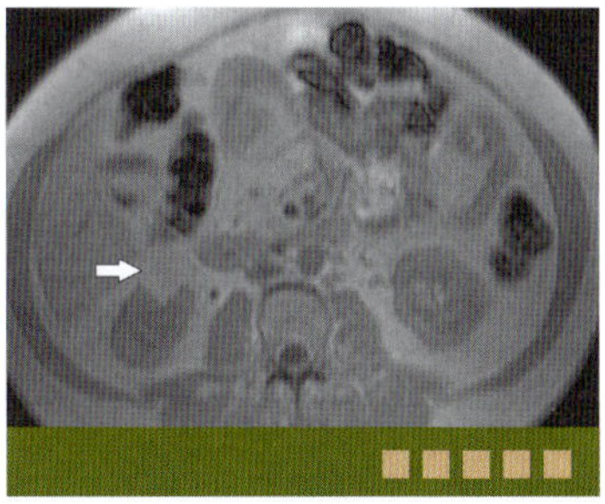

D. Axial in-phase T1-WI in different patient shows that the lesion has high signal intensity and is difficult to distinguish from the adjacent fat but has an adjacent capsule (arrow). On all sequences, it is similar signal intensity to fat.

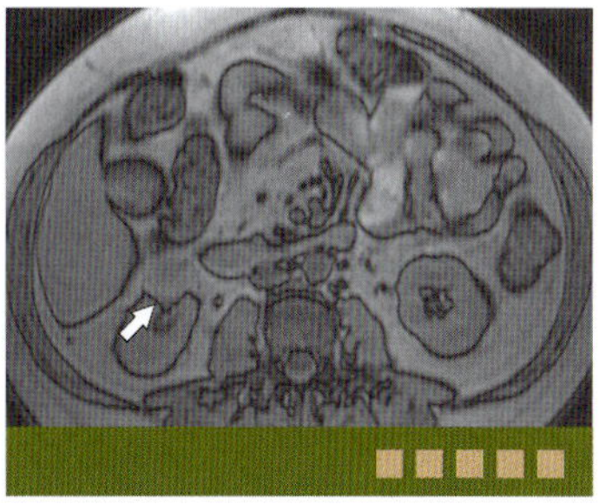

E. Axial opposed-phase T1-WI shows the lesion does not drop in signal intensity relative to Figure D. Note the chemical shift artifact between the fat-containing lesion and the kidney (arrow). No chemical shift artifact is seen with retroperitoneal fat as it is a fat-fat interface. In contrast to clear cell carcinomas, the adipose tissue in this AML is predominately completely lipid, and therefore, does not drop significantly in signal.

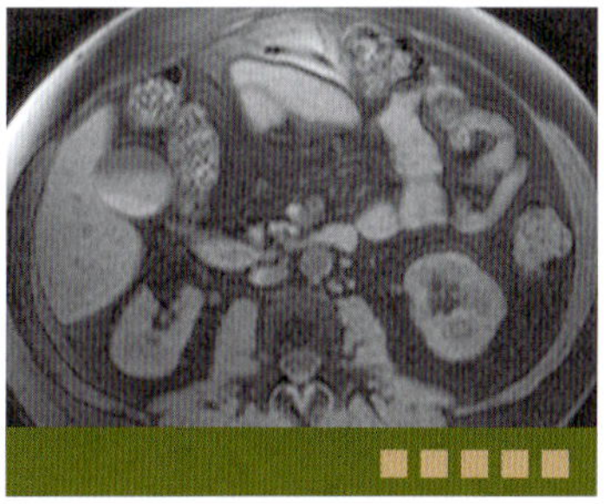

F. Axial frequency selective fat-suppressed T1-WI shows drop in signal intensity because of macroscopic fat in angiomyolipoma. A renal cell carcinoma would not typically show macroscopic fat and drop in signal intensity.

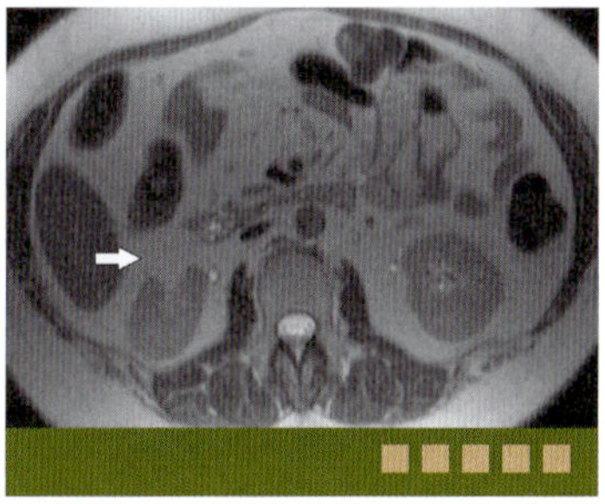

G. Axial T2-WI shows the lesion is similar to adjacent fat on this sequence and all other sequences confirming the presence of fat caused by AML (arrow).

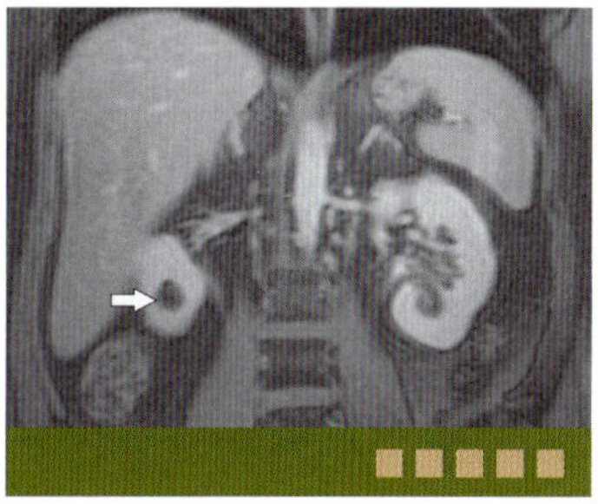

H. Coronal contrast-enhanced T1 fat-suppressed image shows the lesion mimics a cyst as the lesion had fat which is suppressed. To diagnose AML, it is important to look at the nonfat-suppressed images.

DIFFERENTIAL DIAGNOSIS IMAGES (I-K)

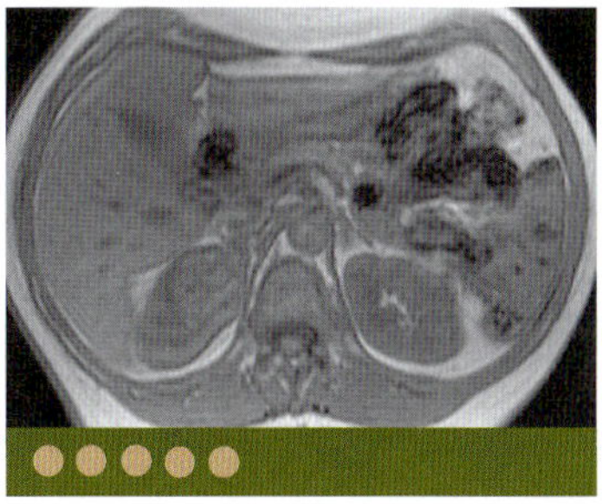

I. Clear cell carcinoma with fat: Axial in-phase T1-WI shows lesion which is intermediate in signal intensity but not high signal intensity as would be seen with angiomyolipoma with macroscopic fat.

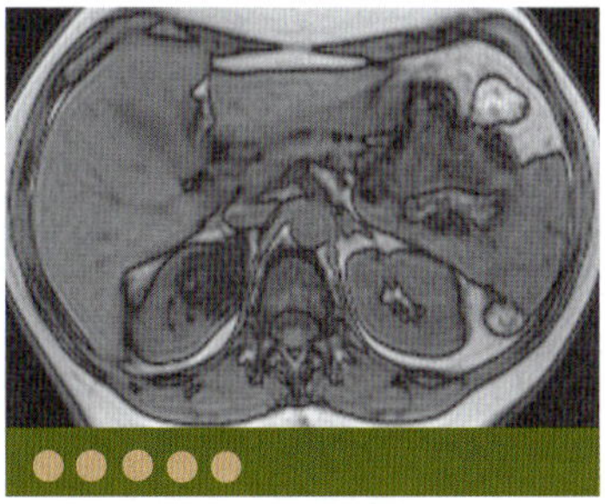

J. Clear cell carcinoma with fat: Axial opposed-phase T1-WI in the same patient as R.H. shows signal drop because of microscopic fat like AML.

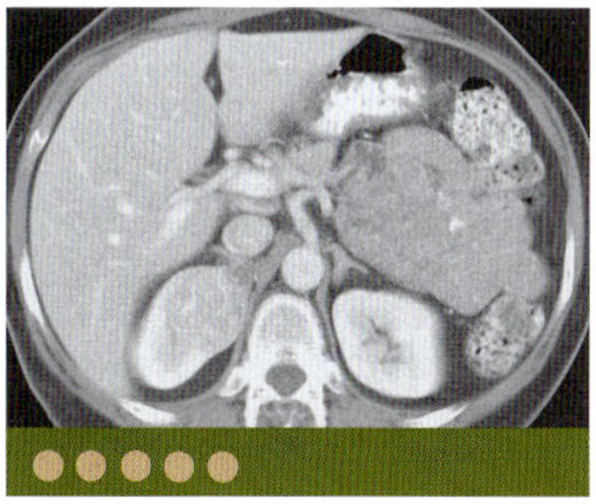

K. Clear cell carcinoma with fat: Axial CECT scan in the same patient does not show macroscopic fat as would be seen with fat-containing AML.

IMAGE KEY

Common

Rare

Typical

Unusual

1–23 Tuberous Sclerosis with Angiomyolipomas

Frank H. Miller

PRESENTATION

Features of tuberous sclerosis including adenoma sebaceum, seizures, and mental retardation. Angiomyolipomas are often incidental but may be associated with pain or hematuria.

FINDINGS

Multiple renal angiomyolipomas (AMLs) caused by tuberous sclerosis.

DIFFERENTIAL DIAGNOSES

- *Renal cell carcinoma (RCC)*: Rare case reports of macroscopic fat in renal cell but tend to be associated with ossification; fat in renal mass without calcification is nearly pathognomonic of AML.
- *Multiple AMLs not caused by tuberous sclerosis*: Similar on imaging; can distinguish by clinical findings.

COMMENTS

Tuberous sclerosis is an autosomal dominant phacomatosis which has the classic triad of adenoma sebaceum, seizures, and mental retardation. Only about a third of the cases are familial. Up to 80% of patients with tuberous sclerosis have angiomyolipomas; however, about 90% of AMLs are seen in patients without tuberous sclerosis. The prevalence increases with age. Angiomyolipomas tend to be detected at an earlier age in patients with tuberous sclerosis. The presence of multiple renal angiomyolipomas suggests tuberous sclerosis. There may also be associated renal cysts, and there is an increased incidence of renal cell carcinoma. AMLs are generally asymptomatic and seen incidentally. The AMLS may become large, and it may be associated with abdominal and flank pain, hematuria, palpable mass, and symptoms from bleeding and mass effect. Patients may present in shock or hypertension or renal failure. Angiomyolipomas especially larger than 4 cm may bleed, and the lesions may develop aneurysms.

Other findings of tuberous sclerosis include multiple renal cysts, lymphangiomyomatosis in the lungs, cardiac rhabdomyomas, and hepatic angiomyolipomas. In the brain, there are characteristically cortical hamartomas or tubers, subpendymal nodules, and subependymal giant cell astrocytomas. A small percentage of patients may develop renal cell carcinoma.

On ultrasound, AMLs are classically well-defined hyperechoic masses. When AMLs replace the kidney in association with tuberous sclerosis, the kidneys may be difficult to identify and may be extremely echogenic. The diagnosis is easy with CT because of the presence of fat attenuation masses seen as less than –10 HU. Some lesions may have minimal or no fat for which thin slices may help to show fat. On MR, the lesions are seen as high signal intensity on T1-weighted images and drop in signal on frequency selective fat suppressed images. They often show the India ink artifact at their margins on opposed phase images. Following contrast, they generally enhance. Color Doppler sonography and contrast-enhanced CT and MR are helpful to show the associated aneurysms. Selective embolization or partial nephrectomy may be required for larger or symptomatic lesions. Total nephrectomy may be required in those patients with nonfunctioning kidney causing uncontrolled hypertension, tumor extension into the renal vein or evidence of renal cell carcinoma.

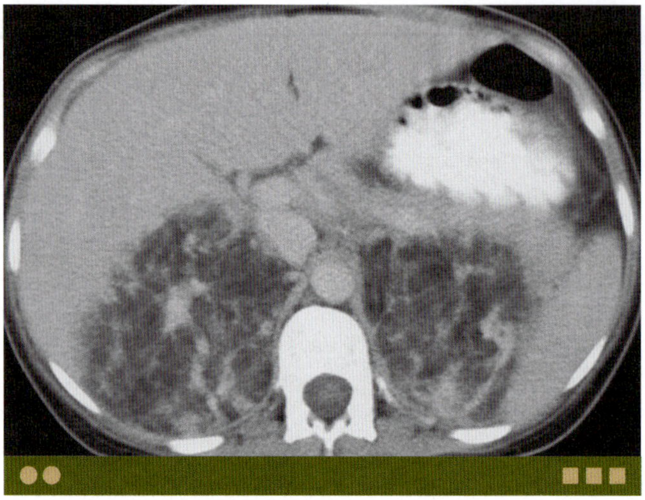

A. Axial CECT shows extensive bilateral AMLs filling both kidneys.

PEARLS

- **Up to 80% of patients with tuberous sclerosis have angiomyolipomas.**
- **Most patients with AMLs do not have tuberous sclerosis.**
- **Bilateral AMLs should suggest possibility of tuberous sclerosis.**
- **AMLs may grow and bleed or develop aneurysms that can rupture.**
- **CT and MR are diagnostic for AMLs by showing macroscopic fat.**

ADDITIONAL IMAGES (B-J)

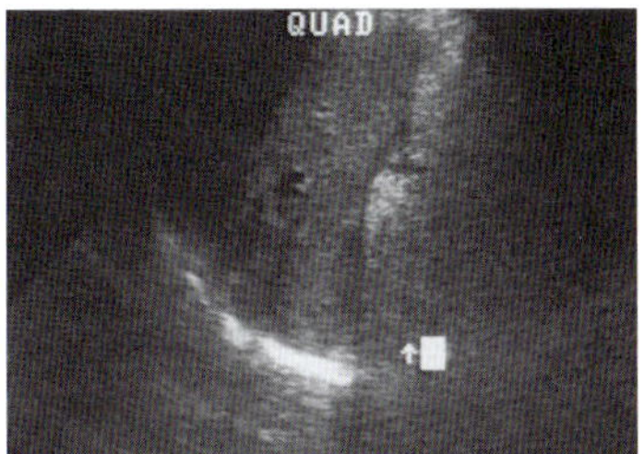

B. On longitudinal sonogram, the kidneys are difficult to identify as they are very echogenic and replaced by AMLs in patient with tuberous sclerosis.

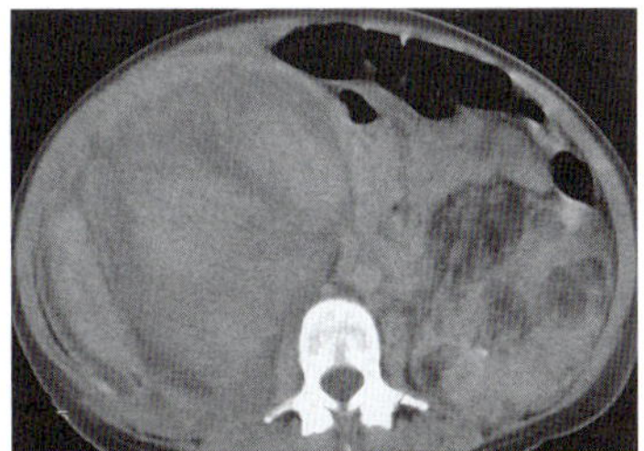

C. Axial NECT in the patient in Figure B a couple years later shows perirenal hemorrhage involving the right kidney.

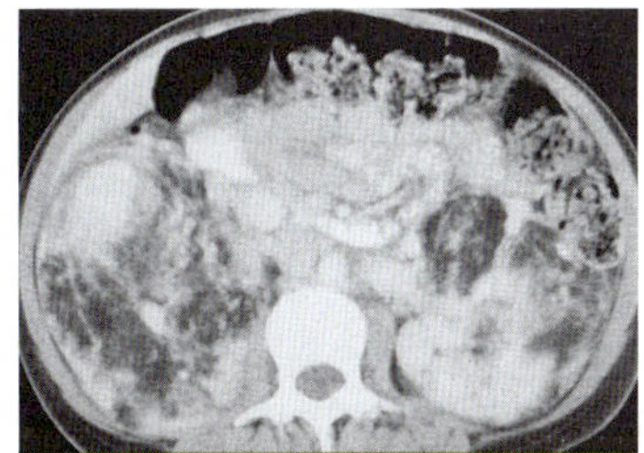

D. Axial CECT in the patient in Figure B shows right renal artery aneurysm.

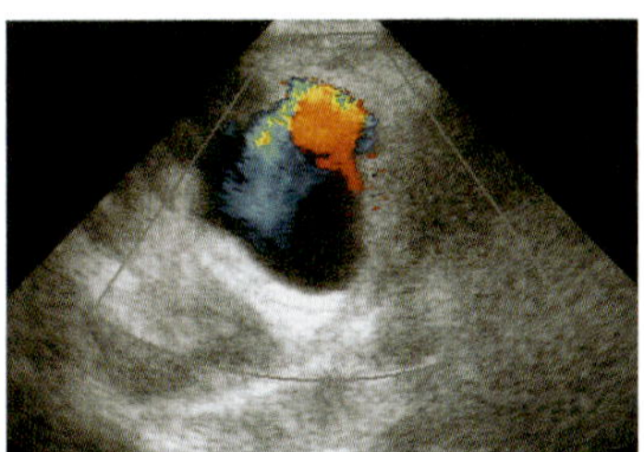

E. Longitudinal sonogram shows color Doppler flow within right renal aneurysm.

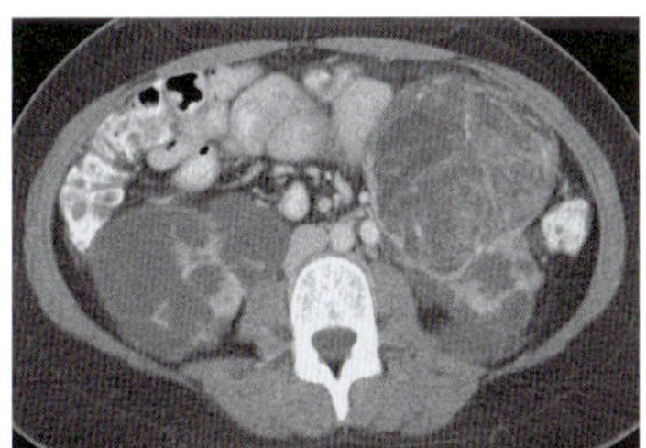

F. Axial CECT shows kidneys replaced with cysts and large AML in left kidney because of tuberous sclerosis.

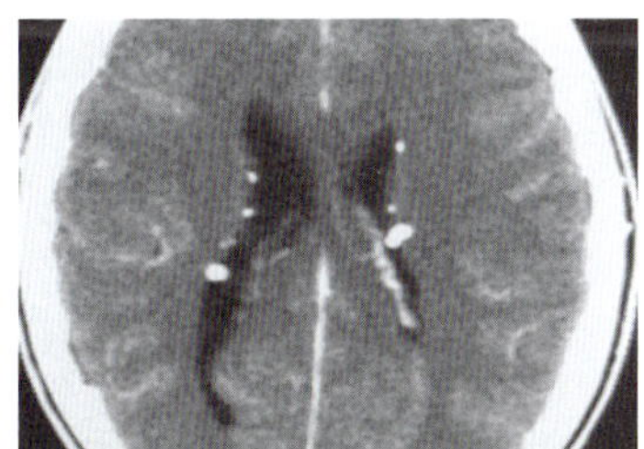

G. Axial head CT shows bilateral periventricular nodules because of tuberous sclerosis.

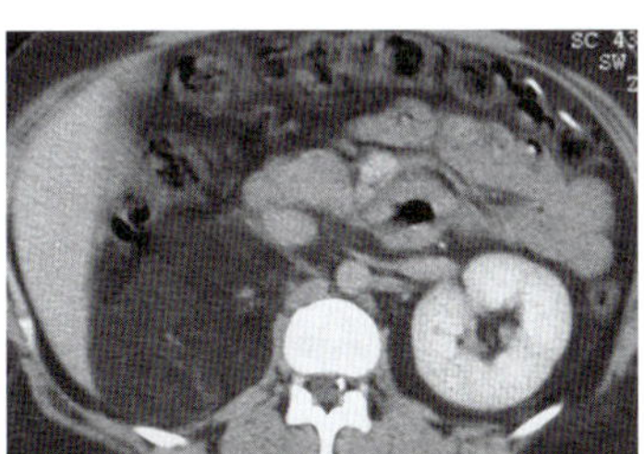

H. Axial CECT shows right kidney replaced with AMLs in patient with tuberous sclerosis.

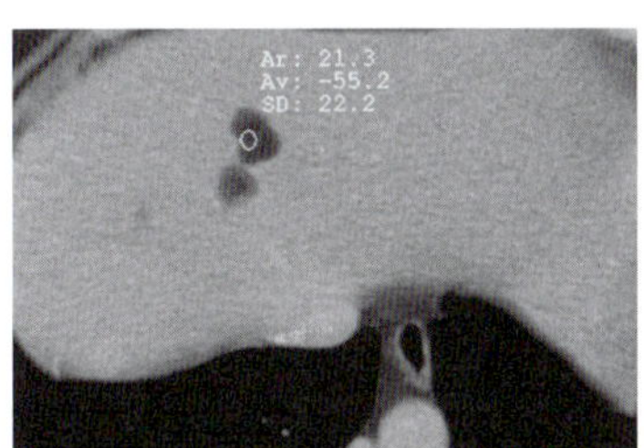

I. Axial CECT with fat density mass in the liver caused by AML.

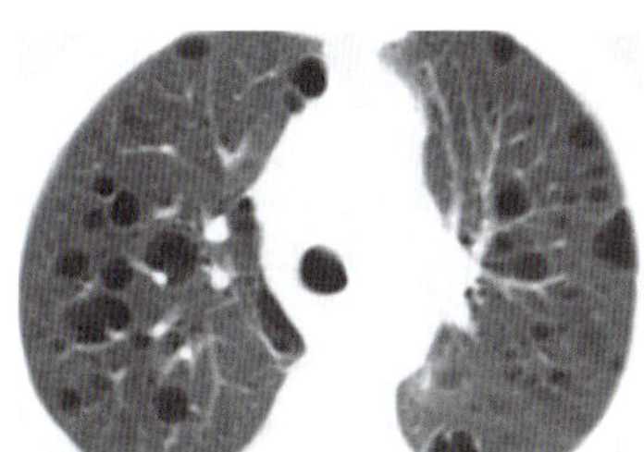

J. Axial CECT using lung window in same patient shows multiple pulmonary cysts in patient with tuberous sclerosis.

Figures B, C, D, and E are the same patient.
Figures F and G are the same patient.
Figures H, I, and J are the same patient.

IMAGE KEY

Common

Rare

Typical

Unusual

1–24 Renal Medullary Fibroma

Paul Nikolaidis

PRESENTATION

Incidental finding on imaging, rare cause of hematuria.

FINDINGS

CT shows a small complex enhancing lesion centered in the medullary portion of the right kidney.

DIFFERENTIAL DIAGNOSES

- *Renal medullary carcinoma*: Usually larger when discovered; associated with sickle cell hemoglobinopathies.
- *Renal cell carcinoma (RCC)*: Generally more cortical in location; usually larger. In advanced cases, there may be tumor extension into the renal vein, nodal, or bone metastases.
- *Transitional cell carcinoma (TCC)*: More typically located in the renal pelvis, but may extend into the medulla; patients may have additional urothelial lesions.

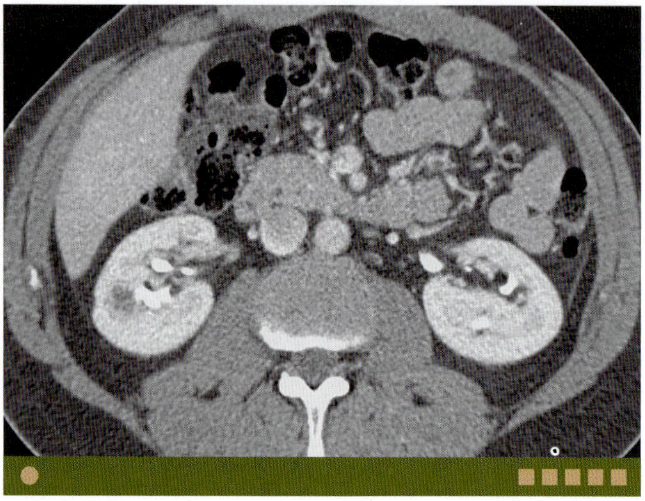

A. Axial CECT shows a small heterogeneous central right renal lesion with enhancing components.

COMMENTS

Renal fibroma, also known as a renomedullary interstitial cell tumor, is a small tumor of the renal medulla comprised of fibrous tissue and small cords of tubular cells. It is a benign lesion, not known to undergo malignant transformation. It is usually solitary and unilateral, and occurs with equal frequency in males and females. Since these lesions are typically quite small, they rarely become clinically apparent. They are often incidental findings on CT or MRI. In some instances, patients may present with hematuria, thought to result from infarction of the fibroma secondary to torsion about its vascular pedicle.

On conventional ultrasound, these small neoplasms may not be well visualized, as they may be isoechoic to the adjacent renal parenchyma. However, they are well seen on intraoperative sonography, which is often used to better delineate the lesion and assist in surgical resection.

On cross-sectional imaging, fibromas are small enhancing soft tissue lesions. Multiphasic, contrast-enhanced CT is the imaging modality of choice. However, there are no specific CT features that effectively distinguish medullary fibromas from other renal neoplasms, in particular transitional cell carcinomas and renal cell carcinoma and tissue diagnosis is usually necessary. Contrast-enhanced MRI is equally capable of detecting these small tumors. They are reported to show low signal intensity on both T1- and T2-weighted sequences, likely because of their fibrous composition.

PEARLS

- **Fibromas are small, benign, usually asymptomatic neoplasms of the renal medulla.**
- **They may not be well visualized on conventional ultrasound, but are well seen on intraoperative sonography.**
- **On CT and MR, fibromas are small enhancing lesions usually indistinguishable from other small renal neoplasms.**
- **Tissue diagnosis is usually necessary.**

ADDITIONAL IMAGE

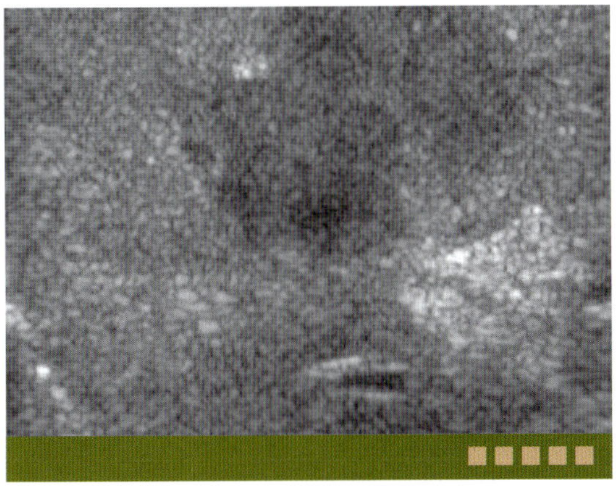

B. Intraoperative sonogram on the same patient shows a solid, mildly hypoechoic lesion in the medullary portion of the right kidney.

DIFFERENTIAL DIAGNOSES IMAGES (C-E)

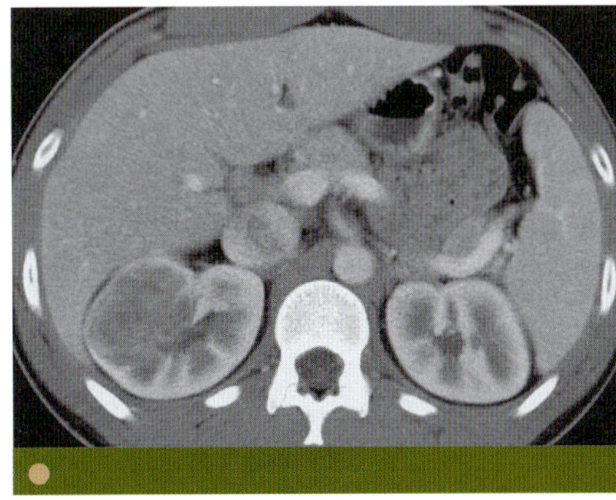

C. Renal medullary carcinoma: Axial CECT shows a large, mildly heterogeneous right renal mass involving the medulla and extending into the cortex. The patient had known sickle cell disease.

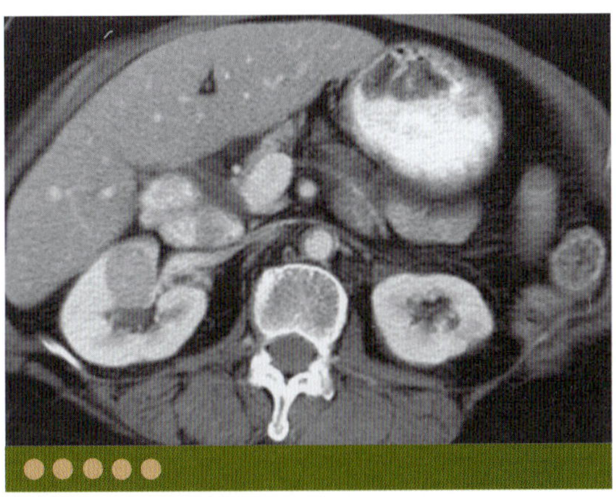

D. Renal cell carcinoma: Axial CECT shows a solid mass in the right kidney, which enhances to a lesser degree than the surrounding renal parenchyma. It is centered in the cortex but extends into the medulla.

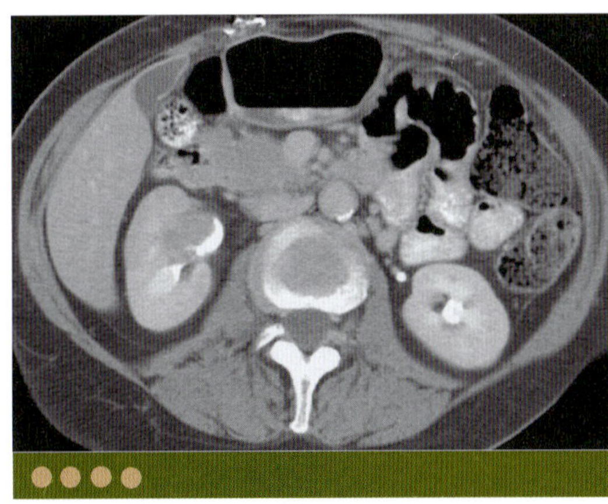

E. Transitional cell carcinoma: Axial CECT shows a solid mass centered in the right renal pelvis, invading into the medulla.

IMAGE KEY

Common

Rare

Typical

Unusual

1–25 Renal Hemangioma

Nancy A. Hammond

PRESENTATION

Intermittent hematuria.

FINDINGS

Small, enhancing mass arising from the superior pole of the right kidney.

DIFFERENTIAL DIAGNOSIS

Benign and malignant solid renal neoplasm; radiographically indistinguishable.

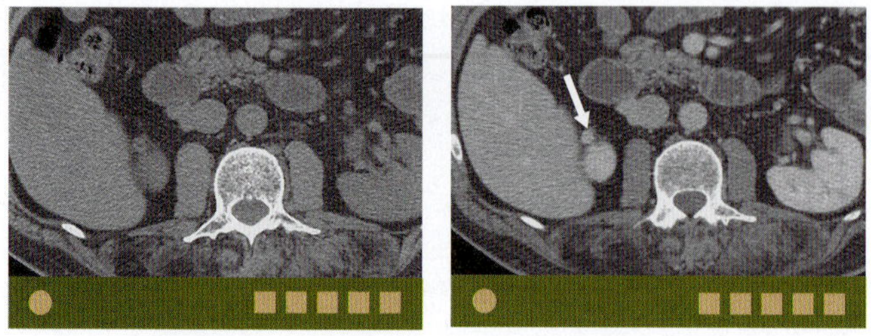

A. Axial NECT shows a small, exophytic soft tissue density mass at superior pole of the right kidney.
B. Axial CECT shows enhancement of the mass.

COMMENTS

Renal hemangiomas are rare benign mesenchymal neoplasms found most commonly in young adults. They are typically solitary but can be multiple (12%). While usually an isolated disease, an association with tuberous sclerosis, Sturge-Weber syndrome and Klippel-Trenaunay-Weber syndrome has been reported. Renal hemangiomas are classified as capillary or cavernous. Ninety percent of cases occur in the submucosal region, the papilla, and medulla, with the remaining 10% located in the renal parenchyma and capsule. While renal hemangiomas are typically small (<1cm), there are reports of larger lesions. Clinically, patients are usually in their 20s or 30s and present with painless or painful intermittent hematuria or renal colic. Hematuria can be microscopic or macroscopic.

Preoperative diagnosis of renal hemangiomas is difficult, and the lesions are commonly mistaken for renal malignancies including (TCC) renal cell carcinoma (RCC). Radiographically, imaging characteristics are not specific. Because of the rarity of these lesions, more common neoplastic entities must be considered in the differential.

Renal hemangiomas are usually not visible on intravenous urogram unless large enough to produce a calyceal deformity or a filling defect. Ultrasound characteristics of renal hemangiomas have been reported as similar to those of hepatic hemangiomas. The tumor is typically hyperechoic but can show variable echogenicity. The absence of posterior acoustic shadowing helps to distinguish from angiomyolipomas. Intratumoral cysts have been reported and may represent blood-filled spaces. With CT and MRI, renal hemangiomas may demonstrate intense arterial enhancement that persists into the venous phase. The degree of enhancement follows that of blood pool. However, there have been reports of renal hemangiomas not demonstrating significant enhancement on CT. On nonenhanced MR images, the lesions are homogeneously hypointense on T1-WI sequences and homogeneously hyperintense on T2-WI sequences.

As preoperative diagnosis of these lesions is difficult, they are typically treated with partial or complete nephrectomy.

PEARLS

- **Rare, benign tumor most commonly found in young patients presenting with hematuria or renal colic.**
- **Pre-operative diagnosis difficult to establish as imaging characteristics can be nonspecific.**
- **On contrast-enhanced CT or MRI, the lesion typically demonstrates arterial enhancement with persistent enhancement on more delayed images.**

ADDITIONAL IMAGES (C-E)

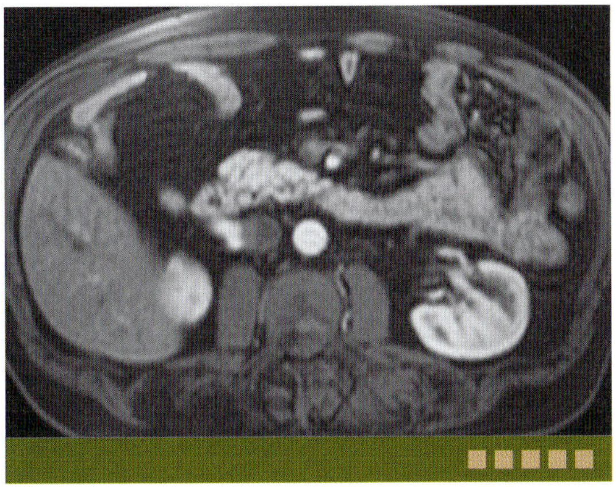

C. Axial contrast-enhanced T1-WI obtained in the arterial phase of enhancement shows avid enhancement of the small lesion at the upper pole of the right kidney.

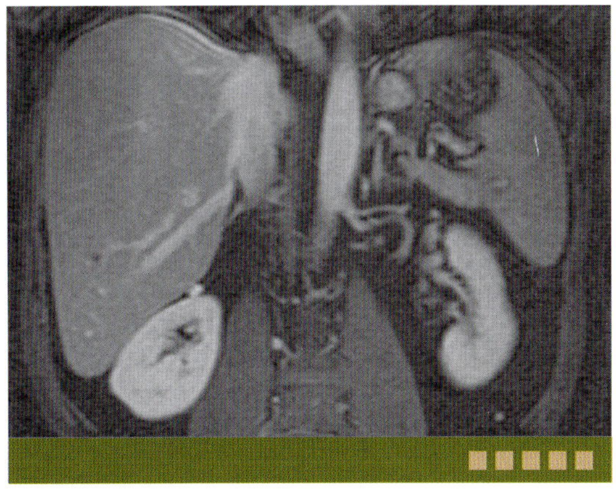

D. Coronal contrast-enhanced T1-WI in the same patient obtained in a later phase of enhancement shows persistent enhancement of the mass.

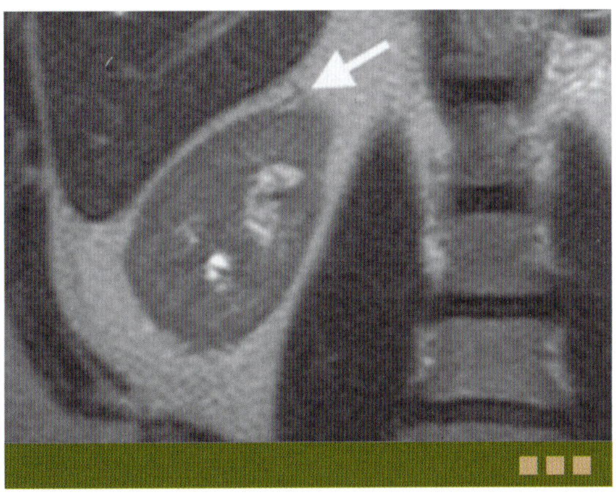

E. Coronal T2-WI shows the mass to be mildly hyperintense (arrow).

DIFFERENTIAL DIAGNOSES IMAGES (F-G)

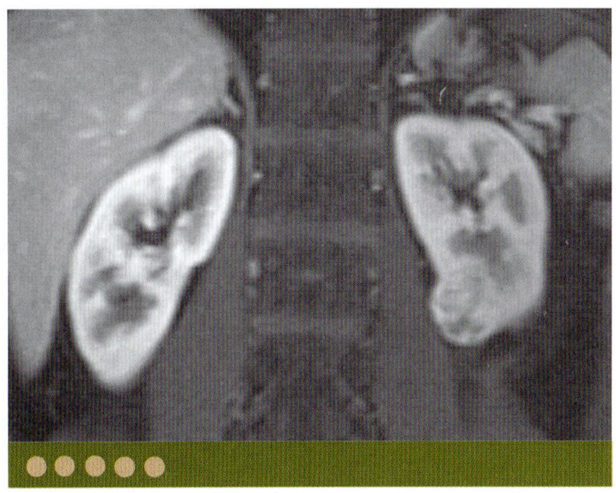

F. Renal Cell Carcinoma: Coronal contrast-enhanced T1-WI shows an enhancing, solid renal mass at the lower pole of the left kidney.

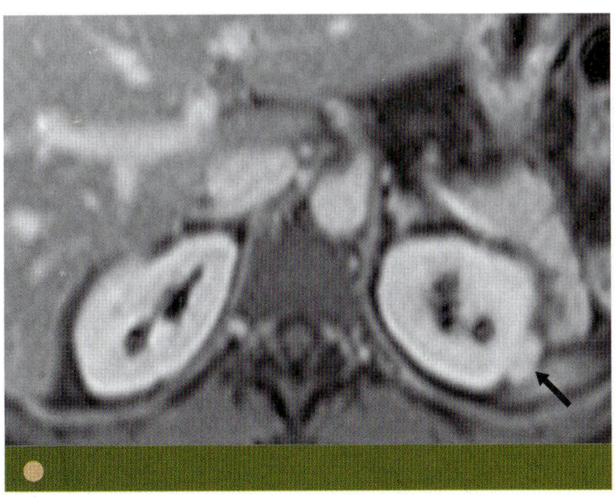

G. Renal capsular leiomyoma. Axial CECT shows an exophytic, enhancing mass arising from the lateral aspect of the left kidney. This lesion was surgically removed and found to represent another rare solid renal neoplasm, a renal leiomyoma.

IMAGE KEY

Common

Rare

Typical

Unusual

1–26 Metanephric Adenoma

Frank H. Miller

PRESENTATION

Asymptomatic; may present as flank mass, hematuria, hypertension, polycythemia, hypercalcemia.

FINDINGS

Enhancing mass on CT and MR.

DIFFERENTIAL DIAGNOSES

- *Renal cell carcinoma (RCC)*: May look identical on imaging studies especially when hypovascular and far more common.
- *Hemorrhagic cyst*: Can be increased density on unenhanced CT but does not enhance.
- *Metastases*: Tend to have known malignancy and may be infiltrative.
- *Oncocytoma*: Can look similar; may have central scar.
- *Angiomyolipoma (AML)*: Typically has fat.

COMMENTS

Metanephric adenoma, which is also referred to as metanephric or nephrogenic adenofibroma or embryonal adenoma, is a rare benign renal neoplasm. It contains stromal and epithelial elements. There is female predominance. It can develop at any age. The size of the tumor ranges from 3 mm to 15 cm. Patients may be asymptomatic or may have hematuria, abdominal pain, or palpable mass. In children, they may be confused with Wilms tumor. They may also be associated with polycythemia.

The lesion is often seen incidentally on imaging studies and may be confused with renal cell carcinoma. The imaging appearance is often similar, and the distinction is made based on pathology.

Metanephric adenoma is a small nonencapsulated solid mass. The appearance can be variable on all imaging modalities. The lesions on pathology can have a high nuclear- to-cytoplasmic ratio with psammomatous calcifications. On ultrasound, it can have variable echogenicity. Occasional increased echogenicity may relate to the presence of psammomatous calcifications and high nuclear-to-cytoplasmic ratio. On unenhanced CT, the lesion may have

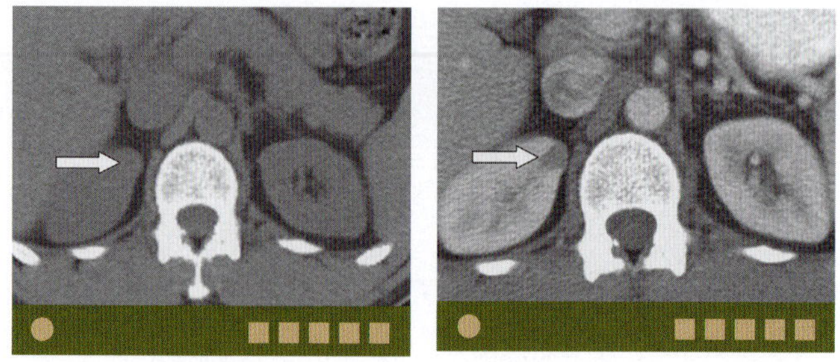

A. Axial NECT shows 12-mm right upper pole lesion which measures 40 HU, which is higher than a simple cyst.
B. Axial CECT shows hypodense lesion that enhances and measures 75 HU.

increased density relative to the kidney but may not show the calcifications as they tend to be small (0.03-0.05 mm). The lesion tends to be hypovascular. It has a nonspecific appearance on MR examinations. It has variable signal intensity and may be hypointense or isointense with the kidney on T1-weighted imaging and hypo-, iso-, or hyperintense on T2-weighted images. It enhances less than the kidney.

The lesions are often surgically resected as they are solid and enhance on imaging studies and suspected to be renal cell carcinoma. Fine needle aspiration may be diagnostic but only rarely performed. The vast majority of solid enhancing lesions will be renal cell carcinoma with the rare diagnosis of metanephric adenoma based on pathology.

PEARLS

- **Metanephric adenoma is a rare benign renal neoplasm.**
- **They can have a high nuclear-to-cytoplasmic ratio with psammomatous calcifications.**
- **On ultrasound, they have variable echogenicity.**
- **On NECT, metanephric adenoma may have increased density.**
- **The lesion tends to be hypovascular following contrast on CT and MR.**

ADDITIONAL IMAGES (C-E)

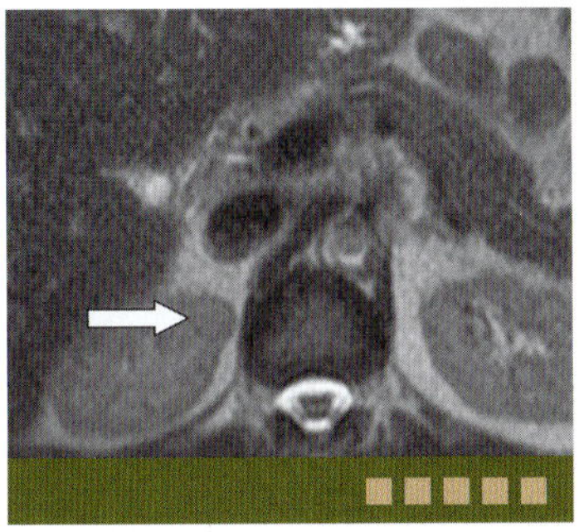

C. Axial T2-WI shows the lesion (arrow) is isointense to the right kidney and difficult to distinguish from the normal parenchyma but shows mild contour deformity.

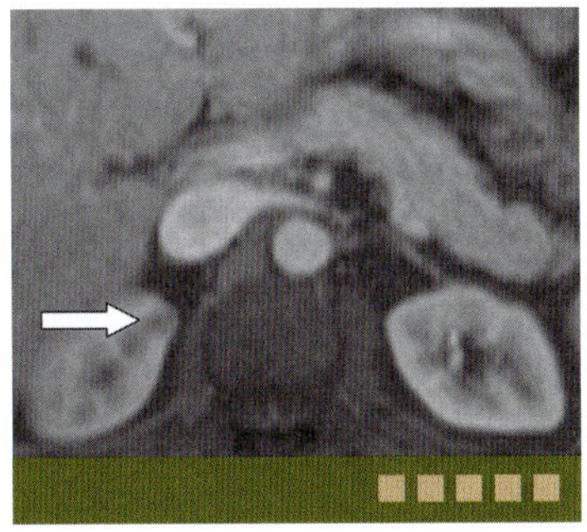

D. Axial contrast-enhanced T1-WI shows lesion (arrow) is hypointense relative to the enhancing kidney.

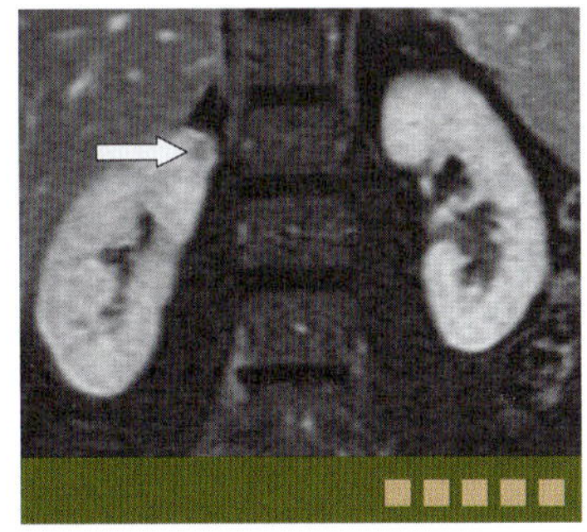

E. Coronal contrast-enhanced T1-WI with subtraction image shows the lesion (arrow) enhances but is hypointense relative to the enhancing kidney.

DIFFERENTIAL DIAGNOSES IMAGES (F-K)

IMAGE KEY

Common

Rare

Typical

Unusual

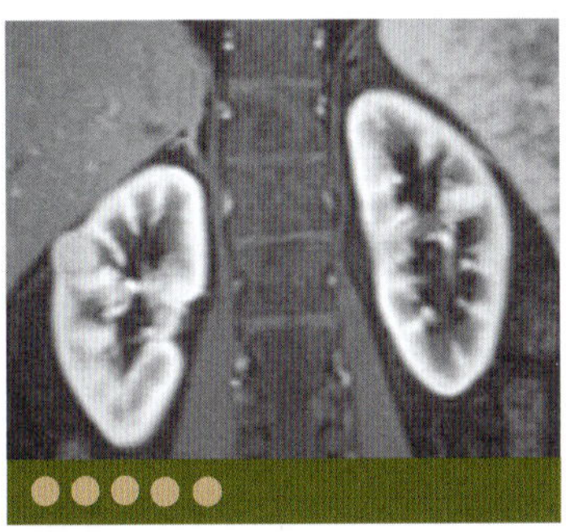

F. Hemorrhagic cyst: Coronal contrast-enhanced T1-WI shows the lesion is hyperintense and it is difficult to determine if the lesion enhanced without putting regions of interest on the lesion or obtaining subtraction images.

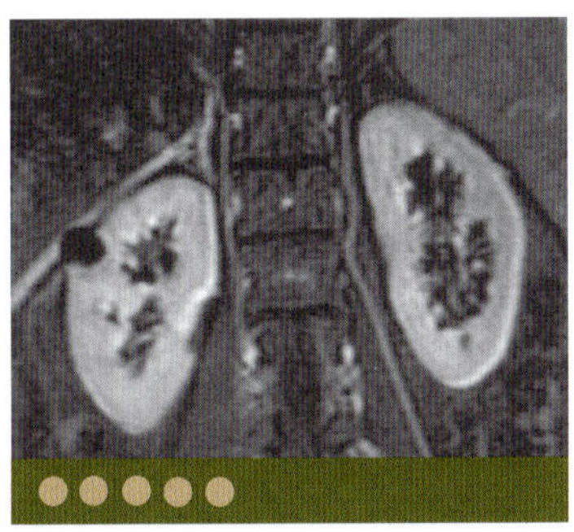

G. Hemorrhagic cyst: Coronal T1-WI with subtraction (unenhanced image is subtracted from the contrast-enhanced lesion) shows lack of enhancement consistent with a hemorrhagic cyst and differs from metanephric adenoma and renal cell carcinoma.

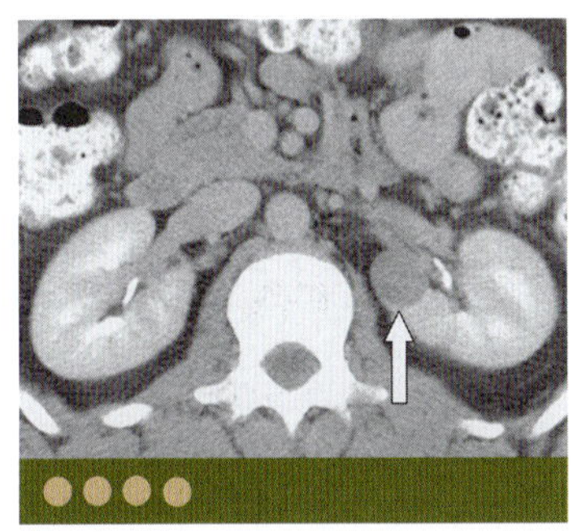

H. Papillary renal cell carcinoma: Axial CECT shows lesion is slightly hypodense to the left kidney (arrow) and is similar to the metanephric adenoma. Papillary renal cell carcinoma is more common than metanephric adenoma but cannot be distinguished on imaging studies.

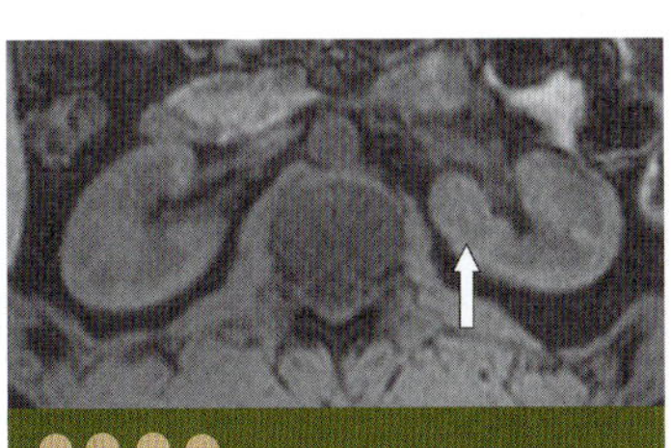

I. Papillary renal cell carcinoma: Axial T1-WI shows left renal lesion (arrow) is similar signal intensity to the kidney.

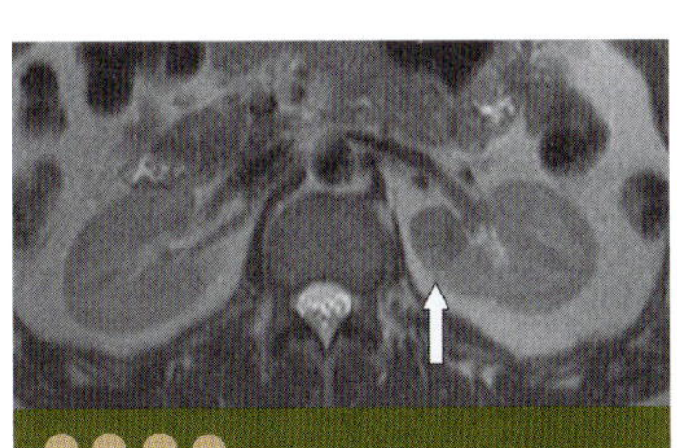

J. Papillary renal cell carcinoma: Axial T2-WI shows lesion (arrow) is hypointense to the left kidney.

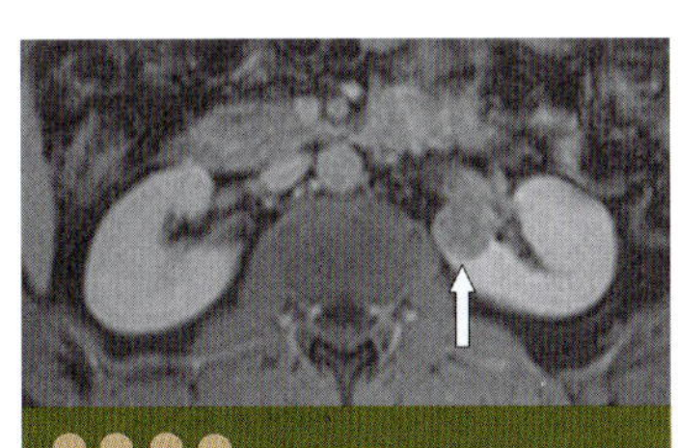

K. Papillary renal cell carcinoma: Axial contrast-enhanced T1-WI shows lesion (arrow) similar to metanephric adenoma. It hypoenhances relative to the kidney.

1–27 Renal Capsule Leiomyoma

Nancy A. Hammond

PRESENTATION

Incidental finding.

FINDINGS

Solid enhancing, exophytic renal mass.

DIFFERENTIAL DIAGNOSES

- *Papillary renal cell carcinoma*: Can be hypointense on T2-WI MR images caused by hemosiderin deposition in the cytoplasm of tumor cells, hypoenhancing on contrast-enhanced images.
- *Angiomyolipoma*: Approximately 5% without macroscopic fat, hyperenhancing on contrast-enhanced images, can be hypointense on T2-WI sequences caused by smooth muscle cells.
- *Renal leiomyosarcoma*: Usually well-circumscribed and peripherally located, cannot be distinguished on the basis of imaging findings unless local invasion or metastases present.
- *Oncocytoma*: Can be indistinguishable on imaging, may have a central scar with spoke-wheeled appearance.
- *Metanephric adenoma*: Hypoenhancing mass on contrast-enhanced images, variable appearance on T2-WI sequences.

COMMENTS

Renal leiomyomas are rare tumors that arise from the smooth muscle cells in the renal capsule, pelvis, calyx, or blood vessels. They are slow growing masses usually found incidentally in asymptomatic patients. Large lesions are rare and can present as a palpable abdominal mass, with abdominal pain or with microscopic hematuria. These tumors are usually seen between the second and fifth decades with a median age of 42. They are more common in women than men. A predilection for either kidney has not been reported; however, an affinity for the lower pole has been reported.

Radiographically, these tumors are difficult to distinguish from other renal neoplasms and can have variable imaging characteristics. Leiomyomas can be solid, solid and cystic, or predominantly cystic. The cystic component depends on the degree of necrosis. Ultrasound findings range from a solid renal mass to a cystic renal mass depending on the internal consistency of the lesion. The vascularity of renal leiomyomas ranges from hypovascular to hypervascular. CT and MRI demonstrate a well-defined, enhancing mass. The mass may be hypointense on T2 weighted images resulting from the smooth muscle component. In cases of capsular leiomyomas, a plane between the kidney and the mass may be present and occasionally a small stalk attaching the mass to the cortex is identified. Although uncommon, calcifications may be present, are typically irregular, and best seen on CT.

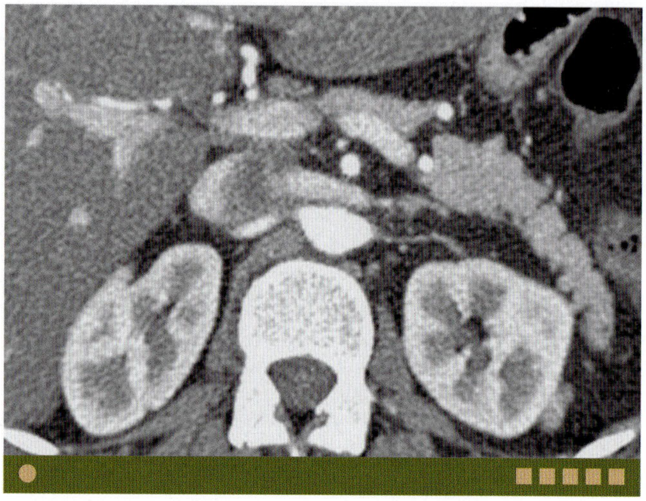

A. Axial CECT shows an enhancing mass arising from the posterolateral aspect of the left kidney. The mass enhances to a slightly less degree than the adjacent renal cortex.

Treatment is typically surgical resection as these tumors cannot be distinguished from renal cell carcinoma on the basis of imaging findings.

PEARLS

- **Rare, benign solid renal masses.**
- **Arise from smooth muscle cells found in the renal capsule, renal pelvis, calyx, or blood vessels.**
- **Difficult to distinguish from other renal neoplasm on the basis of imaging findings.**

ADDITIONAL IMAGES (B-C)

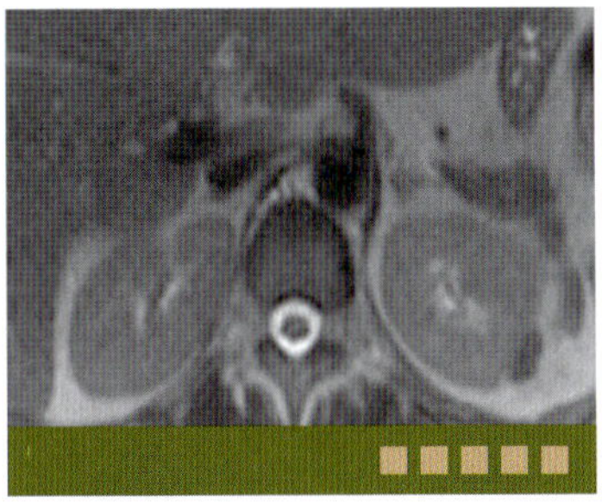

B. Axial T2-WI performed on the same patient shows the mass to be hypointense.

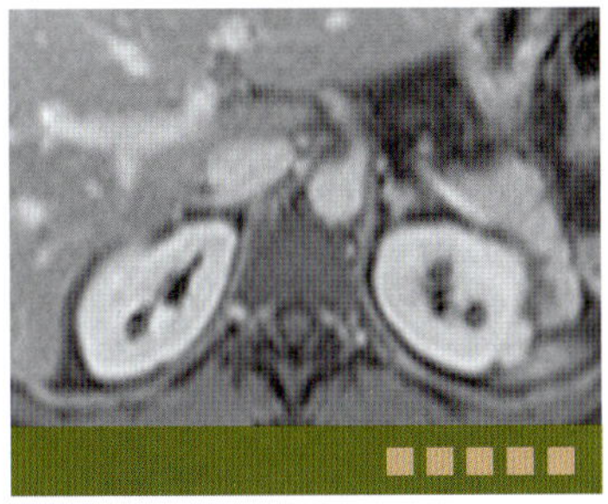

C. Axial contrast-enhanced T1-WI shows avid enhancement of the mass.

DIFFERENTIAL DIAGNOSES IMAGES (D-H)

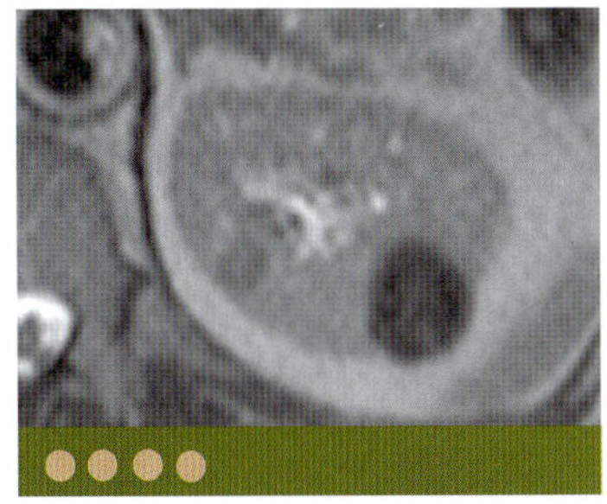

D. Papillary renal cell carcinoma: Axial T2-WI shows a well-circumscribed hypointense mass in the posterolateral aspect of the left kidney.

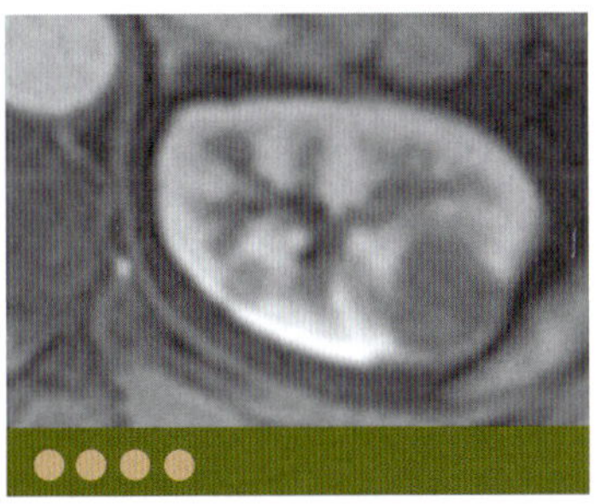

E. Papillary renal cell carcinoma: Axial contrast-enhanced T1-WI in the same patient as in Figure D shows a hypoenhancing mass in the left kidney.

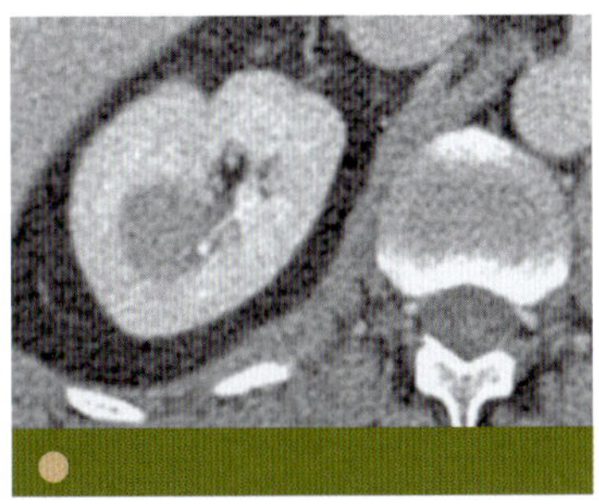

F. Metanephric adenoma: Axial CECT shows a hypoenhancing mass located centrally in the mid pole of the right kidney.

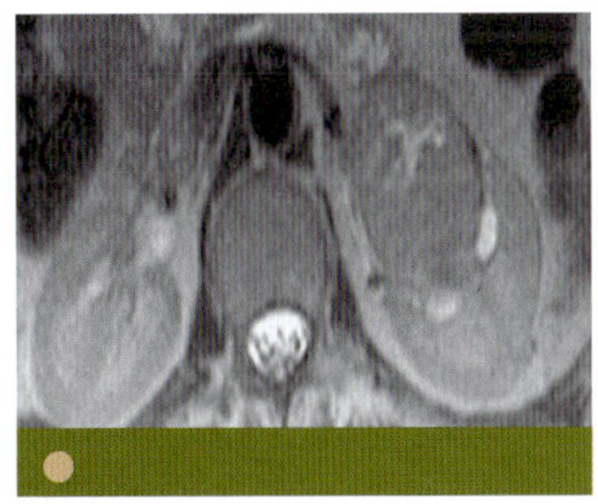

G. Leiomyosarcoma: Axial T2-WI shows a well-circumscribed, heterogeneous arising from the left kidney. The mass is mildly hypointense compared to normal renal parenchyma. T2 bright areas suggest internal necrosis.

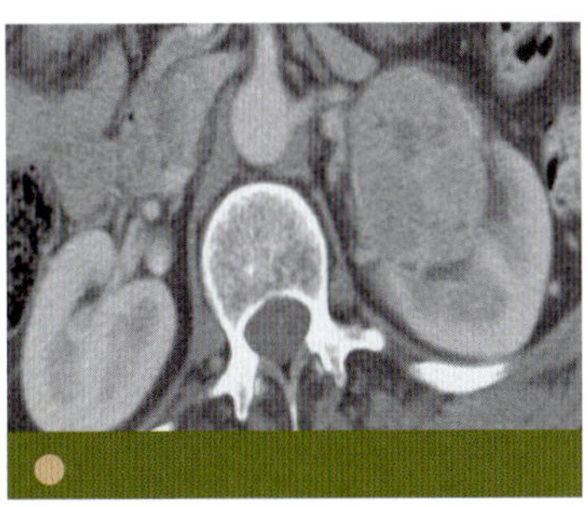

H. Leiomyosarcoma: Axial contrast-enhanced T1-WI shows heterogeneous enhancement of the mass seen in figure G.

IMAGE KEY

Common

Rare

Typical

Unusual

1–28 Perinephric Hemorrhage Caused by Renal Mass

Frank H. Miller

PRESENTATION

Acute flank pain; may have hematuria.

FINDINGS

High-density perinephric hemorrhage.

DIFFERENTIAL DIAGNOSES

- *Perinephric abscess*: Often associated with pyelonephritis and symptoms.
- *Perinephric tumors*: Lymphoma, myeloma, renal cell carcinoma, metastases-generally soft tissue density and enhancing; often history of cancer.
- *Urinoma*: Fluid density; may be associated with stones.
- *Pancreatitis*: Generally distinguished on the basis of a history with pancreatic involvement.

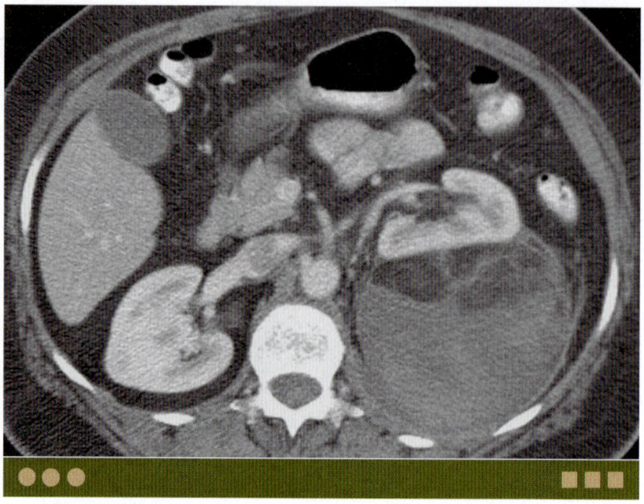

A. Axial CECT shows large mass which contains fat abutting the left kidney with high-density perinephric fluid. The underlying lesion is an AML.

COMMENTS

Causes of perinephric hematoma include spontaneous etiologies (malignant or benign tumors such as renal cell carcinoma or angiomyolipomas, vascular disease, arteriovenous malformations and aneurysms, hemorrhagic cysts or rupture of a cyst, and infections, and infarction), traumatic causes (blunt or penetrating trauma, surgery, percutaneous nephrostomies, extracorporeal shock wave lithotripsy, and biopsy) and anticoagulation or bleeding diathesis. One of the most common causes is tumor, either AML or renal cell carcinoma. AMLs that bleed often are larger than 4 cm while renal cell carcinomas are often small and peripheral and may be difficult to detect in the acute setting. Blood extends into the perirenal and/or subcapsular space.

The treatment of perinephric hemorrhage depends on the identification of the underlying cause. CT and MR scans can be helpful in the diagnosis and can generally diagnose the presence of perinephric blood. On CT, acute hemorrhage is seen as high density. On MR, the appearance of blood depends on its age. Hemorrhage is often seen as increased signal on T1-weighted images because of methemoglobin. The underlying etiology may not be detectable acutely on CT or MR because of the presence of perinephric hemorrhage. The identification of macroscopic fat in a mass is diagnostic of AML. Subtraction images may be helpful to show underlying small enhancing lesions. In patients with perinephric hematomas, it is important to obtain follow-up examinations which may reveal the underlying cause, including renal cell carcinoma. Angiography may be helpful if a mass is not seen especially to show underlying neoplasms and vascular causes, including vasculitis such as polyarteritis nodosa.

PEARLS

- **One of most common causes of perinephric hemorrhage is cancer.**
- **CT and MR are helpful in the diagnosis of perinephric hematomas.**
- **The presence of fat in a mass with hemorrhage should suggest AML.**
- **When cause of perinephric hematoma is not seen, follow-up imaging should be performed to identify underlying cause including malignancy.**

ADDITIONAL IMAGES (B-G)

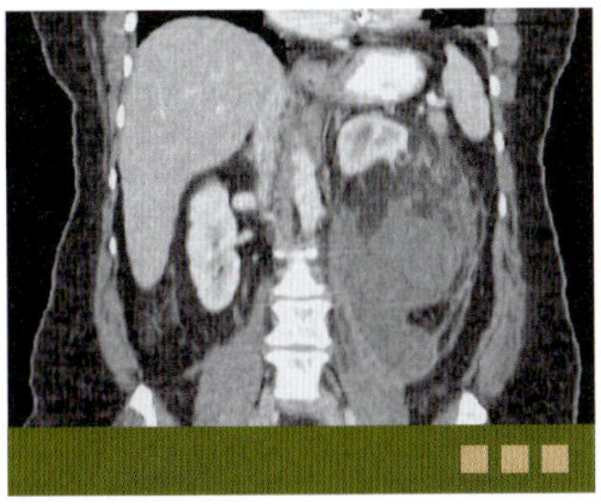

B. Coronal CECT in the same patient shows the lesion arising from the left kidney with "claw-sign" and fat density within the kidney because of angiomyolipoma that bled.

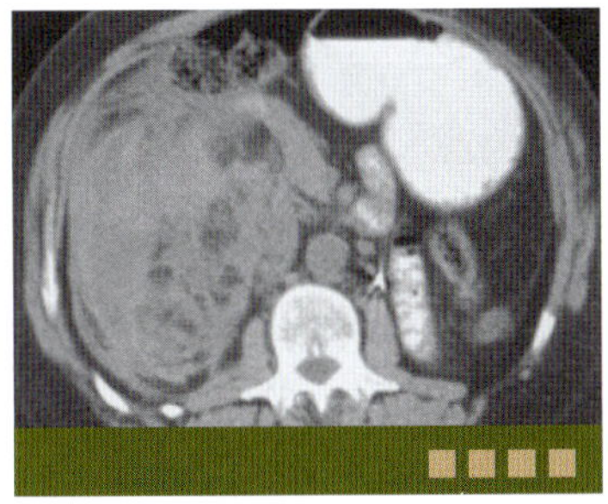

C. Perirenal hemorrhage in patient with tuberous sclerosis. Axial NECT shows right perinephric hematoma with kidney replaced with AMLs. Left kidney had been previously resected with multiple AMLs.

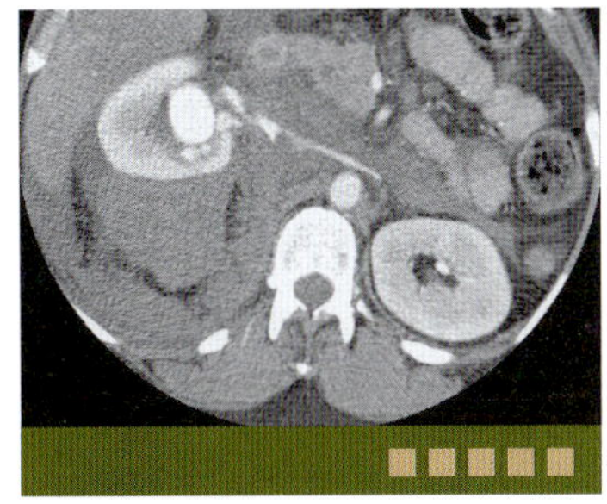

D. Perirenal hemorrhage is caused by renal artery aneurysm. Axial CECT shows large hyperdense lesion with similar density to the aorta resulting from renal artery aneurysm. High-density perirenal hemorrhage is present.

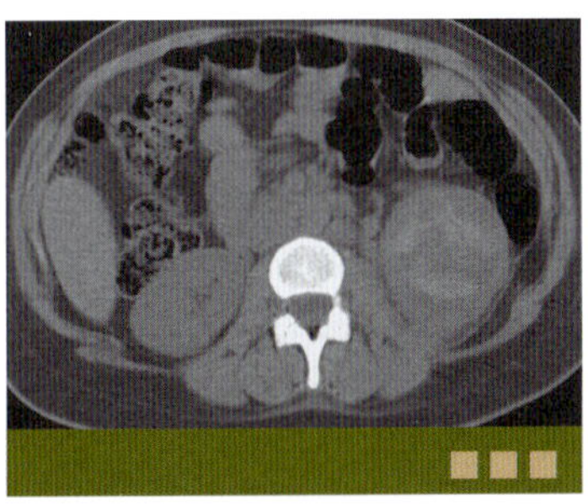

E. Perirenal hemorrhage is caused by clear cell renal cell carcinoma. Axial NECT shows left perinephric hematoma. The patient had post-partum hemorrhage.

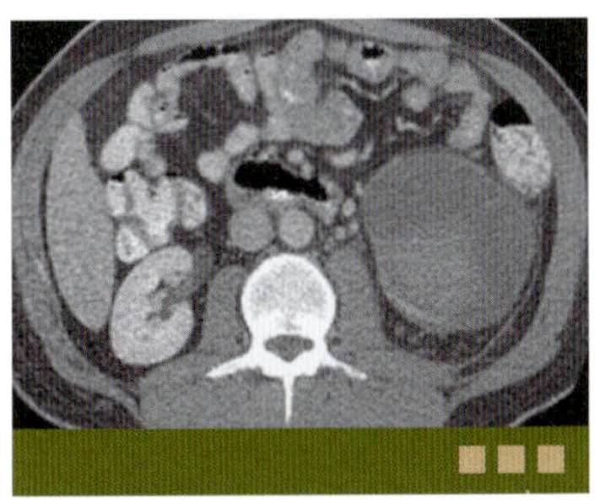

F. Axial CECT showed the perinephric hemorrhage but did not show the cause of the hemorrhage clearly.

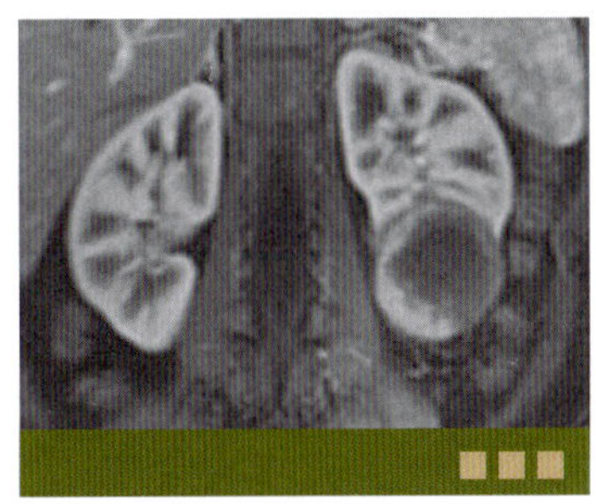

G. Coronal contrast-enhanced T1-WI shows enhancement of the periphery of the mass. Mass was resected and was clear cell carcinoma which had bled.

IMAGE KEY

Common

Rare

Typical

Unusual

DIFFERENTIAL DIAGNOSES IMAGES (H-I)

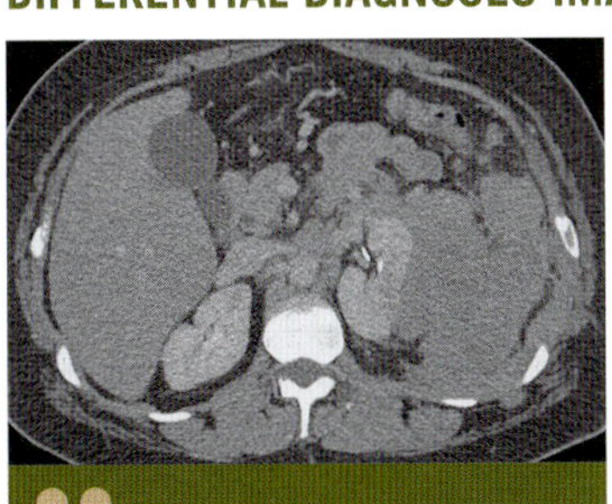

H. Lymphoma: Axial CECT in patient with AIDS shows perinephric soft tissue mass from non-Hodgkin lymphoma. The mass enhances less than the kidney.

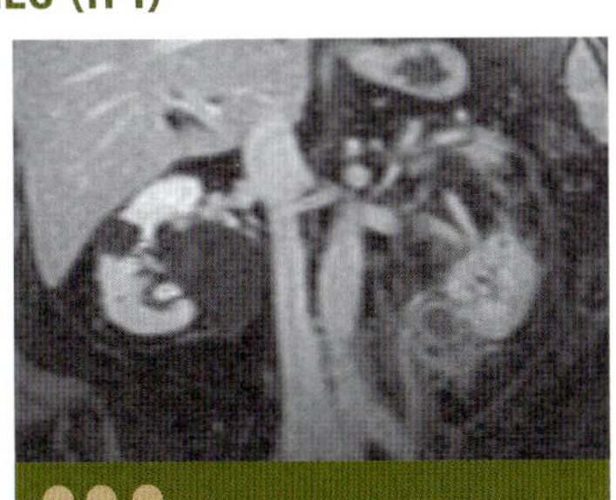

I. Perinephric infection from acute pyelonephritis: Coronal contrast-enhanced T1-WI shows perinephric inflammation from acute pyelonephritis. The clinical history helps distinguish it from other entities.

CHAPTER 2

RENAL CYSTS AND CYSTIC DISEASES

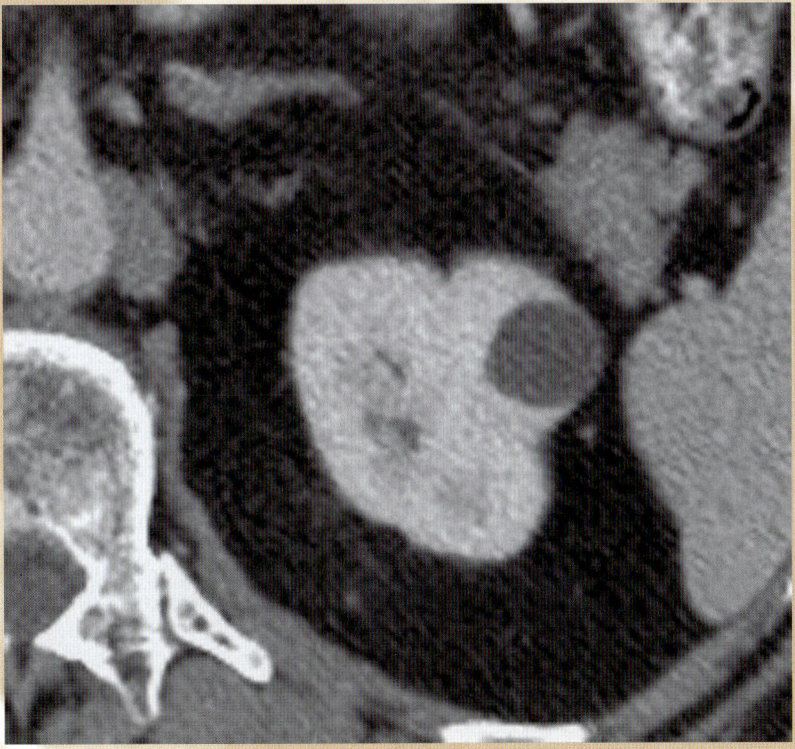

2–1 Simple Cyst

David D. Casalino

PRESENTATION

Asymptomatic.

FINDINGS

Contrast-enhanced CT shows a round, homogeneous, fluid density mass in the lateral cortex of the left kidney.

DIFFERENTIAL DIAGNOSES

- *Calyceal diverticulum*: Structural ectasia from a calyx; may be symptomatic if complicated by stone, hemorrhage, or inflammation; usually fills with contrast on excretory phase imaging.
- *Abscess*: Nonenhancing and may have a rim of less enhancement than the adjacent cortex. Findings of pyelonephritis and symptoms of infection are common.
- *Caliectasis in setting of obstruction*: Typically, there is communication with the rest of the collecting system; not a discrete mass; may fill with contrast.

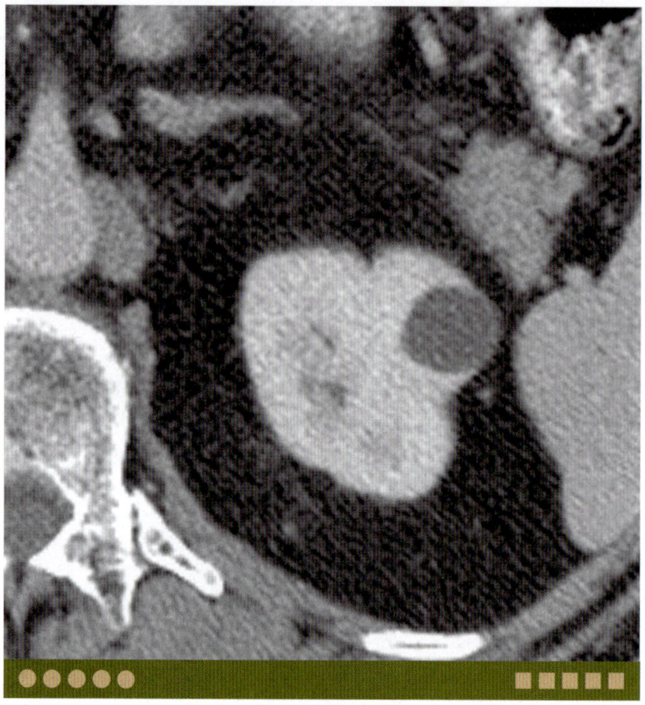

A. CECT shows a round, homogeneous, fluid density mass in the lateral cortex of the left kidney. Its wall is imperceptible.

COMMENTS

Simple cyst is the most common renal mass. Fifty percent of people over the age of 50 years have a renal cyst. Simple cysts are rare in individuals under the age of 30 years. Renal cysts increase in prevalence with age and are presumed to be acquired. The etiology may be obstruction of a renal tubule and the resulting dilatation of the more proximal tubule with serous fluid. Simple cysts more commonly arise in the renal cortex than in the medulla. Simple cysts are usually asymptomatic; however, symptoms may occur because of mass effect.

Bilateral, multiple cysts may be difficult to differentiate from a polycystic kidney disorder. Multiple cysts in a single kidney may be difficult to differentiate from unilateral renal cystic disease (URCD).

On plain radiographs and intravenous urography (IVU), a renal cyst may create a focal contour bulge if peripherally located in the cortex. The interface of such a cyst with normal parenchyma may create a crescentic margin, called "beak" or "claw" sign.

More centrally located cysts may splay or displace the pelvocalyceal system. On ultrasound, simple cysts are anechoic with posterior acoustic enhancement. Simple cysts are fluid density on nonconstrast CT, and they do not enhance. On MR, simple cysts are isointense to fluid, typically low-signal intensity on T1-weighted images (T1-WI) and high-signal intensity on T2-weighted images (T2-WI), and they do not enhance. They have hairline thin walls and do not have septa, calcifications, or solid components.

PEARLS

- **While renal cysts are uncommon in individuals less than 30 years old, they are found in 50% of individuals more than 50 years old.**
- **Simple cysts are anechoic on ultrasound, fluid density on CT, and isointense to fluid on MR.**
- **Simple cysts have hairline thin walls, often imperceptible, and they do not enhance.**

ADDITIONAL IMAGES (B-D)

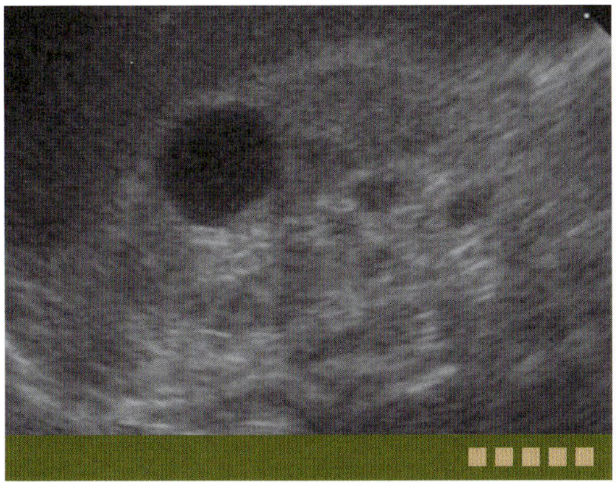

B. Longitudinal sonogram shows an upper pole cyst that is round, anechoic, and creates posterior acoustic enhancement.

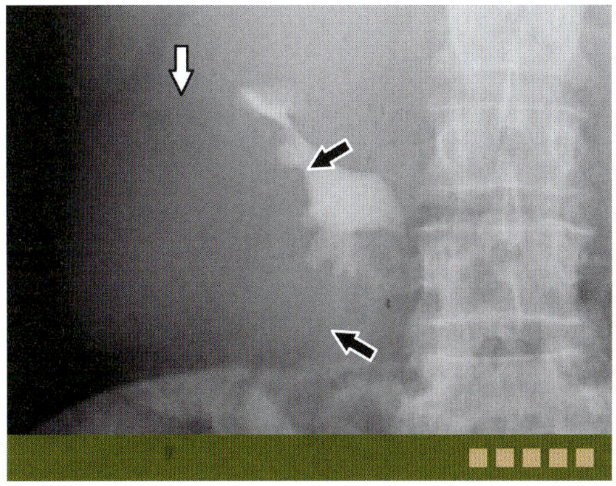

C. IVU shows a beak sign (white arrow) caused by renal parenchyma draping around the upper edge of a 7-cm cyst, which also creates smooth mass effect on the pelvocalyceal system (black arrows).

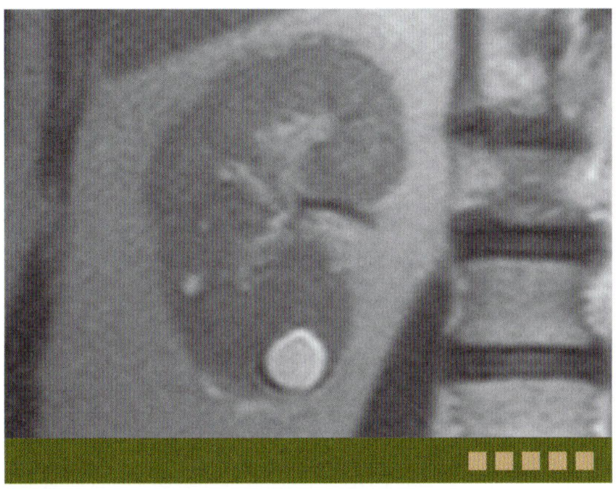

D. Coronal T2-WI shows a homogeneous, hyperintense cortical cyst in the lower pole of the right kidney. A much smaller cyst is seen in the lateral cortex. Both cysts were hypointense on T1-WI and did not enhance.

DIFFERENTIAL DIAGNOSES IMAGES (E-G)

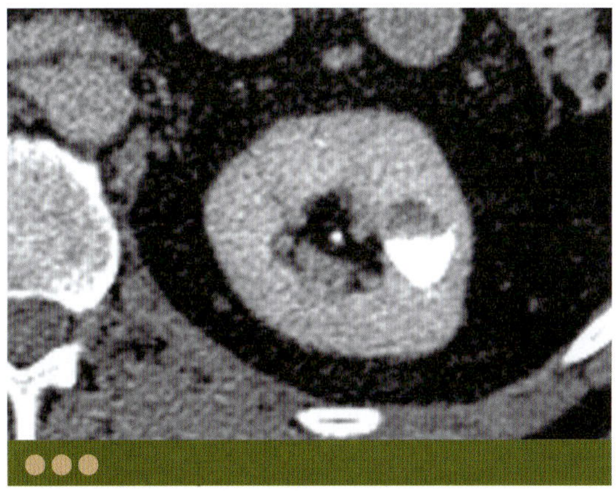

E. Calyceal diverticulum: Axial CECT, excretory phase, shows excreted contrast layering within a round structure that was homogeneous and fluid density on the precontrast and nephrographic phases.

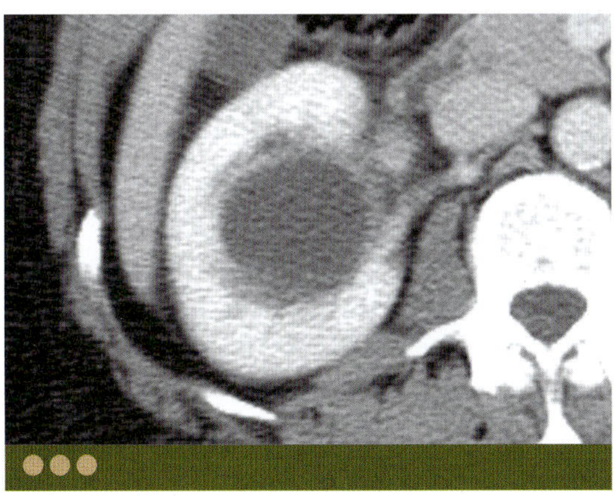

F. Abscess: Axial CECT shows a central, right, renal cystic mass surrounded by a thin rim of hypoenhancing parenchyma. The patient presented with right flank pain, fever, and elevated white blood cell count.

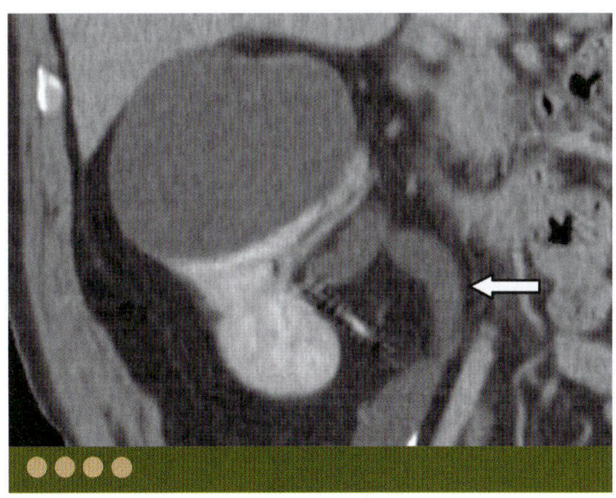

G. Caliectasis: Coronal CECT shows a large upper pole cystic mass that on axial imaging is shown to communicate with the upper pole renal pelvis in this patient with complete duplication. The upper moiety is obstructed distally with dilatation of its ureter (white arrow).

IMAGE KEY

Common

Rare

Typical

Unusual

2–2 Bosniak Category II Cystic Renal Mass

David D. Casalino

PRESENTATION

Asymptomatic.

FINDINGS

CT images prior to and after contrast administration show a large left renal cyst with a single calcified septation. There is no enhancement.

DIFFERENTIAL DIAGNOSES

- *Cystic renal cell carcinoma* (RCC): More complex, as detailed in higher Bosniak categories.
- *Multilocular cystic nephroma* (MLCN): More complex; typically, Bosniak category III or IIF.
- *Abscess*: Nonenhancing and may have a rim of less enhancement than adjacent cortex; findings of pyelonephritis and symptoms of infection are common.

COMMENTS

The Bosniak renal cyst classification system, first introduced in 1986, suggests a patient treatment scheme based on a cystic lesion's morphology and enhancement characteristics. Renal cystic lesions can be classified as Bosniak category I, II, IIF, III, or IV using pre- and postcontrast-enhanced CT or magnetic resonance imaging (MRI).

Bosniak category I cysts are simple cysts. They are fluid density cysts and do not enhance. These cysts have hairline thin walls and do not have septa, calcifications, or solid components. They do not warrant further evaluation.

Bosniak category II cysts are minimally complicated. They may be complicated by fine calcifications or a short segment of slightly thickened calcification in the wall or septa. These cysts may contain a few hairline thin septa, in which there may be "perceived" (as opposed to "measurable") enhancement. Homogeneously hyperdense, nonenhancing lesions measuring lesser than 3 cm that are not totally intrarenal are also included in this category. These hyperdense lesions may be anechoic or hypoechoic on ultrasonography. Category II cysts, in general, do not warrant further evaluation.

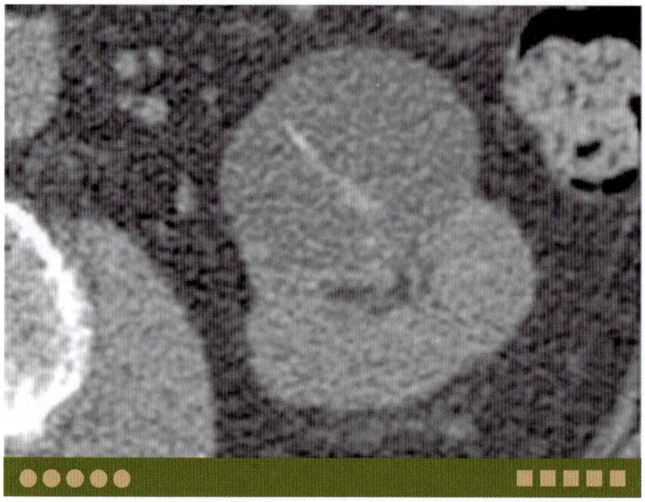

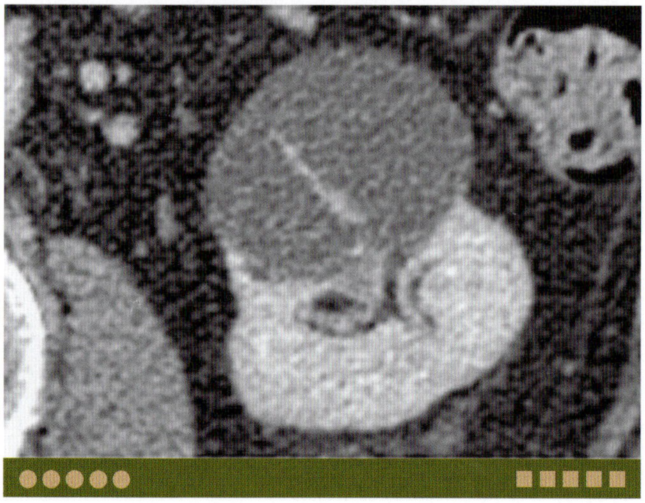

A. and B. Axial NECT and CECT show a large left renal cyst with a single, calcified septation. There is no enhancement of the septation or elsewhere within the lesion.

PEARLS

- **The Bosniak classification system takes into account lesion morphology and enhancement characteristics; therefore, conventional ultrasonography should not be used to categorize a complex cystic lesion.**
- **Bosniak category II cysts may have one or a few septations that are hairline thin, and septations and cyst walls may have fine calcifications or a short segment of slightly thickened calcification.**
- **Some hyperdense, nonenhancing cysts are category II, whereas others are category IIF, depending on the size and assessment of the outer margin.**

ADDITIONAL IMAGES (C-E)

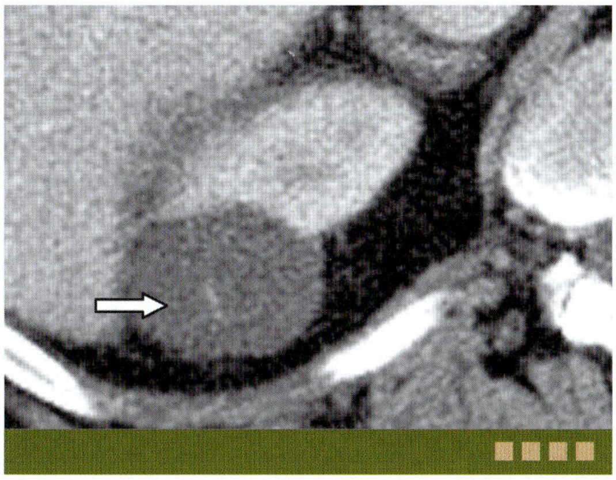

C. Axial CECT shows a right renal cyst complicated by a single hairline thin septation. This septation has "perceived enhancement" because it is neither seen on the NECT nor has measurable enhancement when regions of interest are used to measure changes in density.

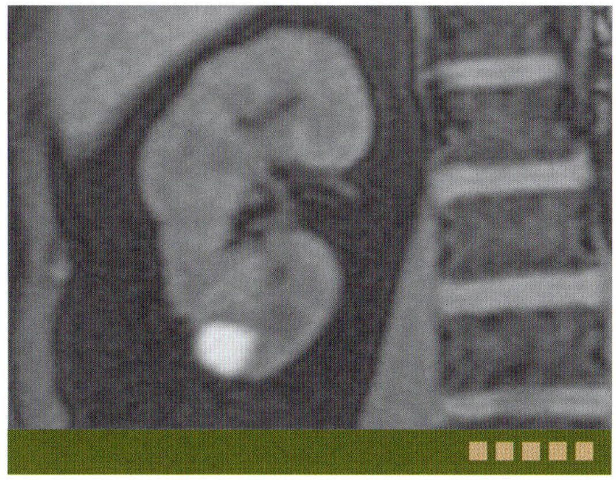

D. Coronal T1-WI shows a round, hyperintense 1.5-cm lesion in the lower pole of the right kidney. This hemorrhagic cyst does not enhance and is homogeneous. On axial imaging (not shown), no mural thickening or enhancement was apparent.

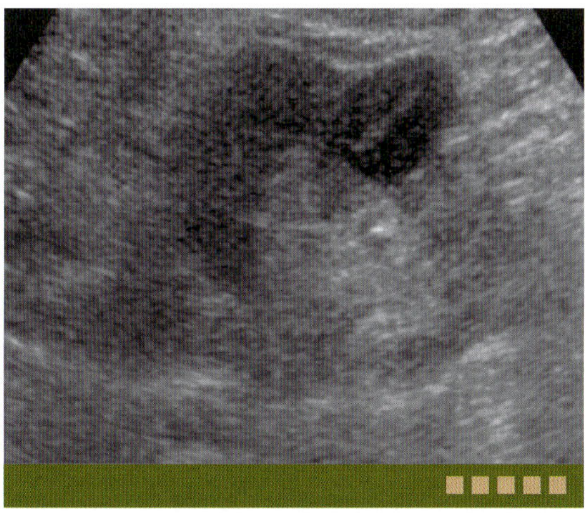

E. Transverse sonogram shows a cortical cyst complicated by a thin septation. CECT (not seen here) showed neither any enhancement of the septation nor any other complicating feature.

DIFFERENTIAL DIAGNOSES IMAGES (F-H)

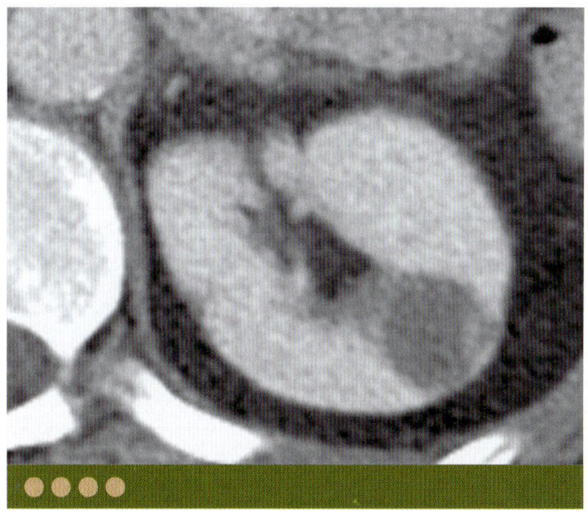

F. Cystic RCC: Axial CECT shows a left renal cystic mass with thick, enhancing septation along its lateral aspect.

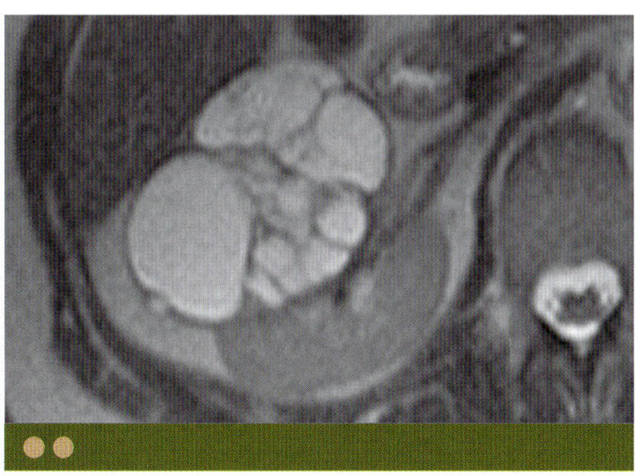

G. MLCN: Axial T2-WI shows a multilocular right renal mass with numerous septations. A few of the septations showed slight measurable enhancement on contrast-enhanced sequences (not shown).

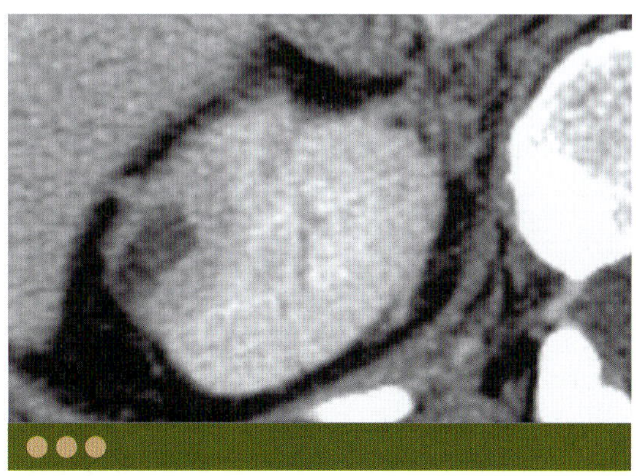

H. Abscess: Axial CECT shows a right renal lesion that is cystic with few thin, perceived septations and surrounded by the cortex. The lesion enhances less than the adjacent cortex. The patient had symptoms and additional right renal findings suggestive of pyelonephritis.

IMAGE KEY

Common

Rare

Typical

Unusual

2–3 Bosniak Category IIF Cystic Renal Mass

David D. Casalino

PRESENTATION

Hematuria.

FINDINGS

Unenhanced CT shows a left kidney cystic mass with nodular septal and mural calcifications. CECT (not shown here) did not show enhancement within the mass.

DIFFERENTIAL DIAGNOSES

- *Complex benign cyst*: Most likely diagnosis, but follow-up imaging warranted.
- *Multilocular cystic nephroma*: May have mural and septal calcifications without measurable enhancement.
- *Cystic renal cell carcinoma*: More often shows mural or septal measurable enhancement.
- *Abscess*: Nonenhancing and may have a rim of less enhancement than the adjacent cortex; findings of pyelonephritis and symptoms of infection are common.

COMMENTS

The Bosniak renal cyst classification system, first introduced in 1986, suggests a patient treatment scheme based on a cystic lesion's morphology and enhancement characteristics. Renal cystic lesions can be classified as Bosniak category I, II, IIF, III, or IV using pre- and postcontrast-enhanced CT or MRI.

Bosniak category IIF cysts may have multiple hairline thin septa or minimal smooth thickening of their wall or septa. They do not show measurable enhancement but may have perceived mural or septal enhancement. Mural or septal calcifications may be thick and nodular. Homogeneously hyperdense, nonenhancing lesions measuring more than 3 cm or totally intrarenal lesions are also included in this category. Bosniak category IIF lesions warrant follow-up imaging, perhaps at 6-month intervals for the first year, and then annually. If on follow-up imaging, there is an increase in the thickness or irregularity of the lesion's wall or septa, surgery, or biopsy at some institutions, is advised. Slight lesion growth or an increase in calcification can occur without indication of malignancy, and follow-up should be continued.

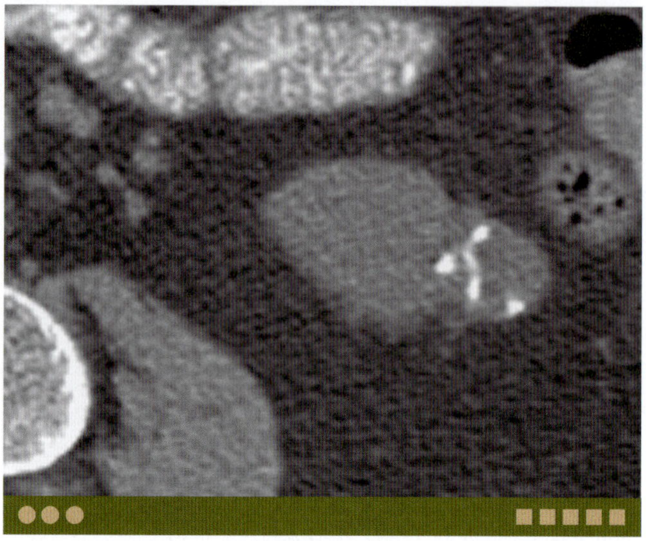

A. Axial NECT shows a 1.5-cm left renal cystic mass with multiple, nodular, septal, and mural calcifications. CECT (not shown) did not show enhancement initially.

In one series (Israel GM, Bosniak MA. *AJR* 2003;181:627–633), 2 of 42 Bosniak category IIF lesions proved to be cystic neoplasms. The average follow-up time was 5.8 years with a median of 5.0 years, though no data are available to suggest when it is safe to discontinue following up IIF lesions. Clinical factors must be taken into account for the most appropriate management of a given patient.

PEARLS

- **Limited data suggest the risk of malignancy in a Bosniak category IIF lesion is approximately 5%.**
- **Bosniak IIF lesions may show perceived enhancement but not measurable enhancement.**
- **Some hyperdense, nonenhancing cysts are category II, whereas others are category IIF, depending on size and assessment of the outer margin.**
- **Histopathologic diagnosis is advised if a Bosniak IIF lesion shows an increase in the thickness or irregularity of its wall or a septation or new enhancement.**

ADDITIONAL IMAGES (B-D)

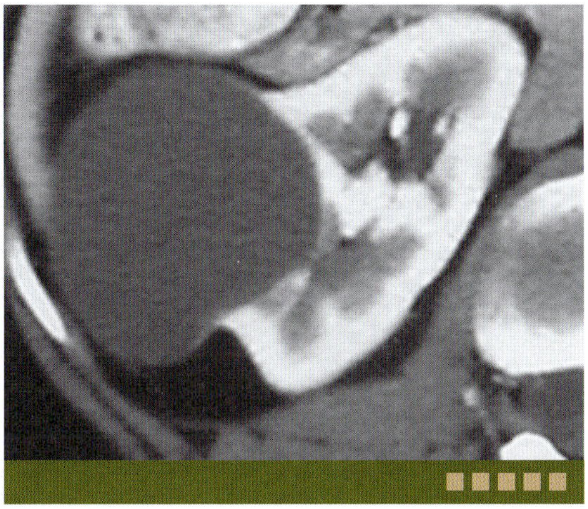

B. Axial CECT shows a 4-cm homogeneous, hyperdense (35 HU) lesion of the right kidney. There was no enhancement, and the lesion has been stable for 4 years.

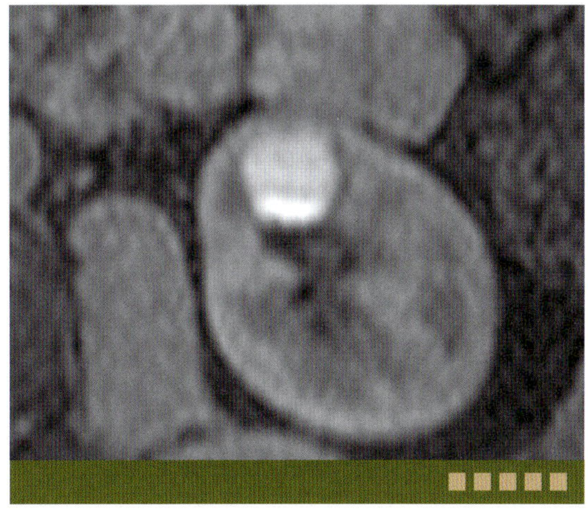

C. Axial T1-WI shows a 1.5-cm hyperintense lesion that is completely surrounded by cortex. There was no enhancement.

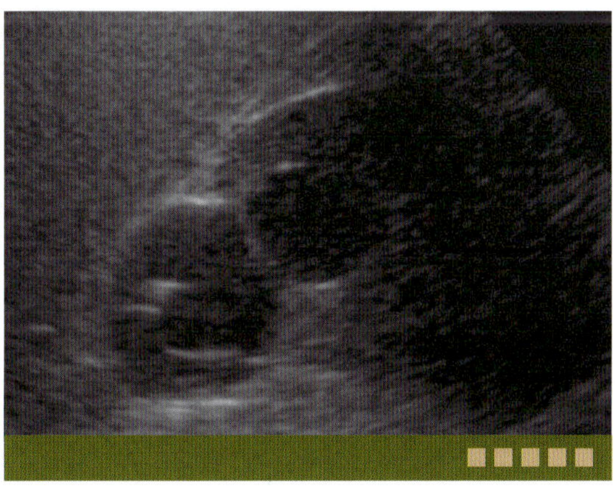

D. Longitudinal sonogram shows a cystic mass with multiple septations. One septation shows minimal smooth thickening. MR (not shown) showed multiple septations but no measurable enhancement.

DIFFERENTIAL DIAGNOSES IMAGES (E-F)

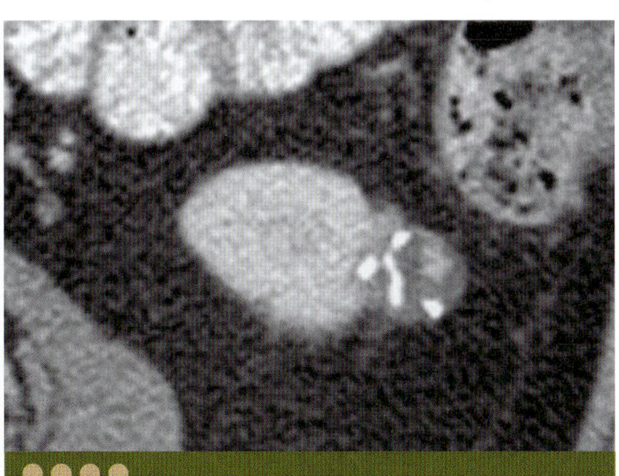

E. Cystic RCC: CECT, from the same patient as first image and performed 18 months after the initial CT, shows a new solid enhancing nodule within the cystic lesion. At surgery, this proved to be a low-grade, cystic papillary RCC.

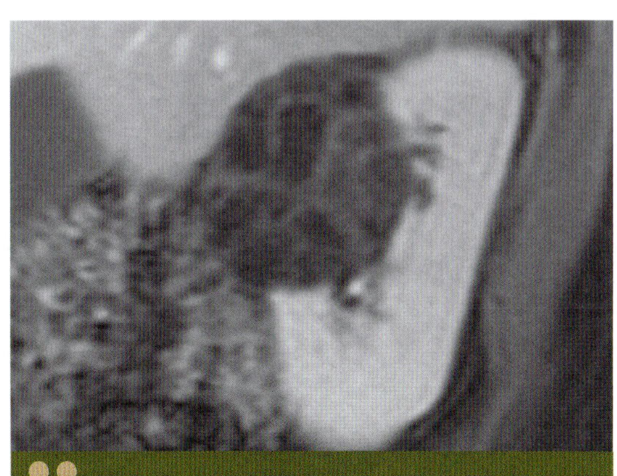

F. MLCN: Sagittal, contrast-enhanced T1-WI shows a multilocular, cystic renal mass with perceived but not measurable enhancement. Because the patient was symptomatic, the lesion was resected.

IMAGE KEY

Common

Rare

Typical

Unusual

2–4 Bosniak Category III Cystic Renal Mass

David D. Casalino

PRESENTATION

Asymptomatic.

FINDINGS

CT images without and with contrast enhancement show a complex left renal cyst mass with multiple thick, irregular septations with measurable enhancement.

DIFFERENTIAL DIAGNOSES

- Imaging cannot reliably differentiate a Bosniak category III cyst that is malignant from the one that is benign.
- The vast majority of malignant lesions in this category are RCCs.
- Benign lesions in this category include benign neoplasms, such as a MLCN, infected cysts, and hemorrhagic cysts.
- A renal artery branch draped around a cyst or coursing between two cysts can mimic a Bosniak category III cyst. Multiplanar reformatted images and higher resolution techniques may allow diagnosis.

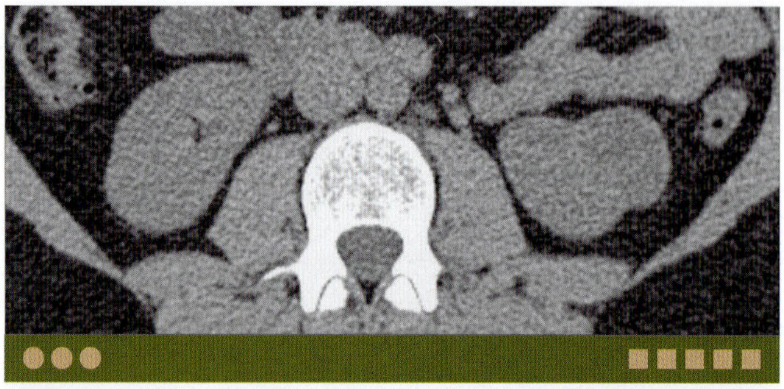

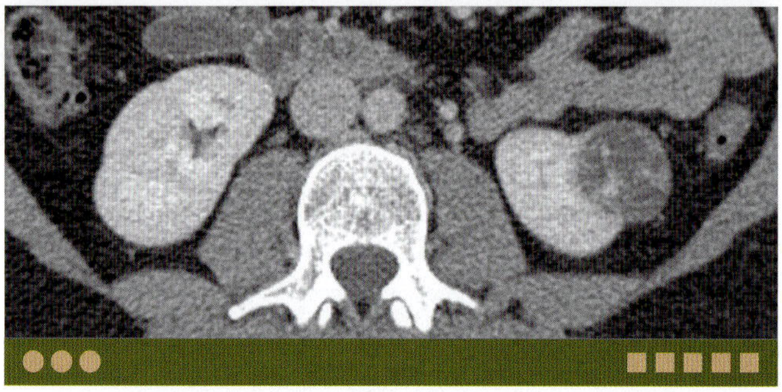

A. Axial NECT shows a left renal cyst that is homogeneous and measures 12 HU throughout.
B. Axial CECT shows the same cyst to have multiple thick, irregular septations with measurable enhancement of the thickest septation, which has a density of 53 HU. This proved to be a cystic RCC.

COMMENTS

The Bosniak renal cyst classification system, first introduced in 1986, suggests a patient treatment scheme based on a cystic lesion's morphology and enhancement characteristics. Renal cystic lesions can be classified as Bosniak category I, II, IIF, III, or IV using pre- and postcontrast enhanced CT or MRI.

Bosniak category III cysts have thickened irregular or smooth walls or septa with measurable enhancement. These should be considered surgical lesions. Data suggest that approximately 50% of lesions in this category will prove to be malignant with the vast majority being cystic RCCs while the other 50% will prove to be benign lesions, such as multiloculated cystic nephroma, infected cysts, and hemorrhagic cysts. Bosniak III lesions are generally regarded as surgical lesions.

The most important criterion used to differentiate surgical lesions from nonsurgical lesions is enhancement, which indicates tissue vascularity. Analysis of enhancement is best done in the nephrographic phase of helical CT imaging. If the postcontrast density of a lesion or component of a lesion is less than 10 Housefield units (HU) more than the precontrast density, there is no enhancement. If the postcontrast density is more than 15 HU more than the precontrast density, most agree there is enhancement. A 10 to 15 HU difference is uncertain for enhancement. Imaging technical factors and lesion size should be taken into account. One may choose to manage a complex cystic lesion with uncertain enhancement as a Bosniak IIF lesion. On MR, enhancement is generally defined as at least a 15% to 20% increase in signal intensity between the pre- and postcontrast T1-WI.

PEARLS

- **The risk of malignancy in a Bosniak category III lesion is approximately 50%.**
- **Enhancement is the most important criterion used to differentiate a surgical renal lesion from a nonsurgical lesion.**
- **Most agree that an increase in density greater than 15 HU is enhancement, and an increase in density of 10 to 15 HU is uncertain for enhancement.**

ADDITIONAL IMAGES (C-G)

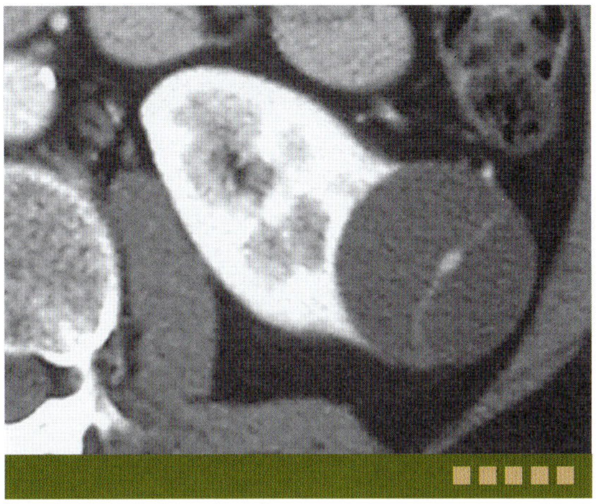

C. Axial CECT shows a left renal cystic lesion complicated by a single septation that has focal thickening with measurable enhancement compared to the precontrast imaging (not shown). This proved to be a cystic RCC.

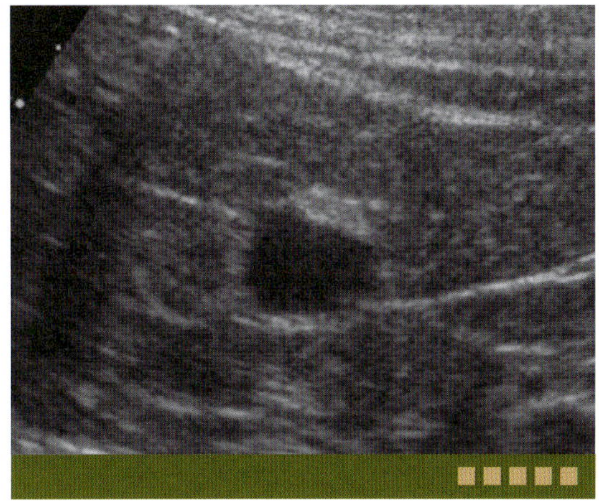

D. Longitudinal sonogram of the left kidney shows a small cystic lesion with focal, hyperechoic mural thickening.

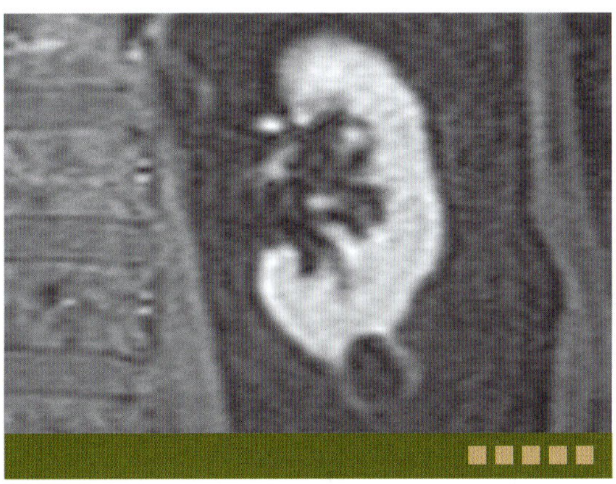

E. Coronal, contrast-enhanced T1-WI from the same patient shows the cystic lesion to have lateral mural thickening with measurable enhancement. This proved to be a cystic, lipid-poor angiomyolipoma.

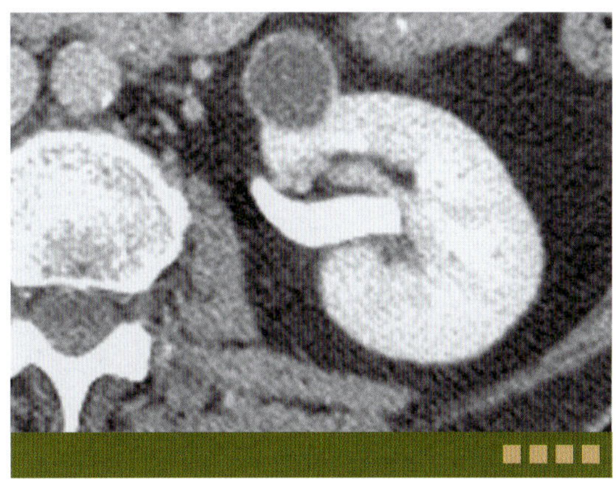

F. Axial CECT shows a left renal cystic lesion with diffusely thickened, enhancing wall. This proved to be a chronic, infected cyst

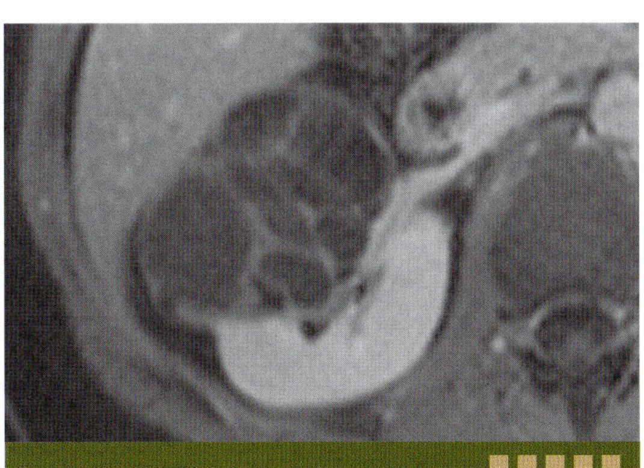

G. Axial contrast-enhanced T1-WI shows a multilocular cystic mass with enhancement of the septations. This proved to be a MLCN.

DIFFERENTIAL DIAGNOSES IMAGE

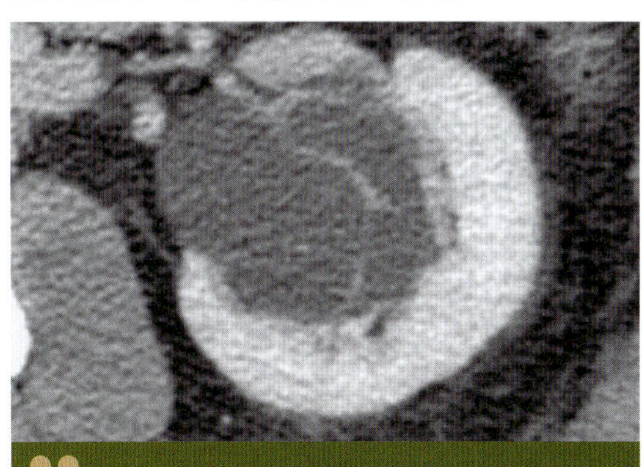

H. Renal artery branch: Axial CECT shows a renal artery branch coursing between a parapelvic cyst and a cortical cyst. On the initial thicker slice images (not shown), the continuity of the vessel was not seen, and the appearance mimicked a Bosniak III lesion.

IMAGE KEY

Common

Rare

Typical

Unusual

2–5 Bosniak Category IV Cystic Renal Mass

David D. Casalino

PRESENTATION

Left flank pain.

FINDINGS

CT images without and with contrast-enhancement show a large left renal cystic mass with enhancing soft-tissue component adjacent to its anterior wall.

DIFFERENTIAL DIAGNOSES

- *Cystic renal cell carcinoma*: The vast majority of Bosniak category IV lesions.
- *Focal xanthogranulomatous* pyelonephritis (XGP): Much more common in women; very often associated with ipsilateral renal calculi and history of chronic urinary tract infection (UTI); symptoms may be nonspecific or absent; usually a surgical lesion.
- *Abscess*: In the early stage of development, an abscess may have nonenhancing cystic and enhancing solid components; findings of pyelonephritis and symptoms of infection are common.

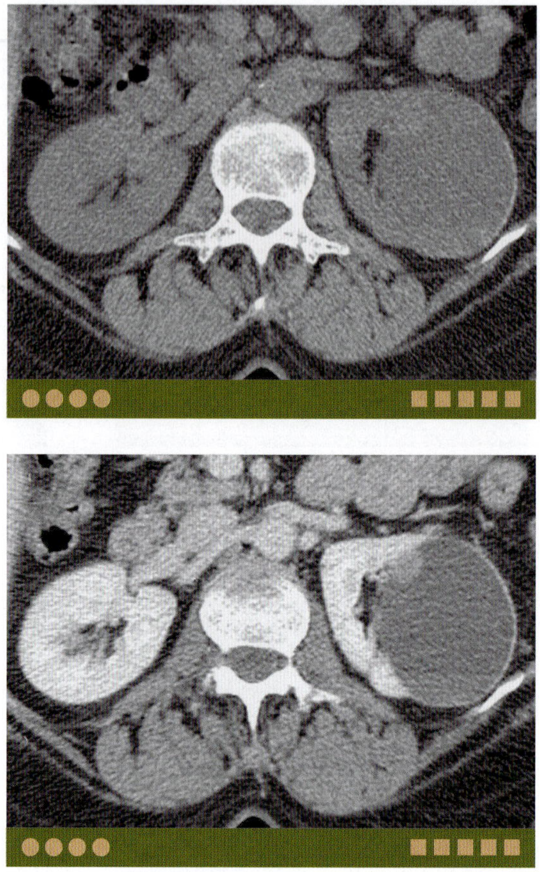

A. Axial NECT shows a large left renal cyst with fine calcifications involving its posterolateral wall.
B. Axial CECT shows a 1.2-cm enhancing soft-tissue component adjacent to the cyst's anterior wall. This proved to be a cystic RCC.

COMMENTS

The Bosniak renal cyst classification system, first introduced in 1986, suggests a patient treatment scheme based on a cystic lesion's morphology and enhancement characteristics. Renal cystic lesions can be classified as Bosniak category I, II, IIF, III, or IV using pre- and postcontrast-enhanced CT or MRI.

Bosniak category IV cysts contain enhancing soft-tissue components adjacent to, but independent of, the wall or septum. These lesions may also have features of category III cysts. Data suggest that approximately 95% of Bosniak category IV cysts are malignant; therefore, these lesions warrant surgical resection.

The most important criterion used to differentiate surgical lesions from nonsurgical lesions is enhancement. It follows that pre- and postcontrast imaging with meticulous technique is critical in evaluating complex cystic renal masses. On CT, there is no enhancement if the increase in density between pre- and post-contrast imaging is less than 10 HU. Most agree that an increase in density greater than 15 HU is enhancement, and an increase in density of 10 to 15 HU is uncertain for enhancement. On MR, enhancement is generally defined as at least a 15% to 20% increase in signal intensity between the pre- and postcontrast T1-WI. While ultrasonography may demonstrate complexity of a renal cyst, it should not be used to assign a Bosniak classification.

PEARLS

- **The risk of malignancy in a Bosniak category IV lesion is approximately 95%.**
- **Enhancement is the most important criterion used to differentiate a surgical renal cystic lesion from a nonsurgical lesion.**
- **Ultrasonography should not be used to assign a Bosniak classification.**

ADDITIONAL IMAGES (C-F)

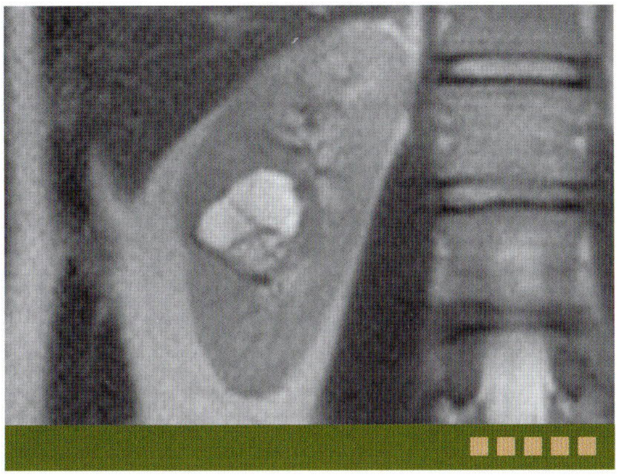

C. Coronal T2-WI shows a right renal complex cystic mass with septations and hypointense, 1-cm nodule in its inferior aspect.

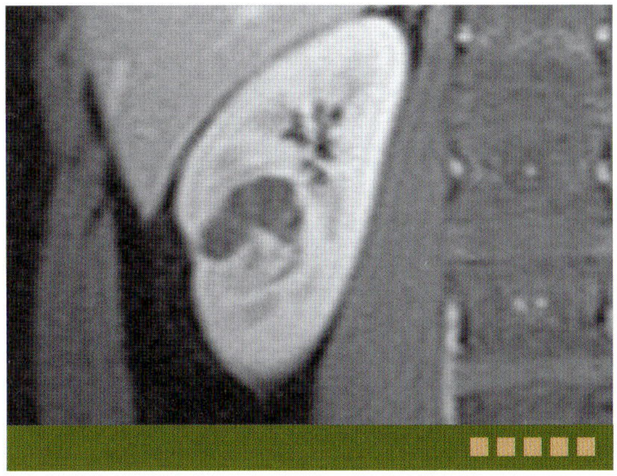

D. Coronal, contrast-enhanced T1-WI from the same patient shows heterogeneous enhancement of the soft-tissue nodule within the cyst. This proved to be a cystic RCC.

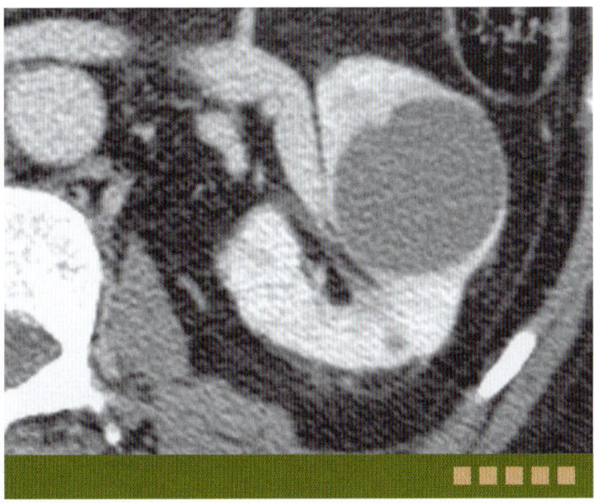

E. Axial CECT shows a left renal cyst with a 5-mm enhancing nodule adjacent to its anterior wall.

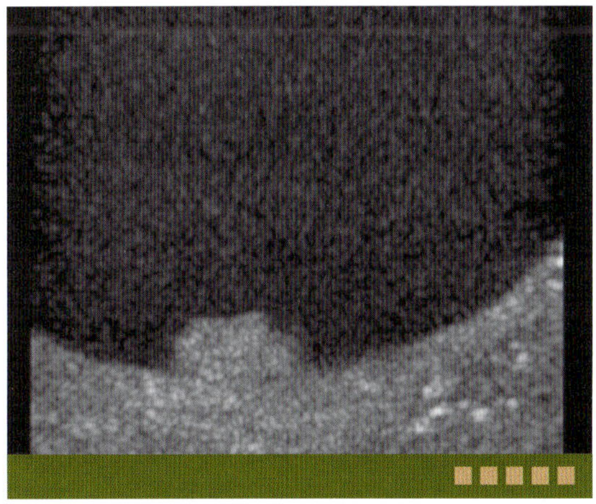

F. Transverse sonogram performed intraoperatively on the same patient shows the nodule within the otherwise simple-appearing cyst. This proved to be a cystic RCC.

DIFFERENTIAL DIAGNOSES IMAGES (G-H)

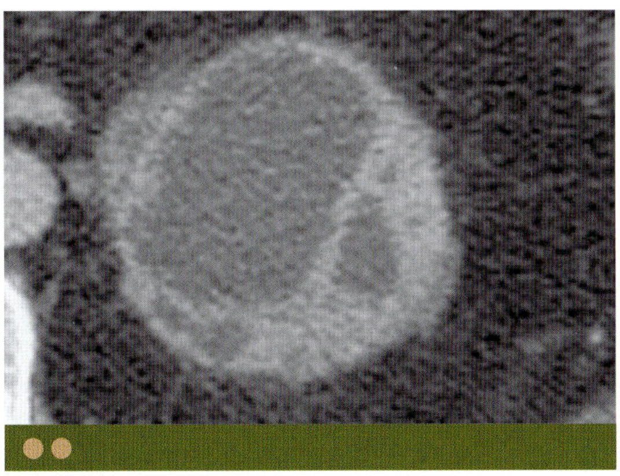

G. Focal XGP: Axial CECT shows an upper pole complicated cystic mass with enhancing septations and mural thickening. The surrounding fat appears normal. The lower pole (not shown) appears normal, and there are no left renal calculi.

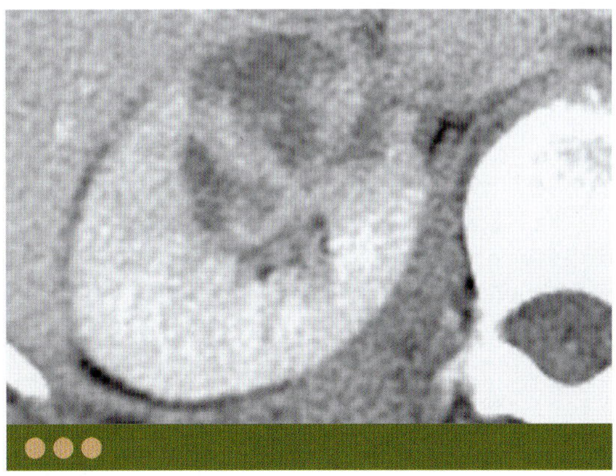

H. Abscess: Axial CECT shows a complicated cystic lesion with thick, enhancing septations and outer rim of enhancement that is slightly less dense than normal cortex. Other areas of cortex (not shown) show heterogeneous enhancement characteristic of pyelonephritis.

IMAGE KEY

Common

Rare

Typical

Unusual

2–6 Autosomal Dominant Polycystic Kidney Disease

David D. Casalino

PRESENTATION

Left flank pain and history of renal disease.

FINDINGS

CT images show both kidneys to be enlarged by numerous cysts, including a large hemorrhagic cyst in the left kidney; there are hepatic cysts as well.

DIFFERENTIAL DIAGNOSES

- *Multiple simple cysts*: Cysts not as numerous; rarely renal enlargement; normal renal function.
- *Acquired renal cystic disease*: Associated with chronic renal failure and dialysis; usually small kidneys with fewer cysts.
- *von Hippel-Lindau* (VHL): Cyst not as numerous; associated with multifocal RCC, pheochromocytomas, pancreatic lesions, central nervous system (CNS) hemangioblastomas, and family history.
- *Tuberous sclerosis* (TS): Associated with renal angiomyolipomas (AMLs), skin lesions, CNS lesions, and family history.
- *Medullary cystic kidney disease*: Cysts are small and in the medulla; kidneys may be small; family history of the disease.

COMMENTS

Autosomal dominant polycystic kidney disease (ADPKD) is the most common genetically transmitted renal cystic disease and is inherited in an autosomal dominant pattern. It is the fourth leading cause of end-stage renal disease (ESRD) in adults.

The PKD1 gene on the short arm of chromosome 16 is most commonly implicated, affecting approximately 85% of patients. The PKD2 gene on the long arm of chromosome 4 is implicated in approximately 15% of patients.

Autosomal dominant polycystic kidney disease most often presents in the third to fifth decade of life with renal disease, perhaps hematuria, hypertension, or renal insufficiency. Renal enlargement caused by cyst growth is associated with decline in renal function. Approximately 50% of patients develop end-stage renal disease. Ultrasound is commonly used to screen the family members of the patients with ADPKD. An individual is unlikely to have the disease if no cysts are detected by the age of 30 years. Patients with ADPKD are not at increased risk of developing a renal malignancy.

Innumerable bilateral renal cysts that massively enlarge the kidneys characterize ADPKD. The cysts are variable in size,

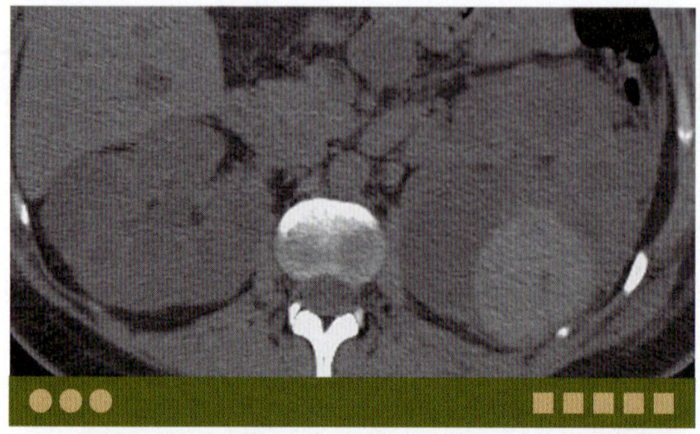

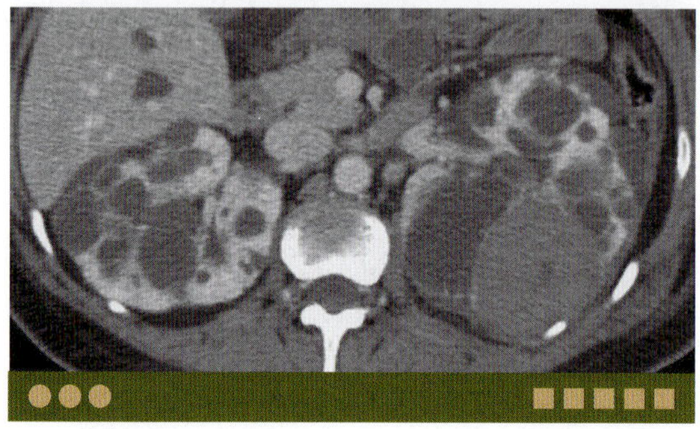

A. and B. Axial NECT and CECT show both kidneys being enlarged with numerous cysts, including a nonenhancing hemorrhagic cyst in the left kidney. The hemorrhage is a new finding since prior study (not shown) and likely accounts for the flank pain. There are hepatic cysts as well.

cortical and medullary in location, and may be complicated by septations, calcifications, and hemorrhage. Cysts are often seen in other organs, including the liver (75% of the patients), pancreas (10% of the patients), spleen, ovaries, and testes. ADPKD may also be associated with intracranial aneurysms in up to 15% of patients, cardiac valvular disorders, hernias, and colonic diverticulosis.

PEARLS

- **Massive bilateral renal enlargement caused by innumerable cysts is characteristic of ADPKD.**
- **Symptoms may relate to renal enlargement or acute hemorrhage into a cyst.**
- **Autosomal dominant polycystic kidney disease is not associated with an increased risk of developing a renal malignancy.**
- **Autosomal dominant polycystic kidney disease is associated with intracranial aneurysms in up to 15% of the patients.**

ADDITIONAL IMAGES (C-E)

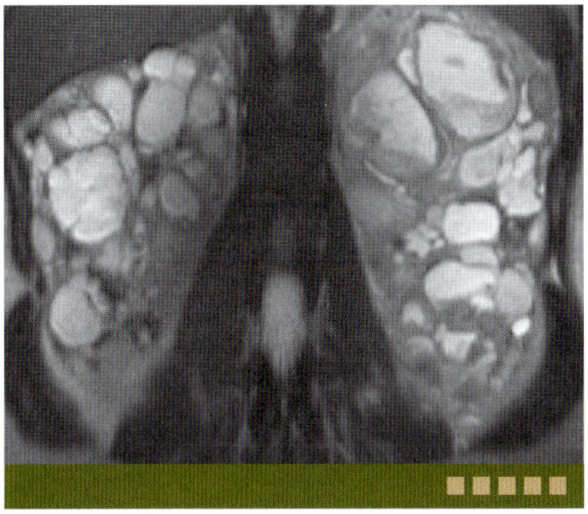

C. Coronal T2-WI shows massive enlargement of both kidneys by multiple cysts of varying size. Several cysts are complicated by hemorrhage.

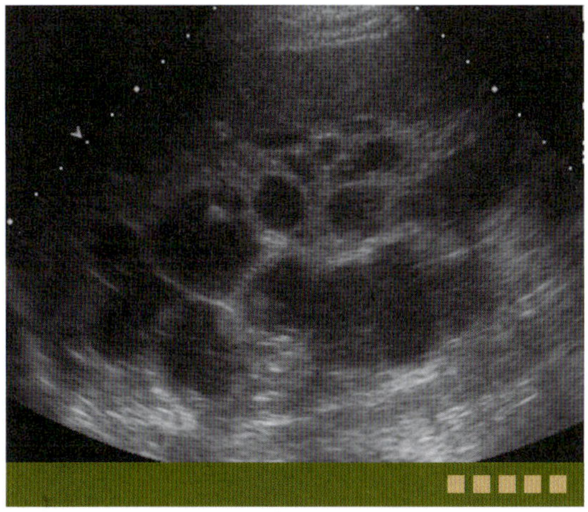

D. Longitudinal sonogram shows the right kidney to be markedly enlarged by numerous cysts. The left kidney had a similar appearance.

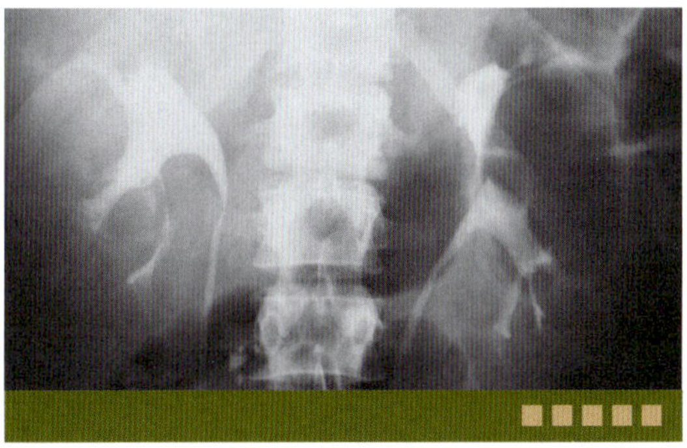

E. IVU shows multifocal enlargement of the kidneys with associated smooth mass effect upon the renal collecting systems.

DIFFERENTIAL DIAGNOSES IMAGES (F-H)

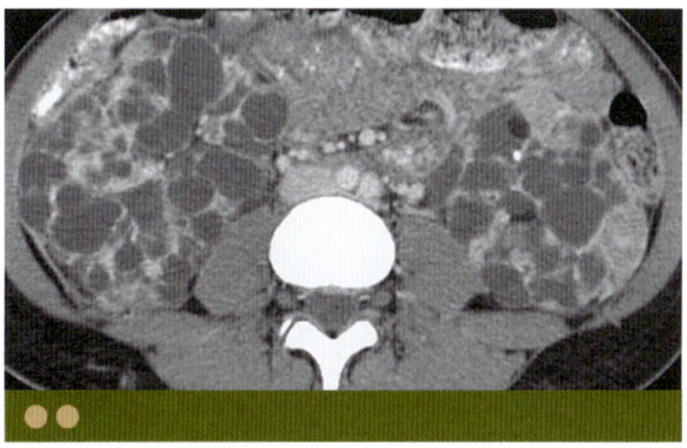

F. TS: Axial CECT shows multiple bilateral renal cysts enlarging the kidneys. There are two fat-density AMLs in the left kidney.

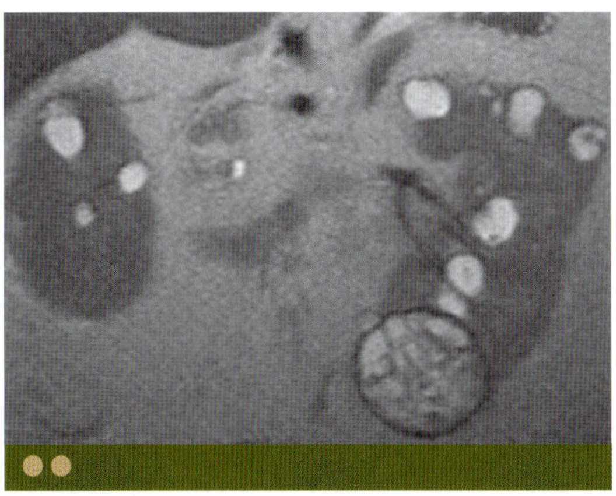

G. VHL: Coronal T2-WI shows several bilateral renal cysts without renal enlargement. Left lower pole complex cystic lesion proved to be a clear cell RCC.

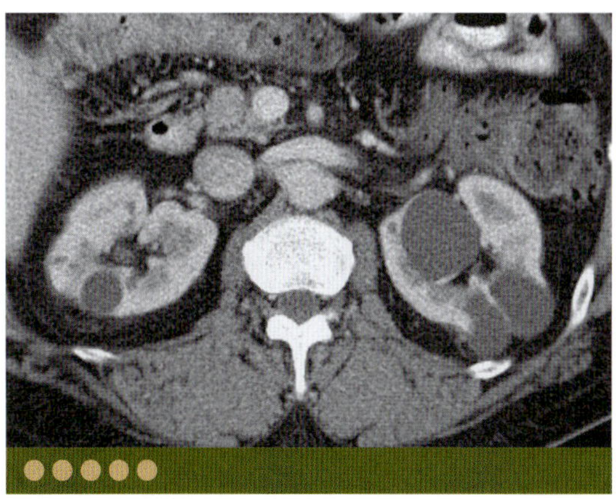

H. Multiple simple cysts: Axial CECT shows multiple bilateral simple renal cysts in normal sized kidneys. The patient had normal renal function and no family history of renal cystic disease.

IMAGE KEY

Common

Rare

Typical

Unusual

2–7 Cystic Kidney in von Hipple-Lindau Syndrome

David D. Casalino

PRESENTATION

Hematuria and recently diagnosed retinal hemangioblastoma.

FINDINGS

MR image show bilateral renal cysts, of which a few are complex. A complex left adrenal gland mass is also demonstrated.

DIFFERENTIAL DIAGNOSES

- *Multiple simple cysts*: Kidneys are usually normal in size and function.
- *Autosomal dominant polycystic kidney disease (ADPKD)*: Kidneys are enlarged by numerous cysts; family history of the disease; other organs with cysts.
- *Tuberous sclerosis*: Associated with renal AMLs skin lesions, CNS lesions, and family history.
- *Medullary cystic kidney disease*: Cysts are small and present in the medulla; kidneys may be small; family history of the disease.
- *Acquired renal cystic disease*: Associated with chronic renal failure and dialysis, usually small kidneys.

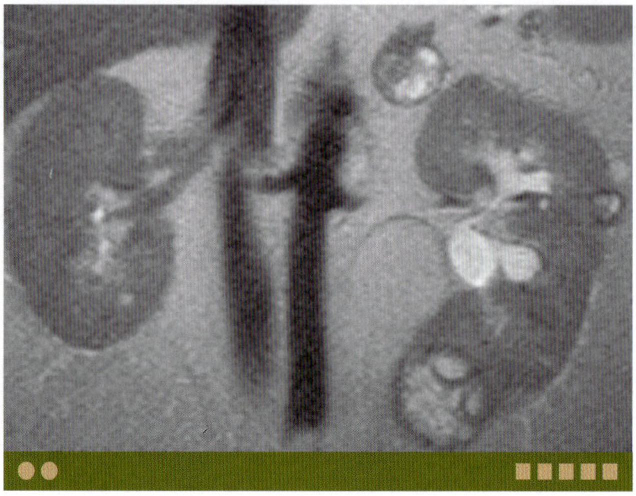

A. Coronal T2-WI shows a few left renal cysts, of which two show mural thickening and septations. These were proven to be cystic RCCs. Complex left adrenal gland mass proved to be a pheochromocytoma.

COMMENTS

von Hippel-Lindau (VHL) syndrome is an autosomal dominant, multisystem preneoplastic disorder linked to the mutation of a tumor-suppressor gene (VHL gene) located on chromosome 3p. The disorder is associated with moderate penetrance and widely variable phenotypic expression. Common manifestations include retinal and central nervous system hemangioblastomas, renal cysts and renal cell carcinomas, pancreatic cysts and pancreatic tumors (serous cystadenomas, carcinomas, and islet cell tumors), and adrenal pheochomocytomas. Patients with VHL most often die from complications of cerebellar hemangioblastoma or metastatic RCCs.

Patients with VHL often present in the third or fourth decade of life with CNS or visual symptoms, though renal cysts may be detected in the late teen years of these patients. Renal cysts occur in two thirds of VHL patients. Simple appearing cysts in these patients are often dysplastic and develop into carcinomas. RCCs, clear cell type, develop in approximately 40% of these patients, may be cystic or solid, and are usually multiple and bilateral. Pheochromocytomas occur in 15% to 20% of VHL patients, are often multiple, bilateral and symptomatic, and are associated with islet cell tumors of the pancreas 20% of the time. Islet cell tumors are rare in VHL patients without pheochromocytoma.

Imaging is used to screen at-risk family members usually in their late teens. CT and MR are superior to ultrasound in diagnosing RCCs as well as extrarenal manifestations of VHL. A solid or cystic renal mass suspected to be RCC may be followed until it is 2.5 to 3.0 cm, the time at which nephron-sparing resection or ablation should be performed. Renal involvement in VHL may result in bilateral renal enlargement by cysts as well as mixed solid and cystic and completely solid tumors.

PEARLS

- **Simple appearing cysts are often dysplastic and may develop into carcinomas.**
- **Routine imaging surveillance is warranted.**
- **Once a solid or complex cystic lesion measures 2.5 to 3 cm, localized resection or ablation should be performed.**

ADDITIONAL IMAGES (B-E)

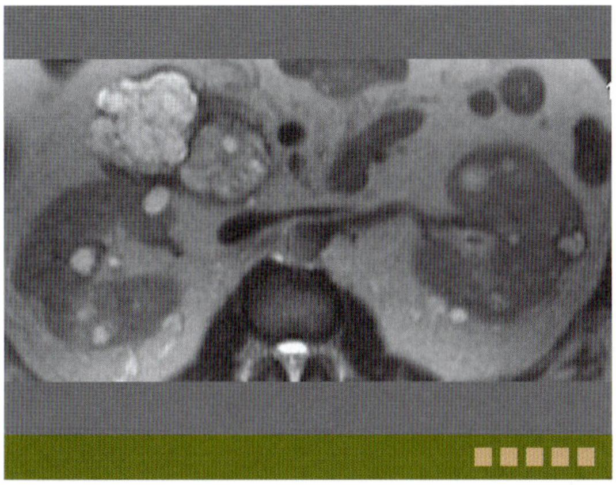

B. Axial T2-WI from same patient shows bilateral renal cysts and two adjacent complex cystic lesions in the pancreatic head. These pancreatic lesions were confirmed to be serous cystadenomas.

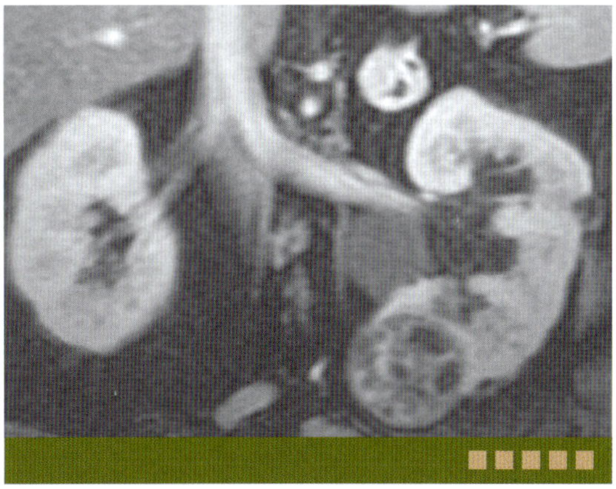

C. Coronal, contrast-enhanced T1-WI shows enhancement within the left lower pole cystic renal cell carcinoma and within the left adrenal gland pheochromocytoma.

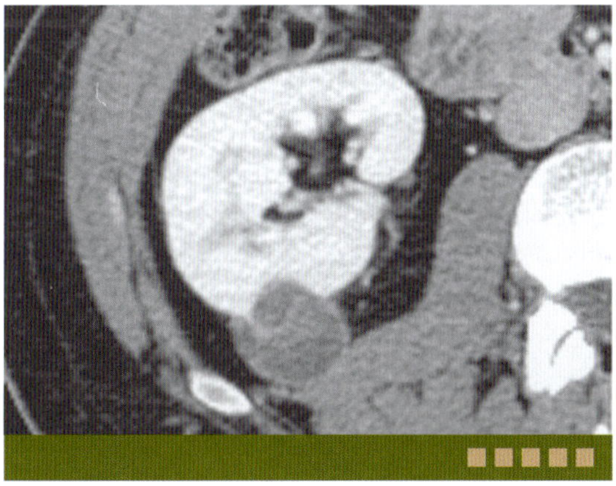

D. Axial CECT shows a right renal cyst with several septations that have measurable enhancement. This cyst showed steady growth and increasing complexity over a few years.

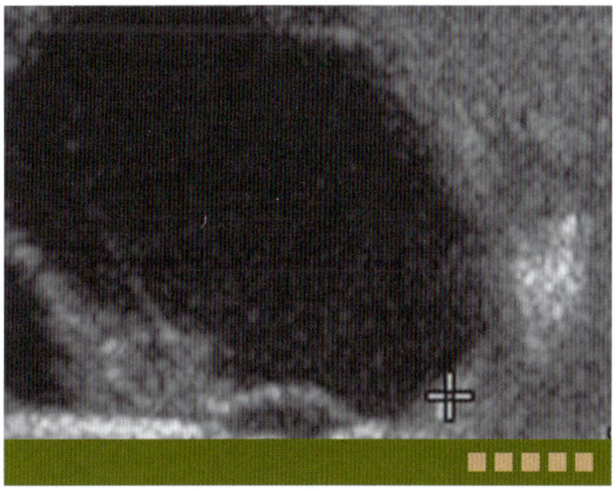

E. Transverse sonogram performed intraoperatively shows a thick irregular septation within the same cyst shown in the previous figure.

DIFFERENTIAL DIAGNOSES IMAGES (F-G)

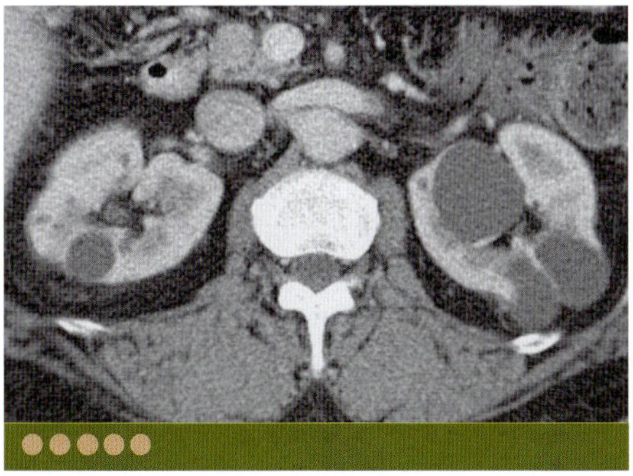

F. Multiple simple cysts: Axial CECT shows multiple, bilateral simple cysts in normal sized kidneys. The patient had normal renal function and no family history of renal cystic disease.

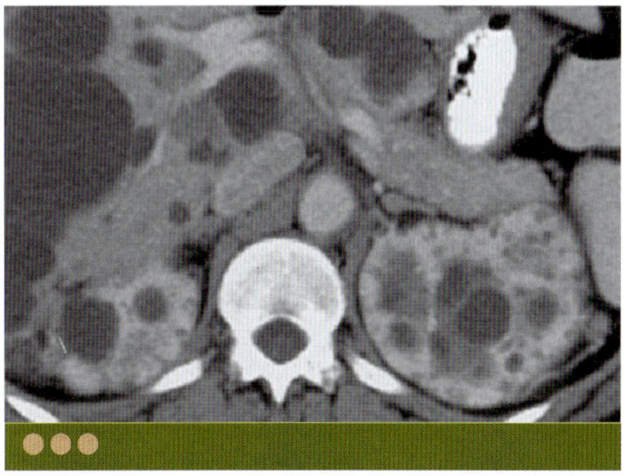

G. ADPKD: Axial CECT shows multiple simple cysts in mildly enlarged kidneys. Multiple simple cysts are also seen in the pancreas and liver. The patient had a family history of ADPKD.

IMAGE KEY

Common

Rare

Typical

Unusual

2–8 Tuberous Sclerosis

David D. Casalino

PRESENTATION

Hematuria and history of lung disease.

FINDINGS

CT shows enlarged kidneys with multiple cysts and a few fat-density lesions; the largest fatty lesion is in the right kidney.

DIFFERENTIAL DIAGNOSES

- *Multiple simple cysts*: Kidneys are usually normal in size and function.
- *Autosomal dominant polycystic kidney disease* (ADPKD)*:* Kidneys are enlarged by numerous cysts; family history of the disease; other organs with cysts.
- *von Hippel-Lindau*: Associated with multifocal RCC, pheochromocytomas, pancreatic lesions, CNS hemangioblastomas, and family history.
- *Medullary cystic kidney disease*: Cysts are small and are present in the medulla; kidneys may be small; family history of the disease.
- *Acquired renal cystic disease*: Associated with chronic renal failure and dialysis, usually small kidneys.

COMMENTS

Tuberous sclerosis (TS), or tuberous sclerosis complex (TSC), is an autosomal-dominantly inherited neurocutaneous disorder that is linked to TSC1- and TSC2-suppressor genes mapped on chromosome 9q and chromosome 16p, respectively. New mutations account for up to 80% of TS cases.

TS is classically characterized by mental retardation, epilepsy, and facial angiofibromas. TS is currently diagnosed on the basis of major and minor features. Major features include certain cutaneous lesions, retinal hamartomas and astrocytomas, cortical tubers, subependymal nodules and giant cell astrocytomas, renal and lymph node angiomyolipomas (AML), cardiac rhabdomyomas, and lymphangiomyomatosis. Minor features include renal cysts and renal carcinomas.

Cysts are found in approximately 50% of the patients with TS. Cysts may be few or numerous, bilateral or unilateral. AMLs are found in up to 80% of the TS patients and are usually bilateral and multiple. CT can detect fat in 95% of AML. Because of the risk of hemorrhage, embolization or resection might be performed on larger (>3-4 cm) AML. RCC, most often clear cell type, occurs in 1% to 2% of the patients with TS. As a result of renal involvement, patients may present with abdominal or flank pain, hematuria, and uremia. 10% to 15% of patients will develop end stage renal disease. AML hemorrhage may mask the fat in the lesion and prevent diagnosis.

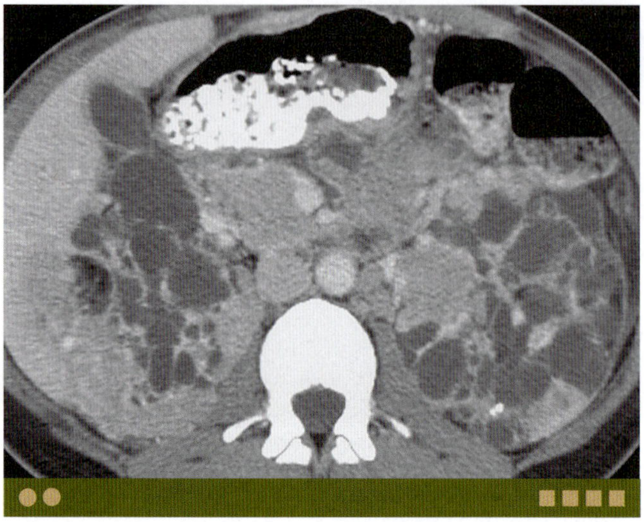

A. Axial CECT shows both kidneys being enlarged by numerous cysts. There are a few fat-density lesions, characteristic of AMLs with the largest one in the right kidney.

Renal imaging characteristics are determined by the number and sizes of renal cysts and AMLs. Both lesions are found in 25% of patients with TS. Usually the kidneys are enlarged. On ultrasound, an AML is usually a hyperechoic mass, which cannot be reliably differentiated from a hyperechoic RCC. On CT or MR, the presence of fat in a mass confirms the diagnosis of AML. A renal mass containing fat and calcification, however, is most likely an RCC. A fat-deficient AML cannot be differentiated from other solid renal masses, including RCC. Angiographic findings of AML include tortuous large vessels, not infrequently with aneurysmal dilatation.

PEARLS

- **In TS patients, the incidences of cysts, AMLs, or both are 50%, 80%, and 25%, respectively.**
- **A renal mass containing fat and calcification is most likely an RCC.**
- **Patients with TS have an increased risk for developing RCC.**

ADDITIONAL IMAGES (B-D)

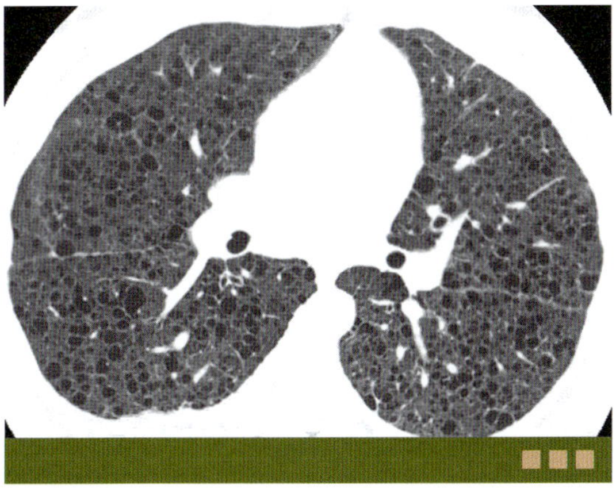

B. Axial NECT in the same patient shows numerous well-defined pulmonary cystic airspaces throughout both lungs, characteristic of lymphangiomyomatosis.

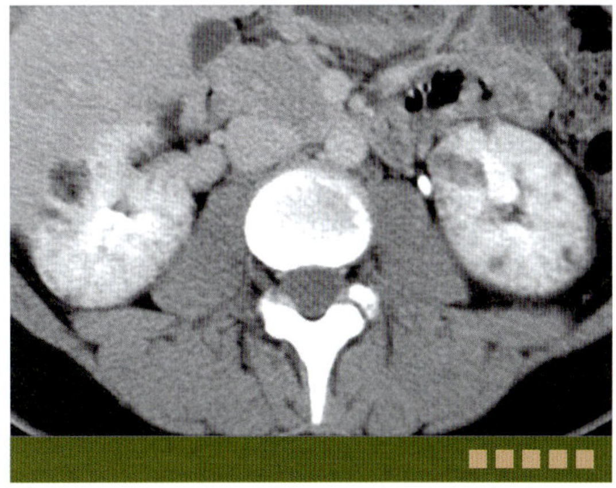

C. Axial CECT in a different patient with TS shows multiple, bilateral AMLs. No renal cysts are seen.

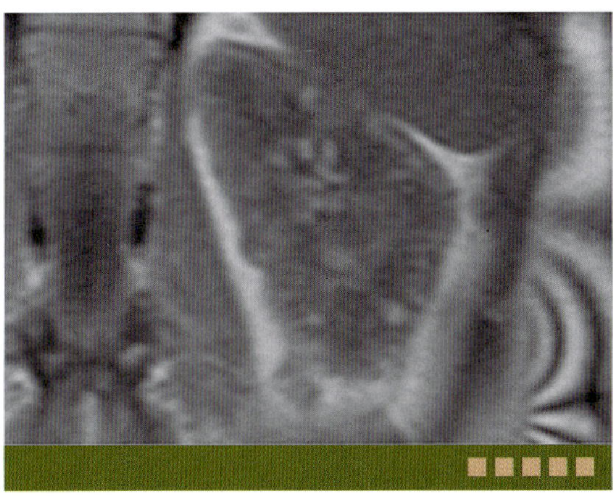

D. Coronal T1-WI, without fat suppression, shows multiple tiny hyperintense cortical lesions that suppress to low-signal intensity on the fat-suppressed TI-WI (not shown), characteristic of AMLs.

DIFFERENTIAL DIAGNOSES IMAGES (E-F)

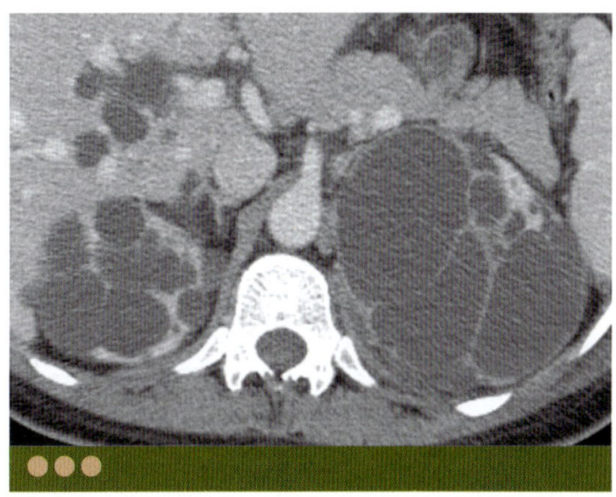

E. ADPKD: Axial CECT shows both kidneys to be enlarged by numerous cysts. There are also multiple hepatic cysts.

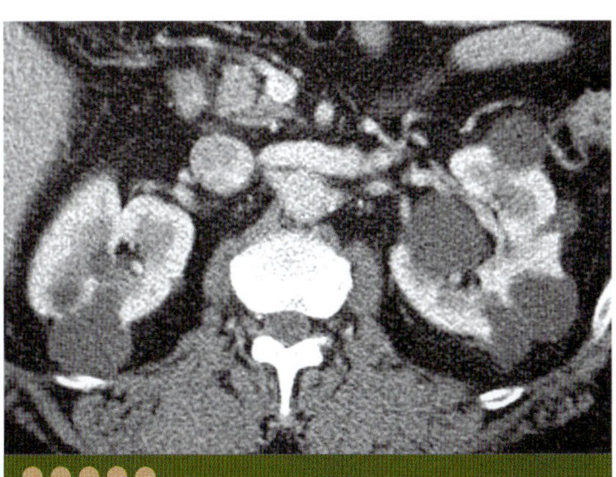

F. Multiple simple cysts: Axial CECT shows multiple, bilateral simple cysts in normal sized kidneys.

IMAGE KEY

Common

Rare

Typical

Unusual

2–9 Multicystic Dysplastic Kidney

David D. Casalino

PRESENTATION

Asymptomatic.

FINDINGS

CT image shows an atrophic left kidney with multiple, peripherally calcified cysts; the right kidney appears normal.

DIFFERENTIAL DIAGNOSES

- *Acquired, complex renal cysts*: Rare in individuals younger than 30 years of age; may be found in otherwise normal or atrophic kidneys; warrant Bosniak classification and appropriate management; unusual for multiple cysts to show peripheral calcification.
- *Unilateral renal cystic disease*: May be diffuse; normal parenchyma is seen between the cysts; renal function is preserved.

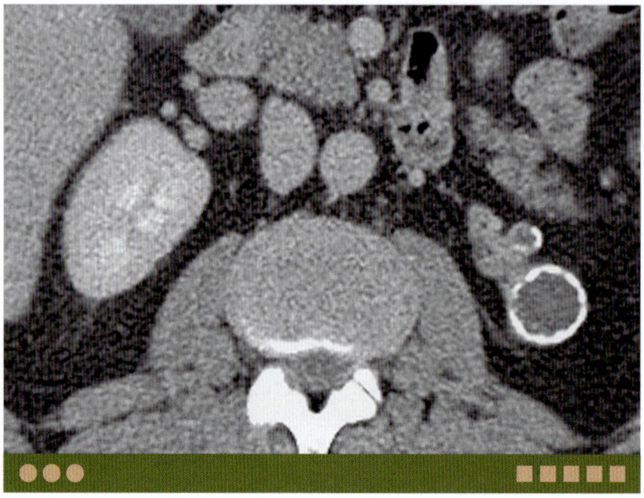

A. Axial CECT shows an atrophic left kidney with multiple, peripherally calcified cysts. Neither internal septations nor enhancing solid components are seen within the cysts. The right kidney appears normal.

COMMENTS

Multicystic dysplastic kidney (MDK) refers to a nonheritable condition of abnormal metanephric differentiation often found in the setting of obstructive uropathy and characterized by the presence of cartilage, undifferentiated mesenchyma, and immature collecting ductules. The dysplastic kidney may vary from extremely hypoplastic to enlarged by multiple cysts with absence of functional parenchyma and resembling a bunch of grapes.

The bilateral form is usually fatal and often associated with other malformations of the urogenital tract and other organ systems. A unilateral form may go undetected for a variable period with 10% found incidentally in adults. Contralateral anomalies, such as ureteropelvic junction obstruction and vesicoureteral reflux, are seen in 40% of patients. MDK is not associated with an increased risk of malignancy.

Most cases of MDK are diagnosed on prenatal ultrasonography or during infancy when a flank mass is palpated. Prenatal diagnosis can be made as early as 20 weeks gestation with ultrasonography showing a large noncalcified mass consisting of multiple, small cysts, little or no parenchyma, and atretic collecting system, ureter, and renal vasculature. Some divide MDK into two forms: pelvoinfundibular type and hydronephrotic type.

In the pelvoinfundibular type, the multiple cysts are variable in size, randomly distributed, and lacking communication. The hydronephrotic type, thought to develop later in gestation, is associated with multiple cysts, which are seen in expected locations of calyces and may intercommunicate, and a dominant cyst in the expected location of the renal pelvis. Over time, the mass may decrease in size as the cysts involute.

In older children and adults, the MDK is usually a nonfunctional, small nonreniform mass with curvilinear calcifications at the periphery of small cysts. The segmental form of MDK is typically confined to the upper moiety of a duplicated collecting system. The upper ureter is ectopic, partially obstructed, and/or injured by vesicoureteric reflux. Reflux nephropathy may also affect the lower moiety.

PEARLS

- **Ten percent of cases are incidentally discovered in adults.**
- **Diagnosis of contralateral abnormalities is crucial.**
- **There is no known increased risk of malignancy.**
- **MDK in adults is typically nonfunctional, small, nonreniform, and contains small cysts with peripheral calcifications.**

ADDITIONAL IMAGES (B-D)

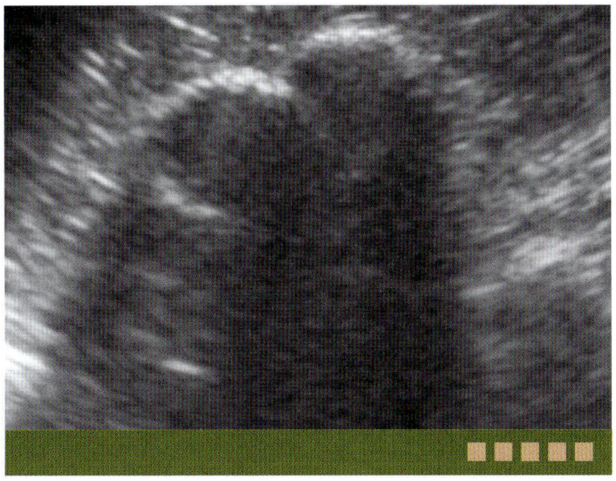

B. Longitudinal sonogram of the left renal fossa shows a small, calcified, and smoothly lobulated mass. The internal features cannot be assessed because of posterior shadowing.

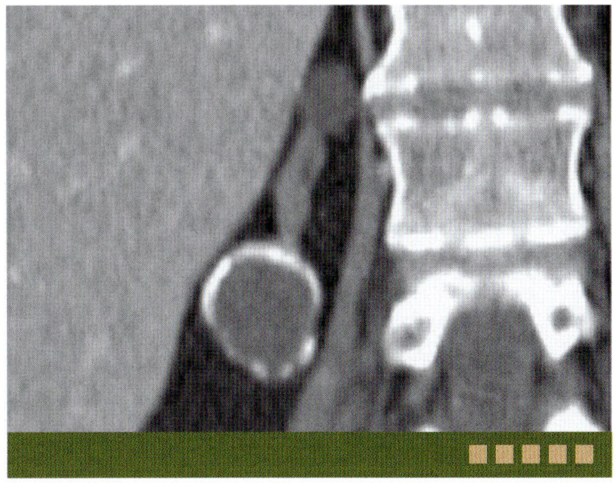

C. Coronal CECT from a different patient shows a non-functional, atrophic right kidney with a tiny superior cyst and larger inferior cyst with peripheral calcification.

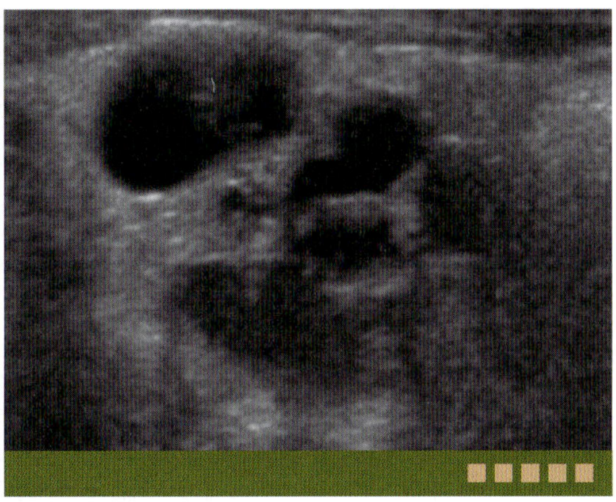

D. Longitudinal sonogram from a newborn shows the right kidney to be enlarged by multiple, noncommunicating, variable-sized cysts. The left kidney (not shown) was normal.

DIFFERENTIAL DIAGNOSES IMAGES (E-G)

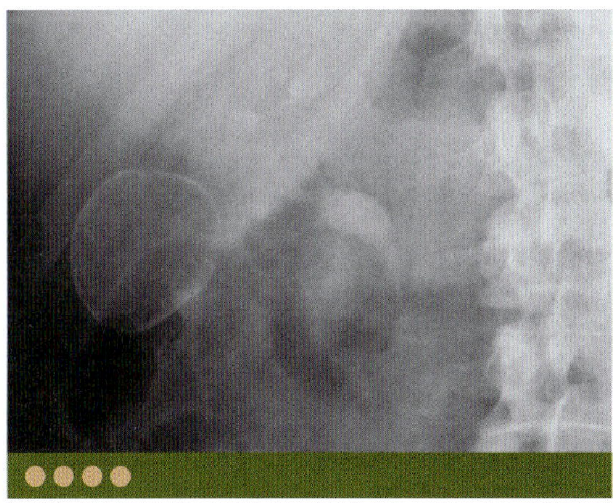

E. Cystic RCC: IVU shows a peripherally calcified mass arising from the lateral cortex of the right kidney.

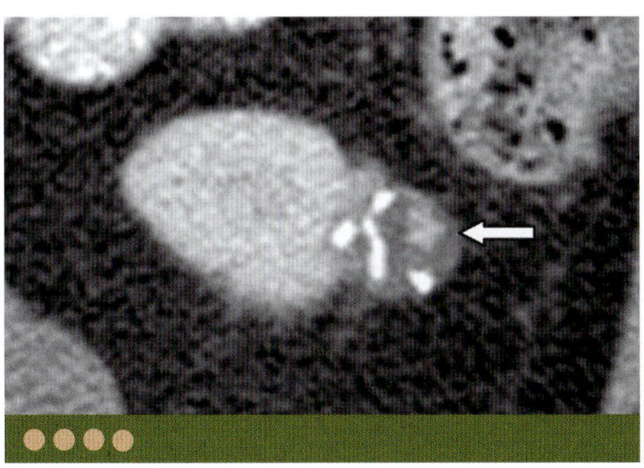

F. Cystic RCC: Axial CECT shows a peripherally calcified left renal cystic mass with a central enhancing nodule (arrow).

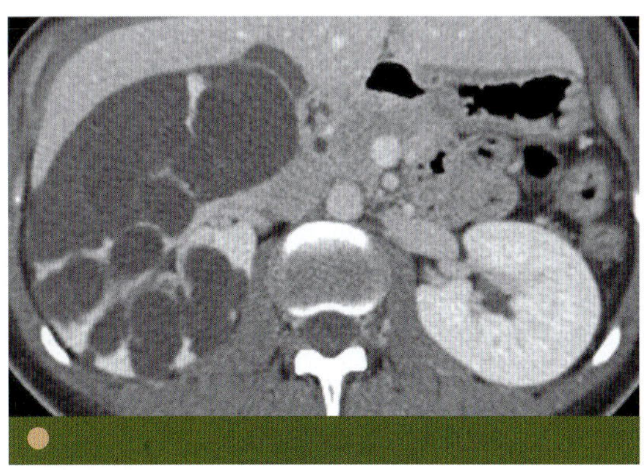

G. Unilateral renal cystic disease: Axial CECT shows enlargement of the right kidney by numerous cysts. Normal parenchyma is seen between the cysts. The left kidney is uninvolved. Both kidneys showed contrast excretion (not shown).

IMAGE KEY

Common

●●●●●
●●●●
●●●
●●
●

Rare

Typical

■■■■■
■■■■
■■■
■■
■

Unusual

2–10 Multilocular Cystic Nephroma

David D. Casalino

PRESENTATION

Right flank palpable mass and hematuria.

FINDINGS

MR images, T2-WI and T1-WI postcontrast, show a large multiloculated cystic renal mass with enhancing septations.

DIFFERENTIAL DIAGNOSES

- *Multilocular cystic renal cell carcinoma*: More common in men; may be associated with solid enhancing components, intravascular extension, metastases, and hemorrhage.
- *Renal abscess*: Thick-walled with rim enhancement; sites of pyelonephritis; perinephric signs of infection; clinical symptoms of infection.
- *Segmental multicystic dysplastic kidney*: Uncommon; usually seen in the setting of renal duplication with minimal, if any, functional parenchyma in the involved region.
- *Cystic oncocytoma*: Rare for oncocytoma to be cystic.
- *Unilateral renal cystic disease*: Rare, cluster of cysts, not encapsulated.

COMMENTS

Multilocular cystic nephroma (MLCN) is an uncommon, nonheritable cystic neoplasm. These benign tumors arise from primitive metanephric blastema and have two peaks of occurrence, with boys less than 3 years old, comprising one half of the cases and middle-aged (fifth and sixth decades) adults, usually women, comprising the other half. These tumors are often asymptomatic but may present with pain, palpable mass, hematuria, or UTI.

On CT and MR imaging, multiple (more than three or four), thin enhancing septa separating epithelium-lined cysts that are noncommunicating, fibrous stroma, and a well-developed capsule characterize MLCN. The septa may be calcified. Tumor herniation into the renal pelvis is a finding suggestive of MLCN and may create a renal pelvic filling defect and caliectasis. These tumors are usually in the Bosniak Category III. Occasionally, protein and blood products may alter density and intensity of the cystic components on CT and MR, respectively. On ultrasound, MLCN appears as a discrete mass consisting of numerous anechoic areas separated by echogenic septations.

In most cases, MLCN cannot be differentiated from a multilocular cystic RCC and, as a result, is generally a surgical lesion.

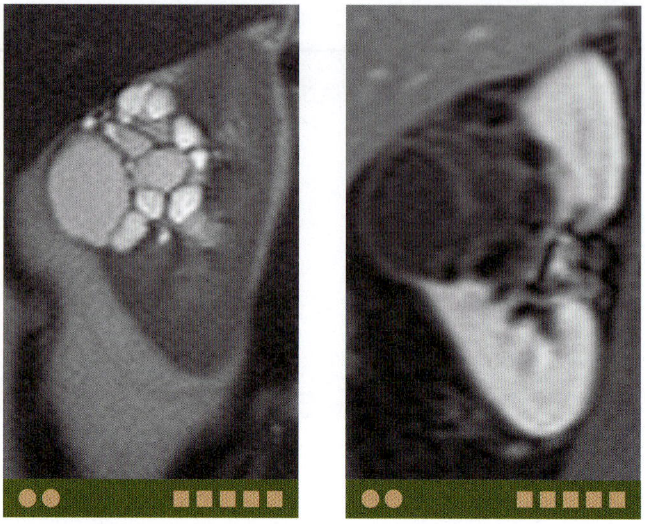

A. and B. Coronal T2-WI shows a well-defined multiloculated cystic mass arising from the right kidney. The internal septations are low in signal intensity.
Coronal contrast-enhanced, fat-suppressed T1-WI shows mild enhancement of the fibrous septations.

PEARLS

- **In adults, MLCN is much more common in women.**
- **A multiloculated cystic mass herniating into the renal hilum is suggestive of MLCN.**
- **MLCN is generally a surgical lesion because it cannot be reliably differentiated from a multilocular cystic RCC.**

ADDITIONAL IMAGES (C-E)

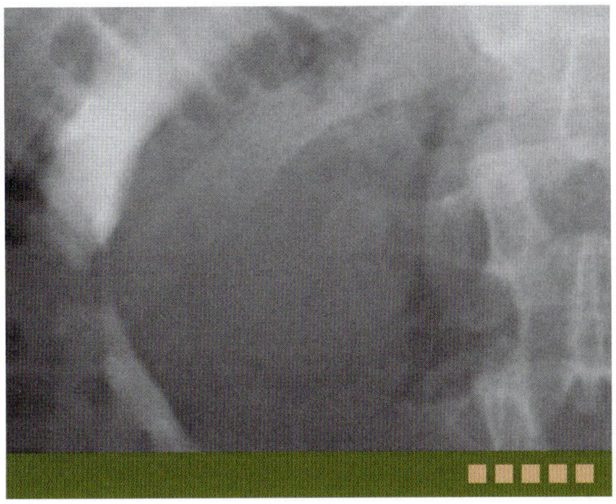

C. IVU from a different patient shows the right renal collecting system to be laterally displaced in a manner suggestive of a large central mass.

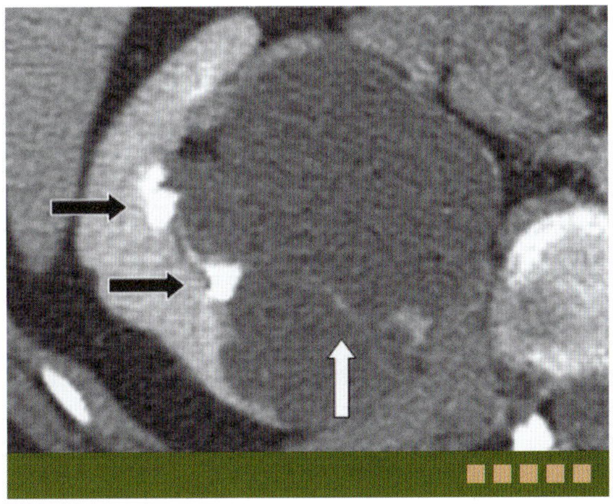

D. Axial CECT in the same patient shows cystic mass with enhancing septations (white arrow), protruding into the renal sinus and distorting the collecting system (black arrows).

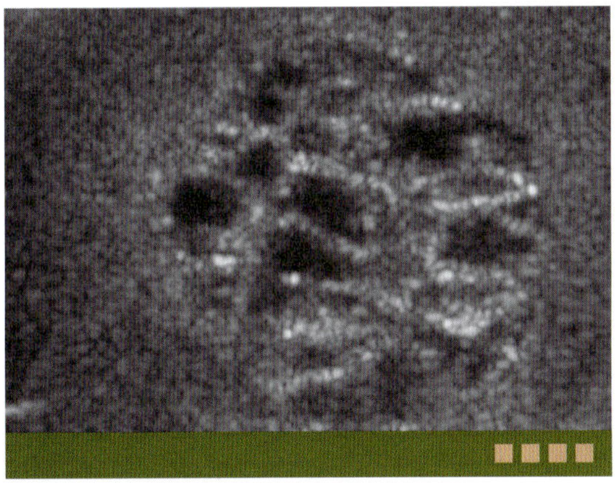

E. Transverse sonogram from a different patient shows a renal mass, containing innumerable cysts separated by echogenic septations.

DIFFERENTIAL DIAGNOSES IMAGES (F-H)

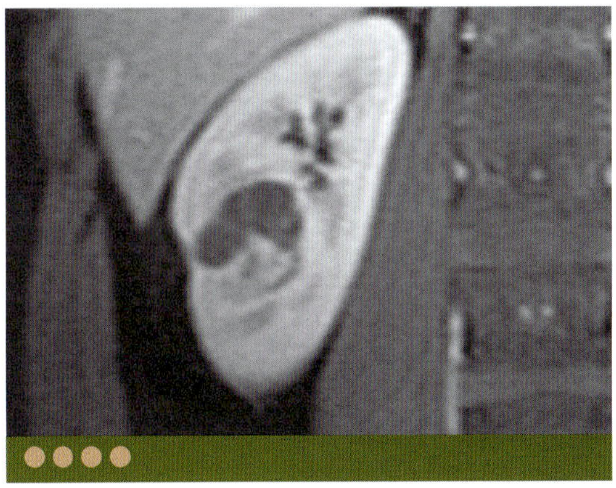

F. Cystic RCC: Coronal contrast-enhanced, fat-suppressed T1-WI shows a multilocular cystic renal mass with an enhancing mural nodule and septations.

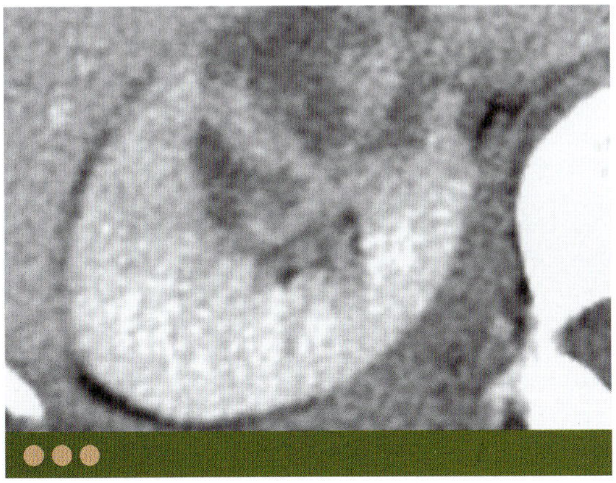

G. Abscess: Axial CECT shows a multilocular cystic lesion with thick septations and outer rim of enhancement that is slightly less dense than normal cortex.

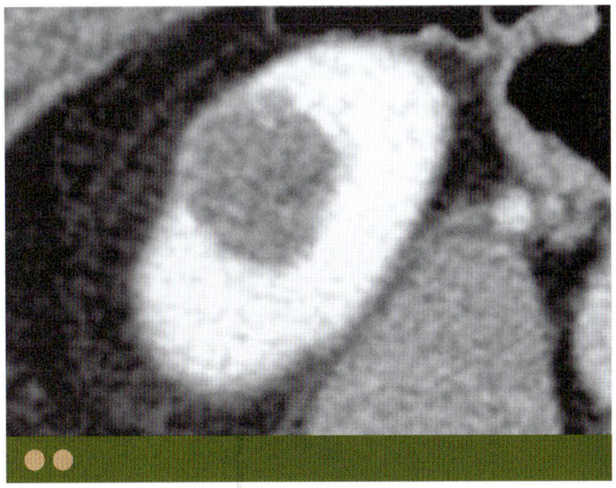

H. Cystic oncocytoma: Axial CECT shows a multilocular cystic renal mass with numerous thin, enhancing septations.

IMAGE KEY

Common

Rare

Typical

Unusual

2–11 Acquired Renal Cystic Disease

David D. Casalino

PRESENTATION

Asymptomatic with end-stage renal disease (ESRD).

FINDINGS

CT shows multiple cysts in atrophic kidneys.

DIFFERENTIAL DIAGNOSES

- *Multiple simple cysts*: Kidneys are usually normal in size and function.
- *Autosomal dominant polycystic kidney disease* (ADPKD): Kidneys are enlarged by numerous cysts; family history of the disease; other organs with cysts.
- *von Hippel-Lindau*: Associated with multifocal RCC, pheochromocytomas, pancreatic lesions, CNS hemangioblastomas, and family history.
- *Tuberous sclerosis*: Associated with renal AMLs, skin lesions, CNS lesions, and family history.
- *Medullary cystic kidney disease*: Cysts are small and in the medulla; kidneys may be small; family history of the disease.

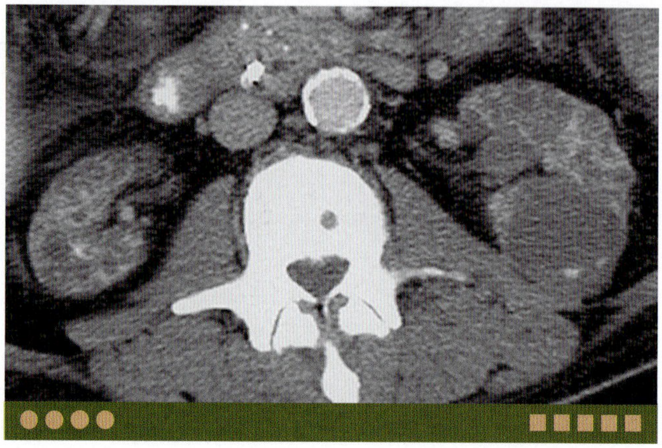

A. Axial CECT shows both kidneys to be small and poorly enhancing with multiple cysts. Several of the cysts are complicated by calcifications.

COMMENTS

Multiple cysts are common in patients on long-term dialysis. The number of cysts increases with duration of peritoneal dialysis or hemodialysis. Up to 90% of patients will acquire renal cysts after 5 to 10 years of dialysis. Cyst formation may be because of an accumulation of growth factors in these patients. Cysts often regress after renal transplantation. Milder manifestations of acquired renal cystic disease may develop in patients with renal function impairment who are not yet on dialysis.

In acquired renal cystic disease, both kidneys are usually small with multiple small cysts. Occasionally, the kidneys enlarge. The cysts usually measure a few millimeters up to 3 cm in diameter and may be complicated by hemorrhage or calcifications. Hemorrhage may be severe and life-threatening.

On ultrasound, these kidneys are often increased in echogenicity and small with multiple anechoic cysts. Whether demonstrated on ultrasound, CT, or MRI, any solid renal mass should be suspected to be RCC because these patients are at a significantly increased risk of developing RCCs (30 times greater risk than the general population). These patients also have an increased incidence of renal adenomas and oncocytomas, lesions that cannot be reliably differentiated from carcinoma by imaging. Hemorrhagic cysts are seen in up to 50% of these patients. On CT, hemorrhagic cysts typically have attenuation values between 40 and 100 HU and do not enhance. Hemorrhagic cysts on MRI are often hyperintense on T1- and T2-weighted sequences and do not enhance.

PEARLS

- **A history of ESRD and dialysis is characteristic.**
- **Both kidneys are involved and are usually small.**
- **The cysts are often complicated by hemorrhage or calcifications.**
- **There is a significantly increased risk of developing RCC.**

ADDITIONAL IMAGES (B-D)

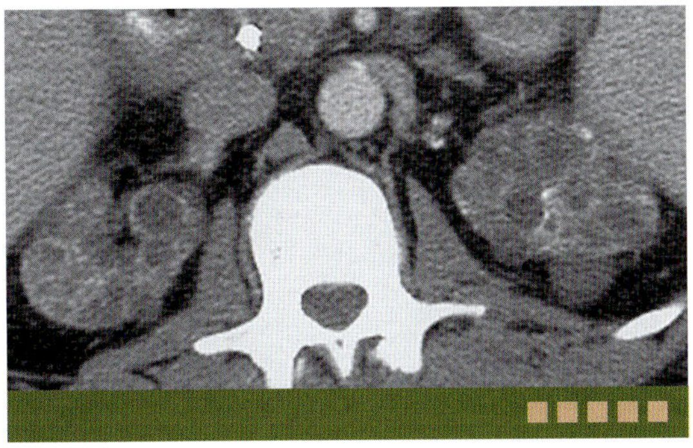

B. Axial CECT in the same patient shows additional small cysts throughout the small kidneys.

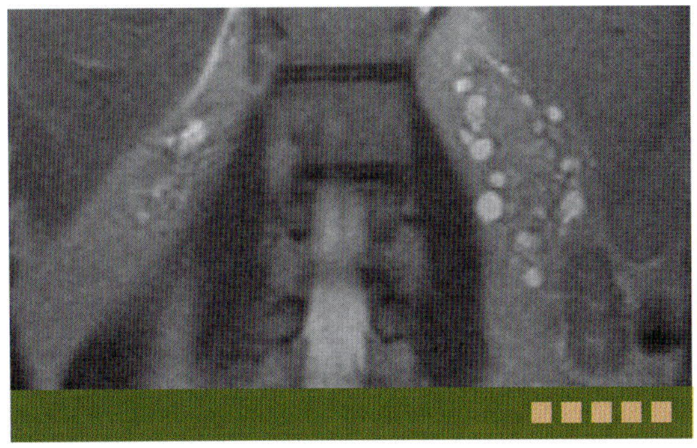

C. Coronal T2-WI shows small kidneys with multiple small hyperintense cysts.

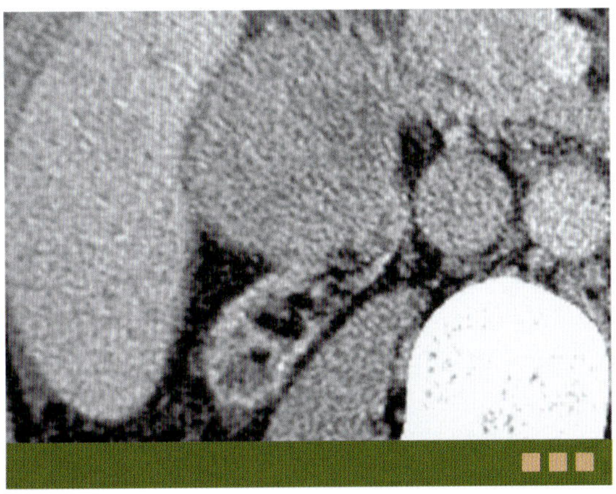

D. Axial CECT shows a large solid mass arising from a small right kidney in a patient on chronic hemodialysis. This mass proved to be a RCC.

DIFFERENTIAL DIAGNOSES IMAGES (E-G)

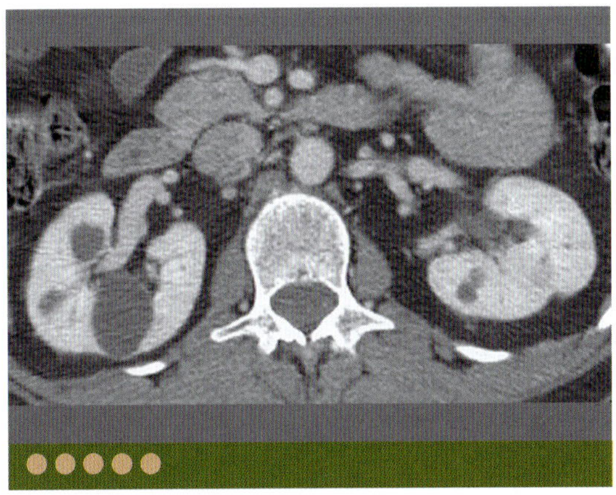

E. Multiple simple cysts: Axial CECT shows multiple, bilateral simple cysts in normal sized kidneys. The patient had normal renal function and no family history of renal cystic disease.

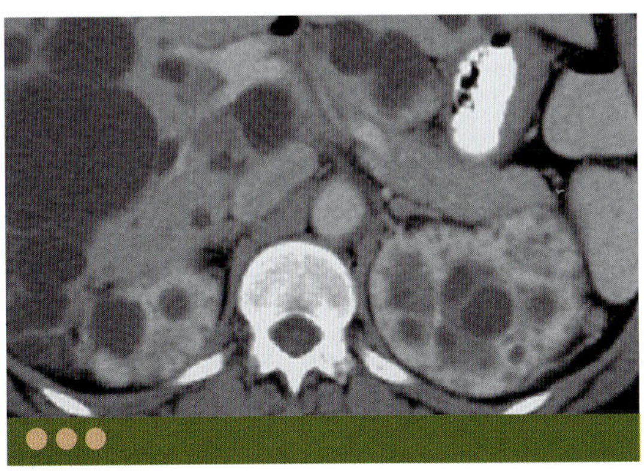

F. ADPKD: Axial CECT shows numerous cysts in mildly enlarged kidneys. Multiple cysts are also seen in the pancreas and liver. The patient had a family history of ADPKD.

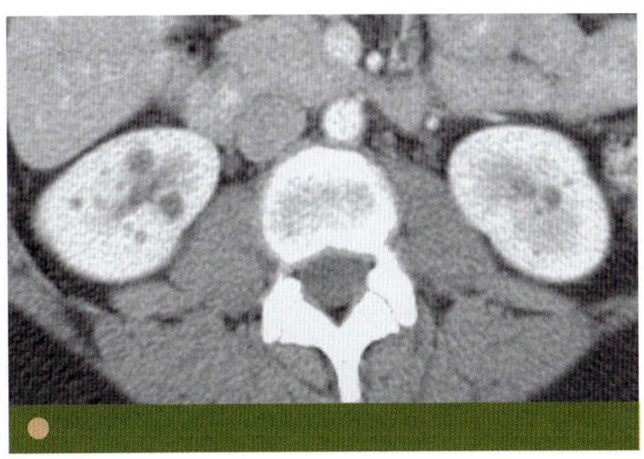

G. Medullary cystic kidney disease: Axial CECT shows a few cysts in normal sized kidneys. The cysts are all located in the medulla.

IMAGE KEY

Common

Rare

Typical

Unusual

2–12 Unilateral Renal Cystic Disease

David D. Casalino

PRESENTATION

Abdominal pain and hematuria.

FINDINGS

CT shows a cluster of simple-appearing cysts arising from the cortex of the left kidney.

DIFFERENTIAL DIAGNOSES

- *Multilocular cystic nephroma*: Encapsulated, multiloculated cystic mass; may herniated into renal sinus.
- *Multiloculated renal cell carcinoma*: Encapsulated, multiloculated cystic mass; may be associated with solid enhancing components, intravascular extension, and hemorrhage.
- *Renal abscess*: May be multiloculated with rim enhancement; sites of pyelonephritis; perinephric signs of infection; clinical symptoms of infection.

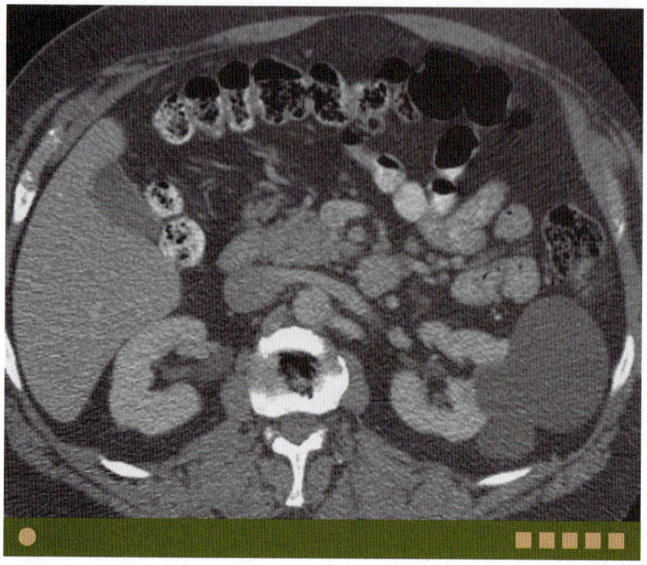

A. Axial CECT shows a cluster of three different size cysts in the lateral cortex of the left kidney. No right renal cysts were identified.

COMMENT

Unilateral renal cystic disease (URCD), or localized renal cystic disease, is a rare, nonfamilial, nonprogressive renal disorder. Patients with URCD typically have multiple variously sized cysts clustered or diffusely distributed in one kidney with the other kidney having no or, rarely, a few simple cysts. Renal function is preserved in the involved kidney. URCD is not associated with cysts or malformations in other organs.

Patients may present with flank or abdominal pain, a palpable mass, hematuria, or hypertension.

Normal parenchymal enhancement between cysts should not be confused with enhancing septations or solid nodules within a solitary mass. Absence of a capsule surrounding a cluster of cysts should aid in diagnosing URCD and differentiating it from multiloculated cystic nephroma, cystic RCC, and Wilms tumor. When diffusely distributed, the involved kidney may have a similar appearance as ADPKD. Discrete cysts are usually apparent on ultrasonography.

PEARLS

- **URCD is a nonprogressive renal disease.**
- **URCD involves multiple cysts clustered or, less commonly, diffusely distributed within one kidney.**
- **Absence of a capsule helps in differentiating it from a multiloculated neoplasm.**

ADDITIONAL IMAGES (B-D)

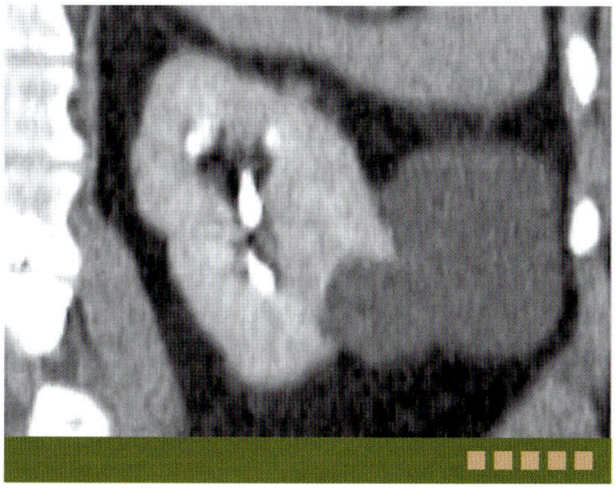

B. Coronal CECT shows a small projection of normal enhancing parenchyma extending between two of the cysts.

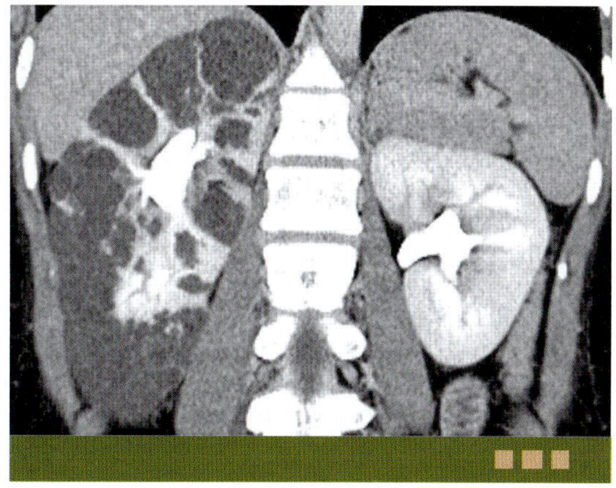

C. Coronal CECT shows diffuse involvement and enlargement of the right kidney by URCD. The left kidney is uninvolved. Both kidneys show contrast excretion.

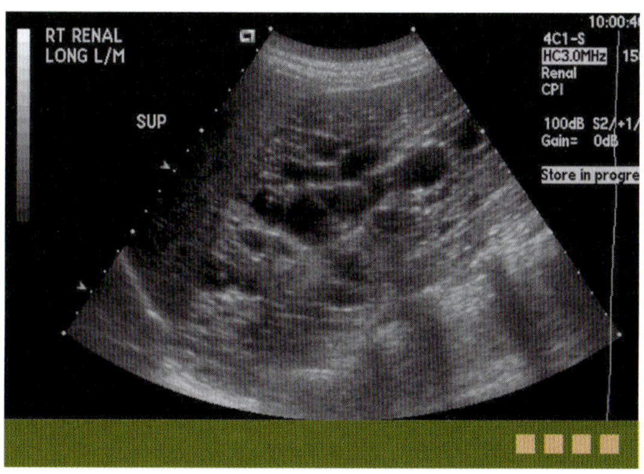

D. Longitudinal sonogram shows numerous cysts enlarging the right kidney of the patient shown in the prior figure.

DIFFERENTIAL DIAGNOSES IMAGES (E-G)

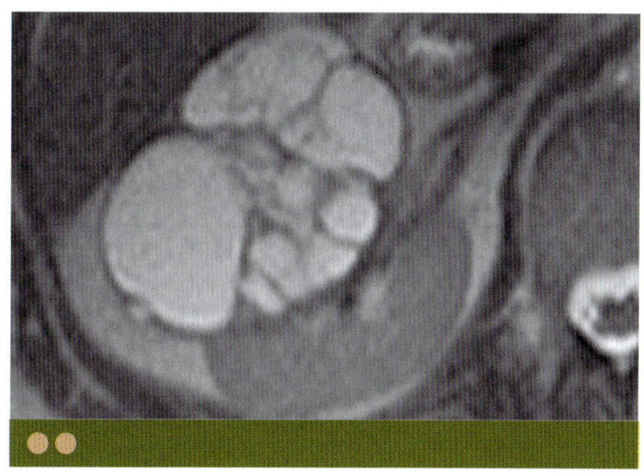

E. MLCN: Axial T2-WI shows a solitary, encapsulated, multiloculated cystic mass of the right kidney. Excision confirmed the diagnosis.

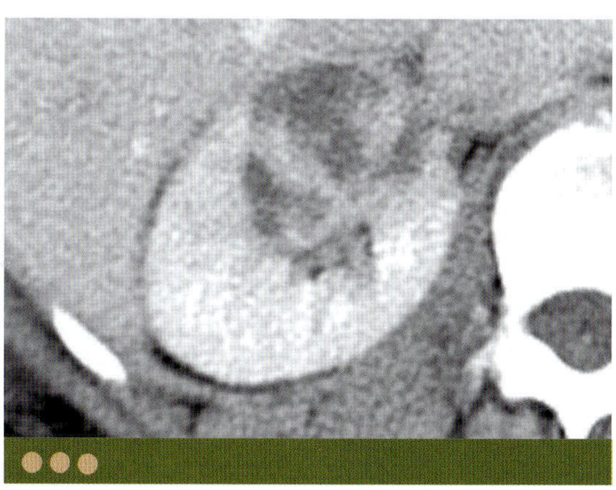

F. Renal abscess: Axial CECT shows a multiloculated cystic mass of the right kidney in a patient with recent history of pyelonephritis and persistent symptoms of infection.

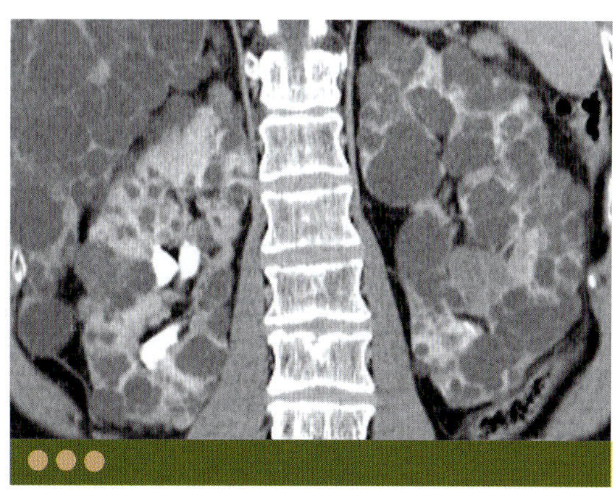

G. ADPKD: Coronal CECT shows bilateral renal enlargement by numerous cysts and numerous cysts within the liver. Excreted contrast is seen in the right collecting system.

IMAGE KEY

Common

Rare

Typical

Unusual

2–13 Medullary Cystic Kidney Disease

David D. Casalino

PRESENTATION

Polyuria and polydipsia.

FINDINGS

CT shows multiple, small medullary cysts in normal size kidneys.

DIFFERENTIAL DIAGNOSES

- *Early Autosomal dominant polycystic kidney disease (ADPKD)*: Cysts are cortical rather than medullary; family history of the disease; other organs with cysts.
- *Multiple simple cysts*: Kidneys are usually normal in size and function with cortical cysts.
- *Acquired renal cystic disease*: Associated with chronic renal failure and dialysis, usually small kidneys.
- *von Hippel-Lindau*: Associated with multifocal RCC, pheochromocytomas, pancreatic lesions, CNS hemangioblastomas, and family history.
- *Tuberous sclerosis*: Associated with renal AMLs, skin lesions, CNS lesions, and family history.

COMMENTS

Medullary cystic kidney disease (MCKD) and juvenile nephronophthisis (JNPHP) are diseases with common pathologic features, including the presence of small cysts at the corticomedullary junction and deeper in the medulla, tubulointerstitial damage, and usually progression to ESRD. The cysts arise from the distal convoluted and collecting tubules. Patients with MCKD and JNPHP usually present with polyuria, polydipsia, anemia, and renal function impairment.

Juvenile nephronophthisis, an autosomal-recessive condition linked to mutations in more than one gene, accounts for 70% of the cases of these two related diseases. It has been mapped to chromosomes 2q, 9q, 3q, and Ip36. Juvenile nephronophthisis is often associated with ophthalmologic and neurologic abnormalities, hepatic fibrosis and skeletal dysplasia. Juvenile nephronophthisis usually presents in the first decade of life.

Medullary cystic kidney disease, an autosomal-dominant condition, accounts for 15% of the cases of these diseases. Two forms of medullary cystic kidney disease are recognized, MCKD type 1 and MCKD type 2, and associated with mutations on chromosome 1q and chromosome 16p, respectively. Medullary cystic kidney disease usually presents in the third to fourth decade of life. MDKD type 2 is associated with a rapid progression to uremia, usually around 30 years of age.

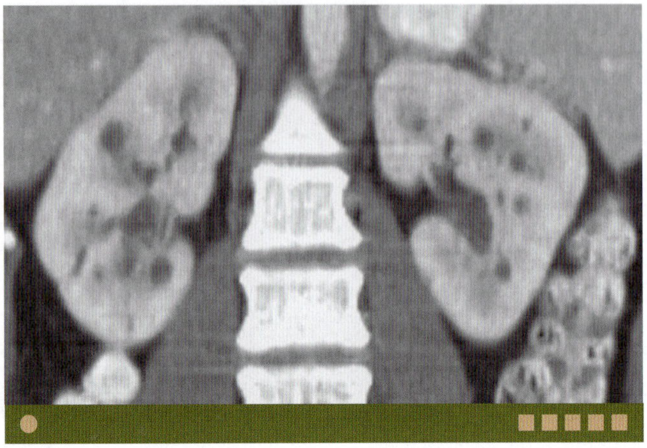

A. Coronal CECT shows multiple, small medullary cysts involving both kidneys, which are normal in size and enhance appropriately.

In approximately 15% of the cases of these two diseases, no family history is identified

The kidneys are of small-to-normal size and have a smooth outer contour. On ultrasound, the kidneys are usually small and hyperechoic, and they demonstrate cortical thinning with medullary cysts. CT and MR will demonstrate the small to normal size kidneys with medullary cysts. Contrast administration may be associated with a striated nephrogram and delayed excretion.

PEARLS

- **Medullary cystic kidney disease is an autosomal dominant condition that may progress to ESRD.**
- **No family history is identified in 15% of the cases.**
- **Characteristic imaging feature is medullary cysts that are bilateral, multiple, and small.**
- **The kidneys are typically small or normal in size.**

ADDITIONAL IMAGES (B-D)

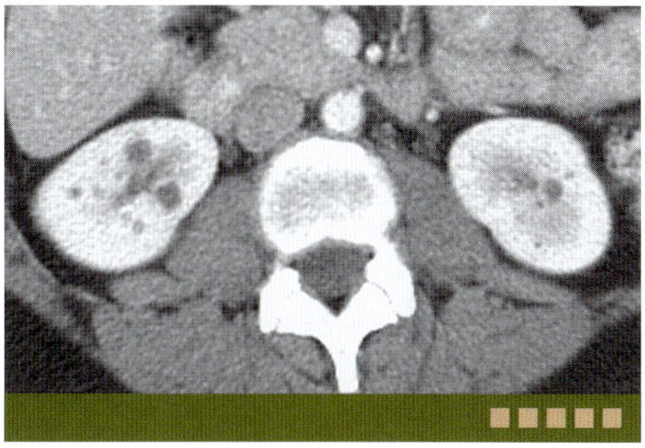

B. Axial CECT in the same patient shows small medullary cysts in both kidneys.

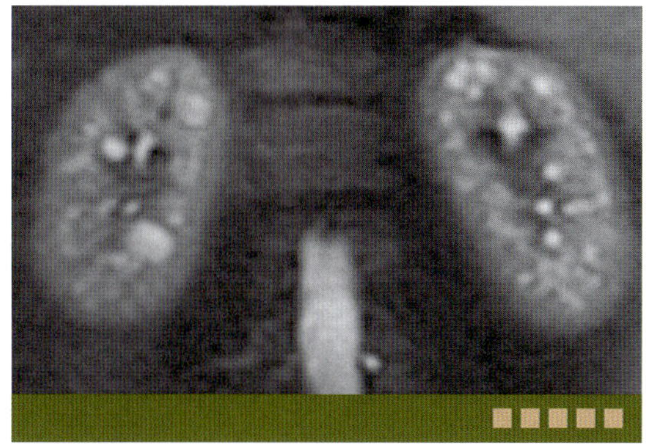

C. Coronal T2-WI in a different patient shows multiple, small round hyperintense lesions that are medullary and bilateral.

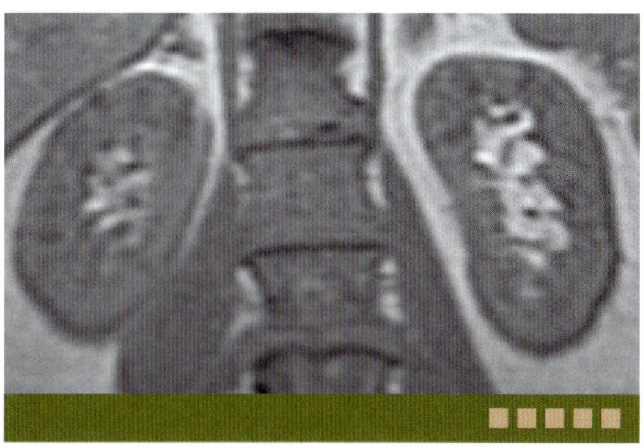

D. Coronal T1-WI, unenhanced, shows these small medullary lesions to be hypointense. They do not enhance (not shown), characteristic of cysts.

DIFFERENTIAL DIAGNOSES IMAGES (E-F)

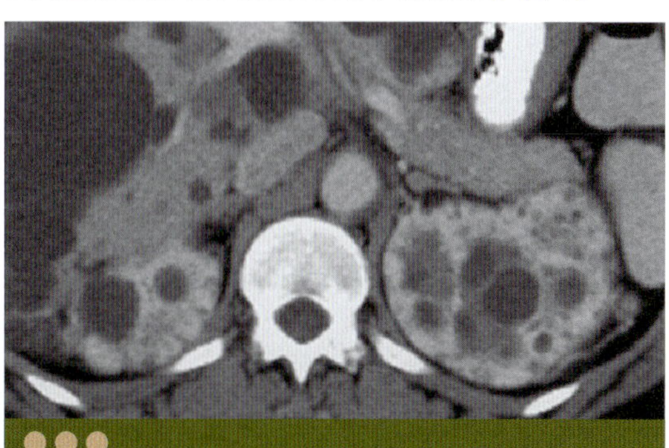

E. ADPKD: Axial CECT shows multiple cortical and medullary cysts in both kidneys, which are normal in size. There are also numerous hepatic cysts.

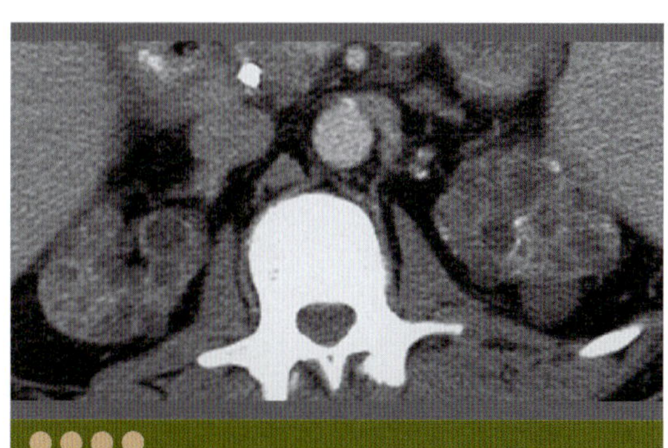

F. Acquired renal cystic disease: Axial CECT shows multiple cortical and medullary cysts in both kidneys, which are small and poorly enhanced. The patient had a history of hemodialysis for past 8 years.

IMAGE KEY

Common

Rare

Typical

Unusual

CHAPTER 3

RENAL INFECTION

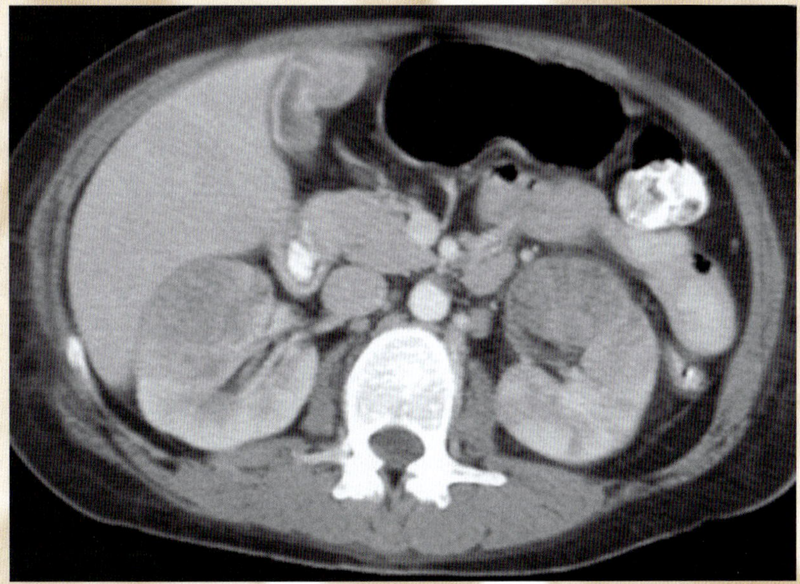

3–1 Acute Pyelonephritis

Frank H. Miller

PRESENTATION

Fevers, chills, and bilateral flank pain.

FINDINGS

Bilateral striated wedge-shaped areas of decreased attenuation involving the kidney on contrast-enhanced CT (CECT).

DIFFERENTIAL DIAGNOSES

- *Renal infarcts*: Different clinical presentation.
- *Acute tubular necrosis* (ATN): Can distinguish based on history. Generally not striated nephrogram following contrast. Often persistent nephrogram.
- *Vasculitis*: Different clinical presentation.

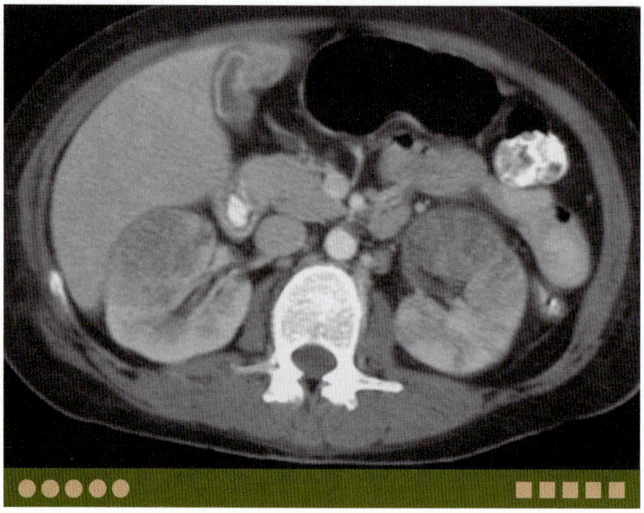

A. Axial CECT shows bilateral striated nephrogram and enlarged kidneys because of acute pyelonephritis.

COMMENTS

The diagnosis of acute pyelonephritis is generally made based on clinical findings and does not require imaging studies. Acute pyelonephritis is generally caused by reflux of infected organisms from the bladder or lymphatic spread from bladder infection. Pyelonephritis is most commonly caused by *Escherichia coli* with other causes including Proteus, Klebsiella, Enterobacter, and Pseudomonas. Imaging studies, especially CT, are helpful in patients with atypical presentations and to assess for causes and complications of acute pyelonephritis. At times, the diagnosis of acute pyelonephritis is not suspected by the referring physicians, and the radiologist is the first to suggest the diagnosis.

Ultrasound is helpful in patients with renal symptoms to assess for hydronephrosis. Acute pyelonephritis can show wedge-shaped areas of hypoechogenicity as well as abnormal color and power Doppler flow with hypoperfusion.

Unenhanced CT scans are helpful to assess renal or ureteral calculi which may be the cause for pyelonephritis. Enhanced CT scans may show enlarged kidneys with multiple wedge-shaped areas of decreased attenuation, following IV contrast or striated nephrogram. Perinephric stranding and inflammatory changes may or may not be seen. The MR imaging findings are similar to CT and include hypoenhancement with striated nephrograms. MR does not show calcifications and gas as well as CT.

Important complications of acute pyelonephritis include renal abscesses for which imaging studies may be helpful and may guide drainage. Abscesses should be suspected when patients do not respond to antibiotic therapy. Follow-up imaging of acute pyelonephritis may show resolution or development of scar with focal atrophy.

PEARLS

- **CT is the best test for the detection of acute pyelonephritis and its complications when the diagnosis cannot be made clinically.**
- **Wedge-shaped striated nephrogram suggests acute pyelonephritis especially in patients with associated clinical findings of acute pyelonephritis.**
- **An abscess should be suspected when patients with acute pyelonephritis do not respond to antibiotic therapy.**

ADDITIONAL IMAGES (B-E)

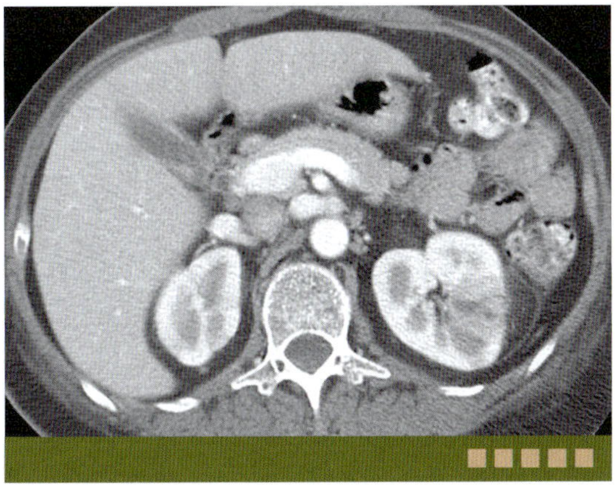

B. Axial CECT shows hypodense left renal lesion from acute pyelonephritis.

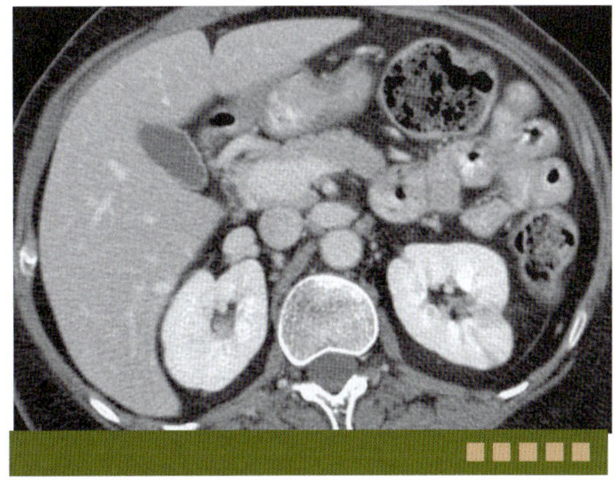

C. Axial CECT performed 7 weeks later shows focal scarring of the left kidney in the same area.

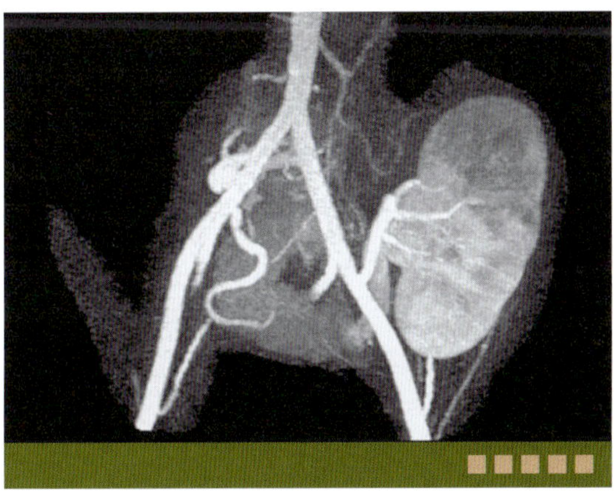

D. Maximal intensity projection MR shows hypoperfusion of upper pole of renal transplant from acute pyelonephritis.

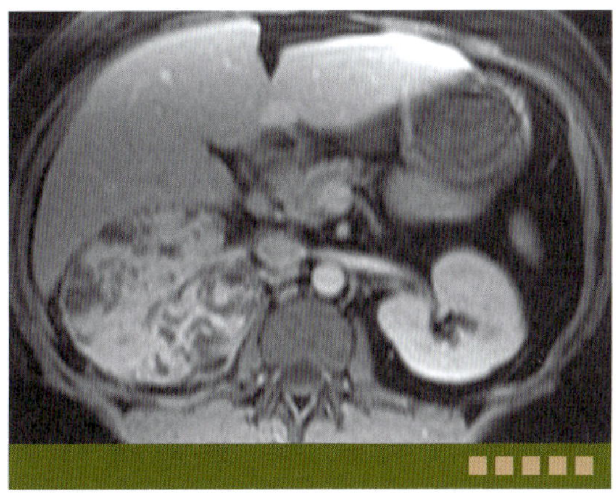

E. Acute pyelonephritis on MR: Contrast-enhanced T1-WI shows enlarged right kidney with heterogeneous enhancement and hypoenhancing areas because of pyelonephritis with developing abscesses.

DIFFERENTIAL DIAGNOSES IMAGES (F-G)

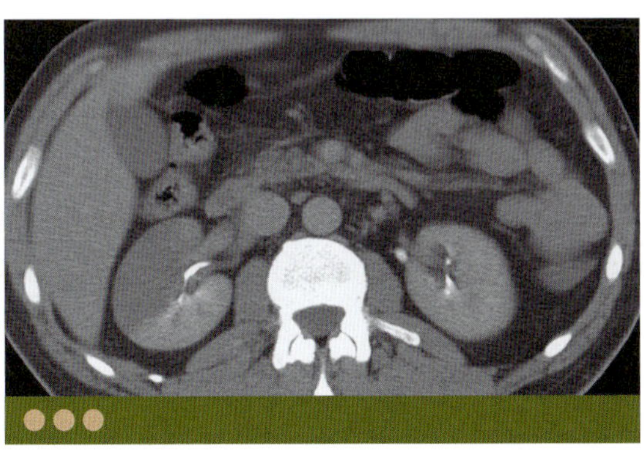

F. Renal infarct: Axial CECT shows large wedge-shaped area of lack of enhancement because of right renal infarct.

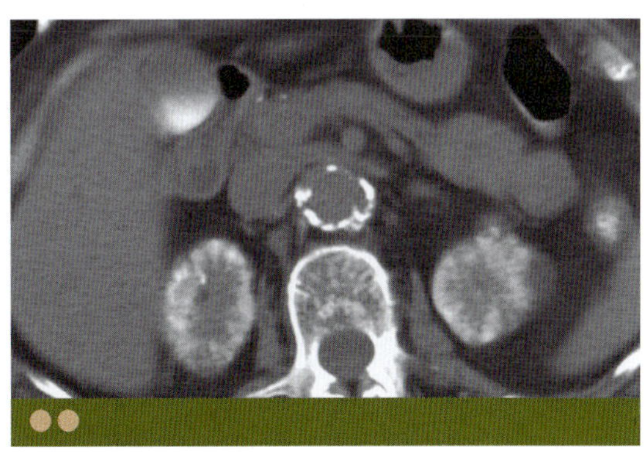

G. Acute tubular necrosis caused by contrast: Axial NECT shows bilateral persistent nephrograms and vicarious excretion into the gallbladder. The patient received intravenous iodinated contrast 24 hours prior to the examination during cardiac catherization.

IMAGE KEY

Common

Rare

Typical

Unusual

3–2 Emphysematous Pyelonephritis

Frank H. Miller

PRESENTATION

Chills, fevers, abdominal pain, diabetes, bacteriuria, and sepsis.

FINDINGS

Air involving the renal parenchyma and extending outside the kidney.

DIFFERENTIAL DIAGNOSES

- *Bilateral angiomyolipomas*: Easily distinguished as the low-density areas are caused by fat and not caused by air.
- *Postprocedure or nephrectomy gas*: Easily distinguished on the basis of clinical history and appearance.
- *Postoperative gas*

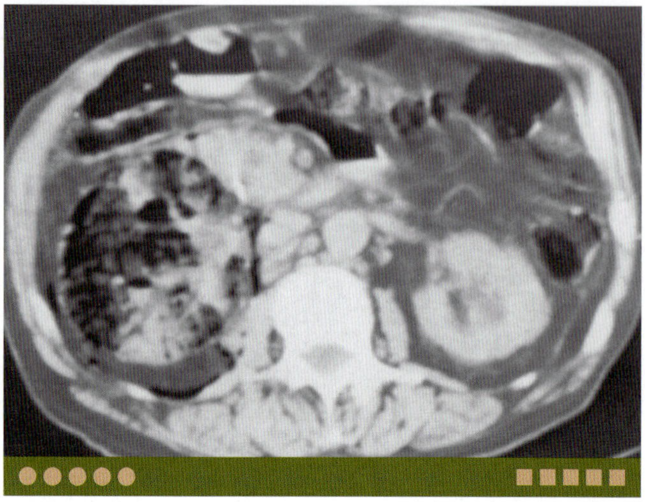

A. Axial CECT in diabetic patient with emphysematous pyelonephritis shows diffuse air involving the renal parenchyma and extending into the perinephric fat.

COMMENTS

Emphysematous pyelonephritis is characterized by gas in the kidney. Emphysematous pyelonephritis has a high morbidity and mortality, if untreated. It is most commonly seen in long-standing diabetes (>90% of cases). There are often multiple associated organisms, most commonly: *E coli*, *Klebsiella pneumonia*, and *Proteus mirabilis* and *Pseudomonas*.

Predisposing factors include stones, calyceal stenosis, cancer, and obstruction.

Emphysematous pyelitis refers to the case when the gas is confined to the renal pelvis and has a better prognosis than true emphysematous pyelonephritis. Perinephric emphysema refers to gas in the perinephric space.

Sonography may be the initial test to evaluate the kidneys, but the diagnosis may be difficult as the gas may mimic renal calcifications based on echogenic foci with reverberation artifacts and shadowing. The gas may be distinguished from calcifications based on "dirty" shadowing. Plain radiographs help distinguish gas from calcifications.

CT is more sensitive and specific in the diagnosis of emphysematous pyelonephritis and will show associated complications and the extent the best of all imaging modalities. MR should not be used in the diagnosis as air is often difficult to identify as it is seen as signal voids on T1- and T2-weighted images. With emphysematous pyelonephritis, the gas is initially seen extending along the renal pyramids. When more severe, the gas becomes more bubbly and extends into Gerota's fascia. Subsequently, the gas extends outside the renal fascia within the retroperitoneum.

It is critical to make the diagnosis early with prompt administration of antibiotics, and surgery may be required.

PEARLS

- **Air within the renal parenchyma is referred to as emphysematous pyelonephritis.**
- **Emphysematous pyelonephritis has a high morbidity and mortality if not treated rapidly.**
- **Emphysematous pyelonephritis is most commonly seen in diabetics and often has multiple associated organisms.**
- **CT is the most sensitive and specific test for emphysematous pyelonephritis.**

ADDITIONAL IMAGES (B-D)

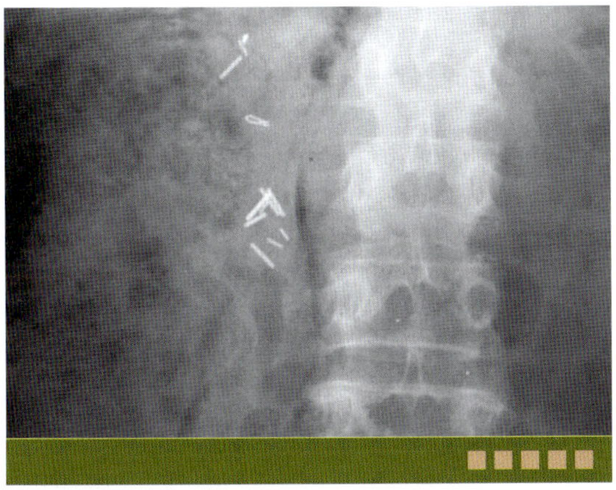

B. Emphysematous pyelonephritis: Same patient as in Figure A. Plain radiograph shows air in the renal fossa and extending along psoas shadow.

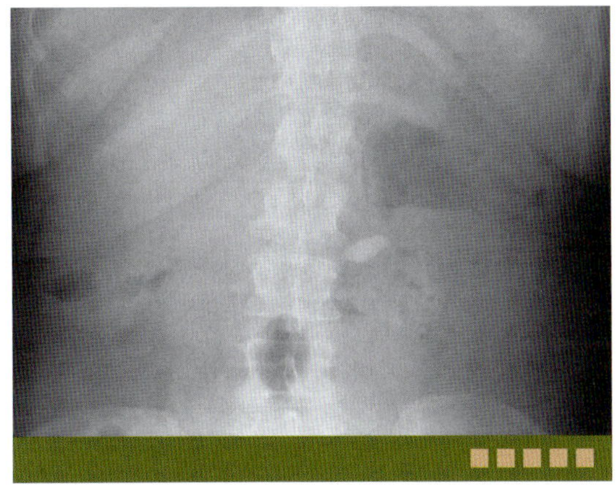

C. Emphysematous pyelonephritis: Plain radiograph in different patient with diabetes and staghorn calculus and air in renal fossa.

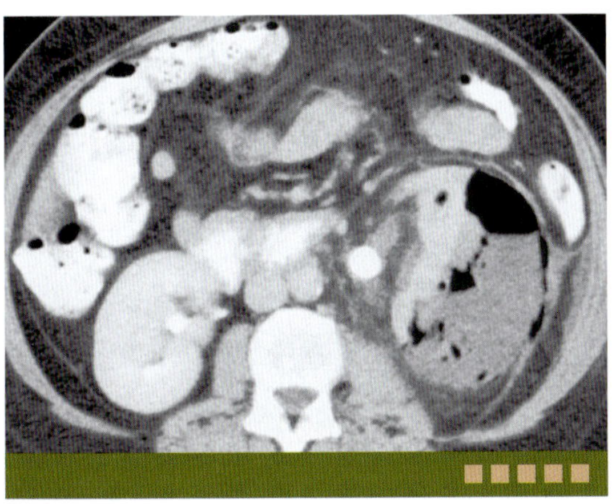

D. Emphysematous pyelonephritis: Axial CECT shows staghorn calculus with air in the kidney and perinephric abscess containing air.

DIFFERENTIAL DIAGNOSES IMAGES (E-F)

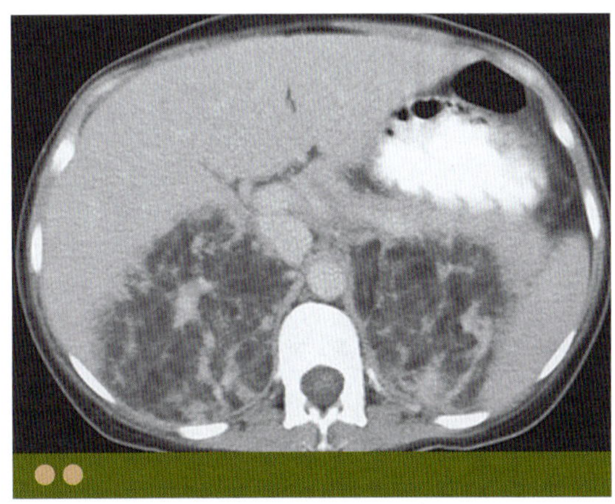

E. Bilateral angiomyolipomas in patient with tuberous sclerosis: Axial CECT shows replacement of the kidneys with angiomyolipomas which are distinguished as fat density and not air unlike emphysematous pyelonephritis.

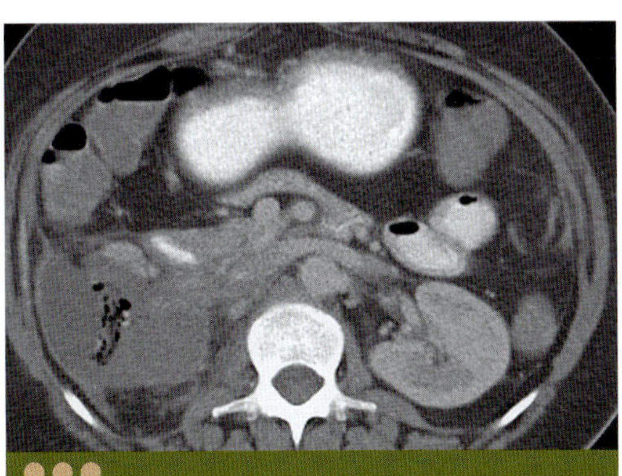

F. Postsurgical air: Axial CECT showed postoperative changes from partial nephrectomy and complications of renal infarction. Gas was seen in the collection which related to recent surgery and Gelfoam placement.

IMAGE KEY

Common

Rare

Typical

Unusual

3–3 Xanthogranulomatous Pyelonephritis

Frank H. Miller

PRESENTATION

Nonspecific chronic symptoms: Abdominal pain, fever, mass, weight loss, and leukocytosis.

FINDINGS

Obstructing staghorn calculus, enlarged kidney, dilated calyces with poor renal function, and perinephric stranding.

DIFFERENTIAL DIAGNOSES

The imaging findings are often specific to make the diagnosis of Xanthogranulomatous pyelonephritis (XGP).

- *Chronic obstruction and inflammation extending into the retroperitoneal fat*: may mimic XGP.
- *Chronic hydronephrosis*: Associated with dilated collecting system but not with other features of XGP.
- *Abscess*: Staghorn calculus more closely associated with XGP, especially in case of poor renal function.

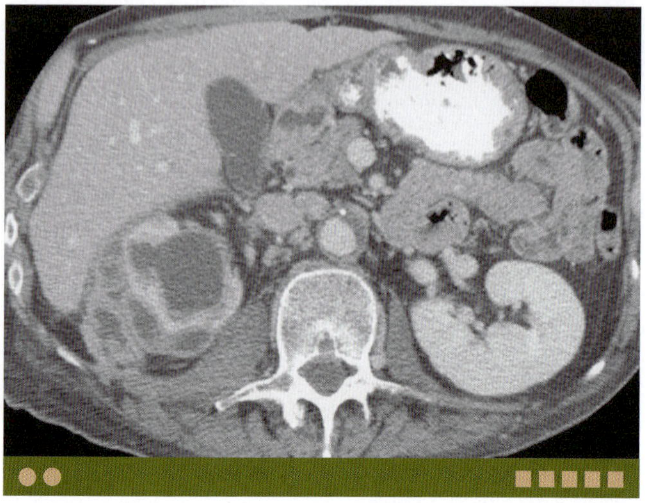

A. Axial CECT shows poorly functioning right kidney with dilated collecting system with extension of low-attenuation areas into the perinephric space.

COMMENTS

XGP is an uncommon chronic renal infection generally caused by an obstructing renal calculus. The infection leads to the replacement of the normal renal parenchyma by the characteristic xanthoma cells, which are foamy, lipid-laden histiocytes. Chronic infection and staghorn calculus is seen in 70% of the cases of XGP, though rarely does chronic upper tract urinary tract infection (UTI) lead to XGP. Proteus mirabilis is the main infectious agent associated but *E coli*, *Klebsiella*, and *Pseudomonas* may also be seen. It is more commonly seen in middle-aged women. XGP is generally unilateral. Despite significant renal function loss of one of the kidneys, the patients often have a normal creatinine as long as the other kidney is normal.

The sonographic findings may consist of enlarged kidney, hypoechoic mass-like areas in the kidney with echogenic central foci from calculi in the renal pelvis. The diagnosis is generally best made with CT scans and the imaging features often are pathognomonic. The triad of diffuse XGP includes a staghorn calculus, unilaterally decreased or more often absent renal excretion of contrast material, and a poorly defined mass or diffuse unilateral renal enlargement. CT findings include calcifications low-attenuation areas (lipid-rich xanthomatous tissue) that are nonenhancing. The kidneys lack function and do not excrete into the collecting systems and ureters. XGP is usually unilateral and diffusely involves the kidney. Involvement may extend beyond the kidney into the perinephric space to the psoas muscle and abdominal wall. Complications include abscess formation and fistulas.

The focal or segmental form of XGP, seen in 15% of the patients, may mimic renal cell carcinoma (RCC) based on imaging studies requiring surgical excision. With the diffuse form, the diagnosis can often be made based on clinical and imaging features, but nephrectomy is usually required for the diagnosis and treatment.

PEARLS

- **Triad of diffuse XGP includes staghorn calculus, decreased or lack of enhancement of kidney, and poorly defined mass or diffuse renal enlargement.**
- **XGT is diagnosed by xanthoma cells or foamy, lipid-laden macrophages.**
- **The diagnosis of XGP is best made using CT scans.**
- **The segmental form of XGP may mimic RCC.**

ADDITIONAL IMAGES (B-E)

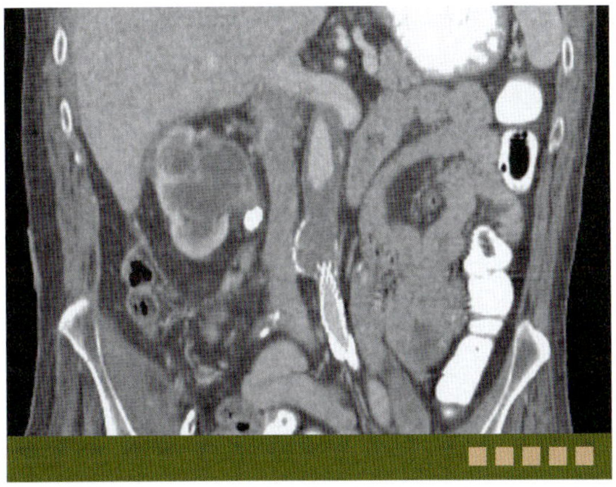

B. The same patient, on coronal CECT scan, has staghorn calculus and hydronephrosis and low-attenuation areas extending into the perinephric space. Stent is seen in the left iliac artery.

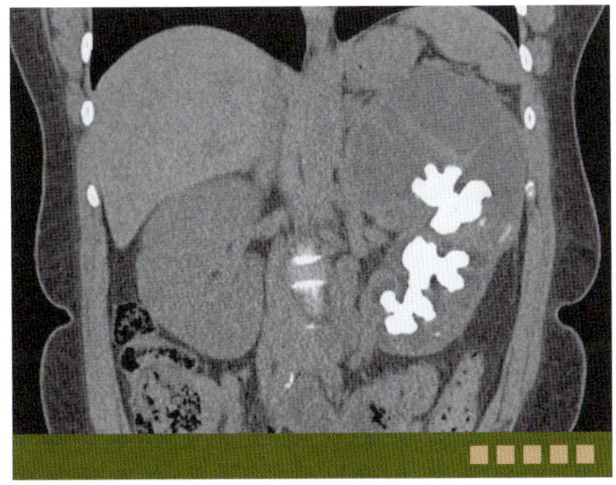

C. Coronal image in different patient shows large staghorn calculi with peripheral low-density areas and enlargement of the left kidney.

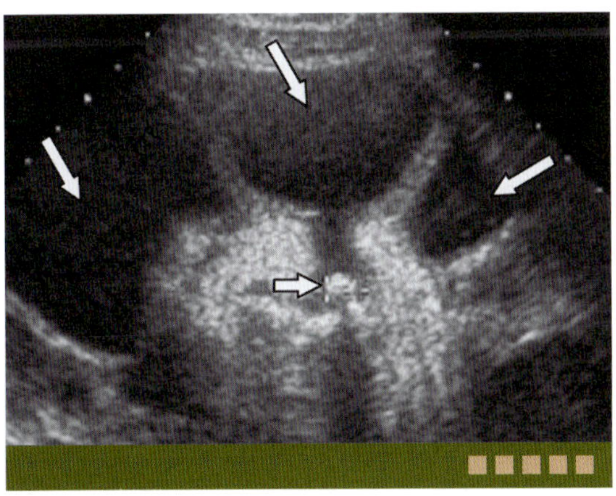

D. Longitudinal sonogram shows enlarged kidney with echogenic focus (short arrow) from staghorn calculus. Large peripheral hypoechoic areas (long arrows) are seen from dilated collecting system and/or inflammatory tissue caused by XGP.

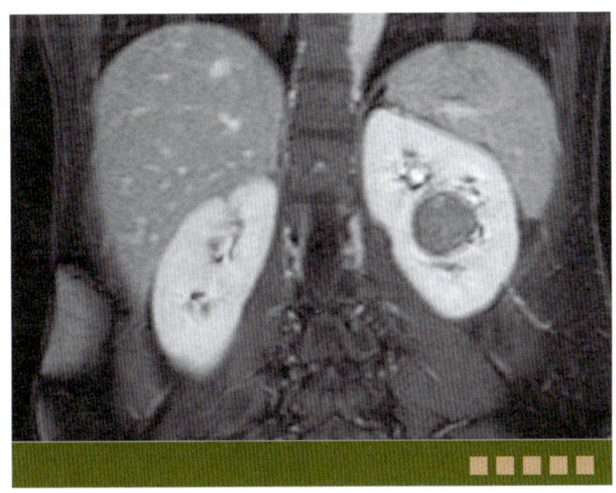

E. Focal XGP: Coronal contrast-enhanced T1-WI shows hypoenhancing left renal mass.

DIFFERENTIAL DIAGNOSES IMAGES (F-G)

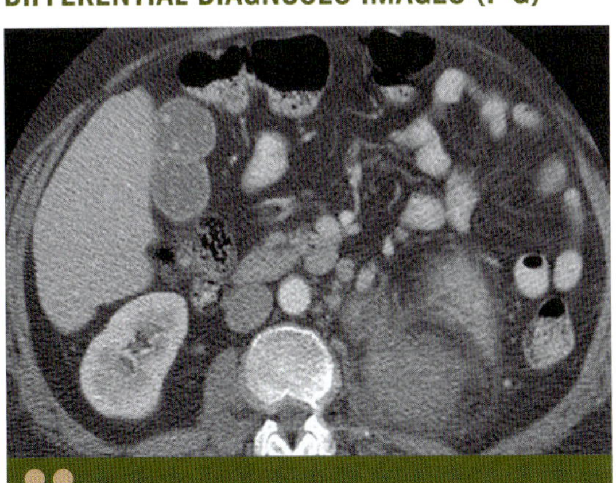

F. Chronic obstructed kidney mimicking XGP: Axial CECT shows fat-containing mass because of perinephric inflammation mimicking XGP.

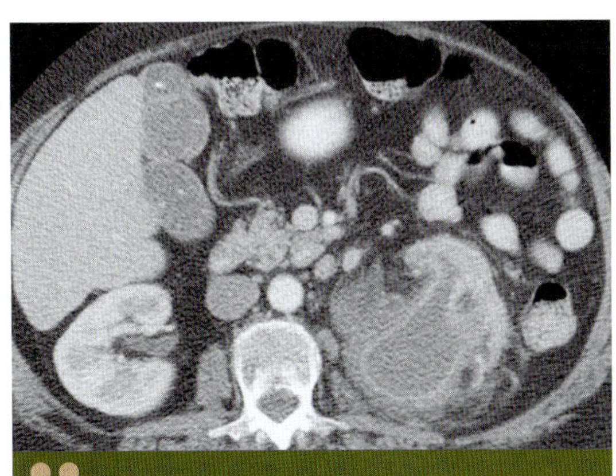

G. Axial CECT in the same patient shows hydronephrosis from chronic obstruction.

IMAGE KEY

Common

Rare

Typical

Unusual

3–4 Renal Abscess

Paul Nikolaidis

PRESENTATION

Fever, chills, and flank pain.

FINDINGS

CECT shows a round, nonenhancing hypodense renal lesion with a thick, irregular outline.

DIFFERENTIAL DIAGNOSES

- *Focal pyelonephritis*: Areas of focal pyelonephritis are usually less distinct and more difficult to separate from adjacent renal parenchyma. However, it is often difficult to distinguish areas of focal pyelonephritis from early abscesses formation.
- *Renal cell carcinoma*: May sometimes mimic a renal abscess, especially when cystic or centrally necrotic. Patients are usually asymptomatic, or present only with hematuria.
- *Lymphoma/leukemia*: Multiple distinct hypodense lesions are one of several manifestations of renal lymphoma or leukemia, and in some cases may be more difficult to distinguish from abscesses. They should enhance slightly and most patients have additional extrarenal sites of involvement.
- *Metastases*: Metastases tend to be multiple small lesions, usually hypodense on precontrast CT with heterogeneous enhancement on CECT; some may be centrally nonenhancing because of necrosis. Patients typically have a known primary malignancy.

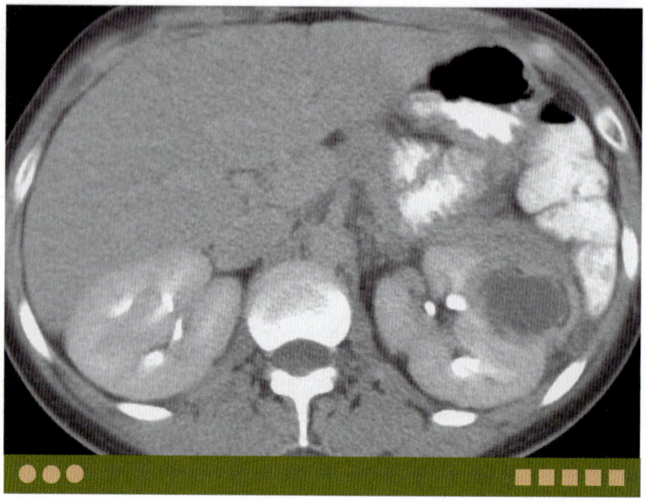

A. Axial CECT shows a large centrally hypodense left renal lesion with a slightly irregular outline.

COMMENTS

Prior to the advent of antibiotics, most renal abscesses were caused by hematogenous spread (usually *Staphylococcus*) from distant sites. With antibiotic therapy now common, renal abscesses are now primarily caused by ascending infections with enteric, aerobic, gram-negative bacilli, including *E coli, Proteus mirabilis,* and *Klebsiella* species. Patients at highest risk have a complicated UTI are diabetic, or pregnant. Clinical presentation includes fever, flank, or abdominal pain, and chills, with or without dysuria, frequency, or urgency. Patients may also have nausea and vomiting.

A contrast-enhanced CT or MR should be obtained if an abscess is suspected, even if the ultrasound is negative. Characteristic CT appearances of a renal abscess include a well-defined, hypoattenuating (0-20 HU) round lesion without appreciable enhancement. There may be adjacent perinephric extension and thickening of the renal fascia. They may demonstrate a sharp demarcation from the adjacent enhancing renal parenchyma, whereas cases of focal bacterial nephritis (focal pyelonephritis) are typically less distinct.

On contrast-enhanced MR, renal abscesses are heterogeneous lesions with central areas of hypo- or isointensity on T1-WI. The central portion of the abscess is usually hyperintense on T2-WI.

Patients with abscesses smaller than 3 cm generally improve with antibiotics. Lesions between 3 and 5 cm are often treated with percutaneous drainage. Any abscess larger than 5 cm may need to be drained surgically.

PEARLS

- **Primarily caused by ascending infection with enteric, gram-negatives aerobes, such as *E coli, Proteus,* and *Klebsiella.***
- **Present with fever, flank or abdominal pain, and chills, with or without urinary symptoms (dysuria, frequency, and urgency).**
- **Well seen on CT as distinct hypodense lesions, sometimes with perinephric inflammation or stranding.**
- **On MR, the abscess center of a renal abscess is usually hypo- or isointense on T1-WI, and hyperintense on T2-WI.**

ADDITIONAL IMAGES (B-D)

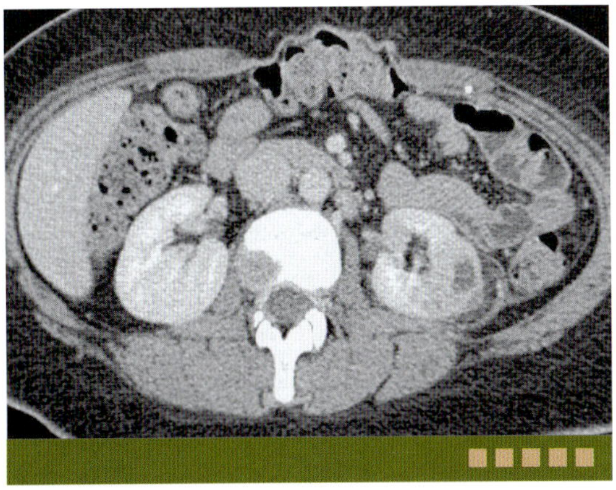

B. Axial CECT on a different patient shows a hypodense left renal lesion. The surrounding renal parenchyma appears shows decreased enhancement related to edema.

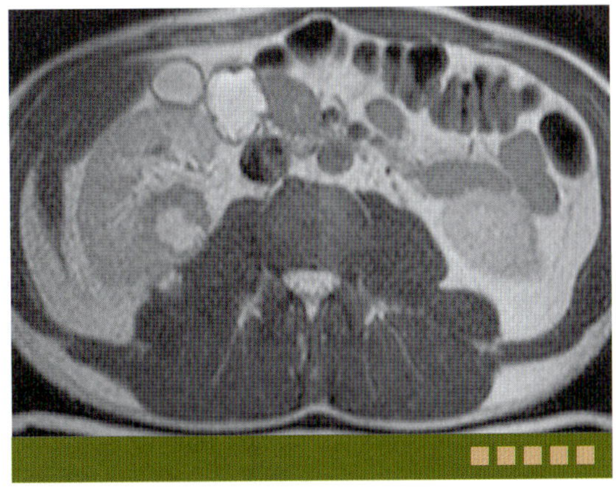

C. Axial T2-WI on a different patient shows a centrally hyperintense left renal lesion with a hypointense rim.

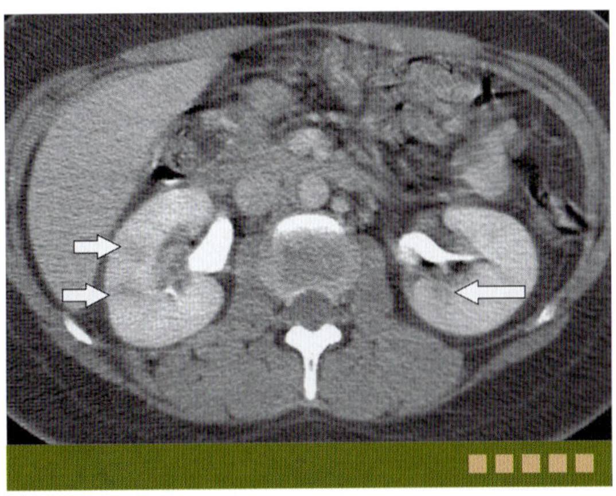

D. Axial CECT on a different patient shows a few ill-defined areas of focal pyelonephritis and very early abscess formation.

DIFFERENTIAL DIAGNOSES IMAGES (E-G)

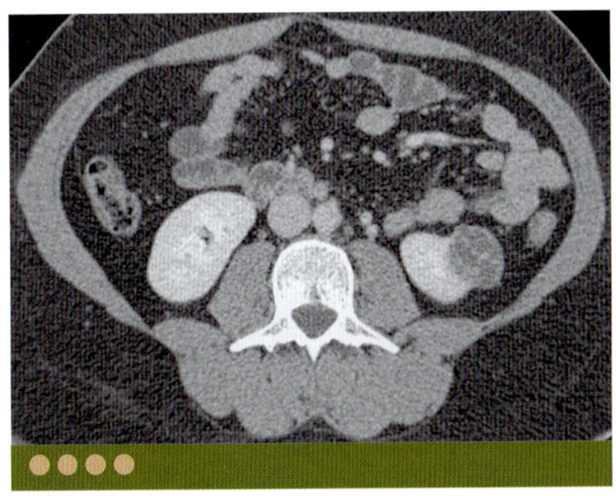

E. Cystic renal cell carcinoma: Axial CECT shows a peripherally located hypodense left renal mass with several enhancing thickened and nodular septations.

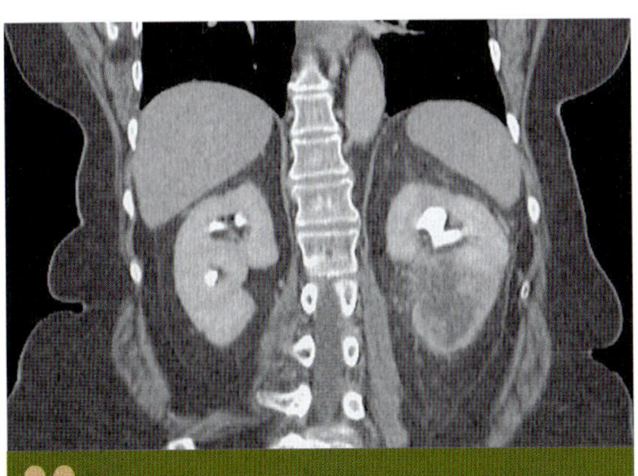

F. Renal metastasis: Coronal CECT reformation shows a large irregular cystic mass in the lower pole of the left kidney, in a patient with known metastatic squamous cell carcinoma.

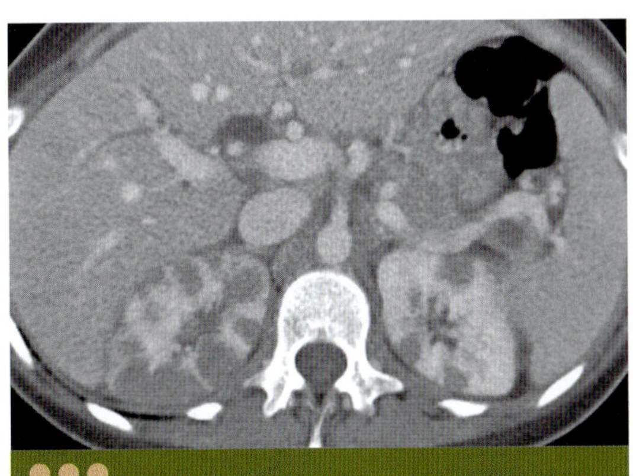

G. Renal lymphoma: Axial CECT shows numerous bilateral hypodense renal masses in a patient with a history of lymphoma. They were hypermetabolic on PET scan.

IMAGE KEY

Common

Rare

Typical

Unusual

3–5 Renal Tuberculosis—Early Reactivation

Nancy A. Hammond

PRESENTATION

Urinary frequency and dysuria.

FINDINGS

Striated nephrogram and focal calyectasis.

DIFFERENTIAL DIAGNOSIS

Pyelonephritis: Striated nephrograms, lacks focal calyectasis seen in tuberculosis.

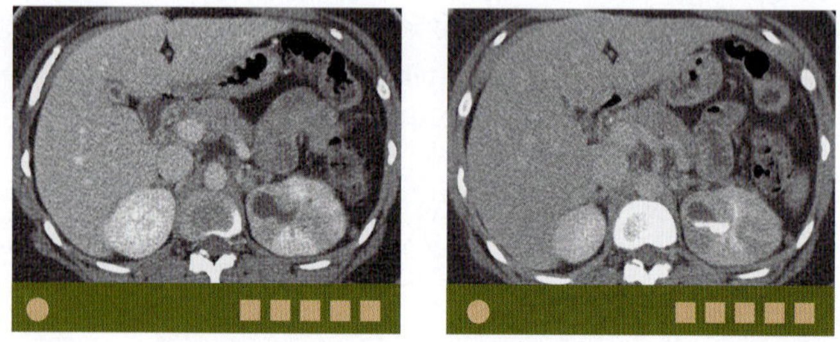

A. Axial CECT shows wedge-shaped areas of hypoperfusion in the left kidney with a focal low-density collection that appears to communicate with the collecting system and was observed to represent focal calyectasis.
B. Axial CECT shows in the same patient obtained in the excretory phase shows contrast material filling the dilated calyx.

COMMENTS

The genitourinary tract is the second most commonly infected site by tuberculosis after the lungs. Approximately 15% to 20% of all new cases of tuberculosis are extrapulmonary. Of these cases, approximately 30% involve the urogenital tract. Renal inoculation usually occurs during the primary exposure via hematogenous spread. Typically, both kidneys are inoculated and tuberculous bacilli are trapped in the periglomerular capillaries with multiple small abscesses developing. In the immunocompetent patient, these foci are suppressed, and they heal to form multiple granulomas. When the host's immune system is compromised, these suppressed foci are reactivated, and they propagate into the renal papillae. Clinically significant and radiographically evident disease is usually unilateral with reactivation. With progression, the reactivated foci can rupture into the collecting system and spread distally and result in multifocal inflammation along the genitourinary tract.

Renal involvement is typically indolent with a latency period of more than 20 years. Clinical symptoms are often absent or minimal until the entire urinary tract is affected. At which time patients present with frequency, dysuria, and nocturia.

Radiographically, genitourinary tuberculosis manifests according to the stage of the disease. Radiographic signs may be absent in about 10% of cases. In the initial stage of dissemination, cortical lesions are too small to be imaged. In early stages of reactivation, the lesions can be seen on CT, MRI, or US. CT and MRI demonstrate hypodense or T1-hypointense cortical nodules. Because of tissue edema and vasoconstriction, areas of hypoperfusion can be seen on contrast-enhanced CT and MR. This finding is similar to that of pyelonephritis. Ultrasound shows hypoechoic cortical nodules. Intravenous urogram (IVU) may demonstrate a moth-eaten, irregular appearance to the involved calyx. With progressive caseation, the tuberculoma enlarges and ruptures into the adjacent calyx resulting in an irregular cavity and papillary necrosis which can be seen on CT, MR, or IVU. The most characteristic cross-sectional imaging finding of urinary tuberculosis is uneven calyectasis. It is caused by the varying degree of fibrosis and obstruction at various sites. Cross-sectional images can show severe calyectasis that is not present on IVU because of its poor opacification. General hydronephrosis can develop when the renal pelvis and ureter are involved. With renal pelvis or ureteral involvement, there is thickening of the wall and enhancement of the involved segment.

Urinary tuberculosis is currently treated with a 6-month regimen of antituberculous drugs. Despite adequate medical therapy, strictures of the infundibula and ureter can still form. In these cases, surgical intervention may be necessary.

PEARLS

- **The genitourinary tract is the second most common site affected by tuberculosis after the lungs.**
- **Hematogeneous dissemination to the kidneys occurs at the time of initial inoculation.**
- **Reactivation is usually clinically and radiographically evident in one kidney.**
- **Early reactivation tuberculosis has a similar appearance to that of pyelonephritis but results in the characteristic uneven calyectasis.**

ADDITIONAL IMAGES (C-F)

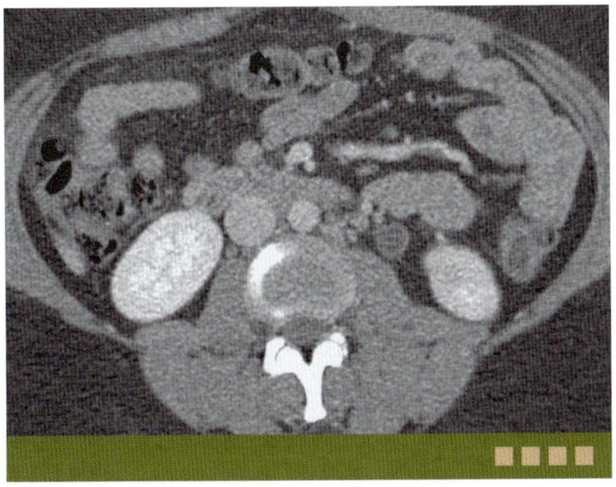

C. Axial CECT in the same patient obtained at the level of the proximal left ureter shows thickening and enhancement of the ureteric wall.

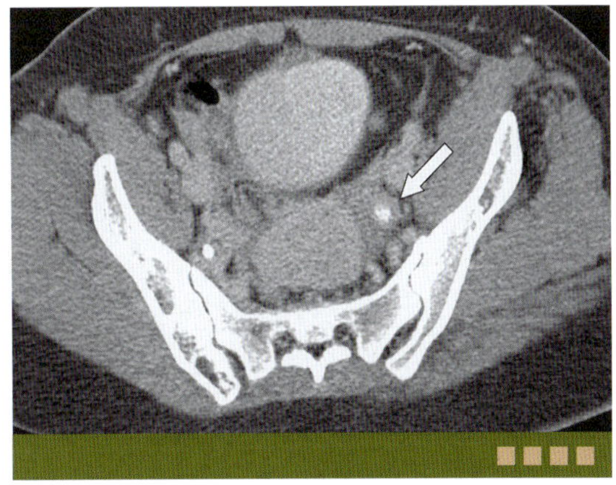

D. Axial CECT further shows tuberculous involvement of the distal left ureter (arrow).

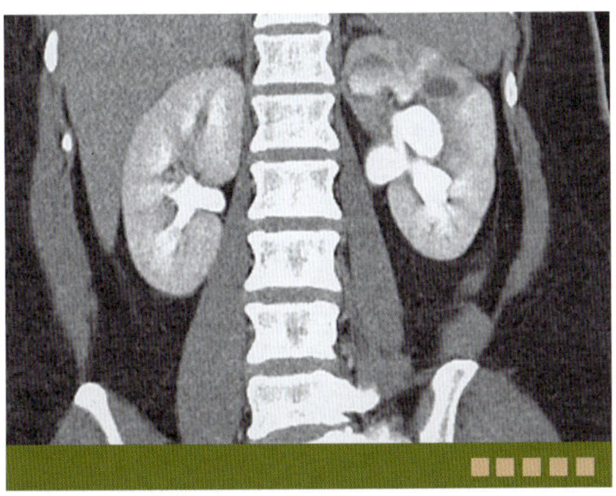

E. Coronal CECT in the same patient obtained 2 months later shows progressive uneven calyectasis to the upper pole of the left kidney with persistent areas of hypoperfusion.

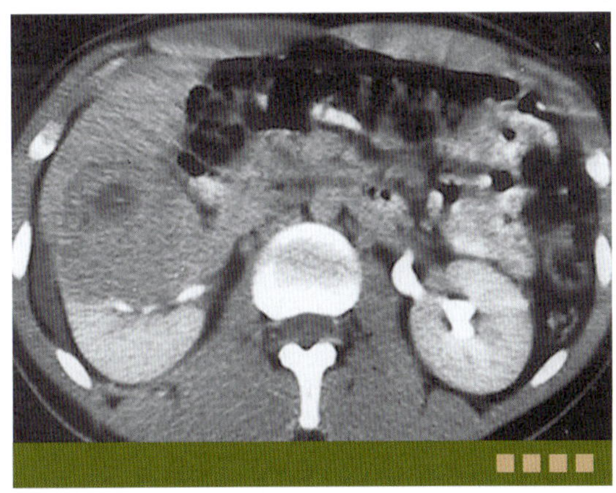

F. Axial CECT in a different patient shows hypoperfusion to the anterior aspect of the right kidney with a central low-density structure consistent with a tuberculoma.

DIFFERENTIAL DIAGNOSES IMAGE

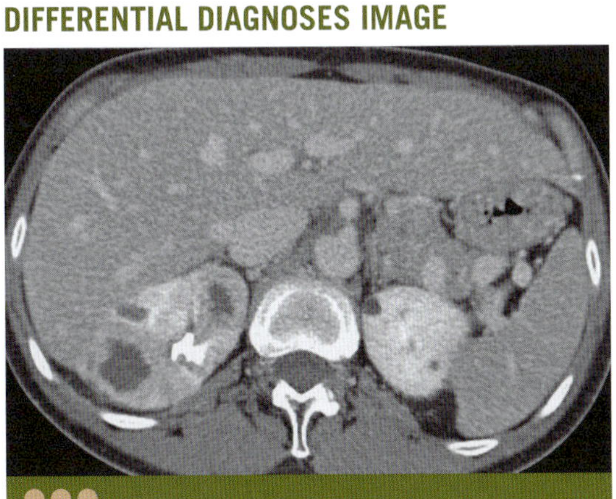

G. Pyelonephritis with abscess formation: Axial CECT shows multiple wedge-shaped areas of hypoperfusion in the right kidney with associated hypodense collections. This image was obtained in the excretory phase. No contrast material was seen filling these collections confirming that these represent abscesses rather than calyectasis.

IMAGE KEY

Common

Rare

Typical

Unusual

3-6 Renal Tuberculosis—Phantom Calyx

Nancy A. Hammond

PRESENTATION

Dysuria.

FINDINGS

Absent opacification of a calyx.

DIFFERENTIAL DIAGNOSES

Transitional cell carcinoma: Cross-sectional imaging or retrograde study demonstrates underlying mass.

COMMENTS

The genitourinary tract is the second most commonly infected site by tuberculosis after the lungs. Approximately 15% to 20% of all new cases of tuberculosis are extrapulmonary. Of these cases, approximately 30% involve the urogenital tract. Renal inoculation usually occurs during the primary exposure via hematogenous spread from the lungs or bones. Reactivation occurs when the host is immunocompromised. While both kidneys are usually initially inoculated, radiographically evident disease is usually unilateral. When reactivation occurs, multifocal inflammation along the entire genitourinary tract can occur. This inflammation results in fibrosis, scarring, and calcifications.

Radiographically, genitourinary tuberculosis manifests according to the stage of the disease. A characteristic cross-sectional imaging finding of urinary tuberculosis is uneven calyectasis. It is caused by fibrosis and obstruction secondary to infundibular stenoses or strictures. Complete infundibular strictures result in the exclusion of the entire calyx from the collecting system or a "phantom calyx." Cross-sectional images can show severe calyectasis that is not present on IVU because of its poor opacification.

Other characteristic findings of genitourinary tuberculosis resulting from fibrosis include corkscrew ureter, resulting from multiple infundibulum and ureteral stenoses, the "purse-string" stenosis of the renal pelvis, and the "pipestem" ureter because of narrow, rigid aperistaltic segment.

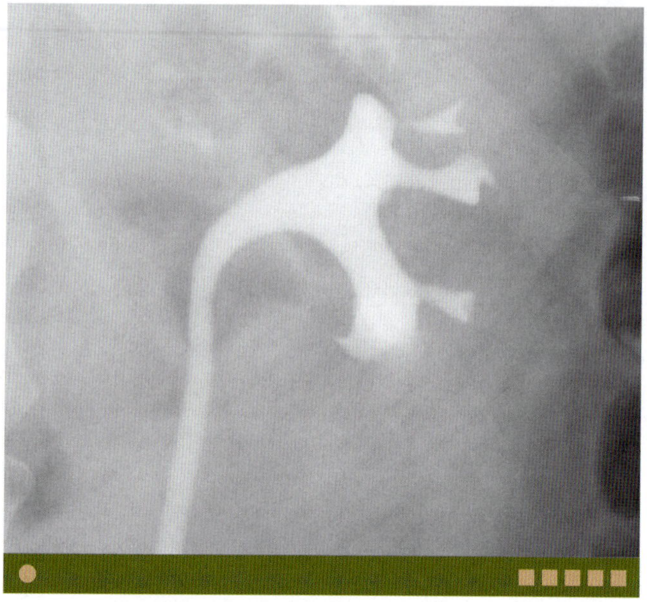

A. Retrograde pyelogram shows absence of filling of the left upper pole calyx in a patient with a history of pulmonary tuberculosis.

PEARLS

- **The genitourinary tract is the second most common site affected by tuberculosis after the lungs.**
- **As a result of the multifocal inflammation and subsequent fibrosis, infundibular stenoses and strictures result in uneven calyectasis. Complete occlusion of an infundibula results in a "phantom calyx."**
- **The phantom calyx caused by stenosis should be differentiated from an underlying neoplasm such as transitional cell carcinoma.**

ADDITIONAL IMAGES (B-C)

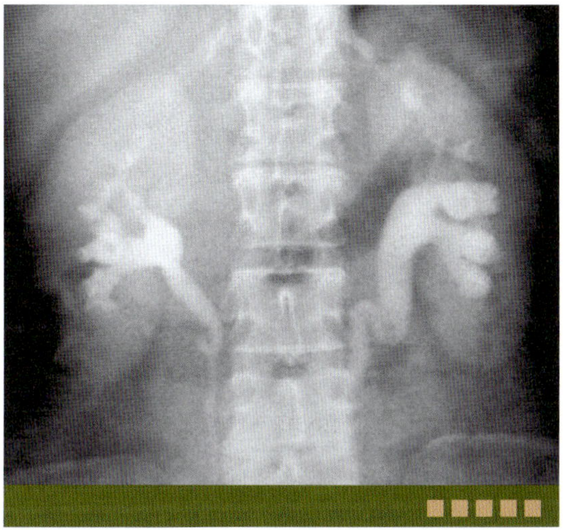

B. Contrast-enhanced IVU shows a stricture involving the upper pole calyx of the left kidney. The remainder of the calyces on the left are clubbed.

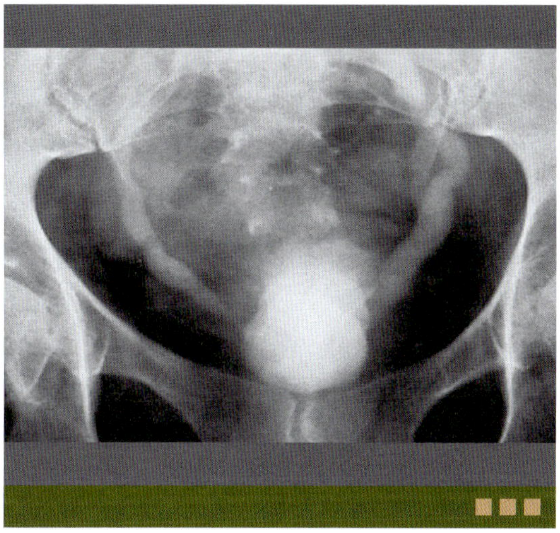

C. Coned down view of the urinary bladder from an IVU in the same patient as Figure B shows a small bladder with an irregular and thickened wall. This finding can be seen in advanced bladder involvement by tuberculosis.

DIFFERENTIAL DIAGNOSES IMAGES (D-E)

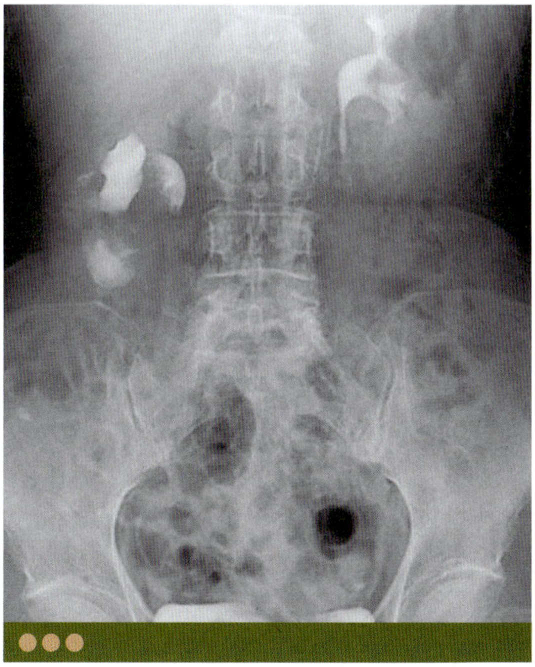

D. Transitional cell carcinoma: Contrast-enhanced IVU shows distortion and dilatation of the right renal calyces.

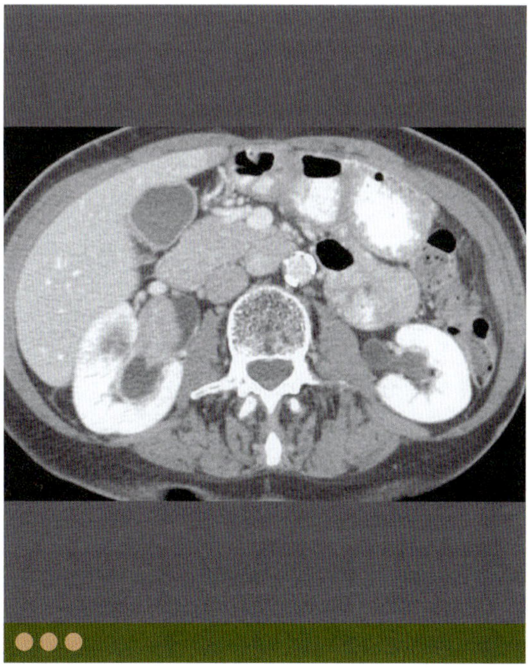

E. Axial CECT in the same patient as Figure D shows an enhancing mass in the renal pelvis as the cause of the calyceal abnormalities.

IMAGE KEY

Common

Rare

Typical

Unusual

3–7 "Putty Kidney" Secondary to Chronic Renal Tuberculosis

Nancy A. Hammond

PRESENTATION

Chronic renal failure.

FINDINGS

Densely calcified kidney.

DIFFERENTIAL DIAGNOSIS

None

COMMENTS

Approximately 15% to 20% of all new cases of tuberculosis are extrapulmonary. Of these cases, approximately 30% involve the urogenital tract. Renal inoculation occurs during the primary exposure via hematogenous spread from the lungs. With progression, the reactivated foci rupture into the collecting system and spread distally resulting in multifocal inflammation along the genitourinary tract. When this inflammation results in fibrosis at the ureteropelvic junction caseous pyonephrosis occurs. In turn, a scarred, atrophic, densely calcified, nonfunctioning kidney develops (autonephrectomy).

With renal involvement, clinical symptoms are often absent or minimal. Presentation is usually associated with lower urinary tract symptoms, including frequency, dysuria, and nocturia. A history of tuberculosis in another site is almost always present, but that site may be inactive at the time of diagnosis. The true prevalence of renal tuberculosis is likely underestimated since radiologic signs may be absent in about 10% of cases.

Radiographically, genitourinary tuberculosis manifests according to the stage of the disease. In patients with chronic or healed tuberculosis, renal calcifications may be present. Calcification can be seen on plain film radiography but CT is more sensitive in detecting them. Punctate calcifications represent healed tuberculomas. When renal tuberculosis is inadequately treated, the kidney atrophies and hydronephrosis progresses. The kidney loses its normal reniform morphology, developing multiple thin-wall cysts and a multiloculated appearance. Eventually, the entire kidney is replaced with a dystrophic calcification resulting in a "putty kidney."

Other characteristic findings of chronic genitourinary tuberculosis include corkscrew ureter resulting from multiple infundibular and ureteral stenoses, the "purse-string" stenosis of the renal pelvis, and the "pipestem ureter" caused by a narrow, rigid aperistaltic segment.

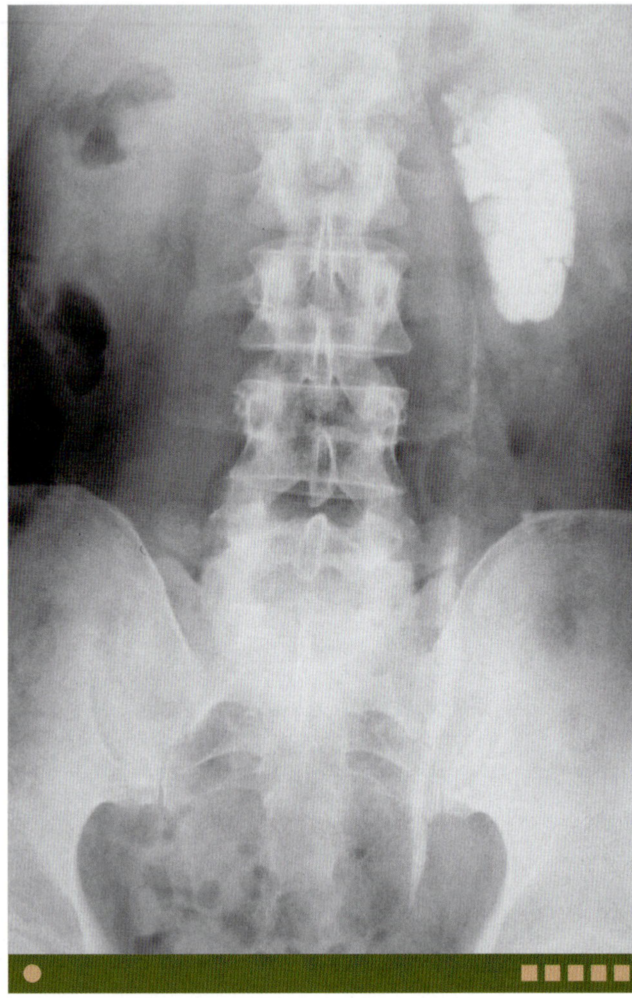

A. AP scout from an IVU shows a densely calcified left kidney. Calcification is also present along the course of the left ureter.

PEARLS

- **Chronic or healed tuberculosis can result in renal calcifications.**
- **Untreated or inadequately treated renal tuberculosis can result in a nonfunctioning kidney or "autonephrectomy."**
- **Putty kidney appears as a densely calcified kidney.**

ADDITIONAL IMAGES (B-E)

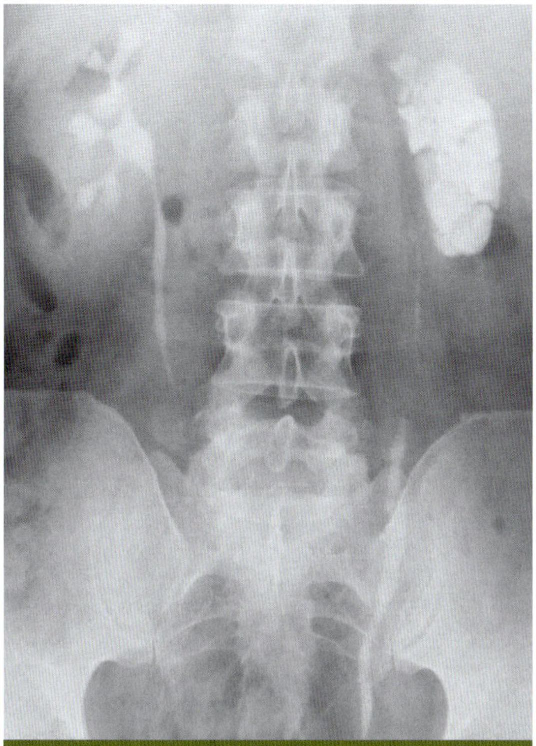

B. Contrast-enhanced IVU in the same patient shows excretion of contrast from the right kidney. No contrast is seen excreted from the left kidney compatible with an autonephrectomy.

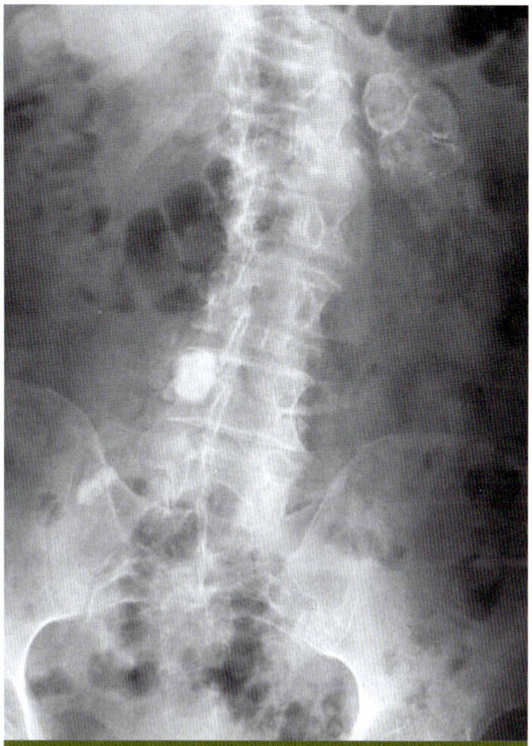

C. AP scout from an IVU in a different patient shows an atrophic left kidney with diffuse calcification. The calcifications appear to conform to a hydronephretic collecting system. Calcifications in the mid-abdomen represent calcified lymph nodes.

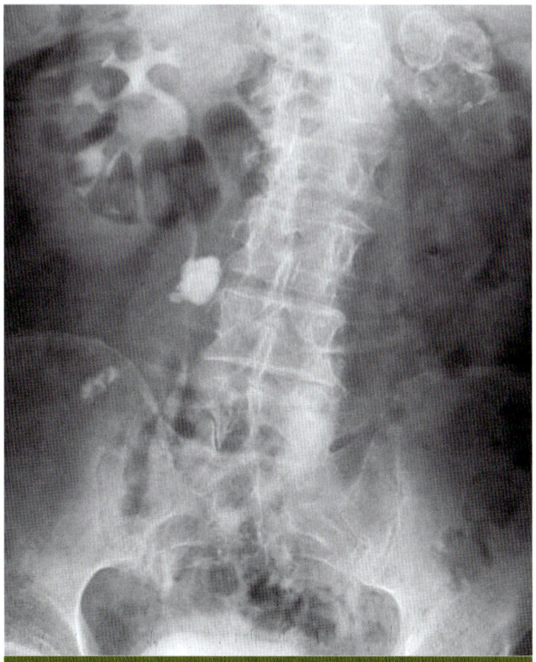

D. Contrast-enhanced IVU in the same patient as Figure C shows excretion of contrast through the right collecting system. No contrast is excreted via the left kidney consistent with loss of renal function.

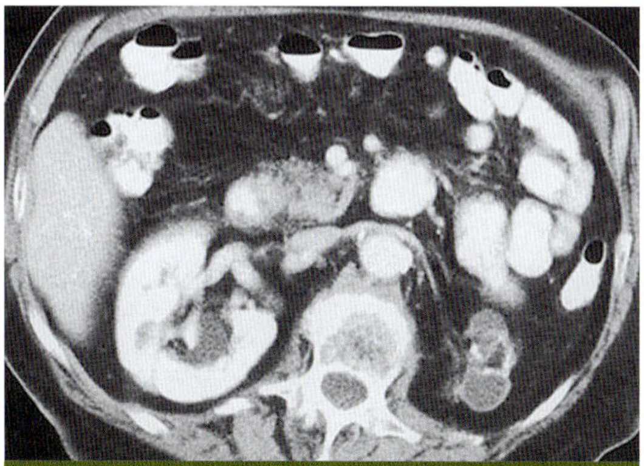

E. Axial CECT in the same patient shows enhancement of the normal appearing right kidney. No enhancing left renal parenchyma is identified. The kidney is replaced by multiloculated cystic spaces some of which are peripherally calcified.

IMAGE KEY

Common

Rare

Typical

Unusual

3–8 Renal Malakoplakia

David D. Casalino

PRESENTATION

Hematuria.

FINDINGS

CT shows a large, enhancing mass with central hypodensity arising from the upper pole of the right kidney.

DIFFERENTIAL DIAGNOSES

- *Renal cell carcinoma*: Much more common; may be complex, cystic, or necrotic mass.
- *Focal xanthogranulomatous pyelonephritis* (XGP): Rare; also more common in women; very often associated with ipsilateral renal calculi and history of chronic UTI; symptoms may be nonspecific or absent; usually a surgical lesion.
- *Abscess*: In the early stage of development, an abscess may have nonenhancing cystic and enhancing solid components; findings of pyelonephritis and symptoms of infection are common.

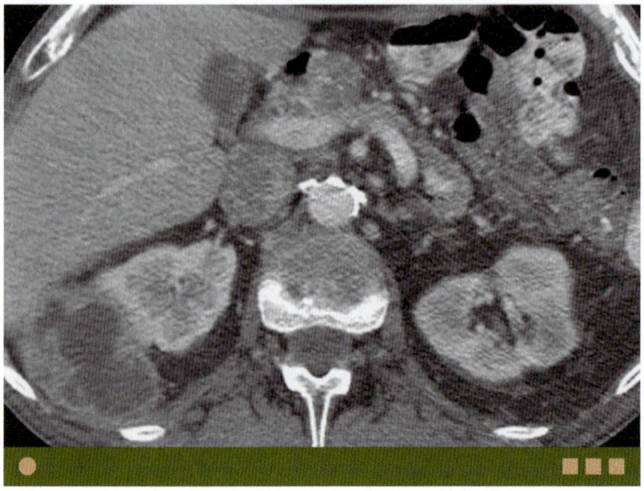

A. Axial CECT shows a large, enhancing mass with central necrosis arising from the right kidney in an elderly man with severe dementia.

COMMENTS

Malakoplakia is a rare, granulomatous response to infection, usually *E coli*, and most often involves the bladder. Much less commonly, malakoplakia may involve the kidney, upper collecting system, testis, prostate, and urethra. The pathogenesis is thought to involve abnormal macrophage function that prevents complete digestion of phagocytosed bacteria. The partially digested bacteria persist in phagolysosomes and become calcified, resulting in intracellular inclusion bodies, known as Michaelis-Gutmann bodies. Malakoplakia is seen most often in immunocompromised individuals and middle-aged women with chronic UTI. Presenting symptoms are those of UTI, such as dysuria, frequency, hesitancy, and bladder irritability. Hematuria is common. A palpable mass may result from renal or testicular involvement. Renal failure may occur because of bilateral renal involvement or obstructive uropathy from bladder or bilateral upper collecting system involvement.

The radiologic appearance of malakoplakia of the kidney usually involves multiple masses that range in size from several millimeters to several centimeters and result in focal enlargement of the kidney, renal contour lobulation, and mass effect on the collecting system. These masses typically enhance less than normal cortex. On ultrasonography, the masses are typically ill-defined and hypoechoic. In less than 25% of cases, malakoplakia may appear as a unifocal mass, which may mimic a cortical neoplasm. The inflammatory process may extend into the perirenal space and renal sinus, and renal vein thrombosis may occur. Hydronephrosis is uncommon. When the bladder is involved there may be diffuse mural thickening or a single or multiple polypoid mural lesions. Malakoplakia may extend into the perivesical space. Malakoplakia of the pelvocalyceal system and ureter may cause multiple, irregular filling defects, dilatation, and urothelial thickening. Malakoplakia of the testis is rare, and imaging cannot reliably differentiate it from a testicular neoplasm and other infectious process. While clinical signs and symptoms of infection may suggest the diagnosis, biopsy or surgical management is usually necessary to differentiate malakoplakia from neoplasm. The treatment may be nonsurgical and involves antibiotics, ascorbic acid, and a cholinergic agonist.

PEARLS

- **Malakoplakia is a rare, granulomatous response to infection that most often involves the bladder, but may also involve the kidney, upper collecting system, testis, prostate, and urethra.**
- **Renal malakoplakia is bilateral in 50% of the cases and more often produces multiple masses than a single mass.**
- **Biopsy or surgical excision is usually necessary to differentiate malakoplakia from neoplasm or other infectious process.**

ADDITIONAL IMAGES (B-E)

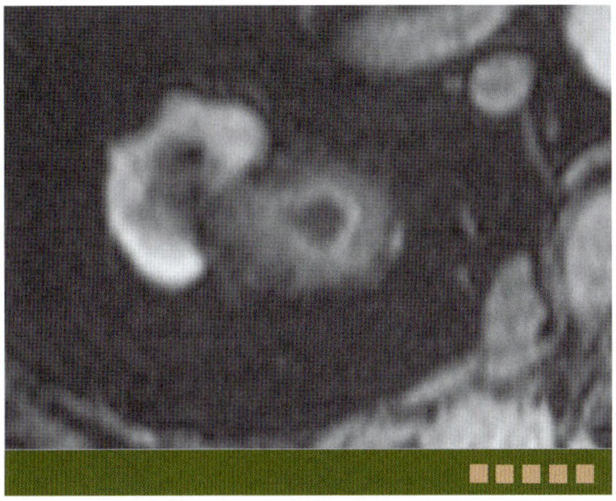

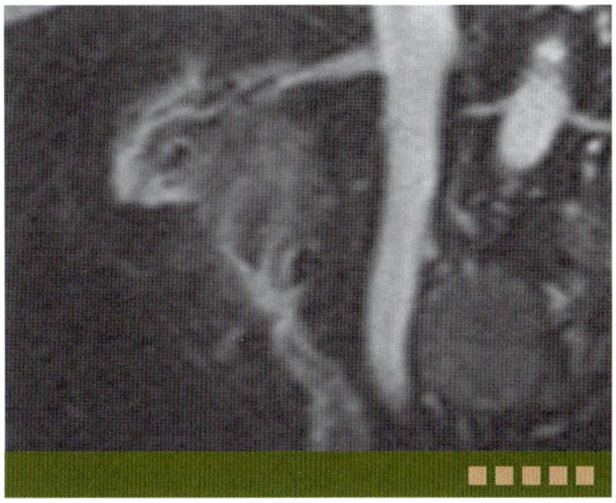

B. and C. Axial and coronal contrast-enhanced T1-WIs from a different patient show mural thickening and intense urothelial enhancement of the right renal pelvis and proximal ureter caused by biopsy-proven malakoplakia. There is mild stranding of the surrounding fat.

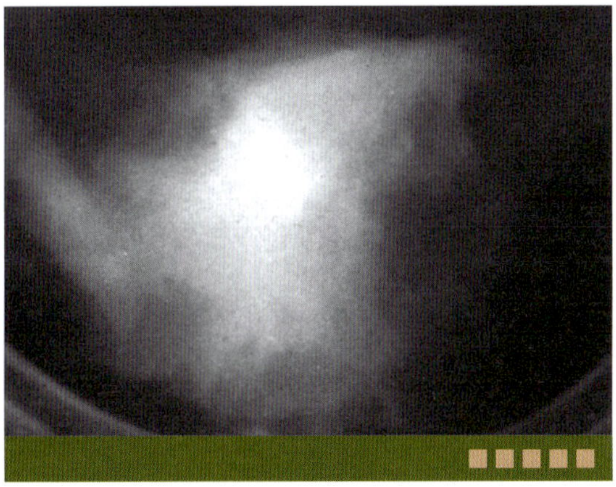

D. IVU shows extensive, irregular filling defects of the bladder due to malakoplakia.

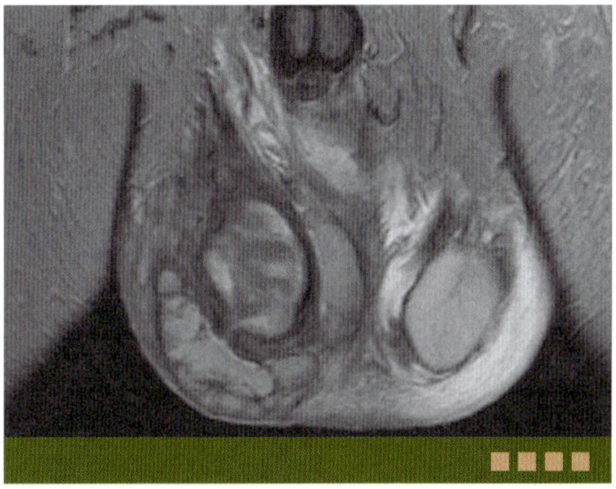

E. Coronal T2-WI of the scrotum shows extensive hyperintense necrosis due to malakoplakia of the right testis, with inferior tunica disruption and an adjacent, hyperintense scrotal collection.

DIFFERENTIAL DIAGNOSES IMAGES (F-G)

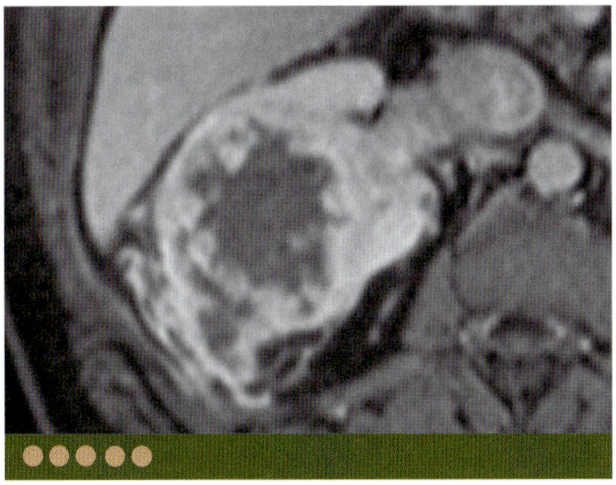

F. Renal cell carcinoma: Axial contrast-enhanced T1-WI shows a large, enhancing mass with central necrosis arising from the right kidney.

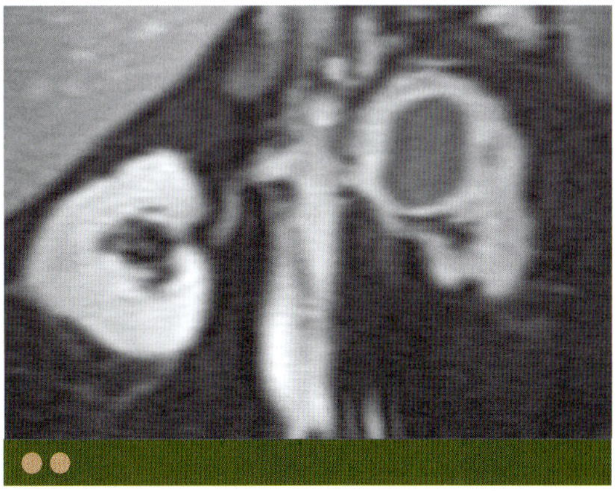

G. Focal XGP: Coronal contrast-enhanced T1-WI shows a complex, mixed solid and cystic, mass arising from the upper pole of the left kidney in a middle-aged woman with low-grade fevers.

IMAGE KEY

Common

Rare

Typical

Unusual

3–9 Reflux Nephropathy

Nancy A. Hammond

PRESENTATION

Recurrent urinary tract infections.

FINDINGS

Atrophic kidney with calyceal dilatation and adjacent cortical thinning.

DIFFERENTIAL DIAGNOSES

- *Hydronephrosis*: Typically involves the entire collecting system.
- *Fetal lobulations*: Irregular renal contours but preserved renal cortex and no associated calyceal dilatation.

COMMENTS

Reflux nephropathy is the consequence of a combination of vesicoureteral reflux (VUR) of infected urine into the kidney via an incompetent ureterovesical junction and intrarenal reflux. Pathologically, the reflux of infected urine into the kidney results in renal parenchymal damage and subsequent scarring. Reflux usually occurs in childhood, but the structural damage is permanent and often detected during early adulthood. It is the primary cause of renal failure in 10% of adults requiring renal transplantation.

Reflux can be caused by primary or secondary causes. Primary reflux occurs because of an abnormality at the UVJ, where there is a shorter than normal intramural portion of the ureter. Secondary reflux is associated with diseases that alter the anatomy of the UVJ, including diverticulum adjacent to the UVJ, posterior urethral valves, ureteral duplication anomalies, and other congenital urinary tract anomalies. Clinically, the most common manifestation of VUR and reflux nephropathy is recurrent UTIs. Adult patients present with UTIs, urinary calculi, hypertension, complications during pregnancy, proteinuria, and renal failure. Risk factors include a family history of reflux, congenital abnormalities of the urinary tract and recurrent urinary tract infections.

Radiographic signs of reflux nephropathy include renal parenchymal scarring, calyceal dilatation at the site of the parenchymal scarring, decreased renal size, and collecting system dilatation. Frequently, the initial signs of reflux nephropathy involve the upper and lower pole and spare the midportion of the disease. Parenchymal scars are broad based with clubbing and dilatation of the adjacent calyx. Because of the irregular parenchymal loss and scarring, the renal contour is typically small and irregular. Findings are typically unilateral but can be bilateral. Unaffected areas may undergo compensatory hypertrophy. This further exaggerates the irregular renal contour seen with reflux nephropathy and may simulate a renal tumor.

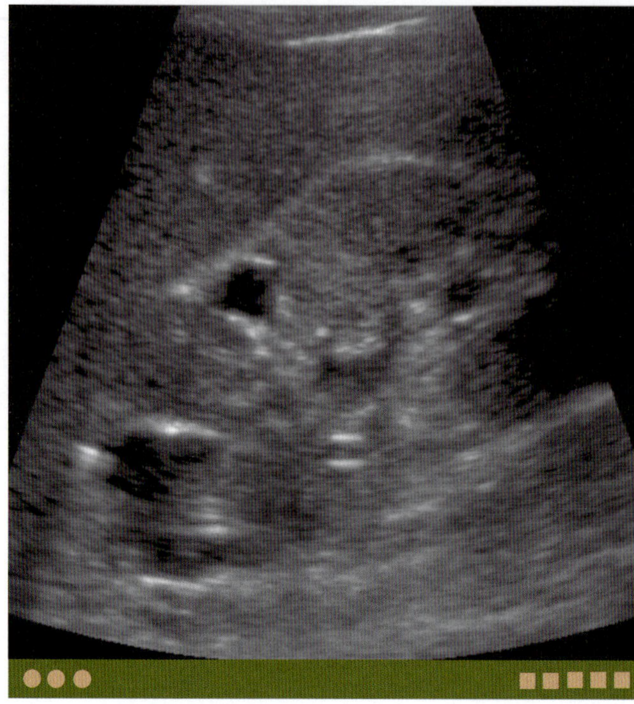

A. Longitudinal sonogram shows focal calyceal dilatation involving the upper pole of the right kidney. There is associated cortical thinning at this level. No central hydronephrosis is identified.

PEARLS

- **Reflux nephropathy is the sequela of VUR, resulting in renal parenchymal scarring.**
- **It is typically a unilateral finding but can be bilateral and is not an uncommon cause of renal insufficiency.**
- **Findings typically involve the upper and lower poles of the kidney and spare the midportion initially.**

ADDITIONAL IMAGES (B-C)

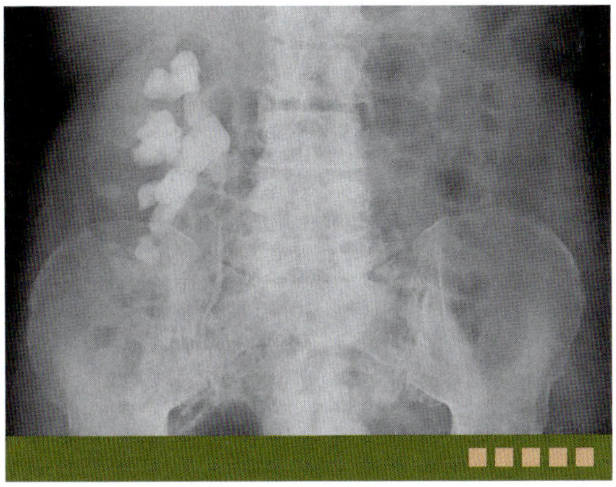

B. Contrast-enhanced IVU shows diffuse broad based clubbing of the right renal calyces with mild cortical thinning most marked at the upper pole. This patient had known history of VUR.

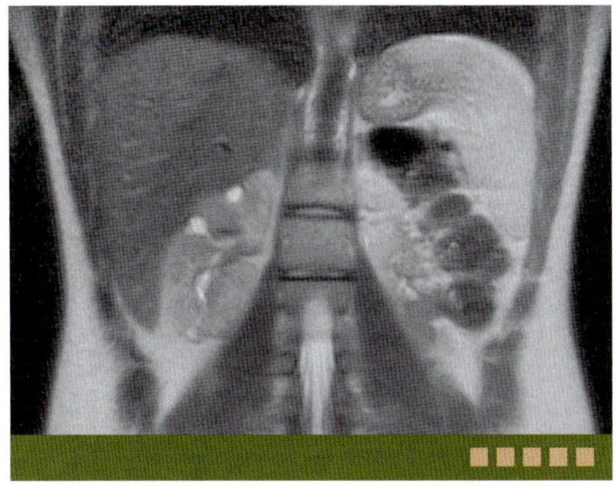

C. Coronal T2-WI shows the equivalent of findings seen in Figure A and are consistent with reflux nephropathy. Areas of calyceal dilatation and associated cortical thinning involving the right kidney are present.

IMAGE KEY

Common

Rare

Typical

Unusual

DIFFERENTIAL DIAGNOSES IMAGES (D-E)

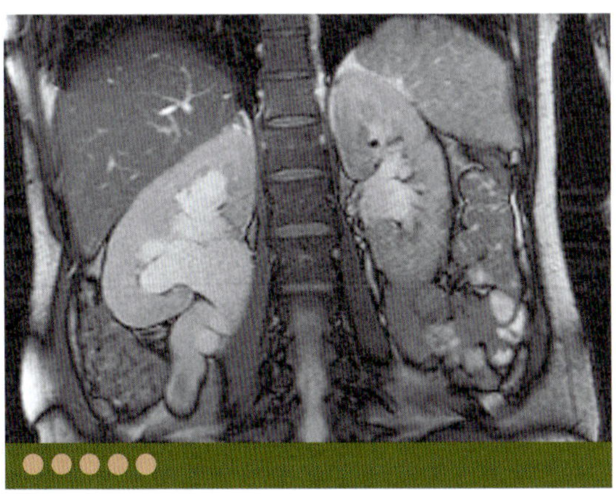

D. Hydronephrosis: Coronal T2-WI shows diffuse dilatation of the right renal collecting system and the visualized proximal right ureter. Note the preservation of the adjacent renal cortex. Hydronephrosis in this patient was secondary to pregnancy.

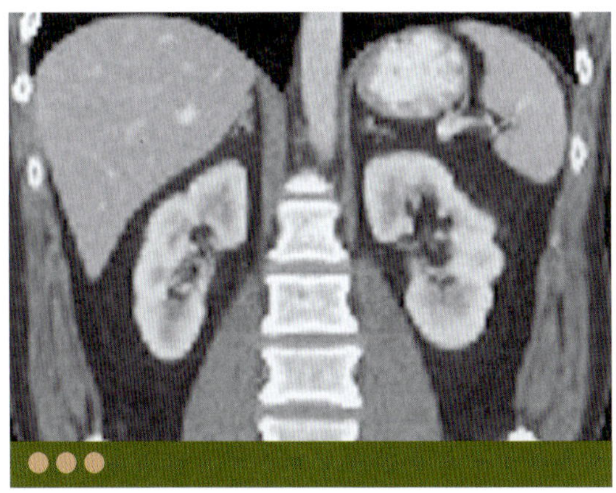

E. Fetal lobulations: Coronal CECT shows irregular renal contours bilaterally. In distinction to reflux nephropathy, there is no associated calyceal dilation or cortical loss.

CHAPTER 4

PARENCHYMAL DISEASE

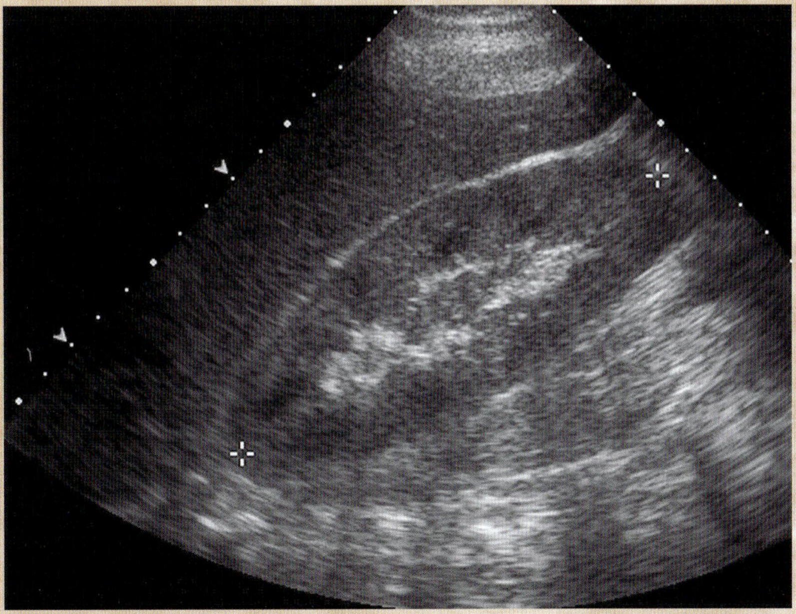

4–1 Diabetic Nephropathy

Nancy A. Hammond

PRESENTATION

Recently diagnosed diabetic.

FINDINGS

Bilateral renal enlargement with normal echogenicity.

DIFFERENTIAL DIAGNOSES

- *HIV nephropathy*: Enlarged kidneys with increased echogenicity.
- *Acute tubular necrosis*: Bilateral nephromegaly with variable appearance of echogenicity, though typically increased.
- *Amyloidosis*: Bilateral renal enlargement with increased echogenicity.
- *Lupus nephritis*: Bilateral renal enlargement with variable echogenicity; may demonstrate cortical hypoechoic areas.

COMMENTS

Diabetic nephropathy is the most common cause of chronic renal failure in the United States. It is more common in patients with insulin-dependent diabetes than noninsulin-dependent diabetic patients. Its development is highly associated with poor glycemic control. Diabetic nephropathy occurs secondary to glomerular hyperperfusion causing glomerular hypertension. This, in turn, results in increased transcapillary pressure and protein leakage into the mesangium causing microalbuminuria and glomerular sclerosis.

The radiographic appearance of diabetic nephropathy depends on the stage of disease. Ultrasound is commonly employed in evaluating renal size and echogenicity. Early in the disease, ultrasound demonstrates bilateral renal enlargement with normal echogenicity. This finding can precede the onset of glycosuria. Diabetic nephropathy is the most common cause of bilateral nephromegaly. As disease progresses, renal atrophy develops. The kidneys demonstrate increased parenchymal echogenicity with variable corticomedullary differentiation. Small, echogenic kidneys are nonspecific and can be seen in other causes of end-stage renal disease. When overt renal failure occurs, the echogenicity of the medulla equals that of the cortex. Small vessel disease resulting in ischemia may lead to papillary necrosis which is nicely demonstrated on intravenous urogram (IVU).

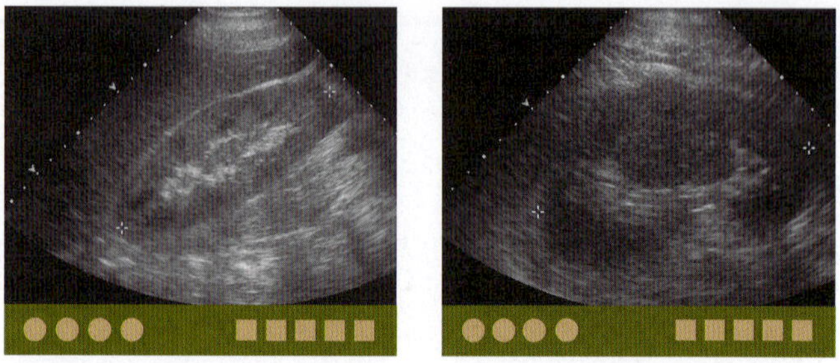

A. and B. Longitudinal sonogram shows bilateral renal enlargement with normal renal echogenicity in this patient recently diagnosed with diabetes. The right kidney measured 13.5 cm and the left measured 13.0 cm.

PEARLS

- **Most common cause of chronic renal failure in the United States.**
- **Early disease commonly presents with bilateral renal enlargement with normal echogenicity.**
- **Early sonographic findings can be seen prior to clinically evident glycosuria.**

ADDITIONAL IMAGES (C-D)

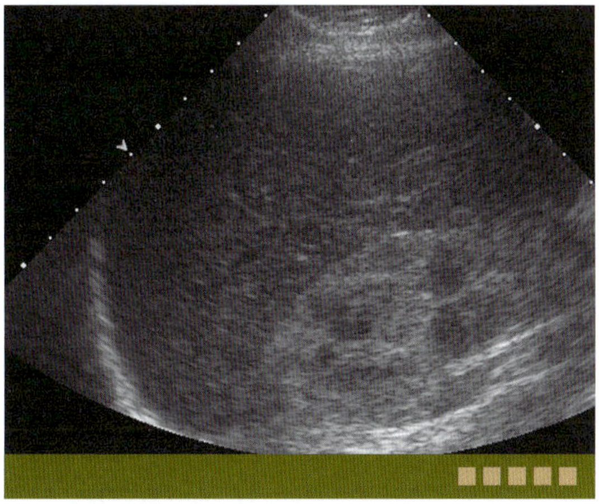

C. Longitudinal sonogram in a patient with longstanding diabetes shows markedly increased parenchymal echogenicity and thinning of the renal cortex. The kidney is atrophic.

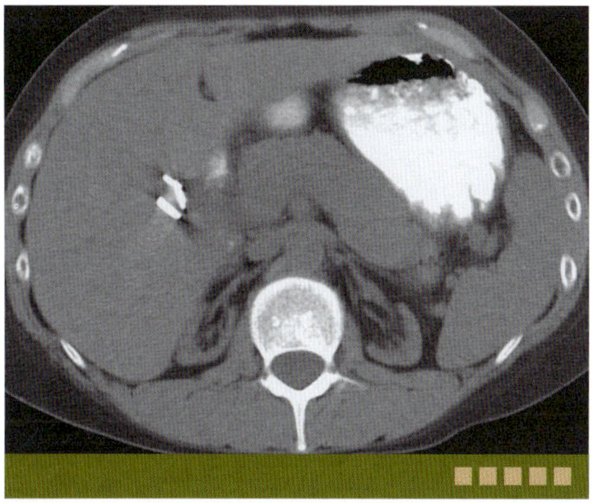

D. Axial NECT in a patient with longstanding diabetes shows bilateral renal atrophy.

DIFFERENTIAL DIAGNOSES IMAGES (E-F)

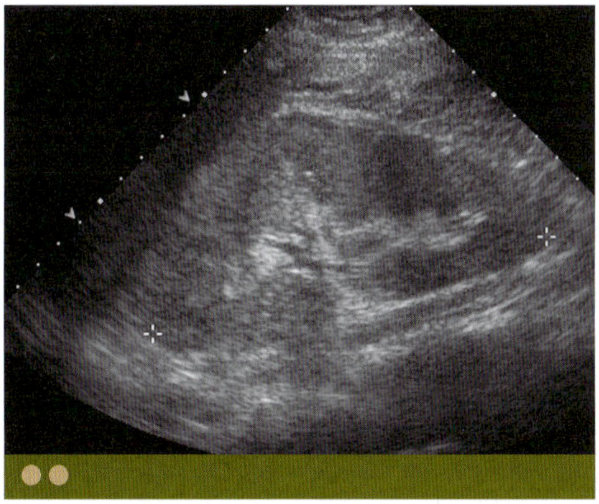

E. Lupus nephritis: Longitudinal sonogram shows renal enlargement with increased cortical echogenicity.

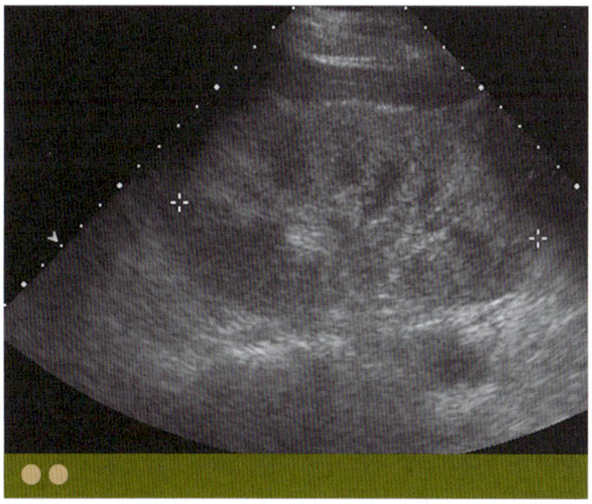

F. HIV nephropathy: Longitudinal sonogram shows renal enlargement with increased cortical echogenicity consistent with HIV nephropathy. Findings were present bilaterally.

IMAGE KEY

Common

Rare

Typical

Unusual

4–2 Lupus Nephritis

Nancy A. Hammond

PRESENTATION

Hypertension and peripheral edema.

FINDINGS

Enlarged and mildly echogenic kidneys.

DIFFERENTIAL DIAGNOSES

- *Pyelonephritis*: Similar CT findings but different clinical presentation, patients present with fever, elevated white count, and flank pain.
- *HIV nephropathy*: Similar sonographic findings of enlarged echogenic kidneys.
- *Polyarteritis nodosa*: Uncommonly, microaneurysms involving the intrarenal arteries as seen in PAN can be present in lupus nephritis.

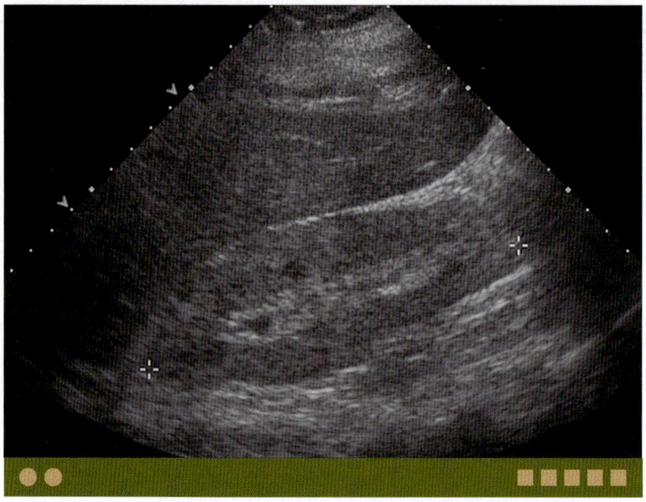

A. Longitudinal sonogram shows an enlarged, mildly echogenic right kidney in a patient with known SLE. The right kidney measured 13.8 cm. The left kidney showed similar findings (not shown).

COMMENTS

Systemic lupus erythematosus (SLE) is a chronic inflammatory disease of unknown cause affecting multiple organ systems. Most patients with SLE have renal involvement that can result in significant morbidity and mortality. Nearly all patients who undergo renal biopsy have microscopic findings of renal disease. Pathologically, immune complex deposition in the glomeruli results in glomerular necrosis and fibrosis. A vasculitis may occur and typically affects the interlobular arteries resulting in areas of infarction and scarring. Demographically, SLE is more common in black people and Hispanic people than in white people. Black people and Asian people may have a higher prevalence of more severe lupus nephritis than other ethnic groups. Lupus nephritis is more common in females, consistent with the overall prevalence of SLE being higher in females. Males with SLE have an increased prevalence of clinical renal disease with a worse prognosis. Clinically, patients with active lupus nephritis present with hypertension and peripheral edema. Proteinuria and elevated serum creatinine are also likely present.

Radiographically, the appearance of lupus nephritis depends on the stage of involvement. Ultrasound is the primary modality for evaluating renal size and echogenicity. Early in the disease, the kidneys can appear normal or enlarged and echogenic on ultrasound. With chronic lupus nephritis, the kidneys become small and demonstrate echogenicity greater than that of the hepatic parenchyma. This appearance is nonspecific and can be seen in other cases of medical renal disease. Intravenous contrast-medium should be used with caution in patients with lupus nephritis as it can aggravate renal failure. However, CT may demonstrate increased size and an abnormal, heterogeneous parenchymal enhancement pattern in lupus nephritis. Renal infarcts are common in lupus nephritis. Sonographically, acute infarcts are hypoechoic, wedge-shaped areas that extend to the renal cortex. Contrast-enhanced MR and CT demonstrate peripheral, wedge-shaped areas of decreased enhancement. Chronically, infarcts result in cortical loss and renal contour abnormalities. With longstanding disease, there may be loss of the corticomedullary differentiation on contrast-enhanced studies. Uncommonly, microaneurysms similar to those of PAN may be present.

PEARLS

- **The kidneys are commonly involved in patients with SLE with the prevalence estimated to be 50%.**
- **Complications of lupus nephritis include nephritic syndrome and renal vein thrombosis (rare).**
- **Imaging findings are nonspecific and depend on the stage of the disease.**
- **Ultrasound is the primary modality in evaluating patients with lupus nephritis.**

ADDITIONAL IMAGES (B-D)

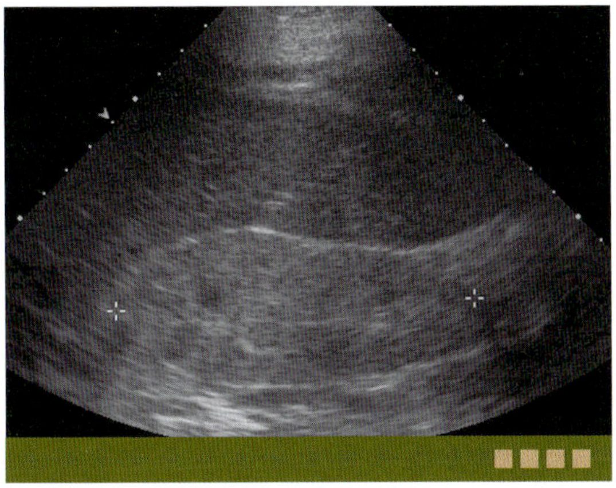

B. Longitudinal sonogram performed in the same patient as Figure A, obtained 4 months later, shows interval decrease in the size of the right kidney (measuring 10.5 cm) and diffusely increasing echogenicity.

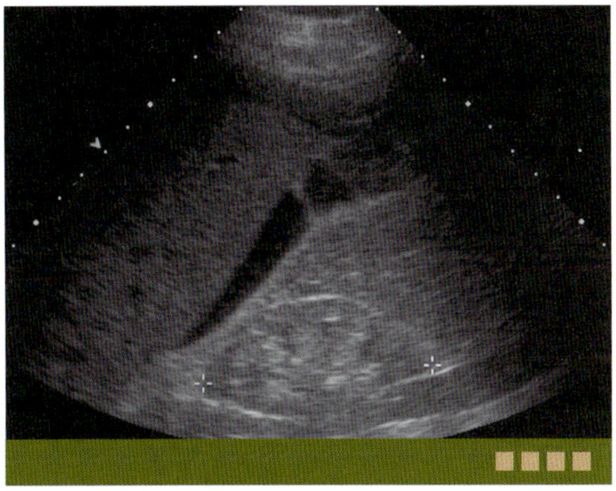

C. Longitudinal sonogram of a patient with chronic renal failure shows an echogenic, atrophic right kidney.

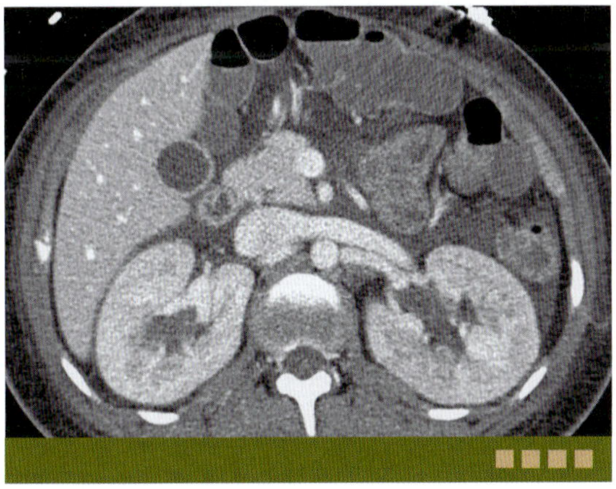

D. Axial CECT shows heterogeneous parenchymal enhancement of the both kidneys as can be seen in active lupus nephritis.

DIFFERENTIAL DIAGNOSES IMAGES (E-F)

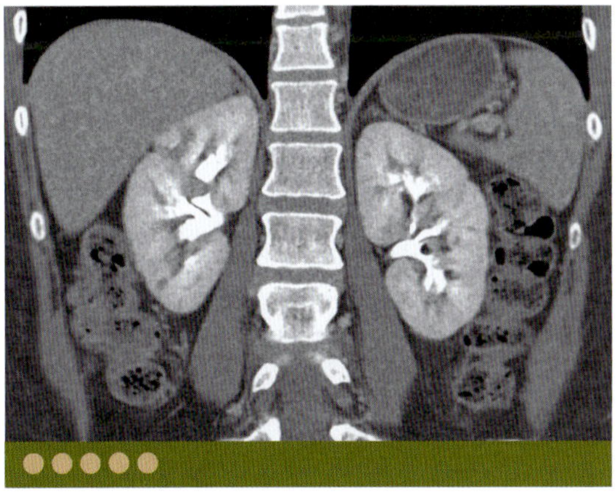

E. Pyelonephritis: Coronal CECT shows bilateral striated nephrograms in a patient with clinically suspected pyelonephritis.

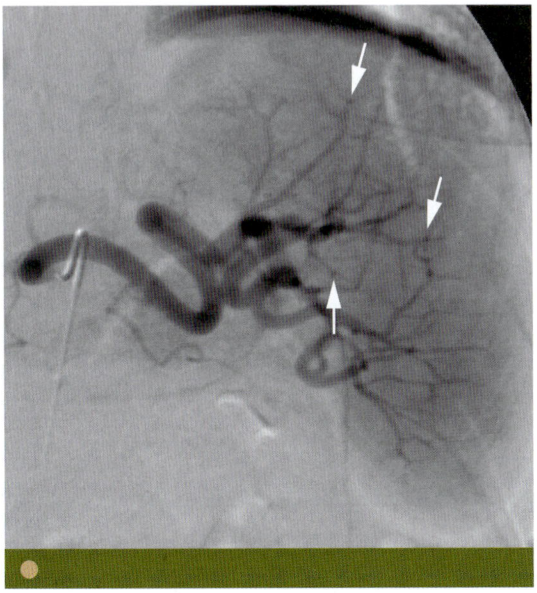

F. Polyarteritis nodosa: Selective left renal artery injection shows microaneurysms of the intrarenal arteries (arrow). This finding can rarely be seen in patients with lupus nephritis but is more characteristic in those with PAN.

IMAGE KEY

Common

Rare

Typical

Unusual

4–3 Human Immunodeficiency Virus Nephropathy

Frank H. Miller

PRESENTATION

Proteinuria, elevated creatinine, and enlarged kidneys.

FINDINGS

Bilaterally enlarged kidneys with increased cortical echogenicity and poor corticomedullary differentiation on ultrasound.

DIFFERENTIAL DIAGNOSES

- *Amyloidosis*: Can have enlarged echogenic kidneys; but rare entity, usually can be distinguished on the basis of history and patient population.
- *Chronic medical renal disease resulting from a number of etiologies*: Generally small kidneys unlike HIV where enlarged.

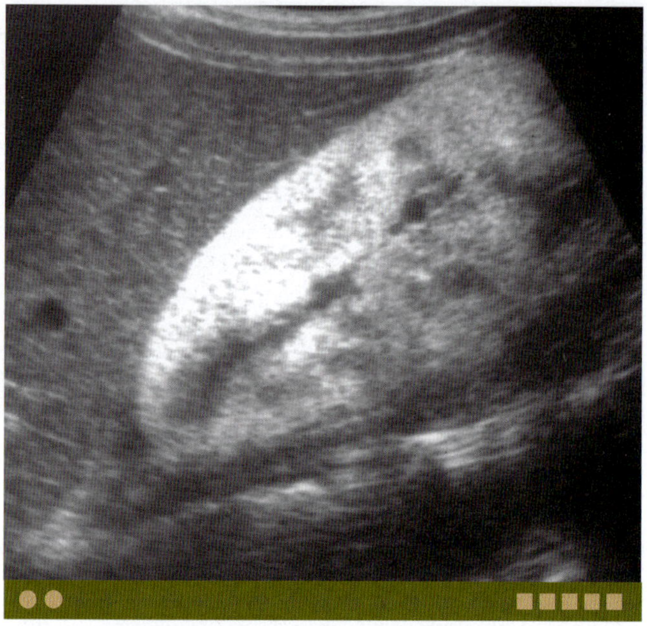

A. Longitudinal sonogram shows very echogenic kidney which is large, measuring more than 12 cm in length, with poor corticomedullary differentiation.

COMMENTS

HIV-associated nephropathy (HIVAN) consists of proteinuria, azotemia, normal pressure, normal-to-large kidneys on sonography, and focal segmental glomerulosclerosis on renal biopsy. HIVAN is more common in IV drug abusers than in the homosexual population. Patients characteristically have heavy proteinuria and large kidneys. Renal disease may be an early, unsuspected manifestation of HIV infection. In the past, patients rapidly progressed to renal failure and end-stage renal disease requiring dialysis. Antiretroviral medication for AIDS has significantly improved the outcome in these patients.

HIVAN is best diagnosed by ultrasound examination. The sonographic findings include bilaterally enlarged kidneys with increased cortical echogenicity. With HIVAN, there is loss of the normal corticomedullary differentiation. These findings are the result of focal and segmental glomerulosclerosis and dilated tubules filled with proteinaceous material. Other types of glomerulopathy have also been described. There is no direct correlation between the extent of disease related to HIVAN and renal echogenicity. In contrast, the kidneys with chronic medical renal disease, although of increased echogenicity, generally become significantly smaller than normal when they become echogenic.

Sonography is preferred for diagnosis to show the findings of HIVAN. The diagnosis is more difficult with CT or MR scans, and the only nonspecific finding may be enlarged kidneys with poor corticomedullary differentiation on unenhanced images and following contrast. These patients may have elevated creatinine for which contrast-enhanced CT and MR studies need to be avoided.

PEARLS

- **HIVAN comprises proteinuria, azotemia, normal pressure, normal-to-large kidneys on sonography, and focal segmental glomerulosclerosis on renal biopsy.**
- **Bilateral enlarged echogenic kidneys should raise suspicion of HIVAN.**
- **Unlike HIVAN, chronic medical renal disease is generally associated with small echogenic kidneys.**
- **Diagnosis of HIV nephropathy is best made on ultrasound compared to CT or MR.**
- **The only finding on CT or MR scans may be enlarged kidneys with poor corticomedullary differentiation following contrast.**

ADDITIONAL IMAGES (B-E)

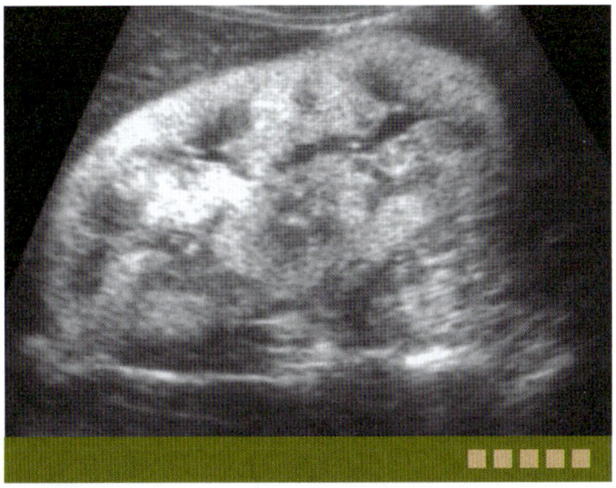

B. HIVAN: Longitudinal sonogram in another patient with HIVAN shows a large echogenic kidney with poor corticomedullary differentiation.

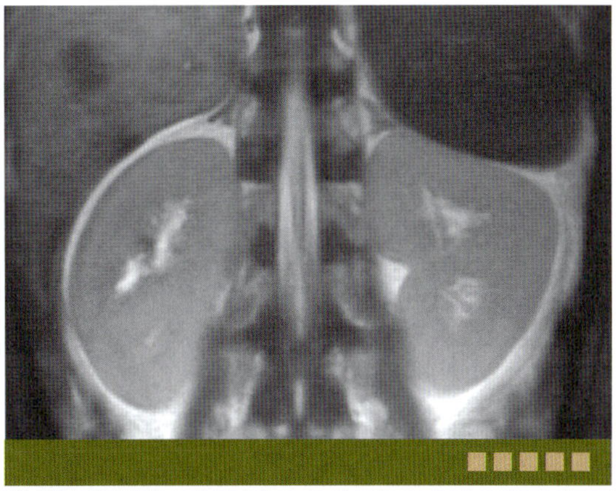

C. HIVAN: Coronal T2-WI shows large kidneys with poor corticomedullary differentiation.

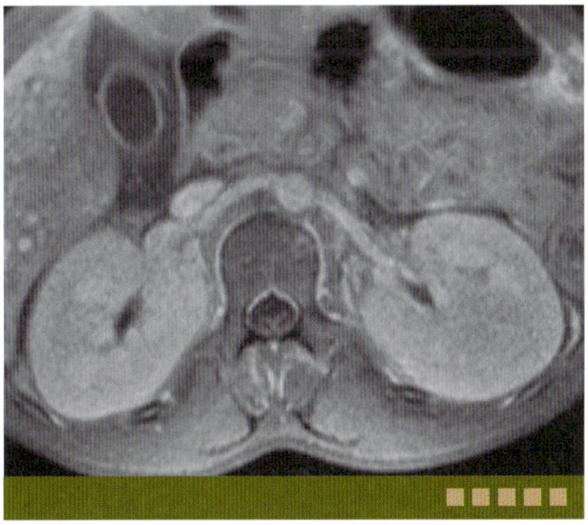

D. Axial contrast-enhanced T1-WI shows edematous kidneys with poor enhancement and corticomedullary differentiation. Note the marked gallbladder wall thickening.

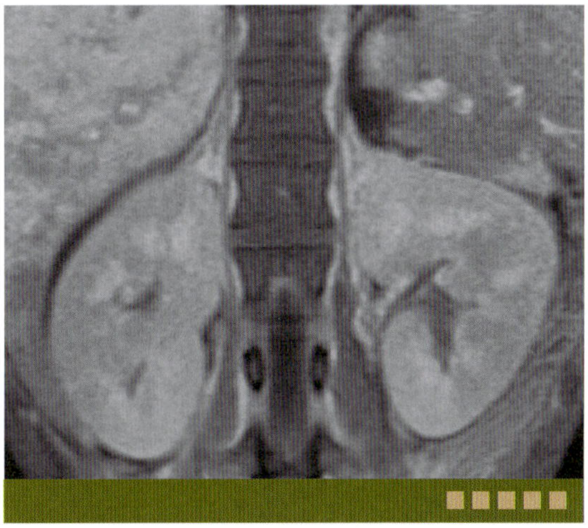

E. Coronal contrast-enhanced T1-WI shows enlarged kidneys with poor enhancement and excretion associated with HIVAN. The patient also had hepatitis.

DIFFERENTIAL DIAGNOSES IMAGES (F-G)

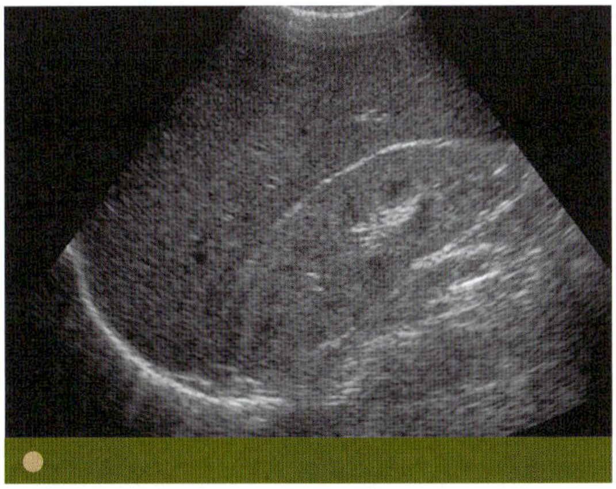

F. Amyloidosis: Longitudinal sonogram shows enlarged echogenic kidneys. This example shows renal corticomedullary differentiation is maintained relative to those with HIVAN.

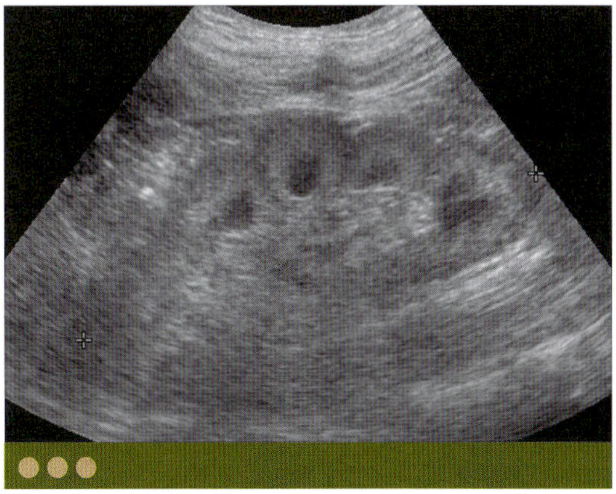

G. Chronic medical disease caused by lupus nephritis: Longitudinal sonogram in patients with SLE shows small kidneys which are echogenic.

IMAGE KEY

Common

Rare

Typical

Unusual

4–4 Paroxysmal Nocturnal Hemoglobinuria

Frank H. Miller

PRESENTATION

Hemoglobinuria, iron deficiency anemia, bleeding, and venous thrombosis.

FINDINGS

Low-signal intensity in the renal cortex on T1-weighted, T2-weighted, gradient-echo images caused by hemosiderin deposition.

DIFFERENTIAL DIAGNOSES

- *Other causes of intravascular hemolysis, such as mechanical hemolysis and hemolytic anemia*: Heavy iron deposition in the liver and spleen, unlike paroxysmal nocturnal hemoglobinuria (PNH).
- *Sickle cell disease*: Unlike PNH, there is low-signal intensity of the spleen because of extravascular hemolysis.

COMMENTS

PNH is a rare disorder associated with abnormal red blood cell breakdown causing hemoglobin to release into the urine. This leads to the urine becoming darker. This is most evident following awakening as the urine concentrates at night, making it appear significantly darker leading to the term, PNH. The clinical triad associated with the condition includes hemolytic anemia, pancytopenia, and thrombosis. It affects men and women evenly and can occur at any age.

PNH is an acquired hematopoietic stem cell disorder characterized by increased sensitivity of the erythrocytes to complement with resultant intravascular hemolysis. Infections, drugs and immunizations, exercise, transfusions, and surgery can precipitate hemolysis, but the cause is often unknown. When there is sufficient intravascular hemolysis to saturate the plasma, the excess hemoglobin is filtered by the renal glomeruli, partially reabsorbed in the proximal tubules, and stored as hemosiderin. The condition is associated with vascular thrombosis. The liver and spleen are spared the iron deposition unless the patient has had significant number of blood transfusions leading to hemosiderosis.

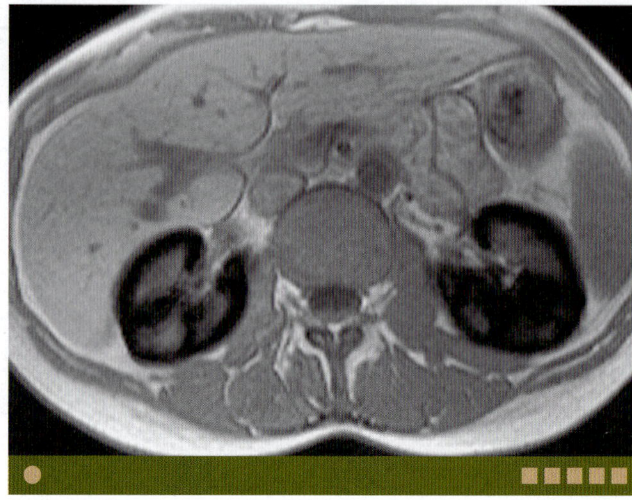

A. Axial T1-WI shows low-signal intensity involving the renal cortex.

Hemosiderin deposition in the renal cortex is best seen on MR imaging, which shows low-signal intensity of the renal cortex on T1- and T2-weighted images, with reversed renal cortex-medulla differentiation on T1-WI. The iron deposition is best seen on T2- and T2-weighted gradient-echo images. When in and opposed phase images are obtained, the signal drop is best seen on the in phase images when these images are of a longer TE than the opposed phase images as these are more T2-weighted than the opposed phase images.

PEARLS

- **PNH is associated with hemolytic anemia, pancytopenia and thrombosis.**
- **MR is the best method to diagnose PNH.**
- **Low-signal intensity on T2-WI involving the renal cortex suggests PNH.**
- **PNH tends not to affect the liver and spleen.**

ADDITIONAL IMAGES (B-E)

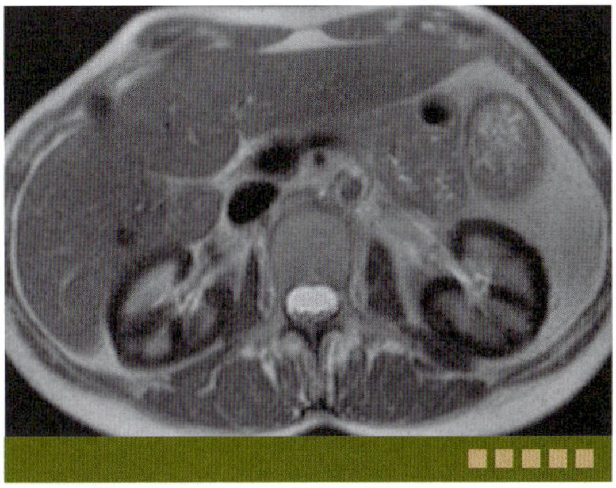

B. Axial T2-WI shows low-signal intensity cortex because of iron deposition. The extensive iron deposition from PNH causes the cortex to be dark not only on T2-WI but also on T1-WI.

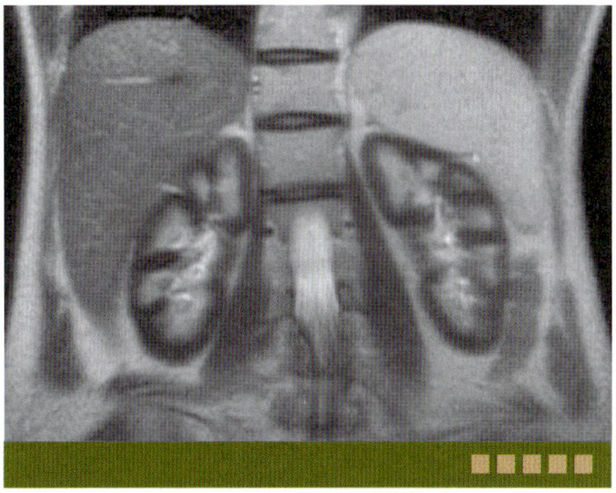

C. Coronal T2-WI nicely shows the extensive iron deposition involving the renal cortex of both kidneys.

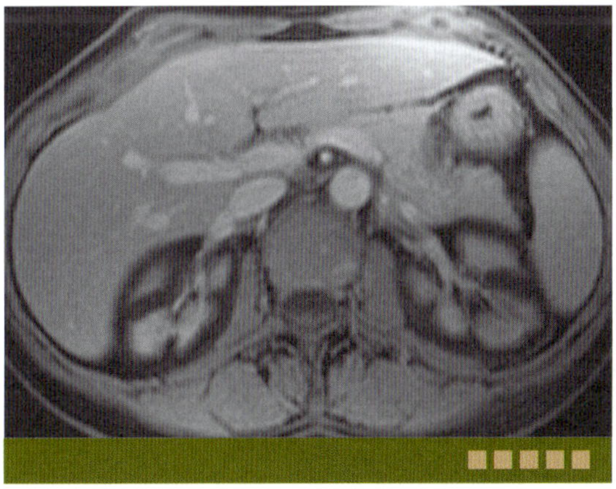

D. Axial contrast-enhanced T1-WI shows enhancement of the kidneys with the cortex remaining dark.

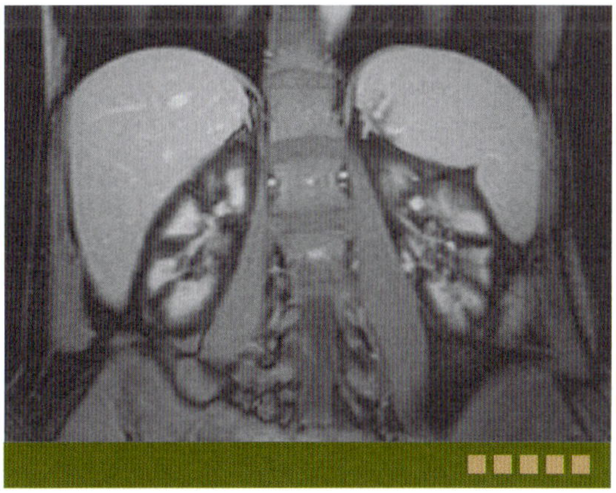

E. Coronal contrast-enhanced T1-WI shows enhancement of the kidneys with the cortex and renal pyramids remaining dark.

DIFFERENTIAL DIAGNOSES IMAGE

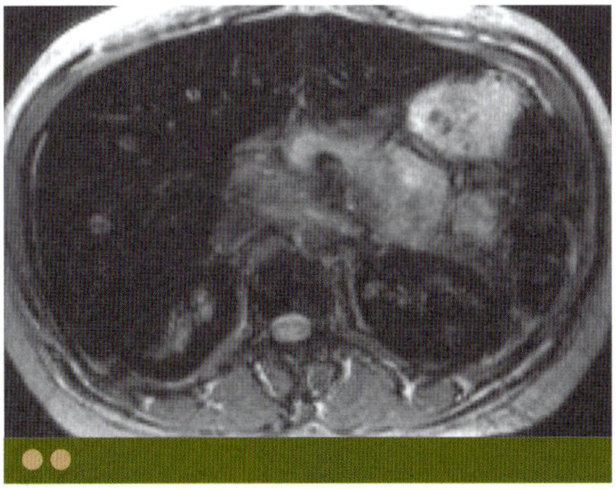

F. Sickle cell disease: Axial T2-WI shows low-signal intensity involving the renal cortex associated with sickle cell disease caused by acute hemolysis with iron deposition in the renal convoluted tubules. The liver and spleen appear dark most likely related to extravascular hemolysis and blood transfusions leading to hemosiderosis.

IMAGE KEY

Common

Rare

Typical

Unusual

4–5 Radiation Nephropathy

Frank H. Miller

PRESENTATION

Hypertension, history of radiation.

FINDINGS

CECT shows atrophy of medial aspect of left kidney with volume loss.

DIFFERENTIAL DIAGNOSES

- *Acute pyelonephritis*: Would not show linear borders because of radiation port; seen as striated nephrogram or mass-like lesion.
- *Renal infarct*: Seen as wedge-shaped lesion or volume loss without linear borders.

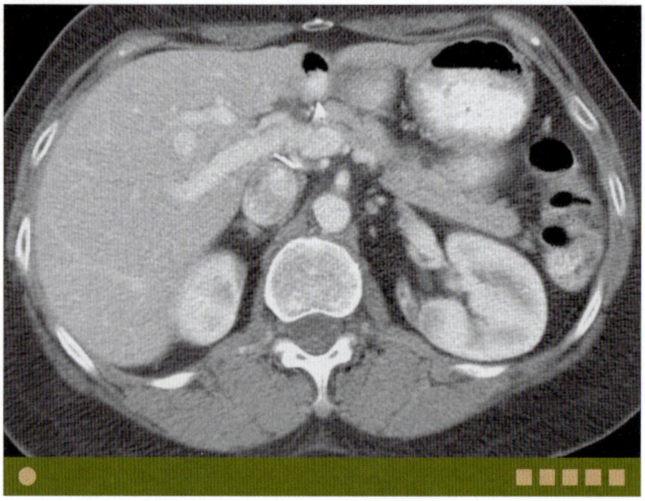

A. Axial CECT shows atrophy of medial aspect of left kidney caused by radiation nephropathy.

COMMENTS

The kidneys are very sensitive to radiation. Radiation-induced injuries occur in proportion to the dose administered and the volume of renal tissue exposed. The threshold dose has been reported as over 2500 rads over 5 weeks. Acute radiation nephritis occurs at 6 months to 1 year after therapy. Despite this term, the condition is neither acute nor does it represent a nephritis with pathologic correlation showing nephrosclerosis. When diffuse and severe, patients may present with anemia, edema, hypertension, proteinuria, uremia, and decreased or absent urination. Deaths may occur because of malignant hypertension. Chronic radiation nephritis typically occurs 1 to 5 years after therapy. Changes are irreversible and progressive. The addition of chemotherapy increases the likelihood of injury. Findings include progressive nephrosclerosis, glomerulosclerosis, tubular atrophy, and interstitial fibrosis.

This case illustrates the CT findings of acute segmental radiation nephritis in patients who received radiation to the spine. Clues to the diagnosis include the geographic linear borders corresponding to the lateral limits of the radiation port. The imaging features include decreased parenchymal thickness and atrophy of the kidney related to the radiation field. Decreased renal enhancement and density may be seen in the portion of the kidney within the radiation port. A similar imaging appearance of linear borders caused by radiation can be seen with involvement of the lungs and the liver.

Patients with radiation nephropathy need to be followed by nephrologists to avoid further renal damage and to undergo hypertension treatment and avoid nephrotoxic medications.

PEARLS

- **Kidneys are very sensitive to radiation.**
- **Chronic radiation nephropathy is seen 1 to 5 years after therapy.**
- **Changes are irreversible and progressive.**
- **Suspect radiation nephropathy when geographic linear atrophy and decreased enhancement of the kidneys.**

ADDITIONAL IMAGE

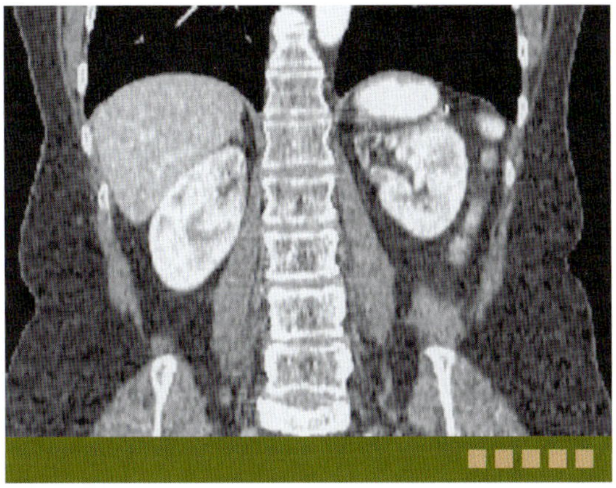

B. Coronal CECT shows atrophy and decreased enhancement of the medial aspect of the left kidney from radiation nephropathy in patient with a history of Hodgkin disease.

DIFFERENTIAL DIAGNOSES IMAGES (C-D)

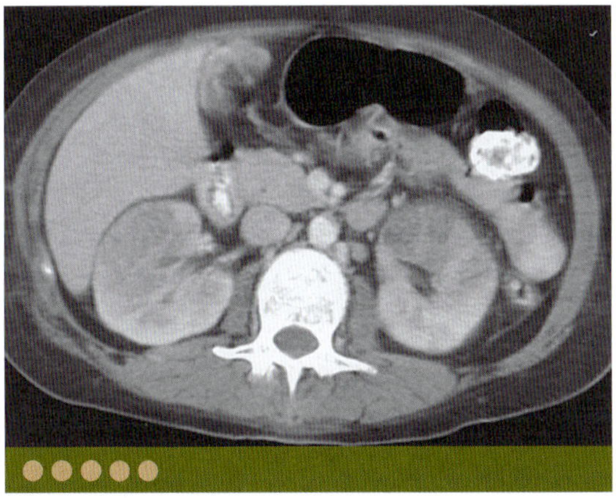

C. Acute pyelonephritis: Axial CECT shows bilateral striated nephrograms from acute pyelonephritis. The involvement is not linear along a radiation port unlike radiation nephropathy.

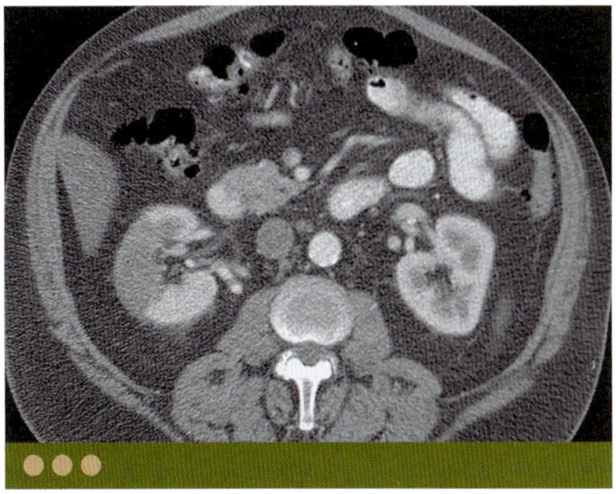

D. Renal infarct: Axial CECT shows right wedge-shaped area of decreased enhancement in kidney from renal infarct.

IMAGE KEY

Common

Rare

Typical

Unusual

4–6 Cortical Nephrocalcinosis

Nancy A. Hammond

PRESENTATION

Asymptomatic patient with history of chronic glomerulonephritis.

FINDINGS

Peripheral calcifications involving the renal cortex on nonenhanced CT (NECT).

DIFFERENTIAL DIAGNOSIS

- *Medullary nephrocalcinosis*: Medullary distribution of calcification.

COMMENTS

The term "nephrocalcinosis" refers to diffuse, fine, renal parenchymal calcification that is radiologically demonstrable and is either cortical or medullary in location. Only 5% of cases of nephrocalcinosis are cortical and the remaining 95% are medullary. No racial or ethnic predilection has been observed in nephrocalcinosis, and both sexes are affected equally. Clinical presentation depends on the underlying cause.

Cortical nephrocalcinosis is caused by the deposition of dystrophic calcification secondary to a prior renal insult. The deposition occurs along the periphery of the kidney and central septa of Bertin but spares the medullary pyramids. The most common entities causing cortical nephrocalcinosis are chronic glomerulonephritis and acute cortical necrosis. Chronic glomerulonephritis can be seen in Alport syndrome, oxalosis, and renal transplant rejection. Acute cortical necrosis is seen with toxic ingestions (ethylene glycol) or exposures (methoxyflurane) and acute vascular insults.

Sonography and CT detect nephrocalcinosis earlier than conventional radiographs. If the attenuation of the affected renal parenchyma exceeds 100 HU on CT, the increased density of the kidneys will be visible on conventional radiographs. Sonographically, the renal cortex appears echogenic and typically does not shadow. NECT shows

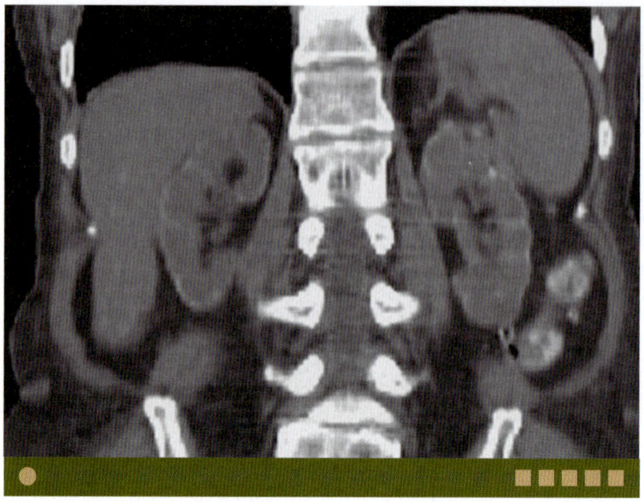

A. Axial NECT shows diffuse peripheral hyperdensity involving the renal cortex with sparing of the medullary pyramids.

high attenuation of the cortex. When visible on conventional radiographs, cortical nephrocalcinosis shows thin peripheral lines of calcification with a "tram-track" appearance when seen in profile or diffuse punctuate calcifications representing necrotic cortical tubules. Most patients with cortical nephrocalcinosis have global renal atrophy with small, smooth kidneys.

Treatment is directed toward the underlying cause of the cortical nephrocalcinosis.

PEARLS

- **Cortical nephrocalcinosis is a rare entity comprising only 5% of all cases of nephrocalcinosis.**
- **Most commonly seen with chronic glomerulonephritis and acute cortical necrosis.**
- **CT and sonography detect findings earlier than conventional radiographs.**

ADDITIONAL IMAGES (B-D)

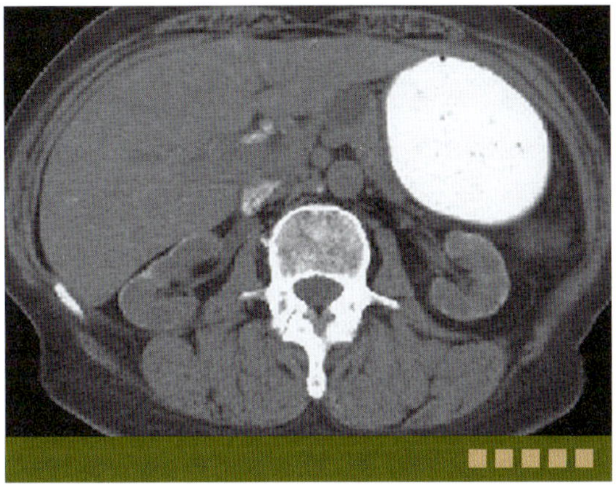

B. Coronal NECT in the same patient further shows the extent of the calcification involving the renal cortex.

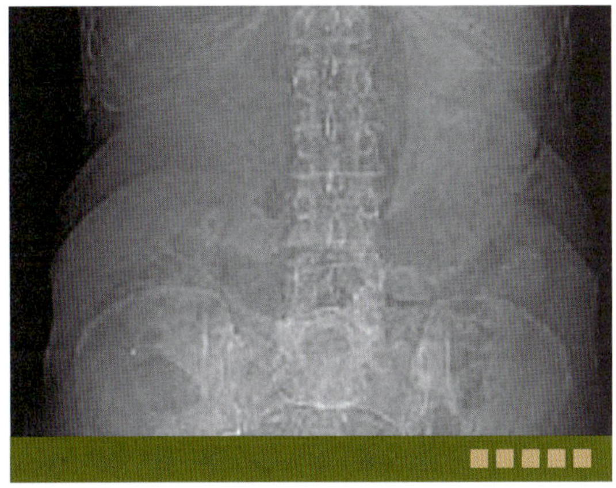

C. Coronal CT scout from the same patient fails to reveal the cortical calcifications seen on CT.

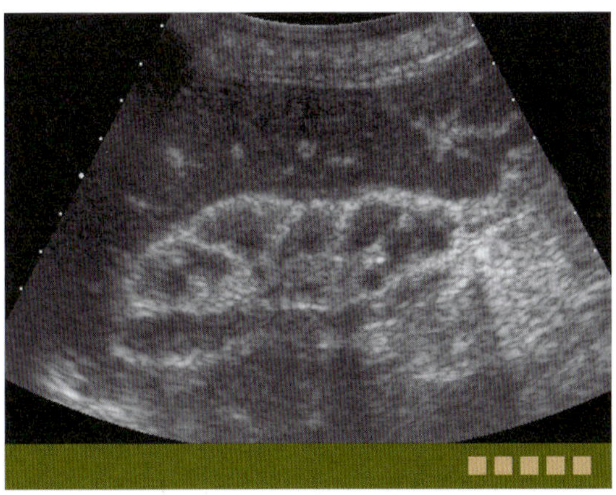

D. Longitudinal sonogram in the same patient shows peripheral hyperechogenicity occupying the renal cortex with sparing of the renal medulla. No associated shadowing is noted.

DIFFERENTIAL DIAGNOSES IMAGES (E-G)

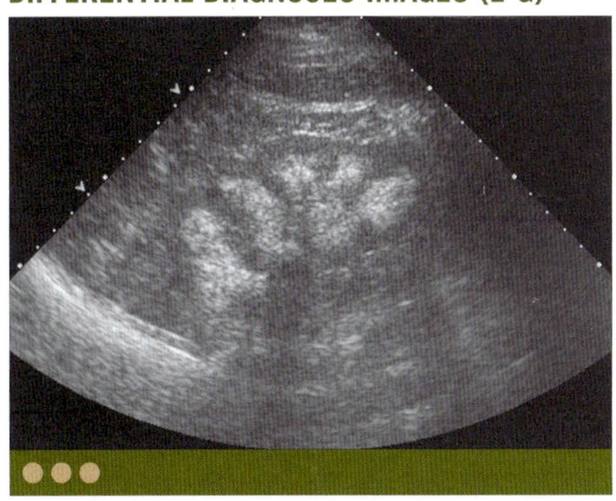

E. Medullary nephrocalcinosis: Longitudinal sonogram shows hyerechoic foci involving the renal medulla compatible with medullary nephrocalcinosis. No posterior acoustic shadowing is present.

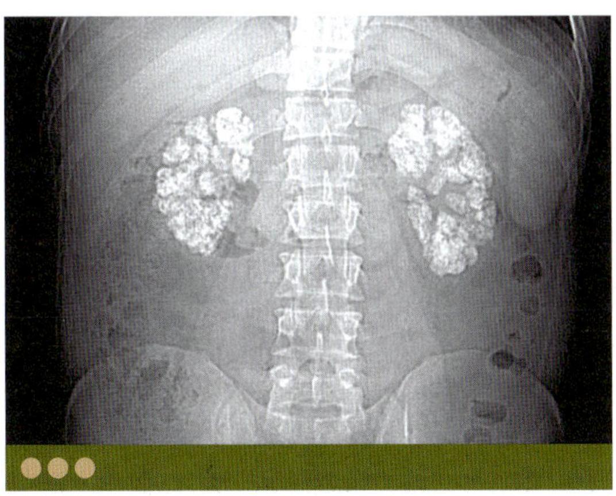

F. Medullary nephrocalcinosis: Coronal CT scout shows dense calcifications in the expected location of the renal pyramids compatible with medullary nephrocalcinosis.

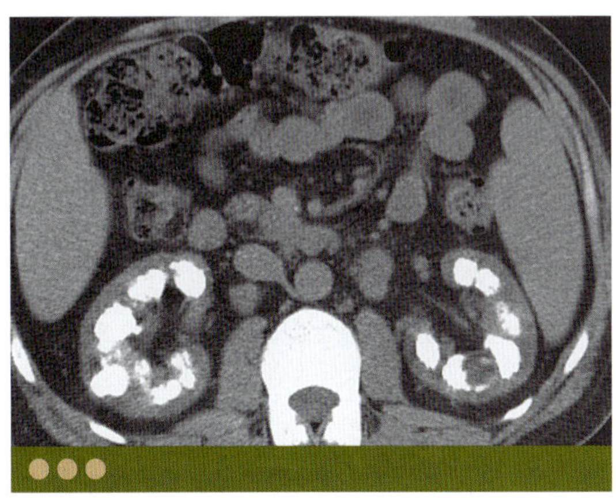

G. Medullary nephrocalcinosis: Axial NECT in the same patient as Figure F shows dense calcification throughout the renal pyramids bilaterally. These images show the different distribution of medullary nephrocalcinosis compared to cortical nephrocalcinosis.

IMAGE KEY

Common

Rare

Typical

Unusual

4-7 Medullary Nephrocalcinosis from Distal Renal Tubular Acidosis

Frank H. Miller

PRESENTATION

May be asymptomatic, showing symptoms of renal colic, hematuria, and urinary tract infections (UTIs).

FINDINGS

Extensive calcifications involving the medullary potions of the kidney.

DIFFERENTIAL DIAGNOSES

- *Other types of medullary nephrocalcinosis*: Generally not as extensive calcifications; medullary sponge kidney (MSK), for example, can be unilateral or segmental; can be associated with brush border appearance after contrast.
- *Cortical nephrocalcinosis*: Affects cortex instead of medullary portion of kidney.

COMMENTS

Medullary nephrocalcinosis is calcification in the tubules of the medullary pyramids. It is generally bilateral and symmetric, as it is associated with metabolic causes. MSK can be unilateral or segmental. Calcifications in the medullary portion of the kidney are much more common than cortical calcifications.

The most common etiologies of medullary nephrocalcinosis are hyperparathyroidism followed by MSK and renal tubular acidosis. Other causes of medullary nephrocalcinosis include causes of hypercalcemia including sarcoidosis, milk alkali syndrome, certain medications such as amphotericin B, and causes of hyperoxaluria. The presence of extensive medullary calcifications should suggest renal tubular acidosis as a cause for medullary calcifications over the other causes.

Renal tubular acidosis is associated with a defect in the renal tubule that prevents the kidneys to excrete acidic urine, leading to the development of stones in the tubules. The presence of extensive calcifications should suggest distal type of renal tubular acidosis. The proximal type of renal tubular acidosis does not typically lead to imaging abnormalities. With distal renal tubular acidosis, the renal function is usually preserved fairly well. Complications include urolithiasis. Renal insufficiency may result from severe longstanding renal tubular acidosis.

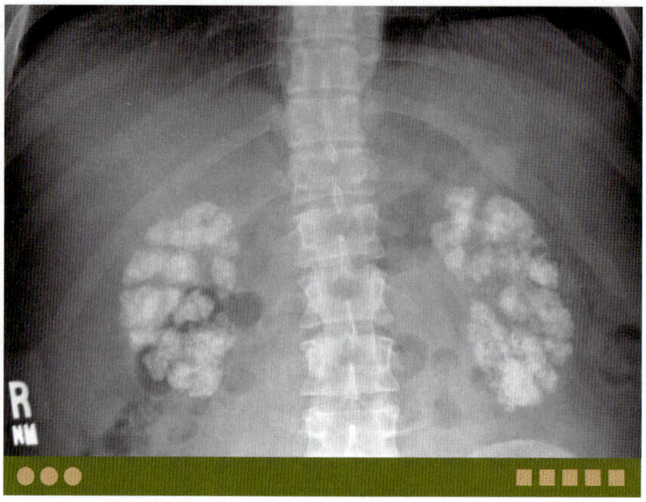

A. Abdominal radiograph shows extensive medullary calcifications which are more extensive than those typically seen in renal MSK or other causes of medullary nephrocalcinosis.

Ultrasound shows that the pyramids are echogenic with shadowing from stones when stones are dense and large enough. Abdominal radiographs show renal medullary calcifications. Unenhanced CT is more sensitive than radiographs in showing the calcifications in the medulla. Associated ureteral stones may be seen well using unenhanced CT.

PEARLS

- **Medullary nephrocalcinosis is calcification in the tubules of the medullary pyramids.**
- **Medullary nephrocalcinosis generally is bilateral and symmetric, as it is associated with metabolic causes.**
- **Most common etiologies are hyperparathyroidism, followed by benign tubular ectasia (MSK) and renal tubular acidosis.**
- **Other causes include the various causes of hypercalcemia.**
- **Extensive medullary calcifications should suggest renal tubular acidosis (distal type).**

ADDITIONAL IMAGES (B-C)

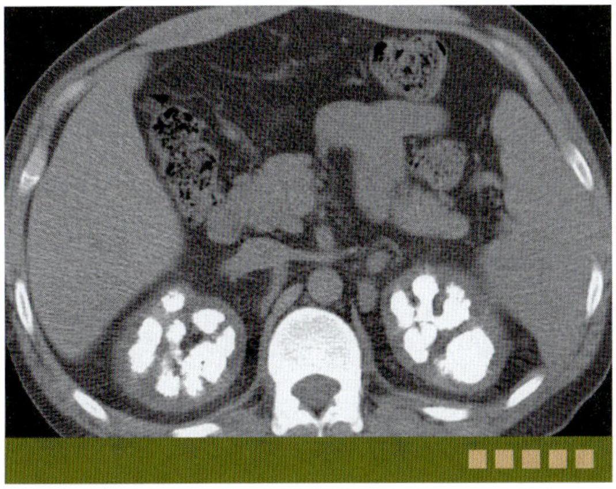

B. Renal tubular acidosis (distal type): Axial NECT shows extensive medullary calcifications from renal tubular acidosis.

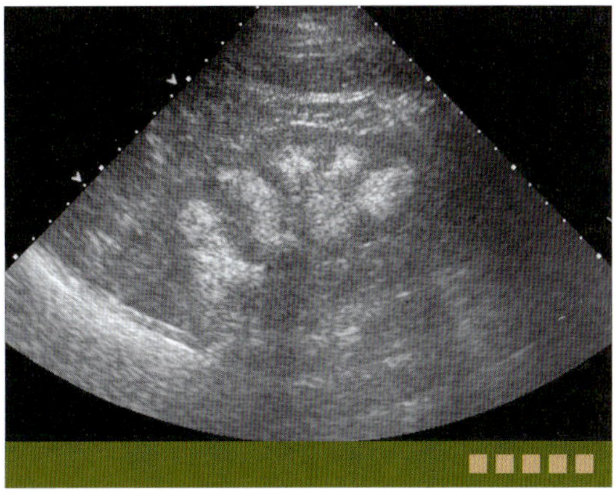

C. Medullary nephrocalcinosis: Longitudinal sonogram shows hyperechoic foci involving the renal medulla compatible with medullary nephrocalcinosis.

DIFFERENTIAL DIAGNOSES IMAGES (D-E)

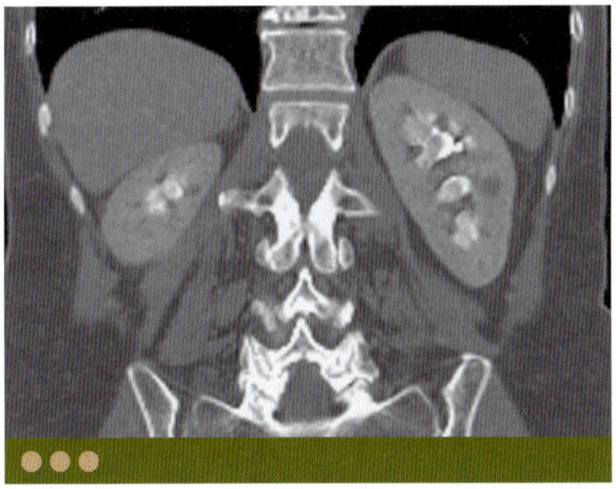

D. Medullary sponge kidney: Coronal CECT shows brush border appearance to the collecting tubules with dilatation.

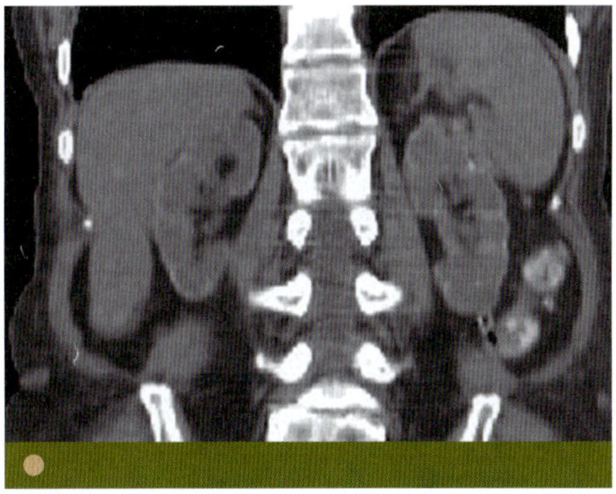

E. Cortical nephrocalcinosis: Coronal NECT shows diffuse peripheral hyperdensity involving the renal cortex with sparing of the medullary pyramids.

IMAGE KEY

Common

Rare

Typical

Unusual

4–8 Renal Medullary Sponge

Frank H. Miller

PRESENTATION

Most patients are asymptomatic; symptoms include renal colic, hematuria, and dysuria.

FINDINGS

Calcifications involving the medullary portion of the kidney with paint brush-like striations following contrast.

DIFFERENTIAL DIAGNOSES

- *Other causes of medullary nephrocalcinosis (hyperparathyroidism, renal tubular acidosis, etc.)*: Can often be distinguished on the basis of history; other causes are more often bilateral and symmetric.
- *Normal variant*: Papillary brush from contrast; lacks nephrocalcinosis and distinct streaks.
- *Cortical nephrocalcinosis*: Affects cortex and not medulla.

COMMENTS

Medullary sponge kidney (MSK), also referred to as renal tubular ectasia, is one of the main causes of medullary nephrocalcinosis. Other causes include hyperparathyroidism and renal tubular acidosis and causes of hypercalcemia. MSK is characterized by cystic dilatation of the renal collecting tubules in the papillae. It is associated with microscopic and large medullary cysts. Bilateral involvement is more common; although may be unilateral and segmental, unlike other causes of medullary nephrocalcinosis which tend to be bilateral and symmetric. Medullary sponge has calcifications generally in the ectatic collecting ducts instead of the renal cortex. The frequency in the general population has been estimated to be 1 in 5,000 to 10,000 people. Patients tend to present between the ages 20 to 50 years, and the prevalence is more common in women. Complications include renal stones, infections, and hematuria.

Most patients are asymptomatic with the diagnosis made on imaging studies. Symptoms relate to UTI and nephrolithiasis and include renal colic, hematuria, and dysuria. MSK is associated with Caroli's disease, autosomal polycystic kidney disease, and Ehlers-Danlos syndrome.

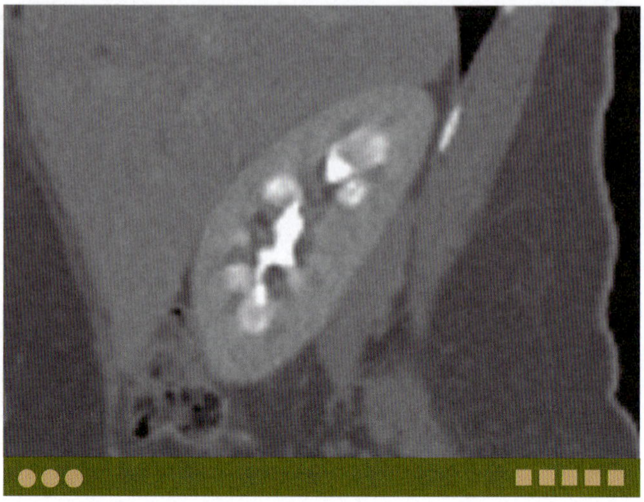

A. Sagittal reformatted CECT shows striations involving the medullary portions of the kidneys with brush border.

On imaging studies, calcifications are seen in the renal papillae. CT is more sensitive than abdominal radiographs to show the calcifications. The calcifications tend to be calcium phosphate or oxalate stones. They tend to be small and multiple. The medullary calcifications may be linear and elongated to suggest the diagnosis. IVU would show the cystic dilatation leading to the appearance of a "paintbrush" with contrast radiating outward toward the calyces with often associated calcification which tend to be small and clustered. On CECT studies, the same findings may be seen with higher sensitivity.

PEARLS

- **MSK is often asymptomatic but may be associated with hematuria, UTIs, or renal colic.**
- **MSK is one of the main causes of medullary nephrocalcinosis. CT is more sensitive to show tiny calcifications than abdominal radiographs.**
- **Following contrast on IVU and CT, dilatation of the collecting tubules with a "paintbrush" appearance is typical.**

ADDITIONAL IMAGES (B-C)

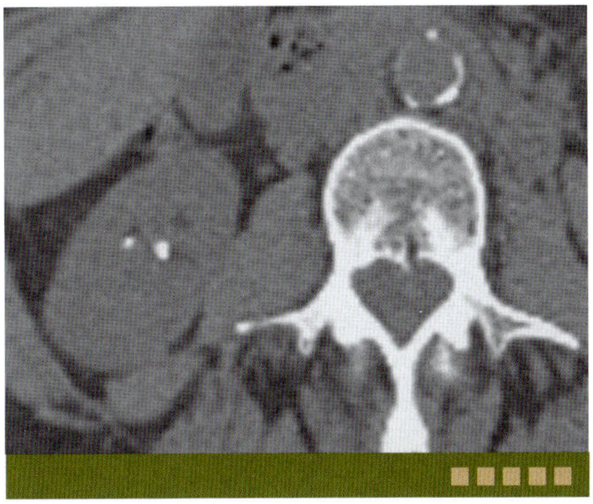

B. Axial NECT shows stones in the medullary portion of the kidney.

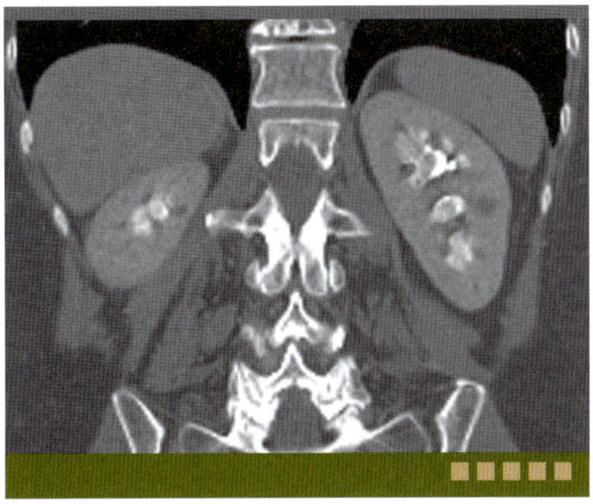

C. Coronal reformatted CECT shows brush border appearance to the collecting tubules with dilatation caused by MSK.

DIFFERENTIAL DIAGNOSES IMAGES (D-F)

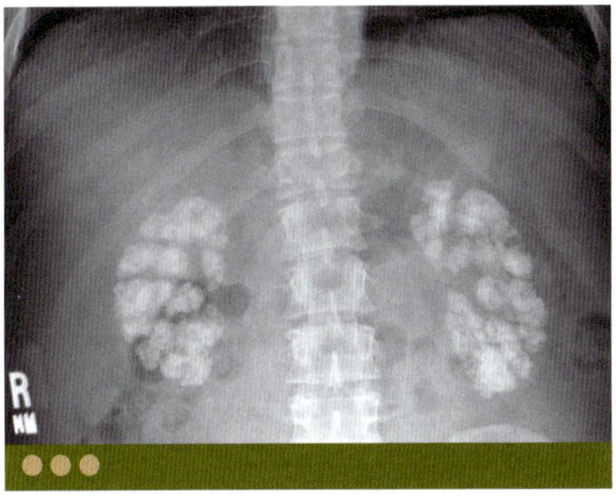

D. Renal tubular acidosis (distal type): Abdominal radiograph shows extensive medullary calcifications which are more extensive than those typically seen in renal MSK.

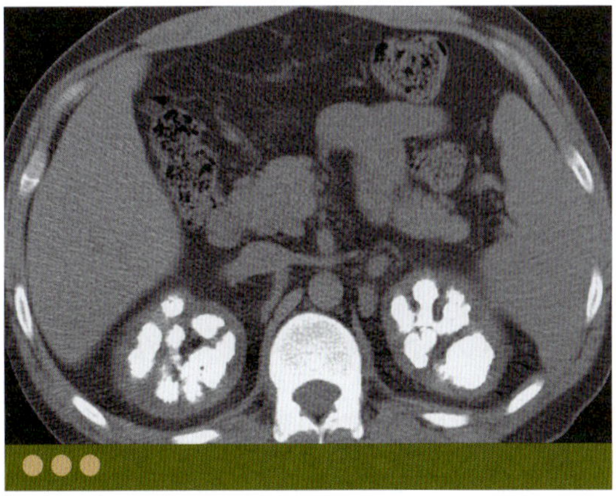

E. Renal tubular acidosis (distal type): Axial NECT shows extensive medullary calcifications from renal tubular acidosis.

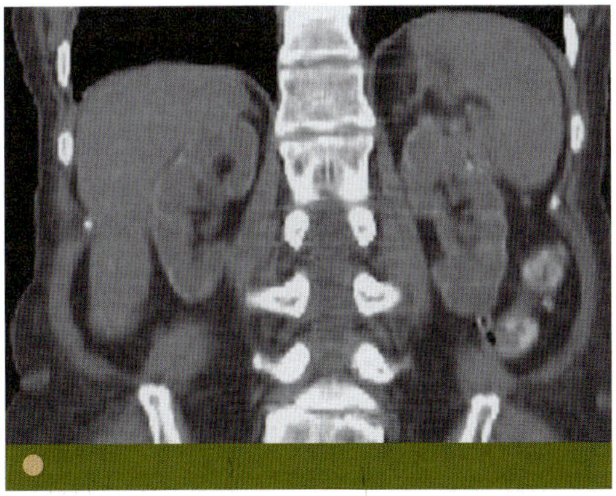

F. Cortical nephrocalcinosis: Coronal reformatted NECT shows diffuse peripheral hyperdensity involving the renal cortex with sparing of the medullary pyramids caused by chronic glomerulonephritis.

IMAGE KEY

Common

Rare

Typical

Unusual

4-9 Acute Tubular Necrosis from Contrast

Frank H. Miller

PRESENTATION

Prior iodinated contrast study and renal failure.

FINDINGS

- Persistent dense nephrograms from contrast during prior cardiac catheterization

DIFFERENTIAL DIAGNOSIS

Acute pyelonephritis: Different clinical findings including fevers, UTI, and different imaging appearance.

COMMENTS

Acute tubular necrosis (ATN) is caused by marked reduction of renal blood flow from elevated arteriolar resistance. There are a number of causes of ATN, including acute ischemic or toxic events involving drugs such as aminoglycosides, major trauma, myoglobinuria, compartment syndrome, transfusion reactions, severe dehydration, and renal transplantation. Iodinated contrast can also cause ATN, especially in patients with poor renal function.

Imaging findings include enlarged edematous kidneys with immediate persistent nephrogram most commonly or increasingly dense nephrograms. Findings include apparent enhancement of both kidneys which appear to be in the corticomedullary phase of enhancement because of prior contrast administration despite the lack of IV contrast administration during the study. No IV contrast, however, was administered as seen by the lack of vascular enhancement. In addition, there is lack of opacification of the collecting system. Other findings include increased density in the gallbladder from vicarious excretion.

Risk factors for contrast-induced nephrotoxicity include preexisting renal insufficiency, decreased renal perfusion (congestive heart failure, diuretics), hypertension, repeated exposure to contrast over short period of time, concurrent nephrotoxic medications, and elderly patients. Methods to prevent contrast-induced nephrotoxicity include vigorous hydration, avoiding iodinated contrast in high-risk patient populations with preexisting renal dysfunction, decreased iodinated contrast administration, and increased interval between contrast examinations. Contrast-induced acute renal failure is diagnosed when azotemia develops more than 24 hours after the use of contrast material. A persistently dense nephrogram on IVU or CT should suggest contrast-induced ATN. The presence of a 30-minute nephrogram that is denser than the 5-minute nephrogram with no evidence of obstruction should suggest contrast-induced ATN.

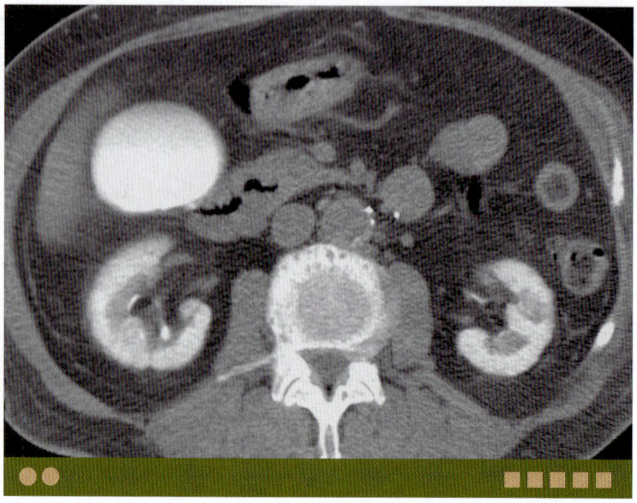

A. Axial NECT shows enhancement of both kidneys in the corticomedullary phase of enhancement (persistent nephrograms) with contrast in the right collecting system caused by ATN from contrast during prior cardiac catheterization. Contrast is seen in the gallbladder from vicarious excretion. No IV contrast was administered during this CT as seen by lack of vascular enhancement.

PEARLS

- **ATN is associated with a number of causes including iodinated contrast.**
- **Persistent dense nephrograms should suggest ATN.**
- **Risk factors for contrast-induced ATN include preexisting renal insufficiency, decreased renal perfusion, hypertension, repeated exposure to contrast over short period of time, concurrent nephrotoxic medications, and increased age of patients.**

ADDITIONAL IMAGE

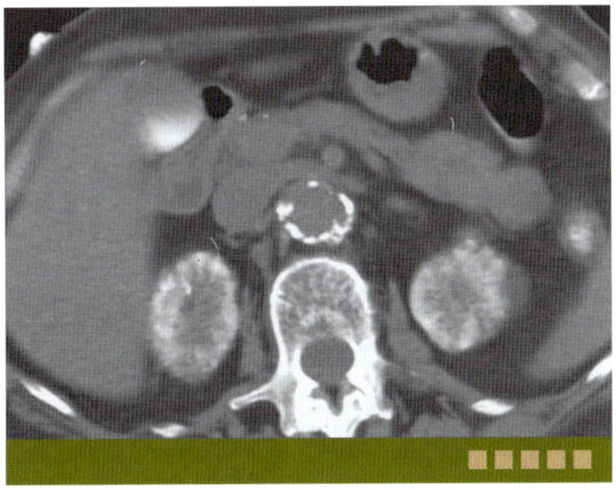

B. Axial NECT in a different patient shows persistent nephrogram in the kidneys over 24 hours after receiving iodinated contrast from cardiac catheterization caused by ATN. The kidneys have a striated nephrogram. Contrast is seen in the gallbladder from vicarious excretion.

DIFFERENTIAL DIAGNOSES IMAGE

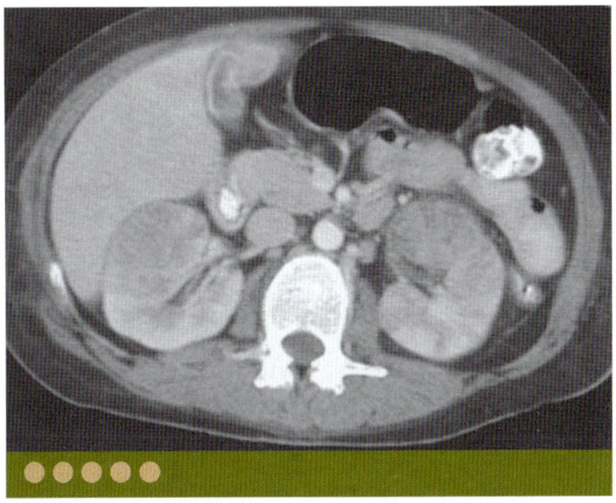

C. Acute pyelonephritis: Axial CECT shows striated nephrogram following contrast. There is not any persistent nephrogram unlike prior examples of ATN. The clinical history differs significantly.

IMAGE KEY

Common

●●●●●
●●●●
●●●
●●
●

Rare

Typical

■■■■■
■■■■
■■■
■■
■

Unusual

4–10 Papillary Necrosis

Nancy A. Hammond

PRESENTATION

Hematuria and flank pain.

FINDINGS

Multiple cavities in the areas of the renal papilla.

DIFFERENTIAL DIAGNOSES

- *Medullary sponge kidney*: Multiple small cystic cavities, medullary calcinosis, linear densities seen in pyramids on IVU.
- *Hydronephrosis*: Dilated pelvicalyceal system.

COMMENTS

Papillary necrosis is a descriptive term referring to disorders causing renal medullary ischemia, resulting in necrosis and sloughing of the papillary tissue. Papillary necrosis occurs in a variety of diseases that cause tubulointerstitial nephropathy. A well-known pneumonic utilized to remember common causes of papillary necrosis is "POSTCARD": Pyelonephritis, Obstructive uropathy, Sickle cell disease, Tuberculosis, Calculi, Analgesics, Renal vein thrombosis, and Diabetes mellitus. Diabetes is the most common condition associated with papillary necrosis. Papillary necrosis varies in its severity and rate of progression ranging from rapid progression to an indolent course. Clinically, patients present with flank pain, dysuria, ureteral colic, pyuria, and hematuria.

The radiographic findings of papillary necrosis are not specific for the underlying cause. IVU and retrograde best demonstrate the classic features of papillary necrosis. Total or partial necrosis of the papilla can occur. Three types of parenchymal involvement have been described; medullary, papillary, and necrosis *in situ*. The medullary type results in central erosions of the papilla, and the papillary type results in necrosis developing at the periphery of the papilla with eventual sloughing of the papilla. A sloughed papilla appears as circular or irregular filling defects in the pelvocalyceal system. Occasionally, the sloughed papilla may cause ureteral obstruction. Necrosis *in situ* is described as necrotic papillae that remain attached, shrink, and frequently calcify. Renal atrophy and cortical thinning is a common sequela of papillary necrosis.

Ultrasound is rarely used for the diagnosis of papillary necrosis. Reported findings include echogenic foci surrounded by hypoechoic rims in early disease. Advanced stages of papillary necrosis demonstrate single or multiple cystic cavities in the medullary pyramids continuous with the calyces. Sloughed papillae appear as echogenic lesions in the collecting system.

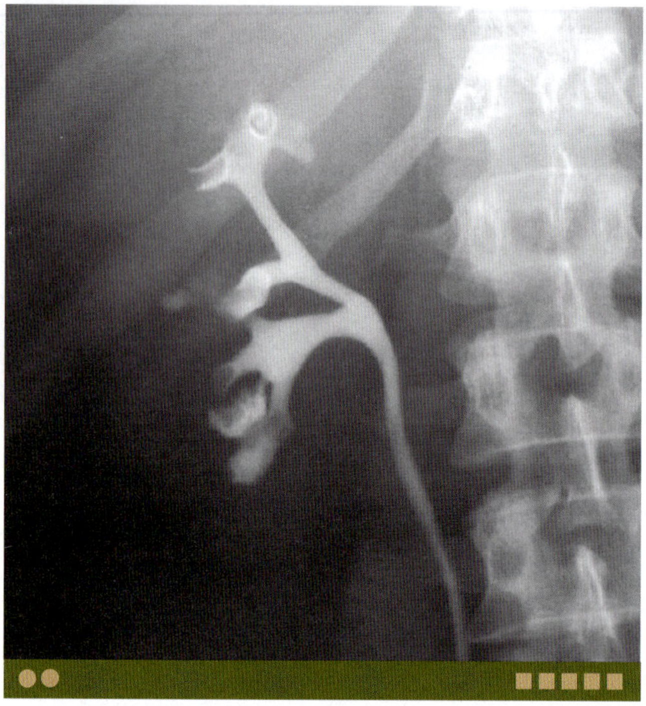

A. IVU shows bulbous cavities involving the mid and lower pole calyces of the right kidney in the region of the renal papillae.

In the early stages of papillary necrosis, CT demonstrates decreased enhancement in the medullary tip with a circumscribed, ill-defined rim. Other CT findings include atrophic kidneys, ring-shaped medullary calcifications, contrast filled clefts in the renal parenchyma, or a filling defect.

PEARLS

- **Not a unique entity but refers to disorders causing necrosis of the renal papillae secondary to interstitial nephritis or ischemia.**
- **POSTCARD is a common pneumonic for etiologies that cause papillary necrosis: Pyelonephritis, Obstructive uropathy, Sickle cell disease, Tuberculosis, Calculi, Analgesics, Renal vein thrombosis, and Diabetes mellitus.**
- **Early stage disease best appreciated on IVP or retrograde study.**
- **Triangular or bulbous cavitation adjacent to calyx on IVP or retrograde study common finding.**

ADDITIONAL IMAGES (B-F)

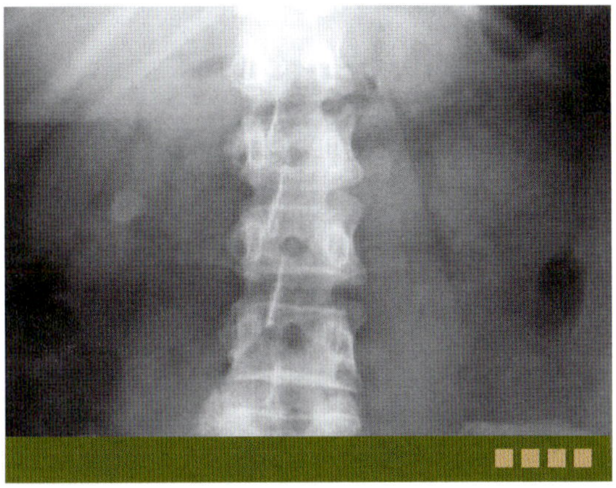

B. AP scout from an IVU shows a round calcification overlying the lower pole of the right kidney in the region of the renal medulla.

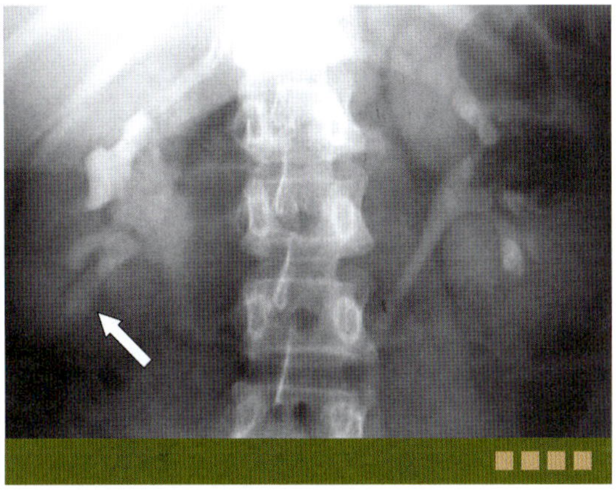

C. Contrast-enhanced IVU shows the calcification to lie in the region of the renal papilla adjacent to a lower pole calyx (arrow).

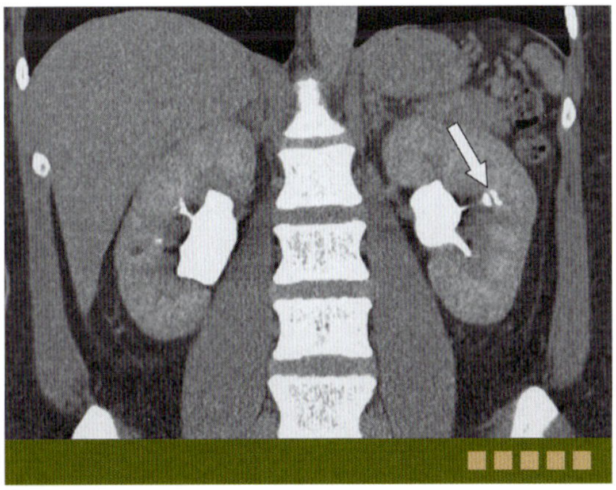

D. Coronal CECT shows a collection of contrast beyond the interpapillary line adjacent to a midpole calyx (arrow).

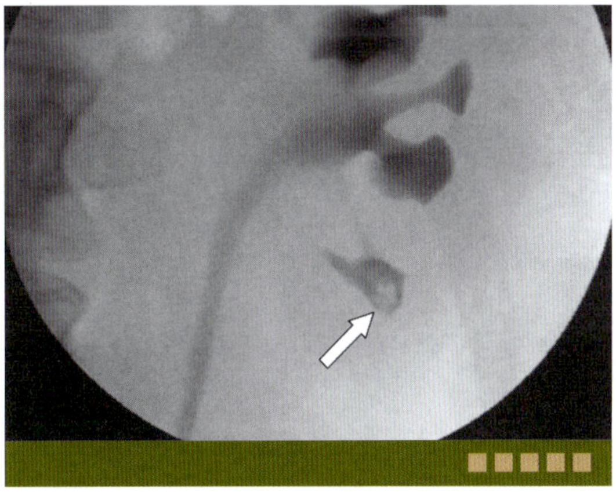

E. Retrograde pyelogram shows a ring-shadow filling defect (arrow) in a lower pole calyx of the left kidney. Calcification was noted in this region on the plain film confirming this finding to represent a calcified sloughed papilla. Clubbing of the upper pole calyces is also present.

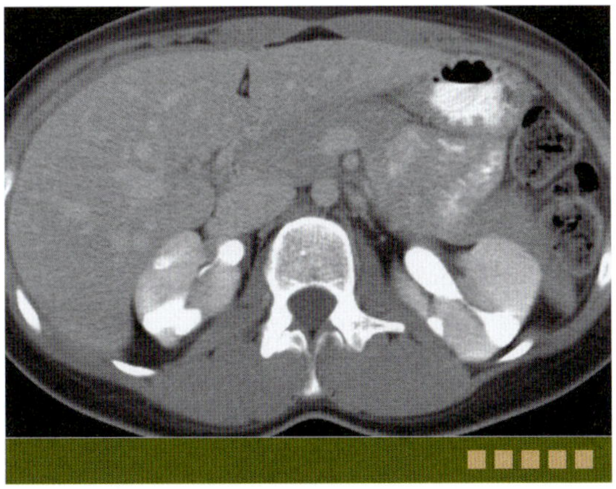

F. Axial CECT shows thinning of the renal cortex with clubbing of the calyces that extend to the periphery of the renal cortex.

DIFFERENTIAL DIAGNOSES IMAGE

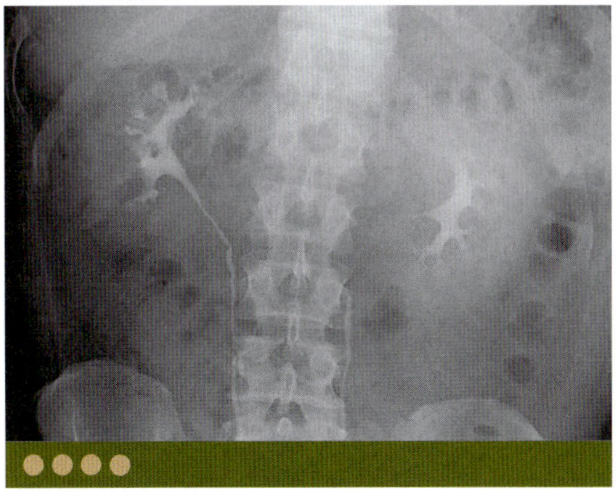

H. Medullary sponge kidney: Contrast-enhanced IVU shows the characteristic "paint brush" appearance of dilated opacified pyramid tubules.

IMAGE KEY

Common

Rare

Typical

Unusual

CHAPTER 5

RENAL VASCULAR DISEASE AND RENAL TRANSPLANTATION

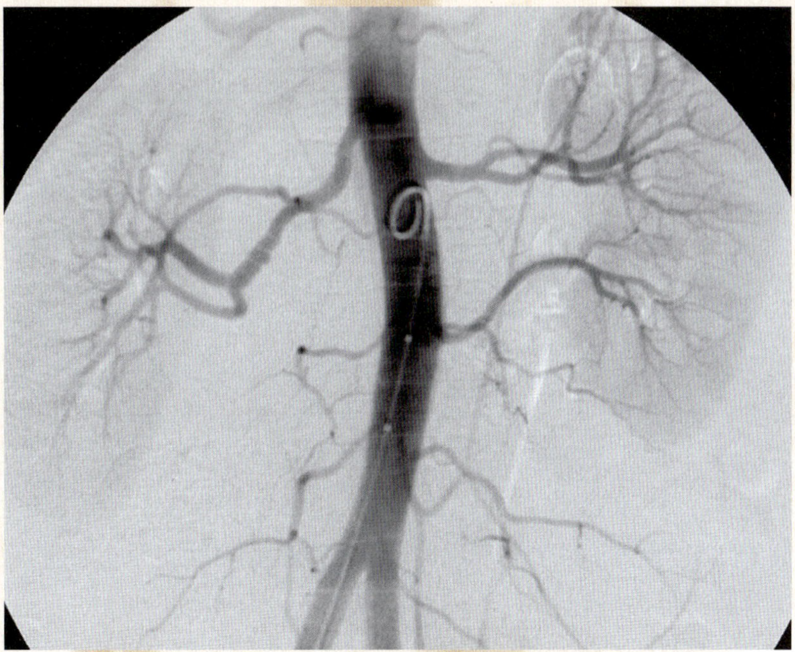

Part 1

Renal Vascular Disease

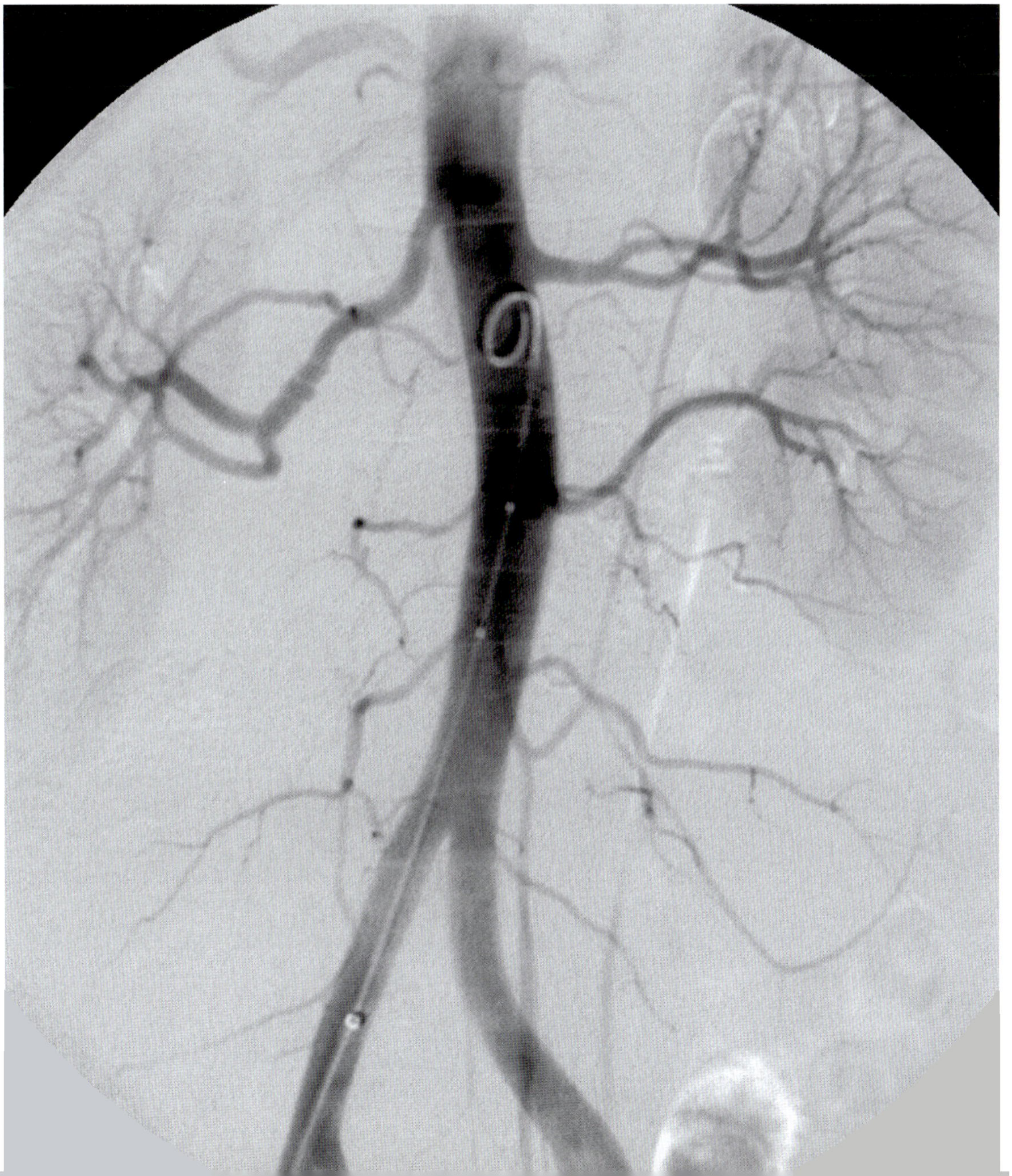

5–1 Renal Artery Stenosis Secondary to Arteriosclerosis

Nancy A. Hammond

PRESENTATION

Hypertension refractory to medical therapy.

FINDINGS

Focal stenosis at the proximal renal artery.

DIFFERENTIAL DIAGNOSIS

- *Renal artery stenosis (RAS) secondary to fibromuscular dysplasia (FMD)*: beaded appearance of the mid and distal renal artery.

COMMENTS

Essential hypertension accounts for the majority of cases of hypertension. Renovascular disease accounts for 1% to 5% of the cases of hypertension. Atherosclerosis is the most common cause of hypertension secondary to renal vascular disease accounting for approximately 66% of all cases. FMD is the second most common cause. Clinically, rapid acceleration, severe hypertension, and hypertensive retinopathy are more indicative of a renovascular cause than essential hypertension. A flank bruit can be found on physical examination, although this is more commonly seen with FMD than with atherosclerosis. Patients with hypertension caused by renal artery atherosclerosis are typically older than those with FMD. Also in distinction to FMD, men are more commonly affected than females.

In hypertension caused by renal artery atherosclerosis, the lesion usually occurs at the origin of the main renal artery or within the first 2 cm. Typically, the lesions are circumferential but can be eccentric. As atherosclerosis is a generalized process, both renal arteries are often affected.

A variety of imaging techniques have been employed in evaluating patients with suspected renovascular hypertension. While conventional angiography is considered the gold standard, its invasive nature makes it an unlikely screening modality. Doppler interrogation evaluates for elevated velocities at the stenotic portion of the artery and changes in the arterial waveform distal to the stenosis. The upper limits of normal for the renal artery velocity is 180 to 200 cm/s. A parvus tardus waveform or delayed systolic upstroke is seen in the distal artery.

Contrast-enhanced MRA is another modality employed in evaluating for RAS. It has been shown to be 88% to 100% sensitive and 83% to 98% specific in evaluating for hemodynamically significant stenoses. However, MRA can overestimate the degree of stenosis in 5% to 10% of renal arteries. CTA has also been shown to be an excellent modality in evaluating for RAS with comparable sensitivity and specificity of MRA. Both have been shown to be superior to ultrasound.

Treatment of RAS secondary to atherosclerosis is stenting of the stenotic segment.

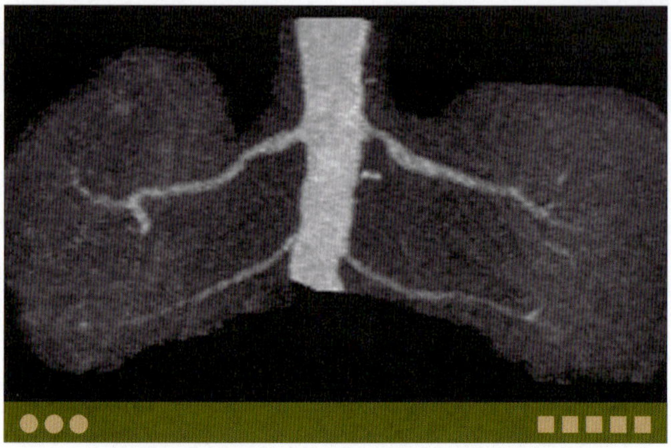

A. Coronal MIP from contrast-enhanced MRA shows a focal narrowing involving the proximal left renal artery. The degree of stenosis is greater than 50% of the luminal diameter and, therefore, hemodynamically significant. Mild narrowing involving the proximal right renal artery is also present.

PEARLS

- **Atherosclerosis is the most common cause of renovascular hypertension accounting for approximately 66% of all cases.**
- **Stenoses caused by atherosclerosis involve the ostial and proximal segments of the renal artery. This is in distinction to FMD which involves the mid and distal arterial segments and results in beaded appearance to the involved artery.**
- **Ultrasound, contrast-enhanced MRA, and CTA are employed in evaluating patients with suspected renovascular hypertension. MRA and CTA have been shown to be superior to ultrasound.**

ADDITIONAL IMAGES (B-D)

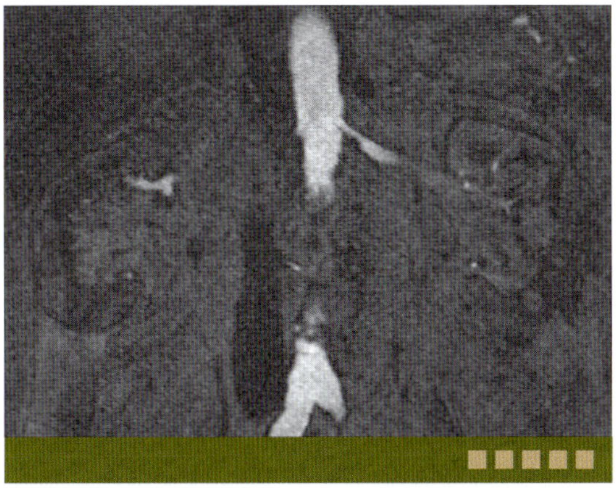

B. Coronal source image from a contrast-enhanced MRA further shows the stenosis of the proximal left renal artery.

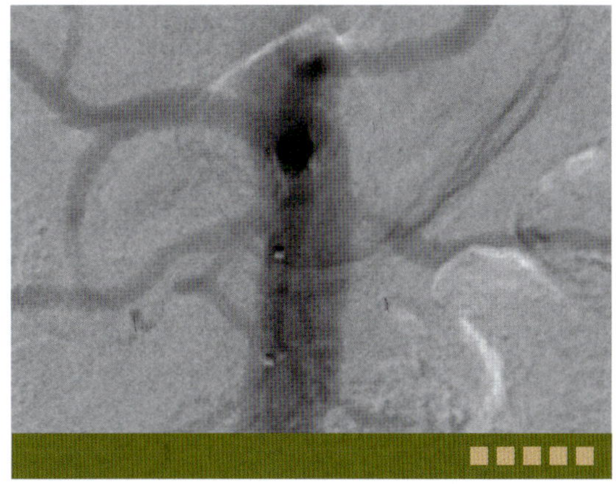

C. Angiogram of the renal arteries from an abdominal aortic injection shows the focal narrowing of the left renal artery.

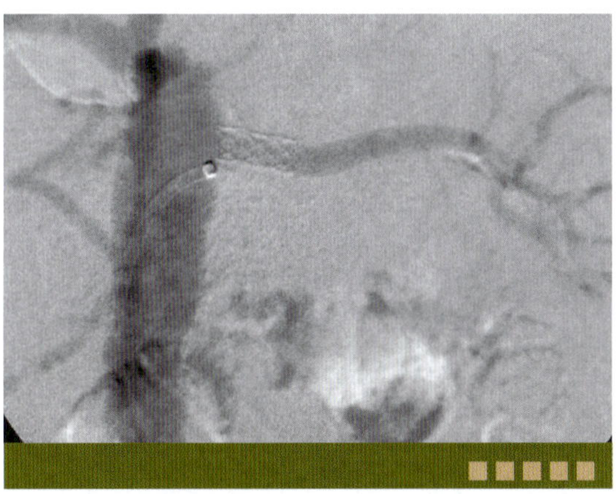

D. Angiogram of the left renal artery after technically successful stent placement shows interval improvement in the narrowing. No hemodynamically significant stenosis is present.

DIFFERENTIAL DIAGNOSES IMAGE

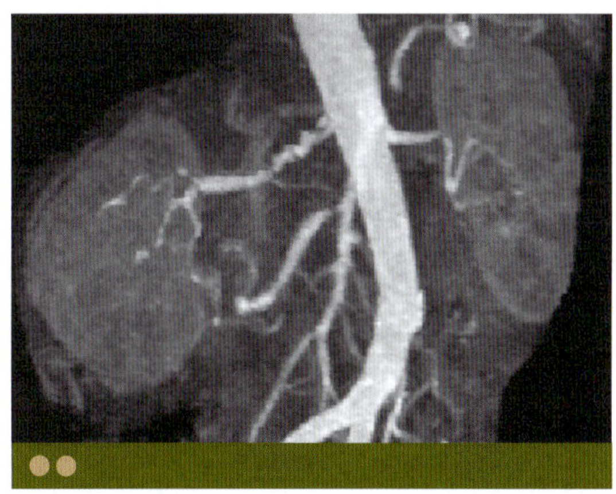

E. FMD: Coronal MIP from a contrast-enhanced MRA shows multiple stenotic foci involving the mid-aspect of the right renal artery creating the characteristic beaded appearance of FMD.

IMAGE KEY

Common

Rare

Typical

Unusual

5–2 Fibromuscular Dysplasia

Nancy A. Hammond

PRESENTATION

Hypertension refractory to medical therapy.

FINDINGS

Beaded appearance to the main renal artery.

DIFFERENTIAL DIAGNOSIS

- *RAS caused by atherosclerosis*: stenosis involves the proximal main renal artery.

COMMENTS

Fibromuscular dysplasia is a nonatherosclerotic narrowing of medium-sized vessels that is most commonly seen in women between the ages 20 and 50. While reported in a variety of vascular beds, it most commonly involves the renal arteries. Second to atherosclerosis, FMD is the most common cause of renovascular hypertension. In distinction to atherosclerotic RAS, FMD tends to involve the mid and distal main renal artery and branch vessels. FMD has been categorized into subtypes based on the vascular layer involved: intima, media, or adventitia. Medial fibroplasia is the most common type accounting for approximately 95% of the cases. Medial fibroplasia results in alternating stenosis and aneurysm formation producing the characteristic "string of beads" appearance. Pathologically, this appearance is caused by the replacement of smooth muscles with collagen, forming thick ridges alternating with small aneurysm formation.

FMD can also involve the cephalic, visceral, and peripheral arteries. While it may involve the carotid and vertebral arteries, it tends to spare the intracranial vessels.

Sonographically, the morphologic changes to the renal artery are not typically visible. Doppler interrogation demonstrates disorganized flow with heterogeneous color assignment typically involving the mid or distal renal artery. Because of its more distal location, RAS secondary to FMD is more difficult to detect sonographically than RAS secondary to atherosclerosis.

While angiography is traditionally considered the gold standard, MR and CT angiography are noninvasive techniques used to establish the diagnosis of FMD. The classic "string-of-beads" is considered pathognomonic for medial fibroplasia.

Percutaneous transluminal angioplasty is considered the treatment of choice with a reported success rate of greater than 90% for stenoses caused by FMD.

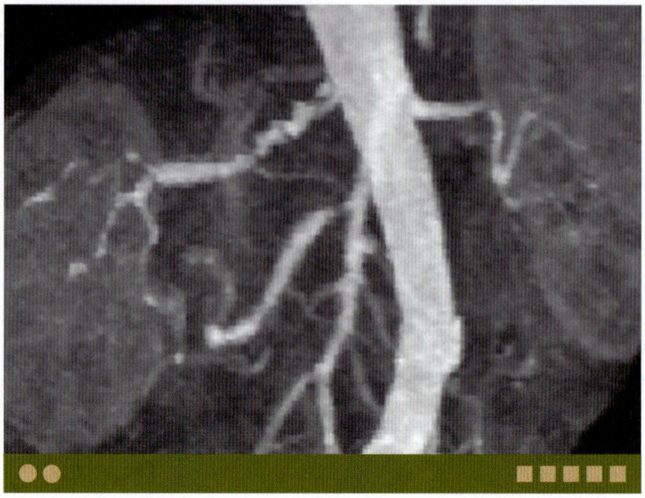

A. Coronal MIP from contrast-enhanced MRA shows multiple areas of narrowing with intervening dilatation involving the mid-aspect of the main right renal artery creating the characteristic "beaded" appearance of FMD.

PEARLS

- **FMD is the second most common cause of renovascular hypertension.**
- **Medial fibroplasia is the most common type of FMD accounting for 95% of the cases.**
- **In distinction to RAS caused by atherosclerosis, FMD involves the mid and distal main renal artery and may extend into the branch vessels.**
- **Percutaneous angioplasty is considered the treatment of choice.**

ADDITIONAL IMAGES (B-E)

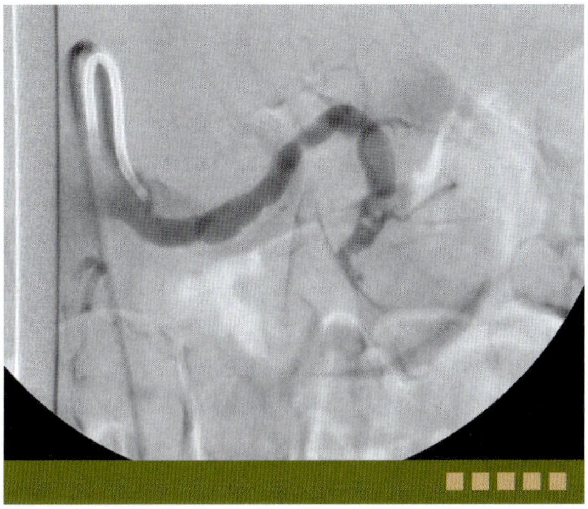

B. Selective left renal artery injection shows the typical beaded appearance of the left renal artery angiographically. Small filling defects are present in the distal renal artery compatible with emboli.

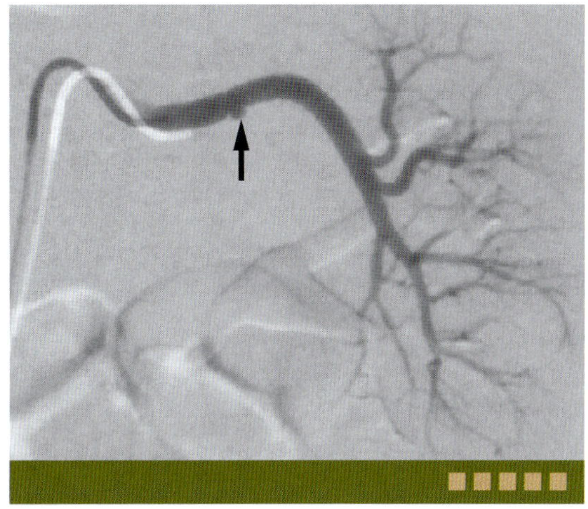

C. Selective left renal artery injection in a different patient shows subtle irregularity consistent with early changes of FMD. Additionally, a small focal aneurysm is present in the mid-left renal artery (arrow).

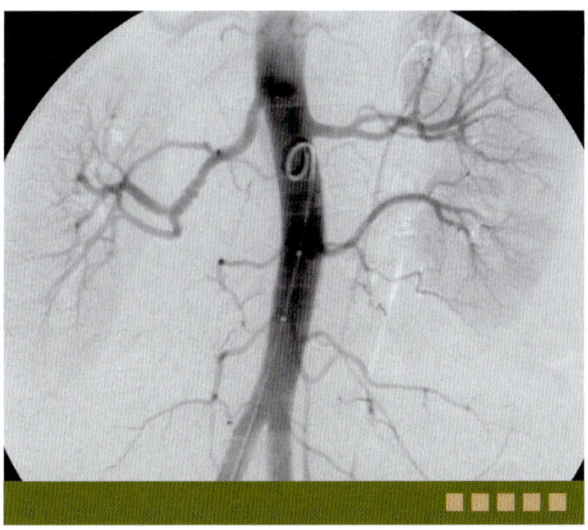

D. Catheter-directed abdominal aortic angiogram shows the characteristic beading of FMD of the right renal artery and an uninvolved left renal artery.

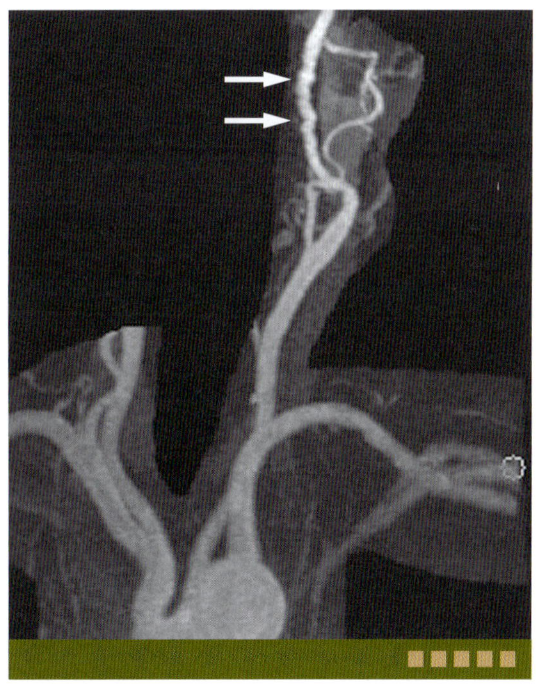

E. Coronal MIP from contrast-enhanced MRA in the same patient as in Figure D shows beading of the left internal carotid artery (arrows).

DIFFERENTIAL DIAGNOSES IMAGE

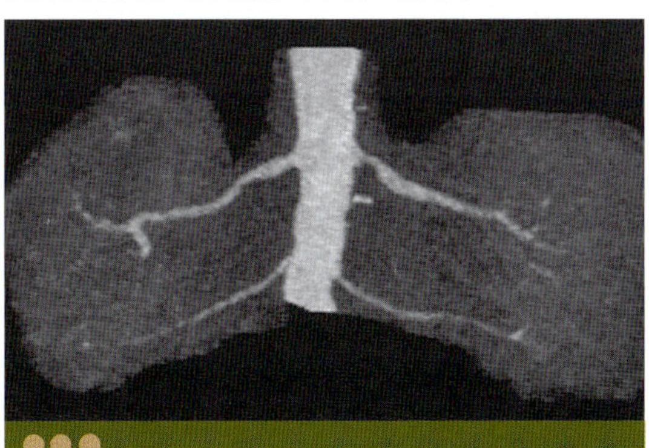

F. Renal artery atherosclerosis: Coronal MIP in a different patient shows narrowing at the origin of the left renal artery consistent with RAS caused by atherosclerotic disease.

IMAGE KEY

Common

Rare

Typical

Unusual

5-3 Renal Artery Arteriovenous Malformation

Nancy A. Hammond

PRESENTATION

Gross hematuria.

FINDINGS

CT shows a serpiginous, arterial enhancing mass. The degree of enhancement follows that of the aorta.

DIFFERENTIAL DIAGNOSIS

Solid enhancing mass: while the distinction can be difficult, the enhancement pattern of neoplasms typically does not follow that of the aorta on all phases. Enlargement of the renal vein should also raise suspicion for an arteriovenous malformations (AVM) rather than neoplasm.

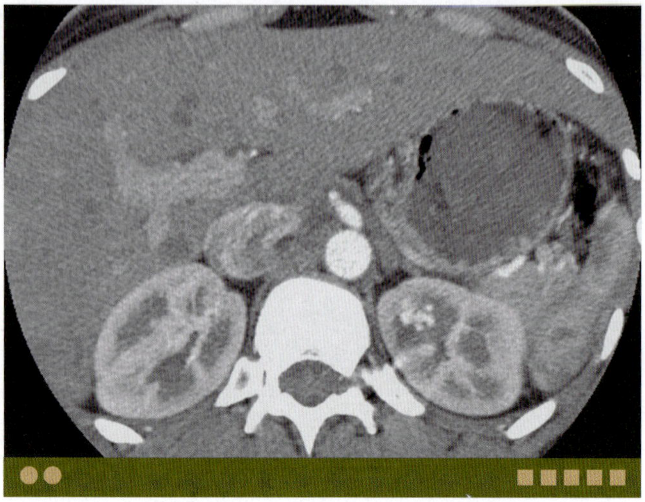

A. Axial CECT shows a renal AVM as a small serpiginous, vascular collection involving the renal medulla of the left kidney. The degree of enhancement is similar to that of the abdominal aorta.

COMMENTS

AVMs of the kidney are most commonly congenital but can also be posttraumatic in origin. The most common types of AVMs are small cirsoid lesions that are seen more frequently in women and occur more commonly in the right kidney. AVMs are also seen in association with syndromes such as congenital telangiectasias (Osler-Weber-Rendu syndrome). Patients usually present with gross hematuria that can be episodic or continuous and mild or massive. In severe cases, this can be life-threatening. When lesions are large, shunting can occur resulting in high-output heart failure.

When small, AVMs may be hard to appreciate on grayscale sonography. Larger lesions appear as complex cystic masses. Color Doppler demonstrates aliasing at the site of the AVM. Vibration of the perivascular tissues may result in color signal outside the true borders of the AVM. Spectral Doppler demonstrates low resistance and high velocity within the lesion. The renal vein can be enlarged with an arterialized waveform.

CTA and MRA demonstrate an arterial enhancing lesion with early filling of a typically enlarged renal vein. Delayed images demonstrate persistent enhancement of the lesion.

Treatment of AVMs is selective embolization of the malformation. However, in some cases when the arteriovenous connection is of large caliber with high flow, embolic occlusion of the malformation may be difficult to impossible.

PEARLS

- **Patients typically present with gross hematuria.**
- **When AVMs are large, they can result in high-output heart failure.**
- **Small lesions may be difficult to detect on grayscale sonography but color Doppler demonstrates aliasing and spectral Doppler shows low resistance and high velocity in the lesion.**
- **Percutaneous selective embolization is the treatment of choice.**

ADDITIONAL IMAGES (B-E)

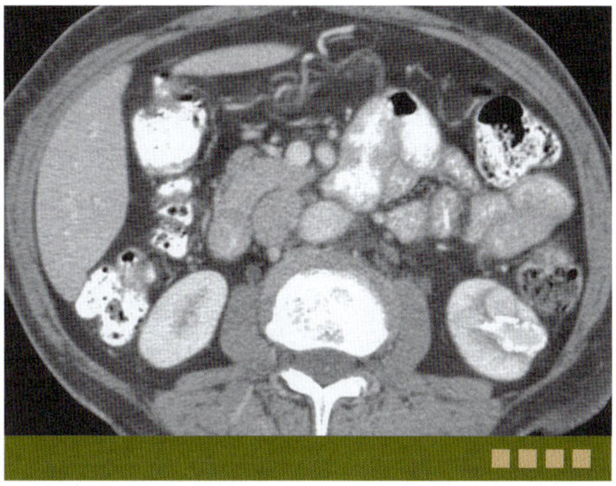

B. Axial CECT shows two lobular foci of enhancement in the lower pole of the left kidney. There is peripheral calcification of one of these foci. The degree of enhancement is similar to that of the aorta.

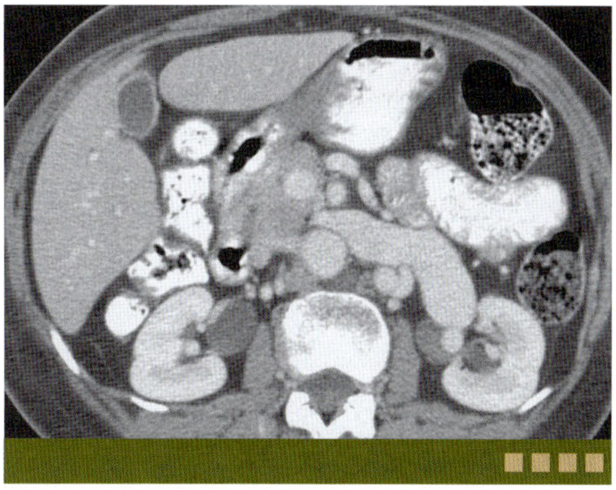

C. Axial CECT in the same patient as Figure B shows enlargement of the left renal vein relating to the presence of the lower pole AVM.

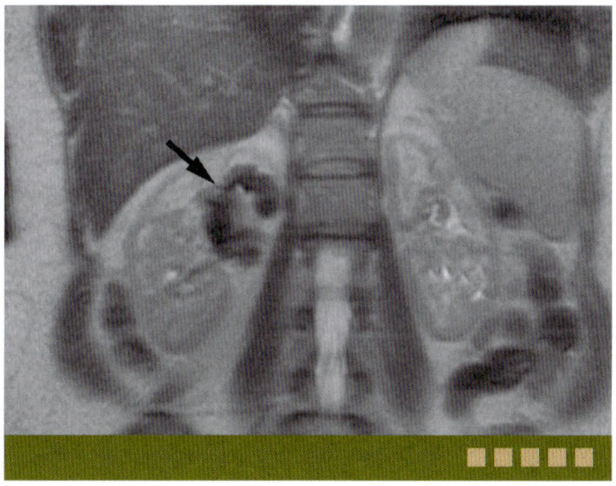

D. Coronal T2-WI in a patient with a large AVM shows a serpiginous, tubular flow void in the upper pole of the left kidney that extends in to the renal pelvis (arrow).

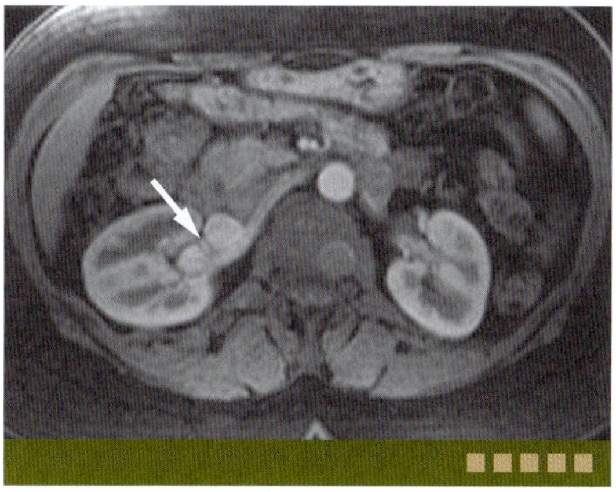

E. Axial contrast-enhanced T1-WI shows enhancement in the location of the T2 flow void (arrow).

DIFFERENTIAL DIAGNOSES IMAGE

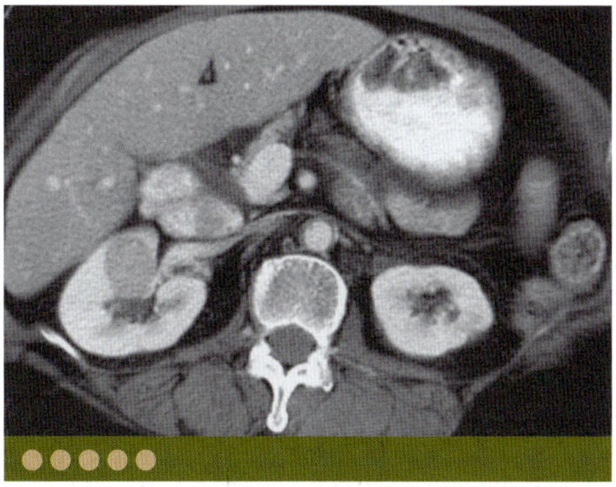

F. Renal cell carcinoma: Axial CECT shows a solid, enhancing right renal mass. The mass enhances to a lesser degree than the surrounding renal parenchyma and the abdominal aorta. Additionally, note the normal appearance and caliber of the right renal vein.

IMAGE KEY

Common

Rare

Typical

Unusual

5–4 Renal Artery Aneurysm

Nancy A. Hammond

PRESENTATION

Typically asymptomatic.

FINDINGS

Focal dilatation of the renal artery, with the degree of enhancement following that of the aorta.

DIFFERENTIAL DIAGNOSIS

- *Renal artery pseudoaneurysm*: Can be difficult to distinguish radiographically. Pseudoaneurysms typically occur in the setting of trauma or prior intervention.

COMMENTS

Renal artery aneurysms occur most commonly in the setting of atherosclerosis. Aneurysmal dilatation of a renal artery is present when the diameter of that segment exceeds twice that of a normal-appearing artery. Aneurysms can be extraparenchymal or intraparenchymal in location with extraparenchymal being more common than intraparenchymal. They can also been seen in patients with renal artery dissection, trauma, vasculitis, and in patients with fibromuscular dysplasia. Intraparenchymal aneurysms are seen with vasculitides, mycosis, tuberculosis, neurofibromatosis, and Ehlers-Danlos syndrome. Renal artery aneurysms are equally as common in men as in women but rupture more commonly in hypertensive and pregnant patients. The diagnosis of renal artery aneurysm is important as they may be the source of emboli to the kidney, resulting in renal ischemia, oversecretion of rennin, and renovascular hypertension.

Clinically, most patients are asymptomatic with the aneurysm detected incidentally on studies investigating other intra-abdominal pathologies. Patients commonly have hypertension and less commonly may present with flank pain or hematuria. Uncommonly, the aneurysm may rupture.

If calcified, conventional radiographs demonstrate curvilinear calcification in the expected location of the renal artery. When left-sided, this can be difficult to distinguish from calcification of the splenic artery. Sonographically, an aneurysm is seen as a hypoechoic mass along the course of the renal artery. Doppler signal may be present, depending on the size of the neck of the aneurysm and the amount of thrombus in the aneurysm; but when present, it is turbulent. CT demonstrates a rounded structure contiguous with the renal artery. Calcifications may or may not be present. Enhancement is variable, depending on the amount of thrombus within the aneurysm, but the degree is identical to the enhancement of the aorta. MR demonstrates similar findings as CT but does not characterize the presence of calcifications.

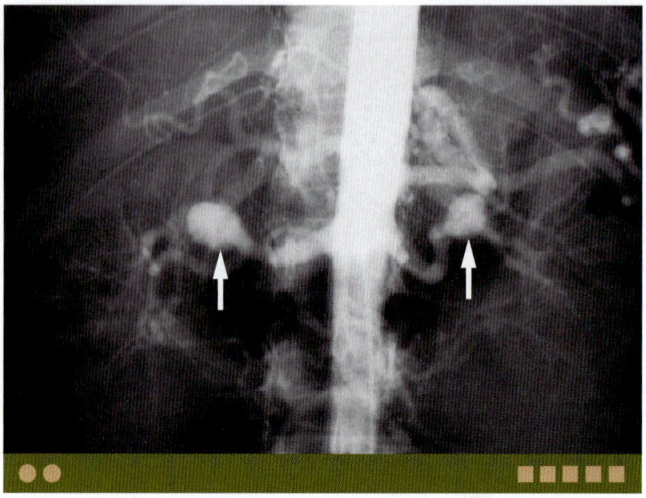

A. Selected image from an abdominal aorta angiogram shows bilateral renal artery aneurysms (arrows).

Potential indications for intervention include rupture of the aneurysm, symptomatic patients presenting with flank pain and/or hematuria, in patients with renovascular hypertension, enlarging aneurysms, aneurysms attributed to acute dissection, and in female patients contemplating pregnancy. While no set criteria exist regarding the size of the aneurysm that necessitates repair, diameters ranging from 1.5 to 3 cm, with the average 2 cm, are generally accepted. When clinically warranted, renal artery aneurysms are treated surgically or with endovascular technology.

PEARLS

- **The renal artery is considered anuerysmal when the diameter of the affected segment is twice that of the nonaffected artery.**
- **Most renal artery aneurysms are extraparenchymal and seen in the setting of artherosclerosis.**
- **Patients are most commonly asymptomatic but may be hypertensive.**
- **When clinically warranted, repair can be surgical or via endovascular technique.**

ADDITIONAL IMAGES (B-E)

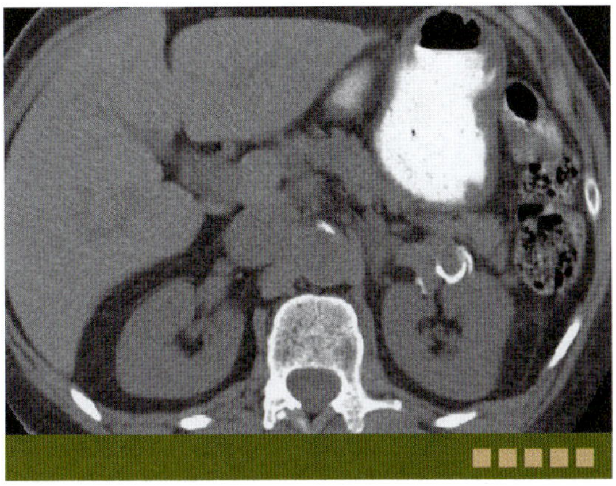

B. Axial NECT shows curvilinear calcification along the course of the main left renal artery suspicious for a small renal artery aneurysm.

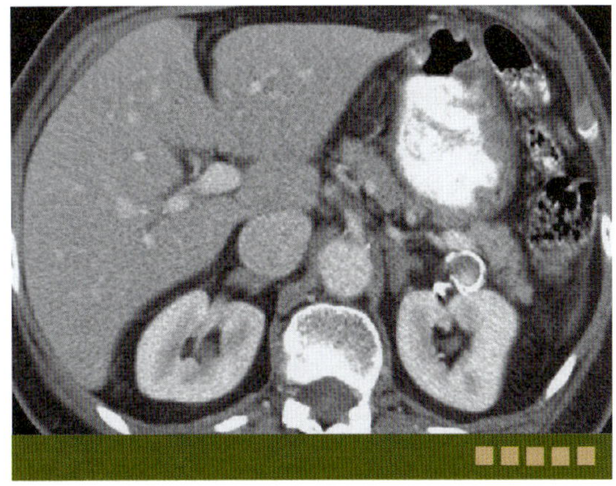

C. Axial CECT in the same patient as in Figure D shows partial enhancement of the renal artery aneurysm with some peripheral mural thrombus present.

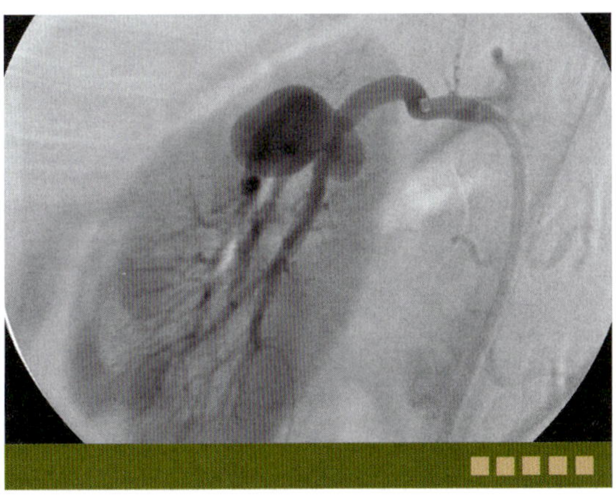

D. Angiogram from a selective right renal artery aneurysm shows a large aneurysm arising from the distal main right renal artery.

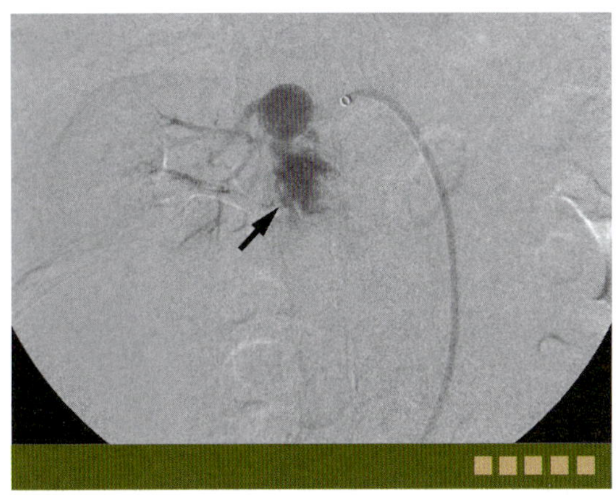

E. Angiogram in the same patient as in Figure F during attempted coiling of the aneurysm shows acute extravasation of contrast material (arrow). Hemostasis was subsequently achieved by coiling the main right renal artery.

DIFFERENTIAL DIAGNOSES IMAGE

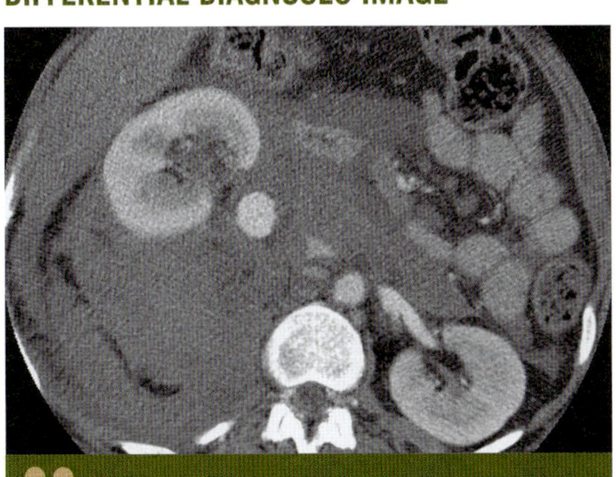

F. Renal artery pseudoaneurysm: Axial CECT shows a hyperenhancing round structure in the right renal hilum and a large perinephric hematoma displacing the kidney anteriorly.

IMAGE KEY

Common

●●●●●
●●●●
●●●
●●
●

Rare

Typical

■■■■■
■■■■
■■■
■■
■

Unusual

5–5 Polyarteritis Nodosa

Nancy A. Hammond

PRESENTATION

Hematuria

FINDINGS

Multiple small aneurysms of the interlobular renal arteries

DIFFERENTIAL DIAGNOSES

- *Microaneurysms can be seen in patients with systemic lupus erythematosus*: Wegener granulomatosis, hypersensitivity angiitis, and intravenous drug abuse
- *Bilateral pyelonephritis*: Clinical scenario consistent with infection

COMMENTS

Polyarteritis nodosa is an uncommon vasculitis affecting the small- and medium-sized vessels. It is a multisystemic disease that most commonly affects the kidney but can involve the liver, gastrointestinal tract, skeletal muscles, skin, joints, and peripheral nerves.

Clinically, patients present with fever, abdominal pain, and weight loss. Arthralgia, retinopathy, subcutaneous nodules, hematuria, elevated erythrocyte sedimentation rate (ESR), and peripheral neuropathy may also be present. Although usually present, hypertension is not typically the presenting feature.

Renal involvement occurs in 90% of the patients with PAN and results in ischemia and small aneurysms (1-12 mm) of the interlobular, arcuate, or interlobar arteries. These aneurysms may rupture producing intraparenchymal or perinephric hematomas. Rarely, the ureter can be involved, resulting in acute ureteral obstruction or development of a stricture caused by ischemia.

Radiographically, renal involvement of PAN is nonspecific. Ultrasound, CT, or urography may demonstrate bilateral renal enlargement. With more advanced disease, contrast-enhanced CT (CECT) demonstrates multiple, small wedge-shaped, low-attenuation areas of infarction. When present, perinephric or intraparenchymal hematomas are best demonstrated on CT. Angiography is the most definitive radiographic examination and demonstrates the small aneurysms that involve the intrarenal arteries.

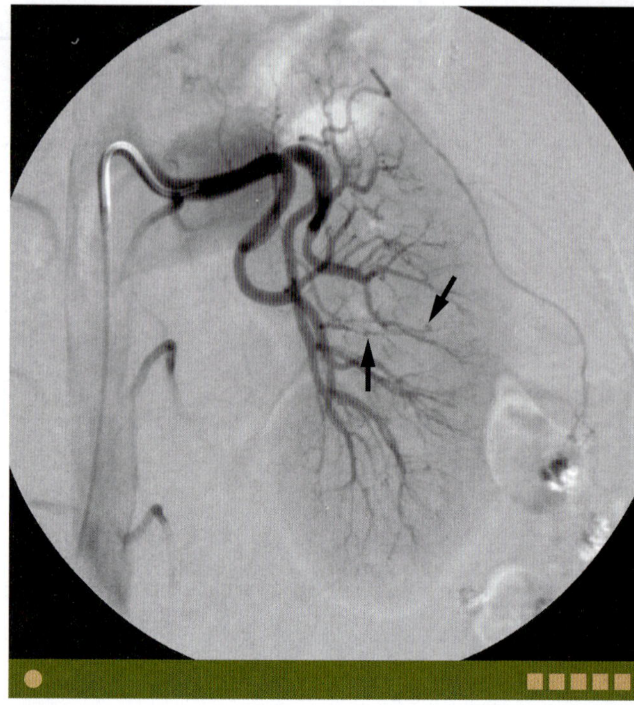

A. Renal artery arteriogram with a left renal artery injection shows multiple small aneurysms of the intrarenal artery branches (arrows).

PEARLS

- **Polyarteritis nodosa is a multisystem vasculitis of the small- and medium-sized arteries most commonly affecting the intrarenal arteries.**
- **Ultrasound and CT findings are nonspecific.**
- **Angiography is an important modality and can be used to establish the diagnosis of PAN by demonstrating microaneurysms involving the interlobar, arcuate, or intralobular renal arteries.**
- **Microaneurysms are typical of PAN but not pathognomonic.**

ADDITIONAL IMAGE

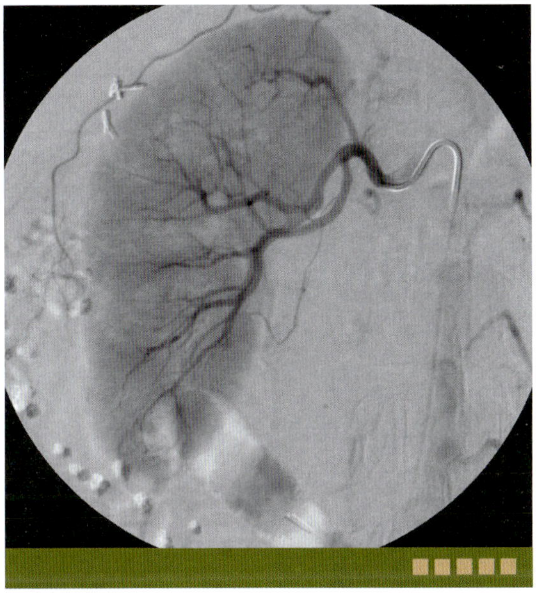

B. Right renal artery injection in the same patient in Figure A further shows multiple microaneurysms involving the intrarenal artery branches

DIFFERENTIAL DIAGNOSES IMAGE

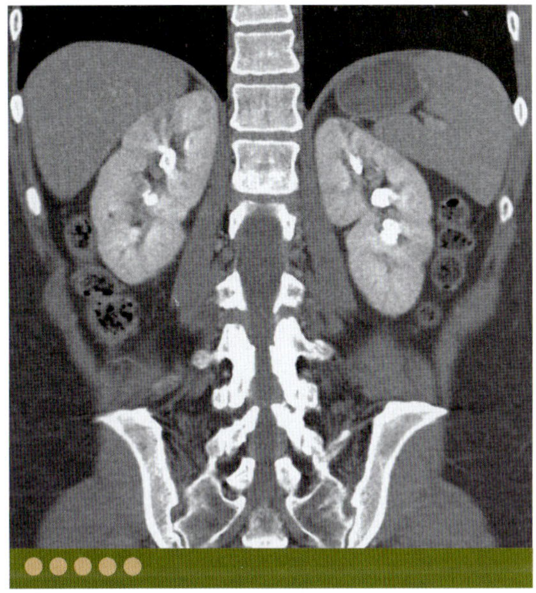

C. Pyelonephritis: Coronal CECT shows wedge-shaped areas of hypoenhancement involving both kidneys in a patient with fever, elevated white count, and bilateral CVA tenderness.

IMAGE KEY

Common

Rare

Typical

Unusual

5–6 Renal Infarction

Nancy A. Hammond

PRESENTATION

Acute flank pain.

FINDINGS

Well-demarcated area of decreased attenuation without mass effect.

DIFFERENTIAL DIAGNOSIS

- *Pyleonephritis*: Clinical presentation and urinalysis distinguishes the two entities.

COMMENTS

Patients with acute renal infarction typically present with nonspecific symptoms including flank pain and hematuria. As the presentation is variable, the diagnosis based on clinical findings is often missed. However, most patients are at risk for thromboembolic disease with factors including atrial fibrillation, previous embolism, and valvular or ischemic heart disease. Bilateral renal infarctions suggest systemic emboli or a vasculitis.

The radiographic appearance depends on the size of the embolus and the location of the arterial occlusion.

Intravenous urogram (IVU) demonstrates absence of the enhancement of the affected segment of the kidney. If the clot is large and involves the main renal artery, there will be no renal function in the kidney. Cross-sectional imaging demonstrates nonenhancement of the affected renal parenchyma. When small, wedge-shaped areas of low attenuation are present in an otherwise normal-appearing kidney. A rim of enhancing cortical tissue may be present because of the preservation of the capsular branches that originate proximal to the main renal artery. The cortical rim sign is virtually diagnostic of renal infarction. Sonographically, the kidney may appear normal on grayscale imaging. Focal and segmental areas of infarction may demonstrate decreased areas of echogenicity indistinguishable from pyelonephritis. Power Doppler imaging is the most sensitive for demonstrating a corresponding area of hypoperfusion.

In the chronic setting, the infarcted tissue contracts resulting in cortical loss and scarring. When the main renal artery is occluded, the entire kidney is affected, resulting in diffuse atrophy and loss of renal function.

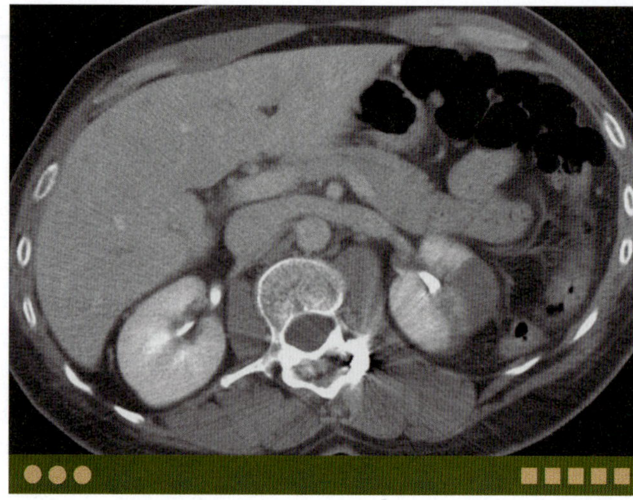

A. Axial CECT shows a wedge-shaped area of nonenhancement in the mid aspect of the left kidney.

Infiltrative lesions may mimic renal infarction and include infiltrative neoplasms, metastases, and pyelonephritis. When bilateral, pyelonephritis and infiltrative metastases should be considered in the differential diagnoses.

Clinical management is guided by the patient's underlying medical condition and function of the contralateral kidney. When clinically warranted, revascularization can be attempted via catheter directed lytic therapy. Many patients are treated conservatively with anticoagulation therapy to prevent further incidents. Early diagnosis is essential in determining clinical management.

PEARLS

- **Clinical presentation is nonspecific.**
- **Patients typically at risk for thromboembolic disease.**
- **Absence of renal parenchymal enhancement best demonstrated by CECT.**
- **Presence of cortical rim sign virtually diagnostic of renal infarct.**

ADDITIONAL IMAGES (B-D)

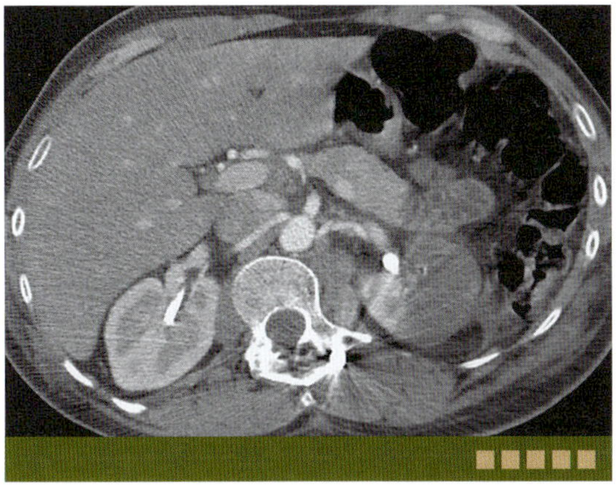

B. Axial CECT further shows the extent of infarct involving the left kidney. A small amount of perinephric fluid is present.

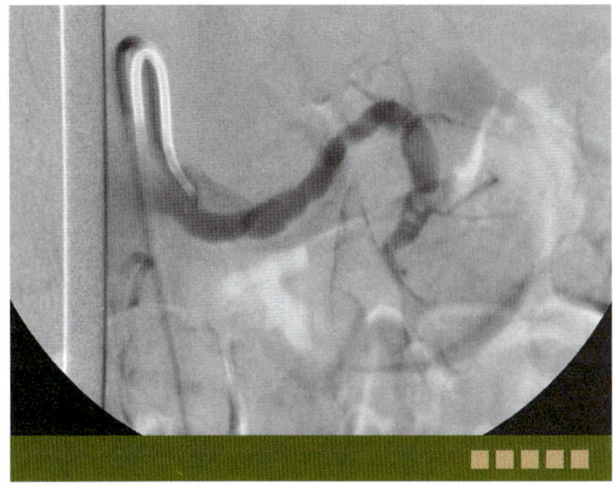

C. Selective catheter injection of the left renal artery shows filling defects distally in the left renal artery compatible with emboli resulting in infarction. Findings consistent with FMD are present in the main renal artery.

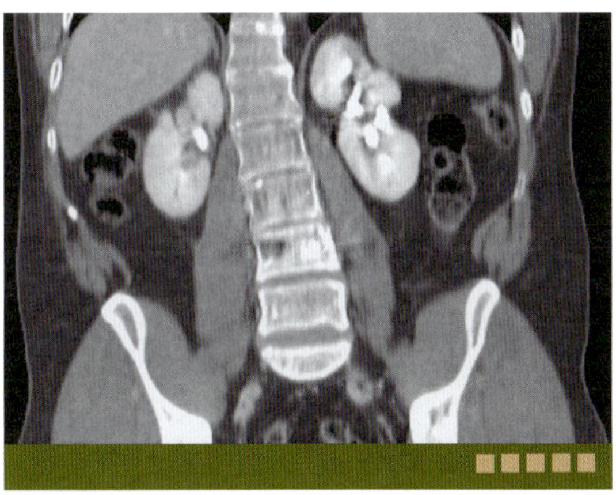

D. Coronal CECT in the same patient performed at a later date shows evolution of the patient's left renal infarct with parenchymal loss and cortical scarring.

DIFFERENTIAL DIAGNOSES IMAGES (E-G)

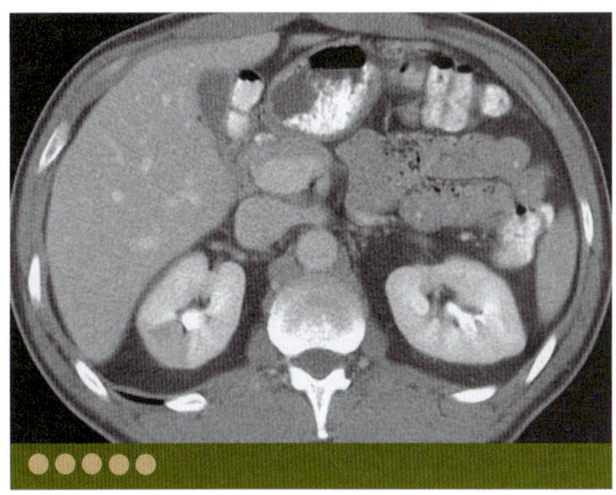

E. Pyelonephritis: Axial CECT shows a wedge-shaped area of decreased attenuation extending to the periphery. This patient presented with fever, elevated white count, and right flank pain.

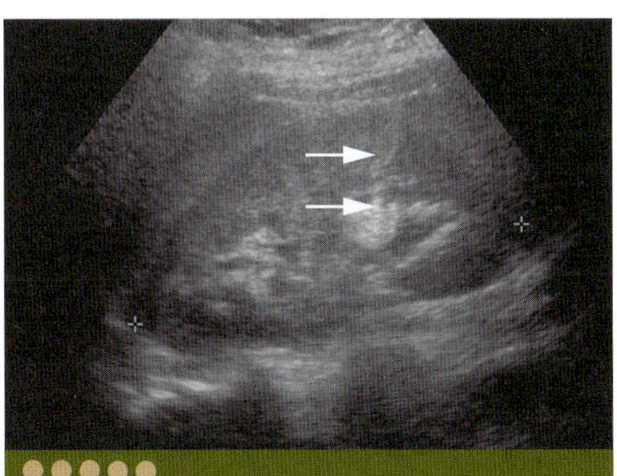

F. Pyelonephritis: Longitudinal sonogram shows subtle decreased echogenicity in the lower pole of the kidney in this patient with clinically suspected pyelonephritis (arrows).

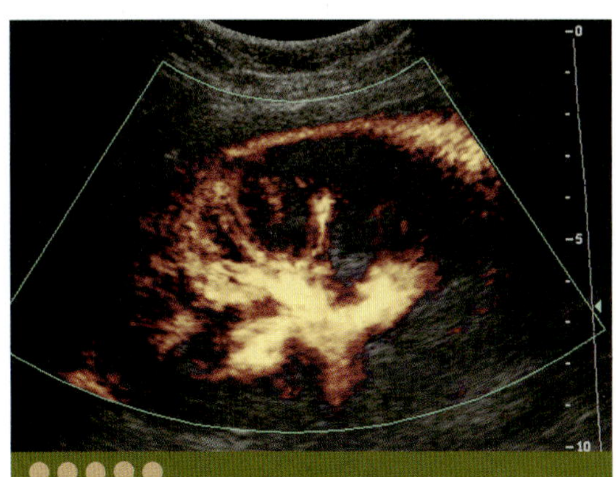

G. Pyelonephritis: Longitudinal power Doppler sonogram in the same patient shows lack of flow to the involved portion of the kidney. Similar findings can be seen with acute renal infarct.

IMAGE KEY

Common
●●●●●
●●●●
●●●
●●
●
Rare

Typical
■■■■■
■■■■
■■■
■■
■
Unusual

5-7 Nutcracker Syndrome

Nancy A. Hammond

PRESENTATION

Microscopic hematuria.

FINDINGS

Compression of the left renal vein in the aortomesenteric angle with collateral vessels.

DIFFERENTIAL DIAGNOSIS

None

COMMENTS

Nutcracker syndrome or left renal vein entrapment syndrome is caused by the compression of the left renal vein by the aorta and proximal superior mesenteric artery (SMA). The elevated renal venous pressure results in the formation of ureteral and renal pelvic venous varicosities and the development of collateral veins. The etiology of nutcracker syndrome has been suggested to be an abnormally branching SMA. The incidence of nutcracker syndrome is not known, but it seems to be equally frequent in males and females and is typically seen in younger patients.

Patients typically present with microscopic or macroscopic hematuria. While the pathophysiology is not entirely understood, this is felt to be the result of the increased pressure in the left renal vein causing rupture of thin walled varices. Physical symptoms are uncommon but include abdominal or flank pain and symptoms of orthostatic disturbances. In male patients, left varicoceles may develop.

CT and MRI demonstrate compression of the left renal vein in the aortomesenteric angle and the development of collateral vessels. CT angiography and MR angiography may demonstrate these findings more clearly. Sagittal images show a small angle of the SMA as it arises from the aorta causing left renal vein compression. Renal venography with measurement of the pressure gradient between the left renal vein and inferior vena cava (IVC) is a reliable method for diagnosing nutcracker syndrome but is invasive. In normal patients, no significant pressure gradient is seen between the left renal vein and IVC. IVU is usually normal but may demonstrate ureteric or pelvic notching because of retroperitoneal collaterals.

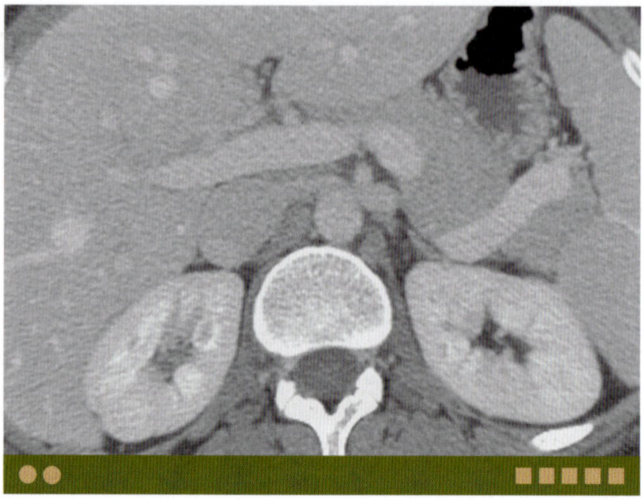

A. Axial CECT shows focal narrowing of the left renal vein as it passes between the SMA and aorta.

Treatment is guided by the severity of the hematuria. Patients with intermittent episodes of hematuria and no anemia are treated conservatively with close follow-up and monitoring. In symptomatic patients with persistent hematuria, surgical intervention may become necessary.

PEARLS

- **Seen more commonly in young patients, present with hematuria.**
- **Cross sectional imaging demonstrates narrowing of the renal vein as it passes between the SMA and the aorta. Collateral vessels develop in the renal hilum.**
- **Venography demonstrates a pressure gradient.**
- **Treatment guided by the degree of symptoms.**

ADDITIONAL IMAGES (B-E)

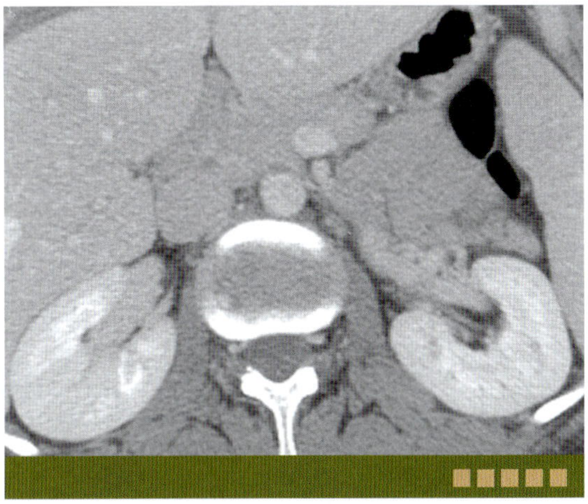

B. Axial CECT shows in the same patient multiple collateral vessels in the left renal hilum.

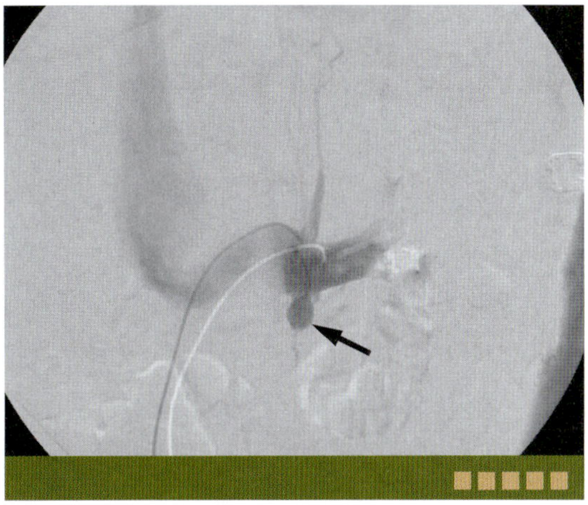

C. Catheter directed venography of the left renal vein shows a band-like compression on the left renal vein at the expected location of the SMA. The pressure gradient was found to be significant measuring 8 mm Hg. Additionally, there is saccular dilatation of the left gonadal vein as it enters the left renal vein (arrow).

IMAGE KEY

Common

Rare

Typical

Unusual

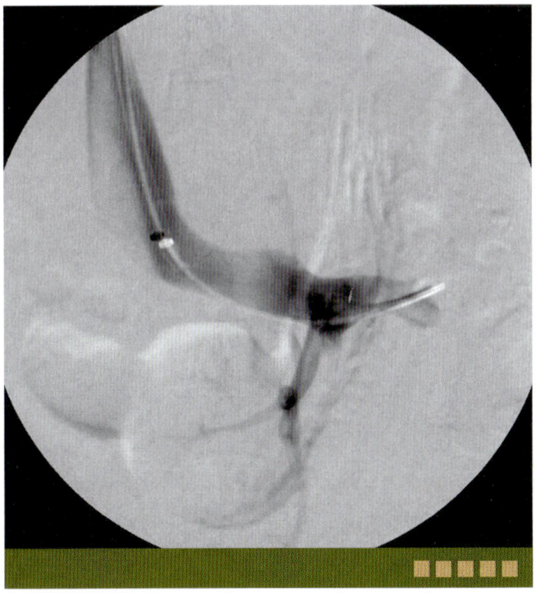

D. Catheter directed venography of the left renal vein in a different patient also shows band-like compression of the left renal vein by the SMA.

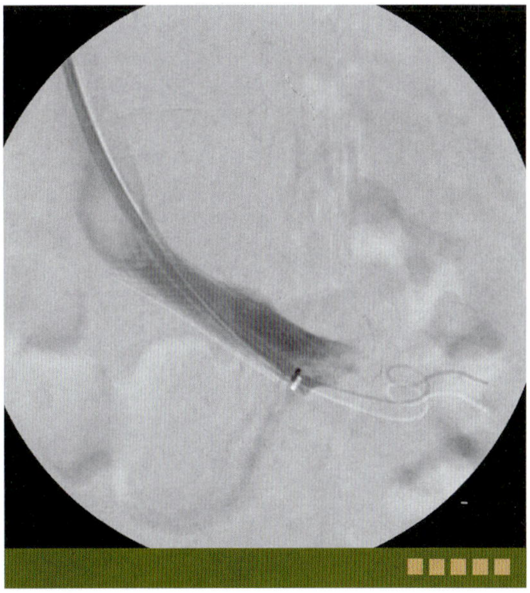

E. Venography after stent placement in the same patient as in Figure D shows resolution of the narrowing of the left renal vein.

5–8 Renal Vein Bland Thrombosis

Frank H. Miller

PRESENTATION

Generally asymptomatic; when acute, may present with acute flank pain and hematuria.

FINDINGS

Filling defect in renal vein because of clot.

DIFFERENTIAL DIAGNOSIS

- *Tumor thrombus*: Tends to be expansile and enhancing and contiguity of thrombus with tumor suggests tumor thrombus. In contrast, bland thrombus does not enhance nor expand the vessel.

COMMENTS

Renal vein thrombosis occurs most commonly with nephrotic syndrome with proteinuria. Renal vein thrombosis is associated with hypercoaguable states. Trauma, renal and adrenal neoplasms, associated use of oral contraceptives, sickle cell anemia, and dehydration are some causes of renal vein thrombus. In adults, it is most often seen with membranous glomerulonephritis. Renal vein thrombosis is most often chronic, and patients are asymptomatic. When acute, it may be associated with flank pain and hematuria. It is more commonly seen on the left side and believed because of the longer course and pathway between the SMA and aorta. There are no specific laboratory tests for the diagnosis, and imaging studies play a critical role in the diagnosis. Complications include renal infarcts and pulmonary emboli. Treatment includes anticoagulation with lytic agents used when thrombus is acute and severe.

Renal ultrasound shows enlarged edematous kidneys, which may be relatively hypoechoic. Color Doppler may show the thrombus. Left renal vein thrombus may be more difficult to identify than right renal vein thrombus because of the longer length of the vein and overlying bowel gas. CT and MR are more sensitive for the diagnosis. In addition, they are helpful in showing associated renal infarcts. When using CT, contrast enhancement is generally required to show the thrombus.

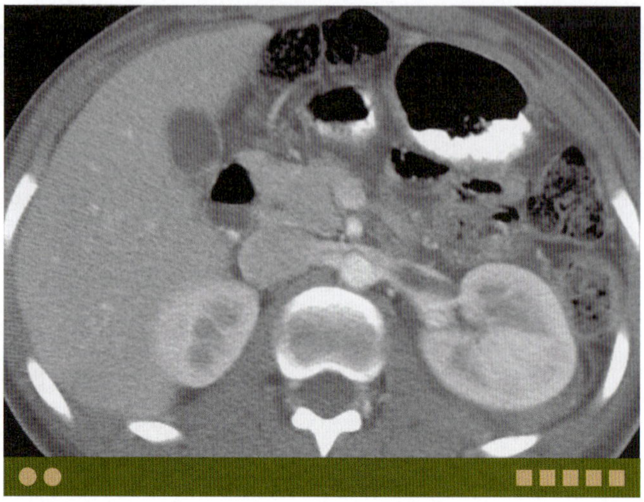

A. Axial CECT shows filling defect in left renal vein from renal vein thrombus in patient with systemic lupus erythematosis.

A filling defect is seen in the renal vein, which may be the only finding especially when nonocclusive. MR has the advantage of lack of radiation and can be used if needed without contrast material. Both CT and MR can be helpful to identify an underlying renal tumor and to assess tumor thrombus.

PEARLS

- **Renal vein thrombosis occurs most commonly with nephrotic syndrome and in adults with membranous glomerulonephritis.**
- **CT and MR are the best tests to assess for renal vein thrombus.**
- **Bland thrombus tends to be nonexpansile and nonenhancing.**
- **Tumor thrombus tends to be expansile and enhancing and may be in contiguity with the primary tumor.**

ADDITIONAL IMAGES (B-C)

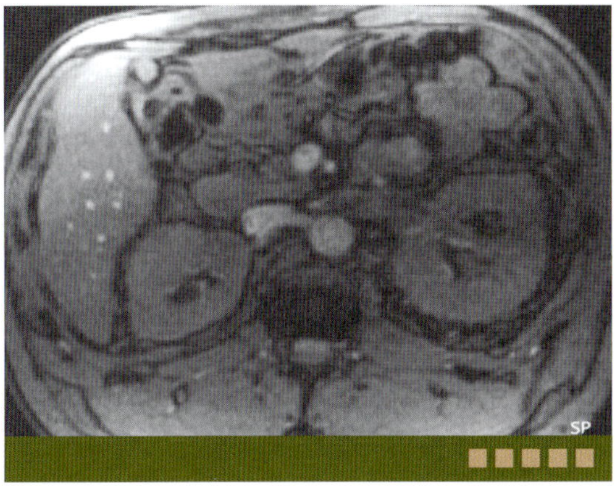

B. True FISP image shows filling defect in different patient with left renal vein clot.

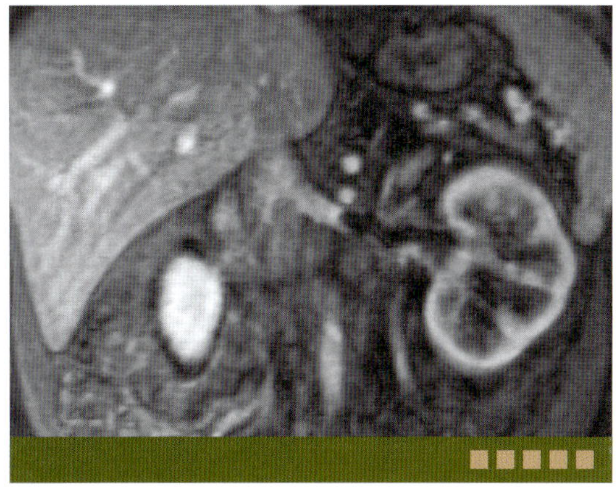

C. Coronal contrast-enhanced T1-WI shows filling defect in left renal vein. Note that the clot does not enhance nor is expansile to suggest tumor thrombus.

DIFFERENTIAL DIAGNOSES IMAGES (D-F)

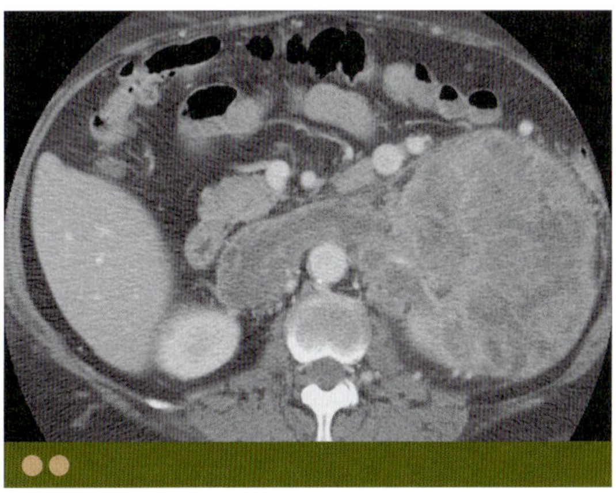

D. Tumor thrombus from renal cell carcinoma. Axial CECT shows large expansile left renal vein thrombus. There is enhancement of the clot and extension from left renal cell carcinoma. Findings are most consistent with tumor thrombus and not bland thrombus.

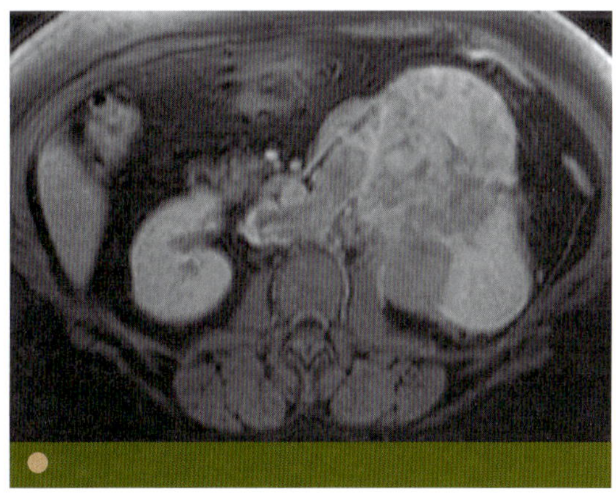

E. Adrenal cell carcinoma with tumor thrombus. Axial contrast-enhanced T1-WI in a different patient shows tumor thrombus seen as expansile enhancing thrombus extending into retroaortic adrenal vein. On this image, it is difficult to determine whether the tumor arises from the kidney or adrenal gland.

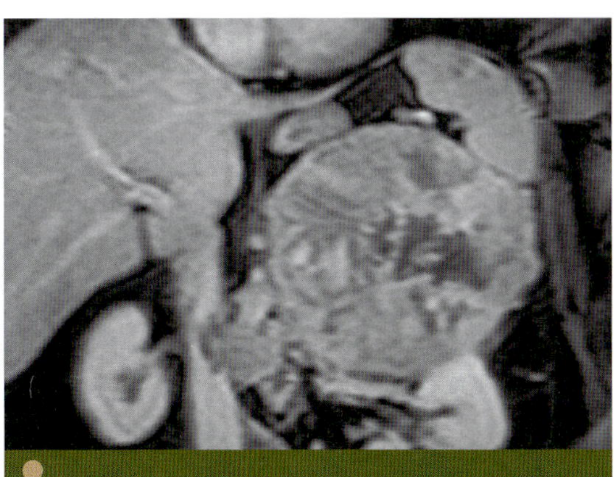

F. Adrenal cell carcinoma with tumor thrombus. Coronal contrast-enhanced T1-WI in the same patient shows that the tumor arises superior and separate from the kidney and arises from the left adrenal gland, and not as a result of renal cell carcinoma.

IMAGE KEY

Common

Rare

Typical

Unusual

5–9 Tumor Thrombus Involving Renal Vein

Frank H. Miller

PRESENTATION

May be asymptomatic or present with leg swelling or rarely shortness of breath as a result of pulmonary embolus.

FINDINGS

Expansile enhancing left renal vein thrombus.

DIFFERENTIAL DIAGNOSIS

- *Bland thrombus*: Does not expand vein nor enhance.

COMMENTS

Tumor thrombus is caused by extension of tumor into the veins. The diagnosis of tumor thrombus involving the renal vein is important as it suggests an underlying tumor as an etiology. Tumors that have a predisposition to invade vessels include renal cell carcinoma, adrenal cell carcinoma, or hepatocellular carcinoma. Those that are seen in the renal vein include most commonly renal cell carcinoma and adrenal cell carcinoma. Angiomyolipoma (AML) rarely can invade the renal vein and IVC. The thrombus may be echogenic on ultrasound or fat-containing on CT and MR.

Tumor thrombus should be suspected when a filling defect is seen within the vein, which is expansile and enhancing. In contrast, bland thrombus neither enhances nor expands the vessel. Another feature suggestive of tumor thrombus includes contiguity of the thrombus with the tumor. The diagnosis can be made with CT, MR, or ultrasound. On ultrasound, Doppler flow may be seen in the thrombus to suggest tumor thrombus.

The presence of tumor thrombus changes the stage of renal cell carcinoma to Robson Stage IIIA from II and using the TNM criteria to T3c when the IVC is involved and T3b with the involvement of the renal vein. In addition, it is important to determine if venous involvement is seen to involve the renal vein, IVC and the right atrium. When it extends to involve the supradiaphragmatic IVC and right atrium, cardiac bypass may be required during surgery.

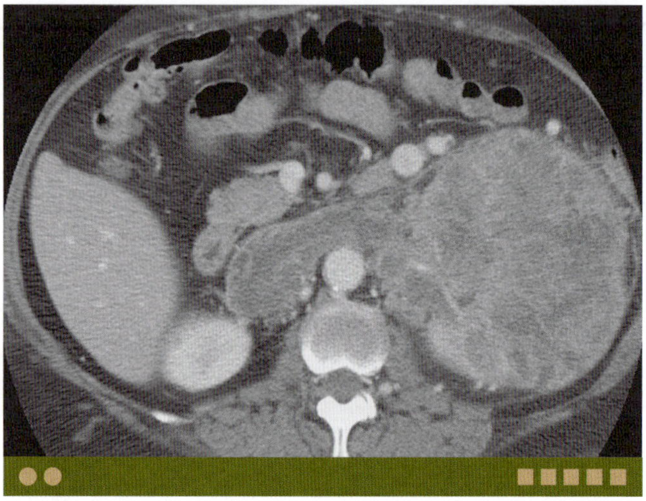

A. Axial CECT scan shows expansile enhancing thrombus within the left renal vein which extends to the IVC as a result of tumor thrombus. Patient has contiguous large left renal cell carcinoma.

PEARLS

- **Tumor thrombus is seen as expansile and enhancing thrombus within the vessel.**
- **Bland thrombus is not expansile and not enhancing.**
- **The presence of tumor thrombus should prompt a search for an underlying tumor.**
- **Tumor thrombus increases the stage of renal cell carcinoma and is important for the surgeons to be aware of prior to surgery.**

ADDITIONAL IMAGE (B-F)

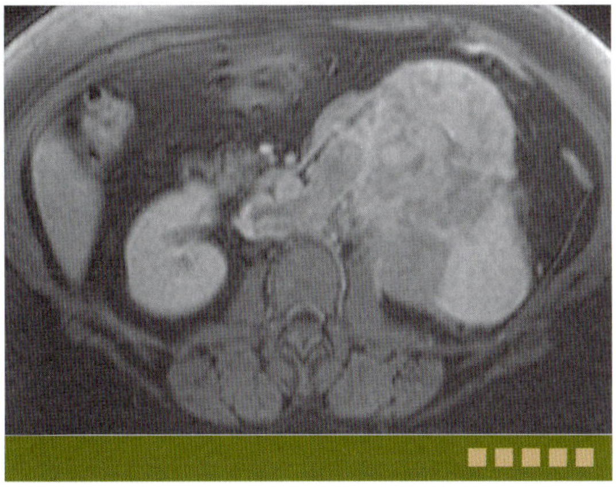

B. Adrenal cell carcinoma with tumor thrombus: Axial contrast-enhanced T1-WI in a different patient shows tumor thrombus extending into retroaortic adrenal vein. On this image, it is difficult to determine whether the tumor arises from the kidney or adrenal gland.

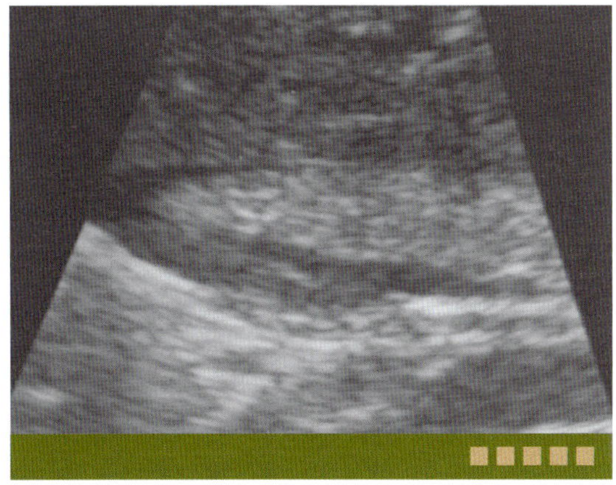

C. AML invading IVC: Longitudinal sonogram in a different patient shows echogenic thrombus within the IVC as a result of the fat-containing thrombus from AML.

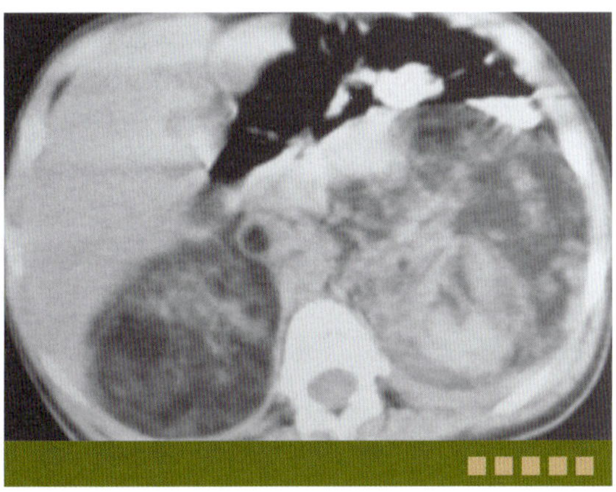

D. AML invading IVC: Axial CECT scan shows that the patient has bilateral AMLs replacing the kidneys from tuberous sclerosis with fat thrombus in the IVC from tumor thrombus. This is a rare complication of AML.

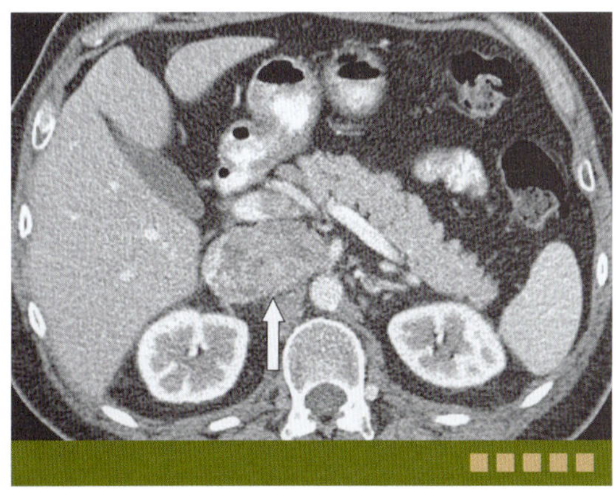

E. IVC leiomyosarcoma: Axial CECT shows enhancing heterogeneous mass expanding the IVC.

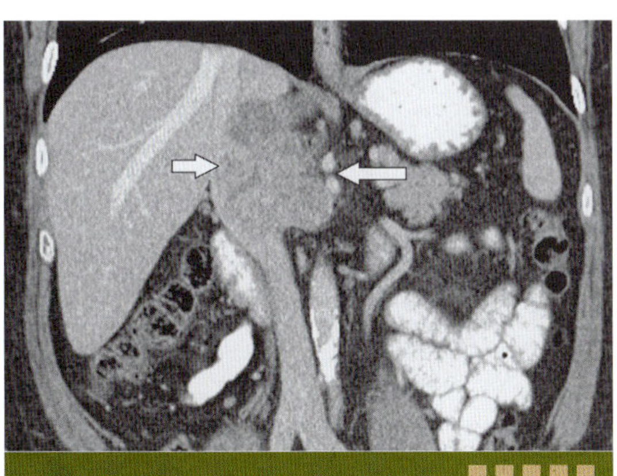

F. IVC leiomyosarcoma: Coronal reformatted CECT in the same patient shows the vein expanded by tumor. The renal vein was not involved, and the mass arose in the IVC and was shown at surgery as a result of because of leiomyosarcoma of the IVC.

DIFFERENTIAL DIAGNOSES IMAGE

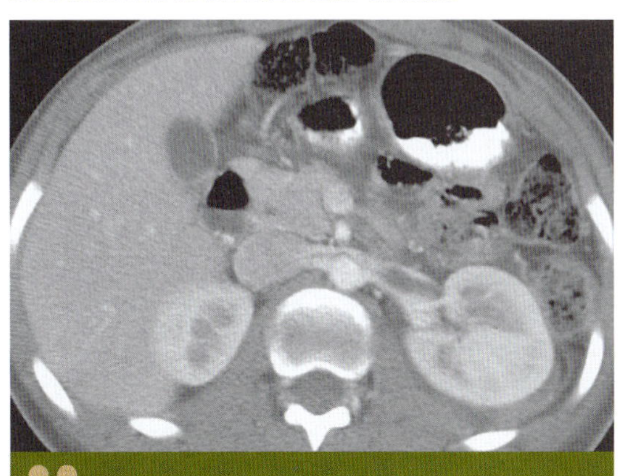

G. Bland thrombus: Axial CECT shows filling defect in left renal vein from renal vein thrombus in patient with systemic lupus erythematosis.

CHAPTER 5
Renal Vascular Disease and Renal Transplantation

PART I
Renal Vascular Disease

CASE

Tumor Thrombus Involving Renal Vein

IMAGE KEY

Common

Rare

Typical

Unusual

Part 2

Renal Transplantation

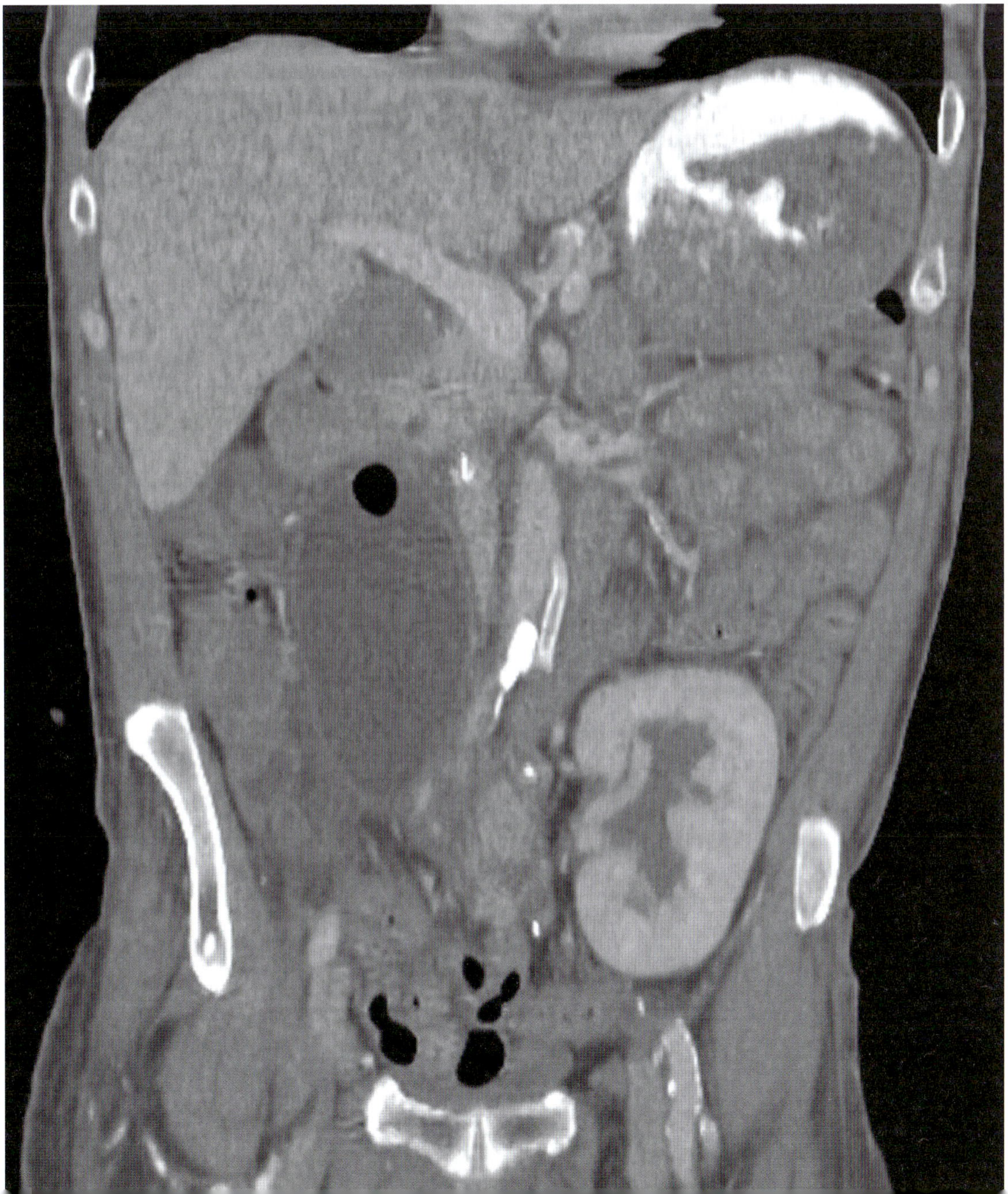

5–10 Posttransplant Renal Artery Stenosis

Nancy A. Hammond

PRESENTATION

Allograft dysfunction and hypertension.

FINDINGS

Aliasing at the level of the renal artery anastomosis with elevation of the velocity above 200 cm/s.

DIFFERENTIAL DIAGNOSIS

- *False positives*: Can occur secondary to kinking or extreme tortuosity of the renal artery.

COMMENTS

Renal artery stenosis (RAS) is the most common vascular complication of renal transplantation occurring in about 10% of transplant recipients. It typically occurs within the first postoperative year. Patients usually present with allograft dysfunction and hypertension not treatable by medical therapy. The most common site for stenosis to occur is at or just distal to the arterial anastomosis. The stenosis is usually as a result of surgical technique. More distal stenoses are felt to be caused by perfusion alterations and some authors have suggested rejection as a cause.

Color Doppler sonography demonstrates focal color aliasing at the stenotic segment with distal turbulent flow. Peak systolic velocities obtained at the involved segment typically measure greater than 200 cm/s. A velocity gradient greater than 2:1 between the stenotic and prestenotic segments is also indicative of a significant stenosis. The intrarenal arteries may show a pulsus tardus-parvus waveform; however, this finding is not always present. Parvus tardus refers to the decreased amplitude of the pulse and delayed time to reach the peak. An acceleration time of the intrarenal arteries greater than 0.07 seconds and an acceleration index less than 300 cm/s are diagnostic criteria for RAS. Acceleration time is measured as the length of time of the systolic upstroke. The acceleration index is defined as the change of velocity divided by the change in time. If indicated, CT or MR angiography can confirm the presence of RAS. False positive may result with MRA because of a clip artifact in the region of the anastomosis. RAS can often by treated by percutaneous transluminal angioplasty.

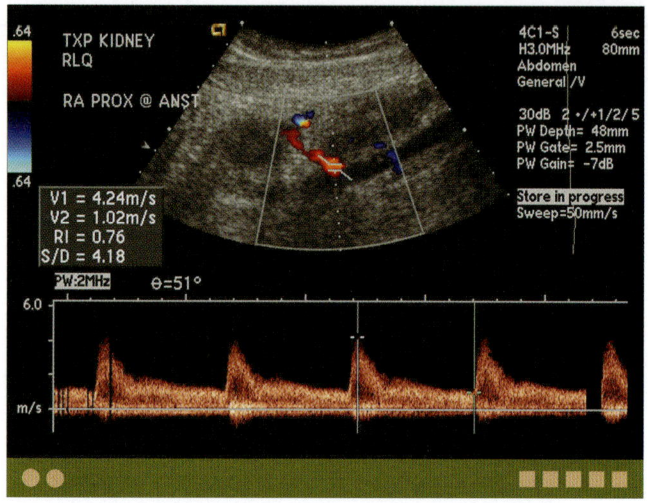

A. Color Doppler sonogram shows a markedly elevated velocity at the level of the renal artery anastomosis with a peak systolic velocity of 424 cm/s.

PEARLS

- **RAS is the most common vascular complication of renal transplantation.**
- **It is most commonly seen at the anastomosis secondary to surgical technique.**
- **Doppler sonography demonstrates an increased velocity of greater than 200 cm/s at the stenotic segment with distal turbulent flow.**
- **RAS may be treated with percutaneous transluminal angioplasty.**

ADDITIONAL IMAGES (B-D)

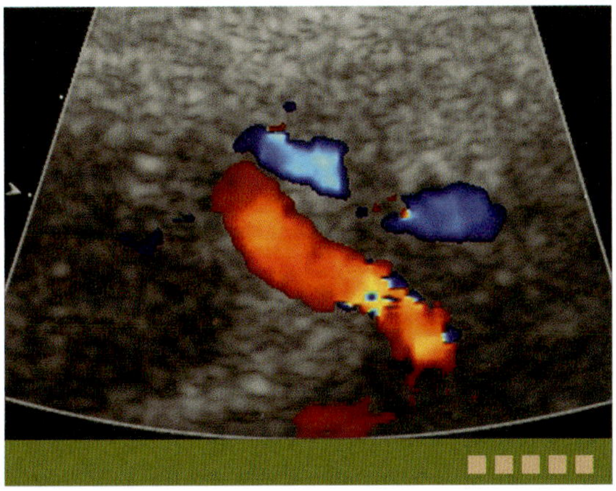

B. Color Doppler shows turbulent flow at the level of the anastomosis supporting the diagnosis of RAS.

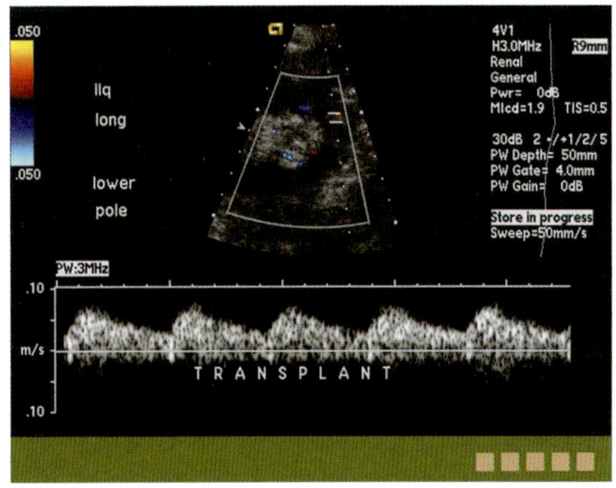

C. Doppler waveform of an arcuate artery in a renal transplant shows delayed systolic upstroke compatible with a parvus tardus waveform. This finding can be seen in RAS, but should not be considered diagnostic.

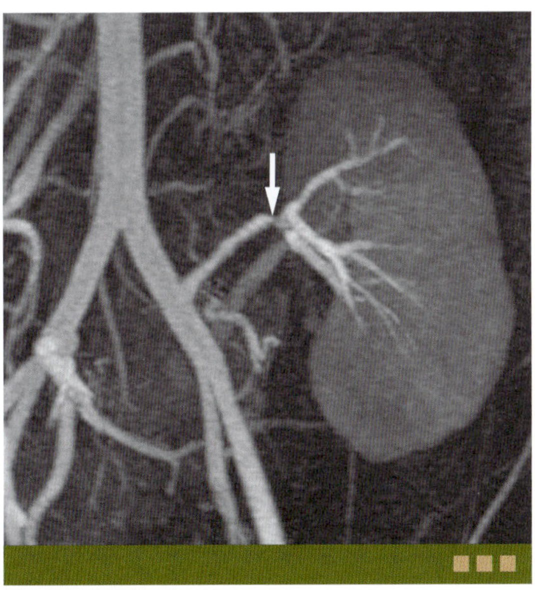

D. Coronal MIP from contrast-enhanced MRA shows focal stenosis in the main renal artery supplying the transplanted kidney (arrow).

IMAGE KEY

Common

Rare

Typical

Unusual

5-11 Transplant Renal Arteriovenous Fistula

Nancy A. Hammond

PRESENTATION

Status renal transplant biopsy.

FINDINGS

Color Doppler demonstrates a focal region of aliasing over the AVF. Turbulent flow is present in the vascular malformation. Spectral Doppler demonstrates low resistance and high velocity within the lesion. If a draining vein is identified, the waveform may be arterialized.

DIFFERENTIAL DIAGNOSIS

None

COMMENTS

In the renal transplant patient, intrarenal arteriovenous fistulas (AVFs) are most commonly the result of arterial and venous laceration during percutaneous renal biopsies. The majority of AVFs are asymptomatic and have little clinical significance. When small, they typically resolve spontaneously. In the rare case of a large AVF, patients may present with bleeding, high cardiac output failure, or renal ischemia because of the shunting.

Intrarenal arteriovenous fistulas can be demonstrated sonographically or with contrast-enhanced MRA or CTA. Sonographically, most AVFs are not apparent on grayscale imaging. When large, they appear as complex cystic structures. Color flow demonstrates turbulence, aliasing, and tissue vibration artifact in the area of the fistula. High-velocity and low-resistance waveforms are present on the arterial side. When identified, the draining vein demonstrates arterial pulsations. Tissue vibration artifact appears as color signal outside of the true borders of the AVF on power Doppler.

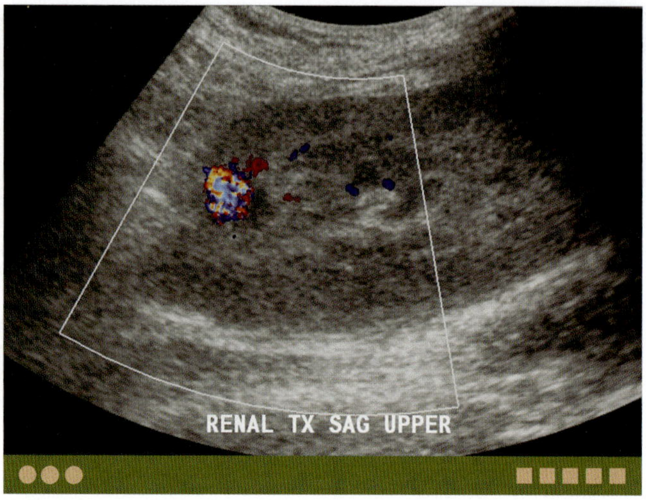

A. Longitudinal color Doppler sonogram shows a focus of abnormal turbulent flow and aliasing involving the upper pole of the transplanted kidney.

MRA and CTA demonstrate an enhancing focus within the kidney corresponding to the vascular nidus and early filling of the renal vein caused by shunting. The vascular nidus remains enhanced on delayed imaging.

When treatment of an AVF is indicated, it is usually embolization.

PEARLS

- **AVFs in the renal transplant patient are typically the consequence of a traumatic renal biopsy.**
- **Most AVFs are small and do not require treatment.**
- **If large, AVFs can be treated with percutaneous embolization.**

ADDITIONAL IMAGES (B-E)

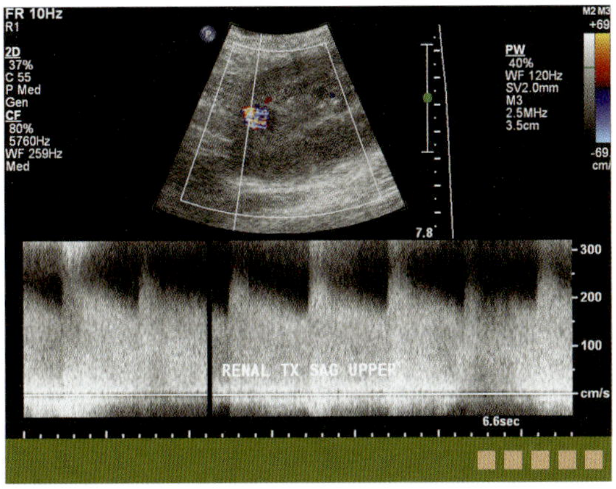

B. Longitudinal spectral Doppler sonogram in the same patient shows a high-velocity, low-resistance waveform over the abnormality consistent with an AVF.

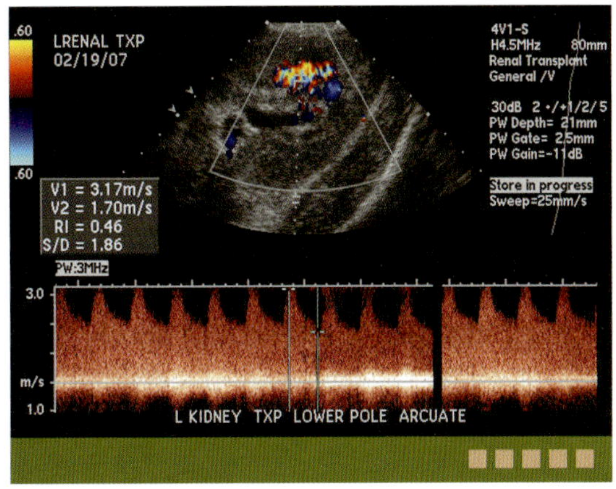

C. Longitudinal color Doppler sonogram in a different patient shows a focus of abnormal turbulent flow in the lower pole of the transplanted kidney. Spectral tracings shows high-velocity (317 cm/s) arterial flow with a low resistance (RI = 0.46).

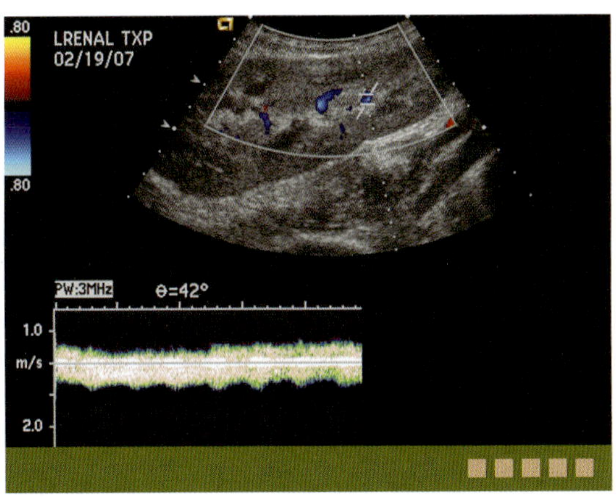

D. Longitudinal color Doppler sonogram in the same patient as Figure C shows arterialization of the venous waveform at the lower pole of the kidney.

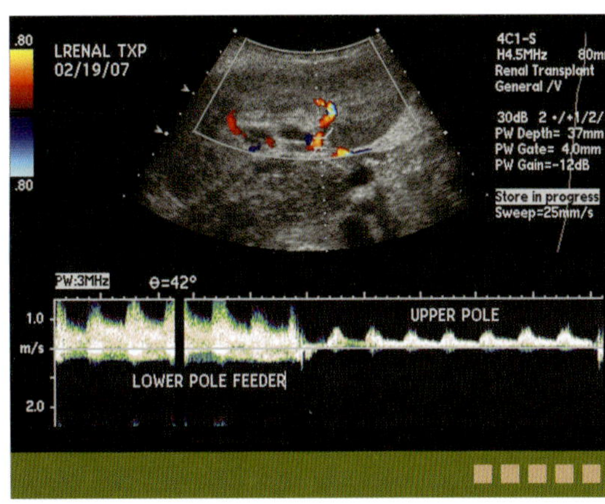

E. Longitudinal color Doppler sonogram shows the feeding vessel to the AVF with high-velocity arterial flow.

IMAGE KEY

Common

Rare

Typical

Unusual

5–12 Transplant Renal Pseudoaneurysm

Nancy A. Hammond

PRESENTATION

Status renal transplant biopsy.

FINDINGS

Grayscale ultrasound demonstrates a cystic structure in the transplanted kidney. Color Doppler typically shows a "yin and yang" appearance.

DIFFERENTIAL DIAGNOSIS

None

COMMENTS

Renal transplant pseudoaneurysms can be intra or extrarenal in location. Intrarenally lesions are the result of vascular trauma to the arterial system sustained during biopsy. Extrarenal pseudoaneurysms typically occur at the anastamosis secondary to the surgical technique and, less commonly, occur as a complication of perivascular infection.

Sonographically, pseudoaneurysms appear as cystic spaces on grayscale imaging and can be mistaken for renal cysts. In the transplant patient, cysts are uncommon, and thus, suspicion for a pseudoaneurysm should be raised. Color Doppler demonstrates a swirling pattern of blood flow within the cystic lesion. Spectral Doppler shows central to-and-fro flow waveform or a disorganized tracing. This "to-and-fro" pattern is because of flow entering the aneurysm during systole and exiting during diastole. Pseudoaneurysms with broad necks may not have the typical Doppler waveform and may show a more disorganized flow, with a high-velocity, low-resistance waveform identified in the neck. Extra and intrarenal pseudoaneurysms have the same ultrasound characteristics.

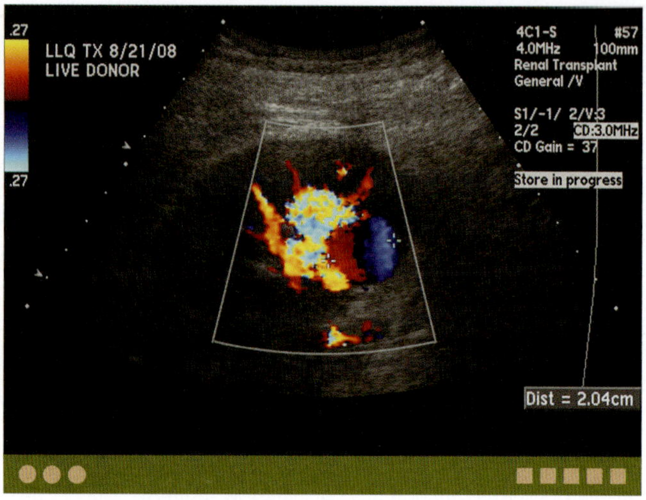

A. Sagittal color Doppler sonogram shows the characteristic yin and yang flow in a pseudoaneurysm.

When treatment of a pseudoaneurysm is indicated, it is usually embolization or surgical.

PEARLS

- **Pseudoaneurysms in the renal transplant patient are typically the consequence of a traumatic renal biopsy.**
- **Pseudoaneurysms occurring at the anastamosis are typically associated with surgical technique.**
- **Appear as cystic spaces on grayscale ultrasound with a characteristic "to-and-fro" appearance on Doppler.**

ADDITIONAL IMAGES (B-E)

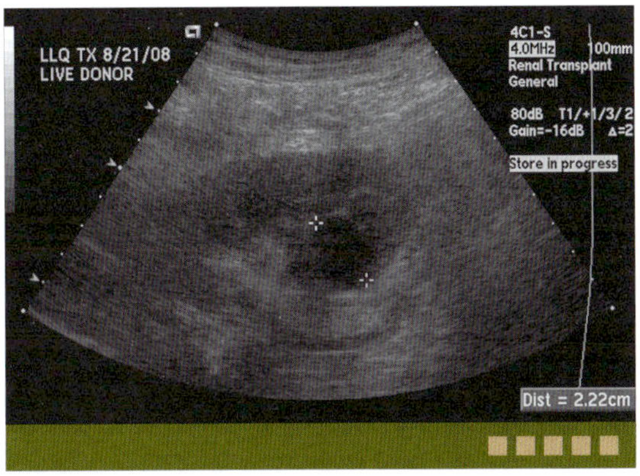

B. Sagittal sonogram shows an anechoic lesion with posterior acoustic enhancement at the site of the above-noted pseudoaneurysm. Without the use of color Doppler, this finding could be easily confused with a cyst.

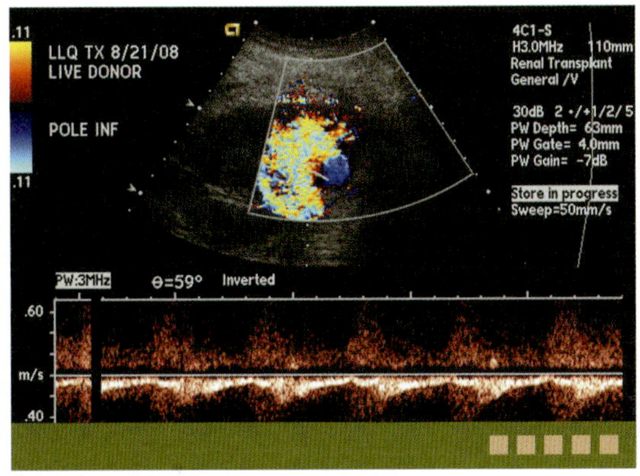

C. Spectral Doppler tracing shows bidirectional flow within the pseudoaneurysm corresponding the apparent cystic space seen in Figure B.

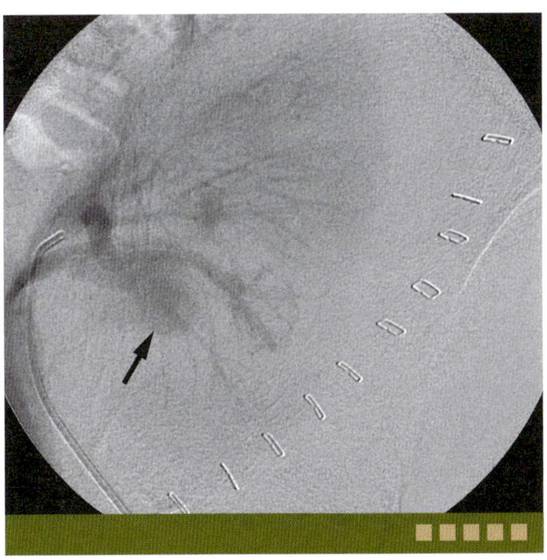

D. Selected angiogram of the transplanted kidney shows a focal collection of contrast (arrow) at the lower pole of the kidney corresponding to the above-noted pseudoaneurysm.

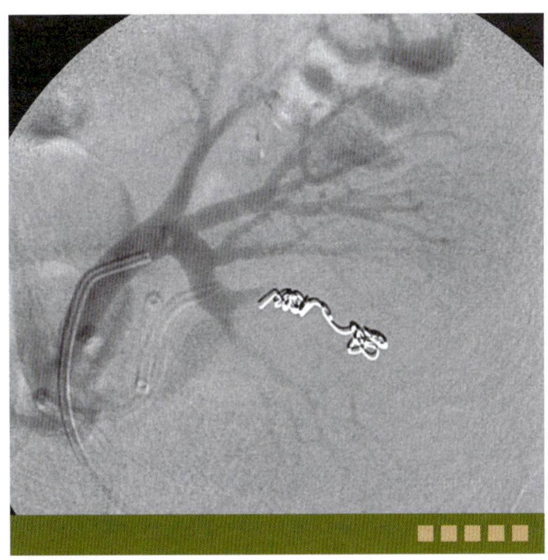

E. Post-therapy angiogram shows resolution of the pseudaneurysm after effective coiling.

IMAGE KEY

Common

Rare

Typical

Unusual

5–13 Renal Vein Thrombosis in Renal Transplant

Nancy A. Hammond

PRESENTATION

Oliguria and graft tenderness.

FINDINGS

Grayscale sonogram demonstrates enlarged and hypoechoic allograft. Doppler interrogation demonstrates absence of flow in the main renal vein and reversal of diastolic flow in the main renal artery.

DIFFERENTIAL DIAGNOSIS

- *Severe rejection and acute tubular necrosis*: These may both demonstrate reversal of diastolic in the arterial waveform.

COMMENTS

Renal vein thrombosis occurs in the early postoperative state in up to 4% of renal transplant recipients. It typically occurs in the first week after transplantation manifesting clinically with oliguria, graft tenderness, and graft swelling. Risk factors include technical difficulties during surgery, hypovolemia, iliac vein thrombosis, and renal vein compression caused by external compression from posttransplant fluid collections.

On grayscale sonography, intra-aluminal thrombus may be seen in a dilated main renal vein but is typically not well demonstrated. The kidney may be hypoechoic and enlarged as a result of edema. Color Doppler demonstrates absence of flow in main renal vein with spectral analysis showing reversal of diastolic flow in the main renal artery. CT may show a dilated renal vein, and if intravenous contrast was administered, a filling defect in the renal vein may be identified on delayed images. A delayed nephrogram and retention of contrast material are indirect signs of renal vein thrombosis on CT. MR demonstrates similar findings.

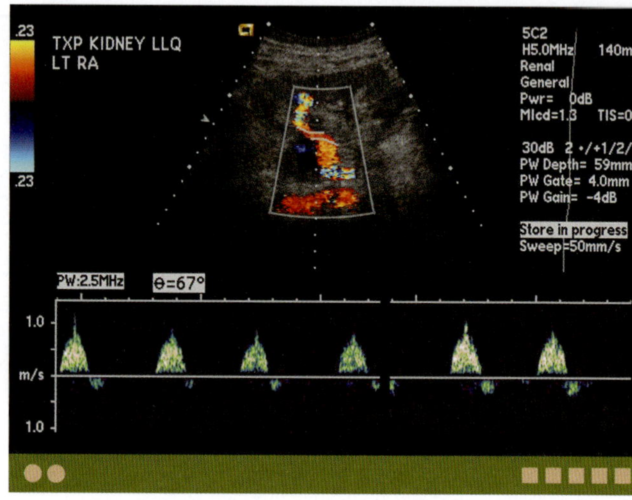

A. Sagittal color Doppler sonogram shows patency of the main renal artery in this transplanted kidney with an abnormal waveform. Reversal of diastolic flow is present.

The treatment is thrombectomy. When left untreated, renal vein thrombosis results in allograft infarction and neccessitates removal of the transplant. Renal vein thrombosis has also been described with chronic rejection. In the chronic setting, treatment is anticoagulation.

PEARLS

- **While reversal of diastolic flow is nonspecific and can be seen with severe rejection and acute tubular necrosis, absence of renal vein flow and reversal of diastolic flow is virtually diagnostic of renal vein thrombosis.**
- **The treatment is thrombectomy.**

ADDITIONAL IMAGES (B-C)

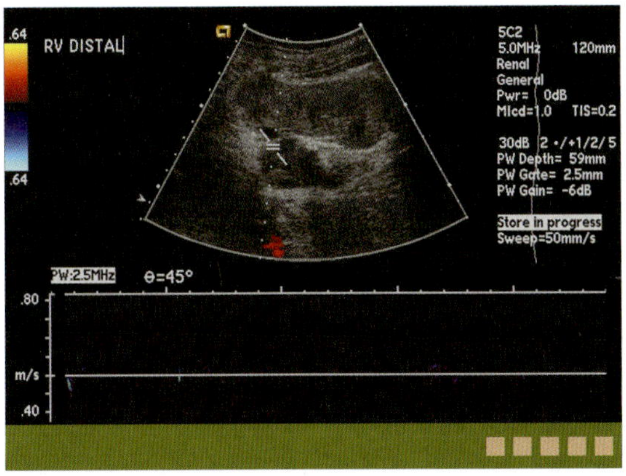

B. Sagittal sonogram through the renal hilum of the same patient shows an enlarged renal vein filled with echogenic material representing thrombus. Doppler interrogation shows absence of flow in the main renal vein confirming the diagnosis of RVT.

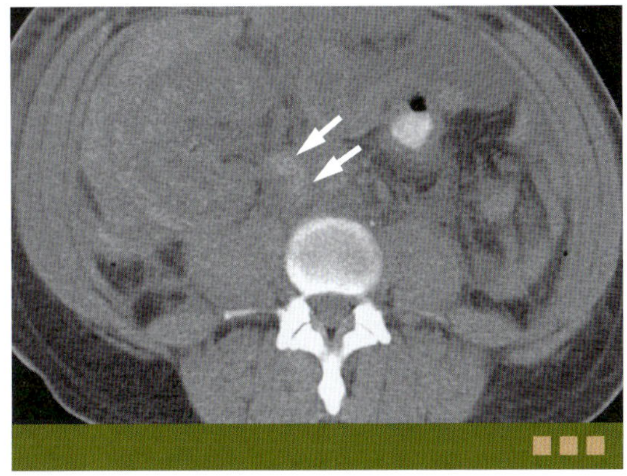

C. NECT in a different patient shows a heterogeneous, enlarged transplanted kidney in the right lower quadrant. Curvilinear hyperdensity (arrow) in the renal hilum in the expected location of the renal vein that was found to represent thrombus in the main renal vein. Perinephric hyperdensity is compatible with a hematoma.

DIFFERENTIAL DIAGNOSES IMAGES (D-E)

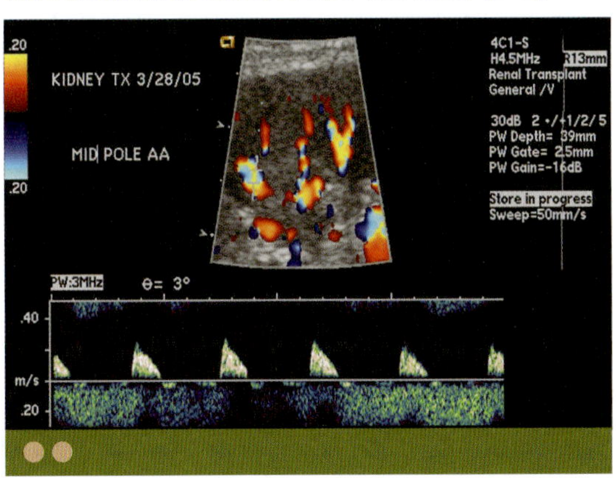

D. Acute rejection: Sagittal color Doppler sonogram in a different patient shows mild reversal of diastolic flow in the arcuate renal artery of a transplanted kidney.

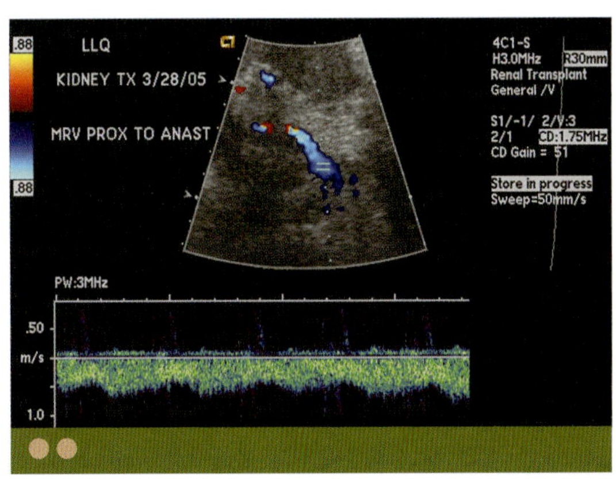

E. Acute rejection: Color Doppler sonogram in the same patient as Figure D shows patency of the main renal vein excluding the possibility of renal vein thrombosis. The patient was subsequently determined to have acute rejection.

IMAGE KEY

Common

Rare

Typical

Unusual

5–14 Acute Rejection

Nancy A. Hammond

PRESENTATION

Status postrenal transplant, elevated renal function test, decreased urine output.

FINDINGS

Increased renal size with variable renal echogenicity. Doppler interrogation demonstrated markedly elevated resistive indices with reversal of diastolic flow.

DIFFERENTIAL DIAGNOSES

- *Acute tubular necrosis*: Considered in the diagnosis as imaging findings overlap but typically occurs earlier than acute rejection; clinical and laboratory findings may be helpful in distinguishing.
- *Cyclosporine toxicity*: Typically occurs at a later stage.
- *Renal vein thrombosis*: Reversal of diastolic flow in renal artery, no flow in renal vein.
- *Urinary tract obstruction*: Presence of hydronephrosis.
- *Perinephric fluid collection*: Abnormal fluid collections present.

COMMENTS

Acute rejection most commonly occurs in the first year after transplantation. It is rare in the immediate posttransplant period and after the first year. Clinically, impaired renal function is manifested as rising serum creatinine levels. Patients can present with malaise, fever, and a painful kidney. Symptoms may be masked by cyclosporine therapy.

Imaging findings of renal complications can be nonspecific, and renal biopsy is often necessary to make the diagnosis. The time of occurrence can help in differentiating among various renal complications. Acute rejection, acute tubular necrosis, and cyclosporine toxicity can be difficult to differenitate based on imaging findings; however, acute tubular necrosis commonly occurs immediately after transplantation, acute rejection typically occurs 1 to 4 weeks postoperatively, and cyclosporine toxicity occurs months to years after transplantation.

Grayscale imaging of acute rejection can demonstrate increased size of the kidney, increased cortical thickness, increased or decreased cortical echogenicity, loss of corticomedullary differentiation, and loss of renal sinus echoes.

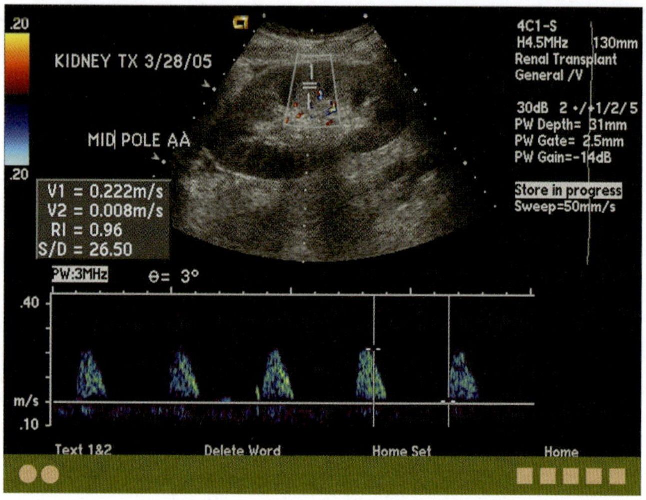

A. Sagittal color Doppler sonogram of the transplanted kidney shows absence of diastolic flow involving the middle pole arcuate artery. The resistive index is markedly elevated measuring 0.96.

Color Doppler ultrasound may be normal or show decreased blood flow and increased intraparenchymal resistive indices. Elevated resistive indices can also be seen in acute tubular necrosis or cyclosporine toxicity. In severe cases of acute rejection, there can be reversal of diastolic flow. This finding can also be seen in entities that cause increased vascular resistance of the allograft such as renal vein thrombosis, urinary tract obstruction, or a perinephric fluid collection.

As imaging findings are nonspecific, renal biopsy is necessary when acute rejection is clinically suspected.

PEARLS

- **Acute rejection most commonly occurs in the first year after transplantation.**
- **Imaging findings of acute rejection, cyclosporine toxicity, and acute tubular necrosis can be identical. The timeframe within which these entities occur varies.**
- **Renal biopsy for diagnosis is necessary when rejection is clinically suspected.**

ADDITIONAL IMAGES (B-D)

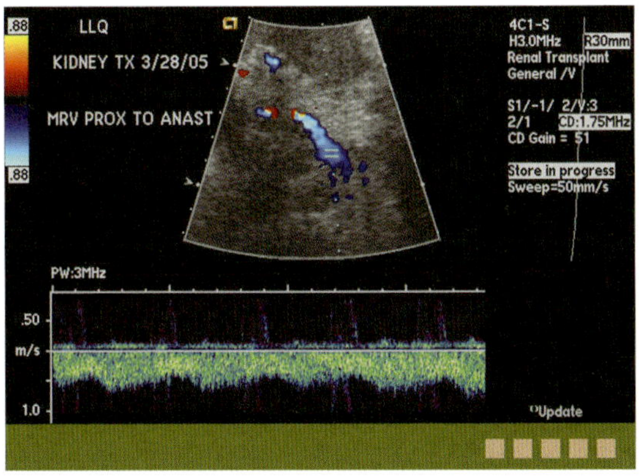

B. Color Doppler sonogram in the same patient shows patency of the renal vein. This excludes renal vein thrombosis as the etiology for the reversal of diastolic flow.

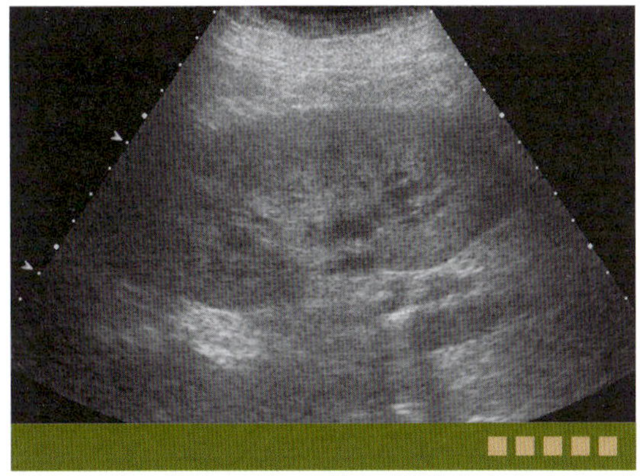

C. Longitudinal sonogram shows a mildly echogenic transplanted kidney with mild loss of corticomedullary differentiation. Findings can be seen in acute rejection.

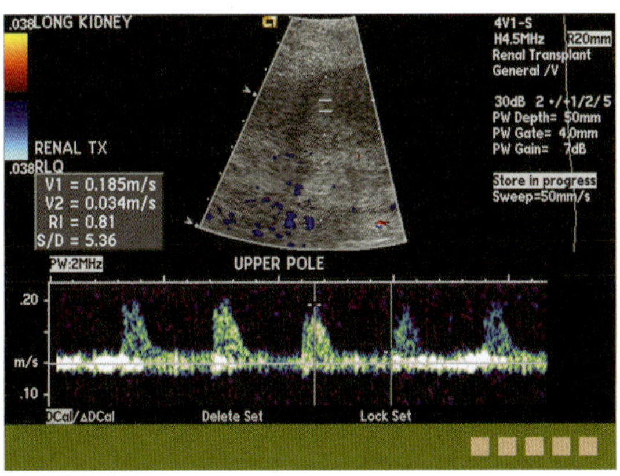

D. Longitudinal color Doppler sonogram in the same patient as in Figure C shows mild elevation of the resistive index measuring 0.81 of the arcuate artery. The RI had increased since the prior study, and the patient presented with decreasing renal function. Renal biopsy was performed confirming the diagnosis of acute rejection.

DIFFERENTIAL DIAGNOSES IMAGES (E-F)

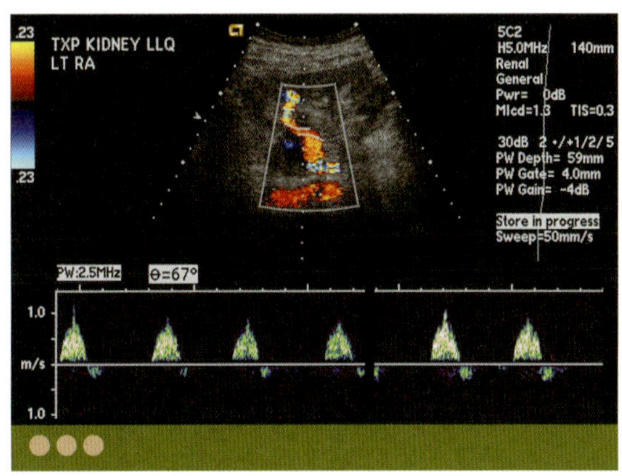

E. Renal vein thrombosis: Sagittal color Doppler sonogram shows reversal of diastolic flow in the transplanted renal artery.

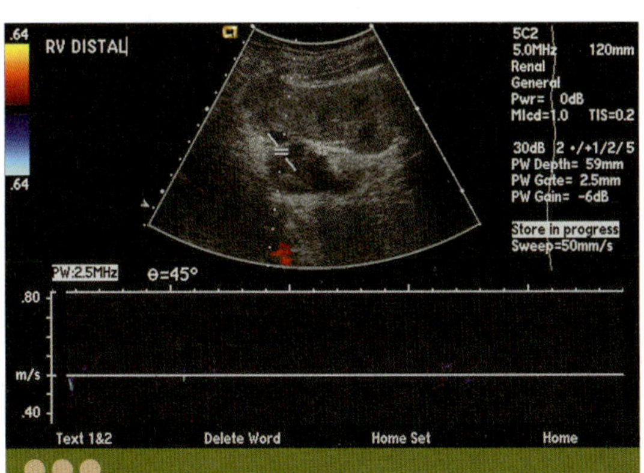

F. Renal vein thrombosis: Color Doppler sonogram through the renal vein in the same patient as in Figure E shows absence of flow in the main renal vein.

IMAGE KEY

Common

Rare

Typical

Unusual

5–15 Hydronephrosis in Transplanted Kidney

Nancy A. Hammond

PRESENTATION

Decreasing renal function.

FINDINGS

Grayscale evaluation of the renal transplant demonstrates hydronephrosis.

DIFFERENTIAL DIAGNOSES

- *Nonobstructive mild pelvocaliectasis*: Can be seen secondary to overhydration, reflux, or diminished ureteral tone. Follow-up imaging may be necessary to exclude progression because of obstructive clauses.
- *Parapelvic cysts*: Nonconverging anechoic structures in the renal pelvis.

COMMENTS

Hydronephrosis from obstruction is uncommon occuring in less than 5% of renal transplant patients. The most common site for obstruction is at the ureteric vesicular anastomosis secondary to edema and ischemia leading to stricture formation. Other causes include infection, extrinsic compression from peritransplant fluid collections, kinking of the ureter and mucosal edema. Calculi are an uncommon cause accounting for less than 2% of the cases. Patients are typically asymptomatic as a result of denervation of the allograft.

Grayscale sonography demonstrates dilatation of the collection system. The presence of echogenic material within the collecting system is significant and should be noted. Hyperechoic masses are suspicious for fungus balls and low-level echoes suggest the presence of pyonephrosis or hemonephrosis. Mild pelvocaliectasis can be seen with nonobstructive causes including overhydration, reflux, diminished ureteral tone resuting from denervation, and secondary to anastamotic edema in the early posttransplant period. If the dilation involves only the renal pelvis without extension to the calyces, the likelihood of obstruction is low.

Treatment options for hydronephrosis in the transplanted kidney are guided by the etiology and include stent placement, balloon dilatation, or correction of the extrinsic compression. When strictures are long or recurrent, surgical reconstruction may be necessary.

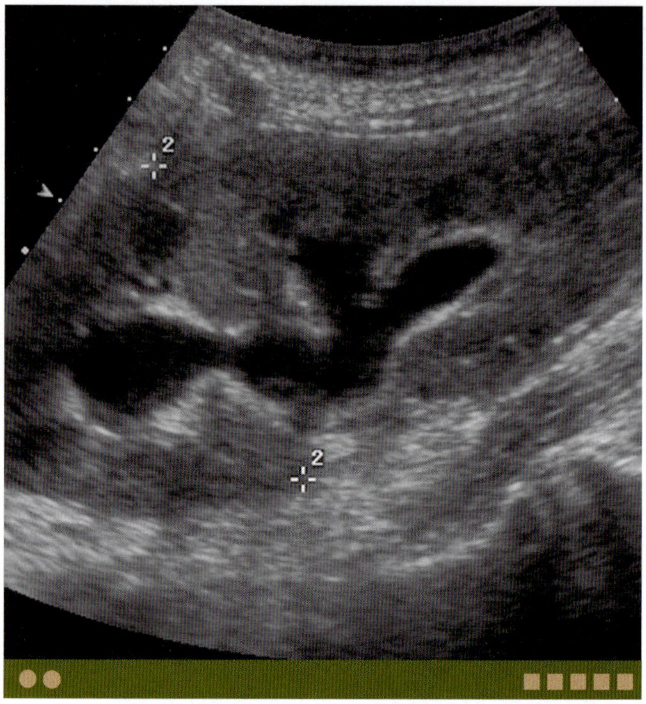

A. Longitudinal sonogram of a transplanted kidney shows moderate hydronephrosis. The etiology was subsequently found to be secondary to narrowing at the ureteric anastamosis.

PEARLS

- **The most common site for obstruction of the renal transplant is at the ureteric-vesicular anastamosis secondary to edema or ischemia resulting in stricture formation.**
- **Mild hydronephrosis can be seen with nonobstructive causes.**
- **The presence of echogenic material within the collecting system should raise suspicion for infection or hemonephrosis.**

ADDITIONAL IMAGES (B-D)

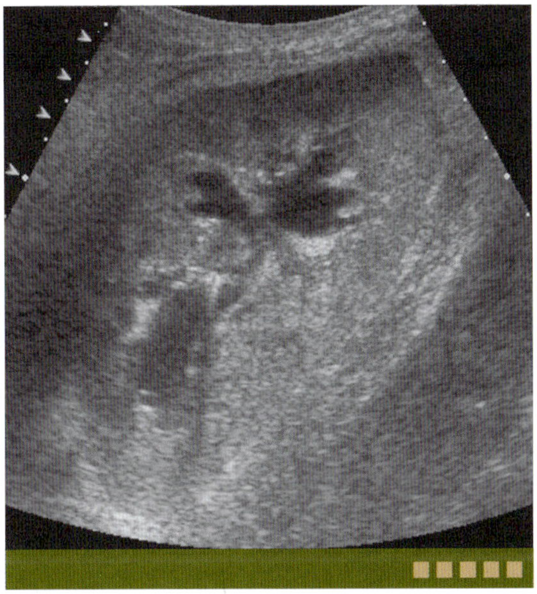

B. Longitudinal sonogram of a transplanted kidney in a different patient shows mild to moderate hydronephrosis.

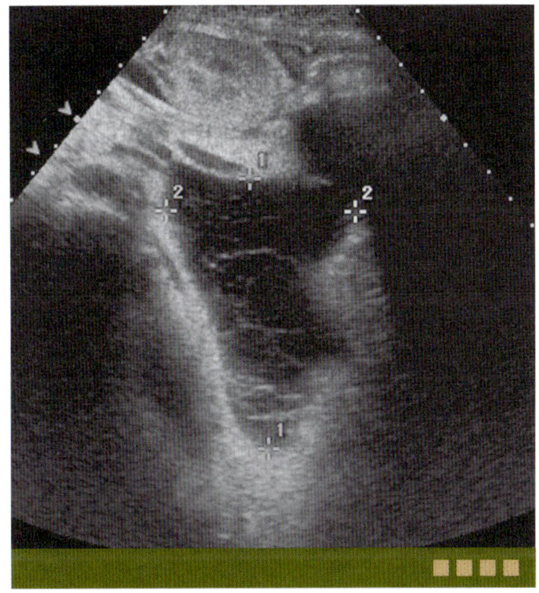

C. Longitudinal sonogram in the same patient as Figure B shows a complex fluid collection inferior to the transplant. The hydronephrosis was secondary to external compression of the ureter by this fluid collection.

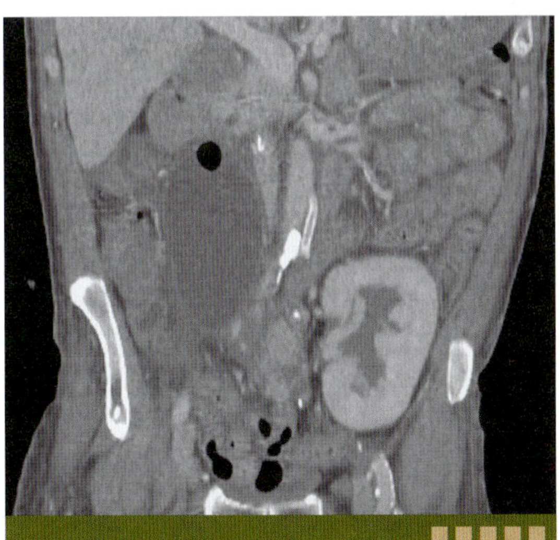

D. Coronal CECT shows mild to moderate transplant hydronephrosis. There was a peritransplant fluid collection, resulting in external compression of the ureter.

DIFFERENTIAL DIAGNOSES IMAGE

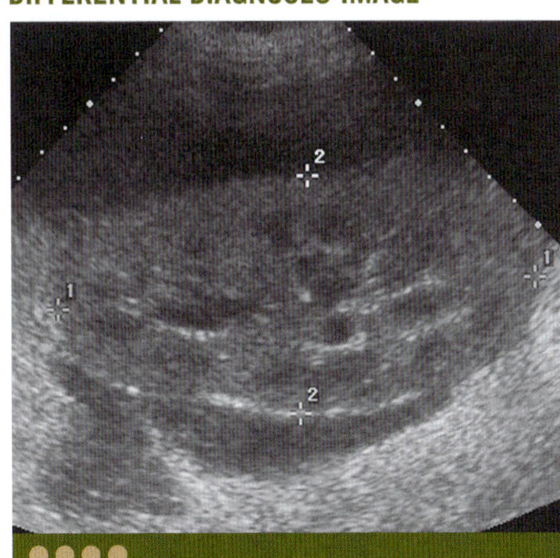

E. Nonobstructive mild pelviocaliectasis: Longitudinal sonogram of a transplanted kidney shows mild pelvicaliectasis without frank hydronephrosis. A small perinephric fluid collection is also present. The mild dilation resolved on subsequent sonograms consistent with a nonobstructive etiology.

IMAGE KEY

Common

Rare

Typical

Unusual

5–16 Posttransplant Urinoma

Nancy A. Hammond

PRESENTATION

Pain, swelling, and discharge from the surgical wound.

FINDINGS

Well-defined, anechoic mass in the region of the transplant.

DIFFERENTIAL DIAGNOSES

- *Hematoma*: Occur in the early postoperative state. Sonographically, hematomas are more complex than urinomas. Acute hematomas appear as echogenic, heterogeneous solid masses. Later, they appear as complex cystic masses with internal echoes and/or septations.
- *Lymphocele*: Occur 4 to 8 weeks after surgery in up to 15% of patients. Sonographically, well-defined, anechoic collections that may contain internal strands.
- *Abscess*: Complex fluid collections in the appropriate clinical presentation.

COMMENTS

Urine leaks are an uncommon complication of renal transplantation that typically occur in the first 2 weeks after surgery. Patients present with pain, swelling, and discharge from the wound. Urine leaks are the result of graft rejection, ureteral necrosis because of ischemia, or inadequate surgical technique. Sonography demonstrates a well-defined anechoic collection that can result in hydronephrosis. On nonenhanced CT, a hypodense mass is identified. After intravenous contrast administration, contrast is seen collecting in the hypodense mass. Delayed images may be necessary to confirm extravasation of contrast material into the fluid collection. Radionuclide studies show progressive radiotracer activity in the abnormal collection.

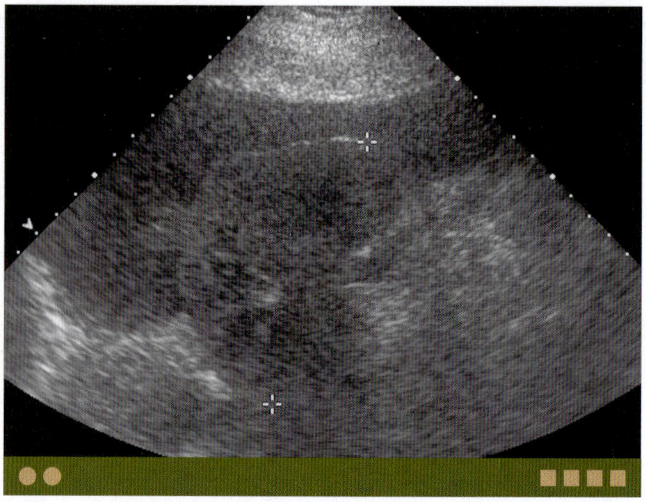

A. Longitudinal sonogram of a renal transplant shows a large perinephric fluid collection. Internal echoes were felt to be artifactual because of a poor acoustic window. Patient was one week postoperative renal transplant.

PEARLS

- **Time of occurrence, clinical presentation, and imaging characteristics discussed above are key factors in distinguishing between the various posttransplant fluid collections.**
- **Urinomas typically occur in the first 2 weeks after transplantation and are the result of graft rejection, ureteral necrosis from ischemia, or inadequate surgical technique.**
- **Imaging demonstrates a well-defined fluid collection. On delayed contrast-enhanced images, intravenous contrast is excreted into and collects in the fluid collection.**

ADDITIONAL IMAGE

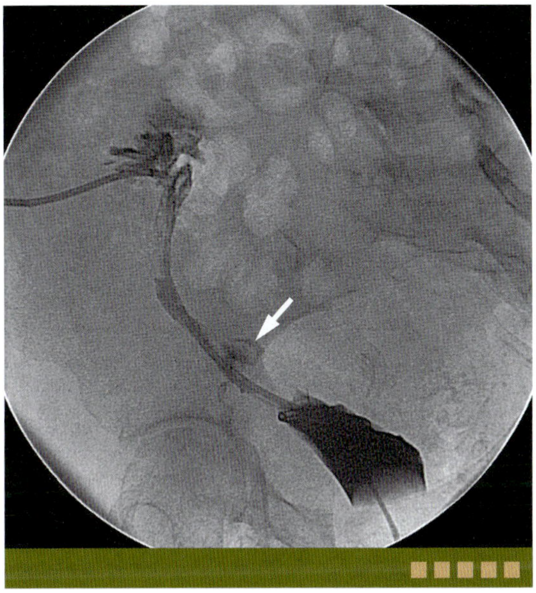

B. Fluoroscopic image in the same patient as Figure A obtained during a nephrostogram after nephroureterual stent placement shows extraluminal contrast. Findings are consistent with a persistent urine leak resulting from ureteral incompetence (arrow).

IMAGE KEY

Common

Rare

Typical

Unusual

DIFFERENTIAL DIAGNOSES IMAGES (C-D)

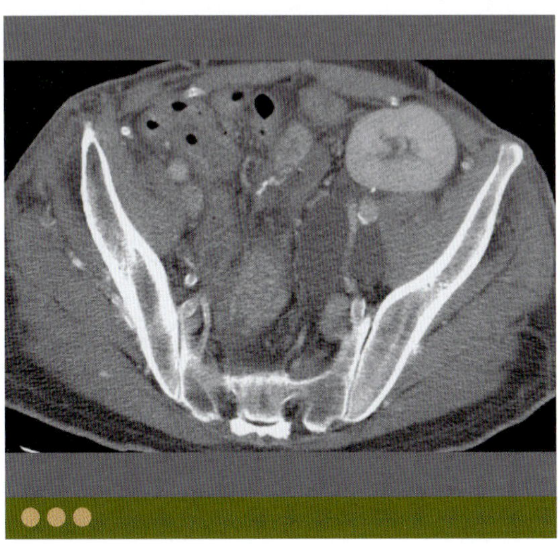

C. Lymphocele: Axial CECT shows two hypodense fluid collections in the left lower quadrant along the course of the external iliac vasculature and at the lower pole of the transplanted kidney.

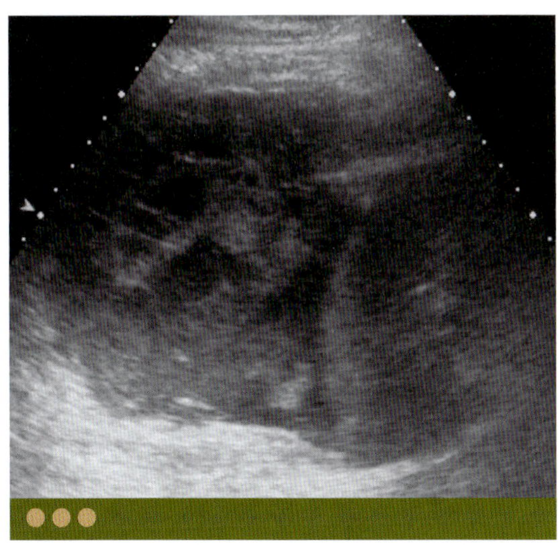

D. Hematoma: Longitudinal sonogram shows a large, complex fluid collection with posterior acoustic enhancement. Along the superior aspect of the transplanted kidney. Internal echoes and septations are noted within the collection.

5–17 Posttransplant Lymphoproliferative Disorder

Nancy A. Hammond

PRESENTATION

Status post renal transplant with fever.

FINDINGS

Hypoechoic mass on renal ultrasound.

DIFFERENTIAL DIAGNOSES

- Focal pyelonephritis or abscess.
- Focal infarction.

COMMENTS

Posttransplant lymphoproliferative disorder (PTLD) occurs in approximately 1% of renal transplant patients. It is associated with the Ebstein-Barr virus and results from the loss of the normal immune mechanisms allowing for the unchecked proliferation of B cells. PTLD can present as localized or disseminated disease and can involve the lymph nodes or solid organs. However, it is less common with renal transplants than with most other organ transplants. The tumors can be aggressive and rapidly progressive. Patients can present with a variety of symptoms including fever, weight loss, anorexia, lethargy, sore throat, swollen glands, diarrhea, abdominal pain, shortness of breath, or neurologic symptoms.

When involving the renal transplant, PTLD appears as a hypoechoic mass involving the renal parenchyma on sonography. Hypoechoic infiltration involving the renal hilum should suggest PTLD. CT findings are nonspecific and include minimally or rim-enhancing hypodense renal masses. On MRI, PTLD typically is hypointense on both T1- and T2-weighted images with minimal contrast enhancement.

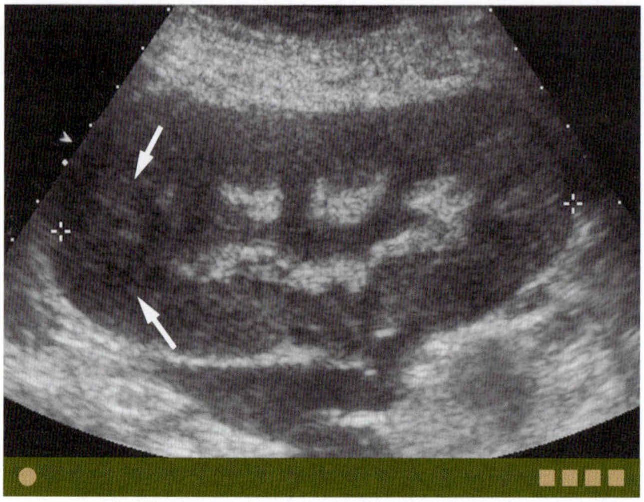

A. Longitudinal sonogram of a transplant kidney shows the suggestion of a hypoechoic mass at the upper pole (arrows).

PEARLS

- **Associated with Ebstein-Barr virus, loss of normal immune mechanism results in unchecked proliferation of B cells.**
- **Can involve lymph nodes or solid organs or both.**
- **Hypoechoic mass on sonography and hypodense mass with minimal or rim enhancement on CT.**
- **Infiltration of the transplant renal pelvis should raise suspicion for PTLD.**

ADDITIONAL IMAGES (B-D)

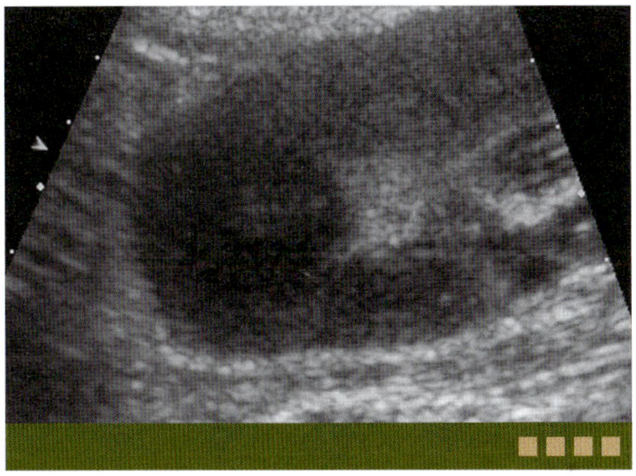

B. Further evaluation of this region with longitudinal sonography confirms the presence of a hypoechoic mass which was subsequently proven to represent PTLD.

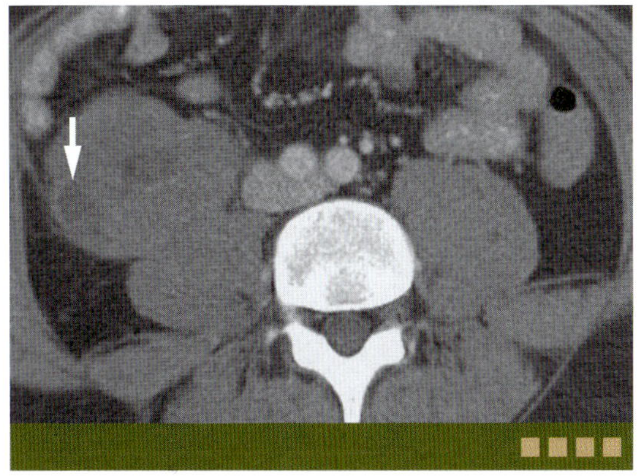

C. Axial CECT shows an additional hypodense mass with mild rim enhancement in the transplanted kidney. The kidney itself enhances poorly without corticomedullary differentiation (arrow).

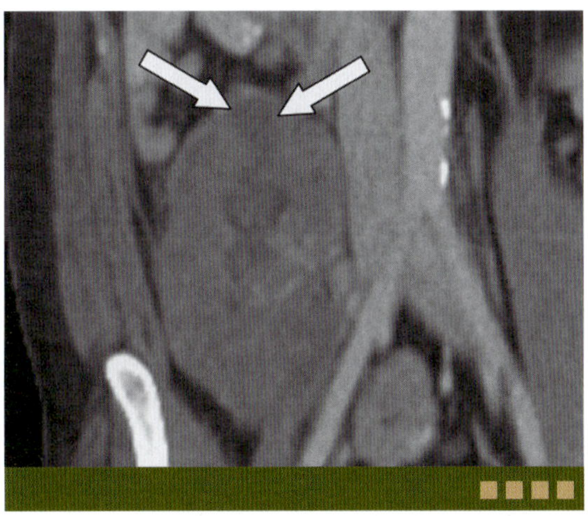

D. Coronal CECT further shows the hypodense mass at the upper pole of the kidney (arrows). Additionally, there is the suggestion of increased density in the renal hilum as can be seen with PTLD.

DIFFERENTIAL DIAGNOSES IMAGES (E-G)

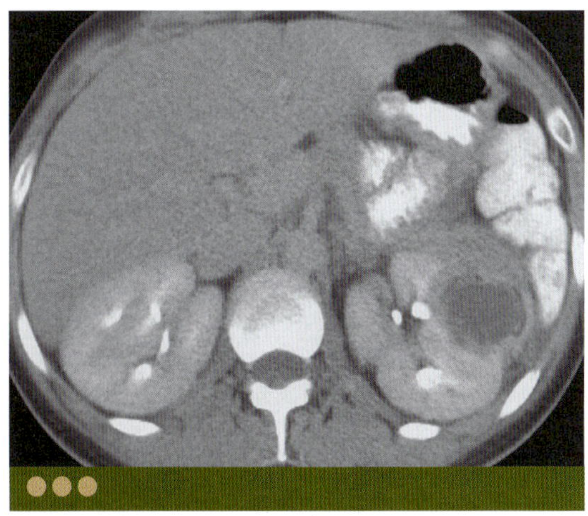

E. Renal abscess: Axial CECT shows a complex cystic mass with a thick enhancing wall in the native left kidney. Patient had a history of pyelonephritis that was not clinically resolving.

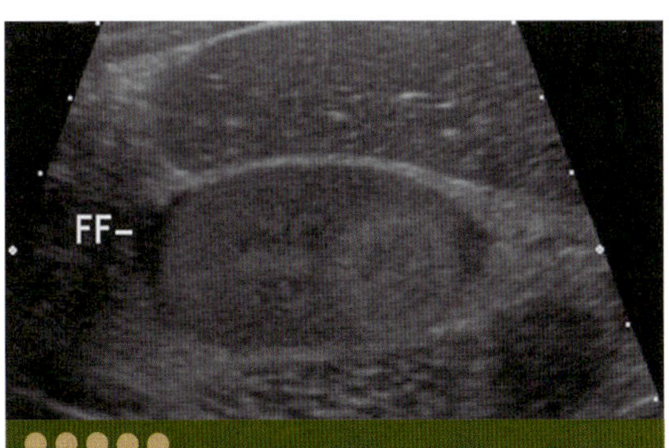

F. Focal pyelonephritis: Transverse sonogram of a native right kidney in a young patient with fever, pyuria, and flank pain shows a hyperechoic mass in the upper pole of the right kidney.

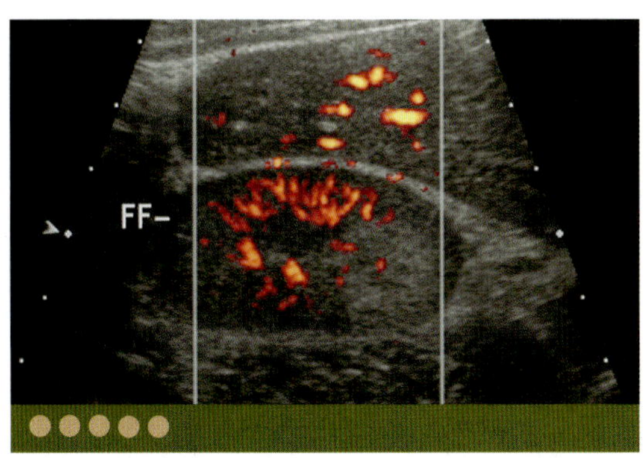

G. Focal pyleonephritis: Transverse power Doppler sonogram the same patient as Figure F shows decreased flow to the region of focal pyelonephritis as is characteristically seen.

IMAGE KEY

Common

Rare

Typical

Unusual

CHAPTER 6

RENAL PELVIS, SINUS, URETER

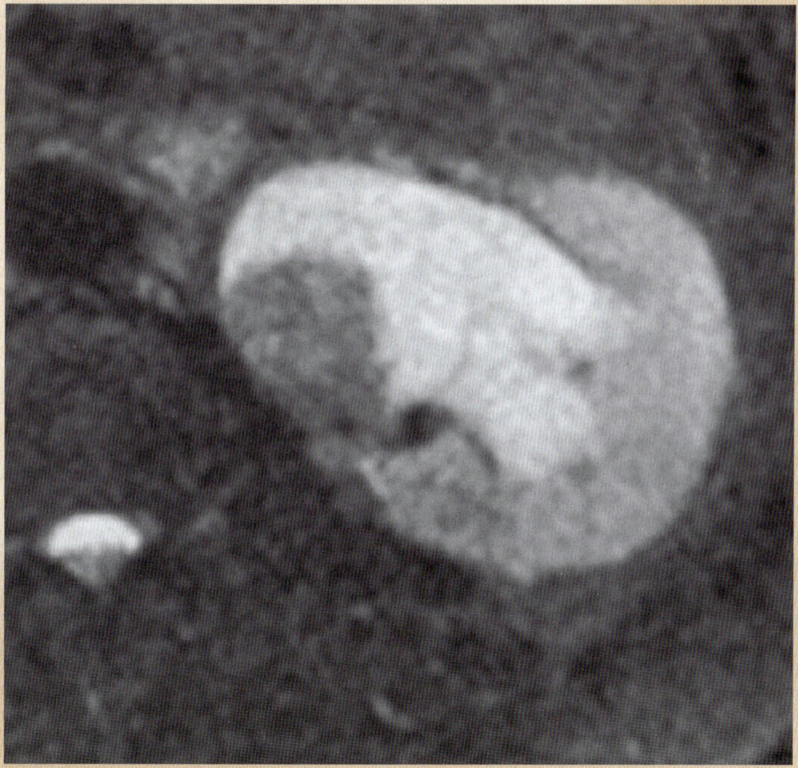

6–1 Pelvocalyceal Transitional Cell Carcinoma

David D. Casalino

PRESENTATION

Gross hematuria and left flank pain.

FINDINGS

MR images show a large filling defect in the posterior aspect of the left renal pelvis.

DIFFERENTIAL DIAGNOSES

- *Calculus*: Most hyperdense (>100 HU) and denser than transitional cell carcinoma (TCC); no enhancement; can be mobile.
- *Blood clot*: Usually hyperdense (40-80 HU) and denser than TCC; no enhancement; can be mobile.
- *Fungus ball*: Usually in immunocompromised patient; no enhancement; can be mobile.
- *Sloughed papilla*: Occasionally triangular; associated with irregular papilla; can be mobile.
- *Renal cell carcinoma (RCC)*: Rarely extends into the renal pelvis; tends to be more hypervascular than TCC.

COMMENTS

TCC, or urothelial carcinoma, accounts for 10% of upper urinary tract neoplasms. Ten percent of TCC occur in the upper urinary tract with 75% being renal, that is, involving the pelvocalyceal system. Upper system TCC is more common in men than in women. Patients usually present in the sixth or seventh decade of life, generally with hematuria. Up to one-third of patients present with flank pain. It is common for TCC to be multicentric. Bilateral upper tract synchronous and metachronous tumors occur in 2% to 5% of cases.

While patients with hematuria have traditionally been assessed by intravenous urography (IVU) and retrograde urography (RU), multiphasic CT urography has become the study of choice at many institutions for assessing patients with hematuria because of its ability to assess the urothelium, renal parenchyma, and surrounding tissues.

On IVU and RU, renal TCC usually appears as a filling defect that may be smooth, irregular, or stippled because of contrast filling tumor interstices. Tumor may fill and dilate a calyx, referred to as calyceal amputation. Tumor may narrow or obstruct portions of the pelvocalyceal system. On unenhanced CT, TCC is usually denser than urine but less dense than a blood clot or a calculus. Calcifications occur in 2% to 7% of urothelial carcinomas and are usually in a diffuse, punctate pattern that may mimic calculi. The tumor enhances. On the excretory phase, the tumor usually appears as a filling defect but may even appear as mural thickening. On MR, TCC will usually appear as a lower signal-intensity filling defect surrounded by high-signal-intensity urine on T2-weighted images (T2-WI). Tumor evaluation should include the use of contrast material. Tumors show moderate enhancement, to a lesser degree than normal parenchyma, on T1-weighted images (T1-WI). On ultrasonography, renal urothelial carcinomas usually appear as central hypoechoic masses.

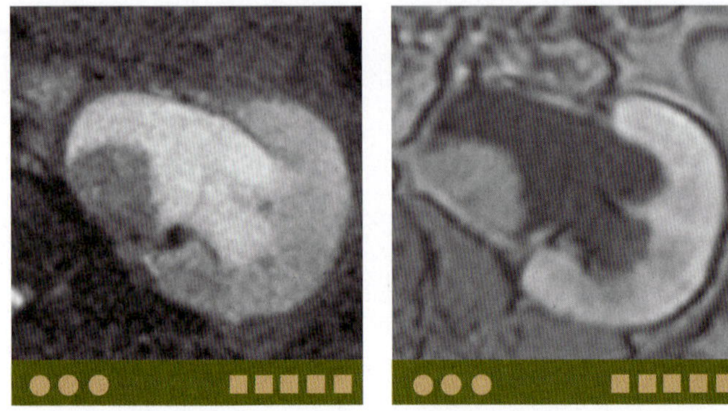

A. and **B.** Axial MRs show a large left renal pelvic filling defect that is hypointense to surrounding urine on the T2-WI (A) and enhances moderately and to a lesser degree than the renal parenchyma on the T1-WI (B).

Management of upper tract urothelial carcinoma is usually surgical. Traditional treatment involves total nephroureterctomy with excision of ipsilateral ureteric orifice and cuff of bladder.

PEARLS

- **Bilateral upper tract synchronous and metachronous tumors occur in 2% to 5% of cases.**
- **Renal TCC may appear as urothelial thickening and irregularity or a filling defect.**
- **TCC is usually denser than urine but less dense than a blood clot or a calculus.**
- **TCC will enhance, typically to a lesser degree than normal renal parenchyma.**

ADDITIONAL IMAGES (C-E)

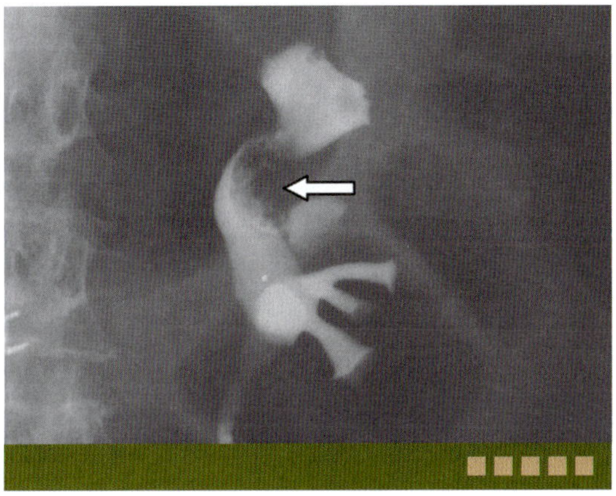

C. RU shows a polypoid filling defect (arrow) in the superior aspect of the left renal pelvis. It is associated with upper-pole caliectasis.

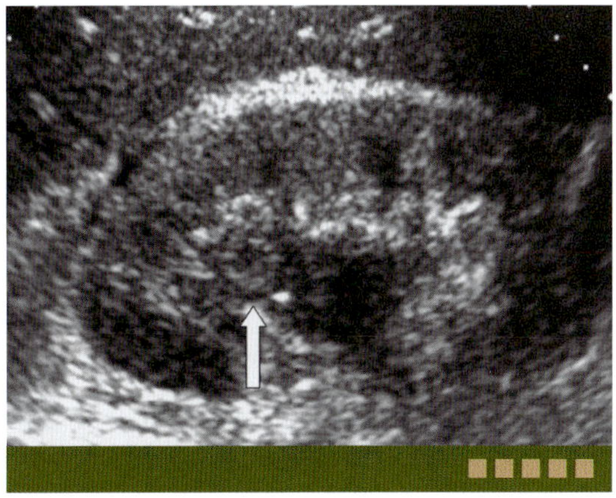

D. Longitudinal sonogram shows a subtle hypoechoic mass (arrow) in the renal pelvis.

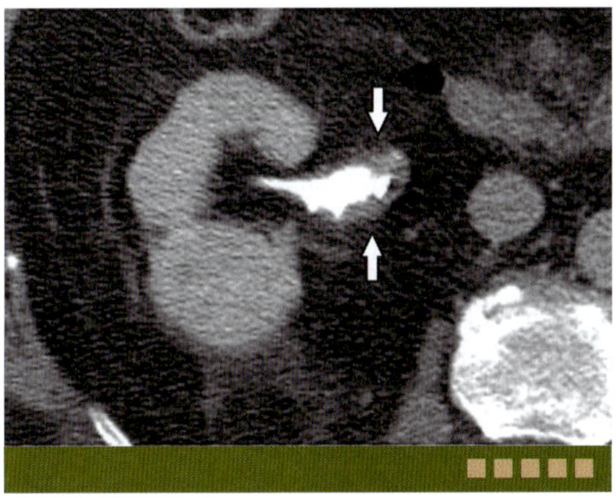

E. Axial CECT during the excretory phase shows irregular urothelial thickening (arrows) of the renal pelvis that proved to be TCC.

DIFFERENTIAL DIAGNOSES IMAGES (F-H)

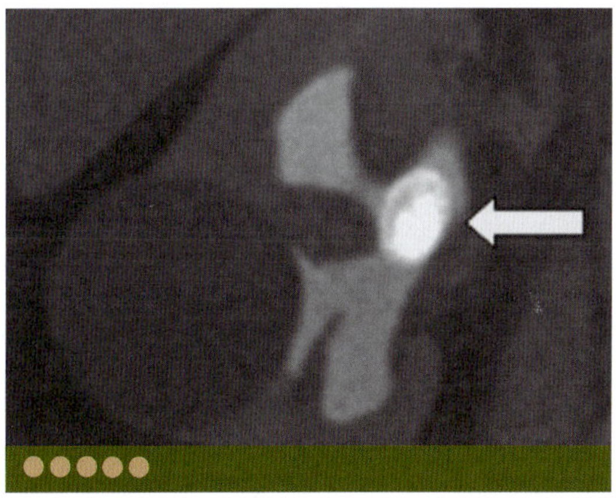

F. Calculus: Coronal CECT during the excretory phase shows a large, dense calculus (arrow) in the renal pelvis, which is filled with contrast-enhanced urine.

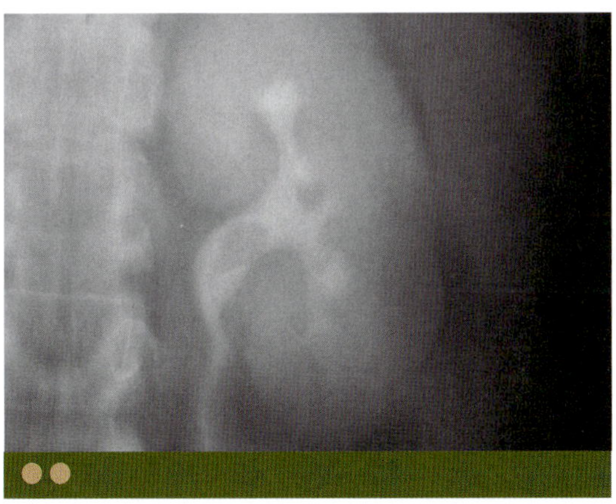

G. Blood clot: IVU tomogram shows a teardrop-shaped filling defect in the renal pelvis of a patient who has recently undergone urinary tract instrumentation.

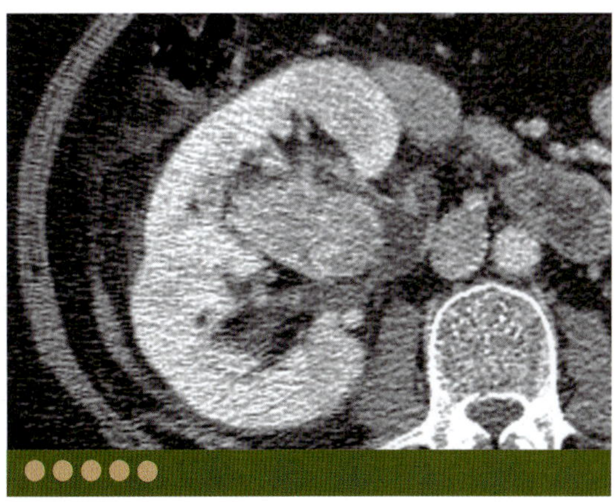

H. RCC: Axial CECT shows an oval, heterogeneously enhancing mass that projects into the dilatated renal pelvis of this patient who has an obstructing stone in the right ureter (not shown).

IMAGE KEY

Common

Rare

Typical

Unusual

6–2 Invasive Upper Urinary Tract Transitional Cell Carcinoma

David D. Casalino

PRESENTATION

Hematuria and left flank pain.

FINDINGS

Axial CT images demonstrate a hypodense, infiltrative abnormality of the left renal parenchyma with soft tissue filling defect in the collecting system and retroperitoneal lymphadenopathy.

DIFFERENTIAL DIAGNOSES

- *Renal cell carcinoma*: Tends to be more hypervascular; more likely to distort the renal contour, displace the collecting system and grow by expansion.
- *Pyelonephritis*: Symptoms of infection are common; can be multifocal and associated with perinephric fat stranding.
- *Renal medullary carcinoma*: Rare; usually occurs in younger patients who are black and have sickle cell trait.
- *Metastasis:* Certain metastases, such as squamous cell carcinoma (SCC), may be infiltrative; usually there is a known primary; multiple lesions are more common.
- *Lymphoma*: Often multiple lesions and lymphadenopathy in the retroperitoneal.

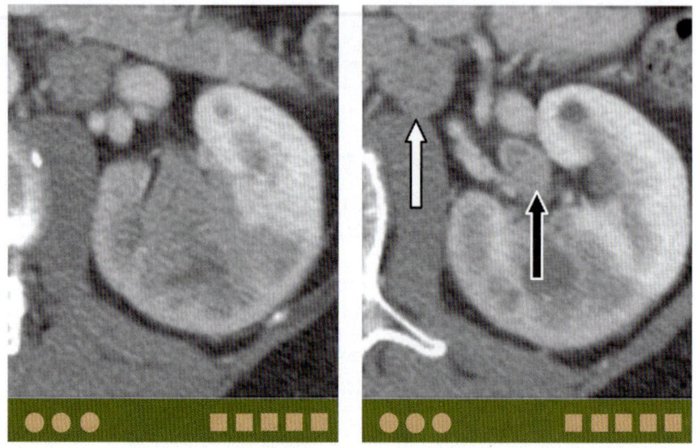

A. Axial CECT shows a soft tissue mass infiltrated the renal parenchyma and renal sinus.
B. Axial CECT shows a component of this mass filling the renal pelvis (black arrow) and lymphadenopathy (white arrow).

COMMENTS

Transitional cell carcinoma (TCC), or urothelial carcinoma, accounts for 10% of upper urinary tract neoplasms. Ten percent of TCC occur in the upper urinary tract with 75% being renal, that is, involving the pelvocalyceal system. Risk factors for developing urothelial carcinoma include cigarette smoking; occupational and environmental chemicals, including aromatic amines; drugs, such as phenacetin and cyclophosphamide; and perhaps heavy caffeine consumption and dietary nitrites and nitrates.

The TNM classification from the American Joint Committee on Cancer is commonly used and is as follows:

TX	Primary tumor cannot be assessed
T0	No evidence of primary tumor
Tis	Carcinoma *in situ*
T1	Tumor invades subepithelial connective tissue
T2	Tumor invades the muscularis
T3	For renal pelvis, tumor invades beyond the muscularis into peripelvic fat or renal parenchyma
T3	For ureter, tumor invades beyond the muscularis into periureteric fat
T4	Tumor invades adjacent organs or through the kidney into perinephric fat
N1	Metastasis in single pelvic lymph node $\leq$2 cm
N2	Metastasis in single pelvic lymph node >2 cm and $\leq$5 cm or multiple nodes $\leq$5 cm
N3	Metastasis in single node >5 cm
M1	Distant metastases

Imaging is important in the diagnosis and staging of upper tract urothelial carcinomas.

Findings of TCC typically include collecting system filling defect(s) and irregularity of the urothelium. In advanced pelvocalyceal TCC, tumor extends beyond the muscularis and may invade the peripelvic fat or the renal parenchyma. Parenchymal involvement typically reflects a centrifugal, infiltrative growth pattern and shows decreased enhancement. The normal architecture is disrupted, yet the reniform contour is maintained.

Management of advanced upper tract urothelial carcinoma is usually surgical. Traditional treatment involves total nephroureterctomy with excision of ipsilateral ureteric orifice and cuff of bladder.

PEARLS

- **If a pelvocalyceal TCC invades the renal parenchyma, it is classified as a T3 tumor.**
- **If the tumor extends through the kidney into the perinephric fat, it is classified as a T4 tumor.**
- **Renal parenchymal invasion typically shows a centrifugal, infiltrative growth pattern that maintains the reniform contour.**
- **If there is absence of sinus fat or excreted contrast between tumor and renal parenchyma, one must consider parenchymal invasion.**

ADDITIONAL IMAGES (C-E)

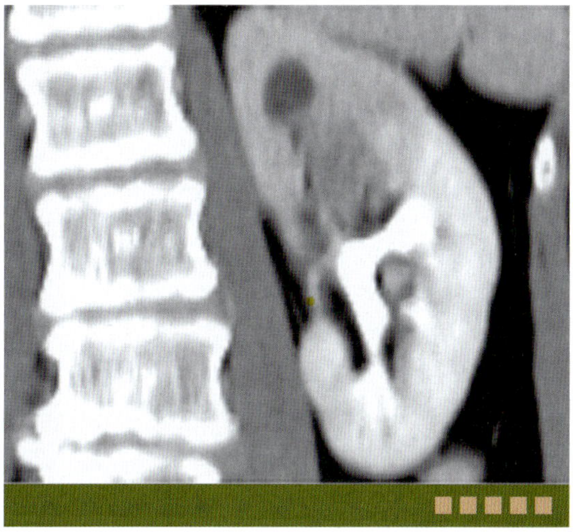

C. Coronal CECT from the same patient shows amputation of the upper-pole collecting system with a dilated calyx.

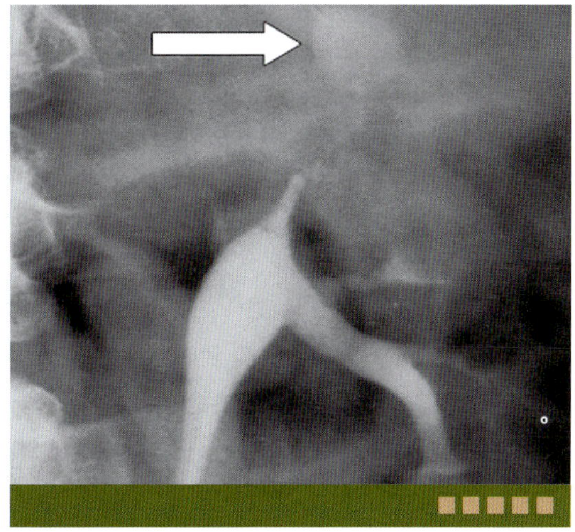

D. RU shows stricturing of the upper-pole infundibulum, amputation of several calyces, and contrast opacification of a dilated calyx (arrow).

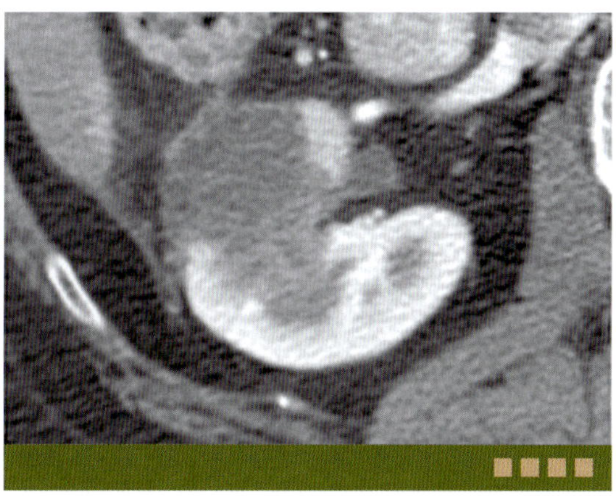

E. Axial CECT shows a hypodense TCC that extends into the perinephric fat and is consistent with a T4 tumor.

DIFFERENTIAL DIAGNOSES IMAGES (F-H)

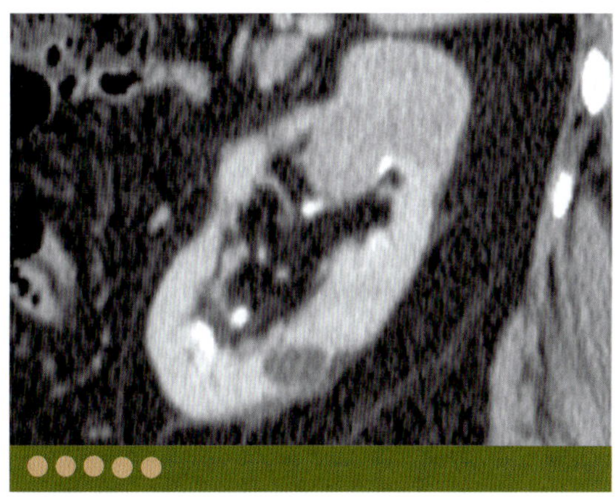

F. RCC: Sagittal CECT shows a moderately enhancing upper-pole mass that bulges the renal contour and displaces the collecting system.

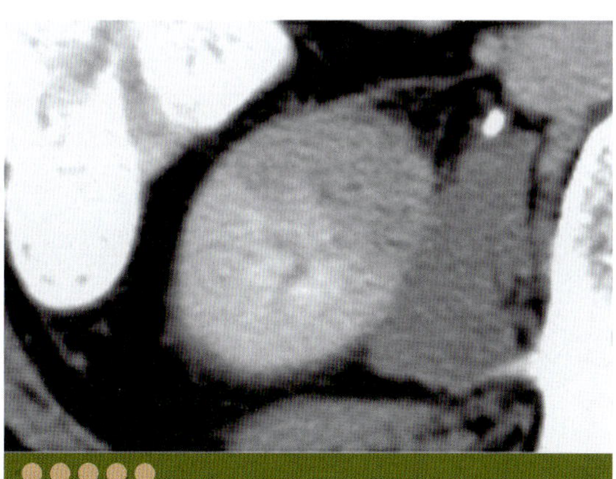

G. Pyelonephritis: Axial CECT shows a wedge-shaped region of hypodensity involving the renal cortex and medulla and mild perinephric fat stranding in a patient with symptoms of infection.

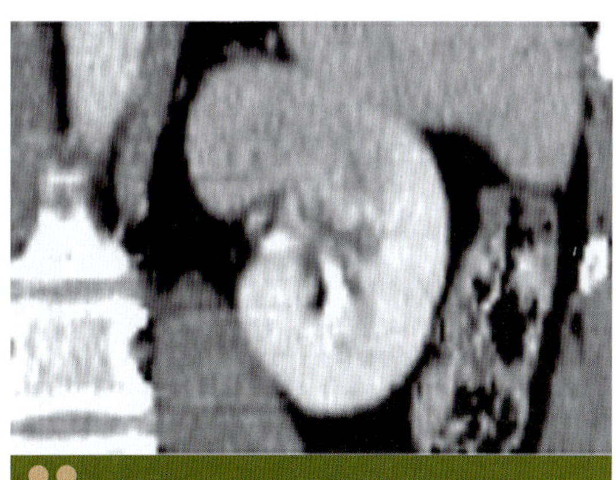

H. Metastasis: Coronal CECT shows an infiltrative hypodense mass that encases the upper-pole collecting system. Biopsy diagnosed a SCC metastasis in this patient with neck SCC.

IMAGE KEY

Common

Rare

Typical

Unusual

6–3 Ureteral Transitional Cell Carcinoma

David D. Casalino

PRESENTATION

Hematuria and intermittent right flank pain.

FINDINGS

RU shows focal narrowing of the distal right ureter.

DIFFERENTIAL DIAGNOSES

- *Traumatic stricture*: Often an abrupt transition in ureteral caliber; often history of stone passage or extraction, ureteral intervention, or radiation therapy.
- *Extrinsic inflammatory or infectious process*: Examples include diverticulitis and appendicitis; usually localized symptoms related to the inflammatory process; typically involves a longer segment of ureter.
- *Retroperitoneal fibrosis*: Ureteral involvement can be bilateral and is usually associated with medial deviation of the mid portion of the ureter, typically at L3 to L5 level.
- *Nontransitional cell carcinoma malignant stricture*: appearance depends on whether malignancy involves the ureter via direct extension, adjacent nodal involvement, or mural metastasis; often a known primary malignancy.

COMMENTS

TCC accounts for 10% of upper urinary tract neoplasms. Ten percent of TCC occur in the upper urinary tract with 25% being ureteral. Upper system TCC is more common in men than in women. Patients usually present in the sixth or seventh decade of life with hematuria and/or flank pain. It is common for TCC to be multicentric. Synchronous bilateral lesions occur in 2% to 9% of cases of ureteral TCC. 11% to 13% of patients with upper tract TCC develop metachronous tumors in the upper tract. Patients with upper tract TCC commonly develop bladder tumors.

On IVU and RU, ureteral TCC usually appears as a filling defect that may be smooth, irregular, or stippled. The filling defect may be single or multiple and may be associated with obstruction. The goblet sign, or Bergman sign, is a cup-shaped collection of contrast adjacent to the distal portion of a ureteral filling defect and suggests ureteral TCC rather than stone. Ureteral TCC may produce an irregular circumferential or eccentric stricture. Nontapering margins, or shouldering, favor the diagnosis of a malignant stricture.

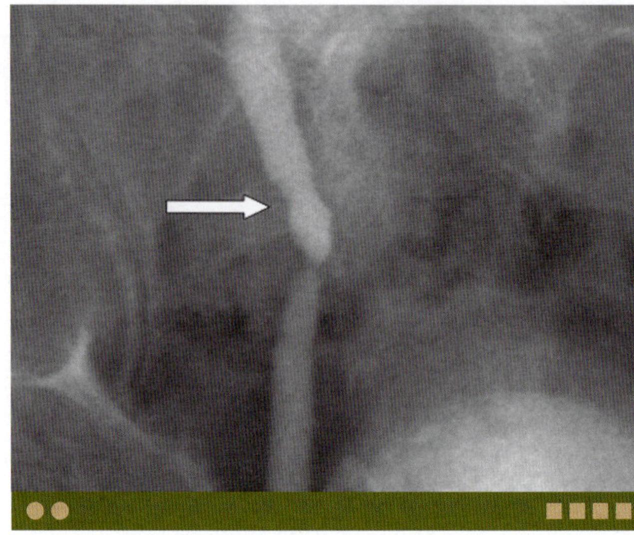

A. Retrograde urogram shows a focal narrowing of the distal right ureter. While the margins are tapered, there is mild mucosal irregularity at the stricture and involving the more proximal urothelium (arrow).

On CT, TCC usually appears as an enhancing mass or ureteral wall thickening. On an excretory phase image, a filling defect may be seen. Periureteric fat stranding suggests tumor invasion beyond the muscularis. On MR, ureteral tumors are usually slightly hyperintense on T2-WI and isointense on T1-WI when compared to muscle. Tumor enhancement is helpful in differentiating it from clot or calculus.

Management of upper tract urothelial carcinoma usually involves total nephroureterectomy with excision of ipsilateral ureteric orifice and cuff of bladder. Endoscopic techniques may be used in selected cases.

PEARLS

- **Ureteral TCC usually appears as a filling defect but may produce an irregular circumferential or eccentric stricture.**
- **Periureteric fat stranding suggests tumor invasion beyond the muscularis.**
- **Tumor enhancement is helpful in differentiating ureteral TCC from clot, calculus, and sloughed tissue.**

ADDITIONAL IMAGES (B-D)

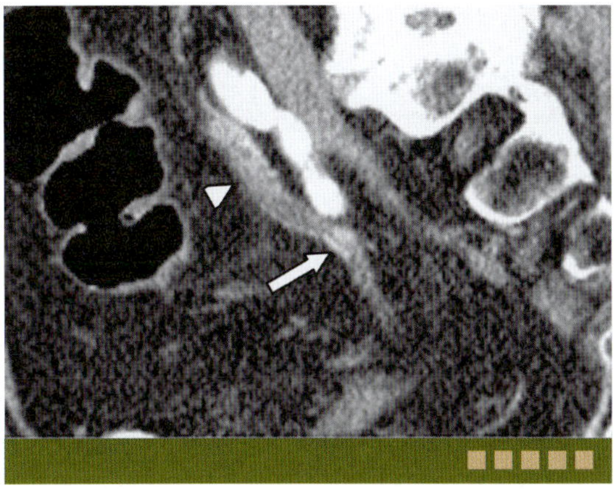

B. Sagittal CECT from the same patient shows an enhancing, focal mass at the site of stricture (arrow) and urothelial thickening and irregularity more proximally (arrowhead).

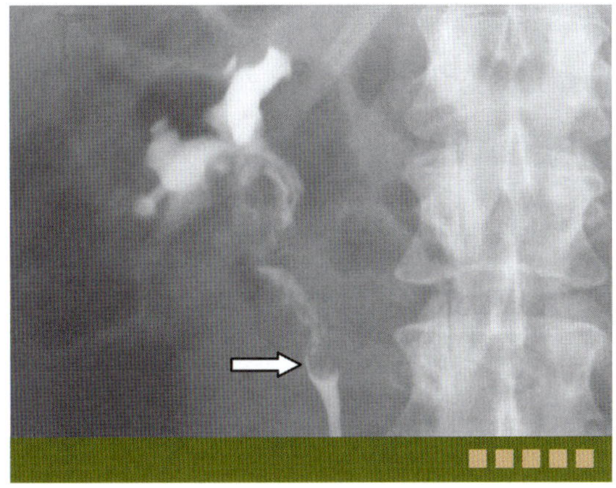

C. RU shows a long filling defect involving the right proximal ureter and renal pelvis. Its irregular appearance relates to contrast extending into tumor interstices. The goblet sign (arrow) is seen at the distal aspect of the tumor.

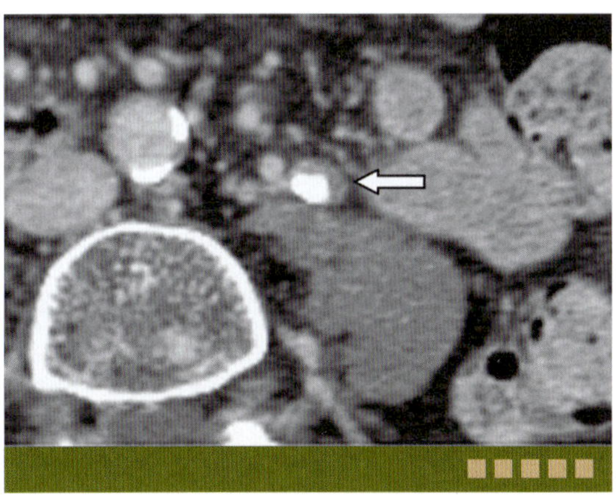

D. Axial CECT shows irregular, eccentric mural thickening (arrow) of the contrast-filled left ureter.

DIFFERENTIAL DIAGNOSES IMAGES (E-G)

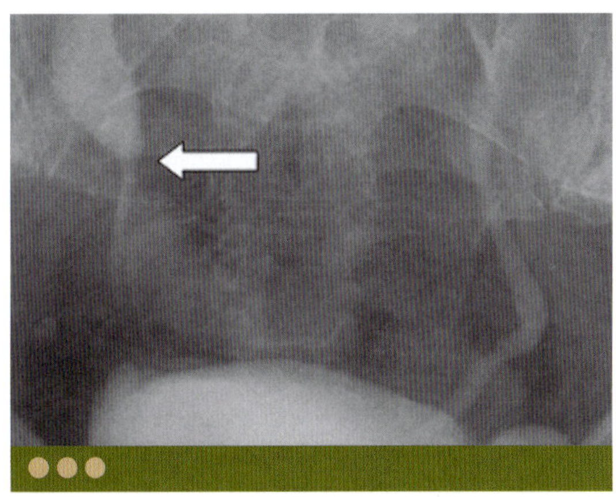

E. Stricture, poststone extraction: IVU shows an abrupt caliber change (arrow) involving the distal right ureter at the site where an 8-mm obstructing stone was extracted 1 year ago.

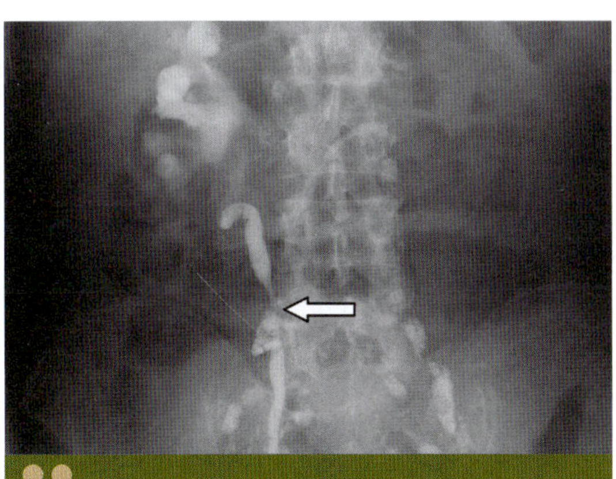

F. Retroperitoneal fibrosis: RU shows right-sided hydronephrosis caused by mid ureteral narrowing (arrow) with medial deviation of the ureter. Note contrast within abnormal lymph nodes from prior lymphogram.

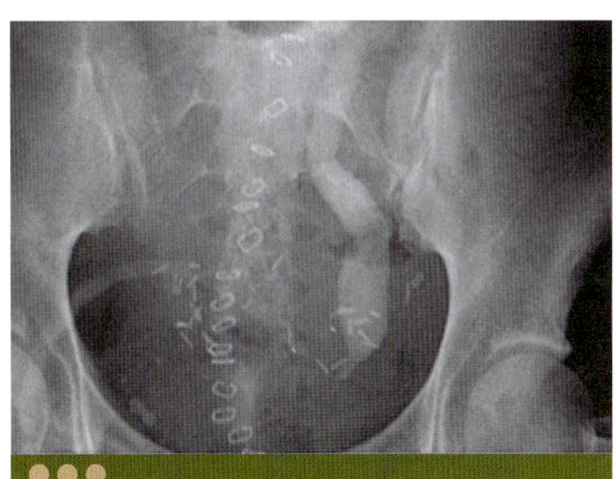

G. Stricture, iatrogenic: IVU shows a focal stricture of the distal left ureter in patient who had undergone emergent cesarean section.

IMAGE KEY

Common

Rare

Typical

Unusual

6-4 Upper Collecting System Squamous Cell Carcinoma

David D. Casalino

PRESENTATION

Hematuria and palpable mass in right upper quadrant.

FINDINGS

RU shows irregular narrowing of the right renal pelvis and proximal ureter and calyceal distortion and mild dilatation.

DIFFERENTIAL DIAGNOSES

- *Transitional cell carcinoma*: Much more common; less frequently associated with calculi; imaging features do not allow differentiation.
- *Postinflammatory, postinfectious processes*: Include malakoplakia and leukoplakia; may be focal or more diffuse; tissue necessary for diagnosis.
- *Pyelitis/ureteritis*: Clinical features may suggest an infectious etiology; often bilateral.

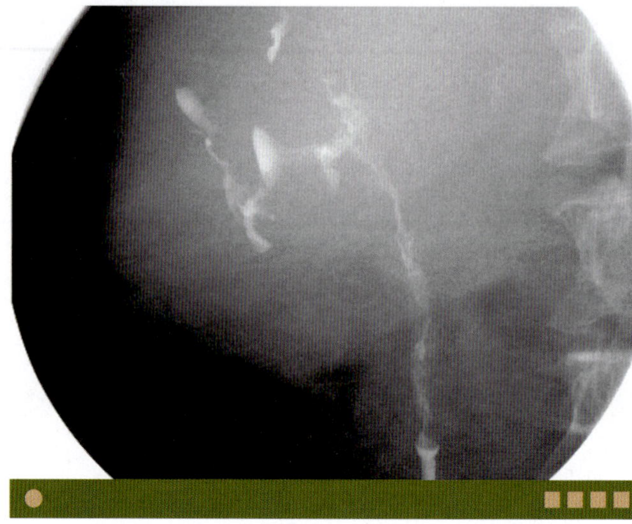

A. RU shows irregular narrowing of the right renal pelvis and proximal ureter and calyceal distortion and mild dilatation.

COMMENTS

Squamous cell carcinoma (SCC) accounts for 1% to 8% of upper tract tumors. It occurs six times more frequently in the renal pelvis than ureter. Chronic irritation of the urothelium and leukoplakia (squamous metaplasia) are associated with an increased risk of SCC. Chronic irritation may be associated with stone disease, a chronic indwelling catheter or chronic infection, such as shistosomiasis. Eighty percent of patients with upper tract SCC will have a calculus. The prevalence of SCC in men is equal to that in women. Patients usually present in the sixth or seventh decade of life. Patients most often present with hematuria, but they may also have signs and symptoms related to chronic stone disease and infection. SCC of the upper urinary tract is usually highly invasive and associated with a poor prognosis. Distant metastases are not uncommon at the time of diagnosis and most often involve lymph nodes, lung, liver, and bones.

Differentiating SCC from TCC is difficult radiologically. SCC should be considered if there are stones, signs of chronic irritation, or in particular, an infected staghorn calculus associated with a central infiltrating tumor. The involved urothelium may have a cobblestone appearance on retrograde pyelography. Lesions are usually single. The kidney may be enlarged by tumor infiltration, and function may be poor. The CT and MR findings of renal pelvic SCC may mimic xanthogranulomatous pyelonephritis (XGP). In contrast to TCC, SCC of the upper collecting system often shows predominantly extraluminal tumor extension, and the perinephric and periureteral spaces are commonly affected.

PEARLS

- **Chronic irritation of the urothelium and squamous metaplasia are associated with an increased risk of SCC.**
- **Eighty percent of the patients with upper tract SCC will have a calculus.**
- **SCC should be considered if there is a central, infiltrating renal tumor in association with calculi or signs of chronic irritation.**
- **Renal pelvic SCC may mimic TCC or XGP.**

ADDITIONAL IMAGES (B-D)

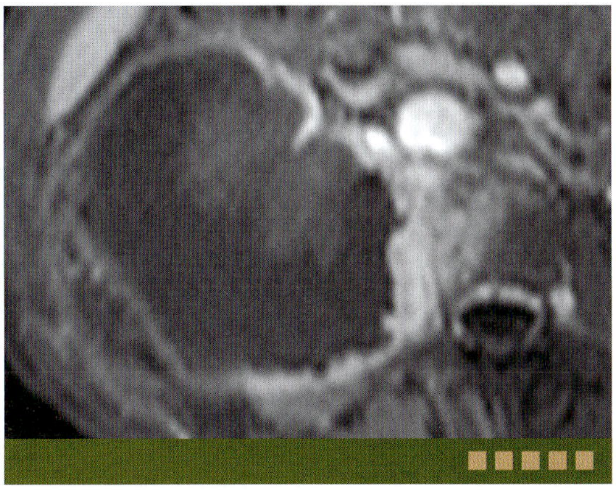

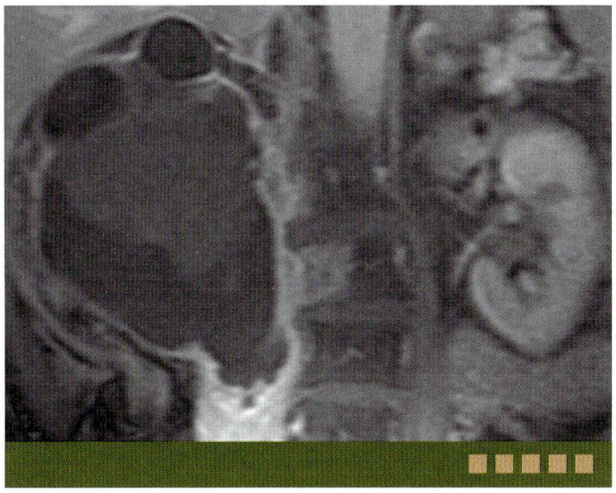

B. and C. Axial and coronal contrast-enhanced T1-WIs from the same patient show a large necrotic mass with peripheral enhancement, replacing the right kidney and invading the adjacent vertebral body.

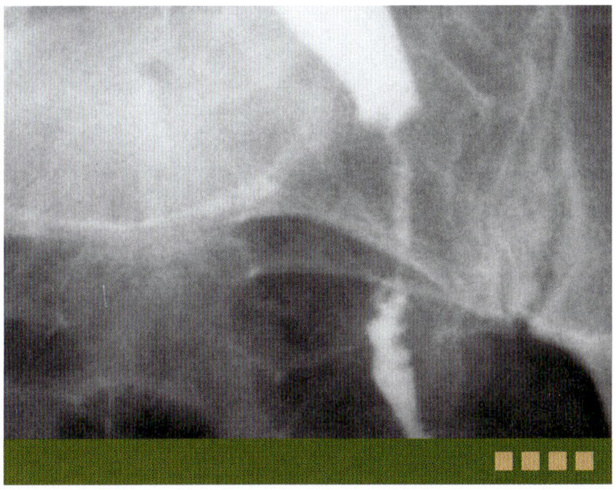

D. RU from a different patient shows abrupt narrowing and mucosal irregularity of the left distal ureter caused by SCC. (*Courtesy of Neil F. Wasserman, MD, Veterans Administration Medical Center, Minneapolis, MN.*)

DIFFERENTIAL DIAGNOSES IMAGES (E-G)

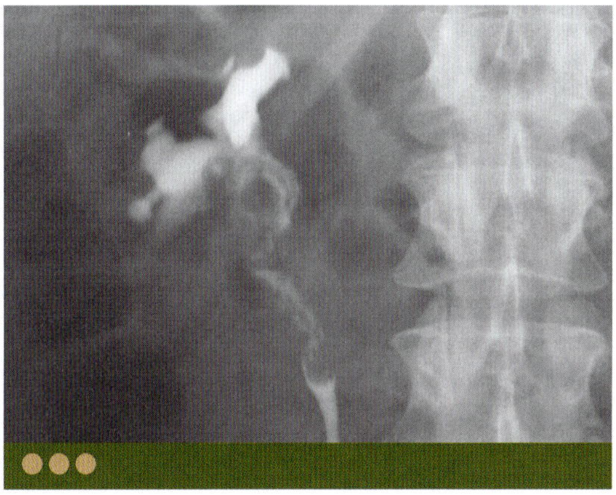

E. TCC: RU shows abnormalities very similar to the original figure with irregular narrowing of the renal pelvis and proximal ureter and mild calyceal dilatation.

IMAGE KEY

Common

Rare

Typical

Unusual

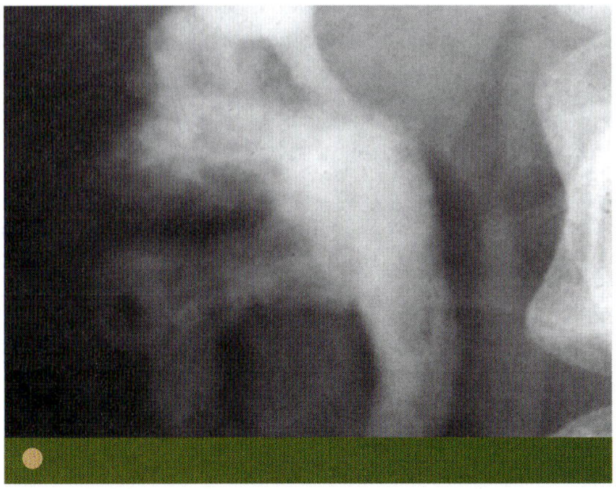

F. Leukoplakia: IVU shows diffuse irregularity of the pelvocalyceal system and proximal ureter.

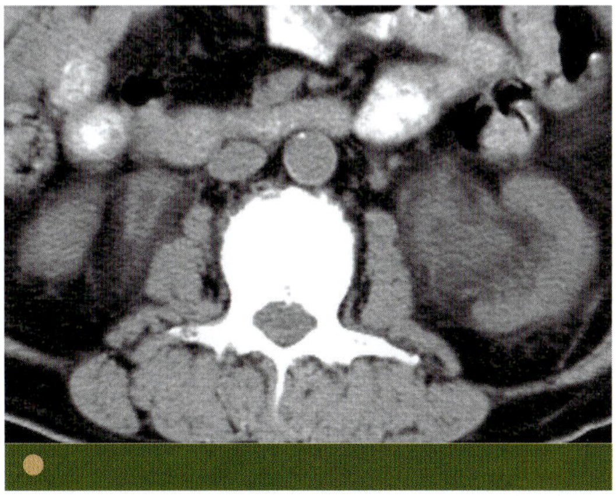

G. Urothelial candidiasis: Axial NECT shows bilateral marked, irregular urothelial thickening in an immunocompromised patient.

6–5 Adenocarcinoma of the Upper Collecting System

David D. Casalino

PRESENTATION

Hematuria and history of recurrent urinary tract infections (UTIs.)

FINDINGS

IVU shows an irregular, radiolucent filling defect involving the right upper-pole collecting system.

DIFFERENTIAL DIAGNOSES

- *Transitional cell carcinoma*: Much more common; imaging features do not allow differentiation.
- *Other neoplasms*: Much less common than transitional cell carcinoma; tissue necessary for diagnosis.
- *Postinflammatory, postinfectious processes*: Include malakoplakia and leukoplakia; may be focal or more diffuse; tissue necessary for diagnosis.
- *Blood clot*: Usually denser than neoplasm on CT; no enhancement; may be mobile.

COMMENTS

Adenocarcinoma of the upper collecting system is rare and less common than urothelial, or transitional cell, carcinoma or SCCs. It accounts for less than 1% of upper tract tumors. Like SCCs, adenocarcinoma is often associated with stone disease and other conditions of chronic inflammation, including infection, of the urothelium. A calculus, usually staghorn, is present in up to two thirds of patients. Patients most often present with hematuria. As with SCC, adenocarcinoma may be associated with signs and symptoms related to chronic stone disease and infection.

Adenocarcinoma may appear as a globular mass or as a flat tumor of the pelvocalyceal system. The mass is often associated with a stone. Hydronephrosis may occur as a result of the tumor and/or a stone. Dystrophic calcifications may be seen in these tumors, which are often mucin-producing.

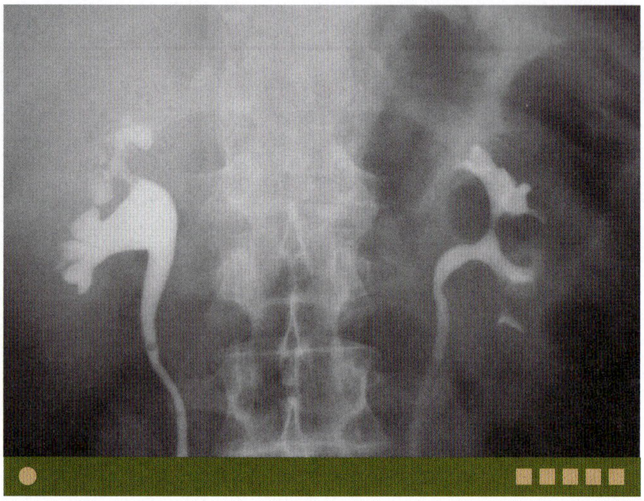

A. IVU shows an irregular, radiolucent filling defect involving the right upper-pole collecting system. No abnormality of the left renal collecting system is seen.

PEARLS

- **Adenocarcinoma accounts for less than 1% of upper tract tumors.**
- **Associated with conditions of chronic inflammation, including infection and stone disease.**
- **May appear as a globular mass or flat tumor of pelvocalyceal system.**

ADDITIONAL IMAGE

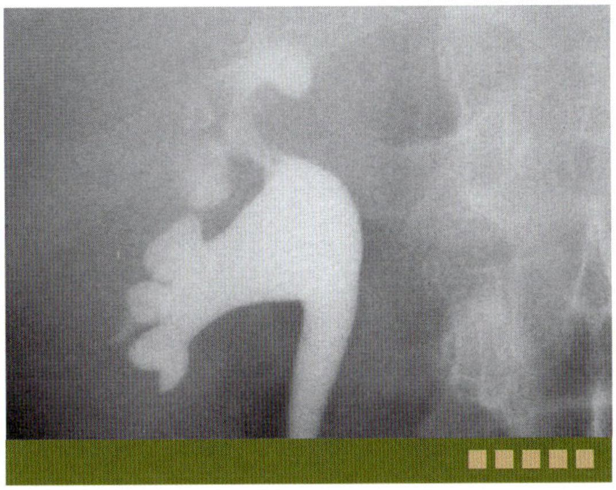

B. IVU (enlarged image) again shows the irregular filling defect in the upper-pole collecting system and blunting of all calyces.

DIFFERENTIAL DIAGNOSES IMAGES (C-F)

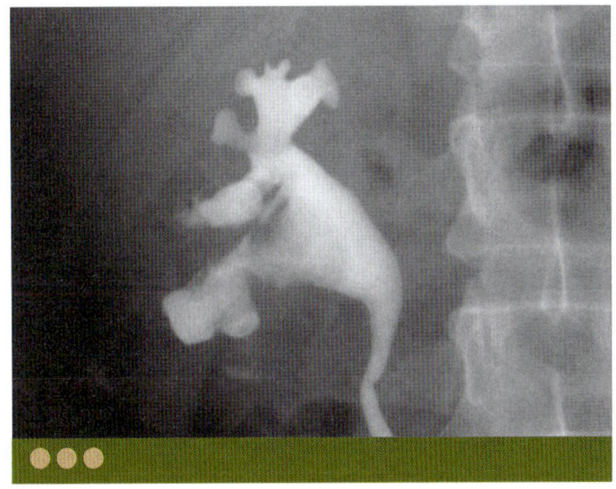

C. TCC: IVU shows an irregular filling defect, involving the lower-pole collecting system.

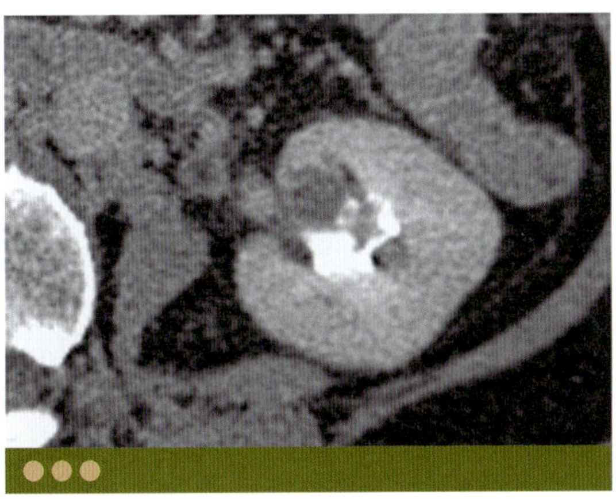

D. TCC: Axial CECT during excretory phase shows an irregular calyceal filling defect that showed slight enhancement compared with NECT (not shown).

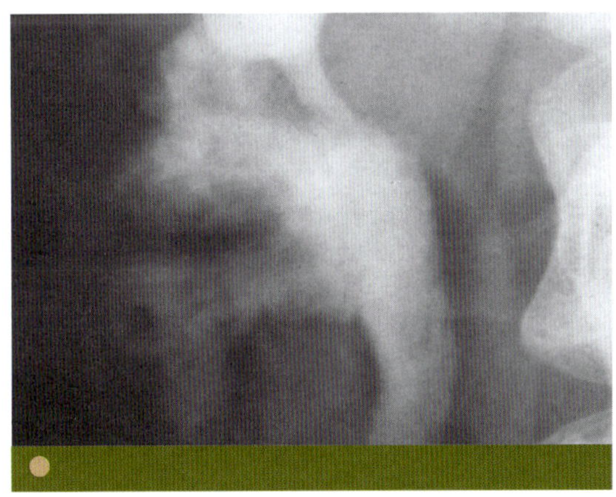

E. Leukoplakia: IVU shows diffuse irregularity of the pelvocalyceal system.

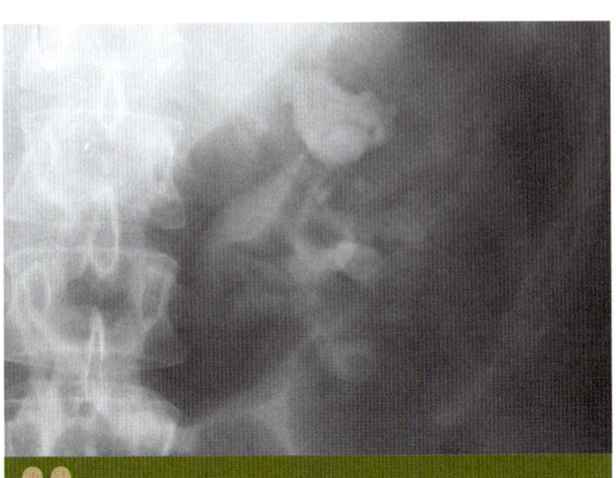

F. Blot clot: IVU shows irregular filling defects, involving the left renal collecting system in a patient taking warfarin.

IMAGE KEY

Common

Rare

Typical

Unusual

6–6 Extraureteral Malignancies Involving the Ureter

David D. Casalino

PRESENTATION

Right flank pain and history of breast cancer.

FINDINGS

RU shows an irregular filling defect in the proximal aspect of the right ureter causing obstruction.

DIFFERENTIAL DIAGNOSES

- *Transitional cell carcinoma*: More common; older patients; enhancement; imaging features may not allow differentiation.
- *Blood clot*: Usually hyperdense (40-80 HU) and denser than tumor; no enhancement; can be mobile.
- *Calculus*: Most hyperdense (>100 HU); no enhancement; can be mobile.

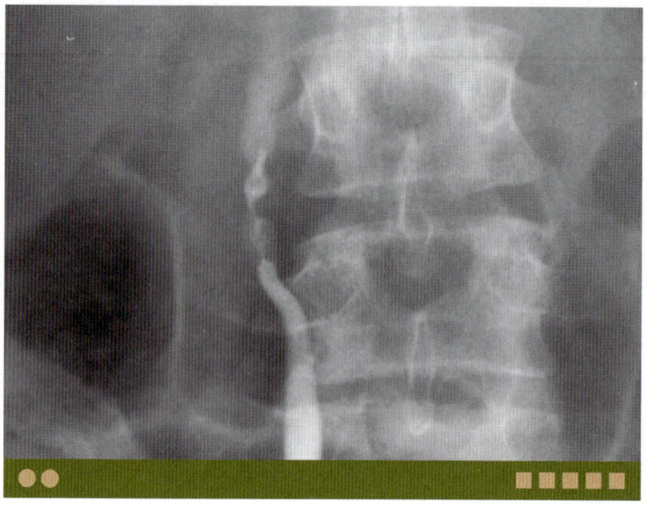

A. RU show an irregular filling defect in the proximal aspect of the right ureter causing obstruction. Biopsy confirmed a breast cancer intramural metastasis.

COMMENTS

Extraureteral malignancies may cause ureteral abnormalities, including stricture, filling defect, and obstruction. Patients usually have a known primary malignancy outside the ureter, and symptoms often relate to obstruction. Ureteral involvement may be the result of a mucosal metastasis, mural metastasis, direct extension, encasement or extrinsic compression. Mucosal metastases are most often from a TCC elsewhere in the urinary tract. Rarely, melanoma and cancers of the kidney, colon, rectum, and prostate may metastasize to the mucosa. Being mucosal, these lesions may form a focal filling defect with acute angles with the adjacent ureteral wall. Intramural metastases most often originate from tumors of the breast, lung, stomach, colon, pancreas, prostate, ovary, and cervix. Being intramural, these lesions may form obtuse angles with the adjacent wall. Direct extension of tumor usually involves the lower third of ureter. Cervical cancer is most common. Carcinomas of the endometrium, ovary, prostate, sigmoid colon, and rectum may also involve the ureter. Tumors may metastasize to periureteral lymphatics or adipose tissue or cause massive adenopathy that results in ureteral encasement. Ureteral encasement by tumor typically produces a stricture that may be smooth or irregular and focal or involve a long segment of ureter. The wall of the ureter is typically thickened on CT. Ureteral angulation and displacement are common. The most common tumors to cause encasement include carcinoma of the breast, lung, stomach, pancreas, and colon and lymphoma. Extrinsic compression of the ureter may be the result of large pelvic, retroperitoneal, or abdominal tumors. The ureter is typically displaced and narrowed without mucosal abnormality. Uterine fibroids are the most common tumor to obstruct the ureter by extrinsic compression.

PEARLS

- **Mucosal metastases most often originate from a TCC elsewhere in the urinary tract.**
- **Intramural metastases and ureteral encasement by tumor most often originate from tumors of the breast and lung.**
- **Prostate cancer may involve the ureter via direct extension, nodal involvement, or mural metastasis.**
- **Mucosal and intramural metastases typically appear as filling defects or focal strictures on imaging.**
- **Ureteral involvement by direct tumor extension, encasement or extrinsic compression typically appears as a stricture, which may be long on imaging.**

ADDITIONAL IMAGES (B-E)

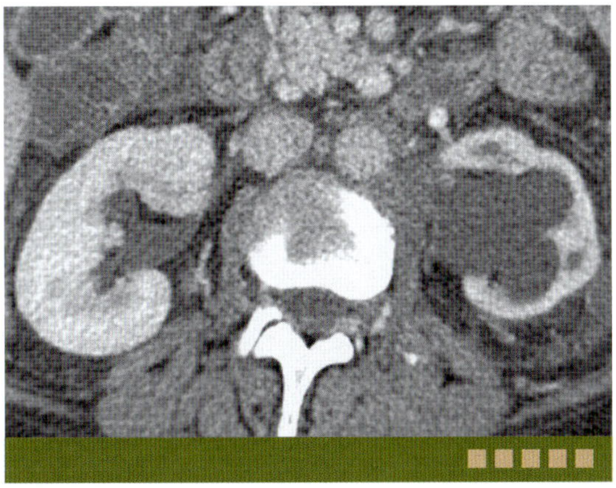

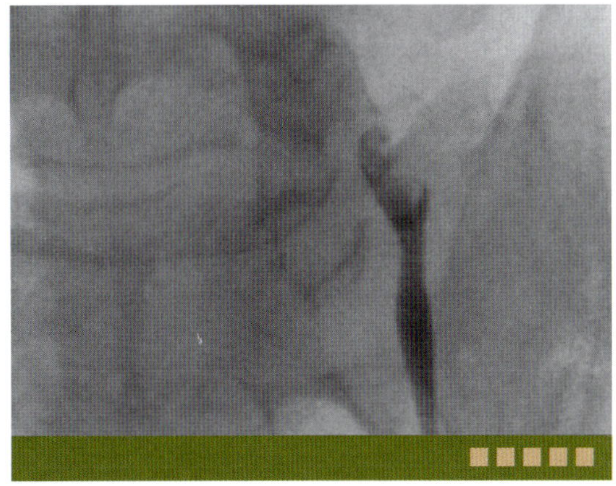

B. and C. Axial CECT and RU show a high-grade, proximal ureteral obstruction caused by encasement by prostate cancer that has extended into the left para-aortic space.

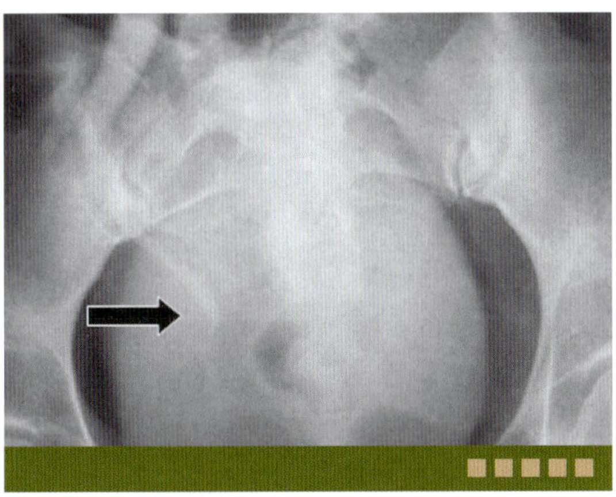

D. IVU shows a focal, smooth ureteral stricture (arrow), involving the distal aspect of the right ureter. This stricture is the result of direct extension of cervical cancer.

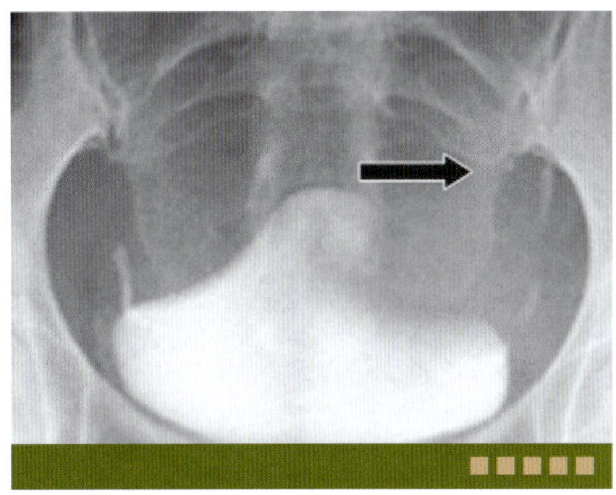

E. IVU shows extrinsic compression and lateral displacement of the distal left ureter (arrow). There is also lobulated mass effect on the bladder. CT (not shown) showed a fibroid uterus.

DIFFERENTIAL DIAGNOSES IMAGES (F-G)

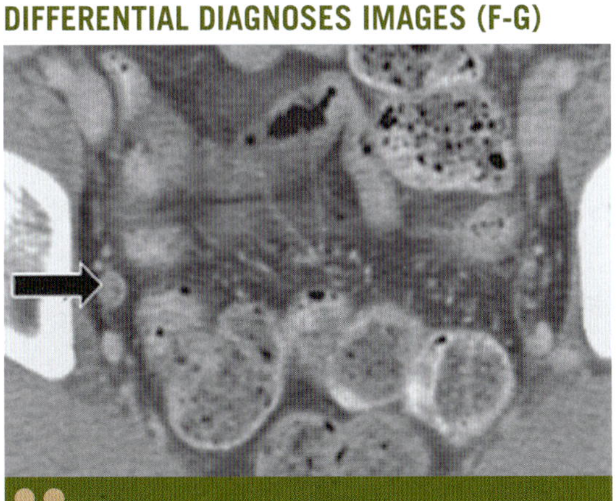

F. TCC: Axial CECT shows an enhancing, round filling defect (arrow) in the distal right ureter.

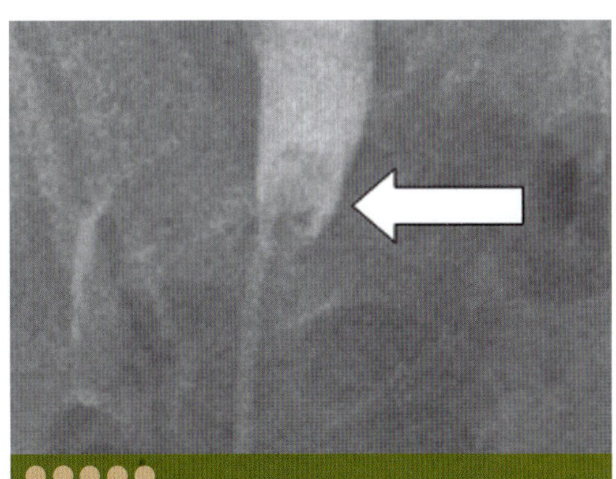

G. Calculus: RU shows a small, round filling defect (arrow) in the right ureter. This calculus was hyperdense on the scout radiograph (not shown).

IMAGE KEY

Common

Rare

Typical

Unusual

6–7 Fibroepithelial Polyp

David D. Casalino

PRESENTATION

Intermittent left flank pain and hematuria.

FINDINGS

IVU shows a large filling defect in the distal left ureter without obstruction.

DIFFERENTIAL DIAGNOSES

- *Transitional cell carcinoma*: More common; older patients, pain less common, more often obstructive; generally immobile.
- *Blood clot*: Usually hyperdense (40-80 HU); no enhancement; can be mobile.
- *Calculus*: Most hyperdense (> 100 HU) and denser than neoplasm; no enhancement; can be mobile.

COMMENTS

Fibroepithelial polyp is a rare tumor and the most common benign mesodermal neoplasm in the upper urinary tract. The core of these lesions consists of loose, edematous fibrous tissue beneath normal urothelium. The stroma is highly vascular. Their etiology is unknown. Fibroepithelial polyps are most often found in males more than 20 years of age but can be seen at any age. Patients usually present with hematuria and pain. The pain is usually intermittent and likely related to partial obstruction.

Imaging findings usually include a long, smooth filling defect (1-13 cm in length), often with a slender pedicle. The pedicle allows free movement of the polyp that may project antegrade or retrograde or prolapse into the bladder. Mobility may be demonstrated on sonography if the tumor is at the ureteropelvic junction (UPJ) or on IVU if the patient positioning is changed. Fibroepithelial polyps are most often seen in the proximal ureter and UPJ. They may be solitary or multiple, and a single stalk may have one tip or multiple smooth finger-like projections. Obstruction is a less common feature of fibroepithelial polyps than TCC. RU may be superior to IVU in defining the polyp. CT and MR findings are nonspecific and cannot reliably differentiate a fibroepithelial polyp from other neoplasms.

Fibroepithelial polyp should be suspected when the patient is a young male with pain and hematuria and imaging demonstrates a tumor on a stalk. This may allow for conservative treatment, perhaps with endoscopic resection, rather than nephroureterectomy.

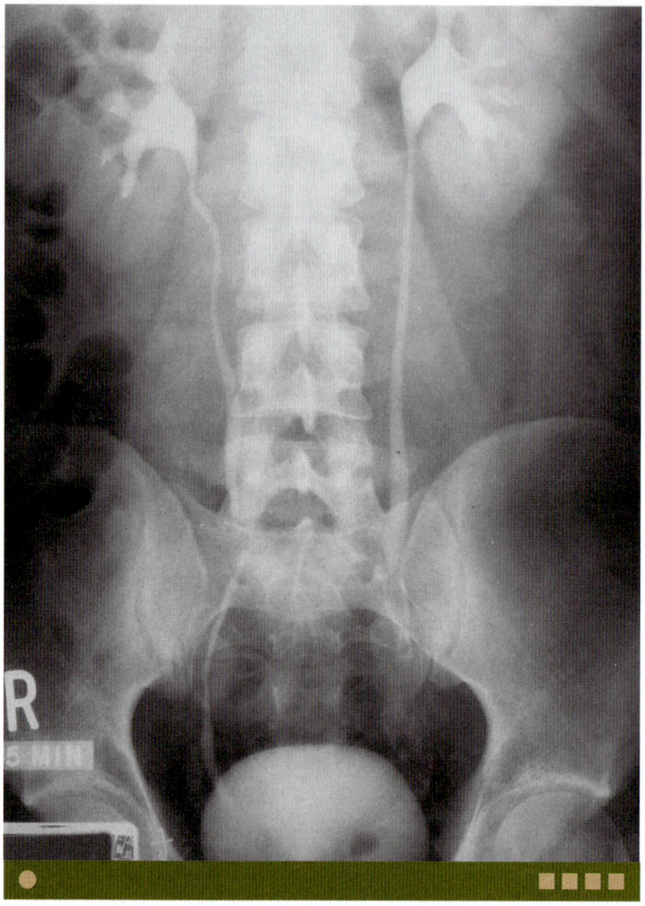

A. IVU during excretory phase shows a long, smooth, multibranched filling defect in the distal left ureter. There is slight extension of the filling defect into the bladder. There is no associated obstruction.

PEARLS

- **Fibroepithelial polyp is a rare, benign tumor that is most often found in children and young adults.**
- **It is most often found in the proximal ureter and UPJ.**
- **Fibroepithelial polyp typically appears as a long, smooth filling defect on a slender pedicle, which allows movement of the polyp.**
- **Imaging features may mimic a TCC.**

ADDITIONAL IMAGES (B-C)

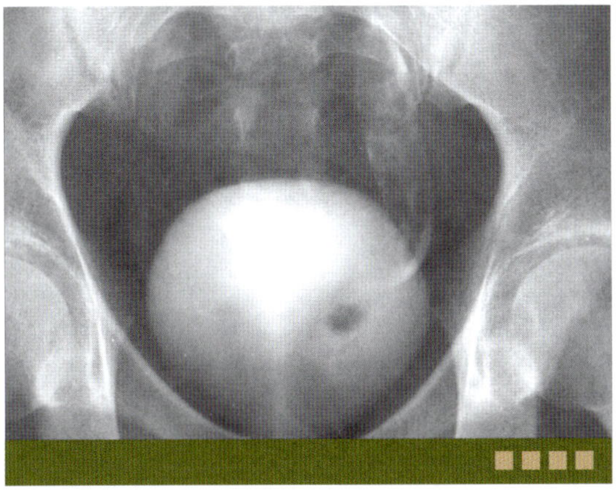

B. IVU bladder image from the same patient again shows a long, smooth, multibranched filling defect in the distal left ureter. There is slight prolapse of tumor into the bladder.

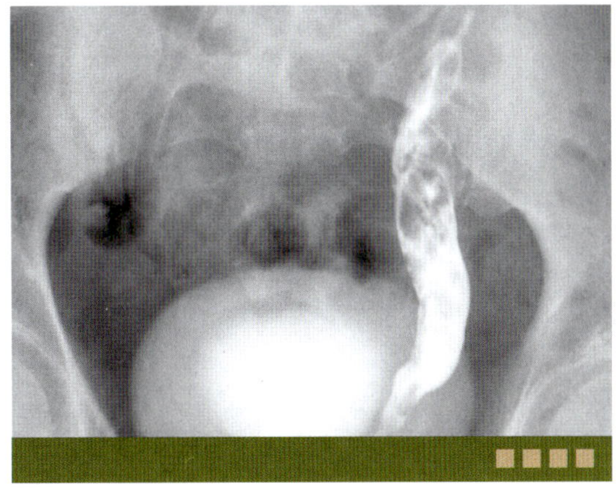

C. RU from the same patient better defines the long, polypoid lesion in the distal left ureter.

DIFFERENTIAL DIAGNOSES IMAGES (D-F)

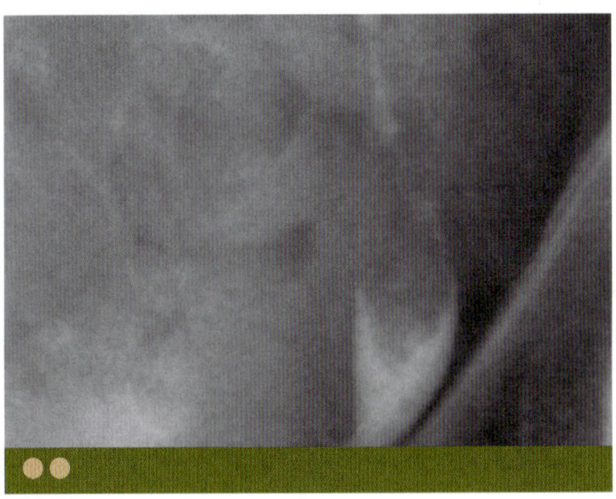

D. TCC: RU shows a focal, slightly irregular filling defect in the left distal ureter without significant dilatation proximal to the mass.

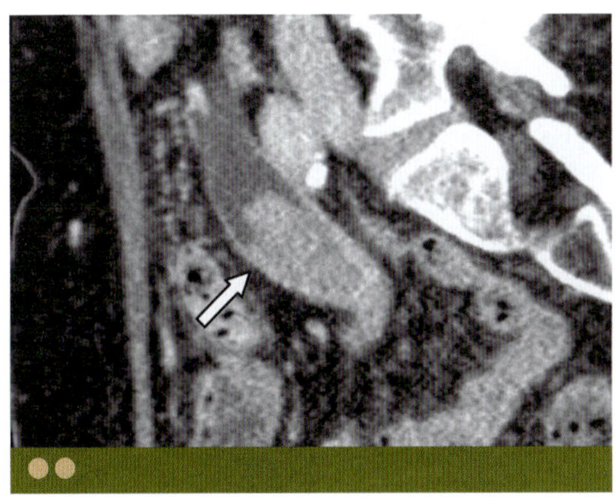

E. TCC: Sagittal CECT shows a large, enhancing mass (arrow) in the left distal ureter. The mass is obstructive.

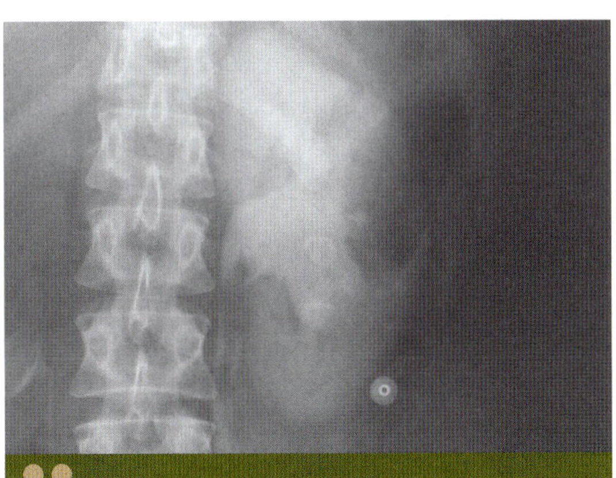

F. Blood clot: IVU shows a long, tubular filling defect, involving the left UPJ and proximal ureter in a patient taking warfarin.

IMAGE KEY

Common

Rare

Typical

Unusual

6–8 Leukoplakia

David D. Casalino

PRESENTATION

Right flank pain.

FINDINGS

RU shows a "goblet" sign and irregular linear filling defects of the renal pelvis and proximal ureter.

DIFFERENTIAL DIAGNOSES

- *Transitional cell carcinoma*: Much more common; less frequently associated with calculi; imaging features do not allow differentiation
- *Blood clot*: Usually denser than neoplasm on CT; no enhancement; may be mobile.

COMMENTS

Leukoplakia and cholesteatoma are uncommon urothelial lesions that can be expressed together under the term keratinizing desquamative squamous metaplasia (KDSM). To be KDSM, there must be no histologic evidence of atypia. While the cause of KDSM is unknown, there is an association with chronic infection, stones, and hydronephrosis. KDSM occurs more commonly in men with a 3:2 male:female ratio and is usually discovered between the third and the sixth decade of life. Patients commonly present with flank pain and passage of cornified material in the urine.

On IVP or retrograde pyelography, the lesion typically appears as a calyceal or renal pelvic filling defect that is typically an irregular, stringy, or laminated plaque. Calcification of the plaque is infrequently seen on conventional radiography. Plaque in the ureter can create a "goblet" sign, mimicking a TCC. KDSM can also assume a complex cystic form, mimicking a cystic RCC.

While KDSM is technically benign, it commonly coexists with SCC of the urothelium, and one series reported that 21% of patients with leukoplakia developed SCC. Because of this association, some chose to consider it a premalignant condition. While the treatment of choice was previously nephroureterectomy, a more conservative approach to management has become more common and may include ureteroscopic treatment and frequent follow-up assessment of the urothelium.

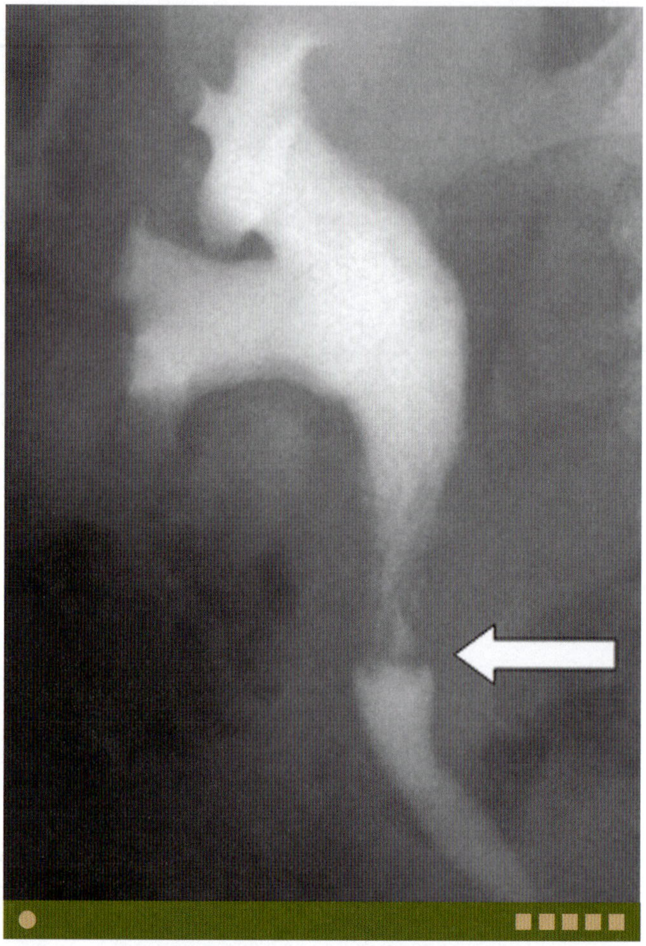

A. RU shows a "goblet" sign (arrow), involving the proximal ureter and irregular linear filling defects of the renal pelvis and proximal ureter. (*Courtesy of Neil F. Wasserman, MD, Veterans Administration Medical Center, Minneapolis, MN.*)

PEARLS

- **KDSM includes leukoplakia and cholesteatoma.**
- **Keratinizing desquamative squamous metaplasia commonly coexists with SCC of the urothelium.**
- **Keratinizing desquamative squamous metaplasia usually appears as a calyceal or renal pelvic filling defect that is typically an irregular, stringy, or laminated plaque.**
- **Keratinizing desquamative squamous metaplasia in the ureter can create a "goblet" sign, mimicking a TCC.**

ADDITIONAL IMAGES (B-E)

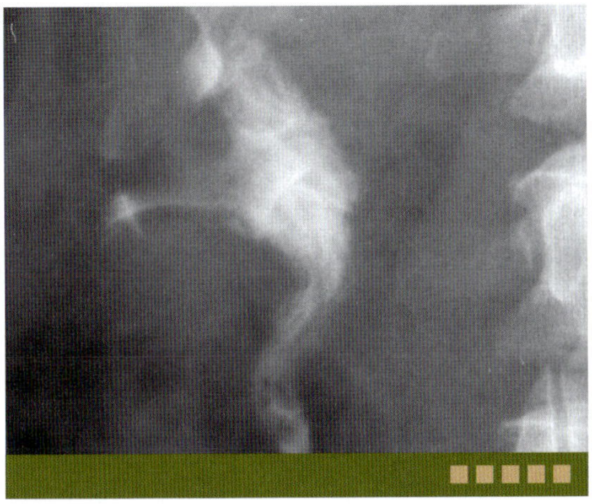

B. RU, decompression view, from the same patient shows the extent of the renal pelvic striations. (*Courtesy of Neil F. Wasserman, MD, Veterans Administration Medical Center, Minneapolis, MN.*)

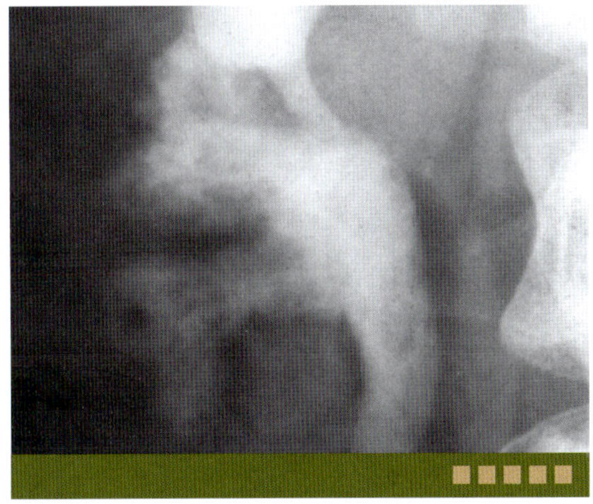

C. IVU from a different patient shows generalized irregularity of the proximal ureteral and pelvocalyceal walls caused by KDSM.

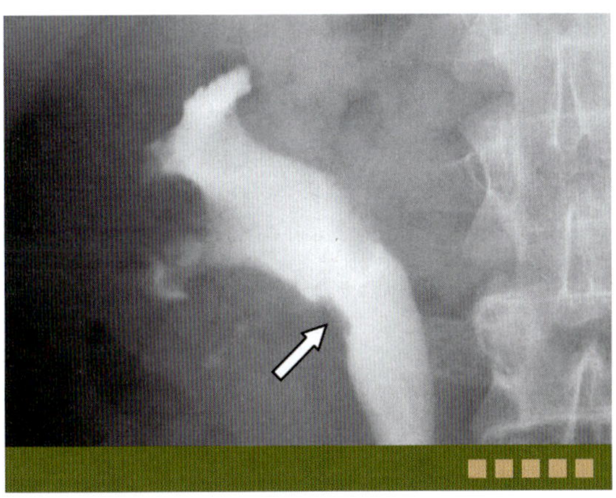

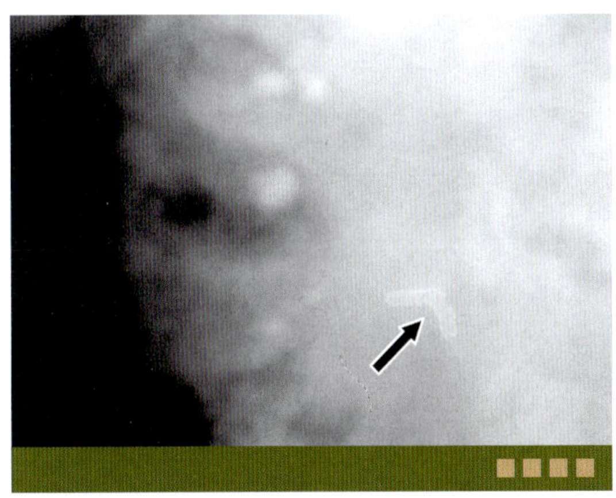

D. and **E.** IVU (excretory phase image and scout tomogram) from a different patient shows a focal filling defect (arrows) in the renal pelvis. It is an irregular, dense mass of desquamated keratin, ie. cholesteatoma. Patient also has multiple renal calculi. (*Courtesy of Neil F. Wasserman, MD, Veterans Administration Medical Center, Minneapolis, MN.*)

DIFFERENTIAL DIAGNOSES IMAGES (F-G)

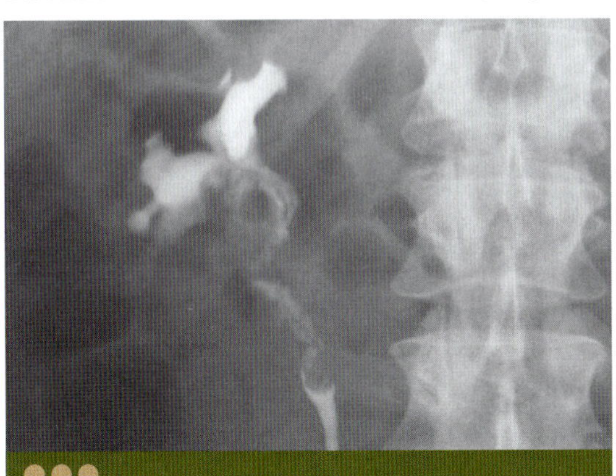

F. Transitional cell carcinoma: RU shows irregular narrowing of the renal pelvis and proximal ureter and mild calyceal dilatation. A "goblet" sign is present.

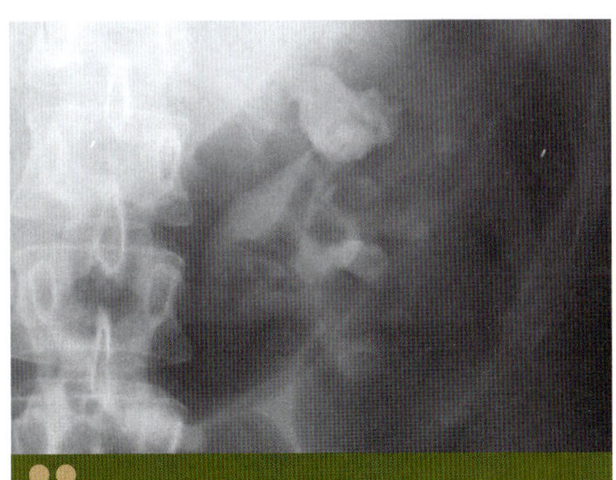

G. Blood clot: IVU shows smooth, linear filling defects in the left renal collecting system in a patient taking warfarin.

IMAGE KEY

Common

Rare

Typical

Unusual

6–9 Pyeloureteritis Cystica

David D. Casalino

PRESENTATION

Hematuria and history of UTIs.

FINDINGS

IVU shows numerous, small filling defects involving the renal pelvis and right ureter.

DIFFERENTIAL DIAGNOSES

- *Multiple calculi*: Denser and less numerous filling defects.
- *Multifocal, urothelial cancer*: Not associated with recurrent UTIs; less numerous filling defects that may be larger and irregular.
- *Clots*: May be mobile; often larger and less numerous.
- *Air bubbles*: Usually related to instrumentation; mobile and less numerous.

COMMENTS

Pyeloureteritis cystica is a condition that usually arises in patients with a history of chronic or recurrent UTIs. Inflamed transitional epithelium extends into the submucosa and forms sterile cysts that are filled with clear proteinaceous fluid. These cysts cause focal elevations of the overlying epithelium. Patients may be asymptomatic or may present with hematuria or UTI. There is no known malignant potential.

On imaging, pyeloureteritis cystica is characterized by numerous, small filling defects involving the renal pelvis and ureter. The filling defects are typically smooth and a few millimeters, but rarely may get as large as 2 cm in diameter. Usually the process is bilateral. Rarely is the condition unifocal. These filling defects persist for at least many months, if not indefinitely.

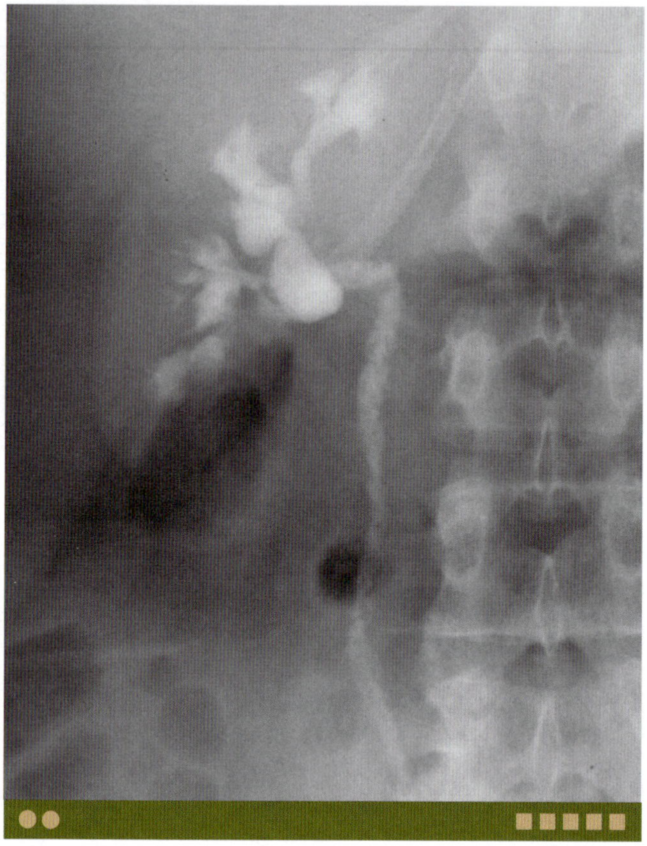

A. IVU shows multiple, small, smooth filling defects in the renal pelvis and ureter. The left kidney (not shown) also showed similar filling defects.

PEARLS

- **No known malignant potential.**
- **Not uncommonly an incidental finding.**
- **The filling defects are typically a few millimeters, smooth, numerous, and bilateral.**

ADDITIONAL IMAGES (B-C)

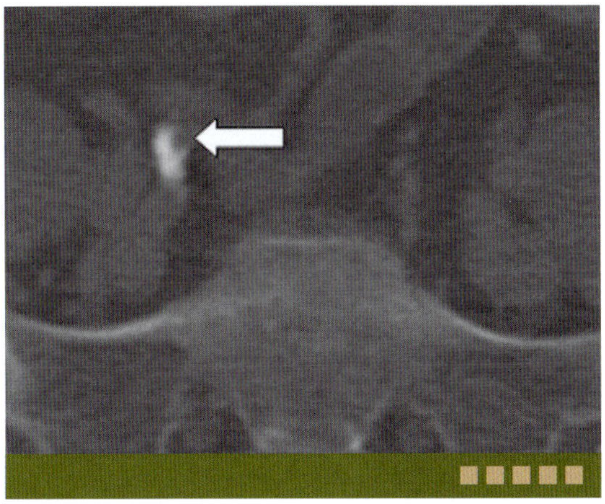

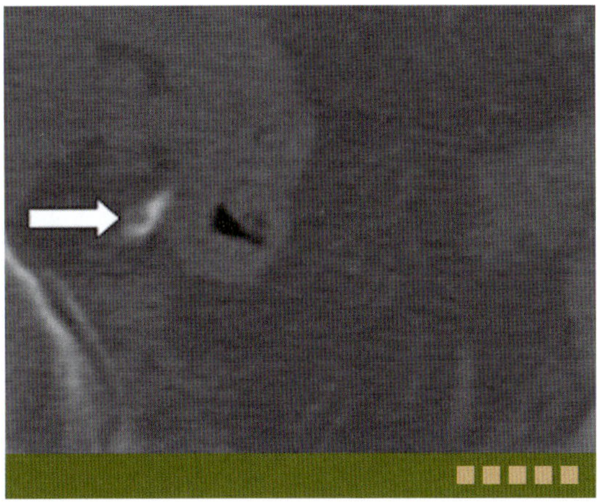

B. and **C.** Axial CECT during excretory phase shows very small, smooth filling defects (arrows) in the right ureter at two different levels.

DIFFERENTIAL DIAGNOSES IMAGES (D-G)

IMAGE KEY

Common

Rare

Typical

Unusual

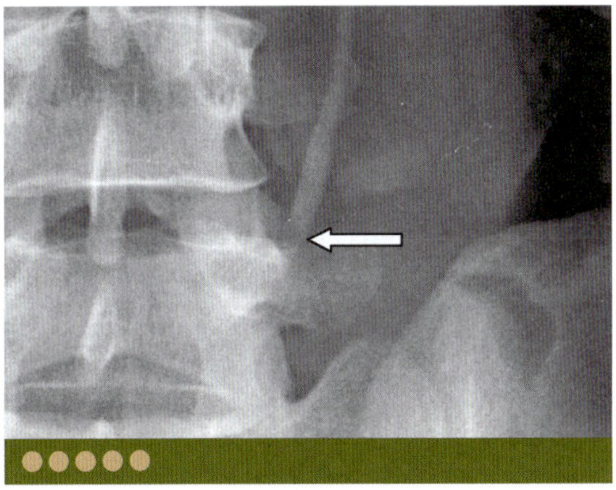

D. Calculus: IVU shows a small smooth filling defect (arrow) in the left ureter. It was dense on the scout radiograph (not shown).

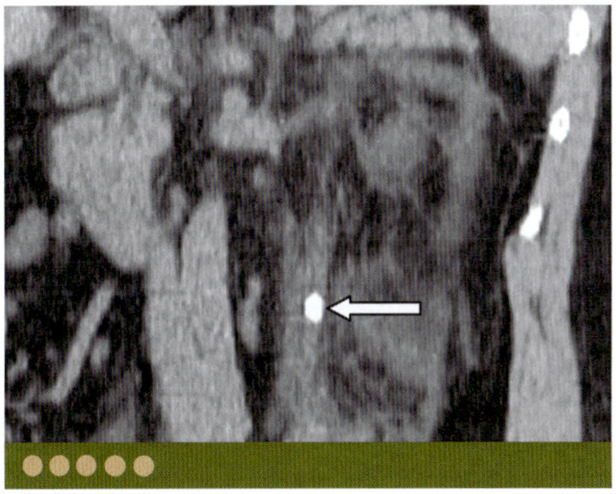

E. Calculus: Coronal CECT shows a small dense calculus (arrow) in the left ureter.

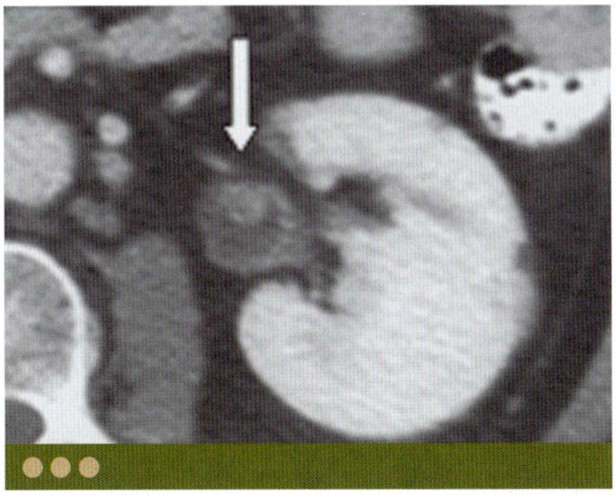

F. Urothelial cancer: Axial CECT shows a small, round filling defect (arrow) in the left renal pelvis. The filling defect showed enhancement when compared to the corresponding NECT (not shown).

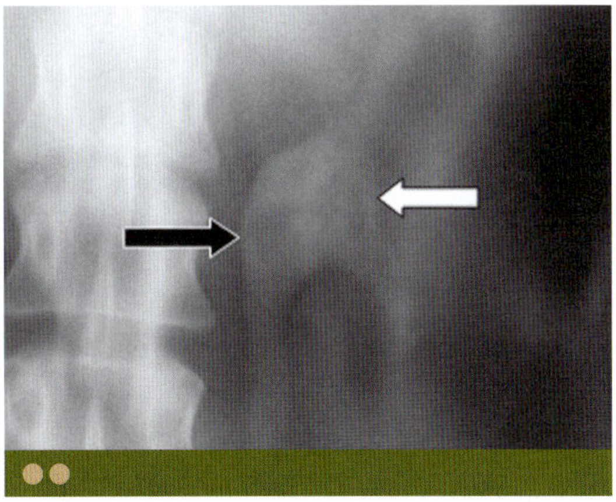

G. Blood clots: IVU tomogram shows two irregularly shaped filling defects (arrows) in the renal pelvis. They were not seen on follow-up imaging.

6–10 Upper Urinary Tract Fungal Infection

David D. Casalino

PRESENTATION

Intermittent flank pain, hematuria, and dysuria.

FINDINGS

Percutaneous urogram shows a slightly lobulated filling defect in the renal pelvis.

DIFFERENTIAL DIAGNOSES

- *Transitional cell carcinoma*: More common; older patients; pain less common; enhancement; immobile.
- *Blood clot*: Usually hyperdense (40-80 HU) and denser than TCC; no enhancement; can be mobile.
- *Sloughed papilla*: Occasionally triangular; associated with irregular papilla; can be mobile.
- *Calculus*: Most hyperdense (>100 HU) and hyperechoic; larger stones will cause acoustic shadowing; no enhancement; can be mobile.

COMMENTS

Upper urinary tract fungal infection and fungal ball, or mycetoma, formation may be the result of blood-borne or ascending infection of the urinary tract. *Candida albicans* is the most common fungus involved. Fungal infection of the urinary tract typically occurs in patients who have weakened immune systems, perhaps because of severe illness, various medications, or AIDS. Patients with diabetes mellitus, drug abuse, or chronic indwelling catheter are also more susceptible to fungal infection. They may present with flank pain if the fungal ball is obstructive. In such cases, dysuria, hematuria, and funguria may be present.

Urothelial candidiasis causes diffuse mural irregularity and thickening of the pelvocalyceal system and ureter. This may be seen in isolation or associated with fungus ball and/or renal parenchymal involvement. A fungus ball will cause a filling defect on imaging. The fungus ball may have irregular margins with contrast filling surface interstices. Gas formation within a fungus ball may create a lacy radiolucent pattern. A fungus ball may be mobile and change its configuration over time. It may cause obstruction, most often at the UPJ. On ultrasound, a fungus ball is hyperechoic compared to the urine in the collecting system. On CT, a fungus ball is usually soft tissue attenuation. Renal manifestation of fungal infection may include papillary necrosis, caliectasis, cortical scarring, and abscess formation.

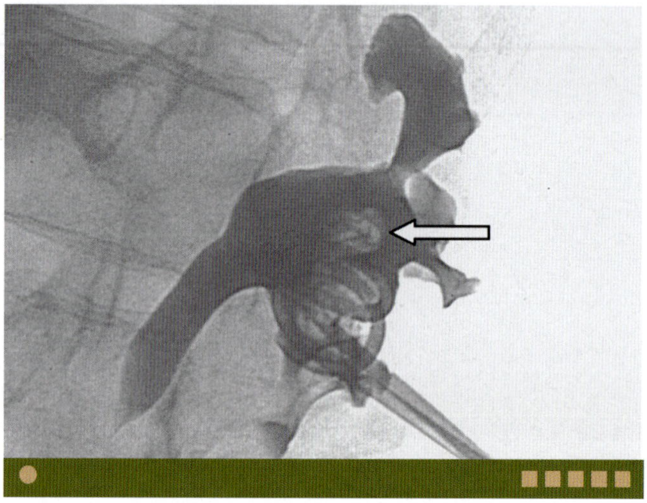

A. Percutaneous urogram shows a slightly lobulated filling defect (arrow) in the left renal pelvis. Contrast fills interstices on the surface of the mass.

PEARLS

- ***Candida albicans*** **is the most common fungus to infect the urinary tract.**
- **These infections typically occur in immunocompromised patients.**
- **Imaging features include pelvocalyceal and ureteral mural irregularity and thickening and fungus ball creating a focal filling defect that may be mobile.**
- **A fungus ball may cause obstruction, most often at the UPJ and occasionally intermittent.**

ADDITIONAL IMAGES (B-D)

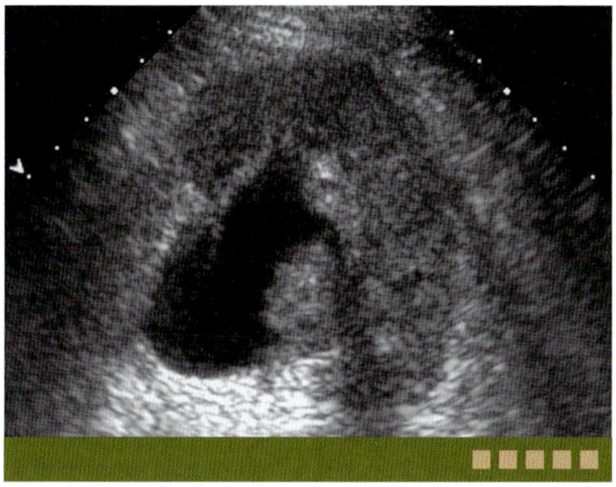

B. Transverse sonogram shows the mass to be hyperechoic without posterior shadowing.

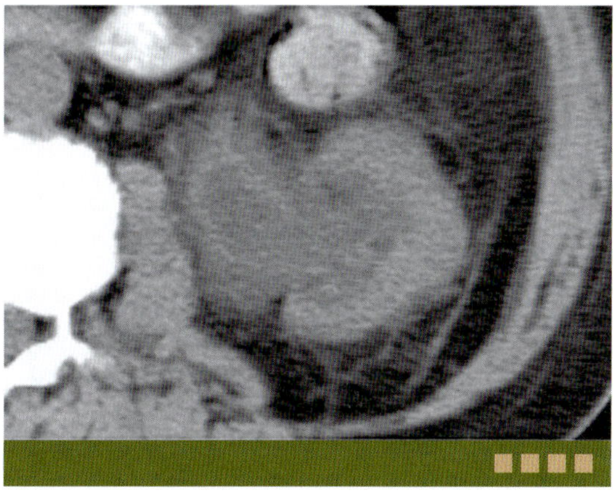

C. Axial CECT shows marked irregular thickening of the left renal pelvis in a different patient. The process was bilateral and also involved the ureters.

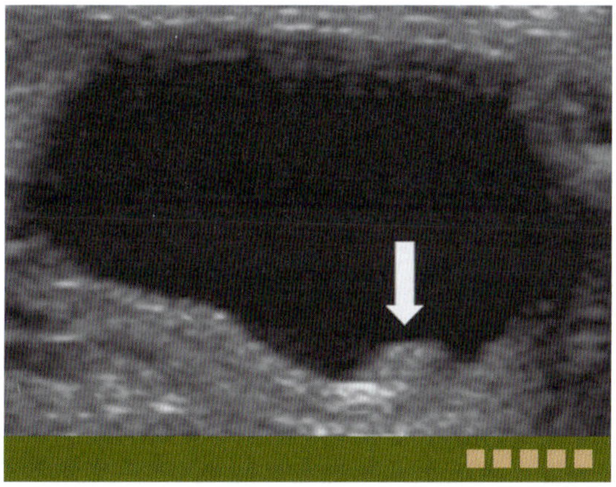

D. Transverse sonogram of the bladder shows a small hyperechoic fungal ball (arrows) in a newborn with fungemia.

DIFFERENTIAL DIAGNOSES IMAGES (E-G)

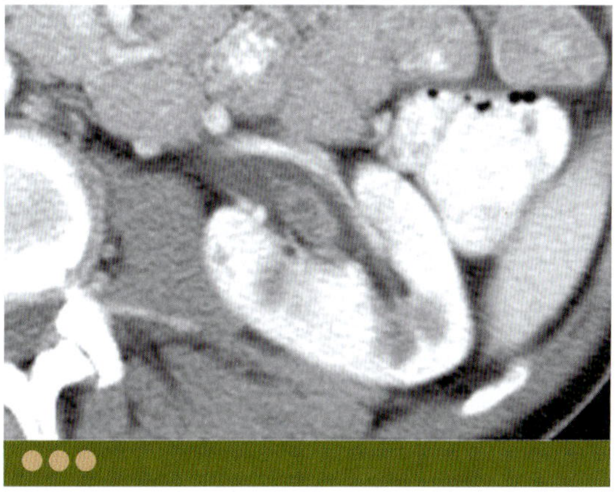

E. Transitional cell carcinoma: Axial CECT shows an enhancing, oval mass in the left renal pelvis.

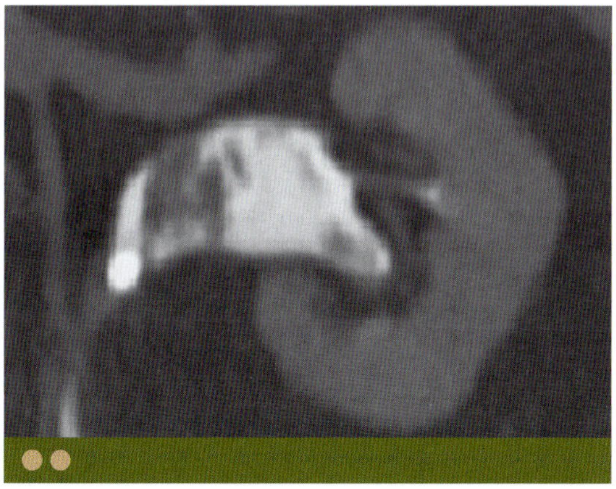

F. Blood clot and calculus: Coronal CECT during excretory phase shows an obstructing calculus at the left UPJ and scattered blood clots in the renal pelvis. The clots were hyperdense on the precontrast imaging and did not enhance.

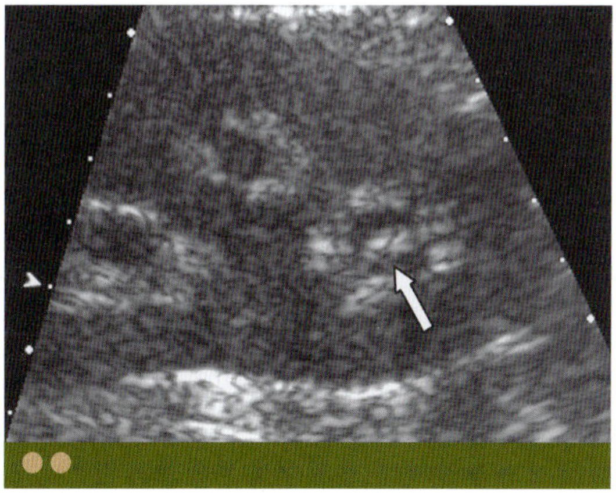

G. Papillary necrosis: Longitudinal sonogram shows a hyperechoic filling defect (arrow) in the lower-pole collecting system of a sickle-cell patient. There is no associated acoustic shadowing.

IMAGE KEY

Common

Rare

Typical

Unusual

6-11 Renal Sinus Cysts

David D. Casalino

PRESENTATION

Asymptomatic.

FINDINGS

CT shows fluid attenuation filling the renal sinus bilaterally.

DIFFERENTIAL DIAGNOSES

- *Pelvicalyceal dilatation*: Can be bilateral because of bilateral ureteral obstruction, bladder outlet obstruction, or reflux; excreted contrast will opacify; ureters may be dilated.
- *Urinoma of renal sinus*: Cavity containing urine caused by ureteral obstruction or trauma; may be symptomatic; may extend into perirenal space; excreted contrast may opacify.
- *Parapelvic cyst*: Typically solitary or few in number.
- *Parapelvic cystic neoplasm*: Includes cystic RCC and multilocular cystic nephroma; usually unilateral and solitary; internal septations and/or enhancing components

COMMENTS

Renal sinus cysts may also be referred to as peripelvic cysts. These fluid-filled cysts are thought to originate from lymphatic tissues in the renal sinus. They are benign with no known malignant potential. They are typically small, bilateral, multiple, and distributed throughout the renal sinus. They are usually asymptomatic, though obstruction of the collecting system or hemorrhage into a cyst may occur.

Parapelvic cysts, in contrast, are typically solitary or few in number and arise from the renal parenchyma with extension into the renal sinus.

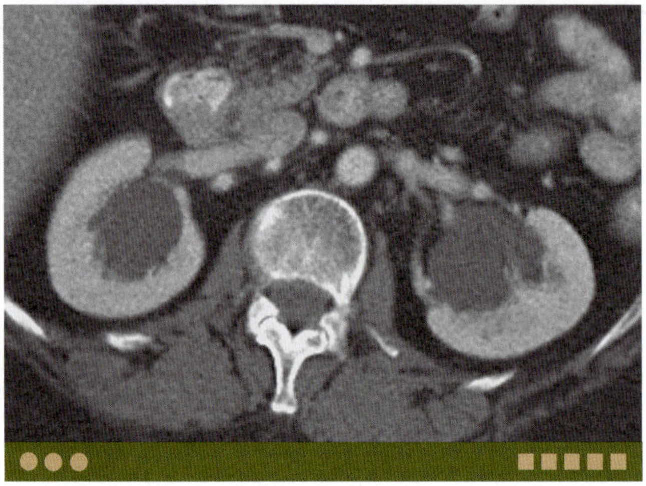

A. Axial CECT, during nephrographic phase, shows fluid attenuation filling the renal sinus bilaterally.

On ultrasound, renal sinus cysts will appear as anechoic with posterior acoustic enhancement. They may appear as discrete small cysts in the renal sinus. The thin walls of these cysts, however, may not be perceptible, and the appearance may mimic pelvicalyceal dilatation. Contrast excretion, whether on excretory urogram, CT, or MRI, allows differentiation of peripelvic cysts from pelvicalyceal dilatation.

PEARLS

- **Renal sinus cysts are usually bilateral, small, multiple, and distributed throughout the renal sinus.**
- **Renal sinus cysts may mimic pelvicalyceal dilatation or, less often, cystic neoplasm.**
- **Excretory phase imaging is most helpful in making the diagnosis.**

ADDITIONAL IMAGES (B-D)

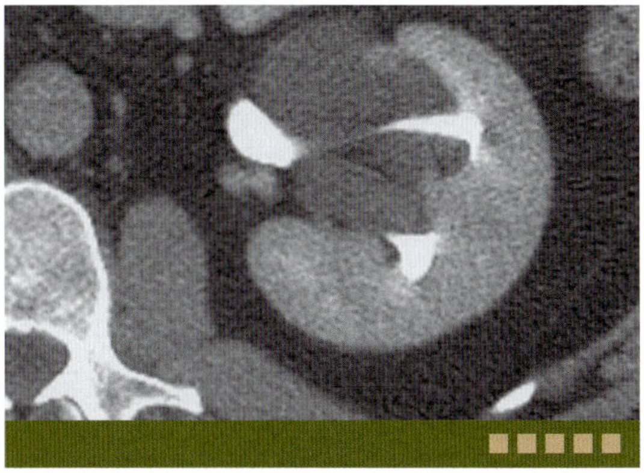

B. Axial CECT, during excretory phase, shows contrast-filled collecting system being stretched and attenuated by the multiple peripelvic cysts.

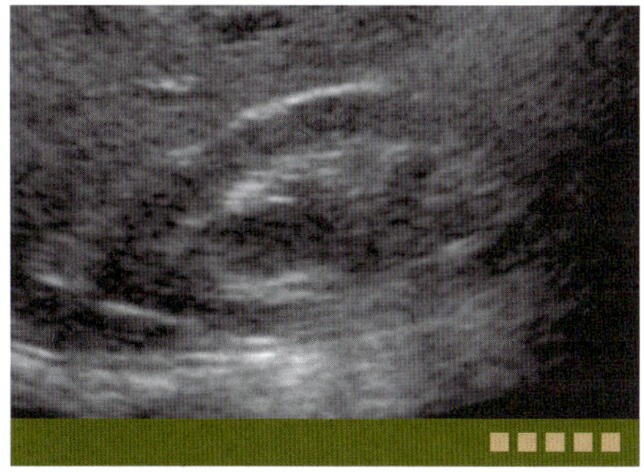

C. Longitudinal sonogram from a different patient shows extensive anechogenicity in the renal sinus suggestive of hydronephrosis. The contralateral kidney had a similar appearance.

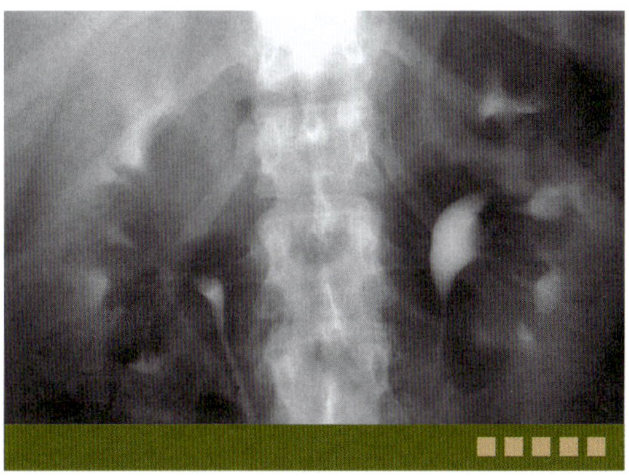

D. IVU, from the same patient as in last figure, shows stretched and attenuated calyces bilaterally. There is no hydronephrosis. Renal sinus lipomatosis can create a similar IVU appearance.

DIFFERENTIAL DIAGNOSES IMAGES (E-G)

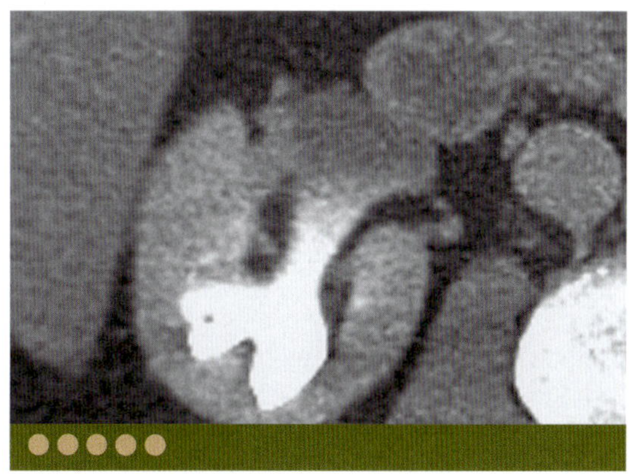

E. Ureteral obstruction: Axial CECT, during excretory phase, shows contrast opacification of the dilated renal collecting system.

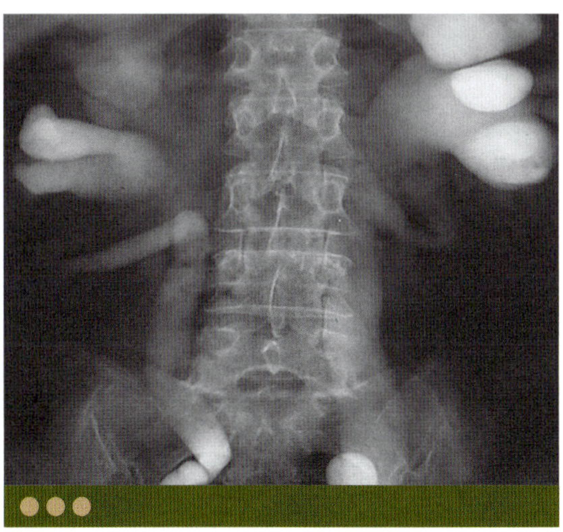

F. Vesicoureteral reflux: Cystogram shows high-grade reflux associated with bilateral massive pelvicalyceal and ureteral dilatation.

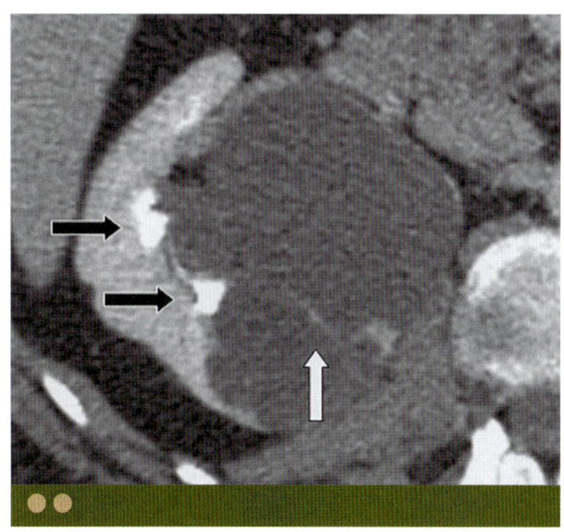

G. Multilocular cystic nephroma: Axial CECT, during excretory phase, shows a well-circumscribed cystic mass with enhancing septations (white arrow), protruding into the renal sinus and effacing the collecting system (black arrows).

IMAGE KEY

Common

Rare

Typical

Unusual

6–12 Renal Sinus Lipomatosis

Paul Nikolaidis

PRESENTATION

Usually asymptomatic.

FINDINGS

CT shows expansion of the renal sinus with nonmass-like proliferation of adipose tissue. There is mild splaying of the vessels that course through the renal sinus.

DIFFERENTIAL DIAGNOSES

- *Replacement lipomatosis of the kidney (fibrolipomatosis)*: An extreme, advanced form of renal sinus lipomatosis with significant parenchymal atrophy and associated inflammation, calculi, and in many cases, hydronephrosis. More typically unilateral.
- *Renal angiomyolipoma*: An angiomyolipoma (AML) extending into the renal sinus may be difficult to distinguish from lipomatosis; however, an AML should be more mass-like and displace the vascular structures of the renal sinus.
- *Renal liposarcoma*: Rare unusual lesions; liposarcomas may get quite large and may be more heterogeneous containing areas of internal stranding or nodularity, septations, or large, solid soft tissue components.
- *Renal sinus (peripelvic) cysts*: May be impossible to differentiate from sinus lipomatosis on IVU; they have a characteristic appearance on all other imaging modalities, however.

COMMENTS

Renal sinus lipomatosis refers to the accumulation and proliferation of adipose tissue in the renal sinus. This process is typically bilateral. It occurs with increasing age, obesity, and steroid use. Patients are usually asymptomatic. In a few instances, excessive proliferation of adipose tissue may cause mass effect on the renal collecting system. This should be distinguished from an advanced form of lipomatosis with an inflammatory component known as replacement renal sinus lipomatosis, where severe parenchymal atrophy, inflammation, calculi, and obstruction are seen.

IVU shows increased radiolucency of the renal sinus along with attenuation and stretching of the infundibula. Ultrasound shows enlargement of the central echogenic renal sinus area.

On CT, hypodense adipose tissue is seen in the renal sinus, which may appear expanded.

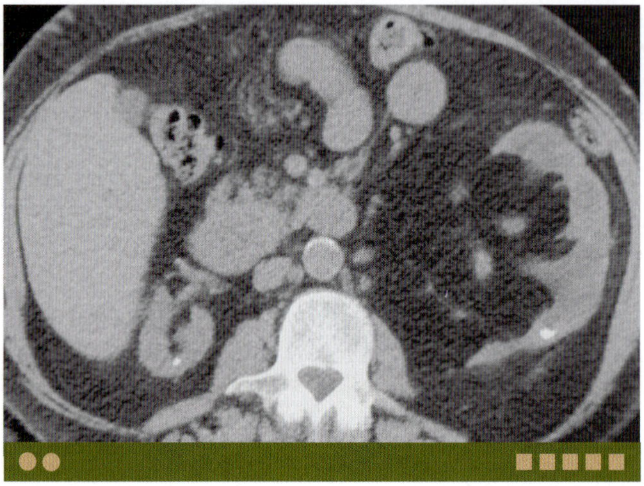

A. Axial CECT shows increased fatty deposition in left renal sinus that surrounds the collecting system. The process is unilateral. A single calcification is seen. There is no evidence of obstruction or inflammation, and the patient is asymptomatic.

On MR, the adipose tissue within the renal sinus follows the signal intensity of fat on all sequences (high on T1-WI and T2-WI and low on fat-saturated T1-WI). Renal sinus lipomatosis should be differentiated from fatty masses extending into or occupying the renal sinus.

There is no specific treatment regimen for renal sinus lipomatosis. Patients are monitored for decreasing renal function or symptoms that may imply progression into replacement lipomatosis of the kidney (fibrolipomatosis).

PEARLS

- **Refers to the accumulation and proliferation of adipose tissue in the renal sinus.**
- **Increased fatty tissue in the sinus is readily identified on imaging.**
- **Should be differentiated from fatty masses extending into or occupying the renal sinus.**
- **May lead to replacement lipomatosis (fibrolipomatosis) with severe parenchymal atrophy and inflammation, calculi, and hydronephrosis.**

ADDITIONAL IMAGES (B-C)

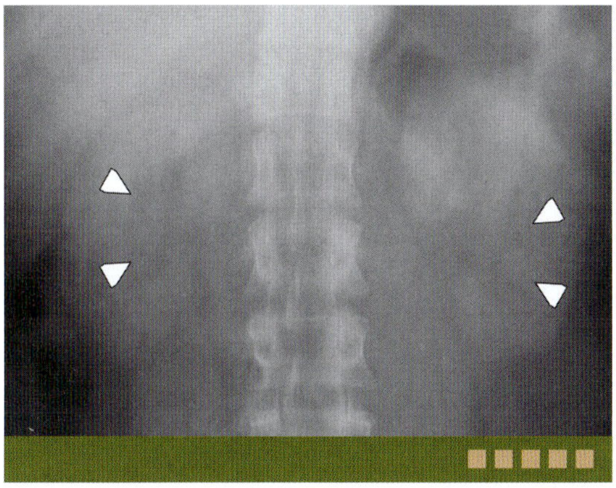

B. IVU tomographic image (at 11 cm) on another patient, obtained 30 seconds after contrast administration, shows central areas of increased lucency in both kidneys corresponding to areas of fatty proliferation/deposition in the renal sinus (arrowheads). This patient had asymptomatic renal sinus lipomatosis. On IVU, lipomatosis may be difficult to differentiate from renal sinus (peripelvic) cysts.

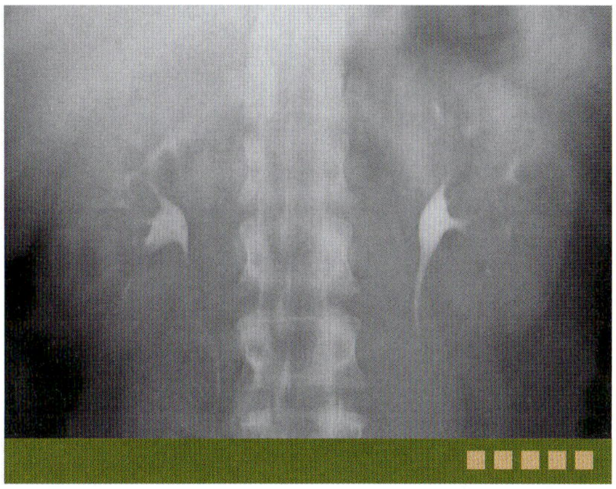

C. IVU on the same patient obtained 5 minutes after contrast administration shows excretion of contrast from both kidneys with diffuse elongation and attenuation of the renal pelves and infundibula. Cortical thickness is maintained. A similar appearance may be seen in cases of bilateral renal sinus (peripelvic) cysts.

DIFFERENTIAL DIAGNOSES IMAGES (D-E)

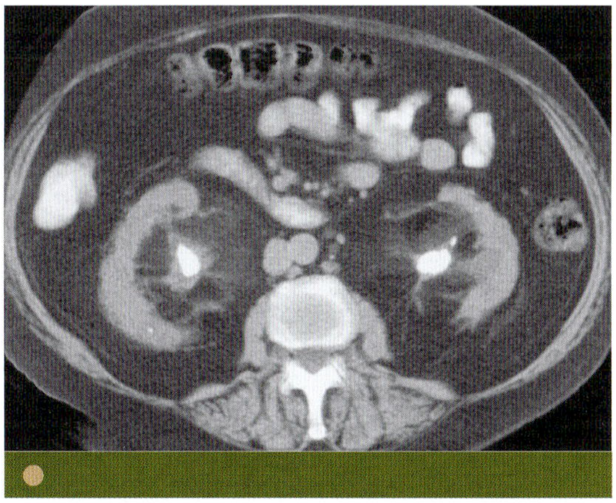

D. Replacement lipomatosis of the kidney (fibrolipomatosis): Axial CECT shows bilateral expansion of the renal sinuses with superimposed inflammatory changes and increased attenuation of the surrounding fat. Note the presence of obstructing calculi. While this process is more typically unilateral, bilateral involvement may sometimes occur. (*Image courtesy of Dr. Akira Kawashima, Mayo Clinic, Rochester, Minnesota.*)

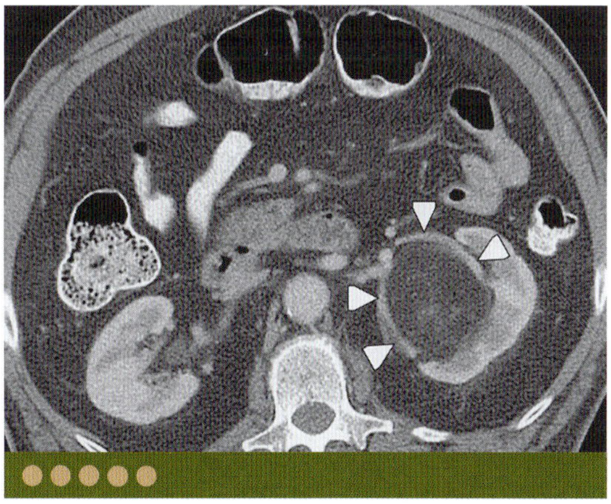

E. AML: Axial CECT shows a rounded fatty mass occupying the renal sinus. Note how the adjacent vessels are displaced outward (arrowheads). In renal sinus lipomatosis, they would be splayed but contained within the fatty mass.

IMAGE KEY

Common

Rare

Typical

Unusual

6–13 Replacement Lipomatosis of the Kidney (Fibrolipomatosis)

Paul Nikolaidis

PRESENTATION

Fever, UTIs and flank pain.

FINDINGS

CT shows the expansion of the renal sinuses fatty tissue, large central obstructing calculi and poor enhancement of the kidneys along with cortical atrophy.

DIFFERENTIAL DIAGNOSES

- *Renal sinus lipomatosis*: Simple adipose tissue is seen expanding the renal sinus, but without any evidence of the severe parenchymal atrophy, calculi, obstruction, or inflammation that accompanies replacement lipomatosis.
- *Renal liposarcoma*: Liposarcomas of the kidney are rare and may be quite heterogeneous and large.
- *Xanthogranulomatous pyelonephritis*: Both processes are classically associated with central calculi and inflammation. Hydronephrosis or pyonephrosis with central cystic changes (closer to fluid, not macroscopic fat attenuation) are a classic finding in xanthogranulomatous pyelonephritis (XGP). Distinction may be difficult as XGP and replacement lipomatosis often coexist.
- *Renal malakoplakia*: Malakoplakia is a rare inflammatory disorder that may affect the kidneys. Calculi and hydronephrosis are typically absent.

COMMENTS

Replacement lipomatosis is a more aggressive and advanced form of renal sinus lipomatosis. This process is also known as replacement fibrolipomatosis. It is associated with more severe parenchymal atrophy and inflammation, calculi, and hydronephrosis. This process is typically unilateral, but may be bilateral at times.

On pathologic examination, the kidney is usually enlarged and has a gross fibrofatty appearance. The reniform shape of the kidney is typically maintained. There is marked proliferation of hyperplastic fat in the renal sinus, with extremely large fat cells that do not permeate the renal parenchyma but merely develop adjacent to it as the renal atrophy progresses. On microscopy, the kidneys show large foci of inflammation, often with areas of necrosis.

CT will best show all the findings of replacement lipomatosis. Hypodense adipose tissue is seen in the renal sinus, which may appear expanded. The renal cortex is atrophied. There may be stranding of the renal sinus fat and perinephric stranding. Central calculi may be present, often causing hydronephrosis.

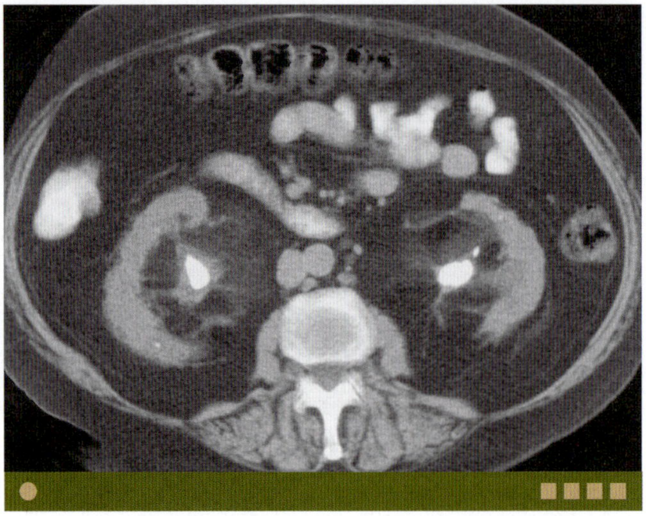

A. Axial CECT shows expansion of both renal sinuses by inhomogeneous fatty tissue that surrounds and mildly compresses the collecting systems. Large central obstructing calculi are present bilaterally. The kidneys enhance poorly, and there is atrophy of the renal parenchyma with some calcifications. (*Image courtesy of Dr Akira Kawashima, Mayo Clinic, Rochester, Minnesota.*)

MR will show inflammation and mass-like proliferation of the renal sinus fat and an atrophied renal parenchyma. CT is superior to MR, however, in demonstrating calcifications.

Treatment options vary but may include percutaneous nephrostomy or drainage and IV antibiotics, when appropriate. Open surgical drainage is sometimes required.

PEARLS

- **An advanced, aggressive form of renal sinus lipomatosis with severe parenchymal atrophy and inflammation, calculi, and hydronephrosis.**
- **Usually a unilateral process.**
- **CT or MR shows inflammatory changes and atrophy of the affected kidney, which may enhance poorly or not at all.**
- **CT is superior to MR in demonstrating calcifications.**

ADDITIONAL IMAGES (B-C)

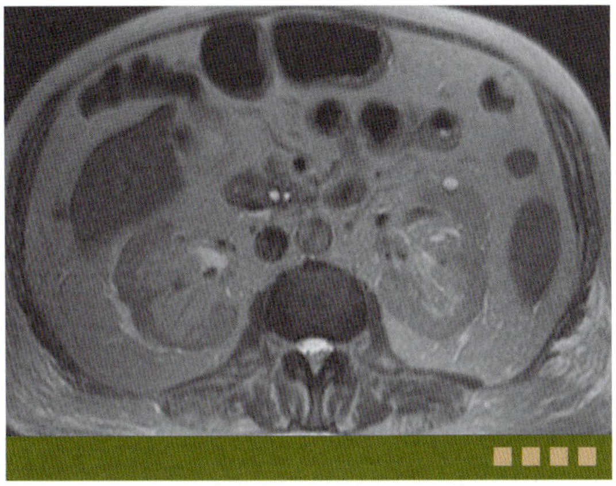

B. Axial T2-WI on another patient with early bilateral replacement lipomatosis shows proliferation of the renal sinus fat. The signal voids in the collecting systems represent small stones. There is mild dilatation of the right collecting system. Perinephric stranding is also present.

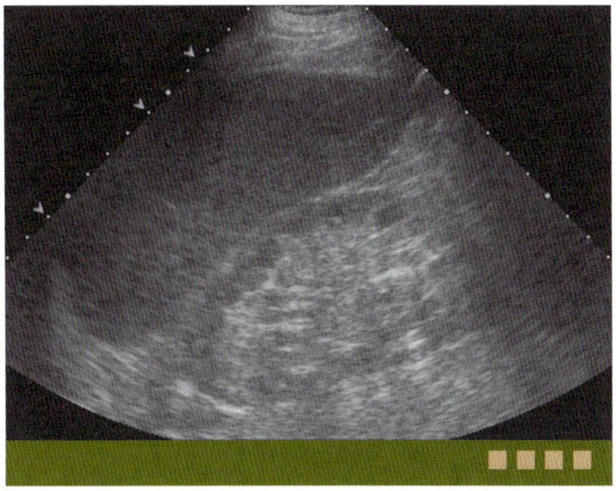

C. Longitudinal sonogram of the right kidney on the same patient shows an expanded, heterogeneously hyperechoic renal sinus. There is also cortical thinning.

DIFFERENTIAL DIAGNOSES IMAGES (D-E)

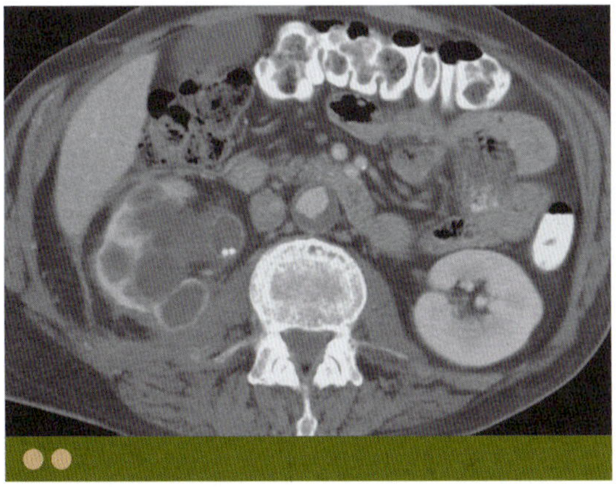

D. Xanthogranulomatous pyelonephritis: Axial CECT shows cortical thinning and obstruction of the right kidney. A few calcifications are also present. Note that renal sinus is occupied by a hypodense (fluid attenuation) inflammatory mass, resulting from collecting system obstruction and infection.

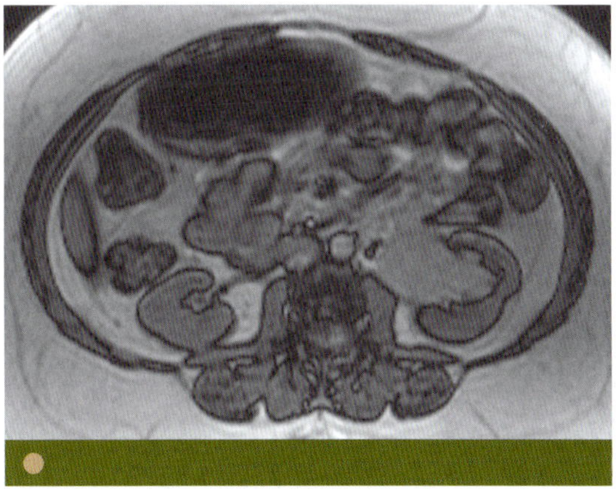

E. Liposarcoma: Axial noncontrast, out of phase T1-WI shows an oval fatty mass occupying the renal sinus. There is slightly increased signal within the mass compared to the adipose tissue elsewhere. No associated atrophy or calculi are seen, as would be expected with replacement lipomatosis.

IMAGE KEY

Common

Rare

Typical

Unusual

6–14 Lymphoma Infiltrating Renal Sinus

Paul Nikolaidis

PRESENTATION

Usually discovered on imaging of patients with lymphoma.

FINDINGS

CT shows bilateral homogeneous, poorly defined soft-tissue masses that extend into and infiltrate the renal sinus fat. They do not cause hydronephrosis. Retroperitoneal lymphadenopathy is present.

DIFFERENTIAL DIAGNOSIS

- *Renal sinus hemorrhage*: Similar ill-defined areas of soft tissue density may be seen; they should be hyperdense on precontrast images, and should not enhance (unless there is active bleeding).

COMMENTS

The kidney is the most commonly involved organ in extranodal dissemination of lymphoma. Typically there is coexistent retroperitoneal adenopathy, which may suggest the diagnosis. Renal involvement by lymphoma usually occurs in patients with known disease.

Involvement of the kidney in lymphoma can have a variety of appearances. The most common appearance is multiple parenchymal masses, often bilateral. Other patterns include a solitary renal mass, a perinephric soft tissue mass and diffuse infiltration of the kidney resulting in nephromegaly. A less common presentation is renal sinus involvement, with extension into, or replacement, of the normal sinus fat by a poorly defined soft tissue mass. Although it encircles the vessels and collecting system, this mass will typically not result in hydronephrosis because of the compliant nature of lymphomatous tissue.

CT is excellent for the diagnosis and staging lymphoma. In cases of lymphoma involving the renal sinus, mild contrast enhancement of an ill-defined lesion is usually seen. CT also helps in identifying additional areas of renal or perirenal involvement, as well as regional lymph node enlargement.

PET-CT studies superimposing fluorine-18-deoxyglucose positron emission tomography (FDG-PET) on traditional CT images are more frequently utilized in the work-up of lymphoma patients. MR should also allow for easy identification of abnormal renal and perirenal soft tissue lesions.

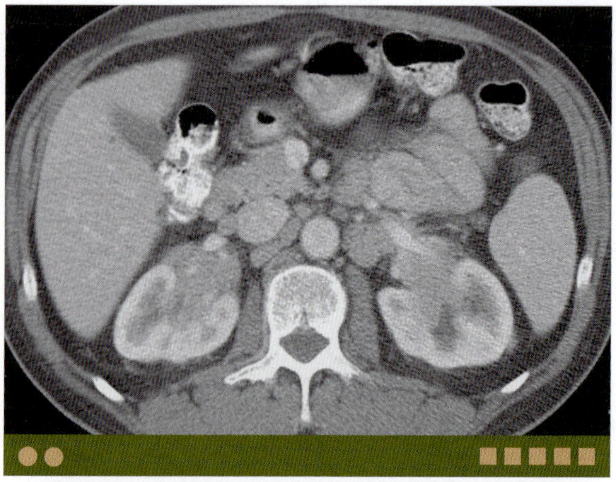

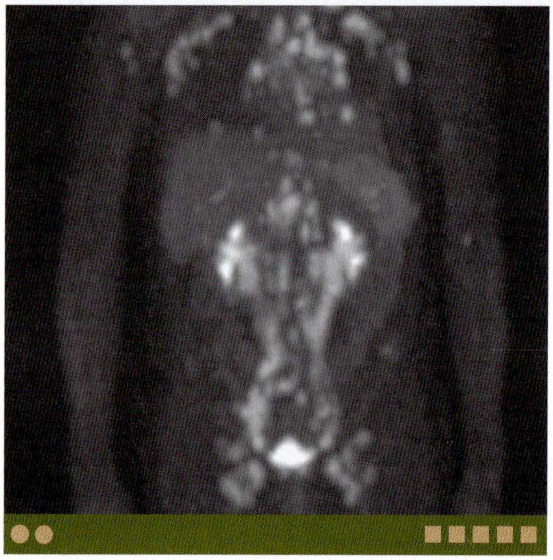

A. Axial CECT shows enhancing, ill-defined, soft tissue lesions infiltrating both renal sinuses. There is retroperitoneal lymphadenopathy.
B. PET scan on the same patient shows areas of increased metabolic activity in both renal sinuses, in addition to extensive lymphadenopathy in the chest, abdomen, and pelvis.

PEARLS

- **The kidney is the most commonly involved organ in extranodal dissemination of lymphoma.**
- **A less frequent presentation is renal sinus involvement, with abnormal soft tissue extending into or replacing the sinus fat.**
- **Because lymphomatous tissue is compliant, there is usually no significant hydronephrosis.**
- **CT should depict an ill-defined lesion, involving the renal sinus with mild contrast enhancement.**

ADDITIONAL IMAGES (C-E)

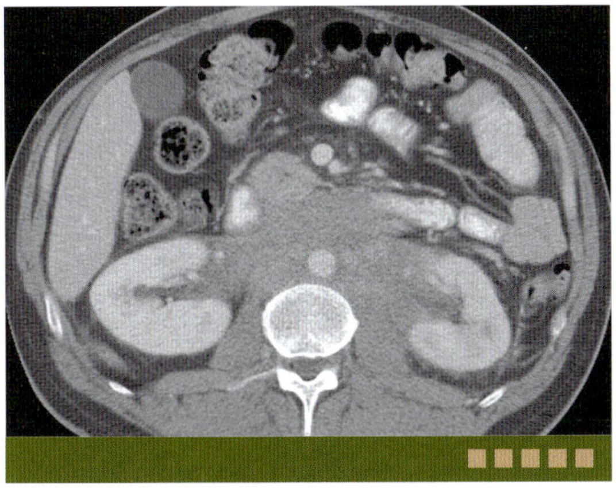

C. Axial CECT shows abnormal confluent soft tissue occupying the retroperitoneum, completely surrounding the aorta, and extending into both renal sinuses. Note the absence of renal obstruction.

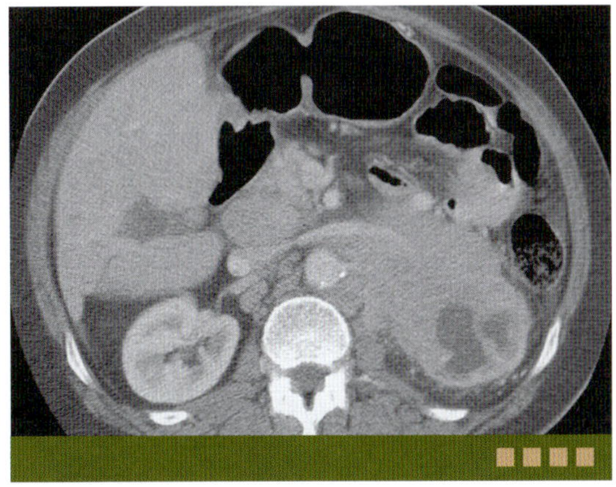

D. Axial CECT on a different patient shows an infiltrative soft tissue lesion occupying the entire renal sinus and extending medially, surrounding the renal artery and left renal vein. In this case, the mass causes mild to moderate caliectasis.

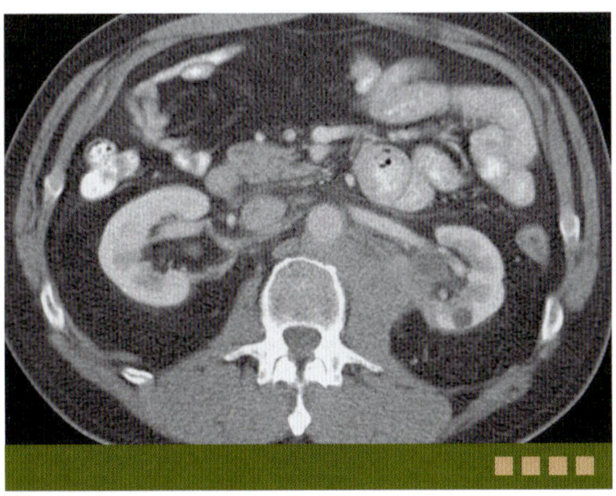

E. Axial CECT on a different patient shows a soft tissue mass that is contiguous with the left psoas and extending into the left renal sinus.

DIFFERENTIAL DIAGNOSES IMAGES (F-H)

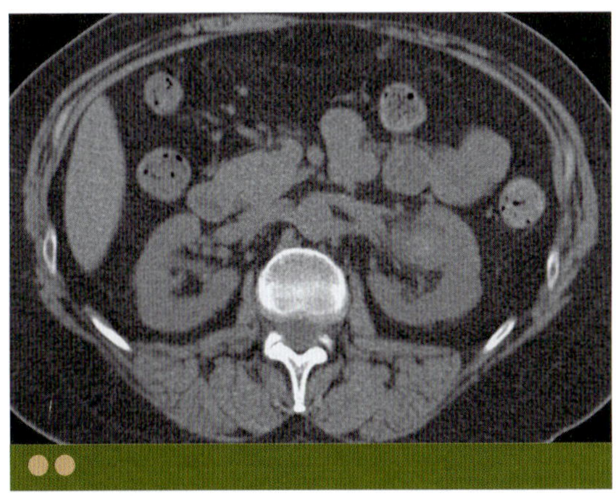

F. Renal sinus hematoma: Axial NECT shows a slightly hyperdense lesion in the left renal sinus.

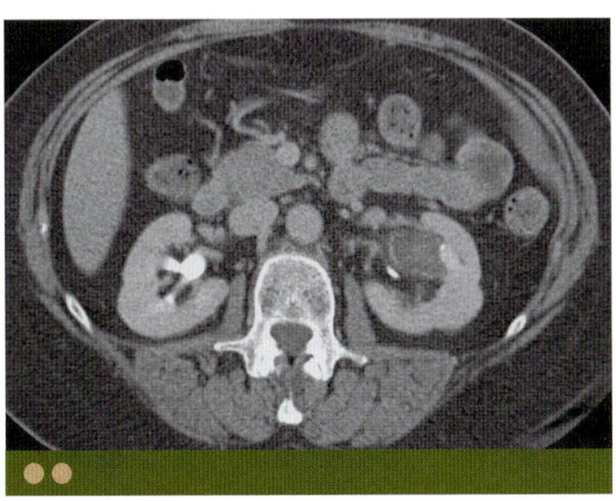

G. Renal sinus hematoma: Axial CECT on the same patient shows that the renal sinus lesion does not enhance. This is compatible with a hematoma.

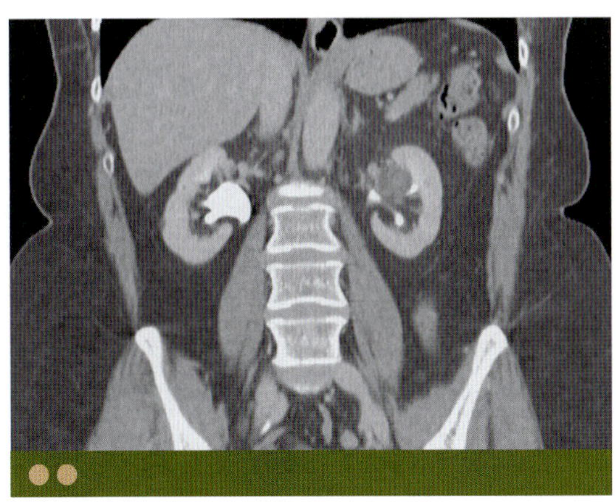

H. Renal sinus hematoma: Coronal CECT reformation on the same patient shows the same round lesion occupying part of the left renal sinus. Note excretion of contrast into the left collecting system surrounding the lesion.

IMAGE KEY

Common

Rare

Typical

Unusual

6–15 Antopol-Goldman Lesion

Paul Nikolaidis

PRESENTATION

Flank pain and hematuria; may be incidental finding.

FINDINGS

NECT shows a central, ill-defined, hyperdense mass in the right kidney that does not enhance postcontrast.

DIFFERENTIAL DIAGNOSES

- *Nonspontaneous renal sinus hemorrhage*: May be the result of trauma, renal infarction, AVM, vasculitis.
- *TCC of the renal pelvis*: May extend into the renal parenchyma; will enhance on CECT.
- *Renal sinus lymphoma*: Similar ill-defined areas of soft tissue density may be seen; lymphoma enhances and is usually a more extensive, multifocal process.

COMMENTS

Subepithelial renal pelvic hematomas are also called Antopol-Goldman lesions. These are rare lesions that usually present with hematuria and flank pain. On histopathology, a small area of subepithelial hemorrhage is seen associated with an organizing hematoma, containing fibroblasts and extravasated erythrocytes. It has been suggested that Antopol-Goldman lesions may be associated with analgesic overuse, which may result in increased renal vascular proliferation and prominent capillary blood vessels in the lamina propria.

On CT, these lesions appear as nonenhancing hyperdense masses in the renal pelvis that may cause extrinsic luminal narrowing. They may be indistinguishable from a renal pelvic malignancy. The presence of hemorrhagic components will often be masked if only a CECT is performed. Unenhanced CT readily should be performed to correctly identify the hyperdense hemorrhagic component of the lesion. High-attenuation material, often along the nondependent surface of the renal pelvis should suggest a subepithelial location. Subepithelial hemorrhage may compress the renal pelvis. Multiphasic CT should be repeated at approximately 4 to 6 weeks after initial presentation and correction of any underlying coagulopathy to confirm resolution.

MR also allows for easy identification of the subepithelial hemorrhage. Precontrast, fat-saturated T1-WI sequences are necessary. Region of interest (ROI) measurements and subtraction images should be obtained to confirm lack of enhancement.

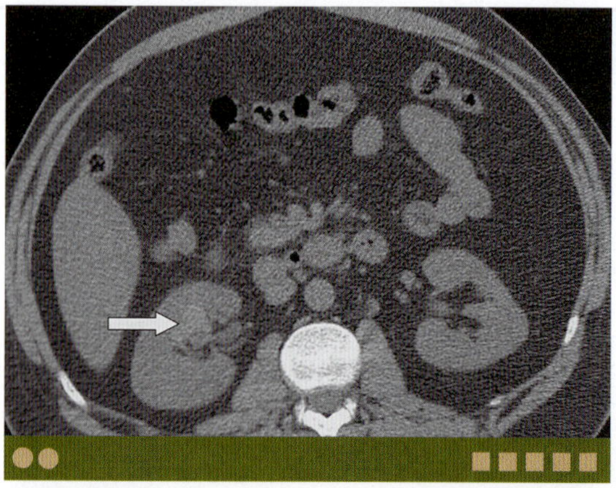

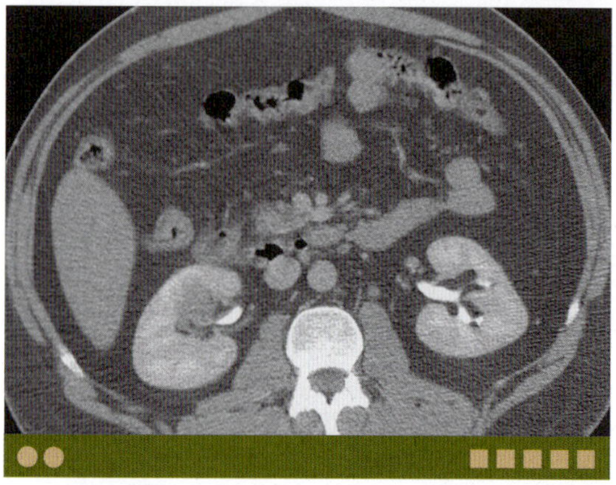

A. Axial NECT shows a central, ill-defined hyperdense mass in the right kidney (arrow).
B. Axial CECT on the same patient obtained during the excretory phase shows that the right renal mass does not enhance. This is compatible with a hematoma, which was shown to resolve on subsequent imaging.

PEARLS

- **Subepithelial renal pelvic hematomas which may extend into the renal sinus are also called Antopol-Goldman lesions.**
- **On CT, they appear as nonenhancing hyperdense lesions in the renal pelvis or adjacent renal sinus.**
- **Pre- and postcontrast CT follow-up examination should be obtained at 4 to 6 weeks to confirm resolution.**
- **On MR, noncontrast FS T1-WI will demonstrate high signal usually in the nondependent surface of the renal pelvis.**

ADDITIONAL IMAGES (C-E)

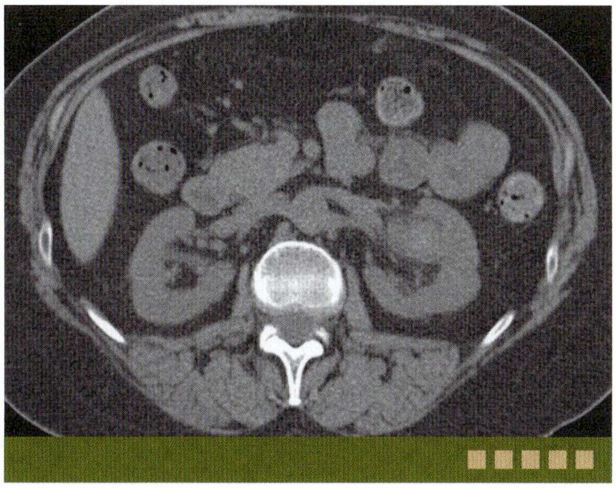

C. Axial NECT on another patient shows an ill-defined hyperdense lesion in the superior portion of the left renal pelvis and sinus.

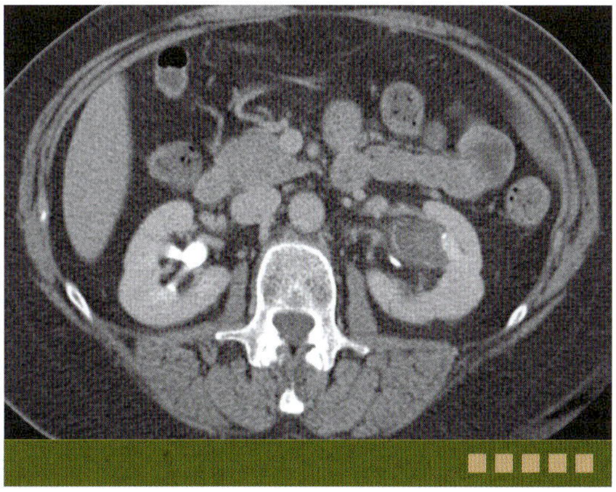

D. Axial CECT on the same patient shows that the lesion does not enhance. Note excretion of contrast into the left collecting system surrounding the lesion.

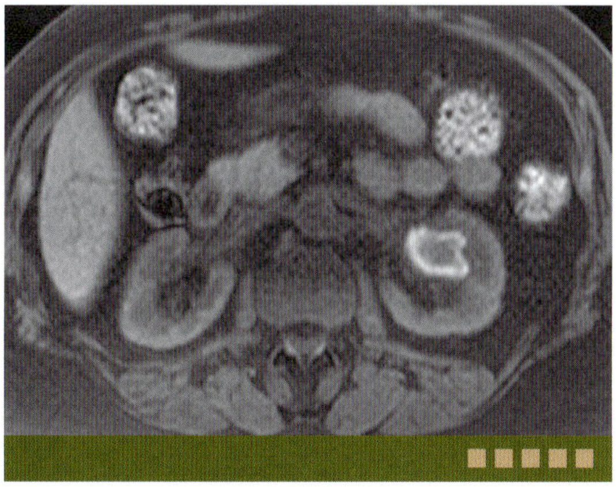

E. Axial fat-suppressed, noncontrast T1-WI on the same patient shows that the renal sinus lesion is hyperintense with similar signal intensity to hemorrhagic products.

DIFFERENTIAL DIAGNOSES IMAGES (F-H)

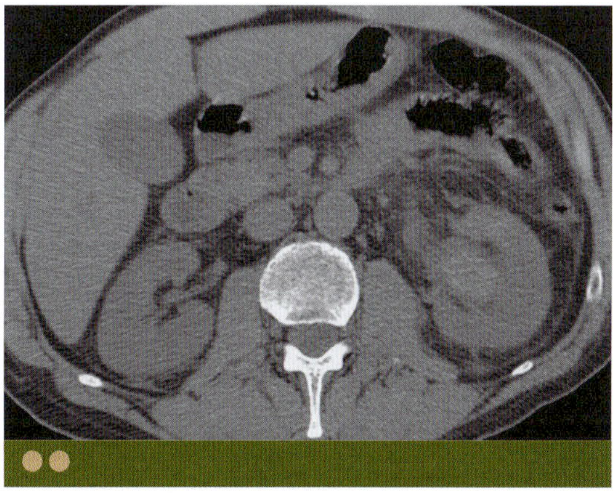

F. Renal sinus hemorrhage from trauma: Axial NECT on a patient who sustained multiple injuries in an MVA shows an irregular hyperdense lesion within the left renal sinus. This represented hemorrhage.

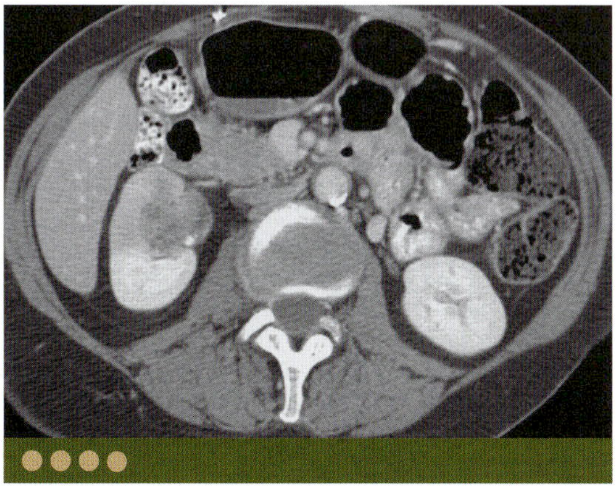

G. Transitional cell carcinoma: Axial CECT on a different patient shows a right renal soft-tissue mass which appears centered in the right renal sinus and renal pelvis.

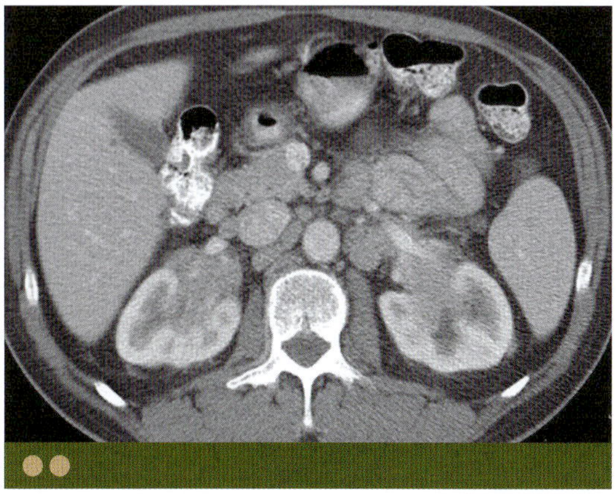

H. Lymphoma infiltrating renal sinus: Axial CECT shows enhancing ill-defined soft tissue infiltrating both renal sinuses.

IMAGE KEY

Common

Rare

Typical

Unusual

6–16 Ureteral Pseudodiverticulosis

David D. Casalino

PRESENTATION

Asymptomatic; history of UTIs and urolithiasis.

FINDINGS

IVU shows a few tiny ureteral outpouchings of contrast.

DIFFERENTIAL DIAGNOSES

- *Multifocal urothelial carcinoma*: Irregular filling defects or adjacent filling defects in profile can create the appearance of outpouchings, but the filling defects are the dominant abnormality.
- *Ureteritis cystica*: Numerous small filling defects; adjacent filling defects in profile can create the appearance of outpouchings, but the filling defects are the dominant abnormality; renal pelvis is often involved (pyelitis cystica).
- *Tuberculosis (TB)*: Often associated with systemic disease; ureteral involvement may include ureteral thickening, irregularity, calcifications, and stricturing, which can create the appearance of outpouchings.

COMMENTS

Ureteral pseudodiverticulosis is an uncommon acquired abnormality characterized by invagination of hyperplastic transitional epithelium into the lamina propria of the ureter. It is usually associated with chronic UTI or urolithiasis. In these patients, there appears to be an increased risk of urothelial carcinoma, perhaps as a result of chronic inflammation rather than the pseudodiverticula. Patients diagnosed with ureteral pseudodiverticulosis should undergo periodic screening, perhaps annually or semiannually, for urothelial carcinoma with urine cytology and imaging. Patients with ureteral pseudodiverticulosis are usually asymptomatic unless there is stone disease or coexisting tumor.

On imaging with IVU or retrograde pyelography, multiple small, smooth luminal outpouchings of contrast are seen. The outpouchings are usually 1 to 4 mm and bilateral. They typically occur in the upper and middle portions of the ureter and become stable over time. Careful assessment for possible coexisting urothelial carcinoma should be conducted. The bladder is the most common site for a coexisting malignancy.

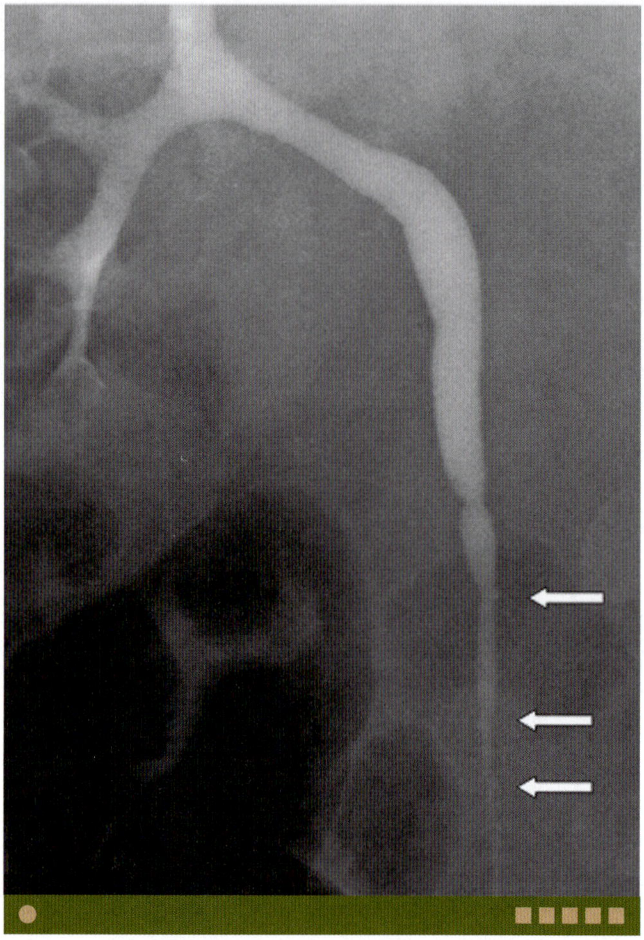

A. IVU shows the right ureter with a few small, smooth luminal outpouchings of contrast (arrows).

PEARLS

- **Up to 25% of patients with pseudodiverticulosis have or will develop urothelial carcinoma within several years.**
- **Pseudodiverticulosis consists of multiple, 1 to 4 mm, ureteral outpouchings of contrast.**
- **Pseudodiverticulosis is bilateral in 70% of cases.**

ADDITIONAL IMAGE

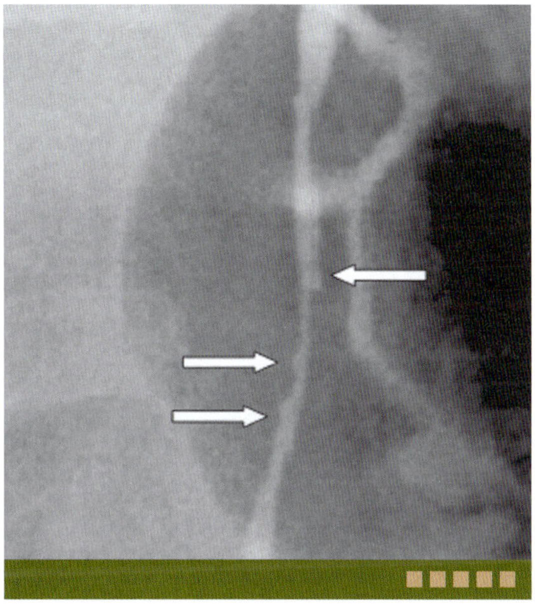

B. IVU shows the left ureter of the same patient to also have pseudodiverticulosis (arrows).

DIFFERENTIAL DIAGNOSES IMAGES (C-E)

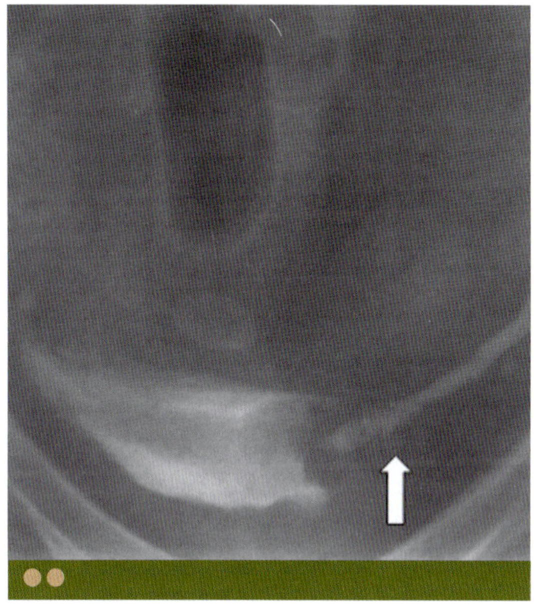

C. Multifocal urothelial carcinoma: IVU shows a cluster of small filling defects in the distal aspect of the left ureter. There is associated subtle luminal outpouching (arrow) of the ureter and prominent mass effect at the left UVJ.

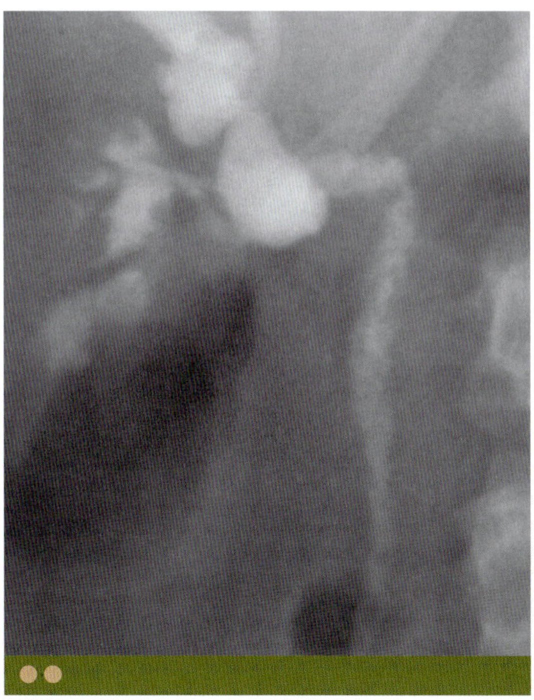

D. Ureteritis cystica: IVU shows multiple, small, smooth filling defects in the right ureter and renal pelvis.

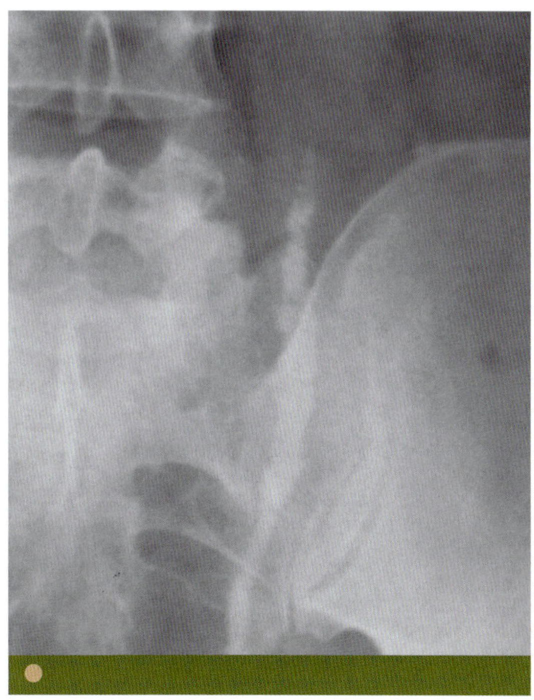

E. TB: IVU shows the left ureter to have an irregular, beaded appearance. On the scout radiograph (not shown), this segment of ureter also showed extensive calcification.

IMAGE KEY

Common

Rare

Typical

Unusual

6–17 Ureterocele

David D. Casalino

PRESENTATION

Asymptomatic, but may develop symptoms because of stones, infection, or obstruction.

FINDINGS

IVU images show fusiform dilatation of the distal ureters with prolapse into the bladder.

DIFFERENTIAL DIAGNOSES

- *Pseudoureterocele, distal ureteral obstruction*: Dilatation of the distal ureter caused by underlying abnormality, such as a stone, tumor, or edema; etiology might be apparent; may have radiolucent outline greater than 2 mm in thickness and irregular on IVU; usually unilateral and associated with dilatation of the upper tract.
- *Primary megaureter*: Typically, fusiform dilatation of the distal ureter proximal to a tapered distal segment that may be up to 4 cm in length; rarely is there caliectasis; unilateral in 75% of the cases.

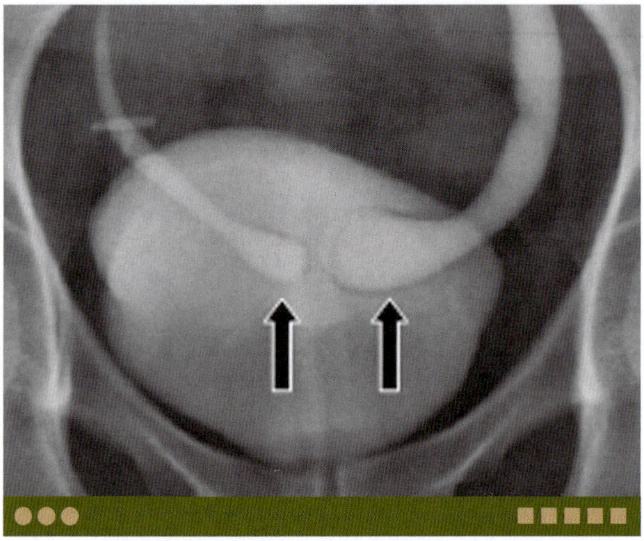

A. IVU shows fusiform dilatation of the distal ureters, which prolapse into the bladder and are outlined by thin lines of radiolucency (arrows). The upper collecting systems are neither duplicated nor dilated (not shown).

COMMENTS

An ureterocele is a focal dilatation of the distal aspect of the ureter. Ureteroceles may be orthotopic or ectopic. An orthotopic ureterocele, sometimes referred to as simple or adult-type, consists of focal dilatation and prolapse of the intramural segment of the ureter into the bladder at the trigone. Orthotopic ureteroceles usually occur in single systems and are small and asymptomatic. They may be either unilateral or bilateral. Patients with larger ureteroceles, greater than 2 cm, are more likely to develop complications, such as stones, infection, and obstruction, and present with associated signs and symptoms. Ectopic ureteroceles are more commonly seen in children and symptomatic, usually caused by obstruction. Ectopic ureteroceles almost always occur in duplicated collecting system and are more common in females and on the left side.

On IVU, the distal ureter has a bulbous configuration that projects into the bladder lumen. When the ureterocele is filled with contrast and surrounded by contrast in the bladder, it is outlined by a uniformly thin (≤2 mm) line of radiolucency that consists of the ureteral wall and bladder epithelium. This gives the ureterocele a "cobra-head" or "spring-onion" appearance. The appearance of an ureterocele is, in part, determined by its size and degree of distention. On cystography, a distended ureterocele will appear as a smooth round or oval filling defect in the location of the ureterovesical junction. It can evert and mimic a bladder diverticulum. The CT and MR appearance will depend on whether the ureterocele is filled with contrast or urine at the time of imaging. On ultrasonography, the ureterocele appears as a thin walled cystic lesion in the bladder base. Continuity with the more proximal ureter can usually be seen.

PEARLS

- **Orthotopic ureteroceles are typically small and asymptomatic and occur in single systems.**
- **Larger ureteroceles are more likely to be complicated by stones, infection, or obstruction.**
- **Ectopic ureteroceles usually occur in duplicated systems and present in children with symptoms of obstruction.**
- **A uniform, thin line of radiolucency should outline the ureterocele on IVU when the ureterocele and bladder are contrast-filled.**
- **A pseudoureterocele must be considered if the radiolucent outline is thicker than or equal to 2 mm or irregular.**

ADDITIONAL IMAGES (B-D)

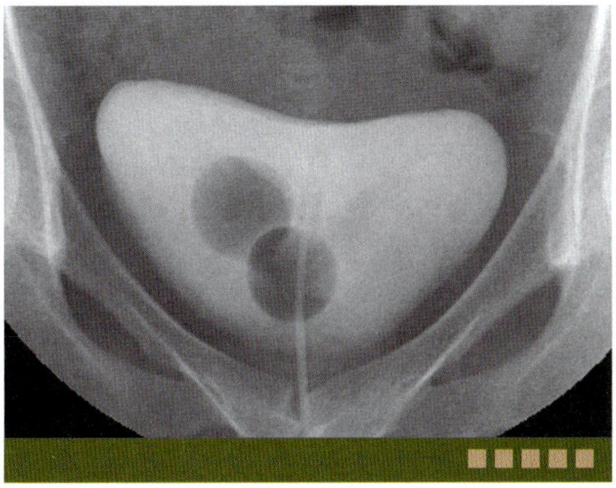

B. Cystogram from a different patient shows a smooth, round filling defect in the region of the right ureterovesical junction and adjacent to the Foley catheter balloon.

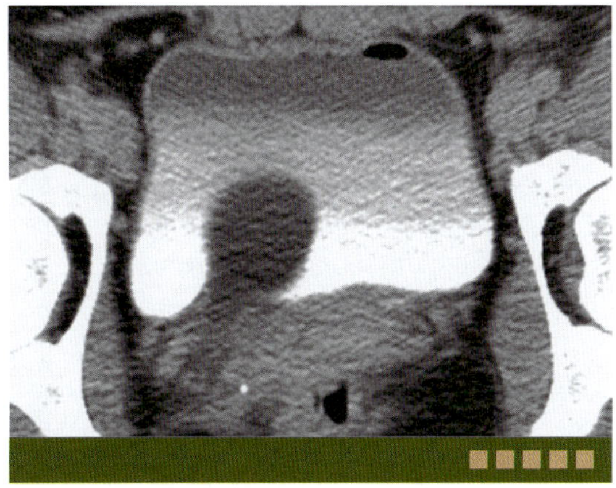

C. Axial NECT cystogram of the same patient shows the ureterocele as thin-walled, fluid-filled, and in continuity with the right ureter.

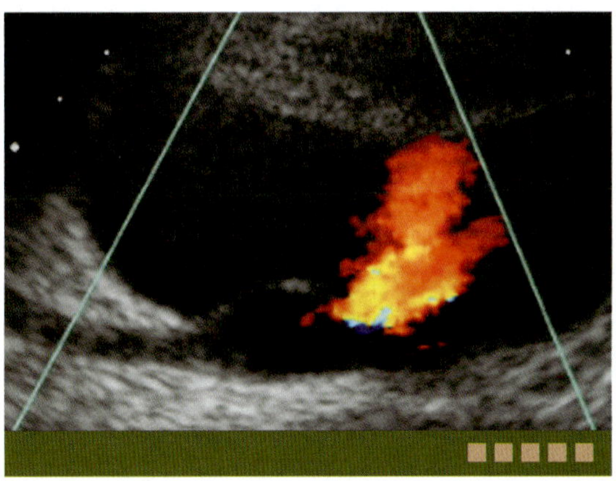

D. Longitudinal color Doppler sonogram shows a thin-walled cystic lesion in continuity with the ureter, in the bladder, and associated with a color jet.

DIFFERENTIAL DIAGNOSES IMAGES (E-G)

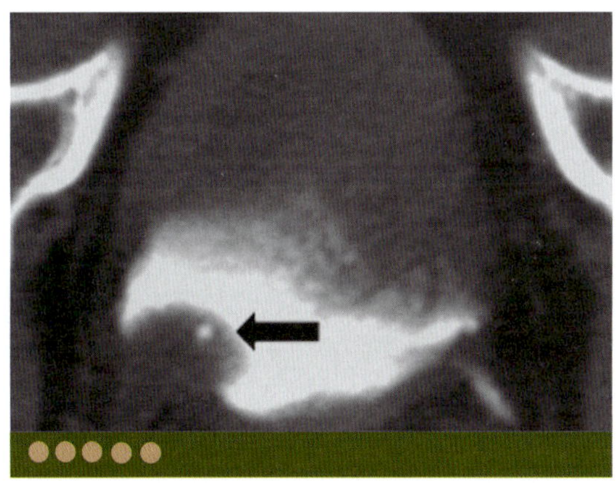

E. Stone disease: Axial CECT shows fusiform dilatation of the distal right ureter caused by an obstructing stone (arrow). Follow-up imaging after stone passage did not show an ureterocele.

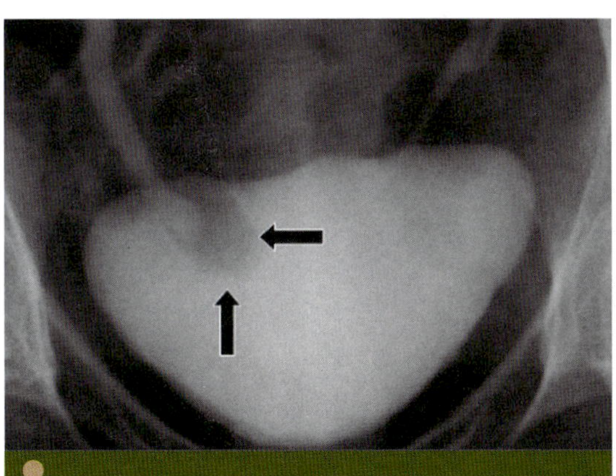

F. Pseudoureterocele: IVU shows dilatation of the distal right ureter surrounded by a thick, irregular radiolucent rind (arrows) that proved to be TCC.

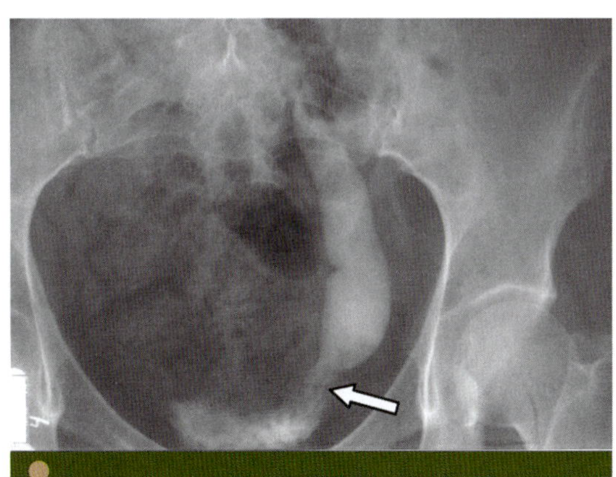

G. Primary megaureter: IVU shows marked dilatation of the lower third of the left ureter with a short segment of distal tapering (arrow). There is mild dilatation of the more proximal ureter and no pelvocaliectasis (not shown).

IMAGE KEY

Common

●●●●●
●●●●
●●●
●●
●

Rare

Typical

■■■■■
■■■■
■■■
■■
■

Unusual

6–18 Pseudoureterocele

David D. Casalino

PRESENTATION

Pain and hematuria.

FINDINGS

IVU shows moderate dilatation of the right collecting system with fusiform dilatation of the distal right ureter, which is surrounded by a rind of lucency.

DIFFERENTIAL DIAGNOSIS

- *Ureterocele*: Usually asymptomatic; when filled with contrast and surrounded by contrast in the bladder, it is outlined by a uniformly thin (≤2 mm) line of radiolucency; "cobra-head" or "spring-onion" appearance.

COMMENTS

Pseudoureterocele is dilatation of the distal, intramural ureter caused by thickening of the bladder mucosa at the ureterovesical junction (UVJ). This thickening of the mucosa may be caused by malignancy of the bladder or invasive from an adjacent organ, stone, or edema from recently passed stone or radiation-induced cystitis.

On IVU, the distal ureter will be dilated with mural thickening and irregularity. There is often asymmetry of the dilated ureteral lumen. The lucent outline between the contrast-filled dilated segment and contrast-filled bladder is greater than 2 mm in thickness or irregular. Other features will depend on the underlying etiology. For example, a filling defect caused by stone or tumor may be seen in the dilated distal ureter. There may be obstruction of the upper tract as well. On cystography, a pseudoureterocele may create a focal filling defect. On CT and MR, mucosal thickening may be seen at the site of the distal dilatation. If present, a stone may be detected.

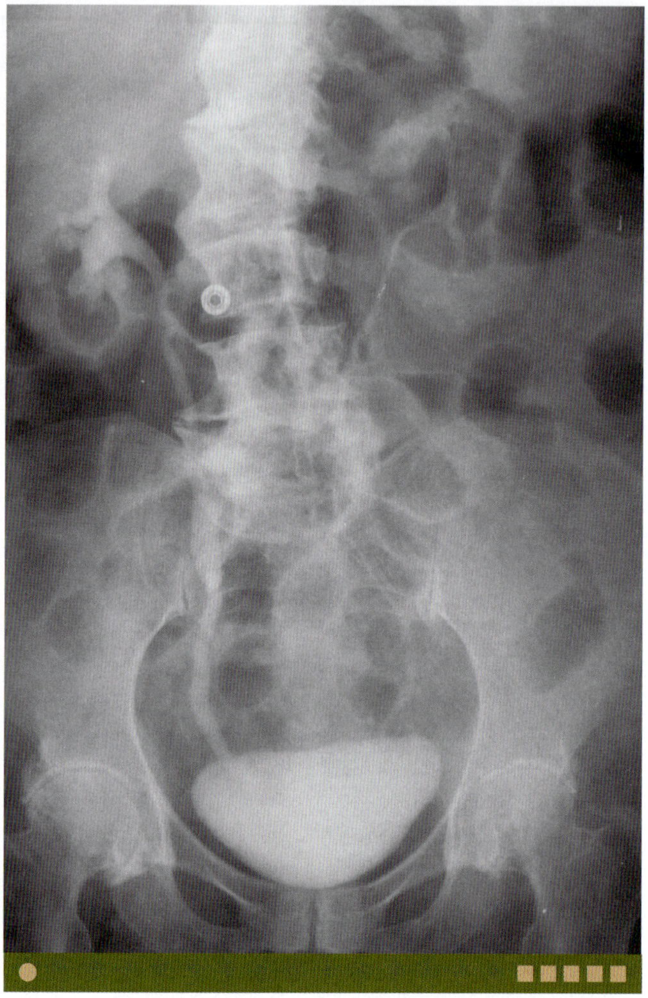

A. IVU shows moderate dilatation of the right renal collecting system and right ureter down to the UVJ. There is fusiform dilatation of the distal aspect of the right ureter, which is surrounded by a rind of radiolucency.

PEARLS

- **Pseudoureterocele is most often the result of an urothelial malignancy or stone.**
- **On IVU, a radiolucency that is greater than 2 mm in thickness or irregular around the dilated distal, intramural ureter is diagnostic of a pseudoureterocele.**
- **Pseudoureterocele may appear as a filling defect on cystography.**

ADDITIONAL IMAGES (B-D)

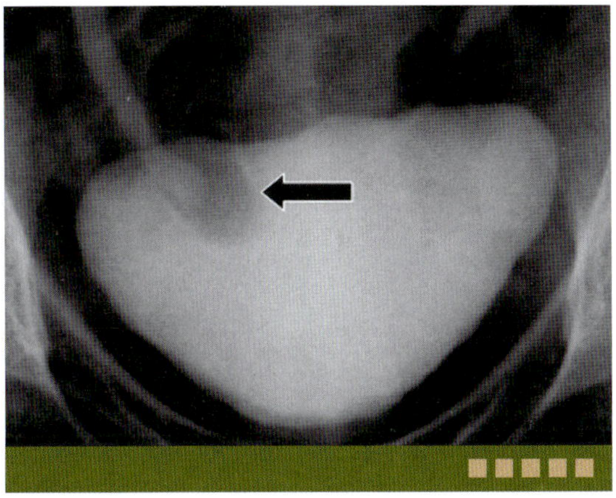

B. IVU, magnified view of the bladder, shows the lucent rind (arrow) to be thick and irregular. The underlying abnormality proved to be a TCC.

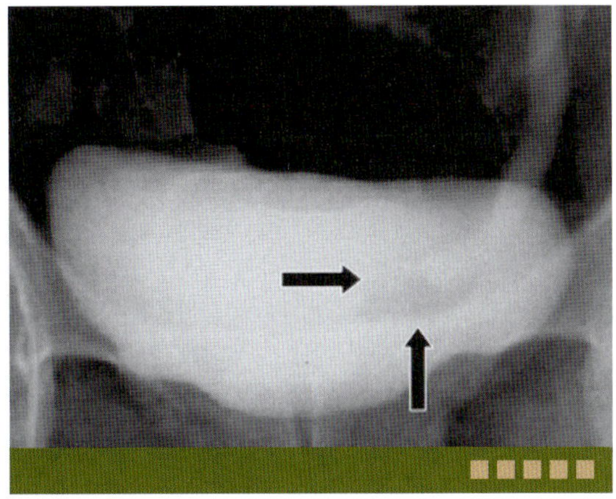

C. IVU, magnified view of the bladder, from a different patient, who presented with left flank pain and gross hematuria, shows dilatation of the left ureter with a thick rind of radiolucency (arrows) at the UVJ.

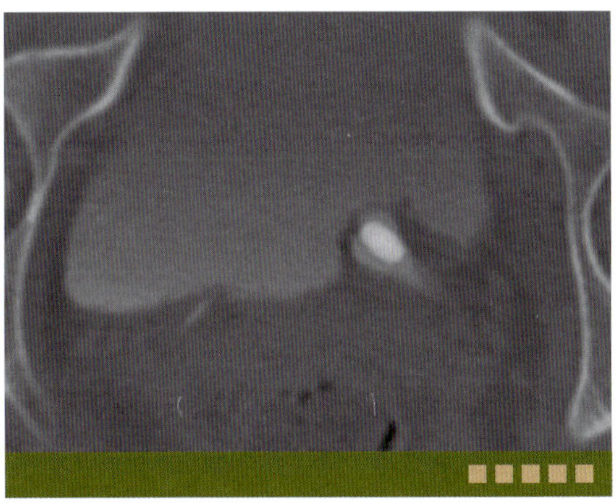

D. Axial CECT excretory phase from the same patient shows the pseudoureterocele is the result of edema associated with a calculus impacted at the UVJ.

DIFFERENTIAL DIAGNOSES IMAGES (E-G)

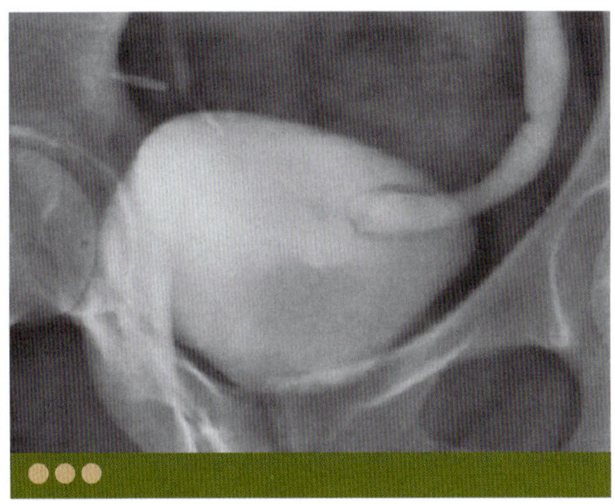

E. Ureterocele: IVU shows fusiform dilatation of the distal left ureter which is surrounded by thin line of radiolucency.

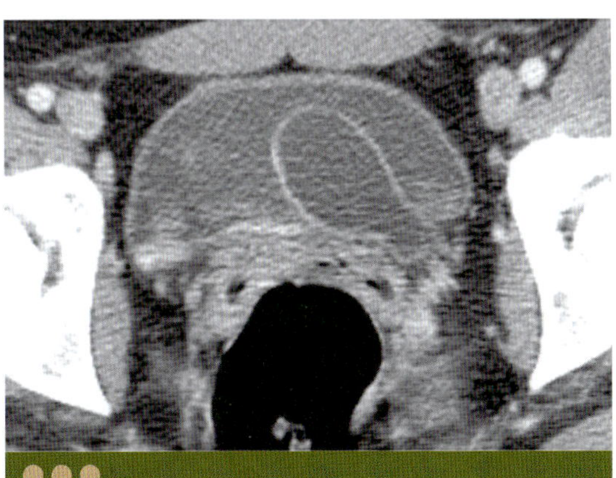

F. Ureterocele: Axial CECT shows a large left ureterocele as an intravesical cystic mass with a thin, regular wall and in continuity with the left ureter.

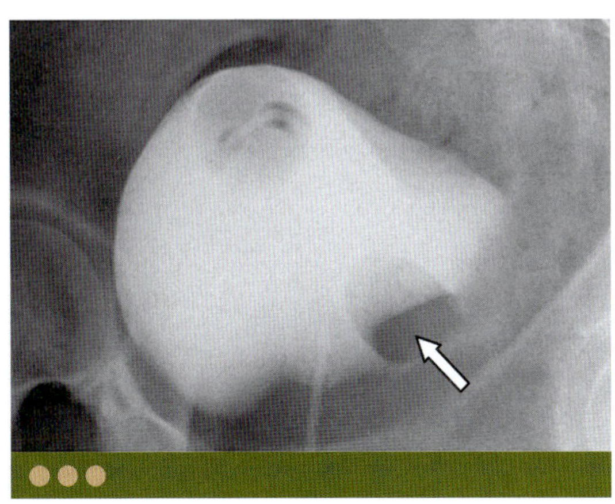

G. Ureterocele: Cystogram, oblique view, shows a smooth filling defect at the left UVJ (arrow) and a Foley catheter.

IMAGE KEY

Common

Rare

Typical

Unusual

6–19 Ureterosciatic Hernia

David D. Casalino

PRESENTATION

Intermittent left flank pain.

FINDINGS

RU shows focal looping of the left ureter into the region of the greater sciatic foramen.

DIFFERENTIAL DIAGNOSES

- The typical appearance is considered pathognomonic.
- A central pelvic mass should be considered if there is less focal, lateral deviation of the lower ureter. Such a mass might impress upon the bladder as well.

COMMENTS

Ureteral herniation is rare. The majority of cases are inguinal, and femoral herniation occurs half as often. Five percent of ureteral herniations are sciatic in location. The sacrospinous ligament divides the sciatic notch into the greater and lesser sciatic foramina. The piriformis muscle subdivides the greater sciatic foramen into the suprapiriformis and infrapiriformis compartments. Ureterosciatic herniation occurs though the suprapiriformis compartment. Any neuromuscular abnormality causing piriformis atrophy may predispose to sciatic herniation.

The left ureter is affected more often than the right. Patients are often asymptomatic with the herniation incidentally discovered on IVU or CT. They may have ill-defined abdominal pain or flank pain if obstruction develops. Symptomatic patients may be treated with stent placement, ureteroureterostomy, or excision and reimplantation.

On imaging, the distal ureter demonstrates a curlicue or loop that is directed horizontally into the sciatic notch. On IVU or RU, the contralateral posterior oblique view is best to demonstrate the posterior course of the hernia. The appearance is considered pathognomonic. CT can demonstrate the position and extent of the ureterosciatic herniation, the herniation of other visceral structures, and aid in planning a surgical approach. The ureter is seen extending posterior and lateral to the ischial spine.

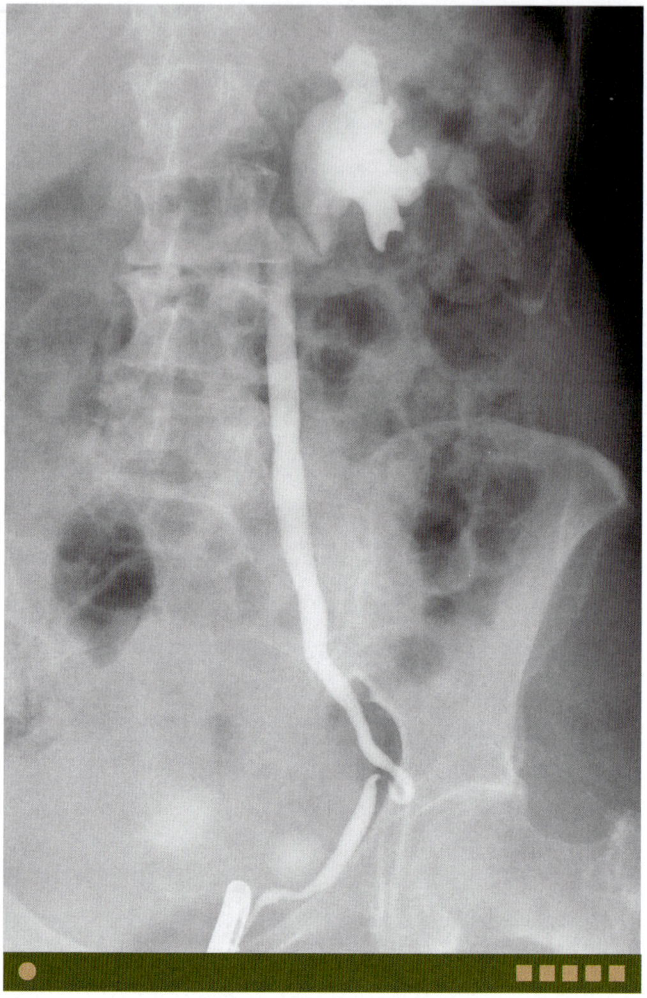

A. RU shows focal looping of the left ureter into the greater sciatic foramen with dilatation of the collecting system proximal to the herniation.

PEARLS

- **Ureteral herniation is rare, with 5% being sciatic in location.**
- **Imaging shows a horizontal looping, or curlicue, of the left ureter into the greater sciatic foramen.**
- **The appearance is considered pathognomonic.**
- **CT may be complementary to IVU by excluding herniation of other structures and aiding in surgical planning, if necessary.**

ADDITIONAL IMAGES (B-C)

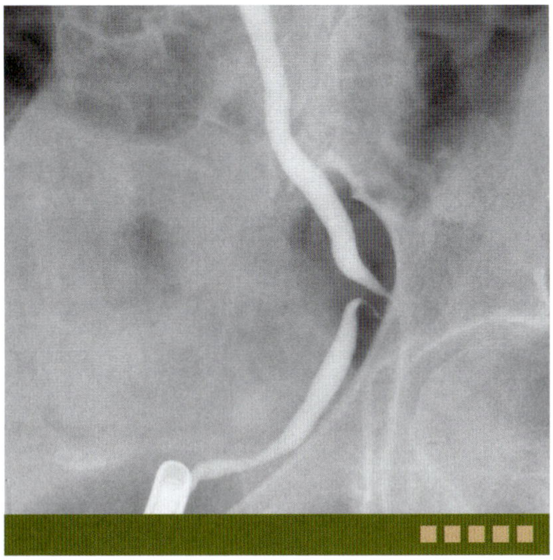

B. RU, right posterior oblique view, best shows the posterior course of the hernia.

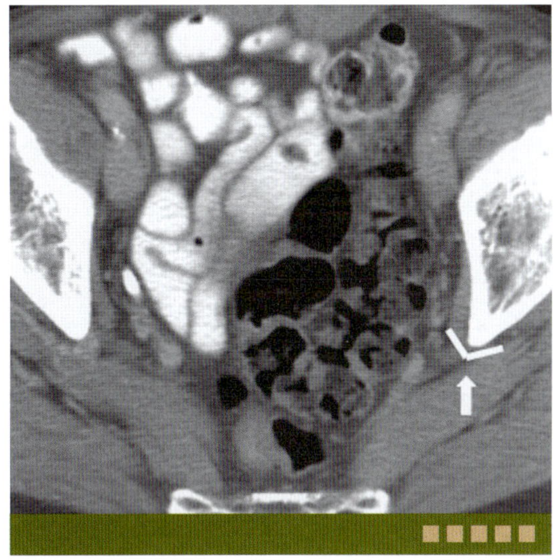

C. Axial CECT shows two joining lines (arrow) drawn to represent the left ureter extending through the greater sciatic foramen, posterior to the ischium.

DIFFERENTIAL DIAGNOSES IMAGES (D-E)

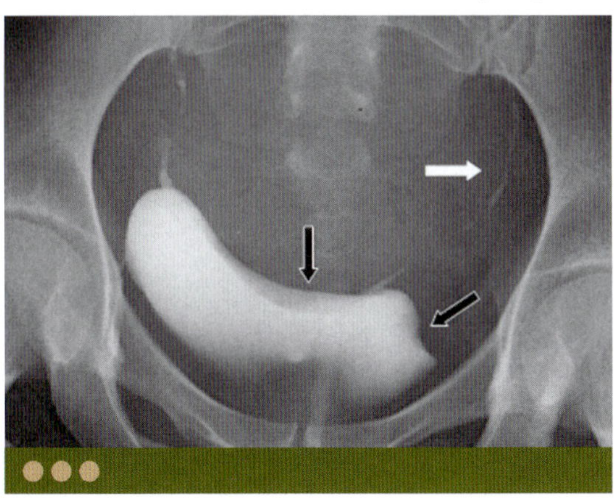

D. Central pelvic mass: IVU shows lateral deviation of the distal left ureter (white arrow) that is not focal. There is focal mass effect upon the superior and left lateral aspects (black arrows) of the bladder.

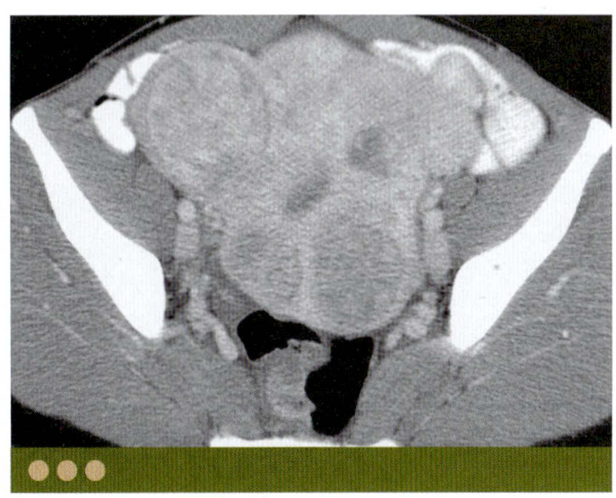

E. Central pelvic mass: Axial CECT from same patient shows the central pelvic mass to be the uterus, enlarged by multiple fibroids.

IMAGE KEY

Common

Rare

Typical

Unusual

CHAPTER 7

UROLITHIASIS, OBSTRUCTION

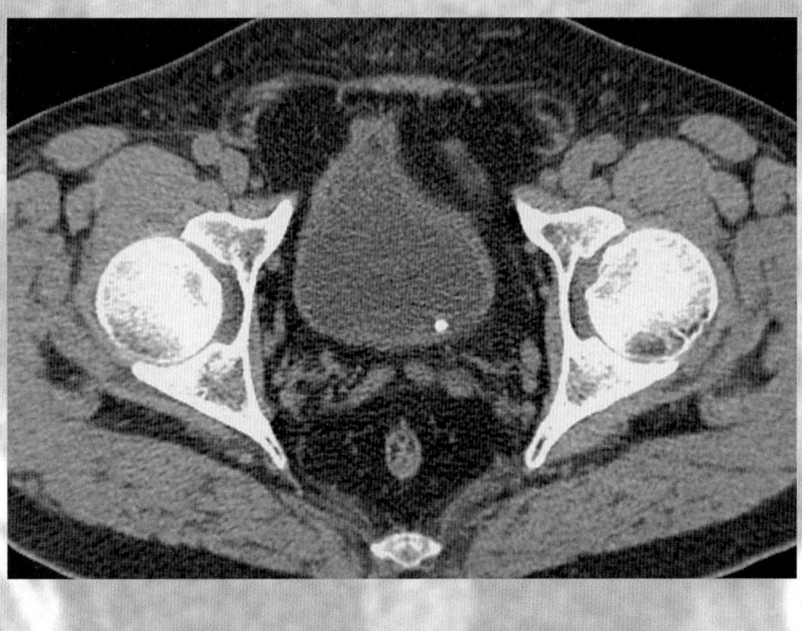

7–1 Obstructive Urolithiasis

Nancy A. Hammond

PRESENTATION

Flank pain and hematuria.

FINDINGS

Calculi within the ureter resulting in hydronephrosis and perinephric and periureteral stranding.

DIFFERENTIAL DIAGNOSIS

- *Phlebolith*: Calcification does not lie within the ureter. Absence of soft tissue rim sign and absence of secondary signs such as hydronephrosis, hydroureter, and perinephric/periureteral stranding may help to distinguish it from a ureteral stone.

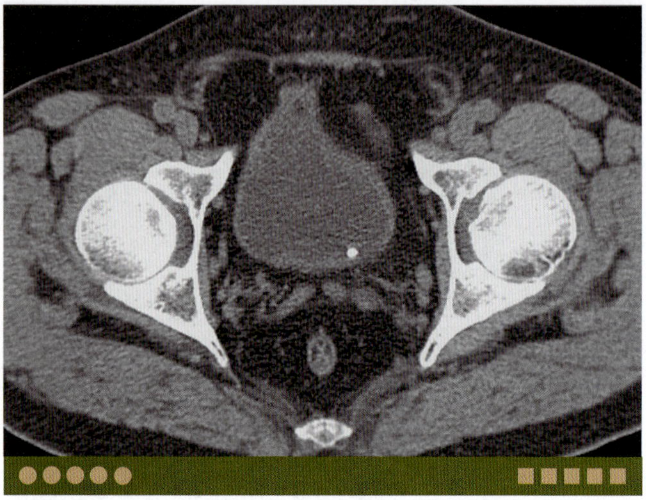

A. Axial NECT shows a calcification in the expected location of the left ureteropelvic junction. Proximal left hydronephrosis and hydroureter confirmed that this stone lied within the UVJ rather than urinary bladder. In cases where it is difficult to distinguish whether findings represent a passed stone or stone in the most distal aspect of the UVJ, the patient can be imaged prone. A passed stone will fall into the dependent portion of the bladder.

COMMENTS

Nephrolithiasis is a common problem with an estimated 5% of females and 12% of males having at least one episode of renal colic secondary to stone disease by 70 years of age. Etiologies for the production of renal stones include a genetic predisposition, occupation, and lifestyle. The peak age for the onset of stone disease is 20 to 30 years. Patients with nephrolithiasis most commonly present with renal colic because of the passage of the stone into the ureter. Renal colic is defined as flank pain radiating to the groin. Hematuria is present in the majority of patients but is absent approximately 15% of the time. The likelihood of stone passage is based on the diameter of the stone. About 90% of stones 4 mm or less will pass spontaneously.

A variety of stone compositions are known including calcium, cystine, struvite, uric acid, xanthine, matrix, oxalate, and indinavir stones. Calcium stones are the most common.

Nonenhanced CT (NECT) is the test of choice to diagnose patients with suspected obstructive urolithiasis. Unlike radiography, virtually all stones are radiodense except those composed of indinavir. With standard radiography, approximately 50% of stones are not detected. Radiolucent stones include those composed of uric acid, xanthine, struvite, and matrix. Sonographically renal/ureteral stones are hyperechoic with posterior acoustic enhancement.

On CT, the course of the ureters should be followed and scrutinized for the presence of calcification within the ureter. The presence of a "soft tissue rim" sign helps to confirm that the stone lies within the ureter and is not vascular in origin. The rim sign results from edema of the ureteral wall.

Secondary signs of obstructive urolithiasis include unilateral perinephric stranding and ipsilateral hydronephrosis. A 90% positive predictive value has been reported for a ureteral stone when both these findings are present and a 90% negative predictive value for ureteral stone has been reported if both are absent. Other findings that may be present include ipsilateral renal enlargement and decreased attenuation of the kidney.

PEARLS

- **Nephrolithiasis is a common problem with the peak age of initial presentation being in the third and fourth decade.**
- **Patients typically present with renal colic and hematuria because of passage of stones.**
- **CT is the first line modality in evaluating suspected stone disease. With the exception of indinavir stones, all stones are radiodense on CT.**
- **Stones measuring 4 mm or less have a 90% chance of passing without medical intervention.**

ADDITIONAL IMAGES (B-E)

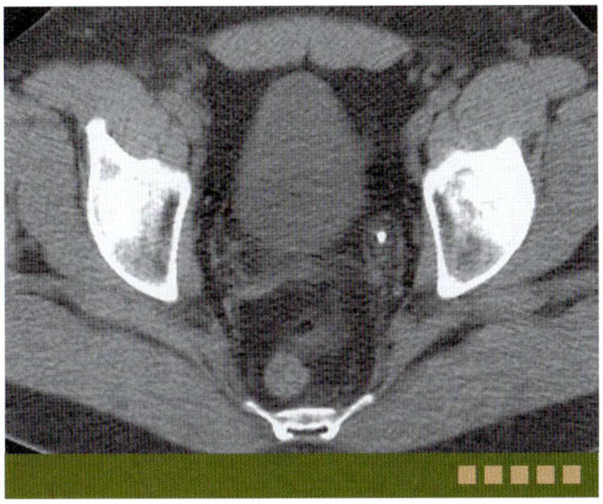

B. Axial NECT shows a small calcification along the course of the distal left ureter. A soft tissue rim sign is present aiding in the distinction between a ureteral stone and a vascular calcification.

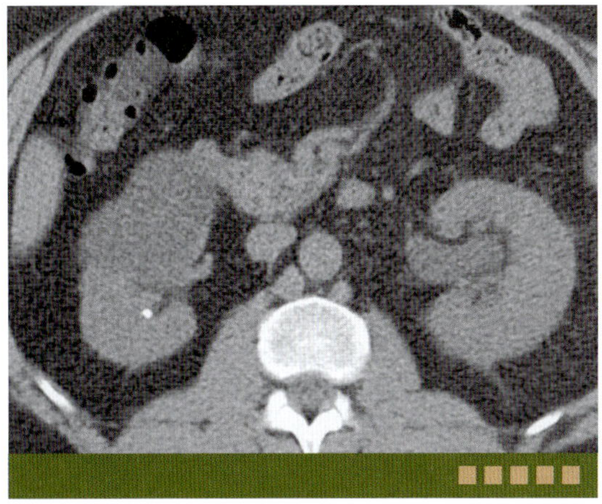

C. Axial NECT in the same patient shows mild hydronephrosis involving the left kidney caused by distal left ureteral stone. A nonobstructing right renal stone and a right renal cyst are also seen in this image.

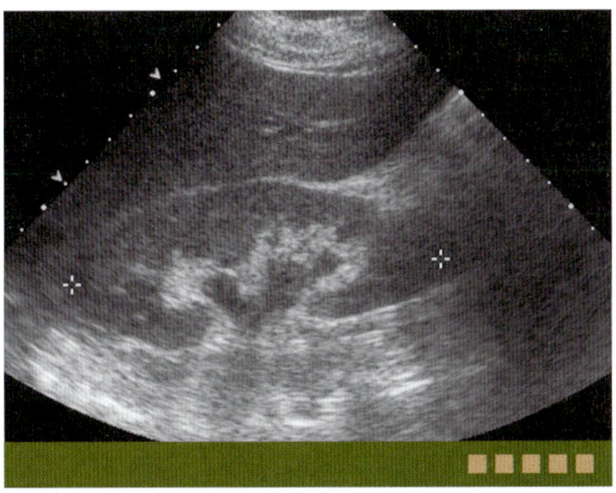

D. Longitudinal sonogram of the right kidney shows mild right hydronephrosis. The etiology of the dilatation was not seen proximally.

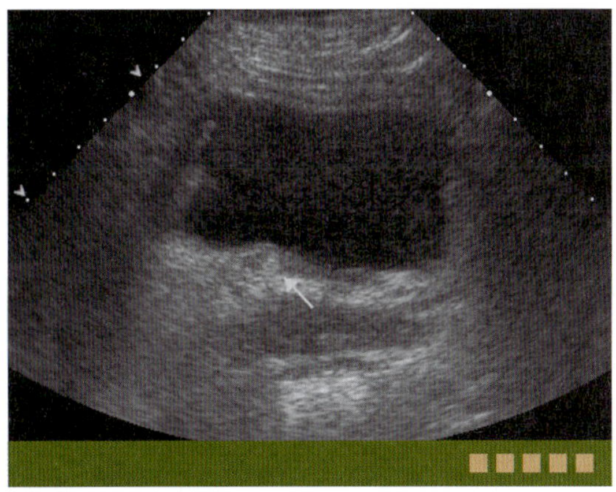

E. Transverse sonogram in the same patient as in Figure D shows a small hyperechoic focus with subtle posterior acoustic shadowing in the region of the right UVJ consistent with an obstructing stone (arrow).

DIFFERENTIAL DIAGNOSIS IMAGE

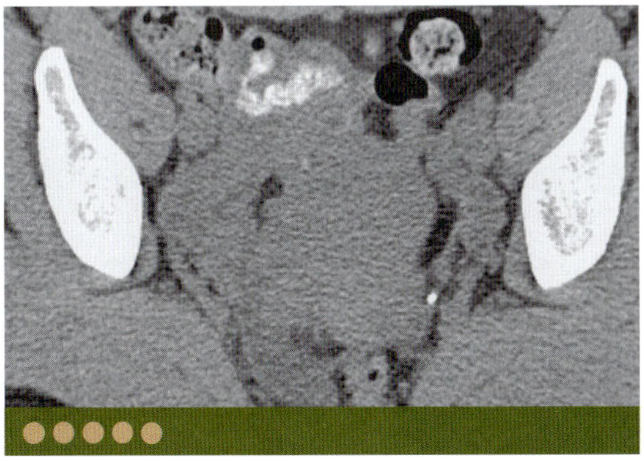

F. Phlebolith: Axial NECT shows a calcification in the left hemipelvis. No soft tissue is seen surrounding the calcification. Additionally, a nondilated left ureter is seen just anterior to the calcification.

IMAGE KEY

Common

Rare

Typical

Unusual

7–2 Forniceal Rupture

Nancy A. Hammond

PRESENTATION

Flank pain and hematuria.

FINDINGS

Hydronephrosis and focal perinephric fluid collection; distal obstructing ureteral stone.

DIFFERENTIAL DIAGNOSES

- *Perinephric stranding*: Less focal, more linear appearance.
- *Perineprhic hematoma*: Hyperdense collection on NECT clinical history of trauma or recent renal biopsy helps direct diagnosis.

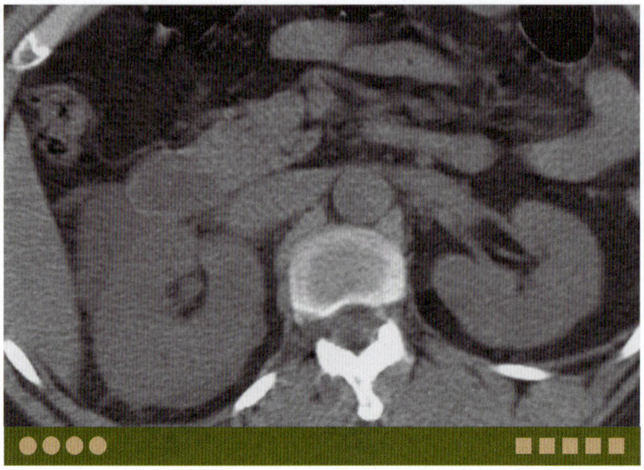

A. Axial NECT shows a focal, low-density perinephric collection adjacent to the right kidney consistent with forniceal rupture.

COMMENTS

Spontaneous forniceal rupture secondary to ureteral obstruction can be seen with obstructive ureterolithiasis. When acutely obstructed, the kidney responds to the increased pressure with the absorption of urine via multiple pathways including pyelosinus, pyelotubular, pyelolymphatic, and pyelovenous backflow mechanisms. In high-grade obstruction when the pressure gradient is too great, a forniceal rupture may occur allowing decompression of the obstructed system and release of urine into the perinephric space. When a fornix ruptures, the increased pressure is rapidly reduced and there is, typically, relief of symptoms.

On NECT forniceal rupture appears as a focal hypodense, nonlinear perinephric fluid collection which represents extravasated urine. In cases when intravenous contrast is administered and delayed images are obtained, extravasation is evident as a hyperdensity within the fluid collection. The CT appearance of forniceal rupture can be distinguished from perinephric stranding commonly seen in obstructive ureterolithiasis because of its focal and nonlinear appearance.

It is important to advise the clinician of possible forniceal rupture, as the patient may be treated with prophylactic antibiotics. Otherwise, forniceal rupture is of little clinical importance and rarely results in urinoma formation.

PEARLS

- **Forniceal rupture occurs when the pressure gradient resulting from acute obstruction is too great for normal mechanisms of urine reabsorption to compensate for the increased pressure gradient.**
- **When forniceal rupture occurs, the patient may be treated with prophylactic antibiotics.**
- **Can be distinguished from perinephric stranding because of its more focal, nonlinear appearance.**

ADDITIONAL IMAGES (B-C)

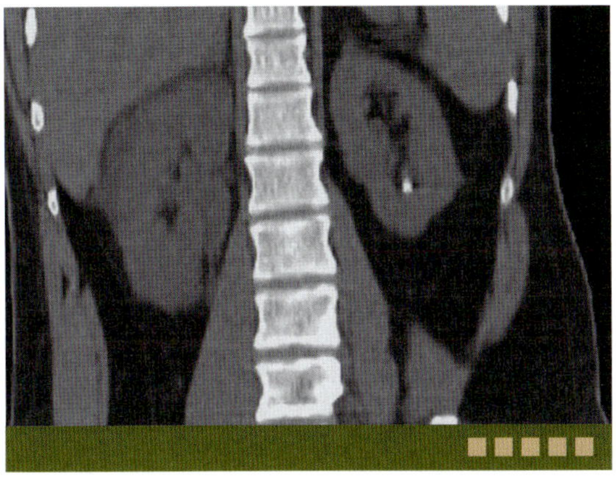

B. Coronal NECT in the same patient as Figure A shows mild dilatation of the right renal collecting system and a small amount of perinephric fluid. Incidental note is made of a nonobstructing stone in the left kidney.

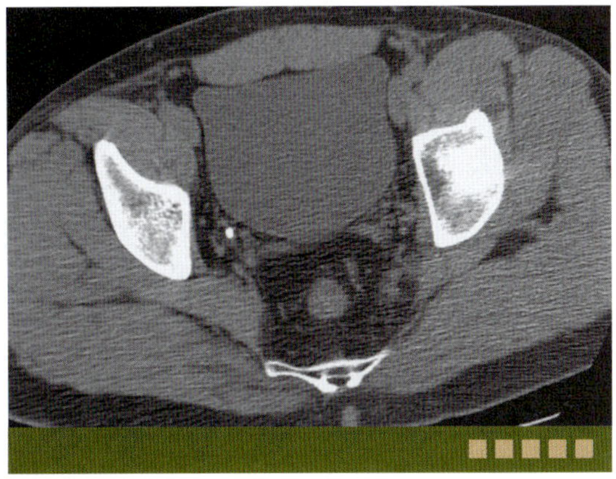

C. Axial NECT confirms the presence of a distal right ureteral stone as the cause of the acute obstruction.

DIFFERENTIAL DIAGNOSES IMAGES (D-E)

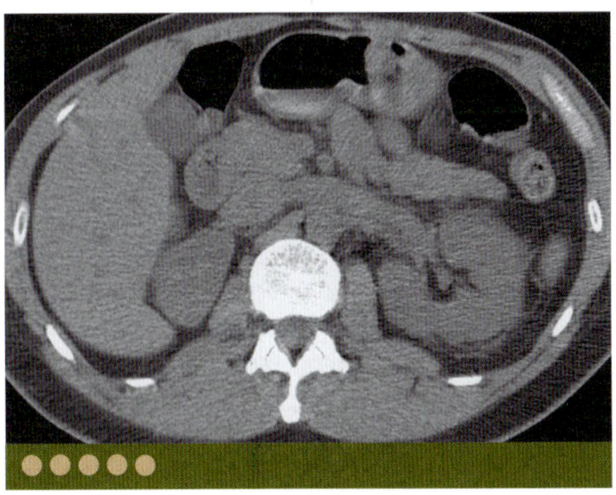

D. Perinephric stranding: Axial NECT shows linear low attenuation surrounding the left kidney.

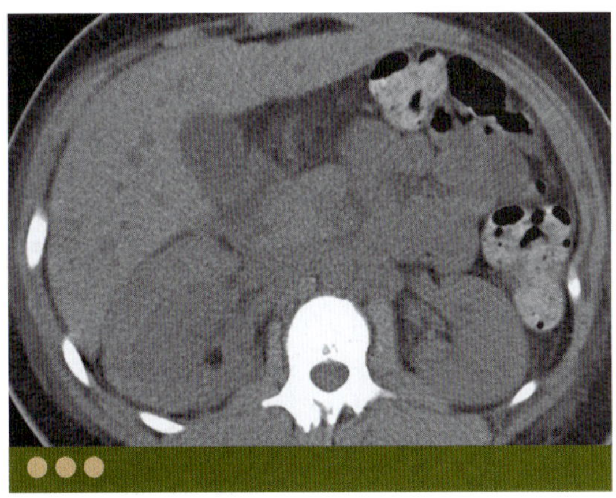

E. Perinephric hematoma: Axial NECT shows a hyperdense perinephric fluid collection consistent with a perinephric hematoma. This is in distinction to the hypodense collection seen in forniceal rupture on NECT.

IMAGE KEY

Common

Rare

Typical

Unusual

7–3 Nephrolithiasis

Nancy A. Hammond

PRESENTATION

Incidental finding on CT, hematuria.

FINDINGS

Renal calcifications on CT.

DIFFERENTIAL DIAGNOSIS

- *Vascular calcifications*: Can be difficult to distinguish from nephrolithiasis; presence of extensive vascular calcifications should suggest diagnosis.

COMMENTS

Nephrolithiasis is a common entity with a lifetime prevalence of urinary tract stone disease in the United Sates estimated to be 10%. The peak age for the onset of stone disease is 20 to 30 years. Nephrolithiasis is seen more frequently in men than in women and in whites and Asians than in other races. Etiologies for the production of renal stones include a genetic predisposition, occupation, and lifestyle. Patients with nephrolithiasis are most commonly asymptomatic but can present with renal colic because of the passage of the stone into the ureter. Renal colic is defined as flank pain radiating to the groin. Hematuria is present in the majority of the patients with a ureteral stone but can be absent approximately 15% of the time.

The development of renal stones is related to decreased urine volume or increased excretion of stone-forming components. A variety of stone compositions are known including calcium, cystine, struvite, uric acid, xanthine, matrix, oxalate, and indinavir stones. Calcium stones are the most common.

Approximately 50% of the stones are detected with standard radiography. Radiolucent stones include those composed of uric acid, xanthine, struvite, and matrix. Sonographically, renal stones are hyperechoic with posterior acoustic shadowing. Small stones may be missed and can be difficult to distinguish from vascular calcifications. A color Doppler artifact called twinkle artifact may aid in identifying small renal stones (<5 mm). It appears as rapidly changing mixture of colors deep to the strong reflector (renal stone). With the exception of indinavir stones, all stones are radiopaque on CT.

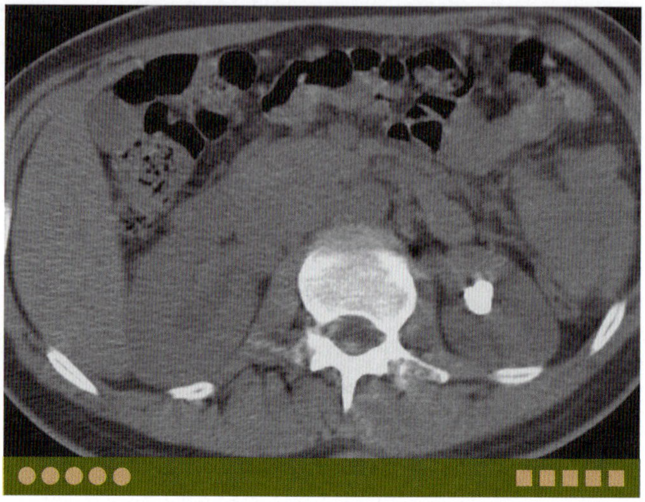

A. Axial CECT shows a large calcification at the lower pole of the left kidney consistent with a nephrolith.

Treatment of nephrolithiasis depends on the size and type of renal stones. While some stones can be dissolved with medical therapy, the most common type, calcium, cannot be dissolved. Prophylactic therapy may be implemented including limitation of dietary components, addition of stone-formation inhibitors or intestinal calcium binders, and increased fluid intake. Uric acid and cystine stones can be dissolved with medical therapy when urgent intervention is not required. Sodium bicarbonate or potassium citrate is used as alkalinizing agents. Extracorporeal shock-wave lithotripsy (ESWL) is used to treat approximately 85% of urinary tract calculi requiring treatment. ESWL is limited by size and location of the stone. ESWL is limited when stones are larger than 15 mm in diameter or located in the lower pole of the kidney. Percutaneous nephrolithostomy is often used in ESWL failures for removal of large renal or ureteral stones.

PEARLS

- **Nephrolithiasis is a common medical condition.**
- **Patients with nephrolithiasis are usually asymptomatic. Presentation is usually renal colic when the stone passes into the ureter resulting in obstruction.**
- **With the exception of indinavir stones, all renal stones are radiodense on CT.**

ADDITIONAL IMAGES (B-E)

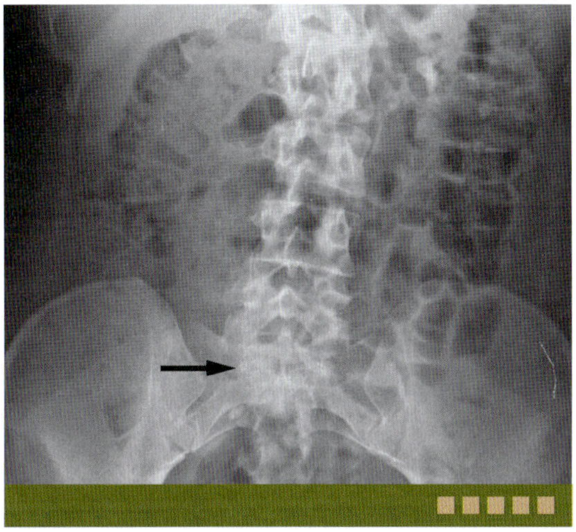

B. Abdominal radiograph in the same patient shows the known renal stone overlying the expected location of the left kidney. A second calcification is seen along the expected course of the right ureter at the level of the inferior aspect of the right sacroiliac joint (arrow).

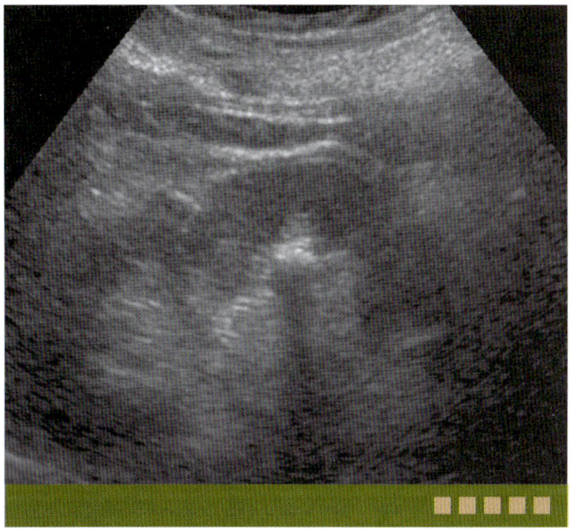

C. Longitudinal sonogram of the left kidney in a different patient shows a hyperechoic focus with posterior acoustic shadowing at the lower pole of the left kidney consistent with a nonobstructing renal stone.

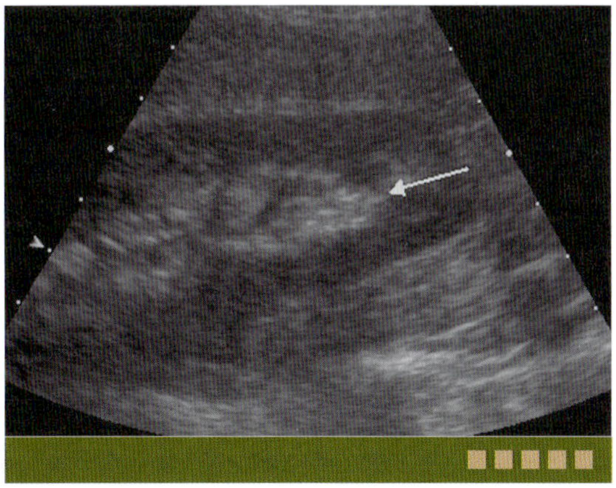

D. Longitudinal sonogram of the right kidney in a different patient shows a tiny hyperechoic focus (arrow) at the lower pole of the left kidney without poster acoustic shadowing. It is difficult to distinguish if this finding relates to a stone or is vascular or artifactual in origin based on this image.

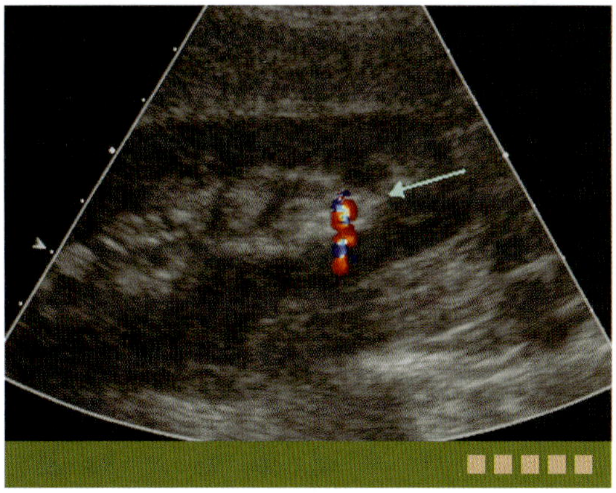

E. Longitudinal color Doppler sonogram in the same patient as Figure D shows twinkle artifact associated with this small hyperechoic focus consistent with a small nonobstructing renal stone.

IMAGE KEY

Common

Rare

Typical

Unusual

7–4 Staghorn Calculi

Nancy A. Hammond

PRESENTATION

Recurrent urinary tract infections (UTIs) and acute flank pain.

FINDINGS

Large radiopaque renal stone involving the renal pelvis and extending into multiple renal calyces.

DIFFERENTIAL DIAGNOSIS

- *Medullary nephrocalcinosis*: Calcifications distributed in the renal medulla.

COMMENTS

Staghorn calculi are defined as upper urinary tract stones that involve the renal pelvis and extend into at least two calyces. Although all types of urinary stones can potentially form staghorn calculi, approximately 75% are composed of a struvite–carbonate–apatite matrix. The remaining 25% are composed of either cystine or uric acid. Struvite stones are associated with UTIs and the presence of urease-producing bacteria, including *Ureaplasma urealyticum* and *Proteus* (most common), *Staphylococcus*, *Klebsiella*, *Providencia*, and *Pseudomonas* species. As women have more UTIs staghorn calculi are seen more commonly in women than in men. They tend to occur in persons older than 50 years of age.

The clinical presentation of patients with staghorn calculi is variable but the diagnosis should be considered in patients with risk factors for developing UTIs. Infections may result in pyelonephritis, pyonephrosis, or perinephric abscess. Symptoms may include flank pain classic for renal colic, fever, urinary symptoms, and hematuria. However, staghorn calculi rarely manifest as a solitary ureteral stone with acute renal colic in the absence of prior intervention.

Radiographs demonstrate a radiopaque structure overlying the renal pelvis and extending into at least two calyces. Sonographically, staghorn calculi appear as large shadowing stones involving the renal pelvis and calyces. Hydronephrosis may be present. NECT further demonstrates the extent of the radiodense stone, whereas contrast-enhanced CT demonstrates the surrounding anatomy and potential complications. Complications include xanthogranulomatous pyelonphritis (XGP) which represents the reaction of the kidney to chronic urinary tract obstruction usually secondary to a calculus (75%) in the presence of UTI.

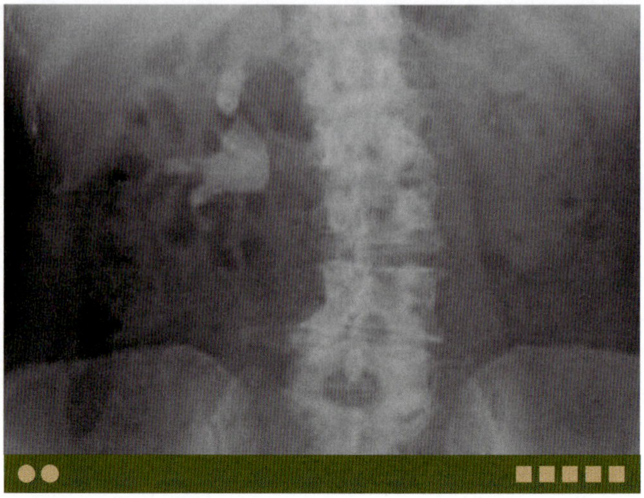

A. Abdominal radiograph shows a radiopaque density overlying the right kidney conforming to the shape of the renal pelvis and extending into three renal calyces.

Treatment of staghorn calculi typically involves surgical removal of the stone. Additionally, the underlying source of infection must be eradicated. Even after complete stone removal, stones recur in approximately 10% of patients; if residual stones or fragments are left after treatment, recurrence rates approach 85%. Staghorn calculi are a potential source of significant morbidity. Studies have demonstrated that 30% of the patients treated conservatively died of renal failure or secondary to pyelonephritis and sepsis.

PEARLS

- **Clinical presentation is variable and patients may be asymptomatic.**
- **More commonly seen in women than in men because of higher propensity for UTI.**
- **Radiopaque stones involving the renal pelvis and at least two calyces.**
- **Removal of stone and eradication of underlying infectious etiology crucial as can result in significant morbidity.**

ADDITIONAL IMAGES (B-E)

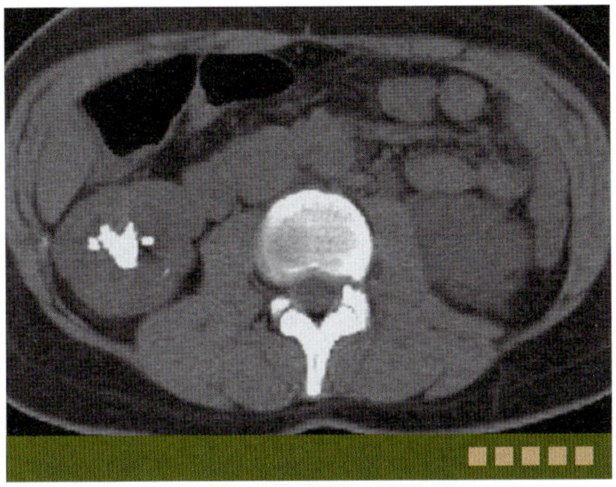

B. Axial NECT in the same patient shows the calcified staghorn calculus involving the right kidney.

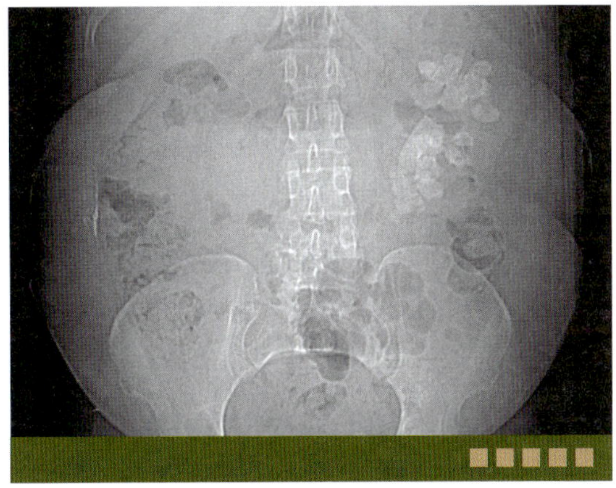

C. Scout image from an abdominal CT shows extensive calcification overlying the left kidney also conforming to the shape of the renal pelvis and extending into multiple calices. There is enlargement of the left kidney.

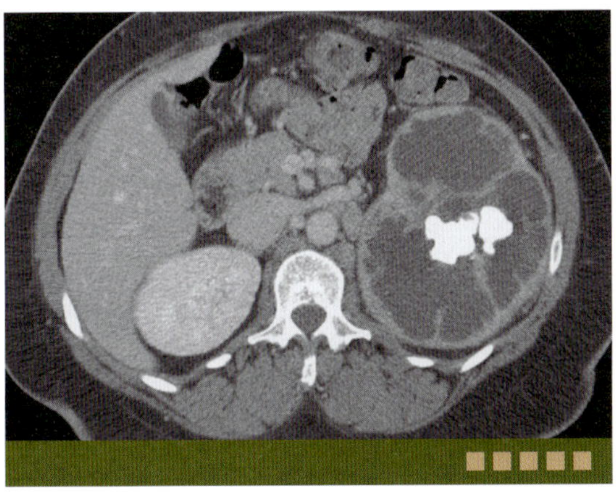

D. Axial CECT in the same patient as Figure C confirms the presence of a staghorn calculus and enlargement of the left kidney. There is delayed excretion of contrast material and associated obstruction of the kidney. Findings are compatible with XGP.

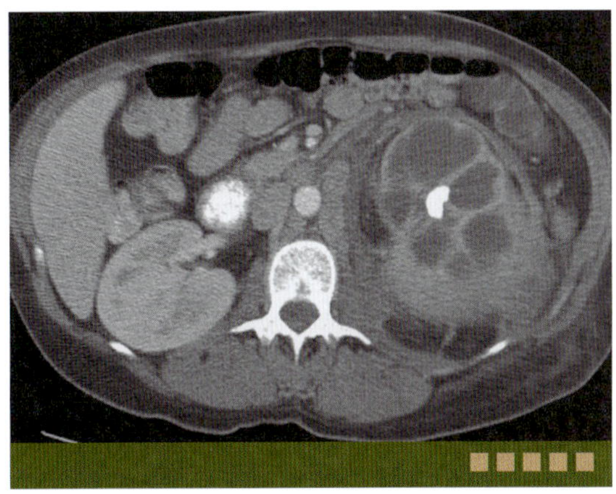

E. Axial CECT in a different patient shows enlargement of the left kidney, dilatation of the collecting system on the left, a staghorn calculus, and extensive perinephric stranding. Findings are compatible with XGP.

IMAGE KEY

Common

Rare

Typical

Unusual

DIFFERENTIAL DIAGNOSIS IMAGE

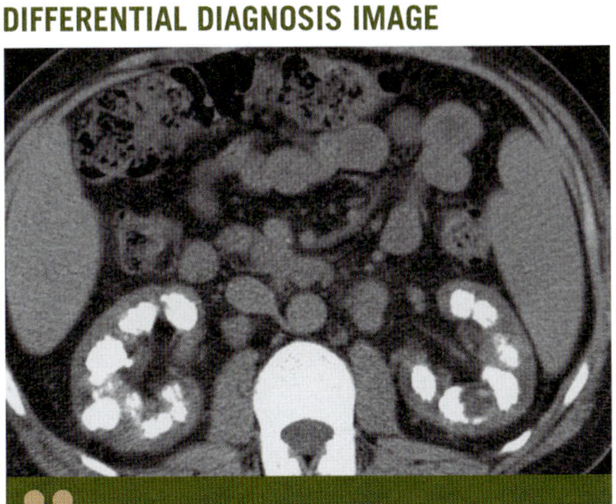

F. Medullary nephrocalcinosis: Axial NECT shows diffuse calcifications involving the renal pyramids compatible with medullary nephrocalcinosis. Note the different distribution of the calcifications and lack of involvement of the renal pelvis compared to that of a staghorn calculus.

7–5 Protease Inhibitor Stones

Nancy A. Hammond

PRESENTATION

Right flank pain and hematuria; HIV positive patient.

FINDINGS

Mild right hydronephrosis and perinephric stranding.

DIFFERENTIAL DIAGNOSES

- *Obstruction secondary to obstructing mass*: Soft tissue lesion identified.
- *Ascending urinary tract infection*: Imaging findings may be similar, clinical history guides diagnosis.
- *Passed stone*: Imaging findings may be similar, clinical relief of symptoms suggests diagnosis of passed stone.

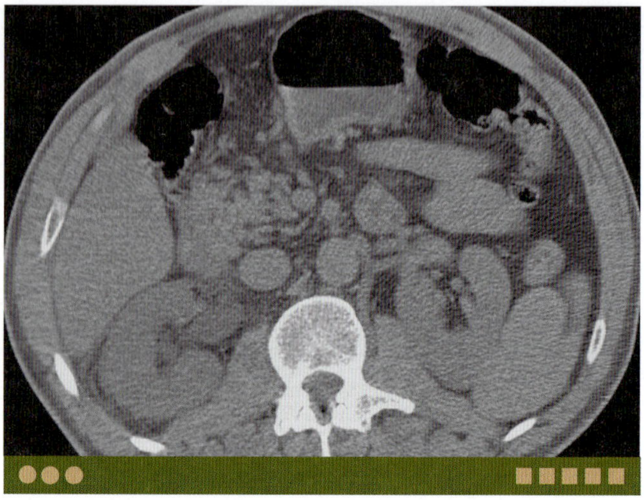

A. Axial NECT shows mild right hydronephrosis and right perinephric stranding. Evaluation of the right colleting system failed to reveal an obstructing stone as a source for the hyrdonephrosis and perinephric stranding.

COMMENTS

As the majority of stones are radiopaque on CT, it is the primary modality in evaluating patients with renal colic. However, patients on protease inhibitors (indinavir) for the treatment of HIV can develop stones that are not visible on CT. These stones are composed of metabolites from indinavir and are radiolucent on CT and plain film radiography. The incidence of stone formation in patients on indinavir is estimated to be between 3% and 13%.

Patients present with typical signs and symptoms of renal colic including flank pain and hematuria. In patients with obstructive uropathy from an indinavir stone, CT demonstrates the presence of secondary signs of obstruction on the symptomatic side in the absence of an identifiable calculus. Secondary signs include hydroureteronephrosis and perinephric and periureteral stranding. While additional diagnoses should be considered, in a patient undergoing therapy with the protease inhibitor indinavir, the findings should suggest the diagnosis of indinavir crystal deposition. Ultrasound may also demonstrate signs of obstructive uropathy including hydroureteronephrosis. The resistive index of the obstructed side may be elevated and there may be absence of the ureteral jet on the affected side. If visualized with US, indinavir stones may have soft tissue echogenicity without shadowing. In cases where an indinavir stone is suspected, intravenous urography or retrograde urography can be used to confirm the diagnosis. On these studies, indinavir crystal depositions will appear as radiolucent filling defects.

Treatment of obstructive uropathy secondary to indinavir stones is typically conservative including hydration and pain control. If surgical intervention is necessary, this typically consists of ureteral stent placement.

PEARLS

- **3 to 13% of patients on indinavir will develop indinavir stones.**
- **Patients present with classic symptoms of renal colic.**
- **Indinavir stones are nonopaque on CT, but secondary signs of obstructive uropathy will be present.**
- **Retrograde urography or intravenous urogram (IVU) can help confirm the diagnosis when clinically suspected.**

ADDITIONAL IMAGES (B-C)

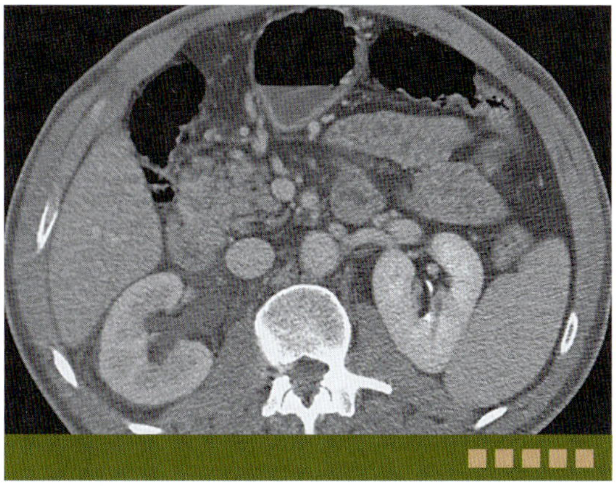

B. Axial CECT in the same patient as Figure A shows a delayed right nephrogram right hydronephrosis and perinephric stranding. No enhancing soft tissue masses were present.

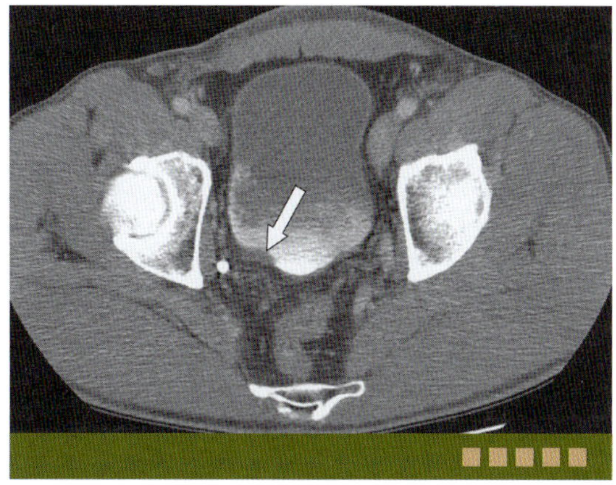

C. Axial CECT in the same patient as in Figure A shows edema at the right ureterovesicular junction (arrow). No opaque stones were identified in this region on nonenhanced images. The patient was on a protease inhibitor and an indinavir stone at the right UVJ was presumed to be the cause of the patient's pain.

DIFFERENTIAL DIAGNOSES IMAGES (D-G)

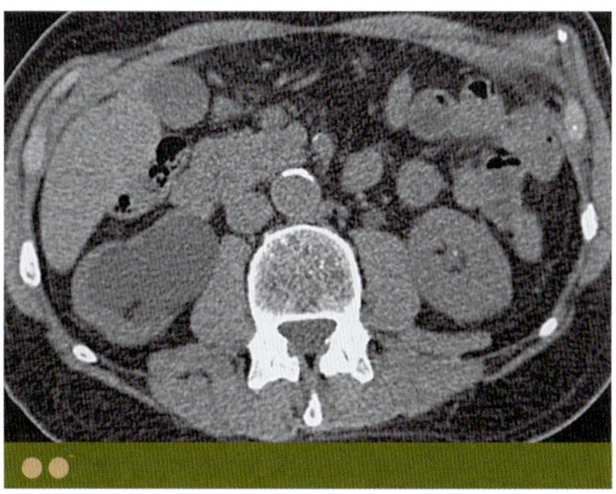

D. Transitional cell carcinoma: Axial NECT shows right hydronephrosis with cortical thinning suggesting a chronic process.

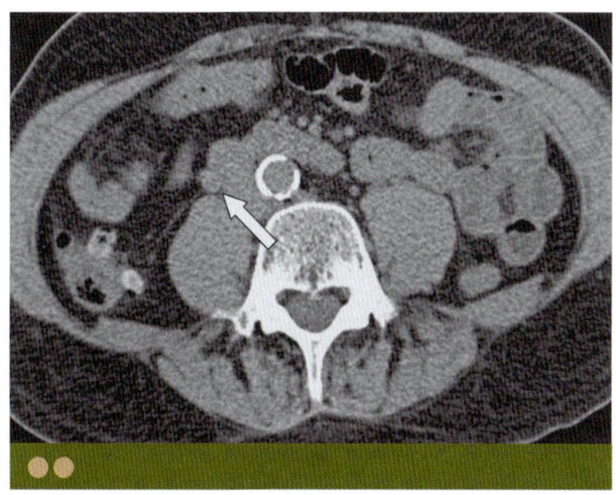

E. Transitional cell carcinoma: Axial NECT in the same patient as Figure D shows focal soft tissue thickening of the right ureter (arrow) as a source for the right hydronephrosis. These findings were confirmed on a retrograde study.

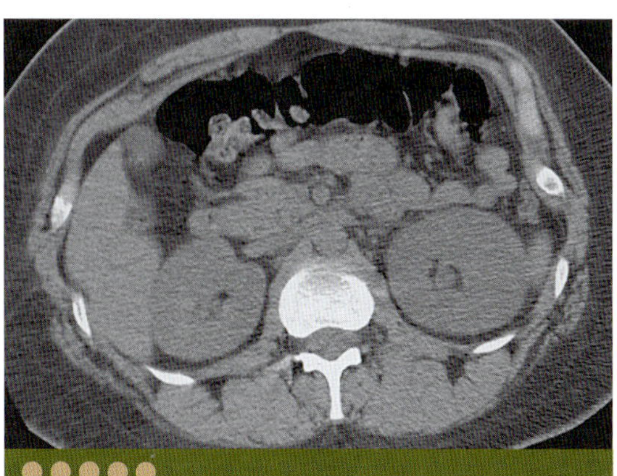

F. Ascending UTI: Axial NECT shows diffuse enlargement of the left kidney with mild dilatation of the collecting system.

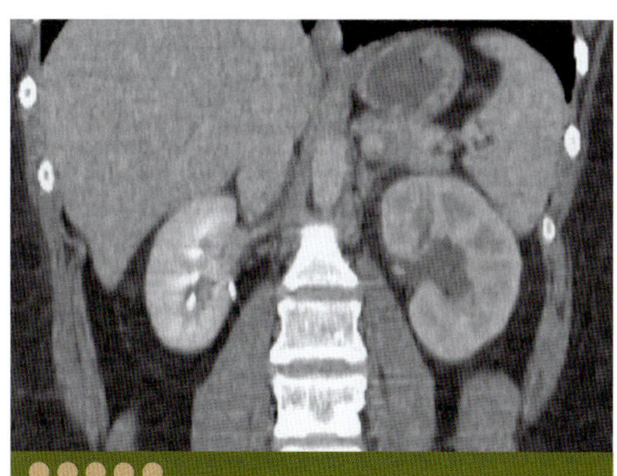

G. Ascending UTI: Coronal CECT in the same patient as Figure F shows mild left hydronephrosis with associated delayed nephrogram.

IMAGE KEY

Common

Rare

Typical

Unusual

7–6 Steinstrasse

Nancy A. Hammond

PRESENTATION

Known kidney stones; status postextracorporeal shock-wave lithotripsy.

FINDINGS

Multiple small calcifications within the ureter.

DIFFERENTIAL DIAGNOSIS

None

COMMENTS

Prior to the development of ESWL, open extraction was the only treatment for stones that could not pass through the urinary tract spontaneously. Currently, ESWL is used to treat approximately 85% of the urinary tract calculi requiring treatment but is limited by size and location of the stone. It is most effective for nonobstructing renal stones measuring less than 20 mm. Although stones in the lower pole of the kidney can be fragmented by ESWL, they can be difficult to pass. ESWL uses shock waves to pulverize larger stones into smaller fragments which can be expulsed spontaneously. The stone fragments typically pass with minimal discomfort. However, in some patients, the comminuted stone fragments may pile up in the ureter and create a column of stones called steinstrasse. Steinstrasse occurs in about 1% to 4% of ESWL cases. As the stone burden increases, the rate of steinstrasse increases. Approximately 40% of patients undergoing ESWL for staghorn calculi develop steinstrasse.

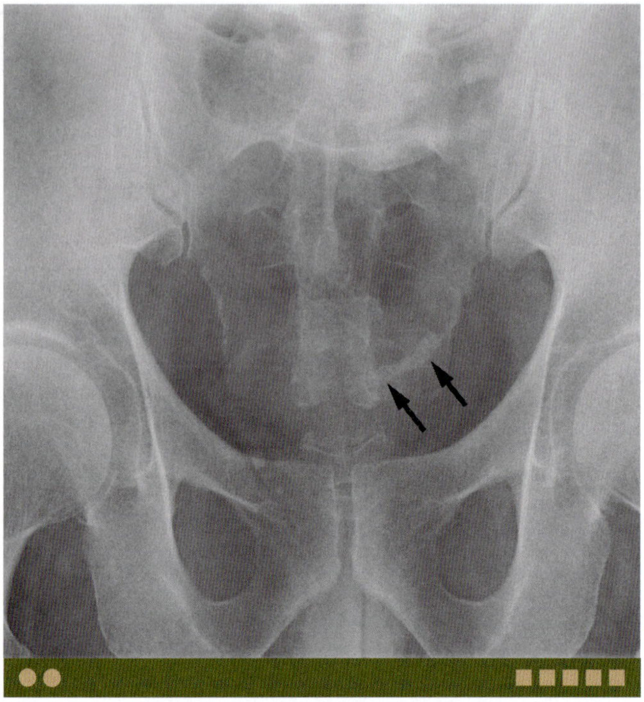

A. Scout conventional radiograph from an IVU coned down over the bladder shows a column of multiple tiny opacities in the distal left ureter consistent with multiple stone fragments (arrows).

Radiographically, steinstrasse can be detected on conventional radiographs as multiple small stones collecting in the distal ureter. When complicated by obstruction, ultrasound, CT, or IVU demonstrates proximal obstruction.

Patients with asymptomatic nonobstructing steinstrasse or mildly symptomatic steinstrasse with mild dilatation of the proximal urinary tract can be managed conservatively and monitored closely with serial imaging. If fragments fail to progress or if the patient develops symptoms of obstruction, endoscopic lithotripsy or percutaneous drainage should be performed. Steinstrasse resulting in high-grade obstruction and concomitant pyelonephritis should be treated with prompt percutaneous nephrostomy drainage and appropriate antibiotic coverage, followed by staged endoscopic removal of stone fragments.

PEARLS

- **Steinstrasse is a German word describing a stone street.**
- **Steinstrasse is the result of multiple small stone fragments collecting in the distal ureter.**
- **Conventional radiographs demonstrate a collection of small stones in the distal ureter.**
- **US, CT, and IVU may be employed to evaluate for obstruction when clinically warranted**

ADDITIONAL IMAGES (B-D)

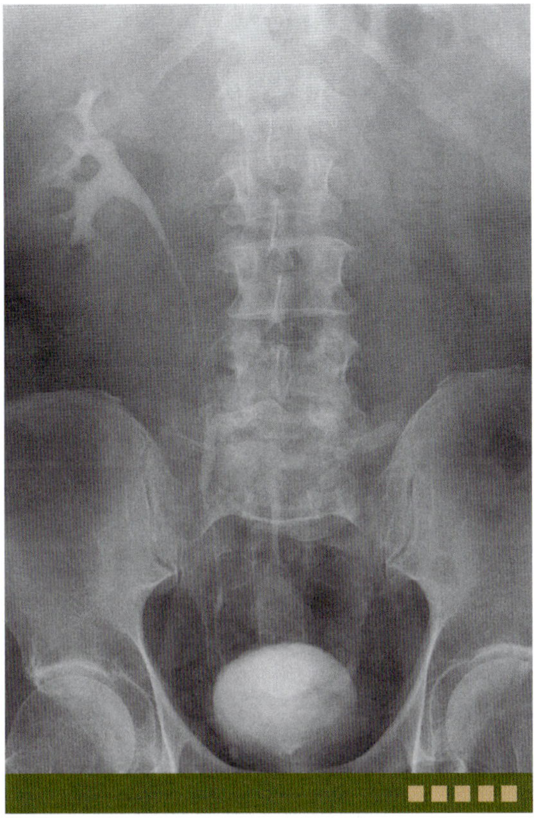

B. Abdominal radiograph from an IVU obtained 15 minutes after injection of contrast showsd normal excretion of contrast from a nondilated right collecting system and no excretion of contrast via the left kidney secondary to the multiple stone fragments in the distal left ureter.

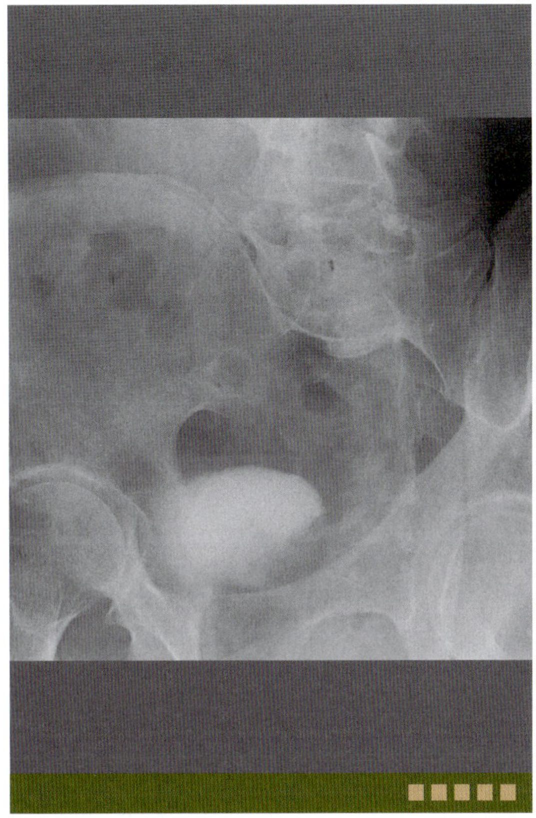

C. Oblique radiograph coned down over the urinary bladder confirms the distal left ureteral location of the stone fragments and edema at the left ureterovesicular junction.

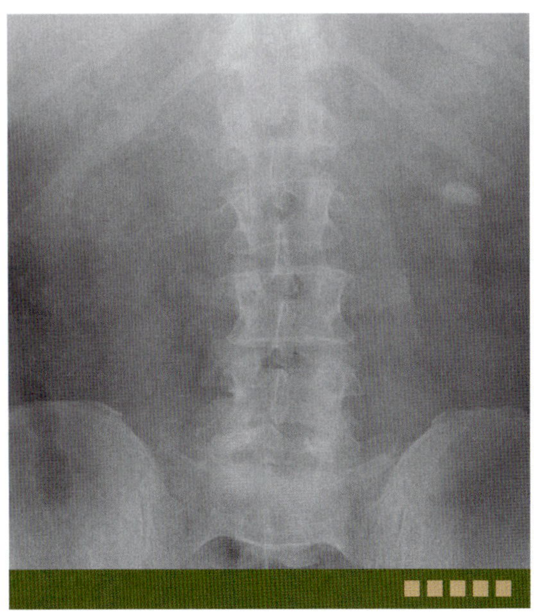

D. Conventional abdominal radiograph shows the 2-cm stone overlying the mid-aspect of the left kidney prior to ESWL.

IMAGE KEY

Common

Rare

Typical

Unusual

7–7 Hydronephrosis of Pregnancy

Nancy A. Hammond

PRESENTATION

Incidental finding.

FINDINGS

Unilateral or bilateral hydronephrosis.

DIFFERENTIAL DIAGNOSES

- *Obstructive uropathy*: Symptomatic patient, source of obstruction may be identified.
- *Parapelvic cyst*: Nonconvergent, centrally located anechoic structures in the renal pelvis.

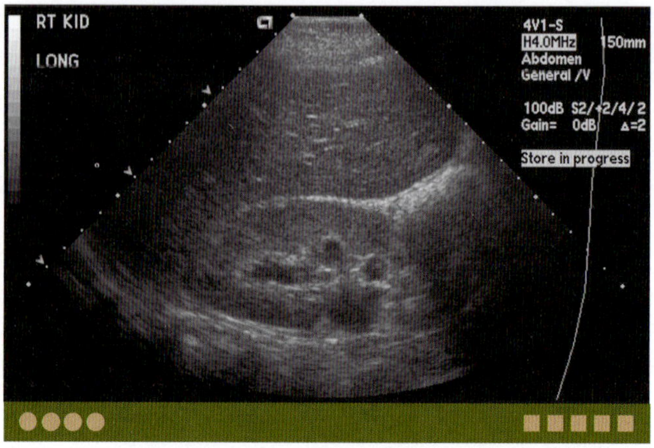

A. Longitudinal sonogram shows mild dilatation of the right collecting system in a 34-week pregnant patient.

COMMENTS

Sixty to eighty percent of women develop physiologic hydronephrosis during pregnancy. Physiologic dilatation usually begins in the first trimester and plateaus at 24 to 28 weeks but can persist 4 to 6 weeks after delivery. A variety of theories have been suggested as a cause for physiologic hydronephrosis during pregnancy. The most accepted theory ascribes hydronephrosis secondary to compression of the ureter at the level of the iliac crests by the enlarging, dextrorotating gravid uterus. As a result of the dextrorotated uterus and engorgement of the right ovarian vein, dilatation tends to be greater on the right than on the left. Approximately 30% of patients have bilateral hydronephrosis. Another theory implicates hormonal factors; high levels of progesterone during pregnancy result in smooth muscle relaxation of the ureteral wall. While usually asymptomatic and typically an inconsequential finding during pregnancy, there are reports of acute renal failure and polyhydramnios, acute pain, hypertension, and spontaneous renal rupture in patients with physiologic hydronephrosis.

Differentiating physiologic hydronephrosis of pregnancy from obstruction resulting from other etiologies including urolithiasis can be difficult. When evaluating the symptomatic pregnant patient with hydronephrosis, other etiologies should be considered. Urolithiasis is the most common cause of nonobstetrical abdominal pain that requires hospitalization in pregnant patients.

Ultrasound is the first line modality in evaluating the pregnant patient as it avoids exposure to ionizing radiation. Gray scale interrogation demonstrates dilatation of the renal pelvis and calyx. Typically the ureter is dilated to the level of the iliac crest. Dilatation of the ureter inferior to the pelvic brim should raise suspicion for other causes of hydronephrosis. In distinction to patients with obstructive uropathy, resistive indices (RIs) in patients with physiologic hydronephrosis are typically symmetric and normal (<0.7). Bilateral ureteral jets can be seen and the degree of dilatation is proportional to the gestational age. In the absence of clinical suspicion for obstructive uropathy, further imaging is not necessary. If a ureteral stone is suspected, ultrasound may be employed to detect the stone with reported sensitivity and specificity ranging from 34% to 95% and 86% to 87%, respectively. If ultrasound is nondiagnostic, limited IUV (scout, 30-s film, and 20-min film) or CT can be utilized. Both CT and IVU expose the fetus to ionizing radiation and, therefore, should be used with caution when the benefits outweigh the risks.

PEARLS

- **Physiologic hydronephrosis of pregnancy is a common entity and requires no further workup in an asymptomatic patient.**
- **The right kidney is most commonly involved but findings can be bilateral. When bilateral, the degree of dilatation is typically greater on the right than on the left.**
- **Ultrasound demonstrates hydronephrosis, symmetric and normal RIs, and bilateral ureteral jets in patients with physiologic hydronephrosis.**

ADDITIONAL IMAGES (B-E)

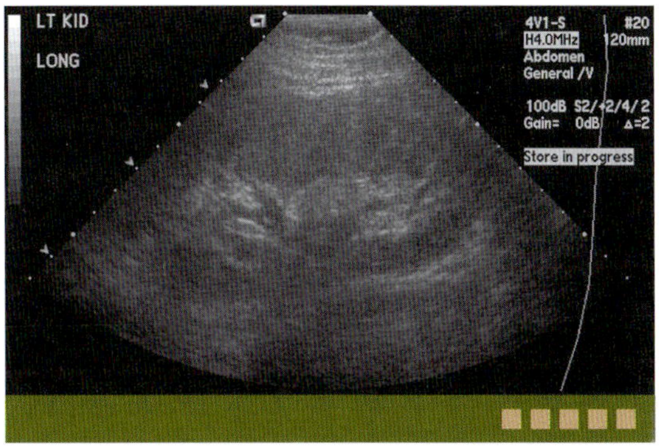

B. Longitudinal sonogram of the left kidney in the same patient as Figure A shows minimal dilatation of the left collecting system.

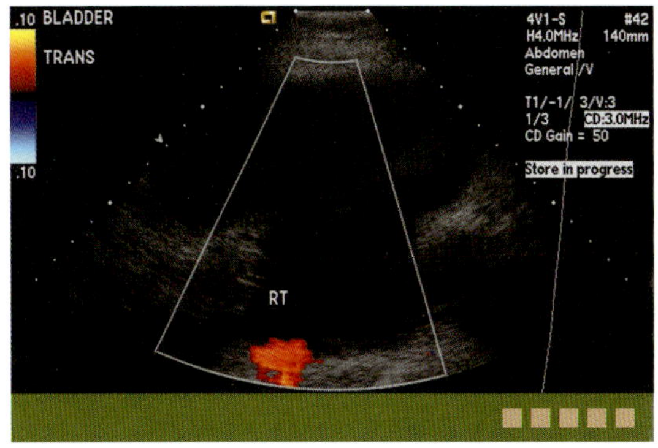

C. Transverse sonogram of the bladder shows a right ureteral jet. A left ureteral jet was also present.

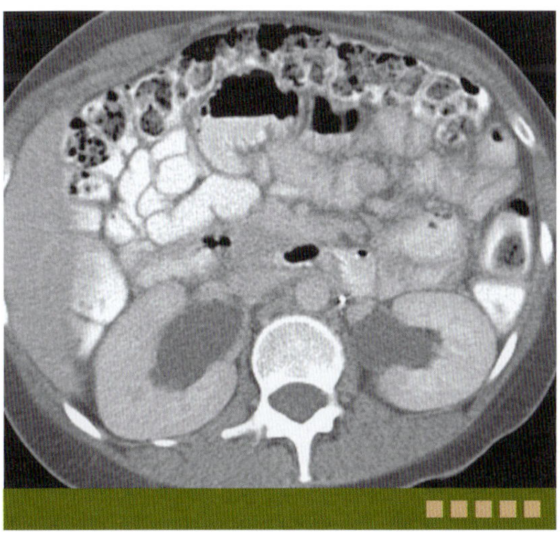

D. Axial CECT in a 27-week pregnant patient shows bilateral moderate hydronephrosis with the degree of dilatation greater on the right than the left.

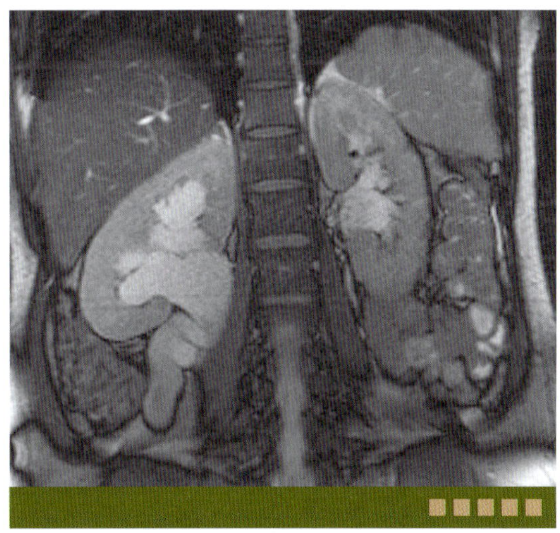

E. Coronal True FISP shows bilateral hydroureteronephrosis in a pregnant patient

DIFFERENTIAL DIAGNOSES IMAGES (F-G)

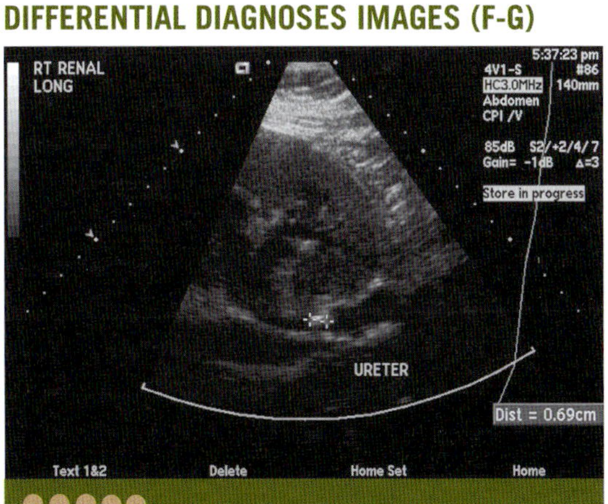

F. Obstructive uropathy: Longitudinal sonogram shows right hydronephrosis and a stone in the proximal right ureter in a 28-week pregnant patient presenting with acute onset of right flank pain.

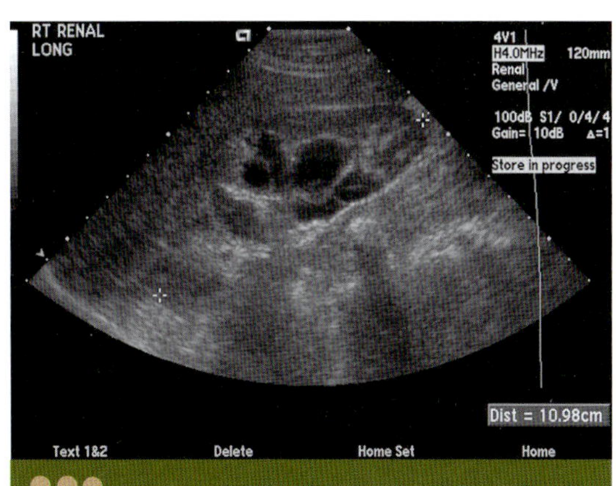

G. Parapelvic cysts: Longitudinal sonogram of the right kidney shows several anechoic structures which do not converge centrally.

IMAGE KEY

Common

Rare

Typical

Unusual

CHAPTER 8

BLADDER

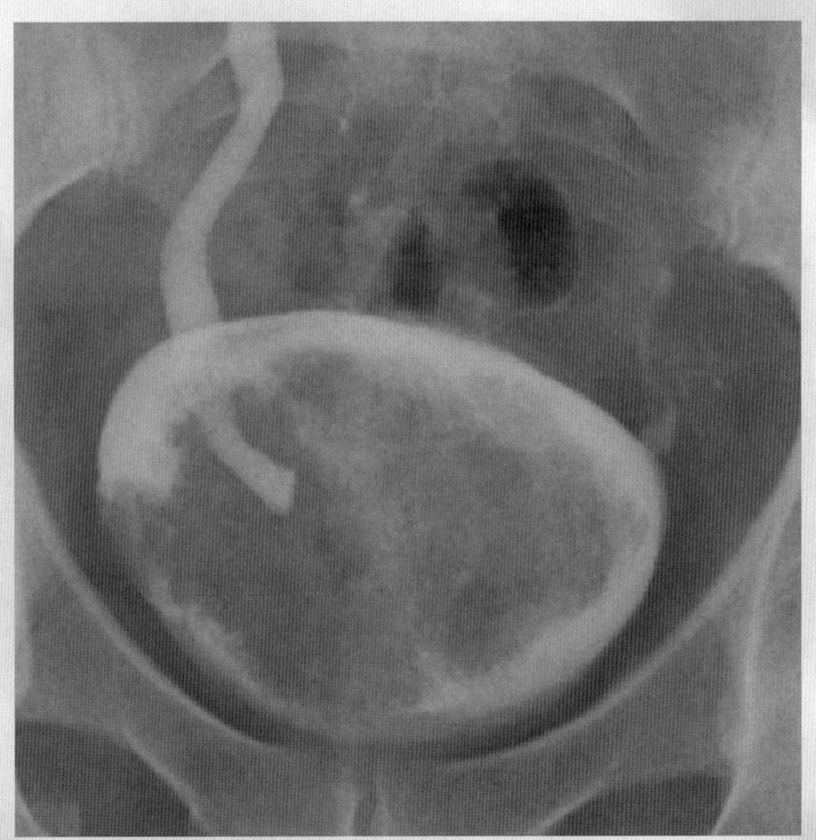

8–1 Urothelial Carcinoma of the Bladder (Part 1)

David D. Casalino

PRESENTATION

Gross hematuria.

FINDINGS

Intravenous urogram (IVU) shows a large, irregular filling defect in the bladder and dilatation of the right ureter.

DIFFERENTIAL DIAGNOSES

- *Other primary bladder neoplasm (malignant and benign)*: Much less common than urothelial carcinoma and less frequently multifocal; tissue necessary for specific diagnosis.
- *Metastases*: Usually known primary; cervical cancer in women and prostate cancer in men not uncommonly involve the bladder by direct extension.
- *Bladder hematoma*: Bladder wall usually normal thickness; clot may move with patient repositioning and will not enhance; etiologies include instrumentation, trauma, stone disease, neoplasm, anticoagulation, and coagulopathy.
- *Cystitis*: More often diffuse than focal; clinical signs and symptoms may suggest an inflammatory or infectious etiology; bladder capacity may be decreased.

COMMENTS

Ninety-five percent of bladder neoplasms arise from the epithelium, with urothelial (transitional cell) carcinoma accounting for 90% of the cases. There will be approximately 71,000 new cases and 14,300 deaths from bladder cancer in the United States in 2009. Risk factors for developing urothelial carcinoma include cigarette smoking, which accounts for up to one-half of all cases; occupational and environmental chemicals, including aromatic amines; drugs, such as phenacetin and cyclophosphamide; bladder stones; and chronic infection and irritation. Urothelial carcinoma is more common in men, with a male-to-female ratio of 3:1. While bladder cancer most commonly occurs in patients older than 65 years, approximately 3% occur in patients under 44 years of age. Patients presenting symptoms are nonspecific. Painless gross hematuria is the most common symptom; although, patients may present with microscopic hematuria or voiding symptoms, such as dysuria, frequency, and pelvic pain.

Pathologic stage is the most important predictor of survival and is important in determining treatment options. The tumor, nodes, metastasis (TNM) classification from the American Joint Committee on Cancer is commonly used and is as follows:

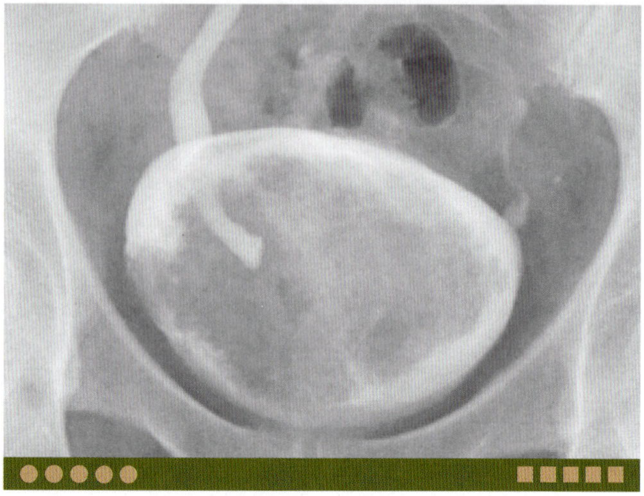

A. IVU shows a large, irregular filling defect in the bladder with dilatation of the right ureter.

TX	Primary tumor cannot be assessed
T0	No tumor
Tis	Carcinoma *in situ*
Ta	Papillary tumor confined to the epithelium
T1	Tumor invades subepithelial connective tissue (lamina propria)
T2a	Tumor invades superficial muscle (inner half)
T2b	Tumor invades deep muscle (outer half)
T3a	Tumor invades perivesical fat, microscopically
T3b	Tumor invades perivesical fat, macroscopically
T4a	Tumor invades surrounding organs
T4b	Tumor invades pelvic or abdominal wall
N1	Metastasis in single pelvic lymph node ≤2 cm
N2	Metastasis in single pelvic lymph node >2 cm and ≤5 cm or multiple nodes ≤5 cm
N3	Metastasis in single node >5 cm
N4	Lymph node metastases above the bifurcations of the common iliac arteries
M1	Distant metastases

Five-year survival for patients is 55% to 80% if the tumor is confined to the lamina propria, 40% if invasion into the muscularis propria, 20% if invasion into the perivesical fat, and 5% if metastatic.

PEARLS

- **Male-to-female ratio is 3:1, and most patients are older than 65 years.**
- **Pathologic staging is important in predicting survival and determining treatment options.**
- **Five-year survival rate is 80%, overall.**

ADDITIONAL IMAGES (B-D)

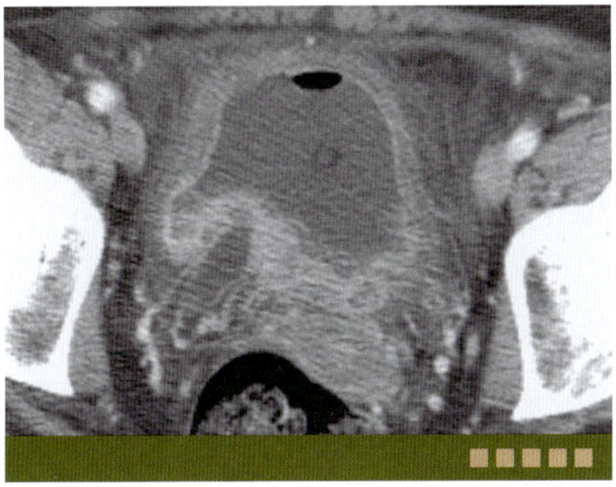

B. Axial CECT from the same patient shows the filling defect is a large, heterogeneous, enhancing mass arising from the posterior wall of the bladder and obstructing the right ureterovesical junction (UVJ).

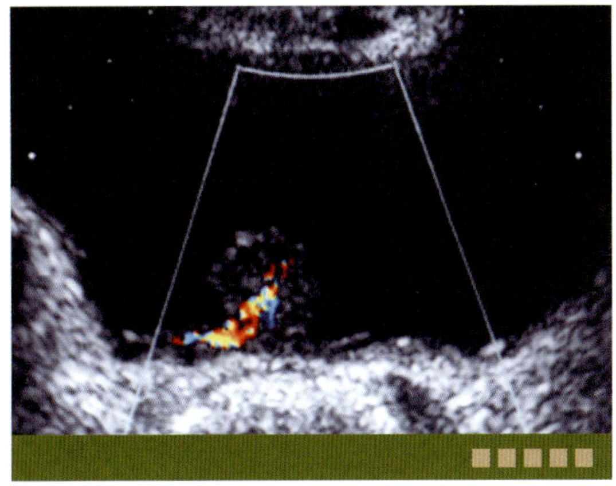

C. Transverse color Doppler sonogram from a different patient shows a polypoid mass with internal color flow arising from the posterior wall of the bladder.

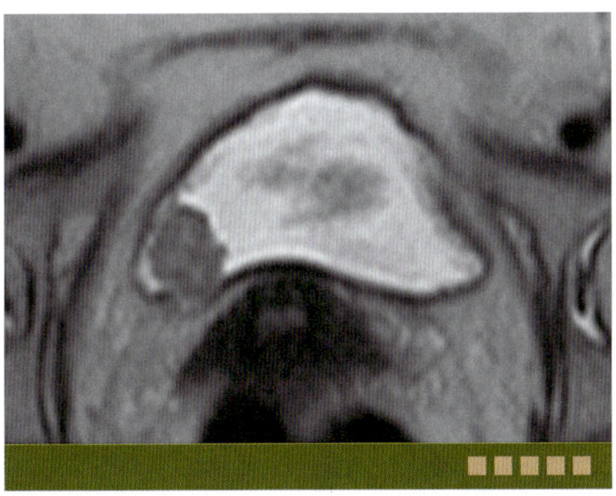

D. Axial T2-WI shows a polypoid mass of intermediate signal arising from the right posterior bladder wall. Note the more hypointense normal wall and hyperintense urine.

DIFFERENTIAL DIAGNOSES IMAGES (E-G)

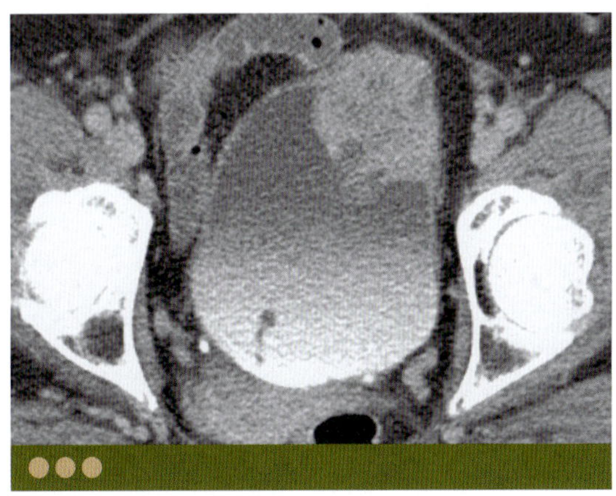

E. Leiomyosarcoma: Axial CECT during excretory phase shows a large, heterogeneous mass of the anterior bladder wall. Biopsy was necessary for diagnosis.

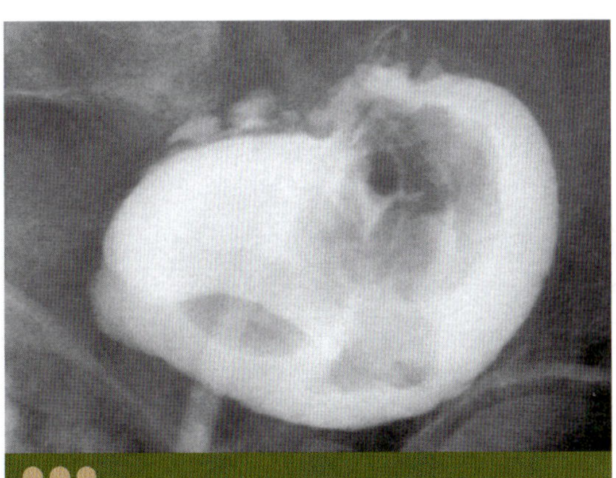

F. Bladder hematoma: Cystogram shows a large, lobulated filling defect in the bladder one day after bladder biopsy. Trabeculation of the superior bladder wall and a Foley catheter are also shown.

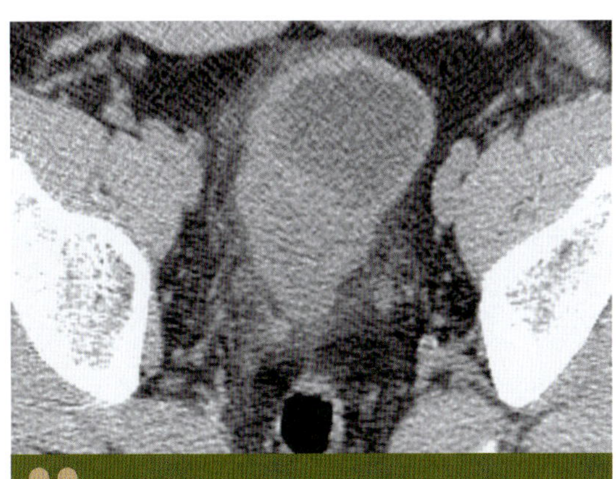

G. Cystitis glandularis: Axial NECT shows a round mass arising from the posterior wall of the bladder and separate from the prostate. Biopsy was necessary for diagnosis.

IMAGE KEY

Common

Rare

Typical

Unusual

8–2 Urothelial Carcinoma of the Bladder (Part 2)

David D. Casalino

PRESENTATION

Gross hematuria and pelvic pain.

FINDINGS

MR shows focal thickening of the left lateral wall of the bladder with associated heterogeneous enhancement.

DIFFERENTIAL DIAGNOSES

- *Other primary bladder neoplasm (malignant and benign)*: Much less common than urothelial carcinoma and less frequently multifocal; tissue necessary for specific diagnosis.
- *Metastases*: Usually known primary; cervical cancer in women and prostate cancer in men not uncommonly involve the bladder by direct extension.
- *Focal inflammatory or infectious process*: Examples include focal cystitis and adjacent diverticulitis; clinical features and associated imaging findings may suggest an inflammatory or infectious etiology.

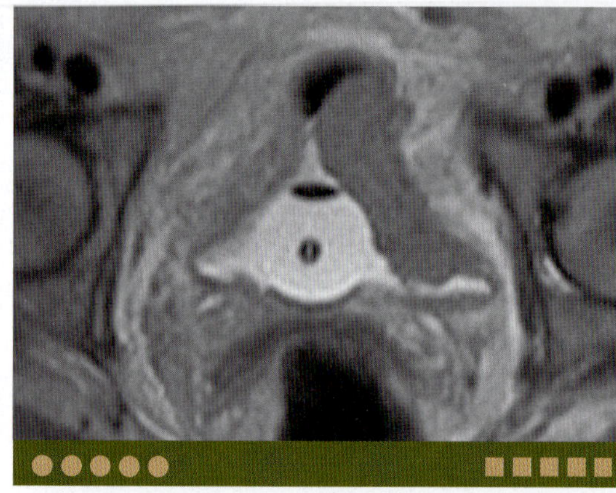

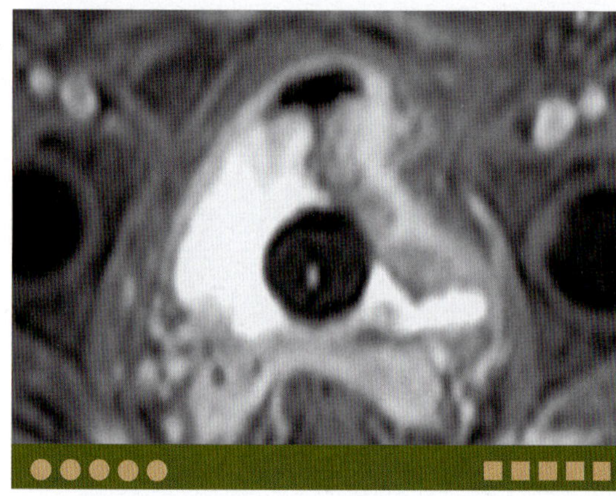

A. Axial T2-WI shows focal thickening of the left lateral wall of the bladder. It is intermediate signal intensity. A Foley catheter is seen centrally in the bladder.
B. Axial contrast-enhanced T1-WI shows intense, heterogeneous enhancement of this area. The bladder lumen is filled by excreted contrast, a Foley catheter, and a small volume of gas anteriorly.

COMMENTS

While cystoscopy with biopsy is the gold standard for diagnosing bladder cancers, imaging is important for accurate staging, treatment planning, monitoring therapy, and evaluating the upper urothelial tract. One-third of urothelial carcinomas are multifocal at time of diagnosis. Synchronous lesions in the upper urinary tract develop in 2% to 4% of patients with urothelial carcinoma, and metachronous lesions occur in 7% of these patients.

CT and MR are the imaging modalities of choice for staging known bladder neoplasms because of their sensitivity for detecting extramural extension and nodal metastases. Contrast-enhanced MR is more accurate than CT in evaluating depth of tumor invasion into the bladder wall. On CT, urothelial carcinoma, or TCC, typically appears as an intraluminal papillary or nodular mass or focal mural thickening. These tumors enhance early, and 5% of lesions will show calcifications. Transmural tumor invasion may manifest as increased attenuation or soft tissue stranding in the perivesical fat. On MR, urine, bladder wall and tumor, and fat are low, intermediate, and high-signal intensity, respectively, on unenhanced T1-weighted imaging. Tumor in intermediate signal intensity on T2-WI, while urine and bladder wall musculature are high- and low-signal intensity, respectively. With gadolinium-based contrast administration, tumor enhances earlier and more intensely than the normal bladder. On ultrasound, bladder tumors appear as papillary masses or focal mural thickening with variable echogenicity. Detection of Doppler flow in a bladder mass can differentiate a neoplasm from hematoma.

PEARLS

- **One-third of bladder carcinomas are multifocal at the time of diagnosis.**
- **Synchronous lesions in the upper urinary tract develop in 2% to 4% of patients with TCC, and metachronous lesions occur in 7% of these patients.**
- **MR is more accurate than CT in evaluating depth of tumor.**
- **TCC typically appears as an intraluminal papillary or nodular mass or focal mural thickening.**

ADDITIONAL IMAGES (C-E)

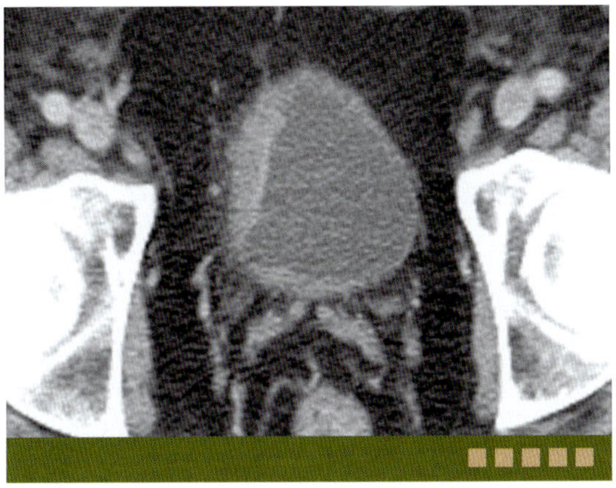

C. Axial CECT shows mild thickening of the right lateral wall of the bladder. Biopsy confirmed TCC.

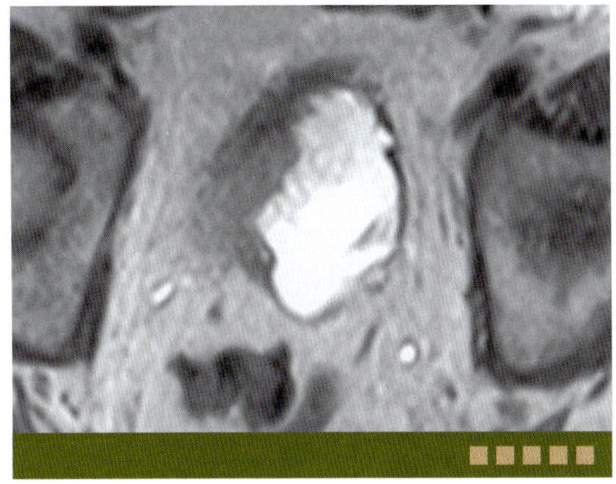

D. Axial T2-WI shows marked thickening of intermediate signal intensity involving the right lateral wall of the bladder. Soft tissue stranding in the adjacent perivesical fat was confirmed to be transmural tumor invasion.

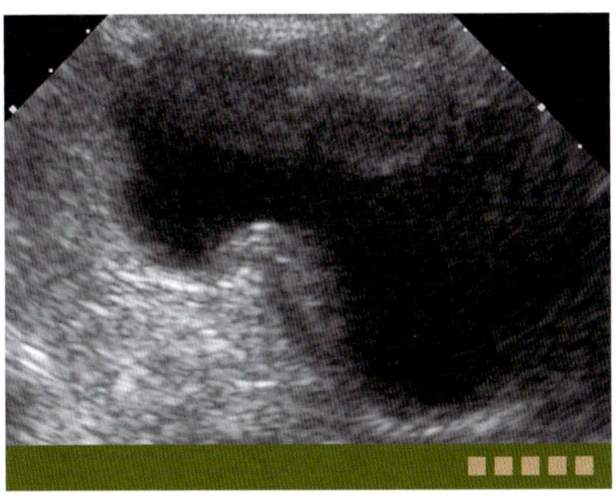

E. Longitudinal sonogram shows focal mural thickening involving the posterior aspect of the bladder.

DIFFERENTIAL DIAGNOSES IMAGES (F-H)

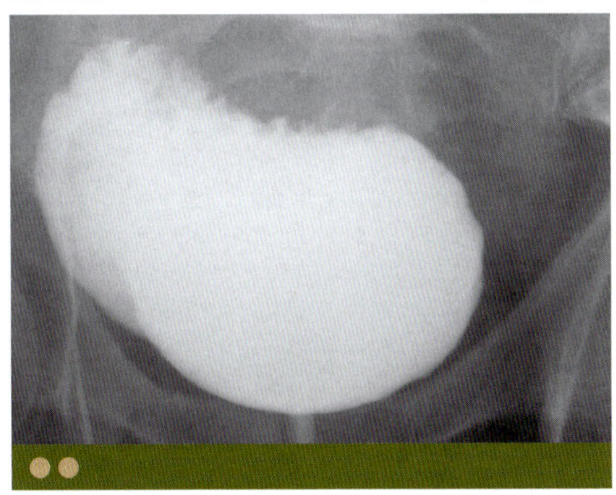

F. Metastasis: Cystogram shows irregular thickening involving the superior aspect of the bladder caused by invasive sigmoid colonic adenocarcinoma.

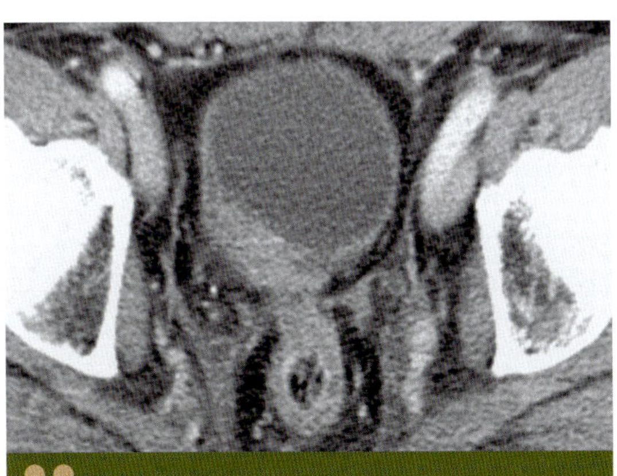

G. Metastasis: Axial CECT shows focal thickening involving the posterior aspect of the bladder caused by prostate cancer. The anterior wall of the rectum is also involved.

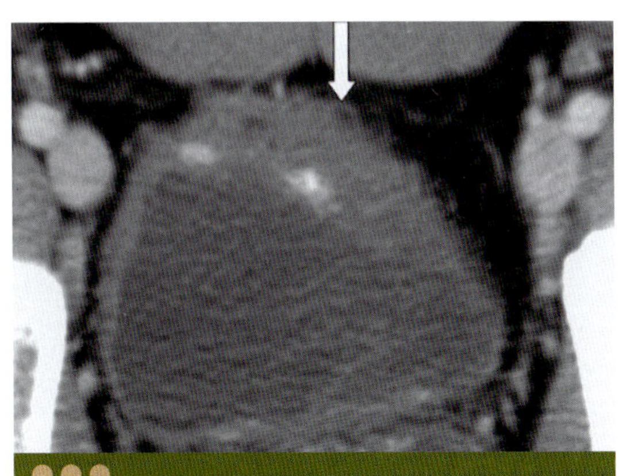

H. Diverticulitis: Axial CECT shows irregular thickening of the anterior wall of the bladder (arrow) caused by adjacent sigmoid colonic diverticulitis.

IMAGE KEY

Common

Rare

Typical

Unusual

8–3 Squamous Cell Carcinoma of the Bladder

David D. Casalino

PRESENTATION

Gross hematuria.

FINDINGS

MR images, pre- and postcontrast, show a large, irregular, enhancing mass arising from the left lateral bladder wall.

DIFFERENTIAL DIAGNOSES

- *Other primary bladder neoplasm (malignant and benign)*: TCC is much more common and more often multifocal and having a papillary growth pattern; adenocarcinoma is less common and may be associated with the urachal remnant; tissue necessary for specific diagnosis.
- *Cystitis*: More often diffuse than focal; chronic cystitis common in patients with bladder squamous cell carcinoma.

COMMENTS

Ninety-five percent of bladder neoplasms arise from the epithelium, with squamous cell carcinoma accounting for 5% to 10% of cases. Prognosis is generally poor because of the tumors often being high grade with muscle invasion and extravesical extension being common at diagnosis. Squamous cell carcinoma of the bladder is seen in increased frequency in patients with neurogenic bladder, chronic indwelling Foley catheter, repeated episodes of cystitis or vesical schistosomiasis. Schistosomiasis accounts for more than 50% of bladder cancers in parts of the world where the parasite is endemic. Presenting symptoms may include gross hematuria and voiding symptoms.

Imaging features of squamous cell carcinoma are nonspecific and may be a solid enhancing mass or focal or diffuse mural thickening. The mass is usually sessile rather than papillary and involves the bladder trigone or a lateral wall. On MR, squamous cell carcinoma, like TCC, is usually intermediate-signal intensity on T1- and T2-WI and enhances. Identifying the tumor may be difficult in a diffusely thickened bladder. Muscle invasion occurs in 80% of the cases, and extravesical spread is common and may be extensive. Squamous cell carcinoma may occur in bladder diverticula and show surface calcifications.

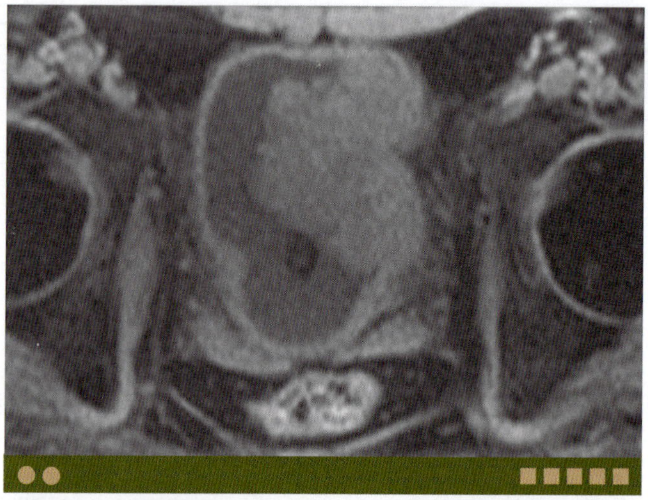

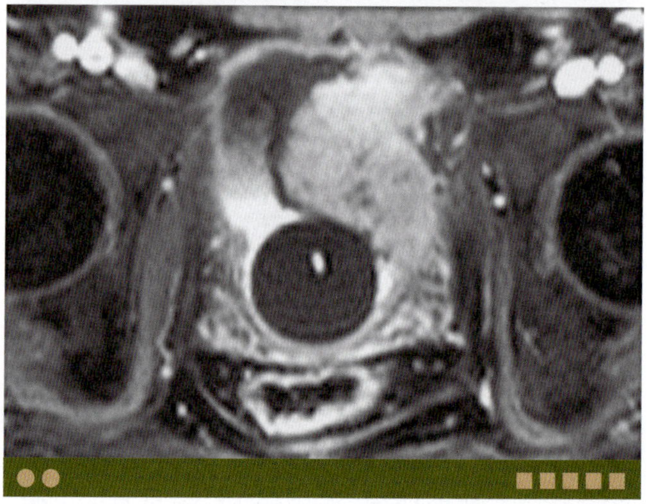

A. and **B.** Axial nonenhanced and contrast-enhanced T1-WI shows a large, irregular, enhancing mass arising from the left lateral wall of the bladder in a patient with chronic indwelling Foley catheter.

PEARLS

- **Chronic inflammation of the bladder is the major risk factor for developing squamous cell carcinoma.**
- **Prognosis is generally poor.**
- **While a sessile mass in a chronically thickened bladder should raise consideration for a squamous cell carcinoma, biopsy is necessary for a specific diagnosis.**

ADDITIONAL IMAGES (C-E)

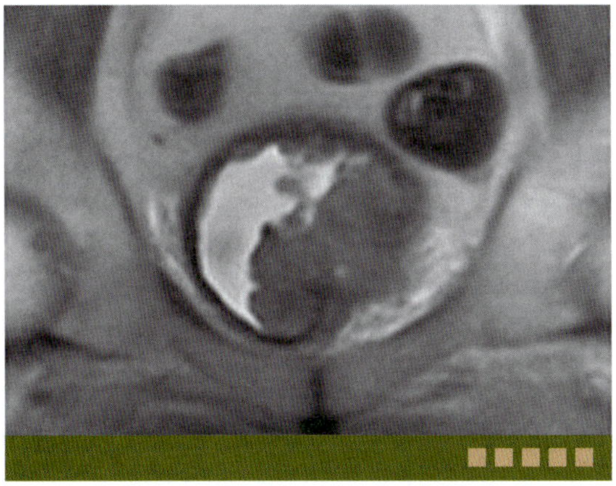

C. Coronal T2-WI from the same patient shows the tumor to have higher signal intensity than the normal wall. The left lateral tumor margin is irregular and extends beyond the normal bladder contour as a result of extravesical tumor spread.

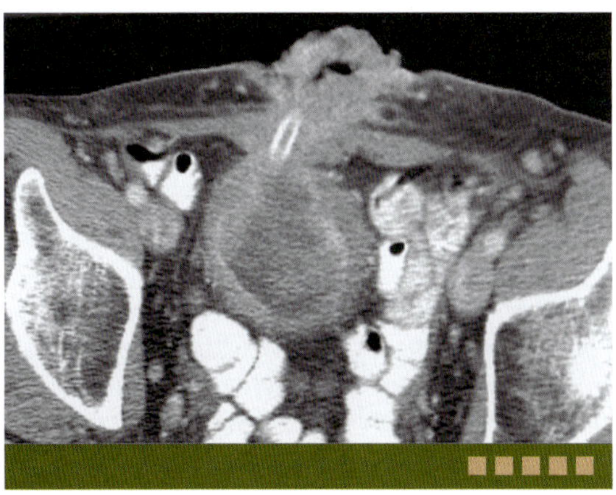

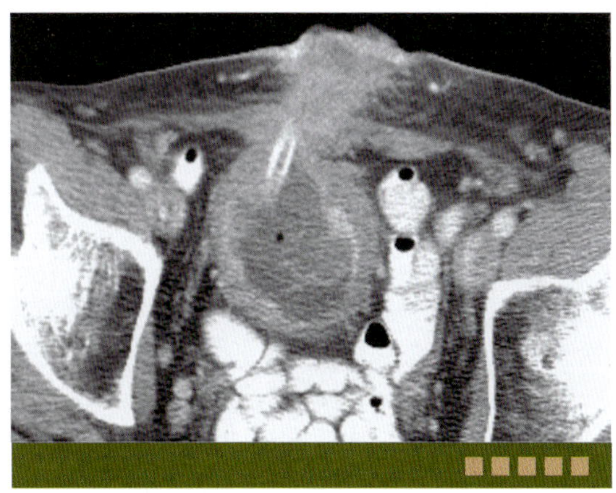

D. and **E.** Axial CECT from a different paraplegic patient show a suprapubic bladder catheter, diffuse bladder wall thickening, and an enhancing tumor extending from the anterior aspect of the bladder to the skin surface.

IMAGE KEY

Common

Rare

Typical

Unusual

DIFFERENTIAL DIAGNOSES IMAGES (F-G)

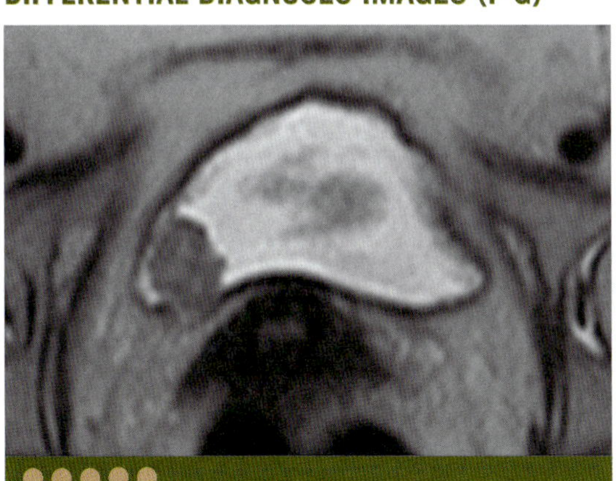

F. Urothelial carcinoma: Axial T2-WI shows a round, hypointense bladder filling defect arising from the posterior bladder wall.

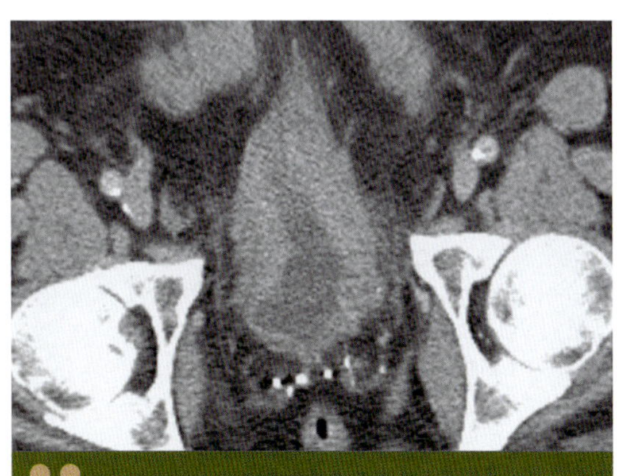

G. Radiation-induced cystitis: Axial CECT shows marked bladder wall thickening that is nonuniform in a patient with a history of prostate cancer treated with brachytherapy seeds.

8–4 Primary Adenocarcinoma of the Bladder (Urachal)

David D. Casalino

PRESENTATION

Painless, gross hematuria.

FINDINGS

CT shows a 3.5-cm enhancing mass with central low attenuation, involving the anterosuperior aspect of the bladder at the midline.

DIFFERENTIAL DIAGNOSES

- *Other primary bladder neoplasm (malignant and benign)*: Transitional cell, or urothelial, carcinoma and squamous cell carcinoma are more common; tissue necessary for specific diagnosis.
- *Metastasis*: Usually known primary; metastatic adenocarcinoma to the bladder is more common than primary adenocarcinoma; direct spread from a colonic, prostatic or rectal primary is more common than hematogeneous or lymphatic spread from a gastric, breast, or lung primary.
- *Focal inflammatory or infectious process*: Examples include focal cystitis, adjacent diverticulitis, and an infected urachal cyst; clinical features and associated imaging findings may suggest an inflammatory or infectious etiology.

COMMENTS

Ninety-five percent of bladder neoplasms arise from the epithelium, with adenocarcinoma accounting for 2% of the cases. Risk factors for bladder adenocarcinoma include persistent urachus, bladder exstrophy, and intestinal metaplasia from chronic mucosal irritation. Adenocarcinoma may also be found in patients with urinary diversions, such as enterocystoplasty, and pelvic lipomatosis because of an association with cystitis glandularis. One-third of primary bladder adenocarcinomas are urachal, while two-thirds are not.

Urachal adenocarcinoma may secrete mucus in the urine or produce an umbilical discharge of blood or mucus. Sixty percent of these tumors are low-attenuation tumors because of mucin, and 70% show dystrophic calcifications. Two-thirds of patients with urachal adenocarcinoma are men between 40 and 70 years of age. The prognosis is much worse than for other bladder carcinomas because of often advanced stage at time of diagnosis. Patients presenting symptoms are nonspecific. Painless, gross hematuria is the most common symptom; but patients may present with microscopic hematuria or voiding symptoms, such as dysuria, frequency, and pelvic pain.

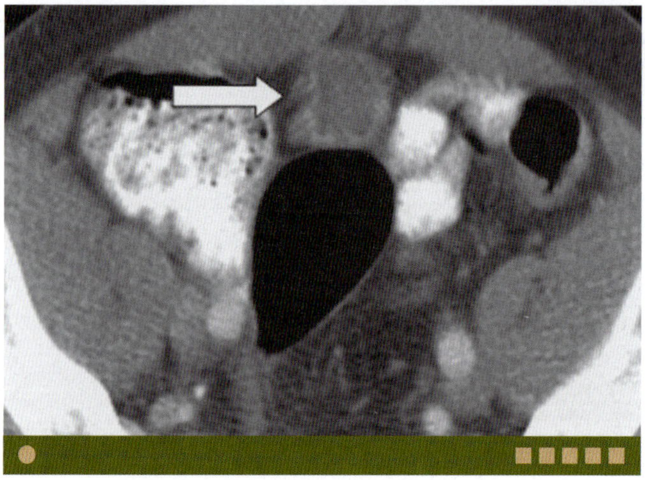

A. Axial CECT shows a 3.5-cm enhancing mass (arrow) with central low attenuation, involving the anterosuperior aspect of the bladder at the midline.

On CT, urachal adenocarcinomas typically appear as soft tissue masses at the anterosuperior aspect of the bladder. They are typically midline and may extend toward the umbilicus. A prominent extravesical component is characteristic. The tumor is often large (>5 cm), and most show calcifications, which are more often peripheral than stippled. On MR, these tumors are typically low-signal on T1-weighted imaging, heterogeneous high-signal on T2-weighted imaging, and enhance. Invasion into adjacent structures is not uncommon.

While radical cystectomy is the treatment of choice for a nonurachal adenocarcinoma, urachal adenocarcinoma warrants cystectomy and en bloc resection of the urachal mass, peritoneum, posterior rectus fascia, and abdominal wall.

PEARLS

- **One-third of primary bladder adenocarcinomas are urachal.**
- **Ninety percent of urachal malignancies are adenocarcinomas.**
- **Urachal adenocarcinomas are typically midline, at the anterosuperior aspect of the bladder, and have a prominent extravesical component.**
- **Urachal adenocarcinomas more frequently show calcifications than urothelial or SCC.**

ADDITIONAL IMAGES (B-D)

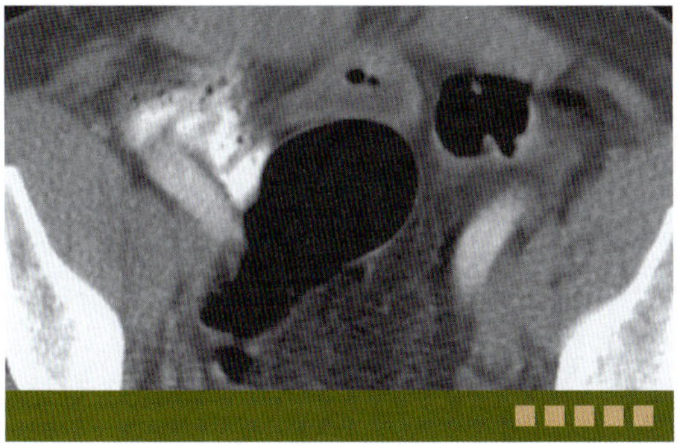

B. Axial CECT more caudad shows the heterogeneous mass in continuity with the bladder.

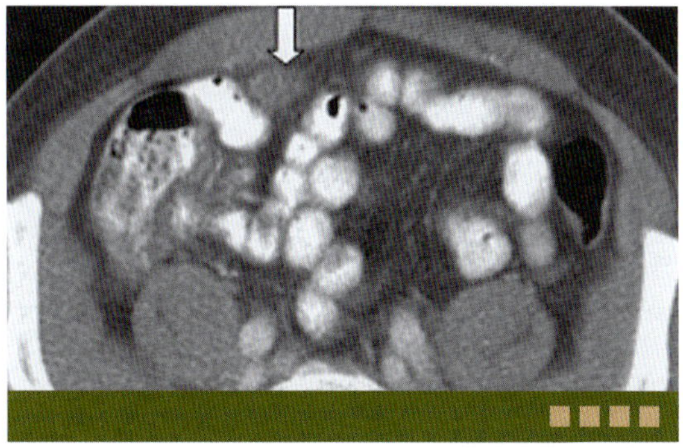

C. Axial CECT more cephalad shows a separate small mass (arrow) in the anterior abdominal fat. This mass proved to be a metastasis from the adenocarcinoma.

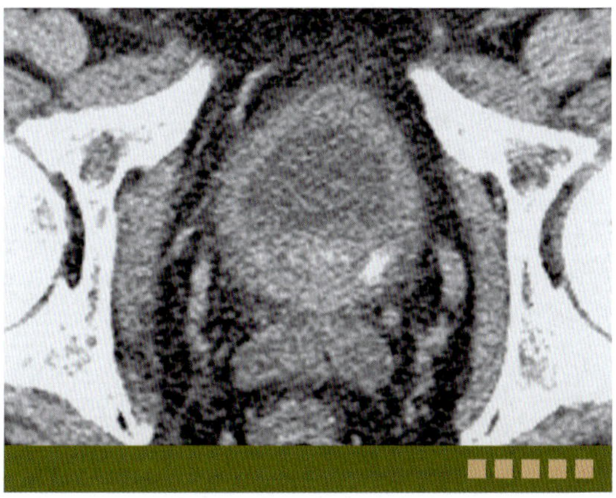

D. Axial CECT from a different patient shows abnormal thickening of the bladder that is greatest along the posterior wall. This proved to be a 3.5-cm primary bladder adenocarcinoma.

DIFFERENTIAL DIAGNOSES IMAGES (E-G)

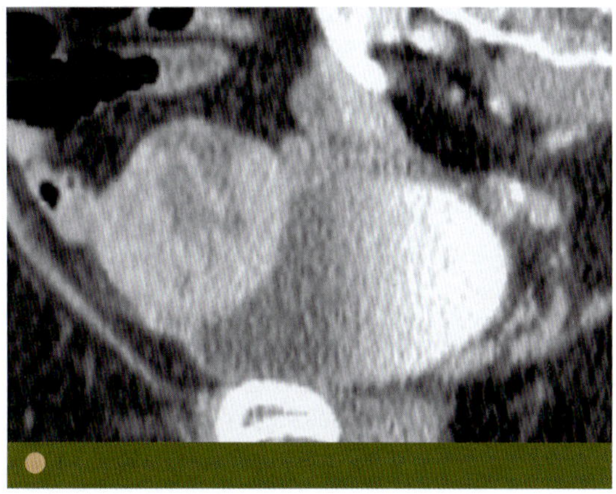

E. Bladder leiomyosarcoma: Sagittal CECT shows a large, heterogeneously enhancing mass arising from the anterosuperior aspect of the bladder. Biopsy was necessary for the diagnosis of a leiomyosarcoma.

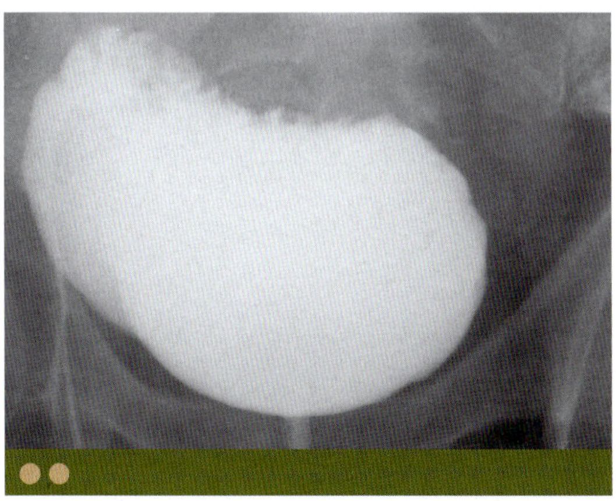

F. Metastasis: Cystogram shows very irregular mural thickening across the superior aspect of the bladder caused by invasion of the bladder by an adjacent sigmoid colon adenocarcinoma.

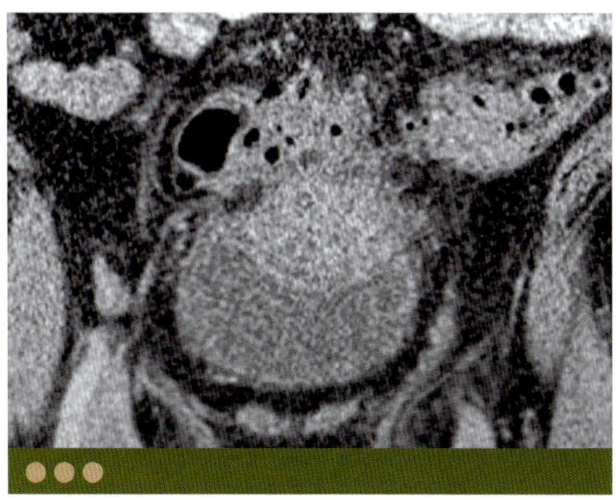

G. Sigmoid colonic diverticulitis: Coronal CECT shows an inflammatory mass involving the superior aspect of the bladder.

IMAGE KEY

Common

Rare

Typical

Unusual

8–5 Urothelial Carcinoma in a Bladder Diverticulum

David D. Casalino

PRESENTATION

Painless hematuria.

FINDINGS

CT shows a large bladder diverticulum with a noncalcified filling defect.

DIFFERENTIAL DIAGNOSES

- *Hematoma*: Will not enhance.
- *Other neoplasm*: Less common; tissue necessary for specific diagnosis.

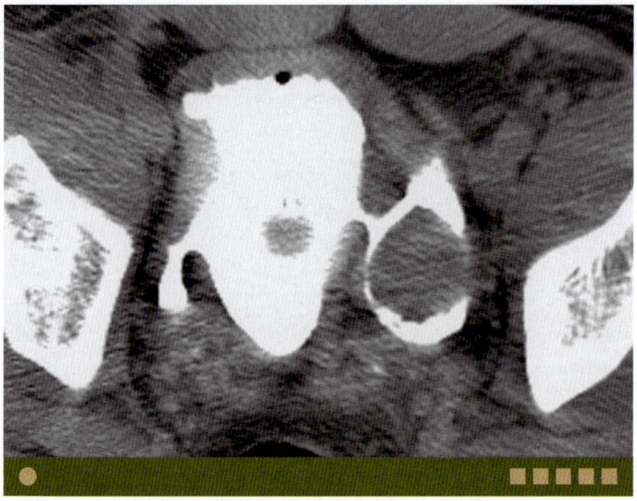

A. Axial CECT during excretory phase shows a large left-sided bladder diverticulum with noncalcified filling defect. There is also a very small, right-sided diverticulum in this patient with benign prostate hypertrophy (BPH).

COMMENTS

Bladder diverticula are common outpouchings that increase in incidence with age. Most are acquired as a result of bladder outlet obstruction and increased intravesical pressure. Acquired diverticula are often multiple but may be single at times. They tend to occur adjacent to the ureteral orifices.

Bladder diverticula have an increased risk of developing cancer. This 2% to 10% risk is thought to be related to urinary stasis within the diverticulum. While all major epithelial type carcinomas have been described in diverticula, urothelial carcinoma, or transitional cell carcinoma (TCC), accounts for 80%. Because diverticula lack a normal muscle layer, diverticular carcinomas have a propensity for early transmural spread into the perivesical fat.

These tumors may appear as a filling defect, mass, or mucosal irregularity on imaging. While cystoscopy is generally considered the gold standard for diagnosing most bladder tumors, a narrow diverticular neck might prohibit cystoscopic assessment for a mass. Diverticular tumors are more reliably imaged by cystography, CT, and MR.

PEARLS

- **Bladder diverticula have an increased risk of carcinoma.**
- **TCCs comprise 80% of these malignancies.**
- **Carcinoma in a diverticulum may appear as a filling defect, mass, or mucosal irregularity.**

ADDITIONAL IMAGES (B-E)

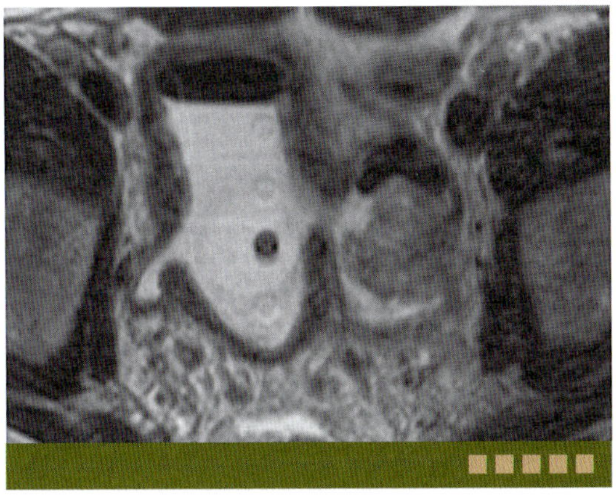

B. Axial T2-WI from the same patient shows the filling defect to be heterogeneous and intermediate-signal intensity. Small amount of gas is seen in the anterior aspects of the bladder and diverticulum.

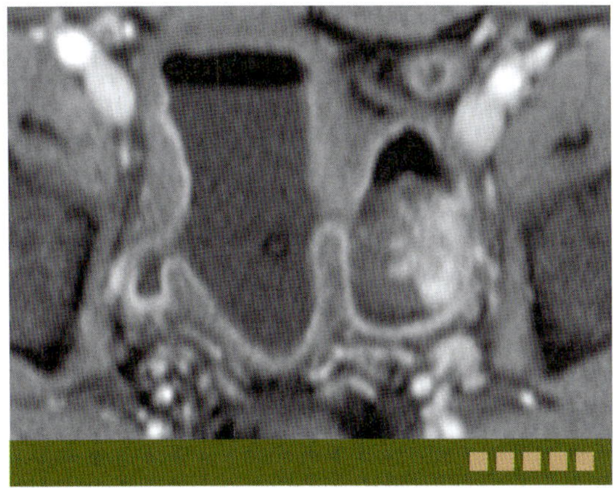

C. Axial contrast-enhanced T1-WI shows intense, heterogeneous enhancement of the mass with irregularity of the lateral margin that proved to be tumor invasion into the perivesical fat.

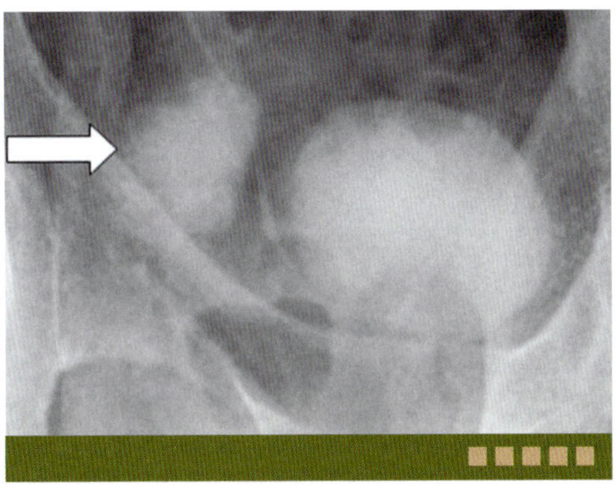

D. IVU from a different patient shows a large, right-sided bladder diverticulum with lateral mural irregularity (arrow).

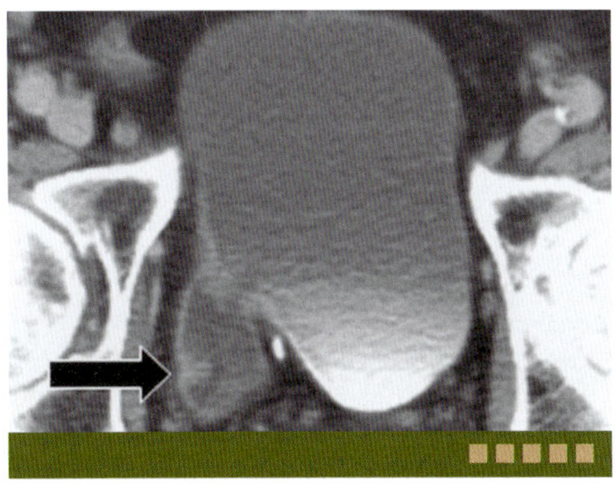

E. Axial CECT from the same patient as in the last figure shows the diverticulum with enhancing mural nodularity (arrow) that proved to be carcinoma.

IMAGE KEY

Common

Rare

Typical

Unusual

DIFFERENTIAL DIAGNOSES IMAGES (F-G)

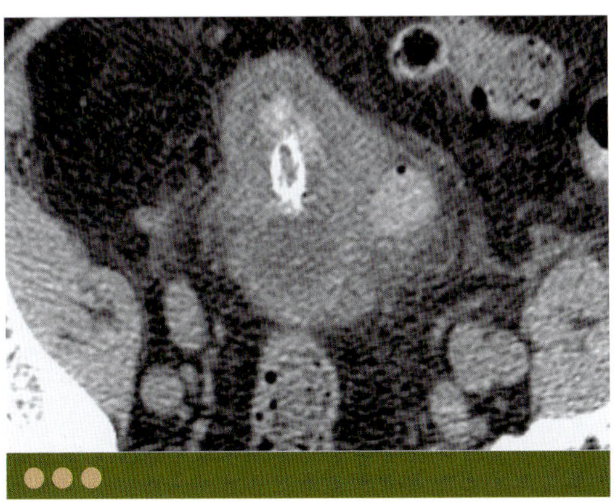

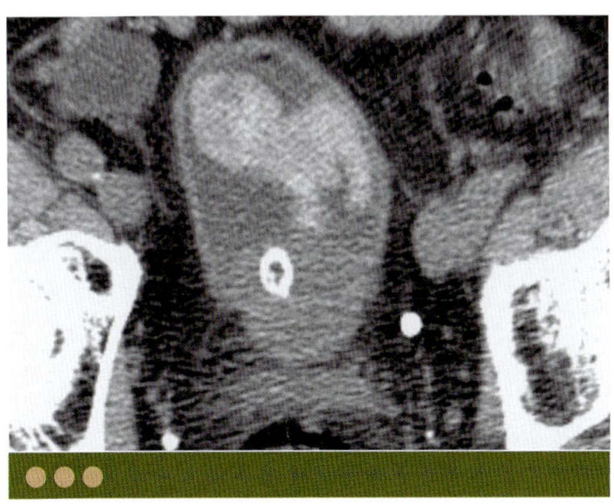

F. and **G. Hematoma:** Axial NECT show hyperdense clot in the bladder and a left-sided diverticulum. A Foley catheter is also seen in this patient who presented with persistent hematuria after recent cystoscopy and bladder biopsy.

8–6 Small Cell Bladder Tumor

David D. Casalino

PRESENTATION

Gross hematuria and history of smoking cigarettes.

FINDINGS

CT shows a large enhancing mass involving the anterior wall of the bladder.

DIFFERENTIAL DIAGNOSES

- *Other primary bladder neoplasm (malignant and benign)*: Urothelial carcinoma is much more common and can also have extravesical extension; urachal adenocarcinoma has a characteristic location; tissue necessary for specific diagnosis.
- *Focal inflammatory or infectious process*: Examples include focal cystitis and adjacent diverticulitis; clinical features and associated imaging findings may suggest an inflammatory or infectious etiology.

COMMENTS

Small cell bladder tumors are rare. They account for less than 0.5% of bladder neoplasms. These tumors originate from dedifferentiated neuroendocrine cells. Small cell tumors are very aggressive tumors, which are almost always invasive at presentation and have a 5-year survival rate of approximately 15%. Patients usually present with hematuria and have a history of smoking cigarettes. These tumors occur more frequently in men with a male-to-female ratio of 4:1. The reported patient age range is 20 to 91 years.

On imaging, the tumors are usually large (3-8 cm), nodular or polypoid, and invasive. Central necrosis, cystic change and heterogeneous enhancement may be seen on CT and MR.

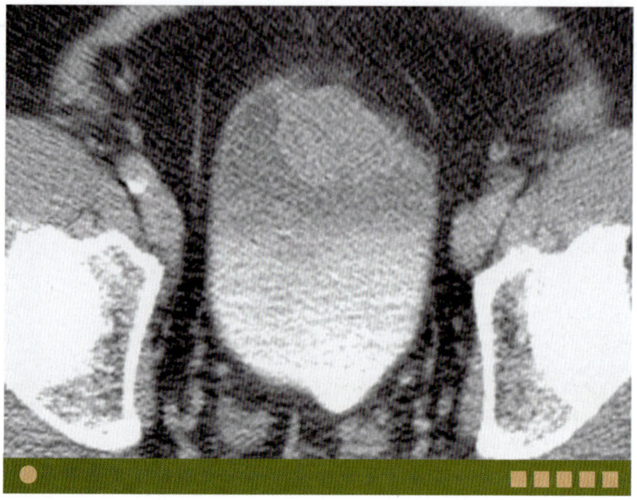

A. Axial CECT shows a large enhancing mass involving the anterior wall of the bladder.

Calcification is not common. These tumors may demonstrate extensive local invasion, peritoneal metastases, lymph node metastases, and distal metastases to the liver, lungs, and bones.

PEARLS

- **Small cell bladder tumors are rare, very aggressive, and associated with a poor prognosis for the patient.**
- **Male-to-female ratio 4:1.**
- **The tumor is typically large, nodular or polypoid, and heterogeneous.**
- **Local invasion and metastatic disease are common.**

ADDITIONAL IMAGES (B-D)

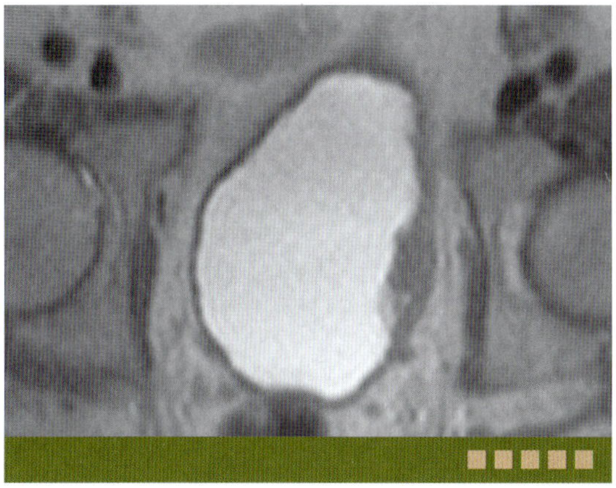

B. Axial T2-WI from a different patient shows a mass involving the left lateral wall of bladder. The mass has intermediate-signal intensity.

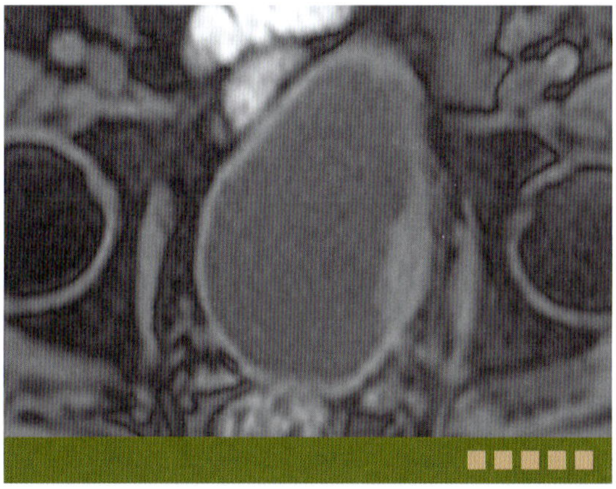

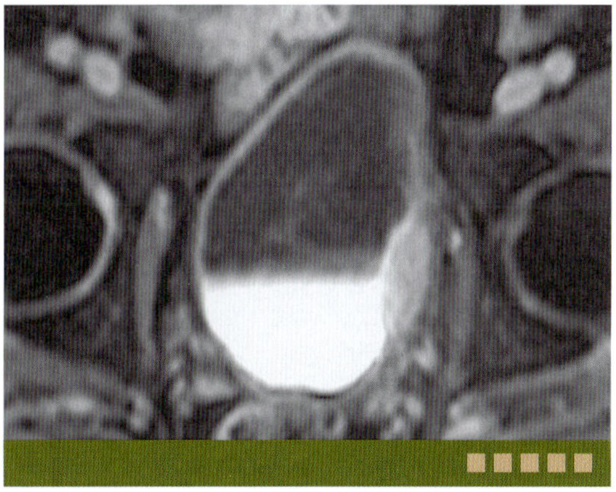

C. and **D.** Axial nonenhanced and contrast-enhanced T1-WI shows that the mass enhances moderately with mild heterogeneity. This is a biopsy proven small cell bladder tumor.

IMAGE KEY

Common

Rare

Typical

Unusual

DIFFERENTIAL DIAGNOSES IMAGES (E-F)

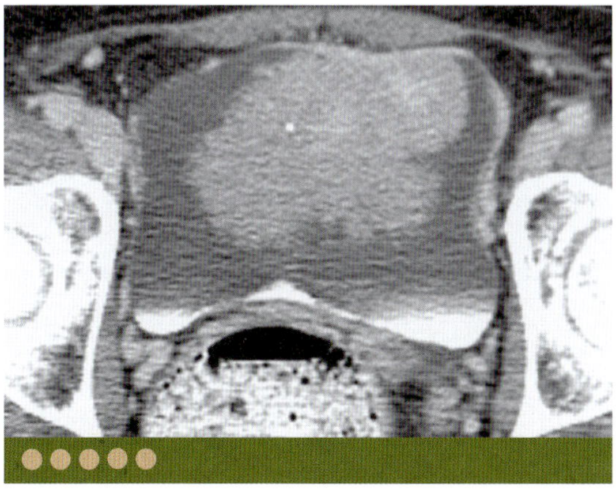

E. Urothelial carcinoma: Axial CECT shows a large, enhancing mass with irregular margins arising from the anterior wall of the bladder.

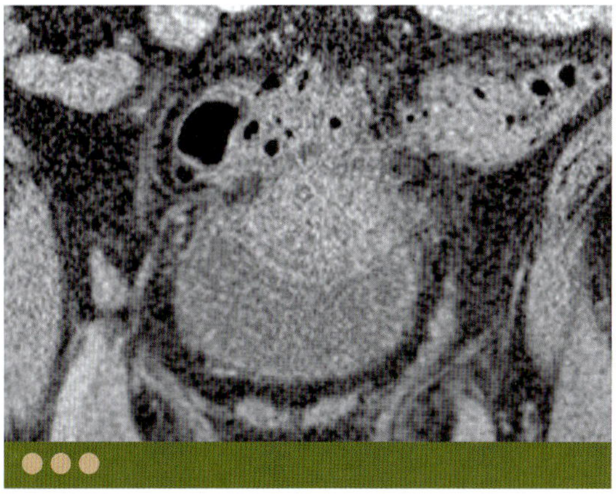

F. Diverticular abscess: Coronal NECT shows sigmoid colonic diverticulitis with an associated abscess involving the superior aspect of the bladder.

8–7 Bladder Lymphoma

David D. Casalino

PRESENTATION

Hematuria and pelvic pain.

FINDINGS

CT shows multiple, enhancing bladder masses.

DIFFERENTIAL DIAGNOSES

- *Other primary bladder neoplasm (malignant and benign)*: Urothelial carcinoma, or TCC, is most common and often multifocal; tissue necessary for specific diagnosis.
- *Metastases*: Usually known primary; cervical cancer in women and prostate cancer in men not uncommonly involve the bladder by direct extension.
- *Cystitis*: More often diffuse than focal; clinical signs and symptoms may suggest an inflammatory or infectious etiology; bladder capacity may be decreased.

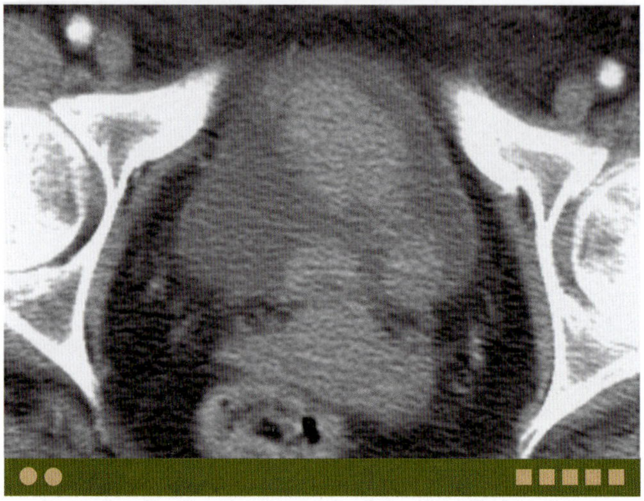

A. Axial CECT shows multiple, focal enhancing bladder masses in a woman with history of breast cancer and lung cancer. Lymphoma was diagnosed by biopsy performed at the time of cystoscopy.

COMMENTS

Primary bladder lymphoma is very rare because there is no lymphoid tissue in the bladder. Secondary involvement is more common, occurring in 10% to 25% of patients with systemic lymphoma and leukemia. The vast majority of bladder lymphoma cases are non-Hodgkin lymphoma (NHL) with diffuse large B-cell-type and low-grade B-cell mucosa-associated lymphoid tissue (MALT) type being most common. Bladder lymphoma is most common in middle-aged women. Presenting symptoms might include hematuria and pelvic pain. Most tumors are low grade and associated with a good prognosis.

Radiographically, bladder lymphoma is indistinguishable from urothelial carcinoma. Well-defined masses are more common than diffuse infiltration and usually involve the dome or lateral walls. On MR, bladder lymphoma is usually intermediate signal intensity on T1- and T2-weighted imaging and shows mild enhancement after gadolinium-base contrast administration.

PEARLS

- **Primary bladder lymphoma is very rare.**
- **Bladder lymphoma is usually secondary involvement in patients with NHL.**
- **Imaging features of bladder lymphoma are indistinguishable from TCC.**

ADDITIONAL IMAGES (B-D)

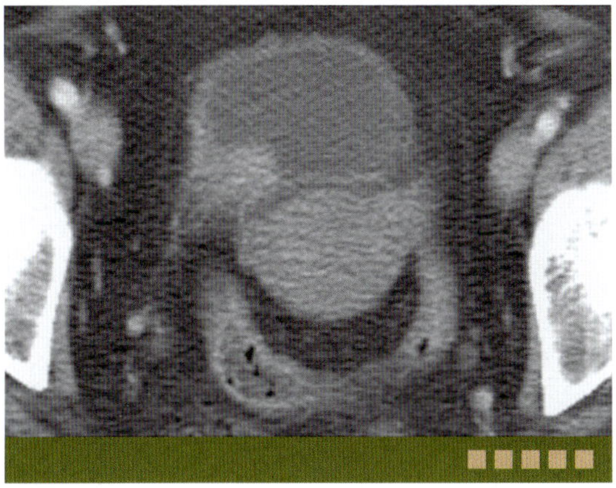

B. Axial CECT more cephalad in the same patient shows an additional bladder mass.

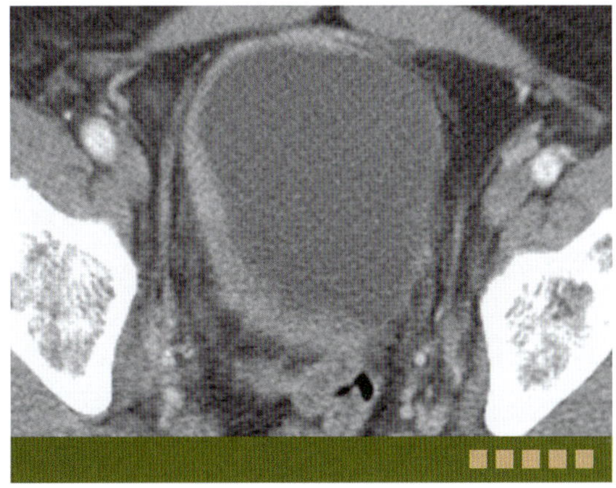

C. Axial CECT shows right lateral and posterior bladder wall thickening that is irregular in a patient with known NHL.

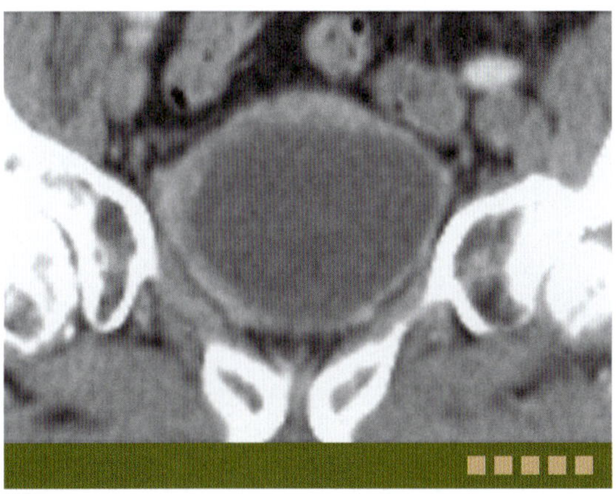

D. Coronal CECT from the same patient shows the bladder wall thickening involves the dome as well with a relatively normal thickness of the left lateral wall.

DIFFERENTIAL DIAGNOSES IMAGES (E-G)

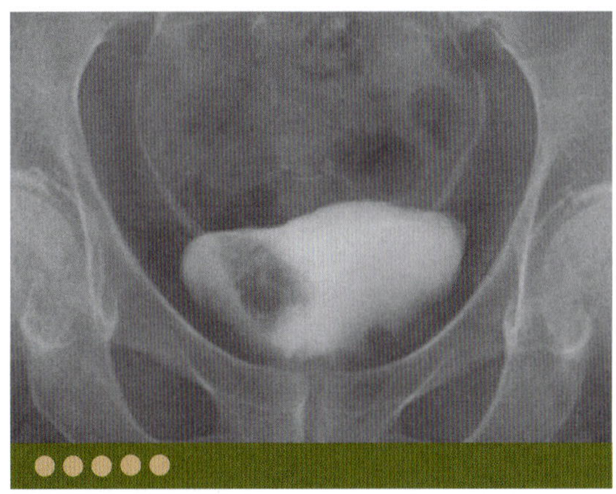

E. Multifocal TCC: IVU shows a large irregular filling defect in the right side of the bladder and multiple smaller filling defects along the inferior wall.

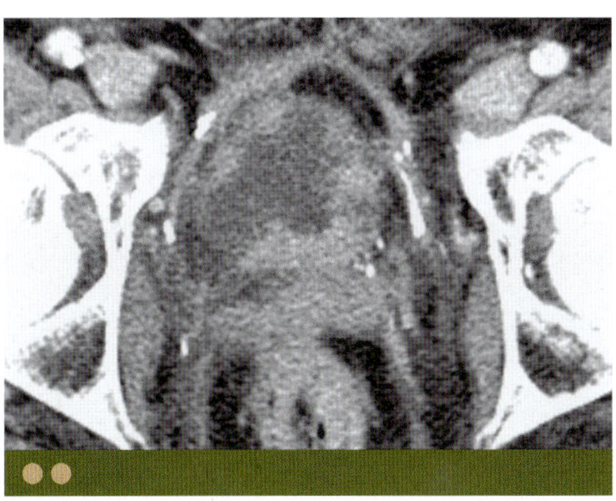

F. Metastases: Axial CECT shows multiple enhancing bladder base masses due to direct extension of patient's known prostate cancer.

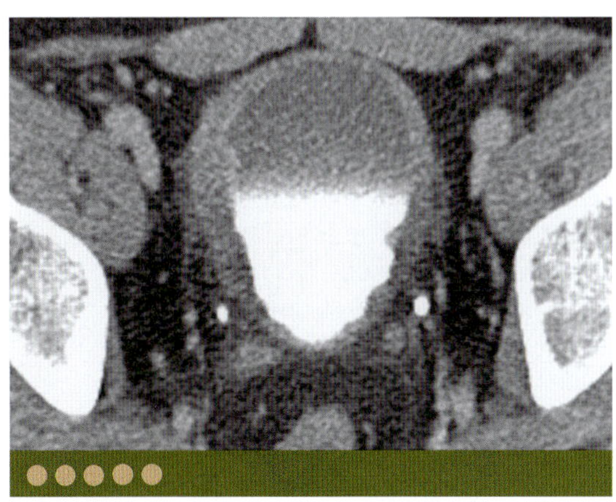

G. Cystitis: Axial CECT shows irregular bladder wall thickening that is more prominent and nodular along the lateral walls in a neutropenic patient with chronic, recurrent urinary tract infections (UTI).

IMAGE KEY

Common
●●●●●
●●●●
●●●
●●
●
Rare

Typical
■■■■■
■■■■
■■■
■■
■
Unusual

8-8 Bladder Leiomyosarcoma

David D. Casalino

PRESENTATION

Painless hematuria.

FINDINGS

CT shows a large, heterogeneously enhancing mass involving the anterior aspect of the bladder dome.

DIFFERENTIAL DIAGNOSES

- *Leiomyoma*: Benign; typically smaller with smooth margins and homogeneous enhancement.
- *Other primary bladder neoplasm (malignant and benign)*: TCC is much more common and can also have extravesical extension; urachal adenocarcinoma has a characteristic location; tissue necessary for specific diagnosis.
- *Metastasis*: Usually known primary.

COMMENTS

Leiomyosarcoma is the most common malignant mesenchymal tumor of the bladder in adults. It accounts for less than 1% of bladder malignancies. The majority of these tumors are high grade and aggressive with rates of local recurrence and metastatic disease reported to be 16% and 53%, respectively. Lung, bone, brain, and liver are the most common sites of distant metastases. The 5-year survival rate is approximately 60%.

These tumors are more prevalent in men with a male predominance of over 2:1. While patients range in age from 15 to 88 years old, most present in the sixth to eighth decades. There is a reported increased risk of developing leiomyosarcomas in patients who have received cyclophosphamide or radiation therapy (RT). Patients most commonly present with gross hematuria and less commonly with obstructive symptoms, pelvic mass, or dysuria.

Leiomyosarcomas most commonly occur in the dome but may involve any part of the bladder. The tumors are often polypoid and large with a mean size of 7 cm. It is not uncommon for these tumors to project into the bladder lumen as well as extend into the extravesical space. On MR, leiomyosarcomas may be low-signal intensity on T2-weighted imaging, similar to leiomyomas. They more often show necrosis and associated heterogeneous signal intensity and enhancement.

When feasible, treatment generally includes surgical excision. Systemic chemotherapy is used for metastatic disease.

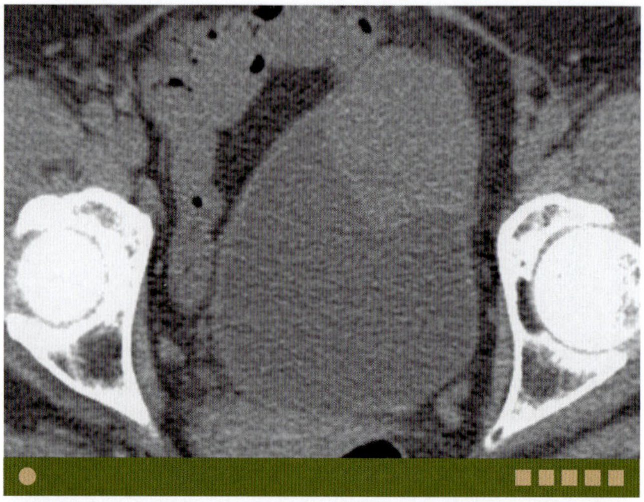

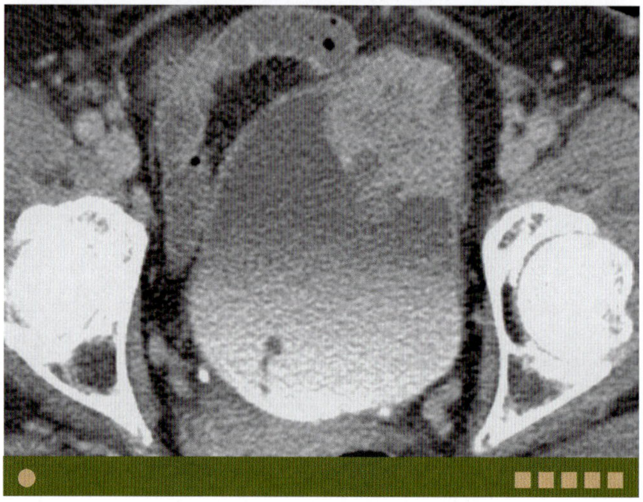

A. and **B.** Axial NECT and CECT show a large, heterogeneously enhancing mass involving the anterior aspect of the bladder dome. The mass extends into the bladder lumen and into the extravesical space.

PEARLS

- **Rare, high-grade, aggressive tumor accounts for less than 1% of bladder malignancies.**
- **Leiomyosarcoma and leiomyoma may have similar imaging characteristics.**
- **Larger size, margin irregularity, and heterogeneity favor a leiomyosarcoma.**

ADDITIONAL IMAGES (C-D)

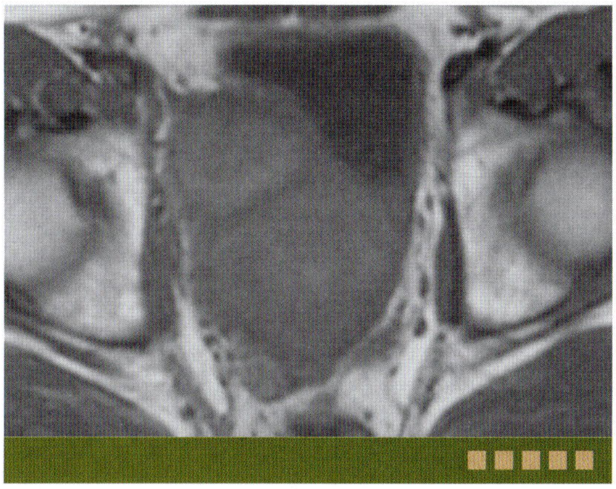

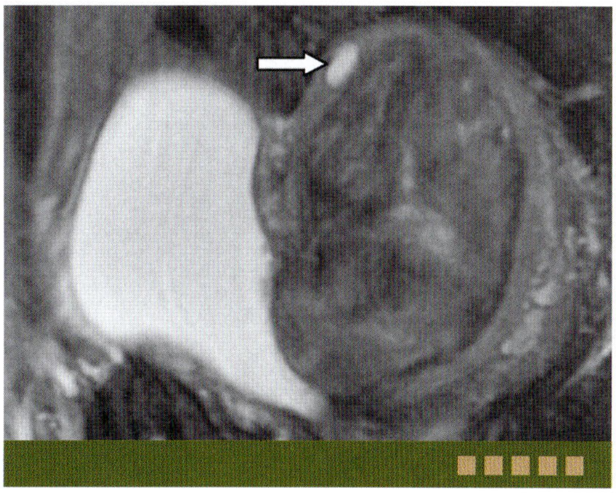

C. and **D.** Axial T1-WI and sagittal T2-WI show a large, heterogeneous mass extending from the posterior aspect of the bladder in a different patient. The tumor is predominantly low-signal intensity on the T2-WI and obstructs the right ureter (arrow).

DIFFERENTIAL DIAGNOSES IMAGES (E-G)

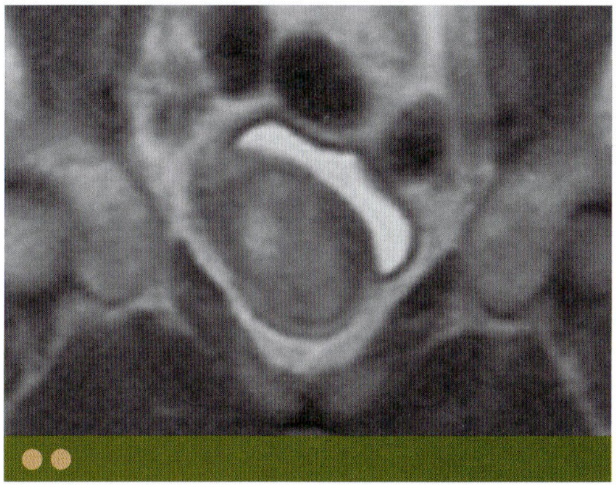

E. Leiomyoma: Coronal T2-WI shows a smoothly marginated, intramural mass of the right lateral bladder wall. It has a low-signal intensity periphery and higher signal intensity central area.

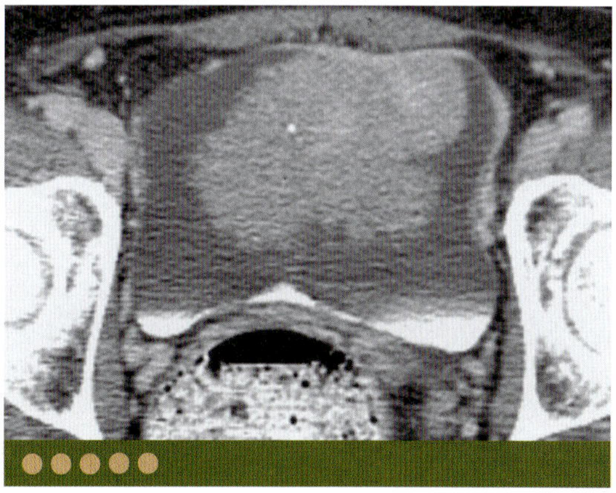

F. Urothelial carcinoma: Axial CECT shows a large, lobulated anterior bladder mass.

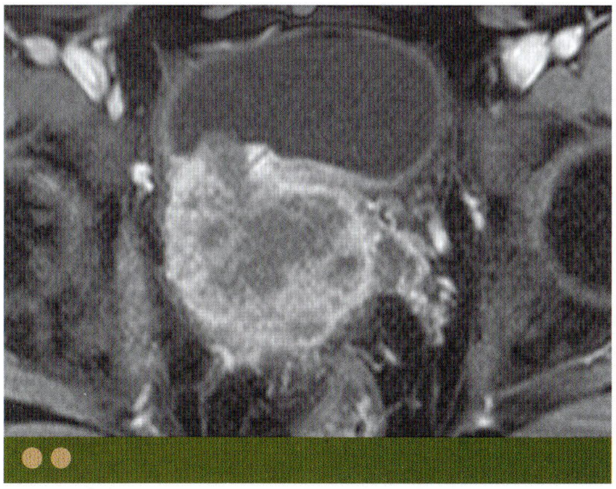

G. Metastasis: Axial contrast-enhanced T1-WI shows a large, heterogeneous mass involving the posterior aspect of the bladder. The mass proved to be an adenocarcinoma drop metastasis in this patient with a history of colon cancer and new hematuria.

IMAGE KEY

Common

Rare

Typical

Unusual

8–9 Paraganglioma of the Bladder

David D. Casalino

PRESENTATION

Hypertension, gross intermittent hematuria, attacks of sweating, headache, and palpitations induced by micturition.

FINDINGS

MR shows an enhancing round mass of the bladder dome.

DIFFERENTIAL DIAGNOSES

- *Other primary bladder neoplasm (malignant and benign)*: The epithelial tumors are much more common; tissue necessary for specific diagnosis.
- *Metastasis*: Usually known primary; direct spread from a colonic, cervical, prostatic, or rectal primary is more common than hematogeneous or lymphatic spread.
- *Focal inflammatory or infectious process*: Examples include focal cystitis, adjacent diverticulitis, and an infected urachal cyst; clinical features and associated imaging findings may suggest an inflammatory or infectious etiology.

COMMENTS

Paragangliomas, the preferred term for extra-adrenal pheochromocytomas, of the bladder account for 0.1% of bladder tumors and less than 1% of all pheochromocytomas. They arise from chromaffin cells and are most often located at the trigone, followed by the dome and lateral walls of the bladder. The age range is wide with a mean of 41 years, and the tumor is slightly more common in women. Most tumors are metabolically active, and patients with such tumors may present with hematuria, hypertension, elevated urine catecholamine levels, and micturition attacks. These attacks occur in 50% of patients, are induced by micturition, and may consist of headaches, anxiety, sweating, palpitations, and syncope with hypertension. While most cases of bladder paraganglioma are sporadic, others are associated with familial syndromes, including neurofibromatosis, von Hippel-Lindau syndrome, tuberous sclerosis, Sturge-Weber syndrome, and multiple endocrine neoplasia. Treatment consists of tumor excision after adrenergic blockage. Lymph node dissection is also performed for invasive tumors. Long-term follow-up is generally recommended because histology is not predictive of malignant behavior that occurs in at least 10% of the cases.

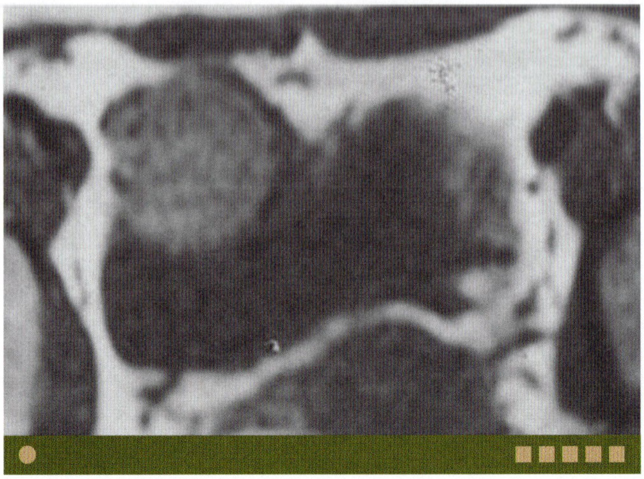

A. Axial contrast-enhanced T1-WI shows a round enhancing mass involving the anterosuperior aspect of the bladder and protruding into the extravesical space right of midline.

On radiologic studies, a bladder paraganglioma usually appears as a solid, homogeneous intramural mass with marked enhancement. Occasionally, the tumor will be heterogeneous because of necrosis or hemorrhage, and ring calcification around the circumference of the lesion is highly suggestive of a paraganglioma. On most imaging modalities, a bladder paraganglioma is indistinguishable from other tumor types; however, characteristic MRI features may help to distinguish this tumor from others. These tumors typically show markedly increased, homogeneous signal intensity on T2-WI and hypointense or isointense signal intensity on T1-WI.

Iodine 131 metaiodobenzylguanidine (MIBG) scanning is highly specific for paragangliomas but less sensitive than MRI.

PEARLS

- **Paragangliomas account for 0.1% of bladder tumors.**
- **Micturition attacks occur in 50% of the patients.**
- **Marked T2-WI hyperintensity is suggestive of the diagnosis.**
- **Iodine 131 MIBG scanning is very specific for paragangliomas but less sensitive than MRI.**

ADDITIONAL IMAGES (B-C)

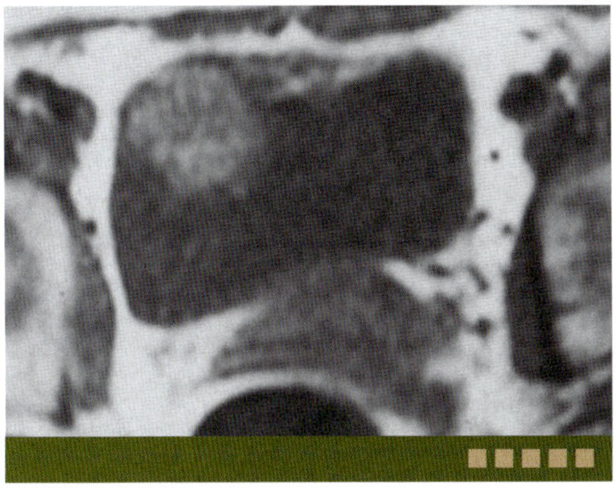

B. Axial contrast-enhanced T1-WI more caudad shows the mass projecting into the bladder lumen.

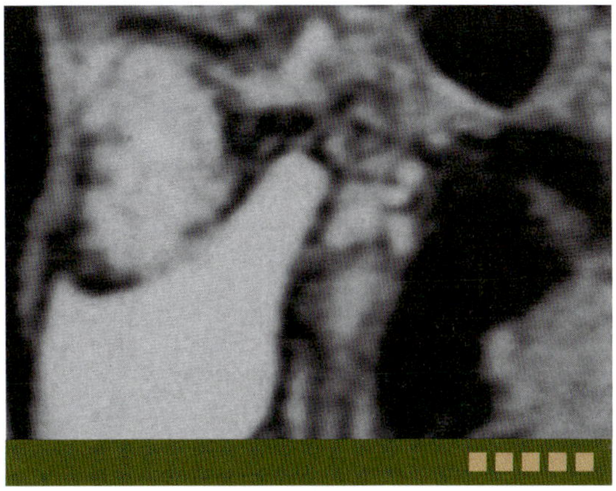

C. Sagittal T2-WI shows the mass to have very high signal intensity.

DIFFERENTIAL DIAGNOSES IMAGES (D-G)

IMAGE KEY

Common

Rare

Typical

Unusual

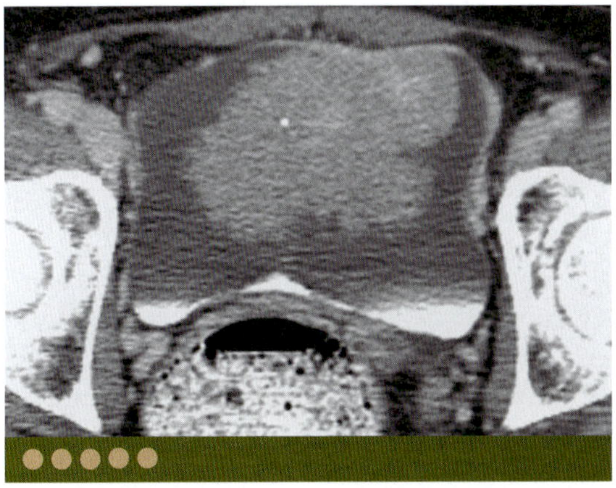

D. Urothelial carcinoma: Axial CECT shows a large, lobulated mass arising from the anterior aspect of the bladder.

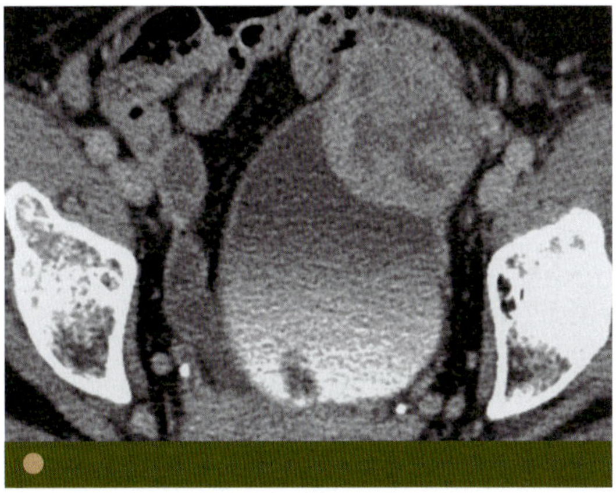

E. Bladder leiomyosarcoma: Axial CECT shows a large, heterogeneously enhancing mass arising from the anterosuperior aspect of the bladder.

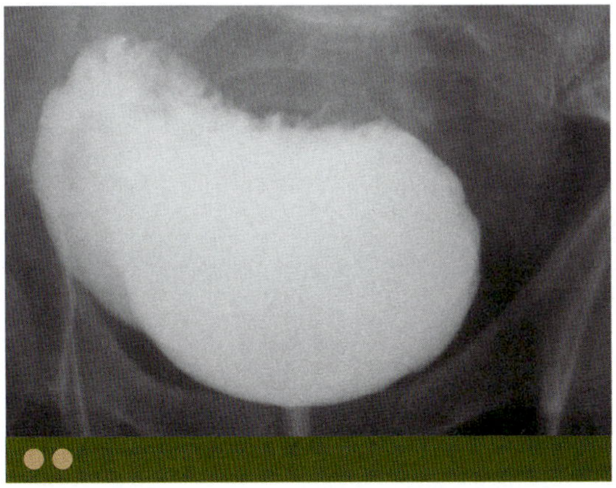

F. Metastasis: Cystogram shows very irregular mural thickening involving the bladder dome caused by invasion by an adjacent sigmoid colon adenocarcinoma.

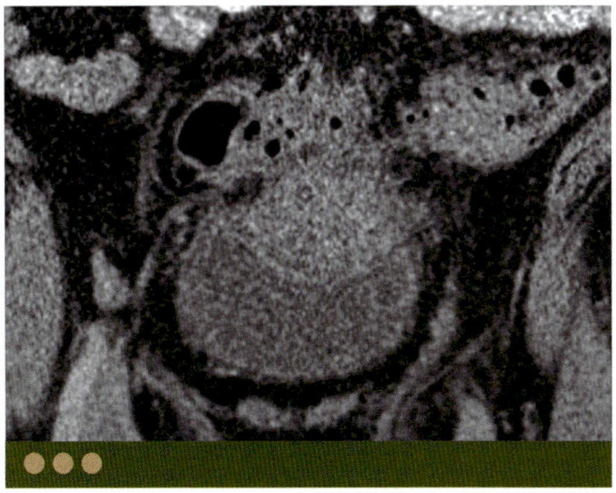

G. Sigmoid colonic diverticulitis: Coronal CECT shows an inflammatory mass involving the superior aspect of the bladder.

8–10 Bladder Leiomyoma

Frank H. Miller

PRESENTATION

Urinary frequency, pressure from mass effect, and hematuria.

FINDINGS

CECT shows smooth intramural mass caused by leiomyoma.

DIFFERENTIAL DIAGNOSIS

- *Transitional cell carcinoma*: Mucosal lesion not submucosal.

COMMENTS

Bladder leiomyomas are rare but are the most common benign bladder tumor. The tumors tend to grow intravesical (73%) but often are extravesical (30%) and less commonly intramural (7%). Most are small and asymptomatic. The lesions are seen on excretory urogram and cystography as well-defined smooth intraluminal masses. They may be detected incidentally on imaging studies such as CT. They tend to be homogeneous and solid masses. They often have smooth compression of the bladder or extend intraluminally. Cystic changes may be seen as the result of degeneration or necrosis. MR tends to be the most specific imaging test. The masses on MR tend to be isointense to the bladder wall. When associated with degeneration, the masses may have cystic components that are high-signal intensity on T2-WI. Following contrast administration, the enhancement pattern is variable: Some may show homogeneous enhancement and others show little or peripheral enhancement especially when associated with degeneration. The distinction between leiomyomas and leiomyosarcomas cannot be easily made at times. Features suggesting leiomyosarcoma include large size, heterogeneous enhancement, and irregular margins. The treatment is generally surgical excision of the masses. Preoperative imaging may help show the nonaggressive features and avoid extensive surgery.

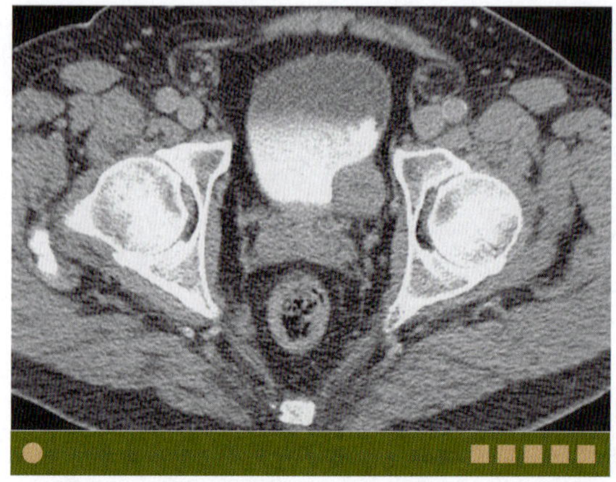

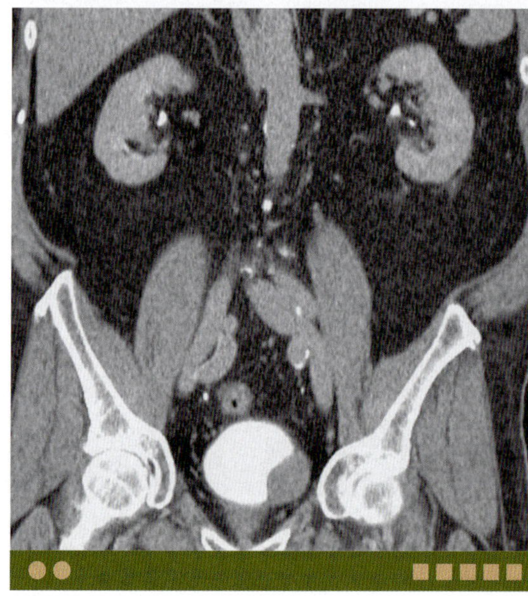

A. Axial CECT shows smooth intramural mass with appearance typical for leiomyoma.
B. Coronal CECT shows the mass along the left lateral aspect of the bladder

PEARLS

- **Bladder leiomyomas differ from more common TCC based on their submucosal location.**
- **Leiomyomas tend to be homogenous and solid masses on CT.**
- **On MR, leiomyomas tend to be isointense to the bladder wall unless when larger, where they may have cystic degeneration.**
- **Leiomyomas tend to have smooth margins.**

ADDITIONAL IMAGES (C-E)

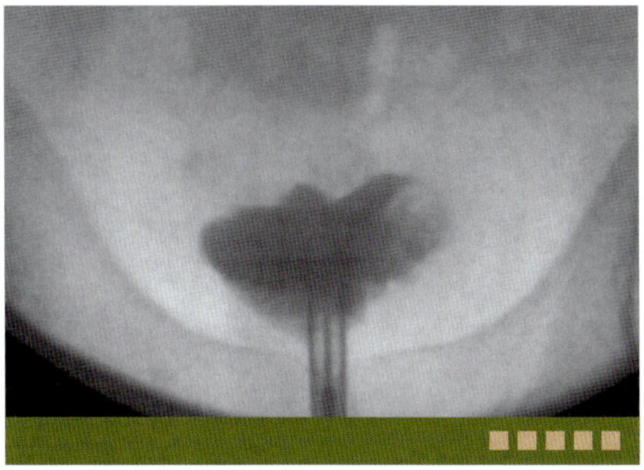

C. Cystogram shows bladder filling defect from leiomyoma.

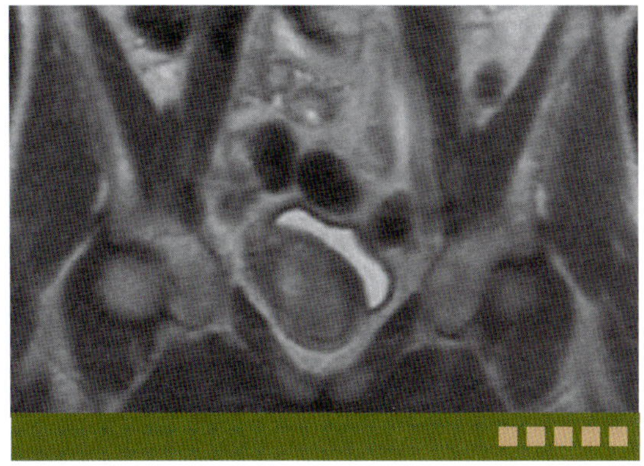

D. Coronal T2-WI from a different patient shows an intramural mass along the right lateral bladder. It has a low-signal intensity periphery and higher signal intensity central area.

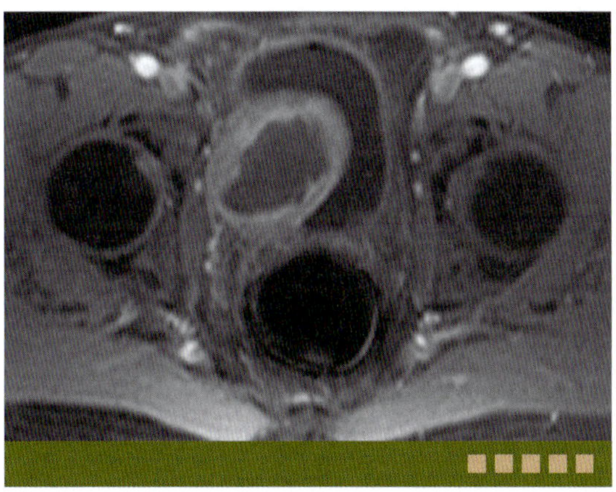

E. Axial contrast-enhanced T1-WI shows lack of enhancement of the necrotic central portion of the mass.

DIFFERENTIAL DIAGNOSIS IMAGES (F-G)

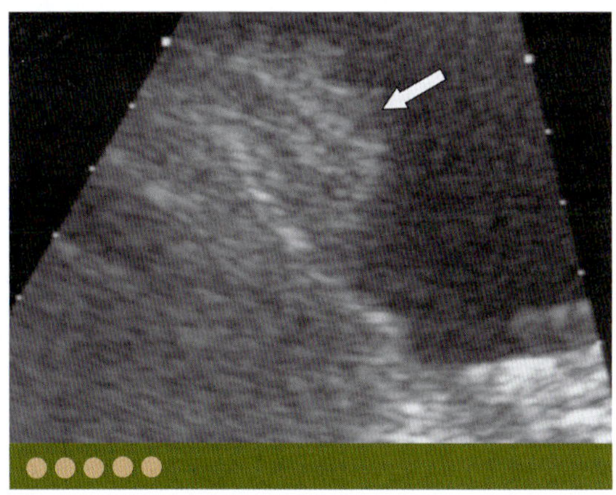

F. Transitional cancer of bladder: Transverse sonogram shows mucosal mass (arrow) caused by TCC.

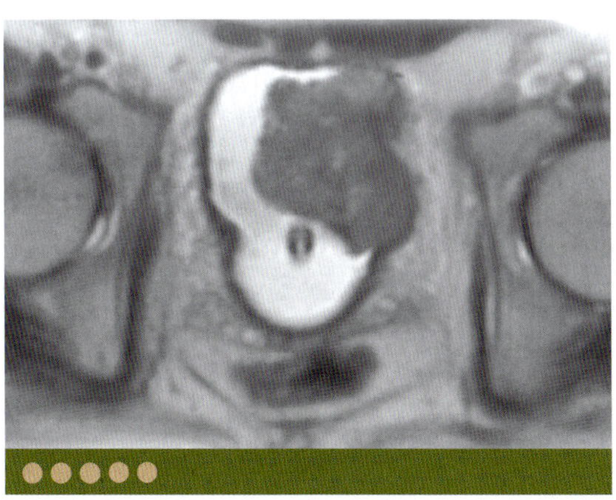

G. Transitional cancer of bladder: Axial T2-WI shows intermediate-signal intensity mass caused by TCC. The margins are ill-defined. The distinction is best made on biopsy with TCC far more common than leiomyomas.

IMAGE KEY

Common

Rare

Typical

Unusual

8–11 Bladder Diverticulum (Acquired)

David D. Casalino

PRESENTATION

Recurrent pelvic pain and gross hematuria.

FINDINGS

IVU images show a large outpouching of contrast along the left side of the bladder and a large, course calcification in the same location on the scout radiograph.

DIFFERENTIAL DIAGNOSES

- *Congenital*: Uncommon, usually single, paraureteral or arising from bladder apex.
- *Cystocele*: Abnormal descent of bladder neck and trigone; urethra may prolapse as well; may be associated with bladder outlet obstruction or hydronephrosis.
- *Bladder hernia*: Uncommon; through the inguinal canal is most common (70%), followed by herniation through the femoral canal (25%).
- *Bladder fistula or contained leak*: Etiologies may be infectious, inflammatory, neoplastic, traumatic, or iatrogenic; often irregular margins; clinical history and associated imaging findings often suggest an etiology.

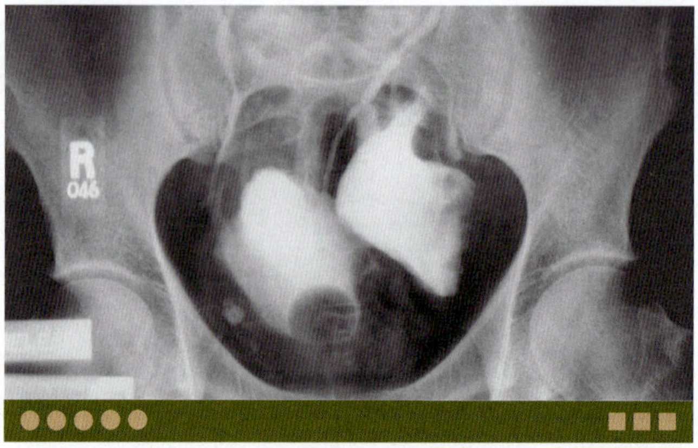

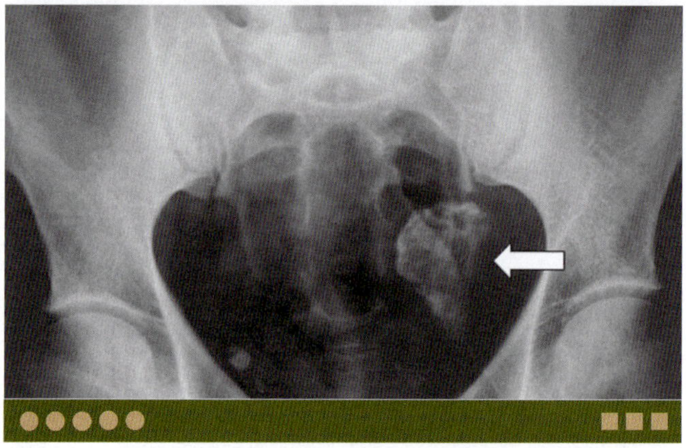

A. IVU shows a large outpouching of contrast from the left lateral aspect of the bladder. This outpouching is associated with medial deviation of the distal left ureter and has an irregular lateral aspect. **B.** IVU scout image shows a large, course calcification (arrow) in the left hemipelvis. It is a stone that has formed in the bladder diverticulum and accounts for the diverticulum's irregularity.

COMMENTS

Bladder diverticula are common and increase in incidence with age. Most are acquired as a result of bladder outlet obstruction and increased intravesical pressure. This increased pressure causes the bladder urothelium and submucosa to herniate through the muscle layer and form an outpouching. When small, these outpouchings are referred to as cellules. When larger and protruding beyond the outer margin of the bladder, they are referred to as diverticula. Acquired diverticula are often multiple but may be single. Congenital diverticula are uncommon and typically single. These include Hutch diverticula, that typically arise from the posterolateral aspect of the bladder (paraureteral), and vesicourachal diverticula that arise from the bladder apex at the midline. Diverticula may be associated with urinary stasis and increased risk of urinary tract infection, stone formation, and chronic irritation and carcinoma. If large, a diverticulum may displace or obstruct the pelvic ureters.

A bladder diverticulum appears as a round or oval outpouching of the bladder wall and usually has a smooth inner wall. A neck connects the diverticulum to the bladder. The narrower the neck, the more likely is the occurrence of urinary stasis and complications. Diverticula are more likely to fill with contrast on a cystogram than on IVU or CECT or MR that includes an excretory phase. On ultrasound, a diverticulum will typically appear anechoic, unless complicated, and communication with the bladder may be apparent. Color Doppler imaging may show signal from urine moving between the bladder and diverticulum.

PEARLS

- **Bladder diverticula are common, increase with age, and are usually acquired as a result of increased intravesical pressure.**
- **Potential complications relate to urinary stasis and include infection, stone formation, and carcinoma.**
- **Uncomplicated bladder diverticula are smooth, round or oval outpouchings of the bladder.**

ADDITIONAL IMAGES (C-E)

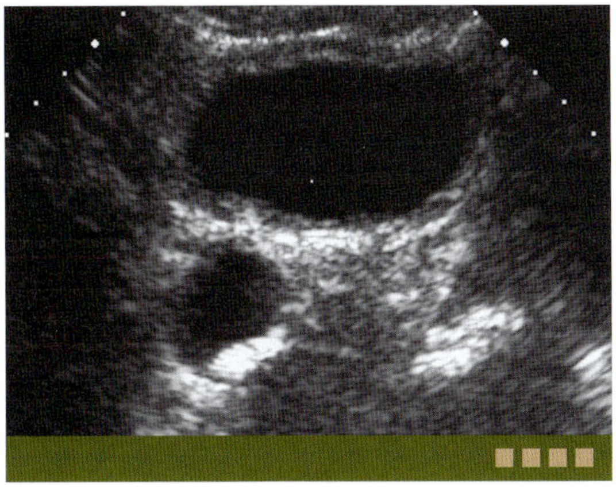

C. Transverse sonogram shows a round, anechoic mass posterior to the bladder. This diverticulum contains two echogenic calculi.

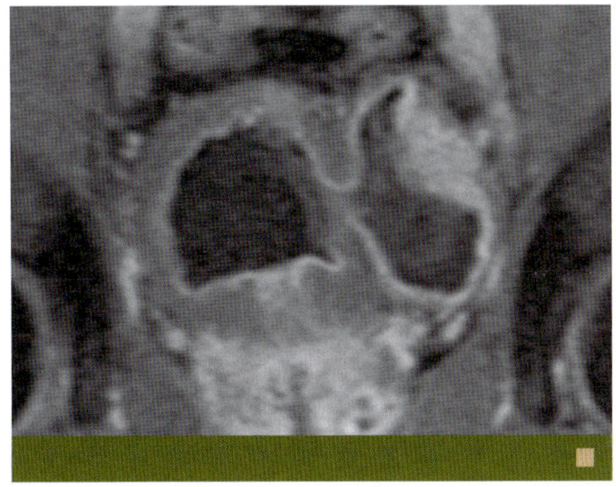

D. Coronal contrast-enhanced T1-WI shows a large, left-sided bladder diverticulum with an enhancing carcinoma arising from its lateral wall.

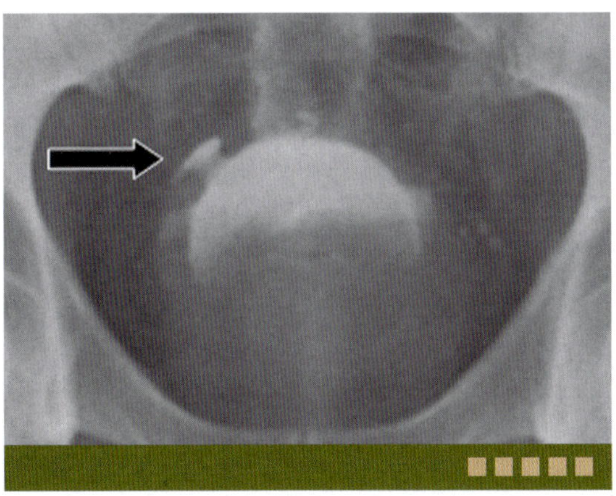

E. IVU shows marked mass effect from an enlarged prostate and several cellules, the largest (arrow) of which extends to but not beyond the outer margin of the thickened bladder wall.

DIFFERENTIAL DIAGNOSES IMAGES (F-H)

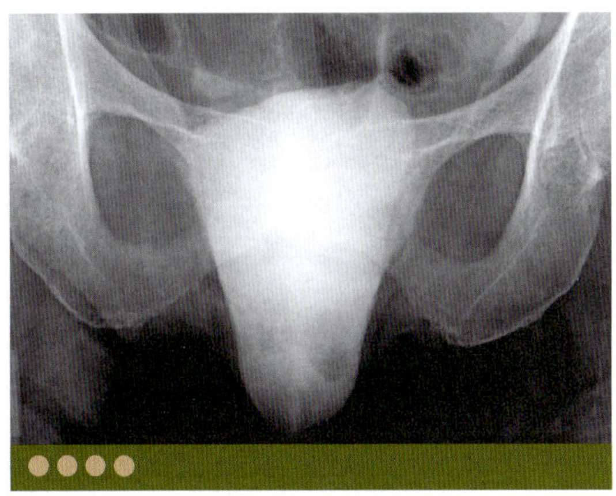

F. Cystocele: IVU during Valsalva maneuver shows prominent, mid-line descent of the bladder well below the level of the pubic symphysis.

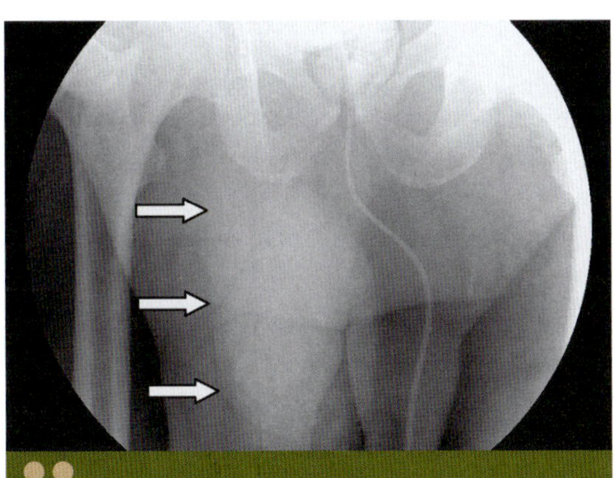

G. Bladder hernia: Cystogram shows the bladder (arrows) extending through the right inguinal canal and into the right hemiscrotum.

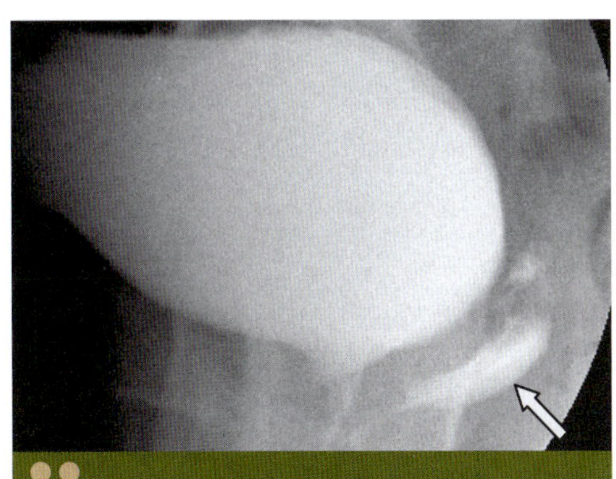

H. Vesicovaginal fistula: Cystogram, sagittal, shows contrast extending from the posterior aspect of the bladder and into the vagina (arrow) in patients with vaginal drainage after emergent cesarean section.

IMAGE KEY

Common

●●●●●
●●●●
●●●
●●
●

Rare

Typical

■■■■■
■■■■
■■■
■■
■

Unusual

8–12 Bladder Diverticulum (Congenital)

David D. Casalino

PRESENTATION

Asymptomatic, but may present with UTI or hematuria.

FINDINGS

NECT shows a small fluid-density mass along the right posterolateral aspect of the bladder.

DIFFERENTIAL DIAGNOSES

- *Acquired bladder diverticulum*: More common; increase with age; often multiple; same potential complications; no typical location.
- *Perivesical fluid collection*: Examples include hematoma, abscess and lymphocele; will not fill with bladder contrast; may be multiple; clinical history may be helpful.
- *Everted ureterocele*: Uncommon; in continuity with ureter.
- *Cystic mass of perivesical organ*: Examples include ovarian or paraovarian cystic mass and paraprostatic cysts; will not fill with bladder contrast.

COMMENTS

Congenital diverticula are uncommon and typically single. Diverticula form as a result of bladder mucosa herniating through the muscle layer of the bladder. Congenital diverticula include Hutch diverticula that typically arise from the posterolateral aspect of the bladder (paraureteral). Hutch diverticula may be small to very large in size and may cause ipsilateral ureteral obstruction or vesicoureteral reflux. Vesicourachal diverticulum is a congenital anomaly because of the failure of closure of the urachus at the bladder. It arises from the bladder apex at the midline. These diverticula may be associated with prune-belly syndrome. Diverticula may be associated with urinary stasis and increased risk of UTI, stone formation, and carcinoma.

A bladder diverticulum appears as a round or oval outpouching of the bladder wall.

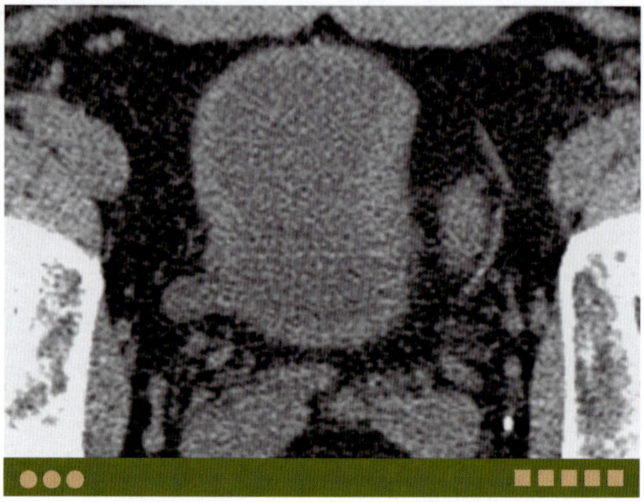

A. Axial NECT shows a small fluid-density mass along the right posterolateral aspect of the bladder.

A neck connects the diverticulum to the bladder. The narrower the neck, the more likely there will be urinary stasis and complications. Diverticula will usually fill with contrast on a cystogram or CT or MR that includes an excretory phase.

PEARLS

- **Congenital diverticula are uncommon and usually single.**
- **Hutch diverticula are typically located slightly above and lateral to the ureteral orifice.**
- **Vesicourachal diverticulum arises from the bladder apex at the midline.**
- **Potential complications relate to urinary stasis and include infection, stone formation, and carcinoma.**

ADDITIONAL IMAGES (B-D)

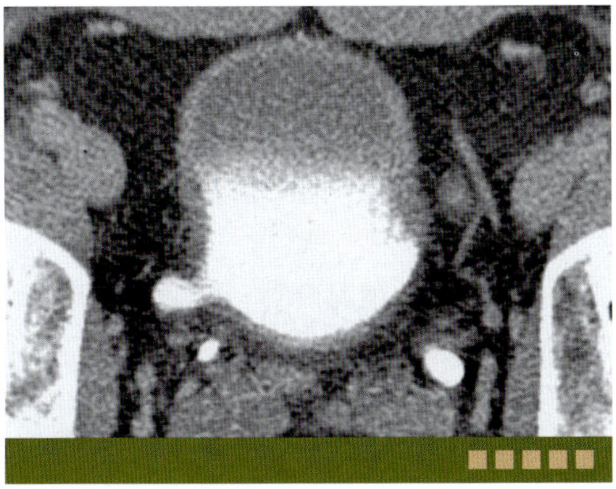

B. Axial CECT during excretory phase shows the mass to be a bladder diverticulum that fills with excreted contrast. The contrast-filled right-sided ureter is separate from the diverticulum.

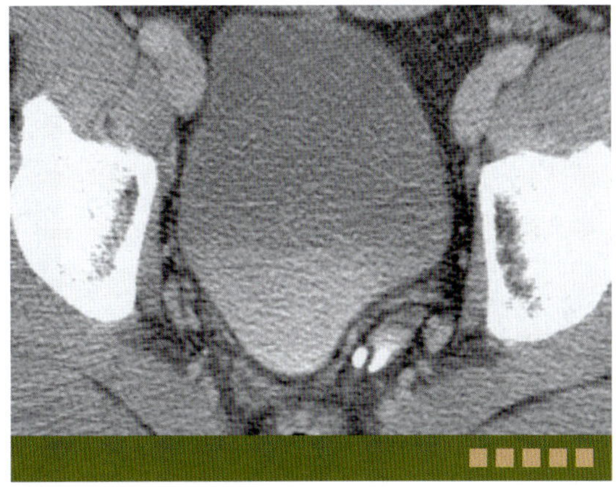

C. Axial CECT during excretory phase from a different patient shows a small left-sided Hutch diverticulum that abuts the anterior aspect of the left ureter.

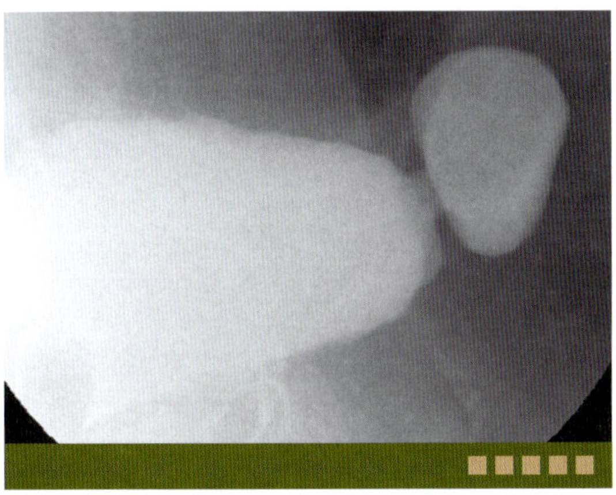

D. Cystogram, lateral view, shows a vesicourachal diverticulum arising from the bladder apex at the midline.

DIFFERENTIAL DIAGNOSES IMAGES (E-G)

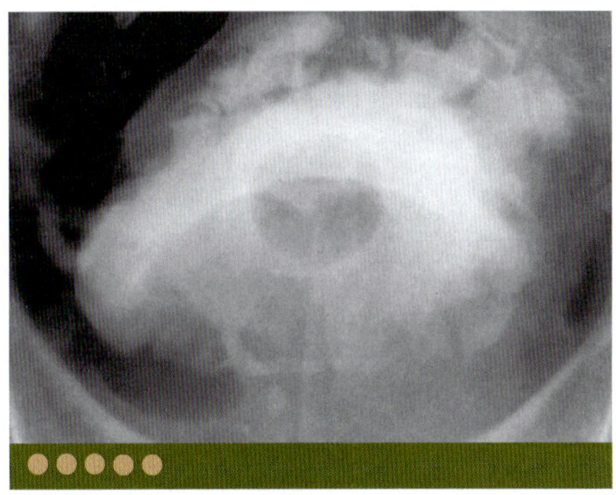

E. Acquired bladder diverticula: Cystogram shows numerous diverticula arising from the superior aspect of the bladder and mass effect from a markedly enlarged prostate.

IMAGE KEY

Common

Rare

Typical

Unusual

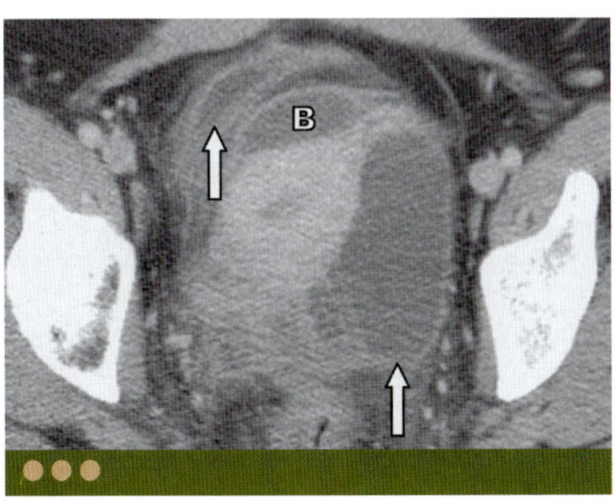

F. Pelvic abscess: Axial CECT shows two abscesses (arrows) adjacent to the bladder (B) in patients with fever, pelvic pain, and a history of pelvic inflammatory disease.

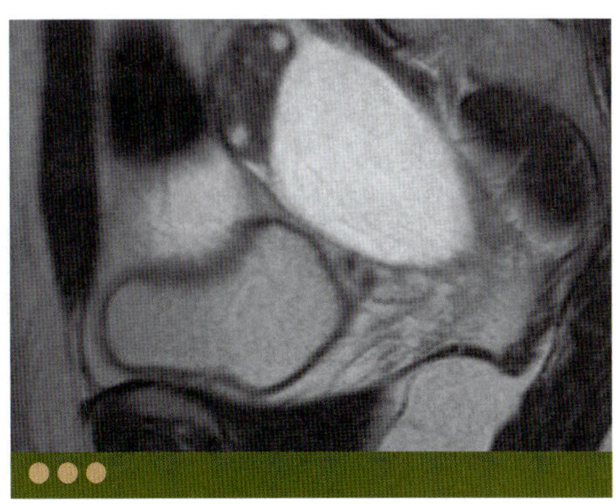

G. Hydrosalpinx: Sagittal T2-WI shows a large cystic mass posterior to the bladder and adjacent to the ovary. Its signal intensity is greater than the bladder content. Continuity with the bladder is not seen.

8–13 Infected Urachal Cyst

David D. Casalino

PRESENTATION

Lower abdominal pain, fever, and dysuria.

FINDINGS

CT shows a round mass with air-fluid level involving the anterosuperior aspect of the bladder.

DIFFERENTIAL DIAGNOSES

- *Diverticular abscess*: Associated with abnormality of involved bowel segment.
- *Bladder diverticulum*: Should have continuity with bladder lumen; usually asymptomatic; typically does not contain gas unless recent instrumentation.
- *Urachal carcinoma*: Solid mass, usually asymptomatic or present with painless hematuria.

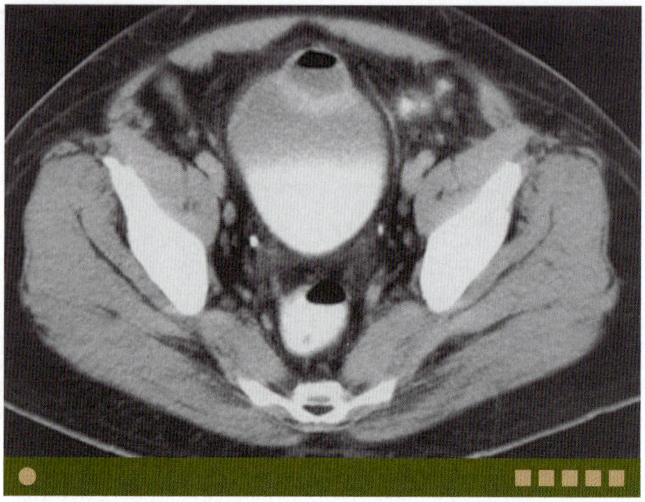

A. Axial CECT shows a thick-walled, cystic lesion with air-fluid level involving the anterosuperior aspect of the bladder. The abnormality is midline and associated with mild stranding of the adjacent perivesical fat.

COMMENTS

In a fetus, the urachus connects the anterosuperior aspect of the bladder to the allantoic duct at the level of the umbilicus. It is an extraperitoneal structure located behind the abdominal wall and anterior to the peritoneum. Before birth, the urachus normally obliterates to form the median umbilical ligament. Anomalies of urachal closure include patent urachus, umbilical urachal sinus, vesicourachal diverticulum, and urachal cyst.

Patent urachus is the most common of these anomalies, is usually diagnosed in the newborn, and may be associated with bladder outlet obstruction caused by posterior urethral valve or urethral atresia. Urachal anomalies retain a mucosal lining that is most often transitional cell urothelium and may give rise to malignancy, most often adenocarcinoma.

An urachal cyst forms when a portion of the urachus remains patent and fluid filled between umbilical and vesical ends that have closed. These cysts tend to form closer to the bladder. Urachal cysts are often asymptomatic until complicated by infection or, rarely, tumor. Pain, fever, dysuria, and palpable mass are clinical findings that might be associated with an infected cyst. Rarely, an infected cyst may drain out the umbilicus.

On imaging, uncomplicated urachal cysts appear as simple cysts in the midline adjacent to or slightly above the anterosuperior aspect of the bladder. When complicated, these cysts are often higher in attenuation than simple fluid and heterogeneous and may show thickened walls or a soft tissue component. Gas formation may be seen in infection as well. Treatment involves antibiotics and excision of the urachal remnant to avoid recurrence of the cyst or occurrence of malignancy in the remnant.

PEARLS

- **Urachal anomalies have characteristic locations.**
- **Urachal cysts may be complicated by infection or malignancy.**
- **Infected cysts are typically heterogeneous and may show mural thickening and contain gas.**
- **Treatment of an infected urachal cyst includes excision.**

ADDITIONAL IMAGES (B-C)

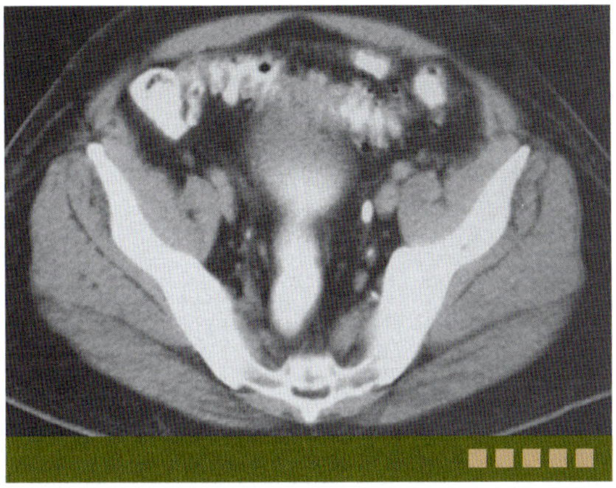

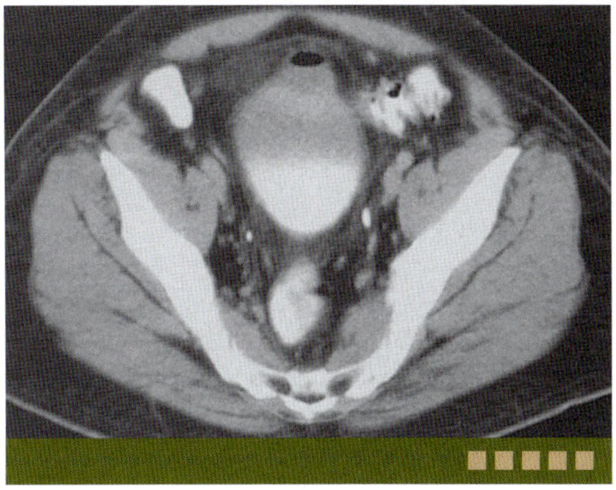

B. and **C.** Axial CECT more cephalad, show a few diverticula of the sigmoid colon, which does not show mural thickening, and additional stranding of anterior perivesical fat.

DIFFERENTIAL DIAGNOSES IMAGES (D-G)

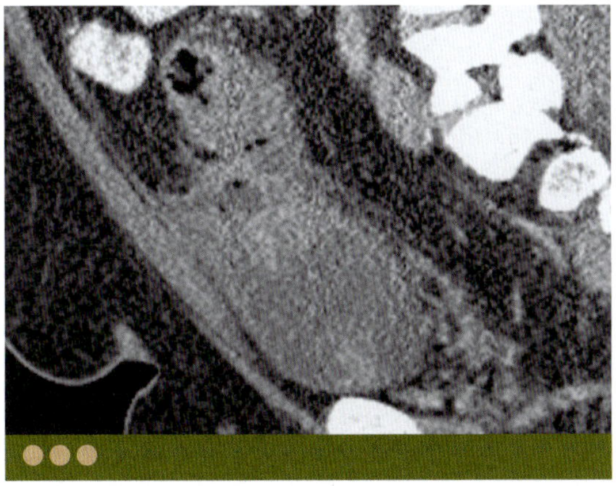

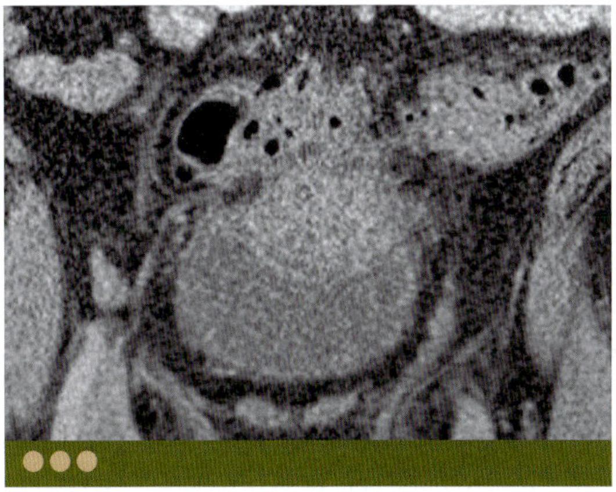

D. and **E. Diverticular abscess:** Sagittal and coronal NECT show sigmoid colonic diverticulitis with an associated gas-containing abscess involving the anterosuperior aspect of the bladder.

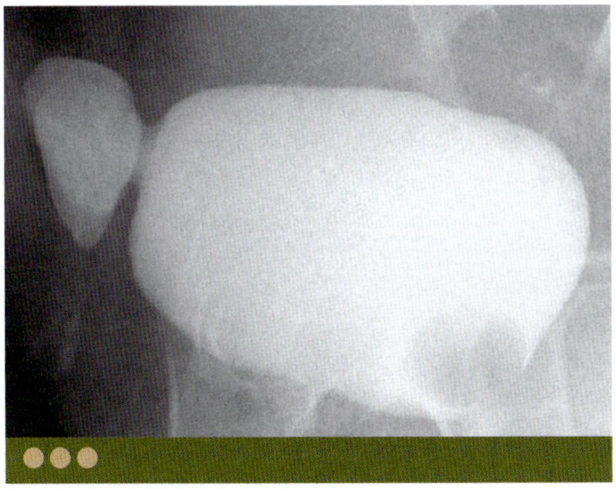

F. Vesicourachal diverticulum: Cystogram, lateral view, shows a diverticulum arising from the bladder apex at the midline.

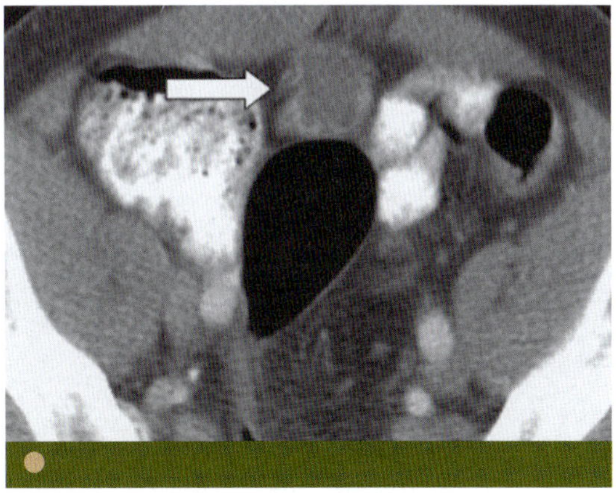

G. Urachal carcinoma: Axial CECT shows an enhancing mass (arrow) with central low attenuation in a patient with gross, painless hematuria. The mass arises from the anterosuperior aspect of the bladder.

IMAGE KEY

Common

Rare

Typical

Unusual

8–14 Infectious Cystitis

David D. Casalino

PRESENTATION

Dysuria, hematuria, and urinary frequency.

FINDINGS

CT shows diffuse bladder wall thickening.

DIFFERENTIAL DIAGNOSES

- *Noninfectious cystitis*: Clinical history and associated imaging findings often suggest the etiology.
- *Bladder cancer*: Often focal; more common in older patients; tissue may be necessary for differentiation.
- *Bladder outlet obstruction*: More common in men and usually because of BPH; cellules and diverticula may be seen.
- *Bladder wall prominence because of limited distention*: Usually an incidental finding.

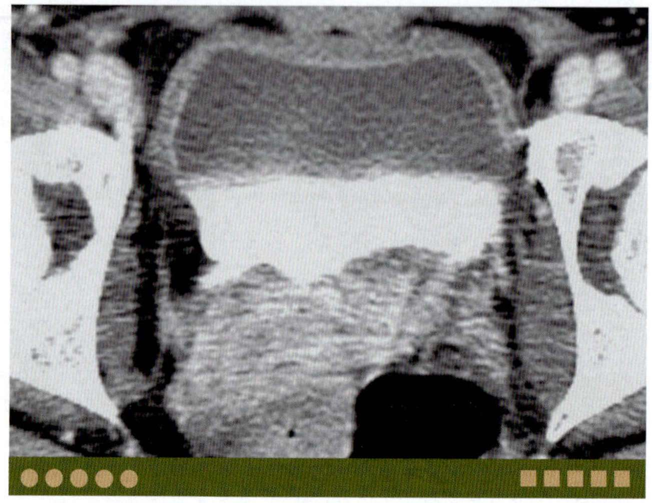

A. Axial CECT during excretory phase shows diffuse, uniform bladder wall thickening in women with a history of chronic recurrent bacterial cystitis.

COMMENTS

Cystitis is inflammation of the bladder. It may involve the entire bladder, referred to as pancystitis, or less commonly, may be focal. Cystitis may have an infectious or noninfectious etiology. Noninfectious etiologies include irritation from foreign body or stone, drug therapy, and RT. Infectious cystitis is most often caused by a bacterial infection which is caused by *Escherichia coli*. *Klebsiella* and *Pseudomonas* are also common pathogens. Bacterial cystitis is most often seen in sexually active women. It is presumed that intercourse causes retrograde spread of the normal bacterial flora of the vagina. Bacterial cystitis in men is usually associated with bacterial prostatitis or bladder outlet obstruction. Other pathogens include viruses, fungi, and parasites. Patients with acute cystitis may present with urinary frequency and urgency, dysuria, hematuria, and pyuria. Potential complications of cystitis include emphysematous cystitis, cystitis cystica and cystitis glandularis, and squamous metaplasia.

Cystitis may be acute or chronic. Acute cystitis refers to inflammation with recent onset of symptoms and shorter duration. Chronic cystitis refers to inflammation of longer duration, usually many months to years. Image of acute cystitis is not uncommonly normal despite mucosal abnormalities being present on cystoscopy. If the cystitis is severe or chronic, the bladder may demonstrate wall thickening that is irregular and appears hypodense on CT, hypoechoic on ultrasound, and hyperintense on T2-weighted MR imaging. The bladder may also show increased post-gadolinium enhancement. Bladder capacity may be decreased. There may also be decreased bladder compliance that may be associated with vesicoureteral reflux and hydroureter. Focal cystitis may mimic a bladder carcinoma.

PEARLS

- **Infectious cystitis is most often caused by *E coli*.**
- **Bacterial cystitis is most often diagnosed in sexually active women.**
- **Imaging of acute cystitis is often normal.**
- **Focal cystitis may mimic a bladder neoplasm.**

ADDITIONAL IMAGES (B-D)

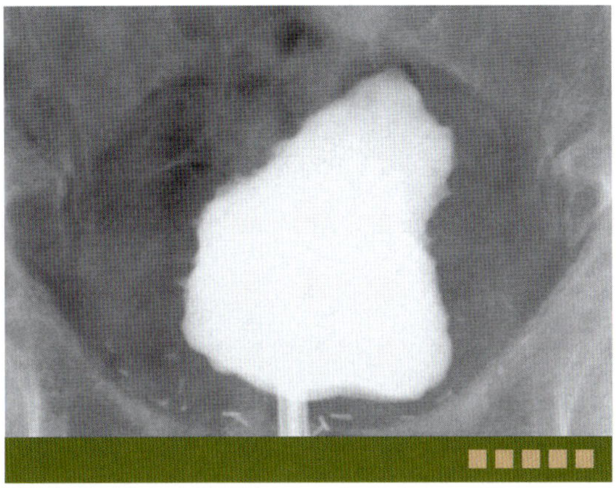

B. Cystogram shows diffuse bladder wall thickening and irregularity. Bladder capacity is also slightly decreased.

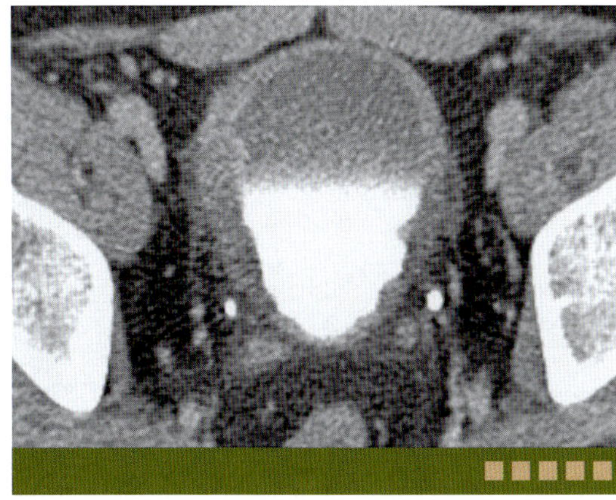

C. Axial CECT during excretory phase shows bladder wall irregularity and thickening that is non-uniform with greater thickening of the posterior and lateral walls. Biopsy confirmed BK virus-associated cystitis in patient status post stem cell transplantation.

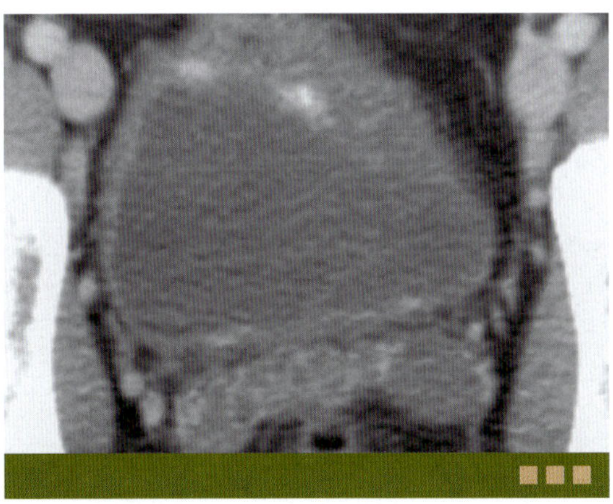

D. Axial CECT shows focal anterior bladder wall thickening and irregularity secondary to adjacent diverticulitis.

DIFFERENTIAL DIAGNOSES IMAGES (E-G)

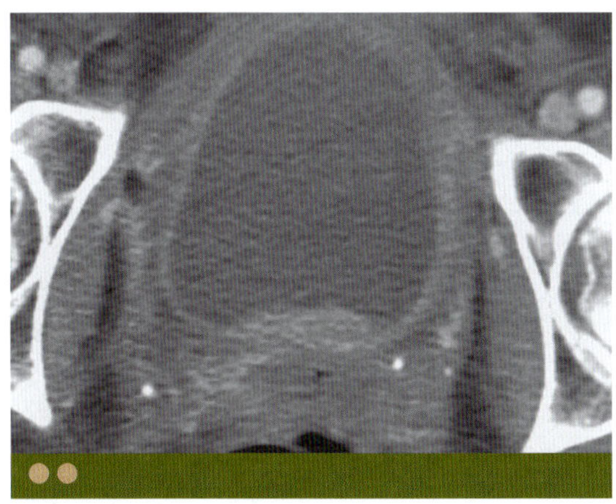

E. Radiation-induced cystitis: Axial CECT shows diffuse bladder wall thickening and increased attenuation of the perivesical fat in patients who received RT for cervical cancer.

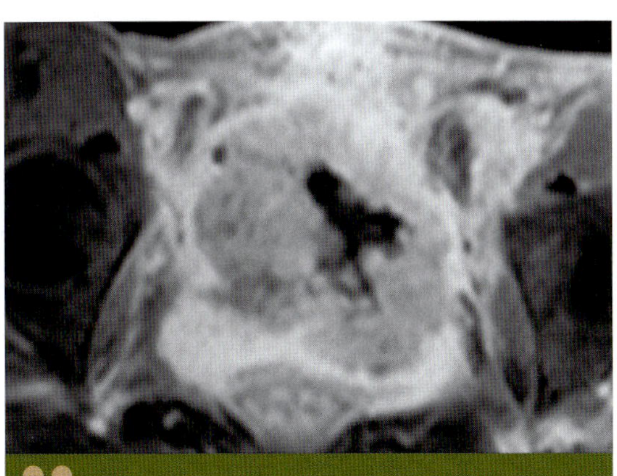

F. Squamous cell carcinoma: Axial contrast-enhanced T1-WI shows marked, heterogeneous bladder wall thickening caused by an infiltrative cancer. The tumor extends into the anterior perivesical space.

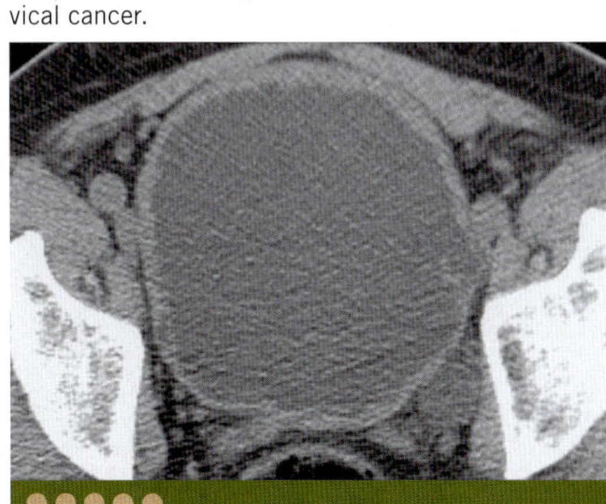

G. Bladder outlet obstruction: Axial CECT shows mild diffuse bladder wall thickening and trabeculation in a patient with BPH.

IMAGE KEY

Common

Rare

Typical

Unusual

8–15 Emphysematous Cystitis

Frank H. Miller

PRESENTATION

Diabetic, dysuria, abdominal pain, hematuria, and fever.

FINDINGS

CT image shows air within bladder wall.

DIFFERENTIAL DIAGNOSIS

- *Air in bladder from recent instrumentation or fistula with small bowel, colon, or vagina*: Air is in lumen and not in bladder wall.

COMMENTS

Emphysematous cystitis is rare form of infection of the bladder associated with gas in the wall of the bladder. It is generally seen in immunosuppressed or elderly and debilitated patients. The majority are diabetics. It is most often a result of *E Coli* infection but can be associated with other gas-forming organisms including *Enterobacter aerogenes*, *Staphylococcus aureus*, *Streptococci* species, *Nocardia* species, and *Candida albicans*. Patients may be relatively asymptomatic or have acute abdominal pain. Unlike emphysematous pyelonephritis, the condition is not life-threatening. The treatment is generally intravenous antibiotics and management of the patient's diabetes and usually the patient responds. If undetected, it can lead to septicemia, bladder rupture, and death.

Conventional radiographs show air within the bladder wall often as curvilinear radiolucencies. The diagnosis is easily made on CT by the presence of air in the wall of the bladder. The bladder wall may appear thickened and irregular because of associated inflammation and edema. Occasionally, the gas can extend into the ureter or area surrounding the bladder. When air is seen within the bladder lumen and not within the wall of the bladder, other causes including recent instrumentation from Foley catheter, cystoscopy, infections, or fistula with the colon, small bowel or vagina should be considered.

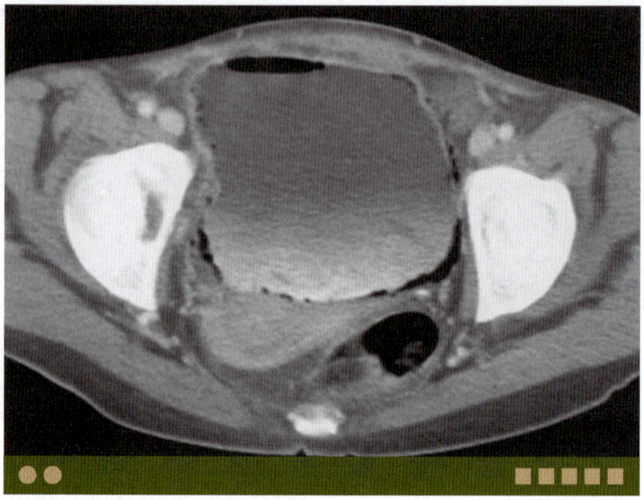

A. Axial CECT shows air within the bladder wall.

PEARLS

- **Emphysematous cystitis should be suspected when air is seen in the wall of the bladder.**
- **It is generally caused by *E coli* infection.**
- **Emphysematous cystitis can be distinguished from recent instrumentation or fistulas as air is in the wall with emphysematous cystitis and in the lumen in the other conditions.**

ADDITIONAL IMAGES (B-D)

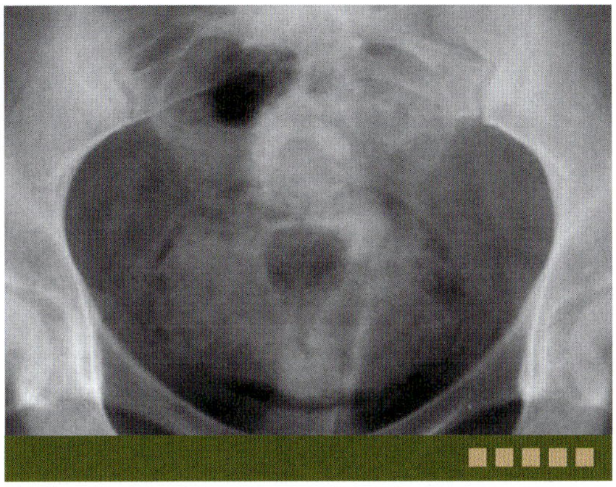

B. Coned-down pelvic radiograph shows air outlining bladder wall in a different patient with diabetes and emphysematous cystitis.

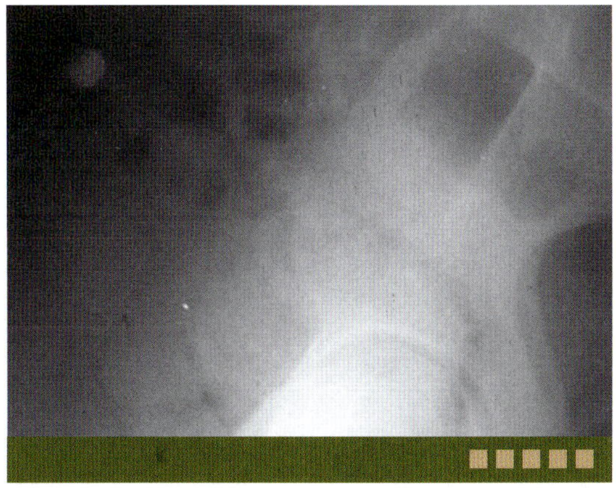

C. Lateral pelvic radiograph of the same patient as in Figure B.

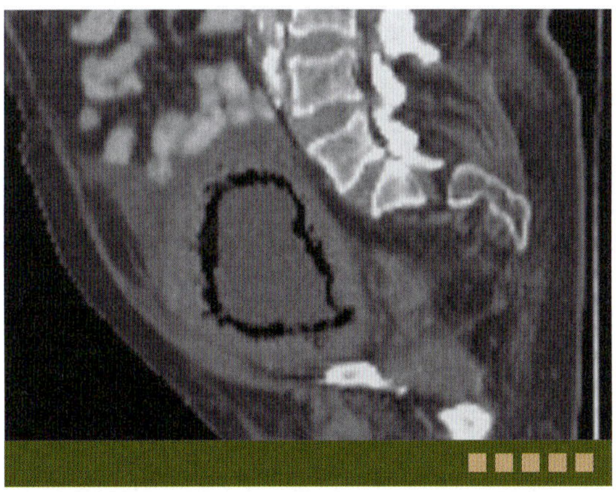

D. Sagittal multiplanar reformatted CECT shows air in the bladder wall in the patient with emphysematous cystitis.

DIFFERENTIAL DIAGNOSIS IMAGE

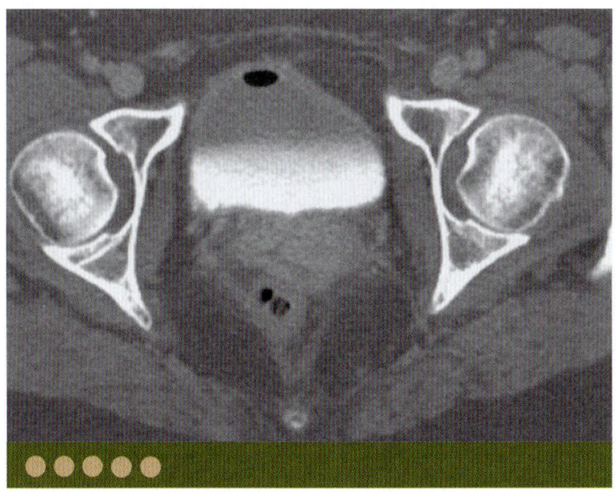

E. Recent Foley catheter in bladder: Axial CECT shows air in the bladder lumen from recent instrumentation.

IMAGE KEY

Common

Rare

Typical

Unusual

8–16 Hemorrhagic Cystitis

David D. Casalino

PRESENTATION

Gross hematuria, dysuria, and frequency.

FINDINGS

T1-weighted MR image shows diffuse bladder wall thickening and hyperintensity in the bladder lumen, consistent with hemorrhage.

DIFFERENTIAL DIAGNOSES

- *Bladder cancer with associated hematoma*: Often focal mass; more common in older patients; tissue may be necessary for differentiation.
- *Bladder hematoma*: Bladder wall usually with normal thickness; clot will not enhance and may move with patient repositioning; etiologies include instrumentation, trauma, stone disease, upper collecting system neoplasm, anticoagulation, and coagulopathy.

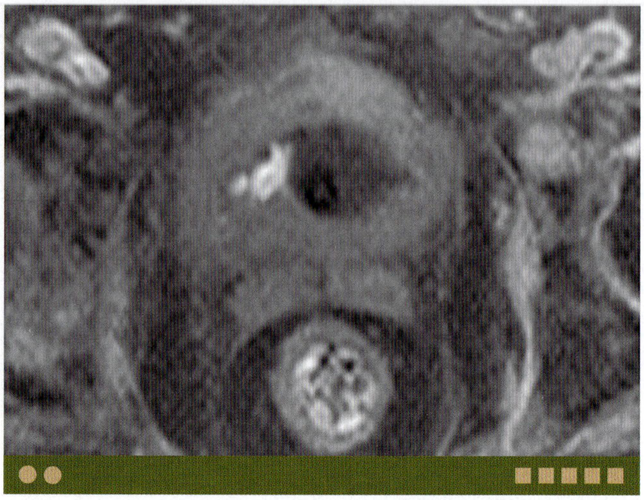

A. Axial T1-WI shows diffuse bladder wall thickening and irregularity and hyperintense hemorrhage in the lumen. There is also a bladder catheter. The patient had a history of pelvic RT for prostate cancer.

COMMENTS

Hemorrhagic cystitis is defined as diffuse vesical bleeding. The most common causes of hemorrhagic cystitis are RT and chemotherapeutic agents. Radiation cystitis most often occurs after external RT for cervical or prostate cancer; although it may occur after RT for rectal or bladder cancers. Twenty percent of patients who receive pelvic RT develop bladder symptoms, including frequency, urgency, dysuria, and hematuria. In acute radiation cystitis, the changes to the bladder are nonspecific in terms of imaging features. Often the bladder wall is thickened and the contour is irregular because of edema and hemorrhage. Mucosal ulcerations may occur as well. Filling defects because of blood clots may be seen. Bladder wall inflammation and edema result in increased signal intensity on T2-weighted images. Delayed radiation cystitis may develop up to 4 years following RT. The imaging features are dominated by extensive fibrosis. The fibrosis results in bladder wall thickening, reduced capacity, and, occasionally, upper tract obstruction. Fistulas may occur. Mural calcifications are rare.

Oxazaphosphorine alkylating agents, such as cyclophosphamide and ifosfamide, are agents most commonly linked to hemorrhagic cystitis. Bladder symptoms usually begin during or soon after chemotherapy is completed. The imaging features are similar to those of acute radiation cystitis. Marked bladder contraction and invasive urothelial carcinoma may develop months or years after therapy. Mural calcifications are more common than in RT and may be similar to those seen in schistosomiasis.

Treatment for hemorrhagic cystitis is supportive and may involve blood transfusion, bladder irrigation to prevent urinary tract obstruction, and instillation of agents such as alum and formalin. In more severe cases, vascular embolization or cystectomy may be warranted.

PEARLS

- **Hemorrhagic cystitis occurs usually as the result of RT or chemotherapy.**
- **Approximately 20% of patients who receive pelvic RT develop bladder symptoms.**
- **Prolonged cyclophosphamide use is associated with a 5% incidence of invasive urothelial carcinoma.**
- **Imaging features may include bladder wall thickening and irregularity, blood clots, reduced bladder capacity, and mural calcifications.**

ADDITIONAL IMAGES (B-D)

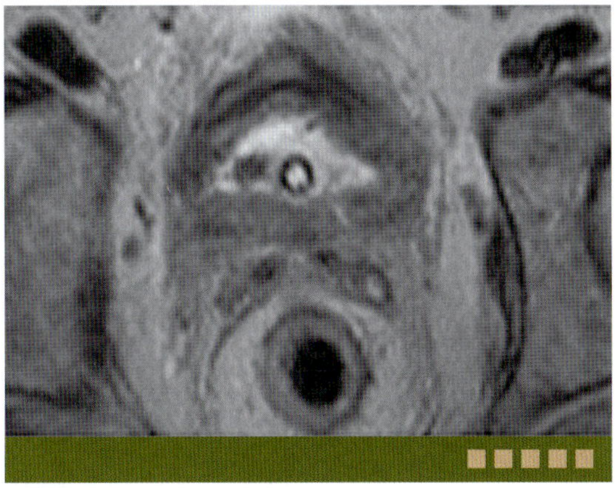

B. Axial T2-WI shows the thickened bladder wall to be hyperintense and heterogeneous.

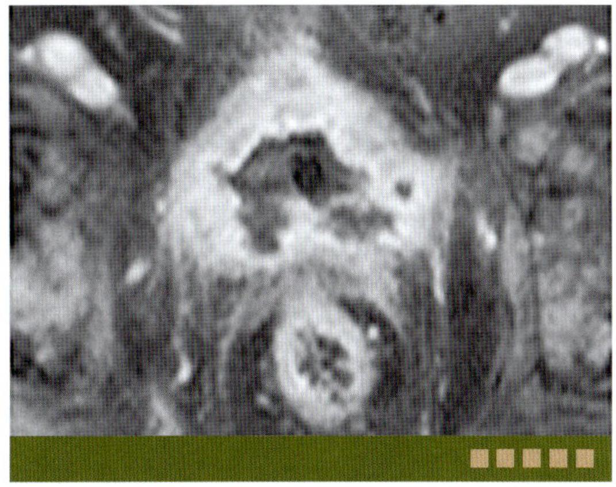

C. Axial contrast-enhanced T1-WI shows heterogeneous enhancement of the thickened bladder wall with areas of ulceration or necrosis involving the posterior wall.

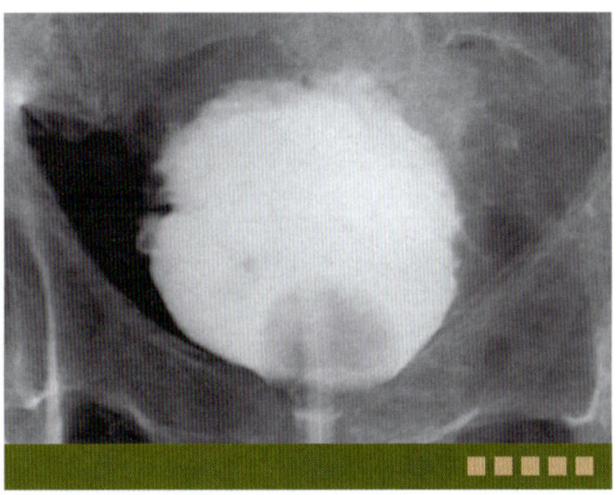

D. Cystogram from the same patient shows a reduced bladder capacity and mural irregularity.

DIFFERENTIAL DIAGNOSES IMAGES (E-G)

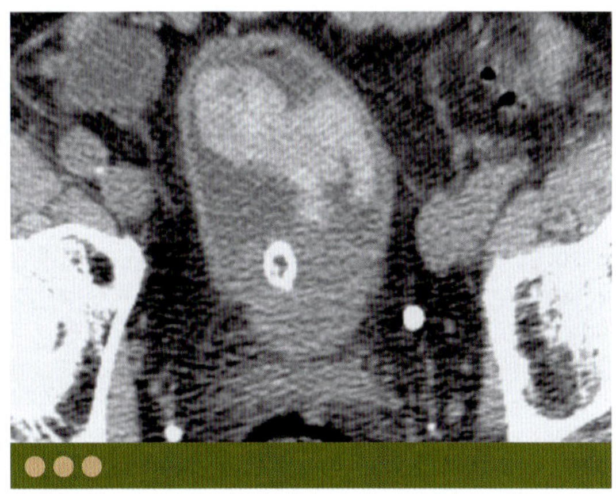

E. Bladder hematoma: Axial NECT shows normal bladder wall thickness and a large hyperdense hematoma in the bladder of a patient who presented with gross hematuria one day after cystoscopy and bladder biopsy.

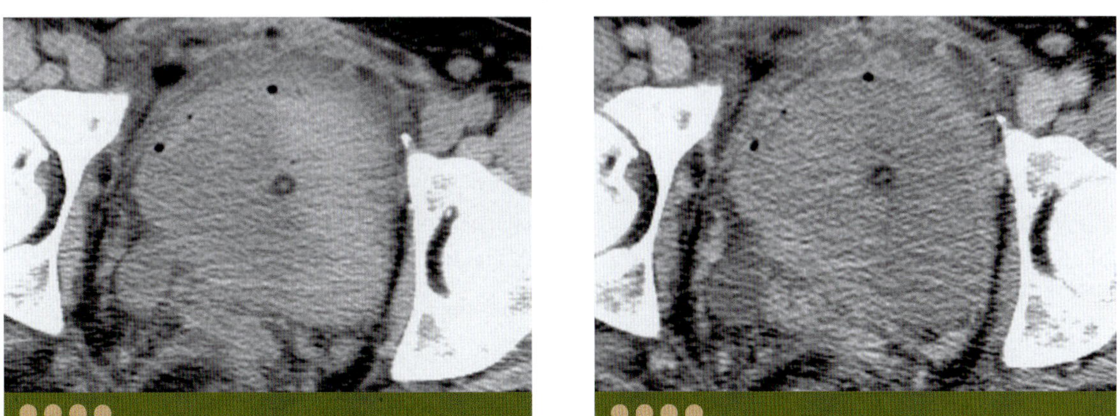

F. and **G. Bladder cancer with hematoma:** Axial NECT and CECT show shifting of bladder content relative density as a result of nonenhancing hyperdense hematoma occupying the left side of the lumen and enhancing bladder cancer occupying the right side.

IMAGE KEY

Common

Rare

Typical

Unusual

8–17 Cystitis Cystica and Cystitis Glandularis

David D. Casalino

PRESENTATION

Dysuria, hematuria, and frequency.

FINDINGS

Cystogram shows mild diffuse bladder wall thickening and mucosal irregularity.

DIFFERENTIAL DIAGNOSES

- *Cystitis*: Clinical features and associated imaging findings may suggest an etiology; bacterial cystitis is more common in women; bladder capacity may be decreased.
- *Bladder cancer*: Often focal; more common in older patients; tissue may be necessary for differentiation.
- *Bladder outlet obstruction*: More common in men and usually caused by BPH; cellules and diverticula may be seen.

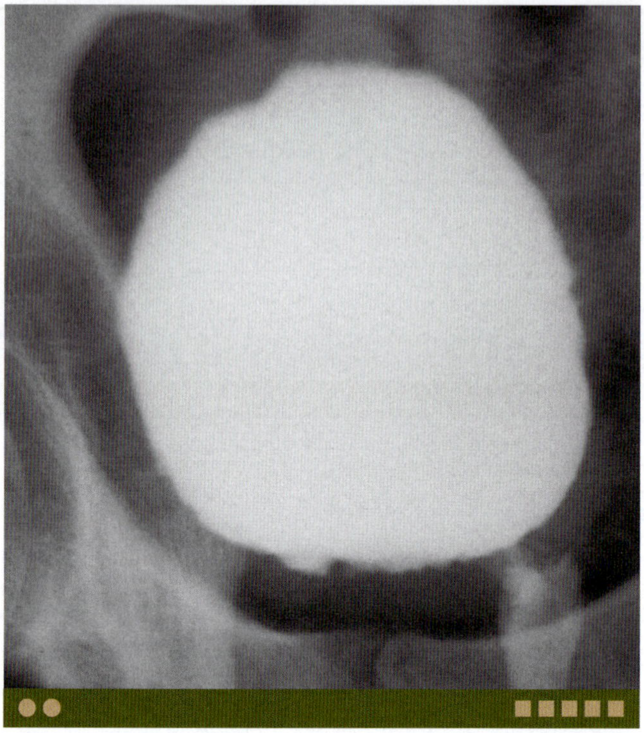

A. Cystogram shows mild diffuse bladder wall thickening and mucosal irregularity.Biopsy confirmed cystitis glandularis. *(Courtesy of Neil F. Wasserman, MD, Veterans Administration Medical Center, Minneapolis, MN.)*

COMMENTS

Cystitis cystica and cystitis glandularis are forms of urothelial metaplasia which develop in the setting of chronic irritation, usually by infection or calculi. The urothelium proliferates into nests of von Brunn, which grow down into the lamina propria. Cystitis cystica results when the nests differentiate into cystic deposits. Cystitis glandularis results when the nests differentiate into intestinal columnar glands. Cystitis glandularis may be seen in association with pelvic lipomatosis and bladder exstrophy, and a rare association with bladder cancer has been reported but is controversial. Cystitis cystica and cystitis glandularis are most often found together in the bladder but similar conditions can also occur in the upper urinary tract, where they are referred to as ureteritis cystica and pyelitis cystica. They can occur at any age. Patients may present with dysuria, hematuria, frequency, and urgency. Sixty percent of the patients with cystitis cystica and cystitis glandularis may have normal bladders, that is, no clinical or radiologic findings.

Radiologic features of both vary and may include a solitary mass, multiple, irregular nodular mucosal lesions, or diffuse bladder wall thickening. Multiple filling defects may create a cobblestone appearance. The lesions are usually hypervascular. On MR, the lesions are usually low-signal intensity on T1-weighted images, low-signal intensity with central hyperintensity on T2-weighted images, and enhance most centrally. These lesions should not invade the muscle layer. The appearance may mimic bladder carcinoma.

Biopsy is necessary for diagnosis. Treatment usually involves surgical excision of the inflamed areas and removal of the source of irritation, if possible.

PEARLS

- **Cystitis cystica and cystitis glandularis are forms of urothelial metaplasia which develop in the setting of chronic irritation and often occur together.**
- **Imaging features may include a solitary mass, multiple mucosal lesions, or diffuse mural thickening.**
- **The appearance may mimic a bladder cancer.**
- **Biopsy is warranted for diagnosis.**

ADDITIONAL IMAGES (B-D)

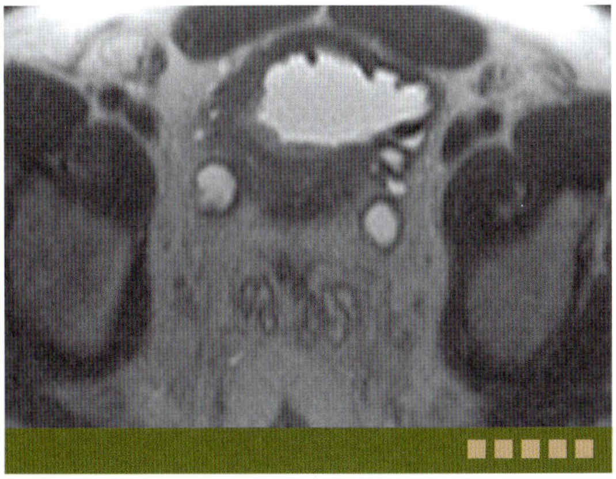

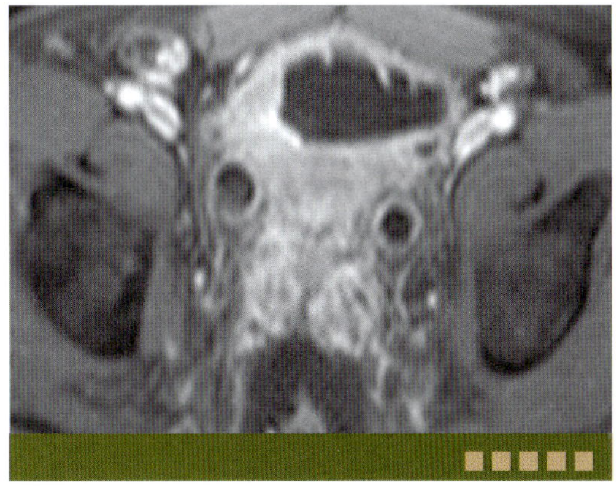

B. and **C.** Axial T2-WI and contrast-enhanced T1-WI show mild diffuse bladder wall irregularity and prominent posterior wall thickening that is hypointense on the T2-WI and shows prominent enhancement. There is also dilatation and thickening of the distal ureters.

DIFFERENTIAL DIAGNOSES IMAGES (E-G)

IMAGE KEY

Common

Rare

Typical

Unusual

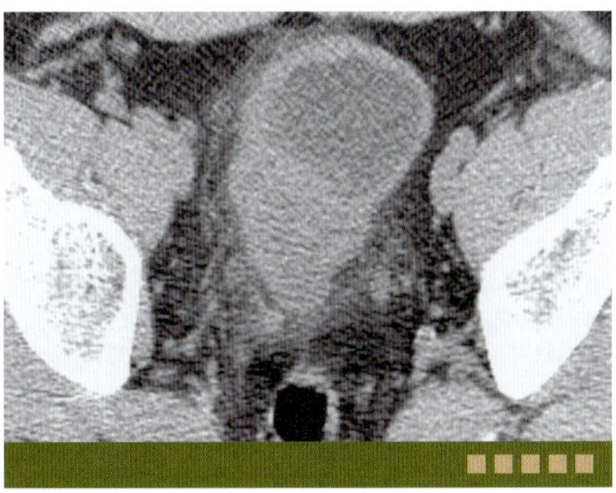

D. Axial NECT shows a large posterior bladder wall mass. Biopsy showed cystitis glandularis.

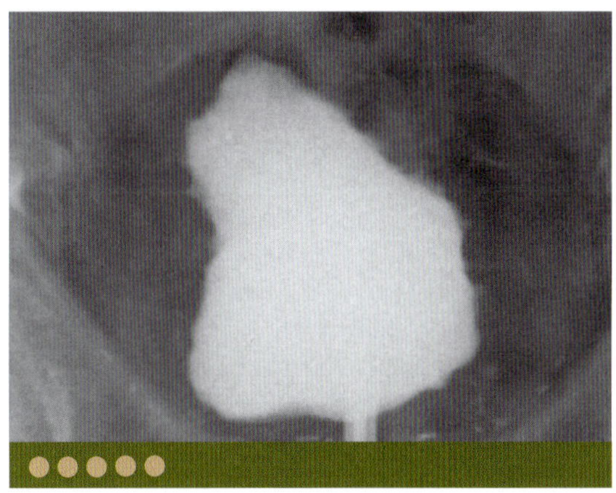

E. Cystitis: Cystogram shows mild diffuse bladder wall irregularity caused by radiation-induced cystitis.

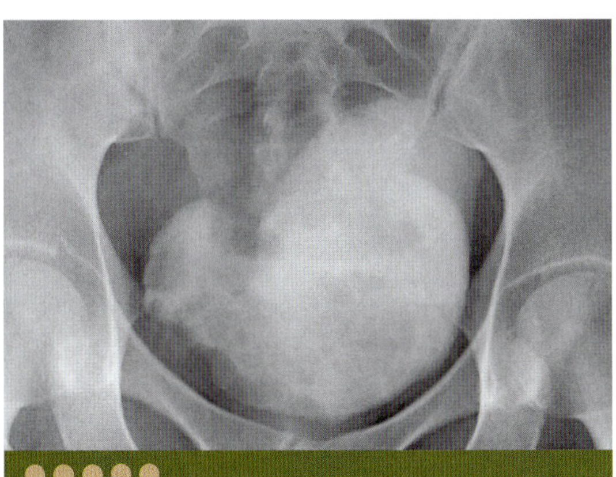

F. Bladder cancer: IVU shows a large, irregular, lobulated filling defect involving the right lateral wall of the bladder caused by urothelial carcinoma.

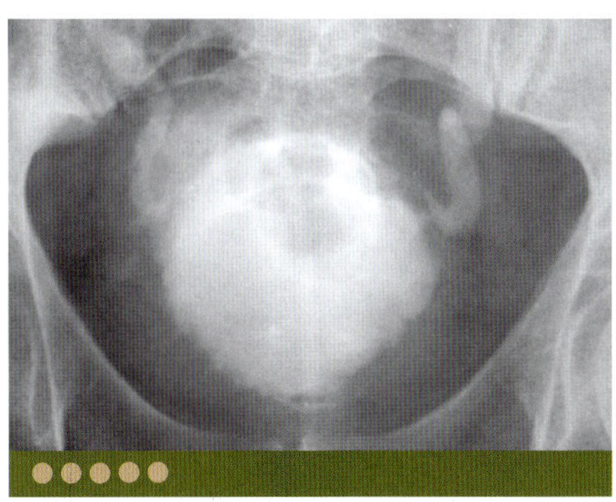

G. Bladder outlet obstruction: IVU shows mild diffuse trabeculation of the bladder and fish hooking of the distal ureters because of BPH.

8–18 Bladder Schistosomiasis

David D. Casalino

PRESENTATION

Hematuria, dysuria, and pelvic pain.

FINDINGS

Conventional radiograph shows sheetlike calcifications involving the bladder wall.

DIFFERENTIAL DIAGNOSES

- *Bladder carcinoma*: Less than 1% of tumors have calcifications that are detectable by conventional radiography; calcifications are typically focal, punctate, coarse or linear, and associated with a mass.
- *Encrustation cystitis*: Usually occurs in the setting of alkaluria and may be secondary to UTI, most often with *Proteus* species or other coliforms, or bladder necrosis caused by RT or cyclophosphamide therapy.
- *Bladder tuberculosis*: Bladder involvement typically occurs after renal and ureteral involvement.

COMMENTS

Schistosomiasis of the urinary tract is caused by *Schistosoma haematobium*, a parasite, and is commonly found in underdeveloped countries. Snails harbor the organism and release the larvae, or cercariae, into water. The larvae penetrate the skin of humans exposed to the infected water, enter the bloodstream, and mature in the liver and lungs of the host. Eggs from adult worms are deposited in the bladder wall vessels, where they trigger a granulomatous inflammatory response. This response results in superficial mucosal ulcerations, polypoid masses, and eventually fibrosis. Eggs in the bladder wall calcify. The diagnosis is made by identifying eggs in the patient's urine. Patients commonly present with hematuria, dysuria, frequency, and pelvic pain. Praziquantel is used to treat patients with schistosomiasis but has no effect on fibrotic changes that have already occurred. Ureteral obstruction may occur and result in obstructive uropathy and renal insufficiency. Patients with schistosomiasis are also at increased risk of developing bladder carcinomas, most often SCC.

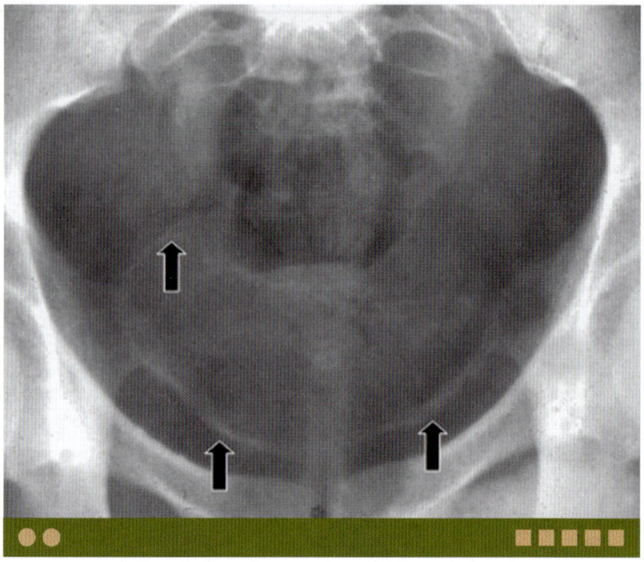

A. Conventional radiograph shows sheetlike calcifications (arrows) involving the bladder wall.

The radiologic findings of bladder schistosomiasis vary with the duration of infection. Early manifestations include bladder wall thickening and irregularity and, on occasion, distal ureteral dilatation. Late manifestations may include a contracted, fibrotic bladder with mural calcification, typically, curvilinear and involving the entire bladder, but occasionally, focal; mural calcifications involving the distal ureters; and focal bladder masses that may be inflammatory or carcinoma.

PEARLS

- **Schistosomiasis is caused by a parasite and is associated with an increased risk of developing bladder carcinoma.**
- **Conventional radiography will demonstrate bladder wall calcifications in approximately 50% of the patients with bladder schistosomiasis.**
- **A focal bladder mass may be inflammatory or carcinoma; therefore, biopsy is generally warranted.**

ADDITIONAL IMAGE

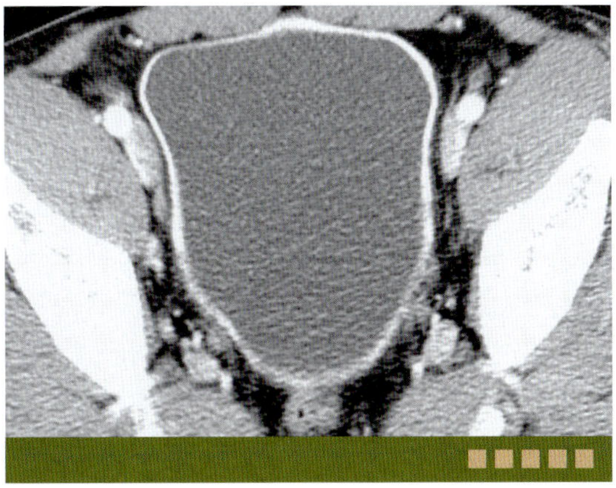

B. Axial CECT shows diffuse bladder wall calcification. No focal mass was present.

DIFFERENTIAL DIAGNOSES IMAGES (C-D)

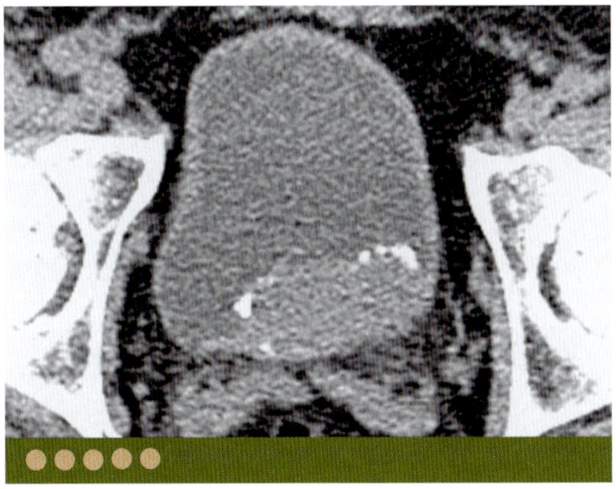

C. Bladder carcinoma: Axial NECT shows a posterior bladder mass with punctate and coarse calcifications. Biopsy confirmed urothelial carcinoma.

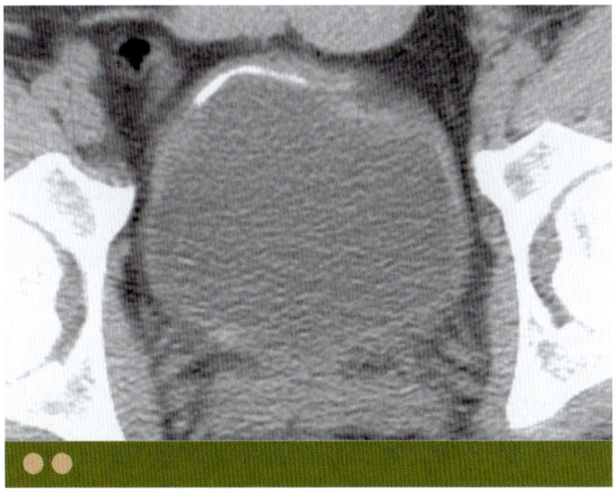

D. Encrustation cystitis: Axial CECT shows mild diffuse bladder wall thickening and curvilinear calcification involving the anterior bladder wall in patients with a history of pelvic irradiation for prostate cancer.

IMAGE KEY

Common

●●●●●
●●●●
●●●
●●
●

Rare

Typical

■■■■■
■■■■
■■■
■■
■

Unusual

8–19 Neurogenic Bladder

David D. Casalino

PRESENTATION

Urinary retention.

FINDINGS

Cystogram shows elongation of the bladder with prominent trabeculation and pseudodiverticula and reflux of contrast into the right ureter.

DIFFERENTIAL DIAGNOSIS

- *Bladder outlet obstruction*: More common in men and usually caused by BPH; cellules and diverticula may be seen; clinical circumstances usually allow differentiation.

COMMENTS

Normal bladder functions require coordination between the detrusor muscle, urethral sphincter, and pelvic floor musculature. A neurogenic bladder is incapable of filling, storing, and expelling urine in a coordinated, controlled fashion because of a neuromuscular disorder. These disorders may involve the cerebrum, spinal cord, or peripheral nerves. Disorders of the central neurons may result in detrusor hyperreflexia and a spastic bladder that has compromised storage function. Disorders of the more peripheral neurons, including the conus, cauda equine, sacral nerve roots, and peripheral nerves, may result in detrusor areflexia and a flaccid bladder. Sphincter dyssynergia refers to inappropriate contraction of the urethral sphincter. The internal, external, or both sphincters may be involved. Patients with a neurogenic bladder may present with urinary incontinence, pressure, urgency, frequency, and urinary retention.

Radiographically, spastic bladders may show serrations of the mucosa during voiding or prominent interureteric indentations. Bladder capacity is small with a rounded, usually smooth contour. In patients with multiple sclerosis and suprasacral spinal cord injuries, the hyperreflexia is usually accompanied by sphincter dyssynergia. This results in chronic bladder obstruction. Bladder trabeculation may occur. There is also increased risk of stone formation, infection, and SCC. Upper tract sequelae may include ureterectasis, reflux, and parechymal loss. A flaccid bladder is usually smooth with a large capacity. Elongation of the bladder with prominent trabeculation and pseudodiverticula is sometimes referred to as a "Christmas tree" or "pine tree" appearance that may occur in the setting of detrusor hyperreflexia or detrusor areflexia.

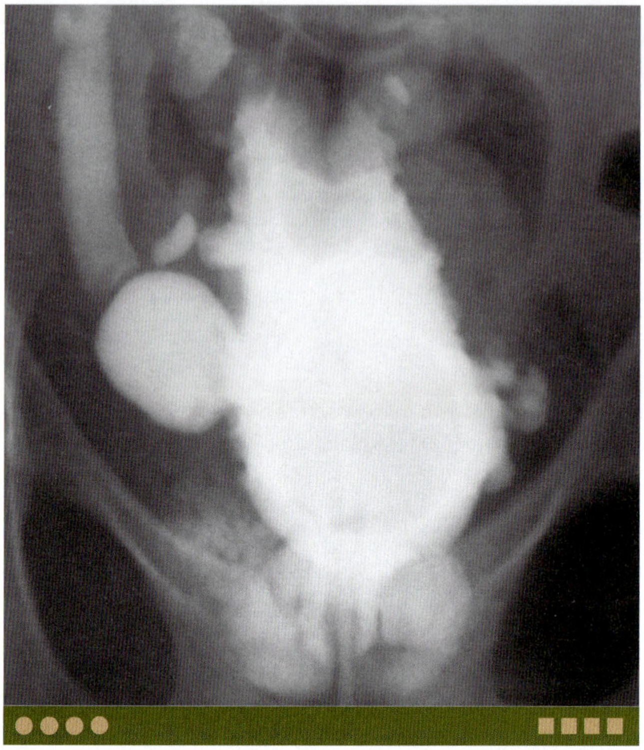

A. Cystogram shows "Christmas tree" appearance of the bladder with prominent trabeculations and pseudodiverticula in a patient with spina bifida. There is distention of the posterior urethra and reflex of contrast into the right ureter and prostatic ducts.

PEARLS

- **Disorders of the central neurons usually result in detrusor hyperreflexia and a spastic bladder.**
- **Disorders of the more peripheral neurons, including the conus, cauda equine, sacral nerve roots, and peripheral nerves, usually result in detrusor areflexia and a flaccid bladder.**
- **The "Christmas tree" appearance of the bladder can be seen in patients with detrusor hyperreflexia or detrusor areflexia.**

ADDITIONAL IMAGES (B-E)

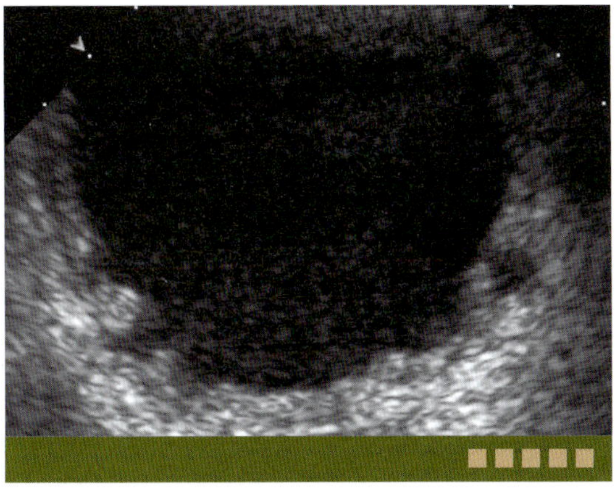

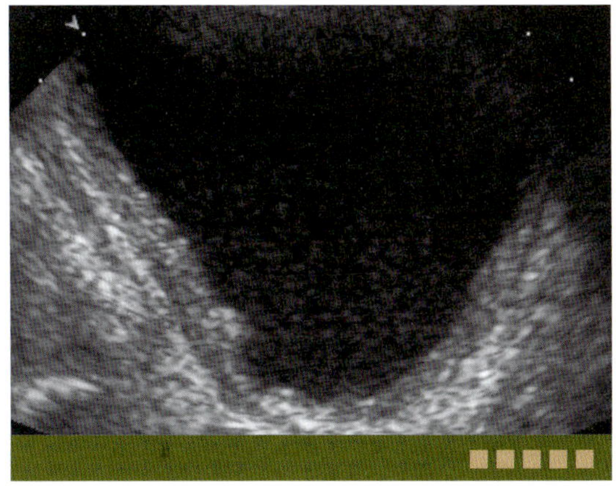

B. and **C**. Transverse and longitudinal ultrasounds show diffuse bladder wall thickening and trabeculation in a patient with multiple sclerosis.

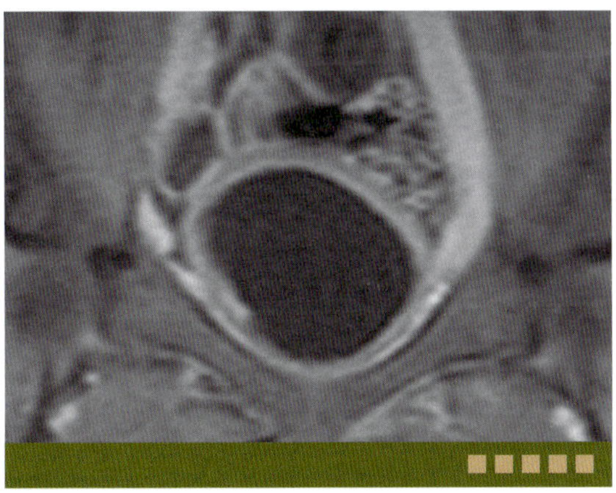

D. Coronal, contrast-enhanced T1-WI shows mild diffuse bladder wall thickening with homogeneous enhancement in a patient with spina bifida.

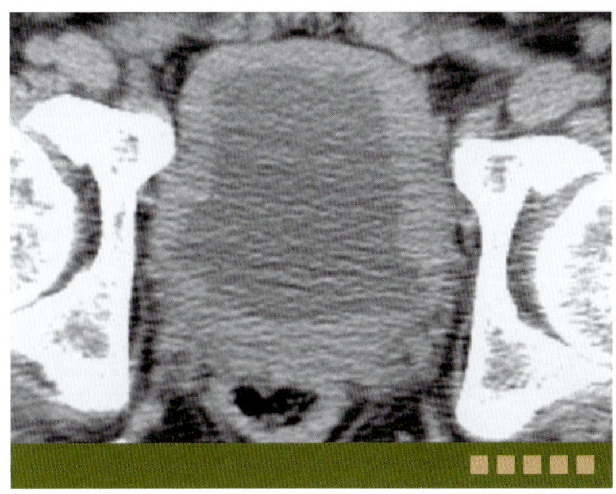

E. Axial NECT shows moderate diffuse bladder wall thickening in a patient with thoracic spine injury from gun shot.

IMAGE KEY

Common

Rare

Typical

Unusual

DIFFERENTIAL DIAGNOSIS IMAGE

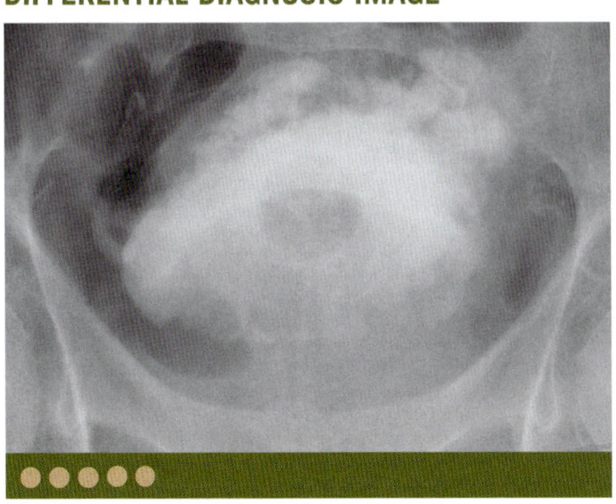

F. Bladder outlet obstruction: IVU shows the bladder to have multiple cellules and diverticula along its superior aspect and prominent mass effect from an enlarged prostate along its inferior aspect. There is also fish hooking of the right distal ureter associated with the BPH.

8–20 Bladder Outlet Obstruction

David D. Casalino

PRESENTATION

Urinary frequency and weak urine stream.

FINDINGS

CT shows an enlarged bladder with diffuse wall thickening and mild trabeculation.

DIFFERENTIAL DIAGNOSES

- *Cystitis*: Clinical features and associated imaging findings may suggest an inflammatory or infectious etiology; bacterial cystitis is more common in women; bladder capacity may be decreased.
- *Bladder cancer*: Often focal; tissue may be necessary for differentiation.
- *Bladder wall prominence caused by limited distention*: Usually an incidental finding.

COMMENTS

Bladder outlet obstruction refers to any condition that reduces or prevents urine flow from the bladder into the urethra. Common etiologies for bladder outlet obstruction include BPH, prostate cancer, bladder neoplasms and stones, and urethral stricture. Bladder outlet obstruction is most common in aging men and caused by BPH. Bladder stones and bladder cancer are also more common in men than women. Symptoms of bladder outlet obstruction may include a weak or intermittent urine stream, urinary hesitancy, urinary frequency, inability to urinate, dysuria, and a continuous feeling of a full bladder. There is an increased incidence of bladder stone formation and infection. Upper urinary tract sequela may include hydronephrosis and hydroureter, vesicoureteral reflux, renal parenchyma loss, and impaired renal function.

Prolonged bladder outlet obstruction is associated with hypertrophy of the detrusor muscle, thickening of the bladder wall, trabeculation (irregularity of the luminal contour of the bladder when filled with urine, because of detrusor instability), and bladder cellules and diverticula. A markedly enlarged bladder may be seen if there is diminished detrusor function. These features of bladder outlet obstruction may be demonstrated on imaging of the bladder. Urodynamic studies are often more reliable than imaging studies, which might include measurement of prevoiding and postvoiding urinary bladder volumes, for the determination of a "significant" bladder outlet obstruction. Treatment of bladder outlet obstruction depends on the etiology.

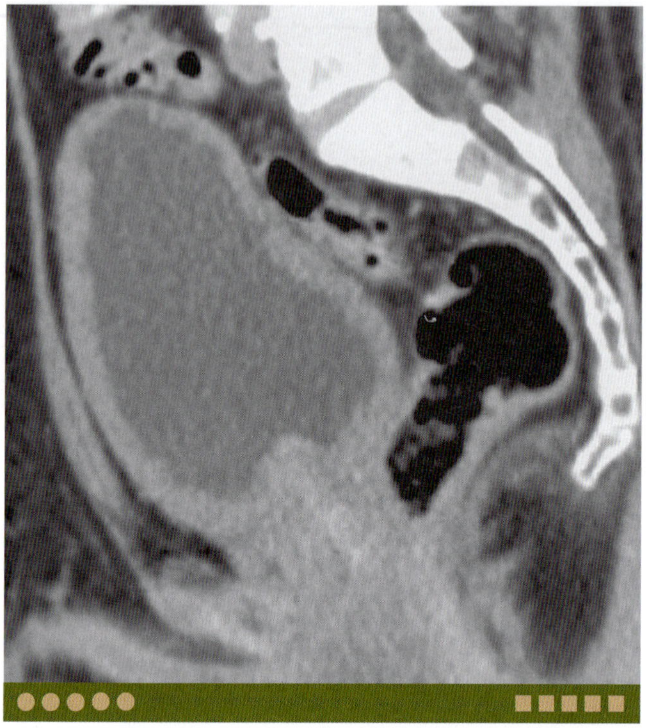

A. Sagittal CECT shows an enlarged bladder with diffuse wall thickening and mild trabeculation, as well as enlargement of the prostate.

PEARLS

- **Bladder outlet obstruction is most commonly caused by BPH.**
- **Common imaging features include bladder wall thickening and trabeculation, cellules, and diverticula.**
- **Bladder enlargement may result from diminished detrusor muscle function.**
- **A normal postvoiding bladder volume does not exclude a significant bladder outlet obstruction nor does an abnormal postvoiding volume necessarily indicate an outlet obstruction.**

ADDITIONAL IMAGES (B-D)

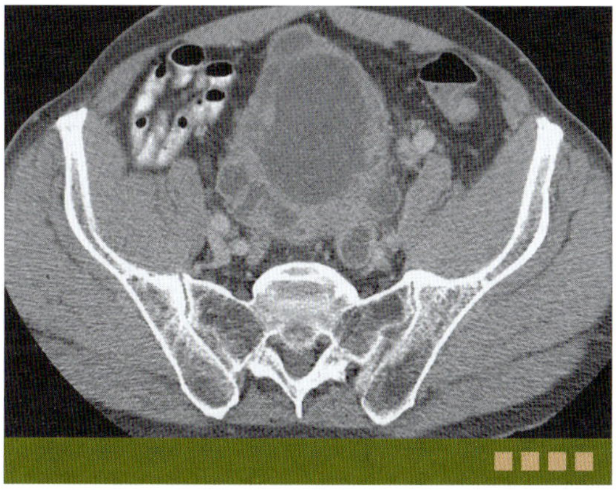

B. Axial CECT from a different patient with BPH shows bladder wall thickening, trabeculation, and multiple cellules and diverticula.

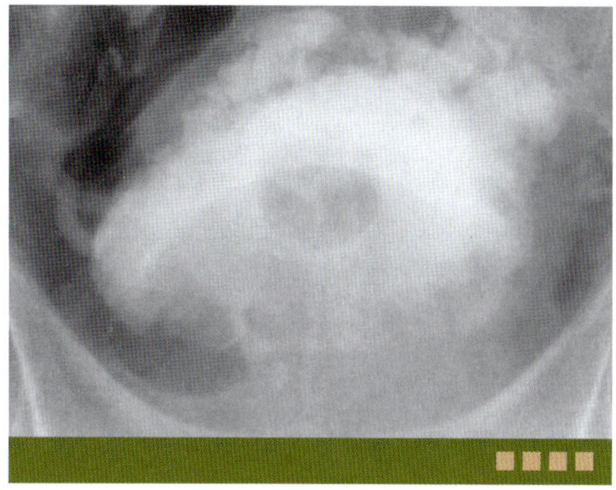

C. IVU shows the bladder to have multiple cellules and diverticula along its superior aspect and prominent mass effect from an enlarged prostate along its inferior aspect. There is fish hooking of the right distal ureter.

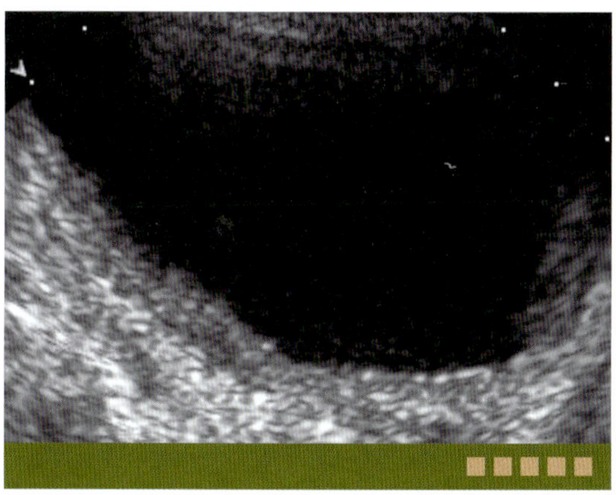

D. Longitudinal sonogram shows thickening of the bladder wall.

DIFFERENTIAL DIAGNOSES IMAGES (E-G)

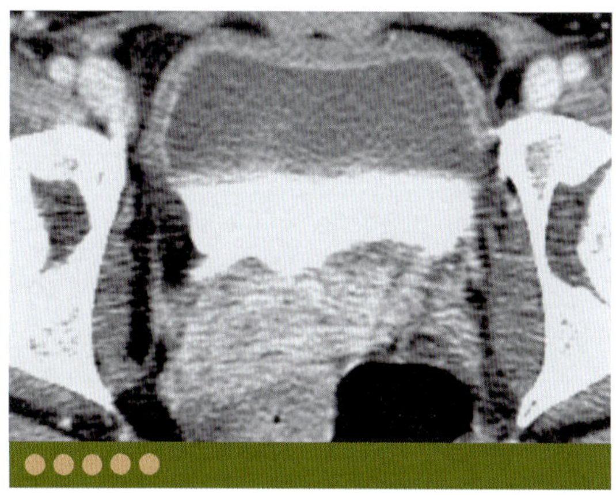

E. Bacterial cystitis: Axial CECT shows diffuse bladder wall thickening in a woman with a long history of recurrent UTI.

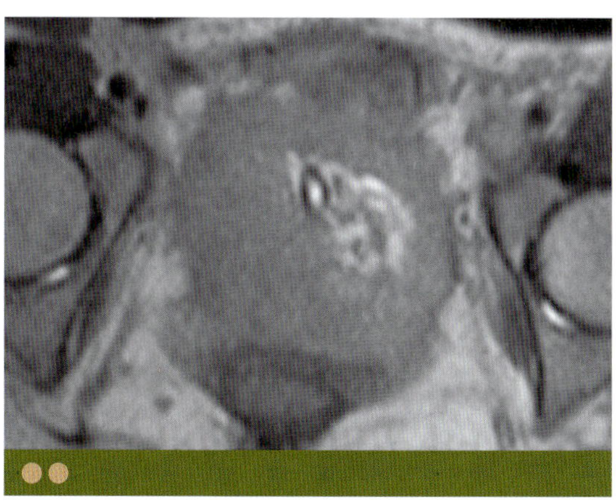

F. Squamous cell carcinoma: Axial T2-WI shows marked diffuse bladder wall thickening that is hyperintense in a patient with a history of neurogenic bladder.

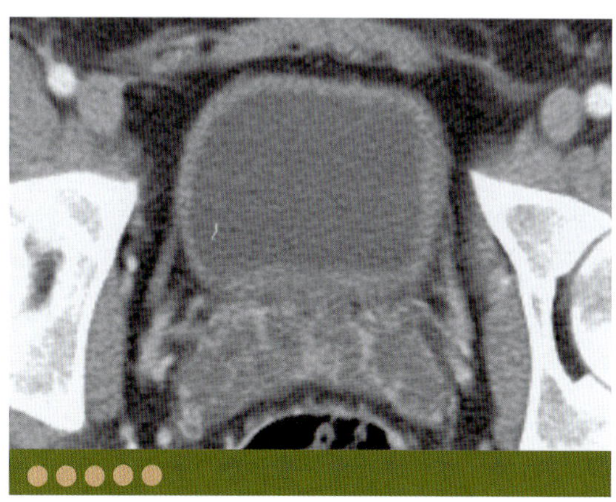

G. Limited distention: Axial CECT shows mild bladder wall prominence, an incidental finding, in a 32-year-old male. Follow-up CT for other indication showed normal bladder wall thickness with greater bladder distention.

IMAGE KEY

Common
●●●●●
●●●●
●●●
●●
●
Rare

Typical
■■■■■
■■■■
■■■
■■
■
Unusual

8–21 Bladder Calculi

David D. Casalino

PRESENTATION

Hematuria and symptoms of BPH.

FINDINGS

IVU images show two round bladder filling defects that are faintly hyperdense on the scout radiograph.

DIFFERENTIAL DIAGNOSIS

- *Calcified neoplasm*: Five percent of urothelial carcinomas, or TCC, will show calcifications; dense rimmed, speckled, irregular, and course nodular calcifications have been described; nonmobile.

COMMENTS

Bladder stones may be the result of urinary stasis and infection or presence of a foreign body, migration from the kidney, or primary endemic stone disease. Urinary stasis is the most common etiology and may be the result of bladder outlet obstruction, for example, in the setting of BPH; neurogenic bladder; cystocele; or diverticulum of the bladder or urethra. Uric acid stones are seen most often in the setting of bladder outlet obstruction, whereas magnesium ammonium phosphate and apatite stones are more commonly associated with UTI. Migrant stones usually pass through the urethra unless the bladder outlet is obstructed. Foreign bodies, such as chronic indwelling catheters, nonabsorbable suture material, sponges, and pubic hair, may serve as a nidus for stone formation and growth. Patients with bladder stones may be asymptomatic or present with hematuria, pelvic pain, or intermittent interruption of urine stream. Chronic bladder irritation as a result of asymptomatic stones is associated with an increased risk of developing SCC of the bladder.

Most bladder stones will be mobile, which is helpful in differentiating them from mural calcifications that may be neoplastic, inflammatory, or metabolic in etiology. Radiodensity of bladder stones varies from very dense to radiolucent. CT is much more sensitive for detecting bladder stones than conventional radiography. On an excretory urogram, stones will usually produce filling defects in the contrast opacified bladder.

In MR, bladder stones show signal void or low-signal intensity and are best demonstrated on T2-weighted images and delayed contrast-enhanced T1-weighted images, in which the urine will have high-signal intensity.

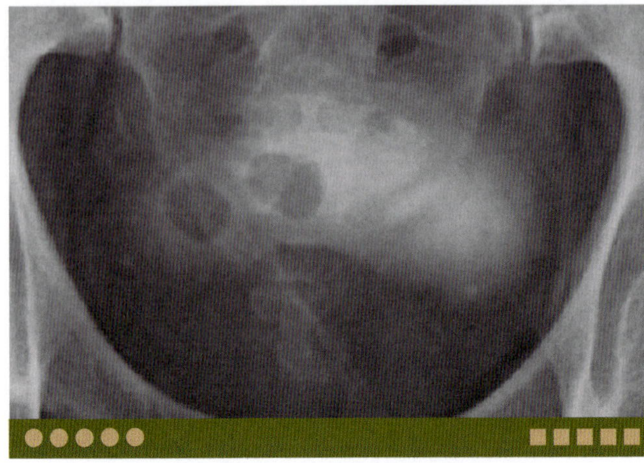

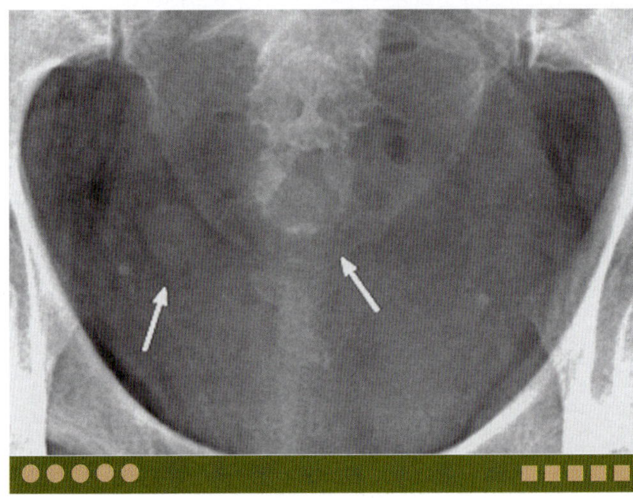

A. IVU shows two round filling defects in the bladder and mass effect from an enlarged prostate caused by BPH.
B. IVU scout shows the filling defects correspond to two faint, homogeneous calculi (arrows).

PEARLS

- **Urinary stasis is the most common etiology for bladder stones.**
- **Most bladder stones are mobile.**
- **CT is much more sensitive than conventional radiography for the detection of bladder stones.**

ADDITIONAL IMAGES (C-F)

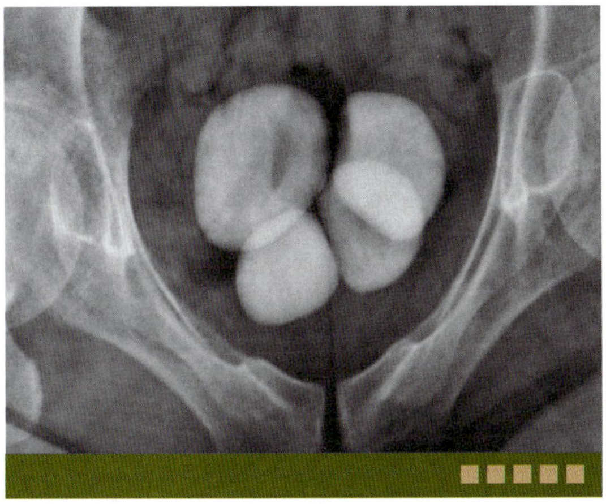

C. Plain radiograph of the pelvis shows four dense bladder stones in a patient with a neurogenic bladder.

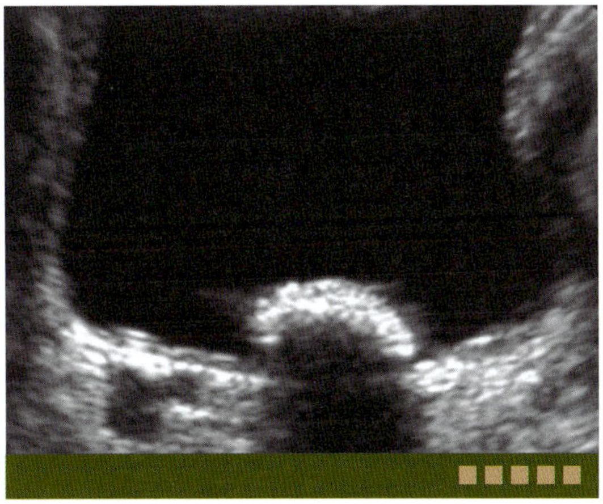

D. Transverse sonogram of the bladder shows an echogenic focus with distal sharp acoustic shadowing characteristic of a stone in a patient with kidney stones as well.

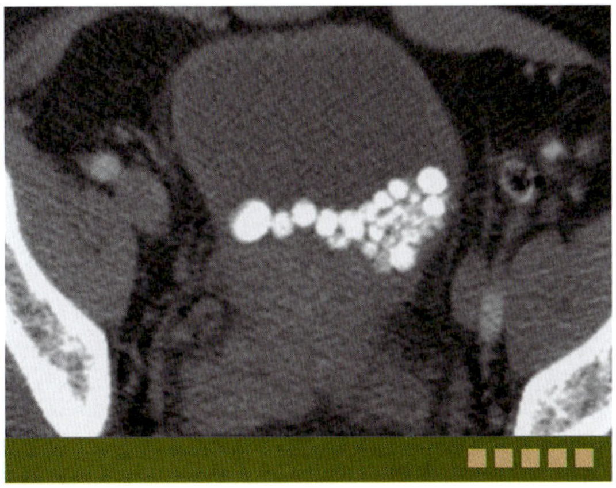

E. Axial CECT shows layering of numerous small bladder stones in a patient with BPH.

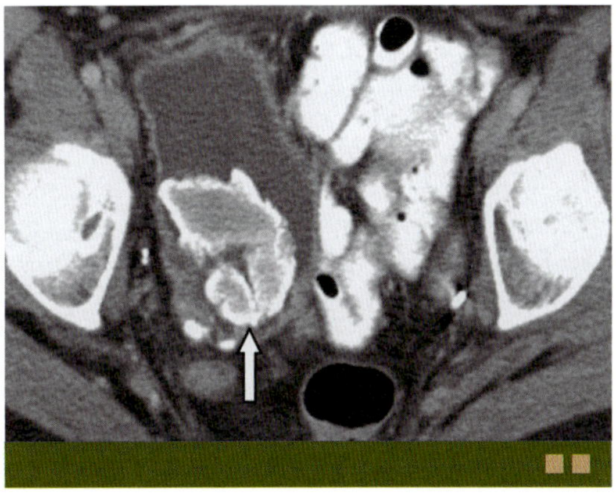

F. Axial CECT shows a foreign body stone (arrow) in an ileal conduit. The foreign body proved to be a gauze sponge.

DIFFERENTIAL DIAGNOSIS IMAGE

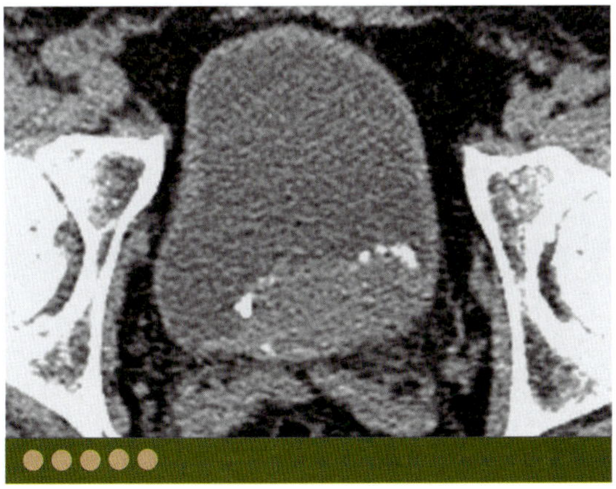

G. Urothelial carcinoma: Axial NECT shows a posterior bladder mass with multiple tiny calcification, most numerous in the tumor periphery.

IMAGE KEY

Common

Rare

Typical

Unusual

8–22 Primary Localized Amyloidosis of the Bladder

David D. Casalino

PRESENTATION

Gross, painless hematuria.

FINDINGS

Ultrasound images demonstrate a small, irregular mural-based mass protruding into the bladder lumen.

DIFFERENTIAL DIAGNOSES

- *Malignant and benign neoplasms of the bladder*: Biopsy or resection necessary for differentiation.
- *Hematoma*: May change position; may clear on follow-up imaging or after bladder irrigation.

COMMENTS

Amyloidosis is a diverse group of diseases that are characterized by extracellular deposition of an insoluble fibrillar protein (amyloid) in one or more organs or tissues.

Primary amyloidosis is associated with an underlying plasma cell dyscrasia, including multiple myeloma or Waldenstrom macroglobulinemia. Multiple organs are typically involved, including the kidneys, heart, joints, gastrointestinal tract, tongue, nervous system, and skin.

Secondary, or reactive, amyloidosis most often is a complication of an underlying chronic inflammatory disease, such as rheumatoid arthritis, osteomyelitis, and inflammatory bowel disease. Patients with certain malignancies, including renal cell carcinoma, may also develop secondary amyloidosis. The most common sites of amyloid deposition include the kidneys, liver, spleen, and adrenal glands.

A less common form of amyloidosis is primary localized amyloidosis, in which there is a localized deposition rather than systemic involvement. Most cases of symptomatic bladder amyloidosis occur as primary localized amyloidosis. Gross, painless hematuria is the most common symptom, and a focal mass protruding into the bladder is the most common imaging finding. Calcifications may be present in these lesions. Resection is usually performed because these lesions cannot be reliably differentiated from a bladder malignancy.

Kidney involvement by amyloidosis, whether primary or secondary, may result in proteinuria, nephrotic syndrome, and renal failure. On imaging, the kidneys are typically smooth and normal in size or slightly enlarged. The nephrogram may be faint. On ultrasound, renal echogenicity may be normal or slightly increased. Over time, the kidneys may become abnormally small, presumably because of ischemia. Renal amyloidosis may be complicated by renal vein thrombosis.

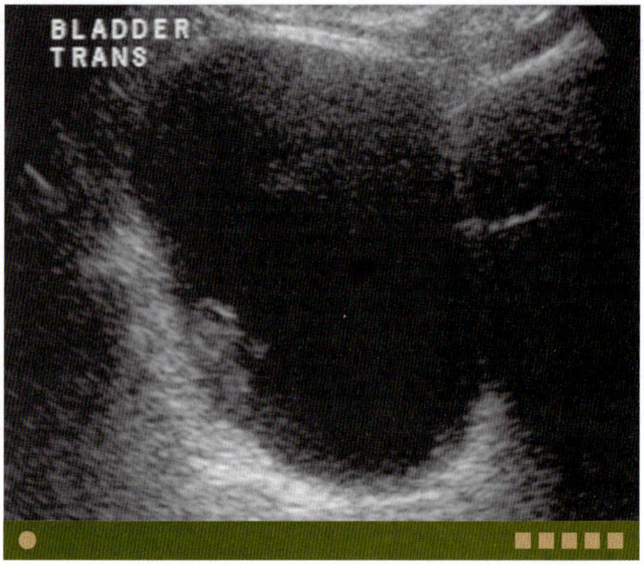

A. Transverse sonogram shows a small, irregular mural-based mass protruding into the bladder lumen. It arises from the right posterolateral wall and did not create a posterior shadow or move when the patient was repositioned.

PEARLS

- **Primary localized amyloidosis is a less common form of amyloidosis yet accounts for most cases of symptomatic bladder amyloidosis.**
- **Imaging cannot reliably differentiate bladder amyloidosis from a bladder malignancy.**
- **Renal involvement by amyloidosis is more common in the setting of secondary amyloidosis and may result in proteinuria, nephrotic syndrome, and renal failure.**
- **Initially, the involved kidneys may appear normal or slightly enlarged.**

ADDITIONAL IMAGES (B-D)

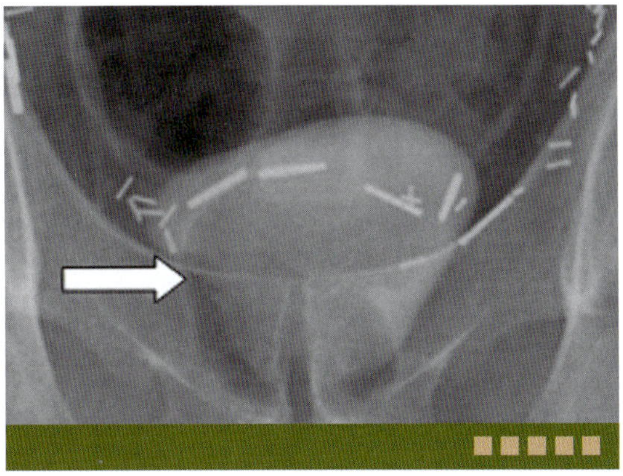

B. IVU from the same patient shows a small filling defect (arrow) of the right lateral wall.

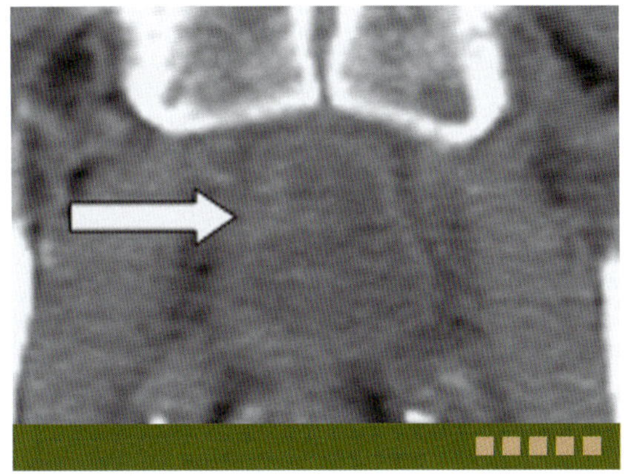

C. Axial CECT from the same patient shows a small enhancing mass (arrow) arising from the right lateral wall.

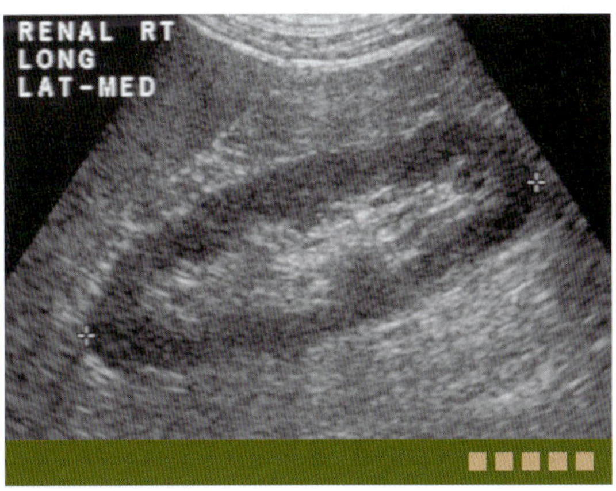

D. Longitudinal sonogram from a different patient with renal involvement by amyloidosis shows a slightly enlarged right kidney, which is otherwise normal in appearance.

DIFFERENTIAL DIAGNOSES IMAGES (E-F)

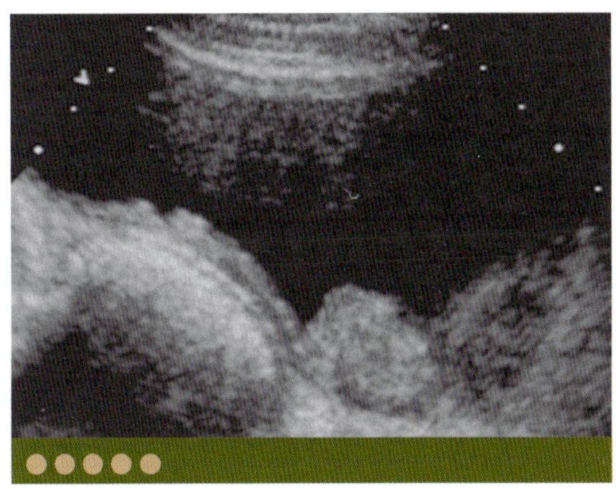

E. Urothelial carcinoma: Longitudinal sonogram shows a slightly irregular mural-based mass. Color Doppler assessment (not shown) showed flow in the mass.

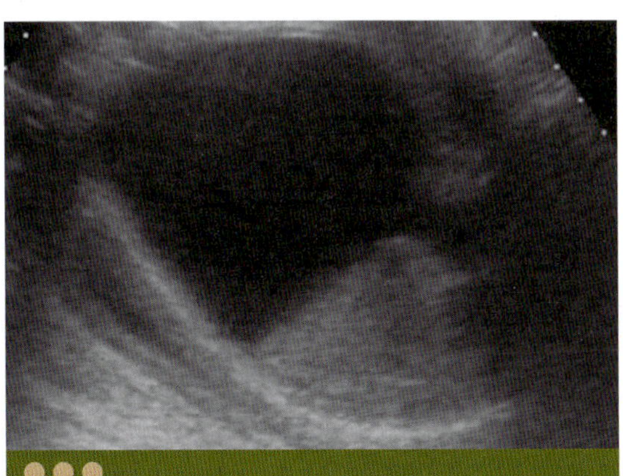

F. Bladder hematoma: Longitudinal sonogram shows a smooth mural-based mass in a patient with a history of hemorrhagic cystitis. The mass did not have color Doppler flow and was not seen on a short-term follow-up sonogram.

IMAGE KEY

Common

Rare

Typical

Unusual

8–23 Bladder Herniation

David D. Casalino

PRESENTATION

Recurrent UTI.

FINDINGS

Cystogram shows contrast filling a small, asymmetric bladder in the pelvis and contrast extension inferiorly and to the right of midline.

DIFFERENTIAL DIAGNOSES

- *Acquired bladder diverticulum*: More common; increase with age and more often in older men; often multiple; no typical location.
- *Cystocele*: Abnormal descent of bladder neck and trigone; urethra may prolapse as well; typically midline; may be associated with bladder outlet obstruction or hydronephrosis; most often in older women.

COMMENTS

Bladder herniation is uncommon and may involve any type of pelvic or lower abdomen opening that usually results from age-related weakening of the abdominal wall supportive structures. Herniation of the bladder through the inguinal canal is most common (70%), followed by herniation through the femoral canal (25%). Up to 3% of inguinal hernias involve the bladder. The inguinal type predominantly affects men, while the femoral type is more common in women. When inguinal, these hernias are most often paraperitoneal (rather than intraperitoneal or extraperitoneal) with a portion of the parietal peritoneum herniating lateral to the bladder hernia, which remains extraperitoneal. Bladder herniation is usually asymptomatic but may present with UTI, hematuria related to stone formation or inflammation, or history of two stage voiding, that is normal voiding followed by manual compression of the herniated bladder.

A bladder hernia should be considered if IVU or cystography shows an asymmetric, small bladder; incomplete visualization of the bladder base; or lateral displacement of the distal ureter. In inguinal canal bladder hernias, the lateral and inferior aspect of the bladder herniates anteriorly and inferiorly. Upright views are generally superior to prone or supine views in demonstrating bladder hernias during IVU or cystography.

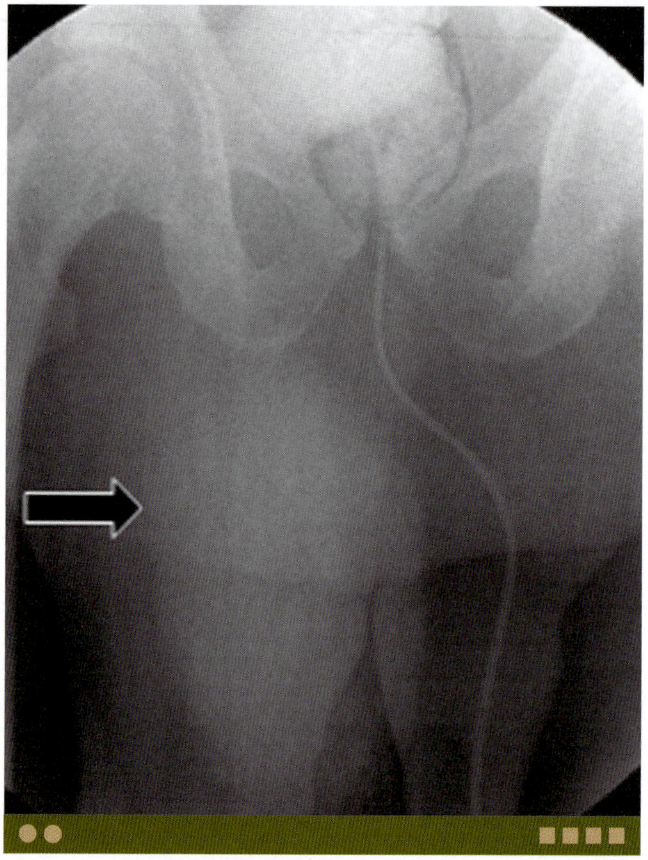

A. Cystogram shows contrast filling a small, asymmetric bladder in the pelvis and contrast extension (arrow) right of midline and inferiorly into the right hemiscrotum.

If the hernia extends into the scrotum and is imaged by ultrasound, other diagnostic considerations would include hydrocele, epididymal cyst, spermatocele, ectopic ureterocele, and intestinal hernia.

PEARLS

- **Bladder herniation is uncommon and most often involves the inguinal canal.**
- **During IVU or cystography, upright views are usually superior in showing a bladder hernia.**
- **In inguinal bladder hernias, the bladder extends anteriorly and inferiorly.**

ADDITIONAL IMAGES (B-E)

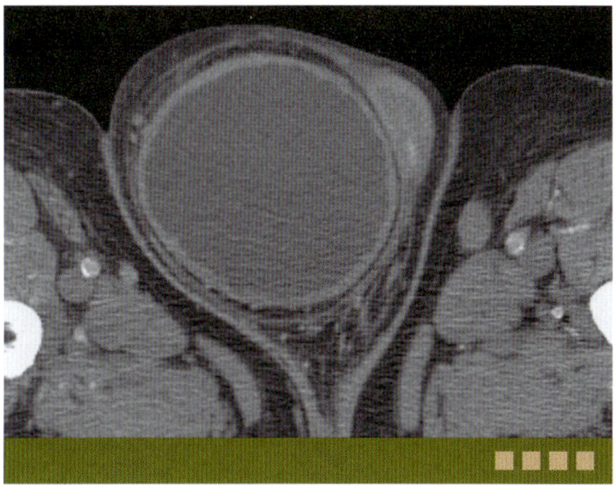

B. Axial CECT shows the large bladder hernia in the right hemiscrotum with mild bladder wall thickening as a result of cystitis.

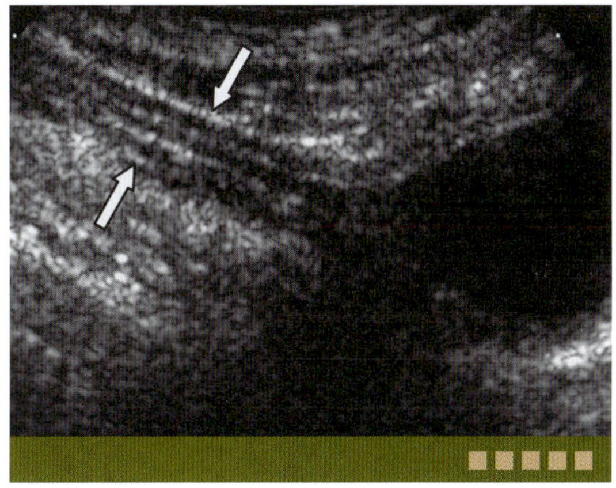

C. Longitudinal sonogram from a different patient shows the bladder hernia in the left inguinal canal. The bladder walls are apposed (arrows) in the superior aspect of the canal.

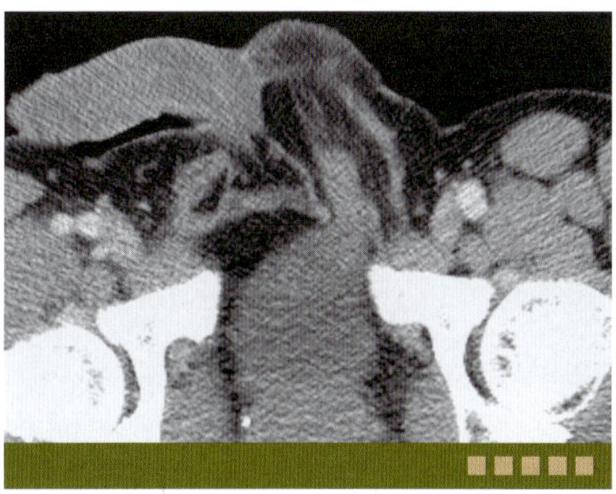

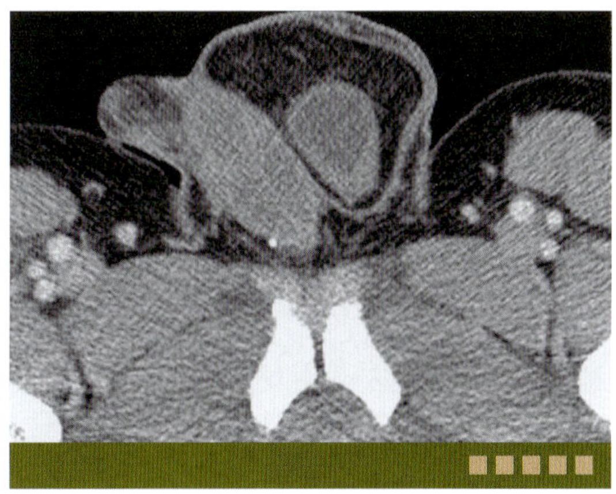

D. and **E.** Axial CECT from the second patient show the bladder herniating into the left inguinal canal.

DIFFERENTIAL DIAGNOSES IMAGES (F-G)

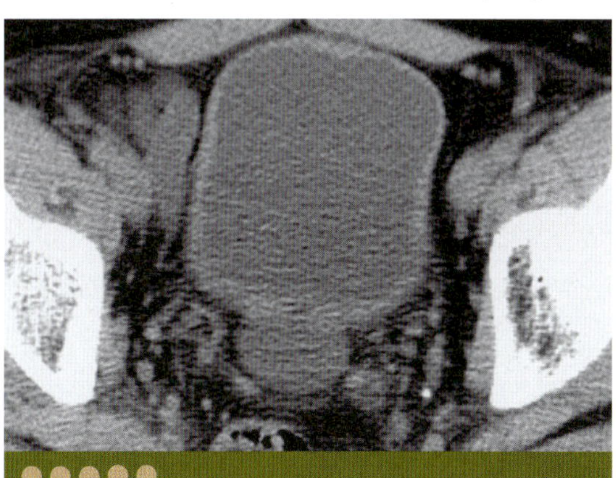

F. Bladder diverticulum: Axial CECT shows a 2.5-cm diverticulum extending from the posterior aspect of the bladder.

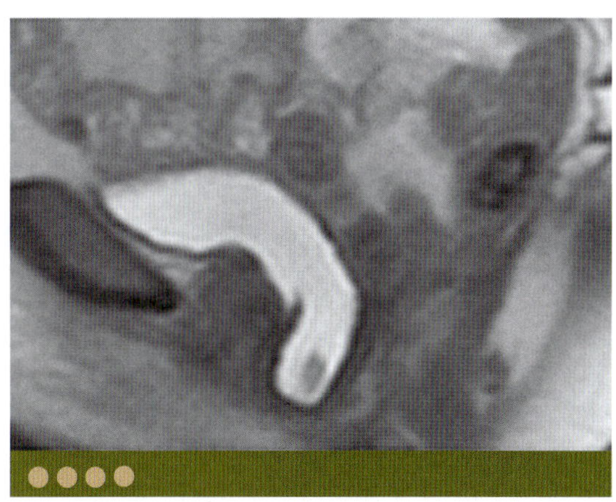

G. Cystocele: Sagittal T2-WI during Valsalva maneuver shows prominent, midline descent of the bladder well below the level of the pubic symphysis.

IMAGE KEY

Common

Rare

Typical

Unusual

8–24 Bladder Fistula

David D. Casalino

PRESENTATION

Fecaluria and pelvic pain.

FINDINGS

Lateral and anteroposterior images from a cystogram show an irregular tract of contrast extending from the superior aspect of the bladder and accumulating in a heterogeneous, rounded pattern.

DIFFERENTIAL DIAGNOSES

- *Bladder diverticulum*: Usually smoothly marginated with a relatively short neck; often multiple; no communication with adjacent structure; etiology for increased intravesical pressure, such as BPH, may be apparent.
- *Bladder injury*: May result from penetrating, blunt, or iatrogenic trauma; no communication with adjacent structure.

COMMENTS

A bladder fistula is an abnormal communication between the bladder and an adjacent structure. They vary greatly in etiology, location, and extent. Etiologies may be infectious, inflammatory, neoplastic, traumatic, or iatrogenic. Diverticulitis is the most common infectious/inflammatory cause. Crohn disease and appendicitis can be associated with fistula formation with the bladder. Advanced malignancies, such as colon cancer or cervical cancer, RT, and pelvic surgeries can be complicated by fistula formation that involves the bladder. The type of fistula will determine presenting symptoms, if any. Patients with vesicovaginal fistulas typically present with continuous urinary incontinence, while those with enterovesical fistulas may present with fecaluria or symptoms of cystitis.

Initial imaging of a patient with suspected bladder fistula is often with cystography or voiding cystourethrography (VCUG), which should include lateral and steep oblique views. The most common imaging finding is contrast extension beyond the normal confines of the bladder. Fistulas are not uncommonly unidirectional, that is they may only be imaged from one side, or viscus. Occasionally, a fistula may intermittently occlude and not be detectable by imaging from either side. The bladder may also show extrinsic mass effect or mural irregularity. CT can identify fistulas. Attention to CT technique is critical. CT cystography might be used and typically involves imaging the pelvis with the bladder initially empty, then fully distended with contrast via a Foley catheter, and finally post drainage. Alternatively, in patients with suspected enterovesical fistulas, CT might be performed with only oral and rectal contrast.

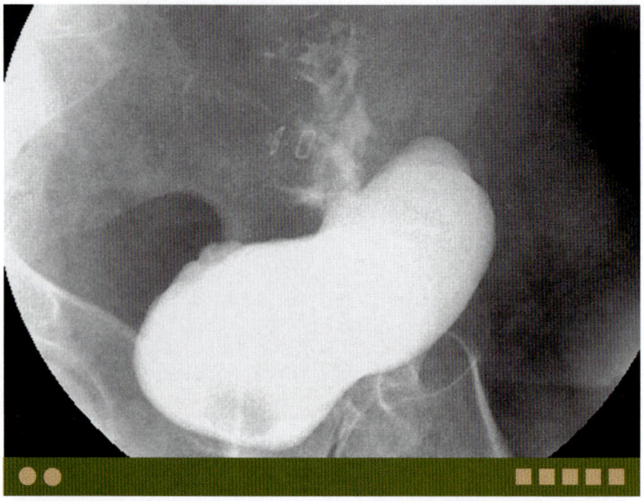

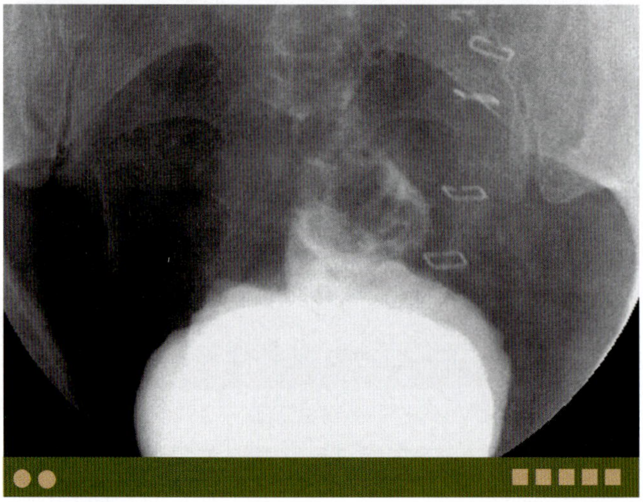

A. Cystogram lateral view shows an irregular tract of contrast extending from the superior aspect of the bladder. **B.** Cystogram AP view shows contrast accumulating in a heterogeneous, rounded pattern, conforming to the lumen of the sigmoid colon, which contains gas and stool. This is a colovesical fistula complicating diverticulitis.

Intravesical contrast or gas may be identified as well as abnormality of the involved bowel and paravesical fat.

PEARLS

- **Etiologies for bladder fistulas may be infectious, inflammatory, neoplastic, traumatic, or iatrogenic.**
- **Cystography or VCUG performed for suspected bladder fistula should include lateral and steep oblique views.**
- **Fistulas are not uncommonly unidirectional.**
- **CT technique should be tailored to the type of fistula suspected.**

ADDITIONAL IMAGES (C-F)

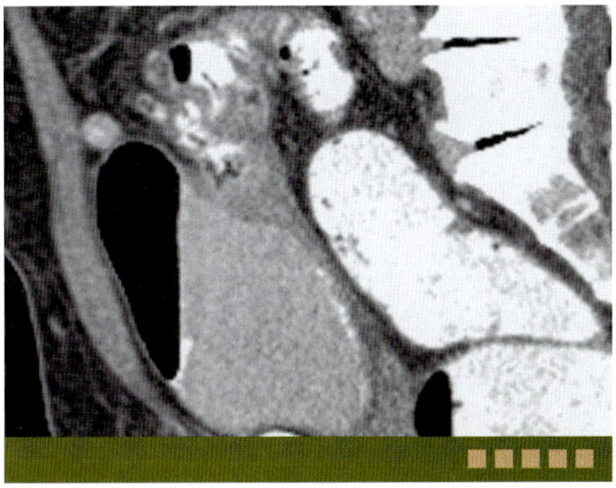

C. Sagittal CECT shows another colovesical fistula complicating diverticulitis. There is thickening of the inflamed sigmoid colon and gas and enteric contrast accumulation in the bladder.

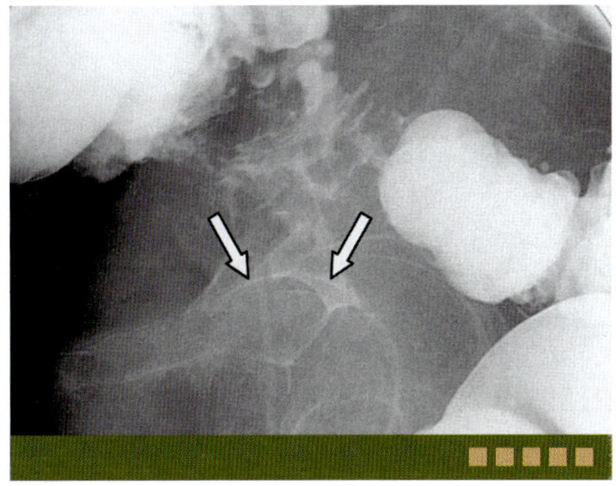

D. Oblique image from an enema with water-soluble contrast shows contrast extending from the sigmoid colon to the bladder with accumulation along the superior aspect of the Foley balloon (arrows).

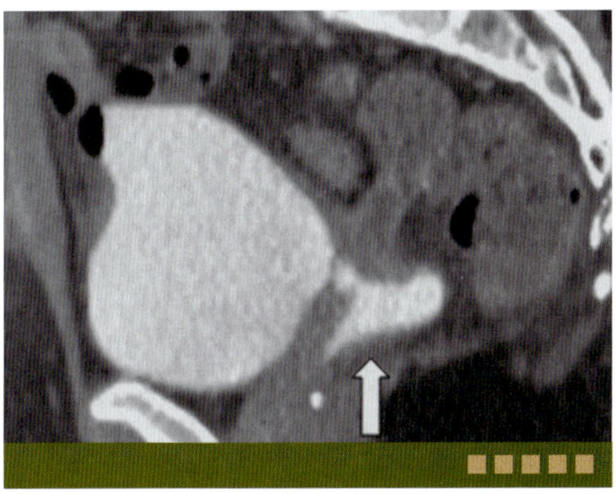

E. Sagittal CT cystogram shows contrast extending from the posterior aspect of the bladder into the vagina (arrow). This vesicovaginal fistula was iatrogenic.

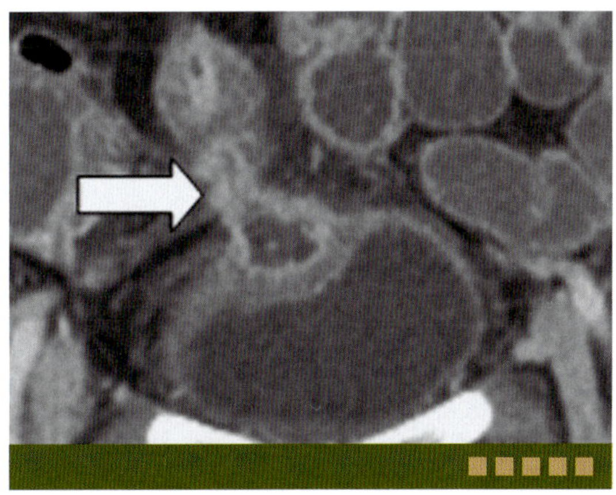

F. Coronal CECT shows a fistula (arrow) from the distal ileum to the superior aspect of the bladder. The patient had a history of Crohn disease and presented with recurrent UTI.

IMAGE KEY

Common

Rare

Typical

Unusual

DIFFERENTIAL DIAGNOSES IMAGES (G-H)

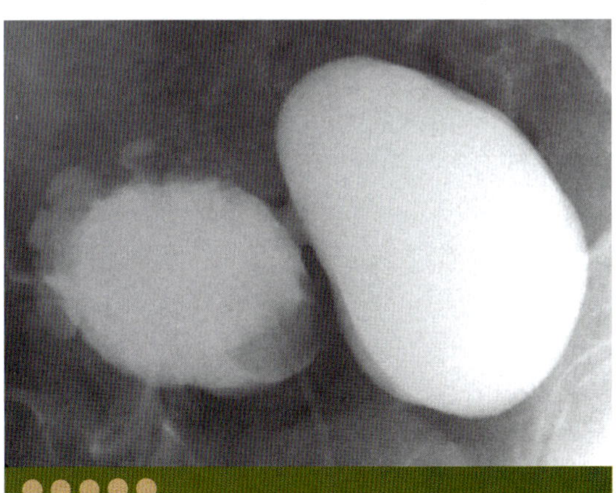

G. Bladder diverticulum: Cystogram shows a large, smoothly marginated diverticulum arising from the left lateral bladder wall. Smaller bladder diverticula and cellules are also shown.

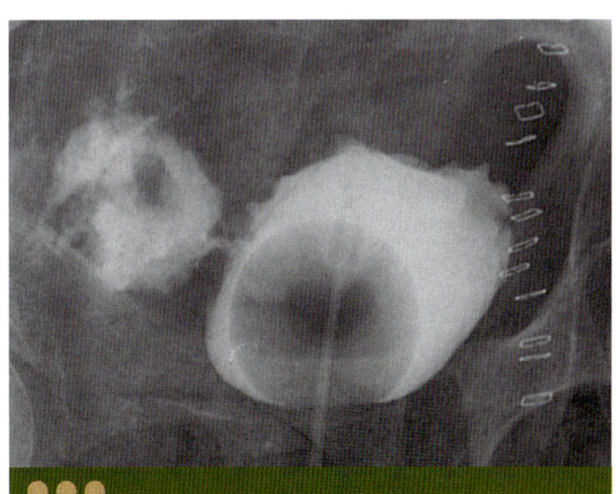

H. Bladder injury caused by gunshot wound: Cystogram shows an irregularly marginated, heterogeneous collection of contrast extending from the right lateral bladder wall. This collection did not accumulate in a pattern suggestive of it being within bowel.

8–25 Cystocele

David D. Casalino

PRESENTATION

Recurrent bladder infections, pelvic pressure and discomfort when straining.

FINDINGS

IVU shows marked bladder prolapse below the level of the inferior pubic rami during straining.

DIFFERENTIAL DIAGNOSES

- *Acquired bladder diverticulum*: More common; increase with age and more often in older men; often multiple; no typical location.
- *Bladder herniation*: Uncommon and most often involves the inguinal canal with the bladder extending anteriorly and inferiorly.
- *Bladder fistula or leak*: Etiologies may be infectious, inflammatory, neoplastic, traumatic or iatrogenic; often irregular margins; clinical history and associated imaging findings often suggest an etiology.

COMMENTS

Cystocele is an abnormal downward bulge of the bladder into the vagina as a result of weakening and stretching of the wall between these structures. This may also be referred to as bladder prolapse. The base of the bladder, trigone, and urethra may be involved.

Cystoceles are seen most often in older women, those who have given birth to multiple children, and those that have had a hysterectomy. There is an association with decreased estrogen after menopause and excessive straining, as in childbirth, chronic constipation, chronic cough, and heavy lifting. A cystocele may be asymptomatic. It may present with a feeling of fullness or pressure in the pelvis; discomfort when straining, lifting, or coughing; recurrent bladder infections; pain or urinary leakage during intercourse; or stress incontinence, that is loss of urinary control with coughing, laughing, or change of posture. When severe prolapse occurs, patients may present with protrusion of soft tissue through the vaginal opening, bladder outlet obstruction, or hydronephrosis. For those patients warranting treatment, options include activity modification, estrogen replacement therapy, use of a pessary, and surgery.

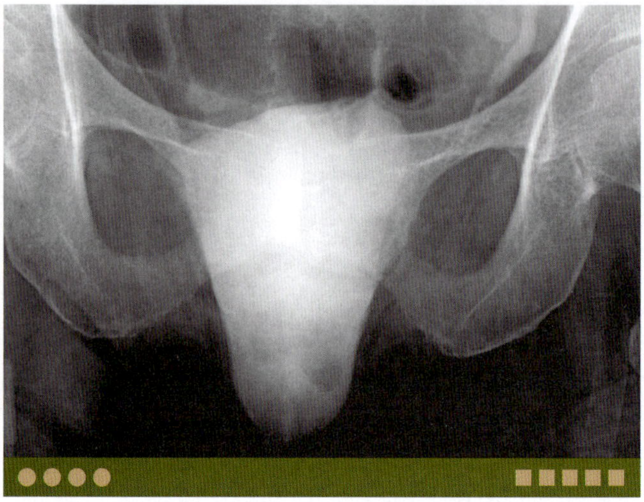

A. IVU shows marked bladder prolapse below the level of the inferior pubic rami during straining

The diagnosis can often be made by a pelvic examination. The diagnosis can be made on cystography when any portion of the bladder extends to or below the level of the inferior pubic rami during straining. This is often best seen on a standing lateral view. Several systems of classification are in use that grade cystoceles based on degree of descent. MRI with patients imaged at rest and straining can also be used to diagnose cystoceles.

PEARLS

- **Cystocele, or bladder prolapse, is a downward bulge of the bladder into the vagina.**
- **Cystocle may result in stress incontinence, bladder outlet obstruction, or hydronephrosis.**
- **The diagnosis can be made on cystography, MRI, or CT when the bladder extends to or below the level of the inferior pubic rami during straining.**

ADDITIONAL IMAGES (B-D)

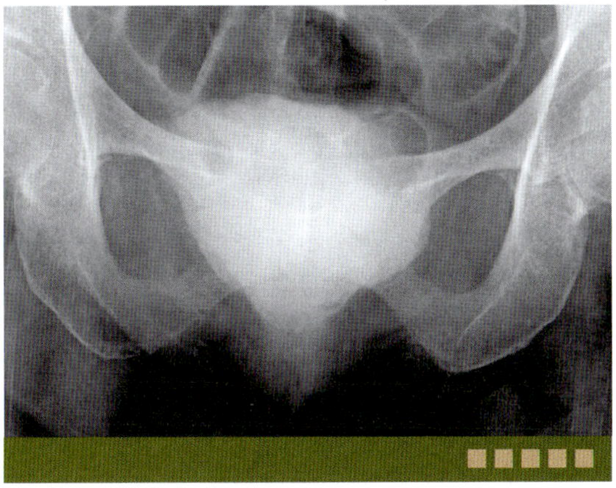

B. IVU from the same patient shows only mild bladder prolapse at rest.

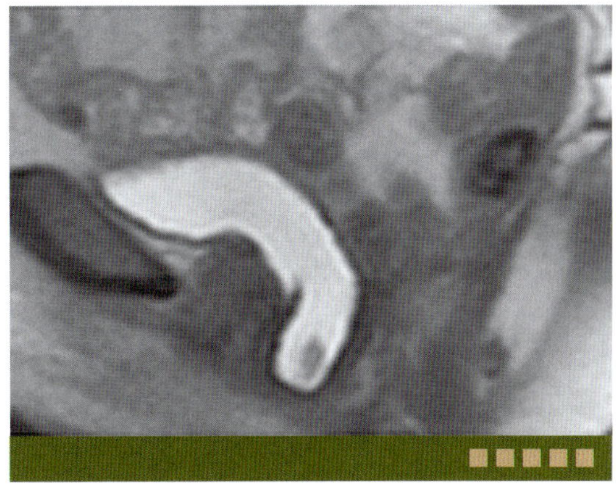

C. Sagittal T2-WI during straining shows prominent, midline descent of the bladder well below the level of the pubic symphysis.

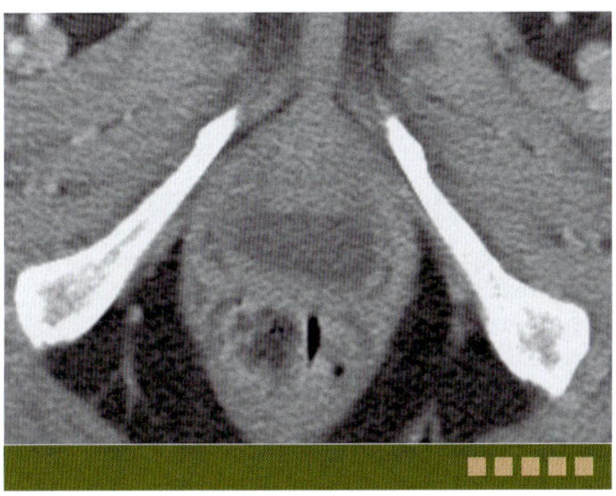

D. Axial CECT shows prolapse of the bladder to the level of the ischial tuberosities.

DIFFERENTIAL DIAGNOSES IMAGES (E-G)

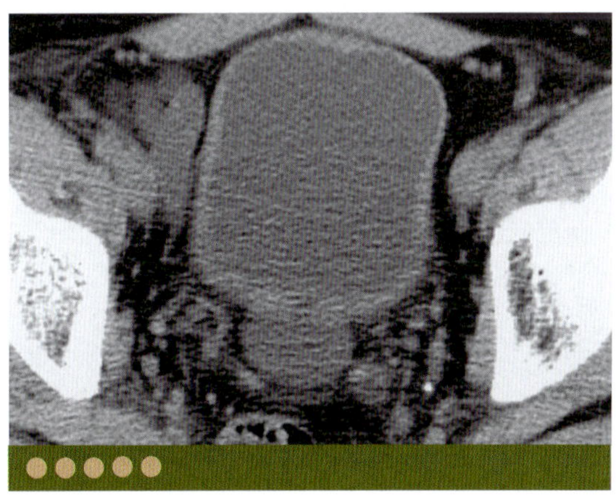

E. Bladder diverticulum: Axial CECT shows a 2.5-cm diverticulum extending from the posterior aspect of the bladder.

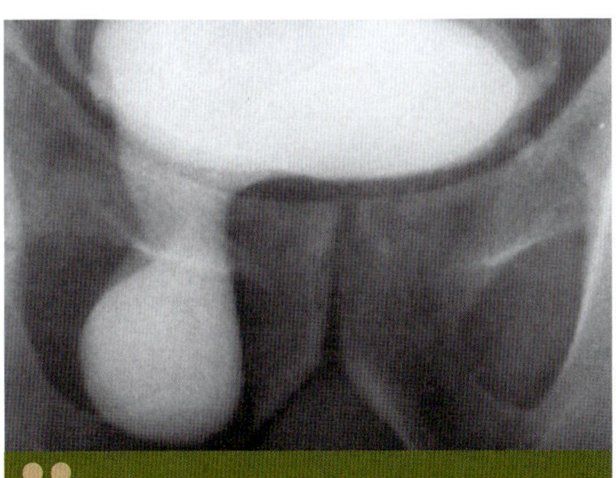

F. Bladder herniation: IVU shows downward protrusion of the inferolateral aspect of the bladder into the right inguinal canal.

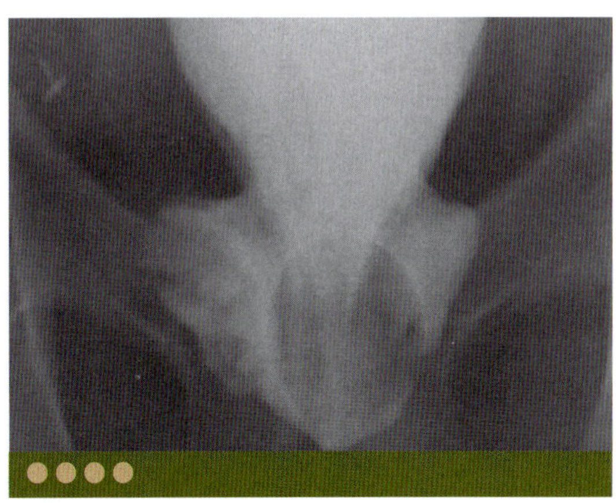

G. Iatrogenic bladder leak: Cystogram shows an irregular contrast collection at the base of the bladder. The Foley balloon is within the collection.

IMAGE KEY

Common

Rare

Typical

Unusual

8–26 Chyluria after Partial Nephrectomy

Frank H. Miller

PRESENTATION

Partial nephrectomy 2 months prior to CT; milky urine caused by chyluria.

FINDINGS

Fat in bladder in patients with partial nephrectomy.

DIFFERENTIAL DIAGNOSIS

- *Recent instrumentation or fistula to bladder*: Associated with air-fluid level and not fat-fluid level.

COMMENTS

Chyluria is a rare condition that is attributed to a lymphatic connection with the urinary tract. Most commonly chyluria has been previously reported to be secondary to infection and obstruction of the renal lymphatics caused by filariasis. More common causes in western countries include tumor, abscess, tuberculosis, congenital conditions, and pregnancy. These causes are generally associated with obstruction and disruption of the lymphatic vasculature into the collecting system. Another cause as illustrated in this example is surgery with resultant lymphatic injury and fistulous communication with the pyelocaliceal system. As partial nephrectomies are being performed more frequently for renal cell carcinoma, this finding may be seen more frequently. We have recently reported these findings in 4 of 125 patients following partial nephrectomy in the *American Journal of Roentgenology*. The radiologist may be the first person to suspect chyluria based on the detection, as in this case, of fat within the bladder. This finding should be differentiated from air-fluid levels in the bladder, typically after recent instrumentation. Prior imaging tests to evaluate chyluria included invasive tests such as lymphangiography.

As a result of chronic chyluria, patients may develop hypoproteinemia; however, our patients did not experience hypoproteinemia nor require surgical treatment for chyluria. Most patients are relatively asymptomatic. Microscopic evaluation of the urine shows granules of fat. None of our patients were suspected to have chyluria prior to the detection of fat in the bladder on CT, although in retrospect some reported cloudy urine. The finding of chyluria may persist for several years.

CT shows a fat-fluid level caused by the supernatant being hypodense relative to the denser fluid in the bladder. This should be distinguished from air-fluid levels, which are more commonly seen, and a result of instrumentation, infection, or fistula with bowel.

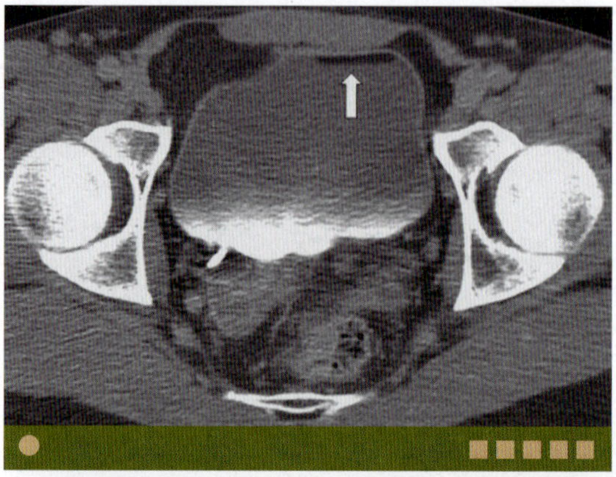

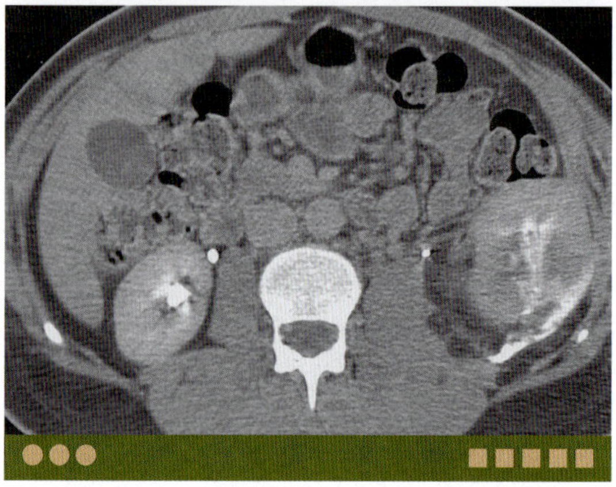

A. Axial CECT 3 months after surgery shows fat-fluid level in bladder with supernatant fat (arrow) hypodense relative to dependent nonfatty urine.
B. Axial CECT shows changes from left partial nephrectomy with contrast material within perinephric collection suggestive of communication with the collecting system.

PEARLS

- **Fat in the bladder on CT because of chyluria needs to be distinguished from the more common air-fluid level from instrumentation.**
- **Chyluria following partial nephrectomy can be suggested by radiologists and suggests lymphatic injury in connection with the collecting system.**
- **Additional imaging is generally not required.**
- **Surgical therapy was not needed, and no significant symptoms were seen after conservative management.**

ADDITIONAL IMAGES (C-D)

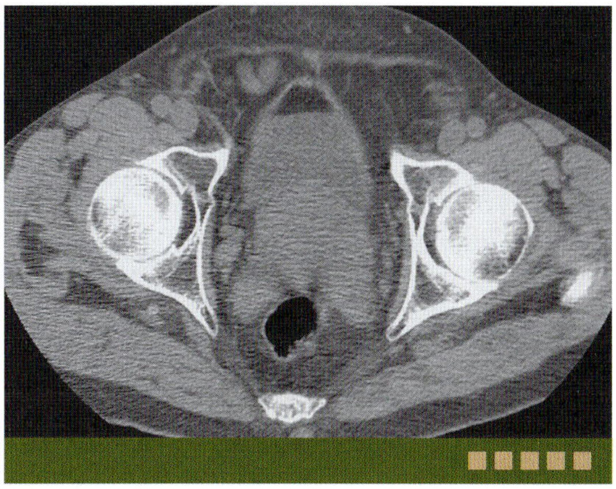

C. Axial NECT in another patient with chyluria and partial nephrectomy shows a fat-fluid level in bladder.

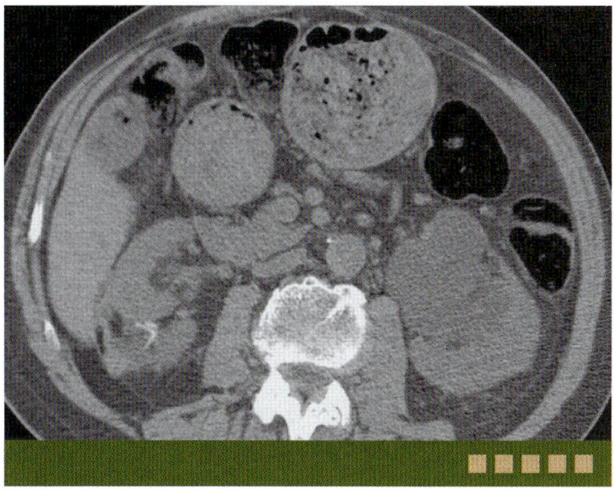

D. Axial NECT shows perinephric stranding surrounding the right kidney that had partial nephrectomy.

DIFFERENTIAL DIAGNOSIS IMAGE

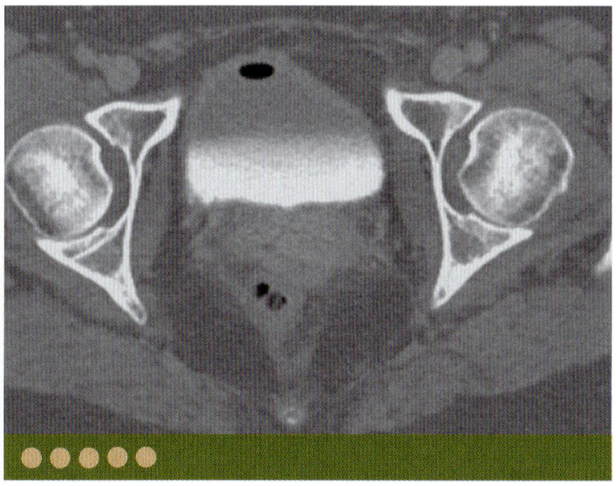

E. Air in bladder: Axial CECT shows focus of air in the anterior, nondependent aspect of the bladder in patient with a history of recent bladder instrumentation.

IMAGE KEY

Common

●●●●●

●●●●

●●●

●●

●

Rare

Typical

■■■■■

■■■■

■■■

■■

■

Unusual

8–27 Pelvic Lipomatosis

David D. Casalino

PRESENTATION

Urinary frequency.

FINDINGS

IVU shows a pear-shaped bladder and mild dilatation of the left ureter.

DIFFERENTIAL DIAGNOSES

- *Pelvic hematoma*: Most common; may be iatrogenic or traumatic with pelvic fractures and/or urinoma; clinical history helpful.
- *Bilateral pelvic lymphadenopathy*: May be associated with adenopathy elsewhere or history of malignancy.
- *Iliac artery aneurysms*: May show peripheral calcifications.
- *Bilateral lymphoceles*: Typically related to lymph node dissection; surgical clips present.
- *Iliac vein varices caused by IVC obstruction*: May be associated with bilateral peripheral edema or visible abdominal wall venous collaterals.
- *Iliopsoas hypertrophy*: As with pelvic lipomatosis, most often seen in young men with narrow pelvis.

COMMENTS

Pelvic lipomatosis is the deposition of excess adipose and fibrous tissue in the extraperitoneal space of the pelvis. It is usually an idiopathic process.

The majority of patients with pelvic lipomatosis are male, mostly black, and usually in early adulthood or middle age. Most patients are between 25 and 55 years of age.

Patients with pelvic lipomatosis are often asymptomatic. On occasion, symptoms may relate to associated bladder inflammation, diminished bladder capacity, outlet obstruction of the bladder or rectum, or ureteral obstruction. Urinary tract obstruction may result in renal failure.

Typical imaging findings include symmetric, external compression and elevation of the bladder resulting in a pear-shaped or gourd-shaped configuration. The bladder mucosa may be irregular, particularly in patients with coincidental cystitis glandularis. The rectum is compressed as well, and there is usually medial deviation of the distal ureters. The abundance of fat in the pelvis will cause increased lucency on standard radiography. An increased amount of fat density or fat signal intensity will be seen in the perivesical soft tissues on CT or MR, respectively. CT is usually the study of choice for a patient found to have a pear-shaped bladder on IVU or cystography.

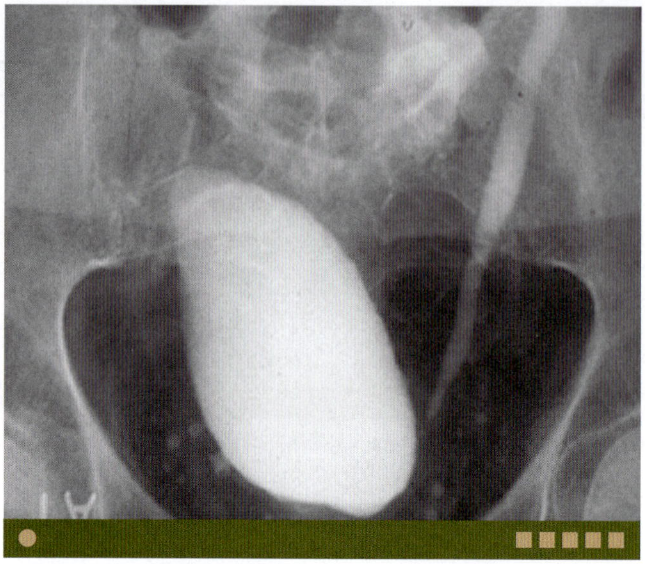

A. IVU shows a pear-shaped bladder with its superior aspect slightly deviated to the left of midline and mild dilatation of the left ureter.

PEARLS

- **Pelvic lipomatosis is an idiopathic process that occurs most often in males between 25 and 55 years of age.**
- **Patients are usually asymptomatic, but some may develop symptoms related to urinary tract obstruction, bladder inflammation, or rectal compression.**
- **The abundance of fat will cause increased pelvic lucency on radiography and have a characteristic appearance on CT and MR.**
- **CT is usually the study of choice for evaluating a patient found to have a pear-shaped bladder.**

ADDITIONAL IMAGES (B-D)

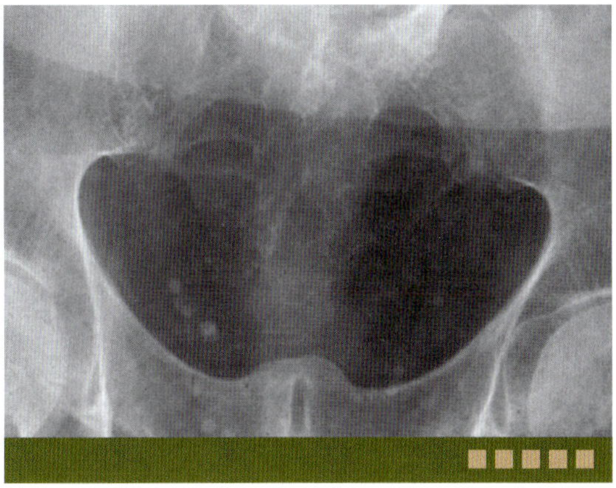

B. Conventional radiograph of the pelvis shows marked pelvic lucency caused by excess fat deposition. The lucency is more apparent on the left side.

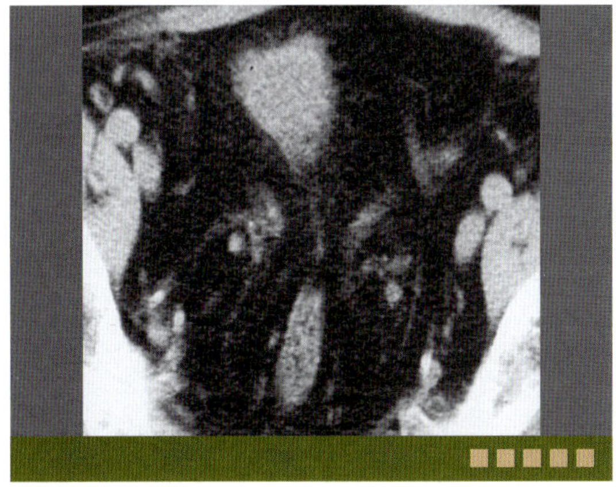

C. Axial CECT shows extensive perivesical and perirectal fat deposition compressing the bladder and rectum.

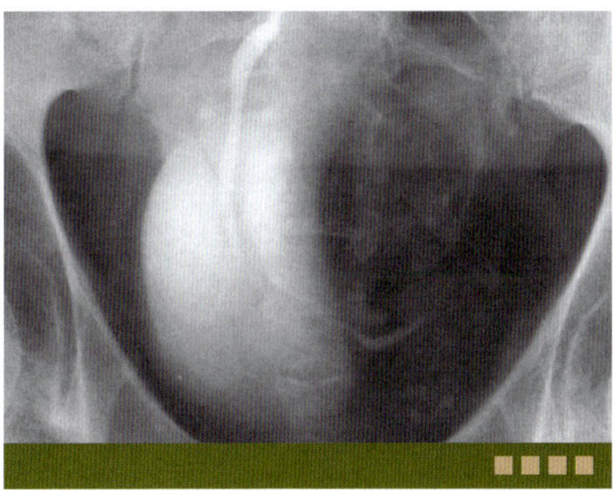

D. IVU from a different patient shows pronounced bladder deformity, medial deviation of the left ureter, and marked left hemipelvic lucency. *(Courtesy of Neil F. Wasserman, MD, Veterans Administration Medical Center, Minneapolis, MN.)*

DIFFERENTIAL DIAGNOSES IMAGES (E-G)

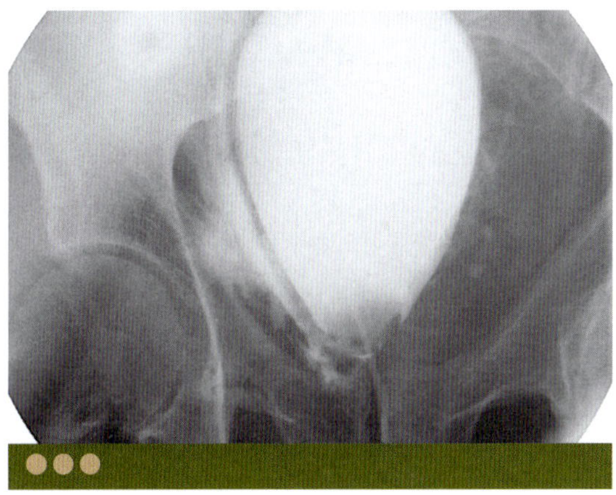

E. Pelvic hematoma: Cystogram shows pear-shaped bladder, extraperitoneal bladder leak, and pubic fracture in patient who fell 30 feet.

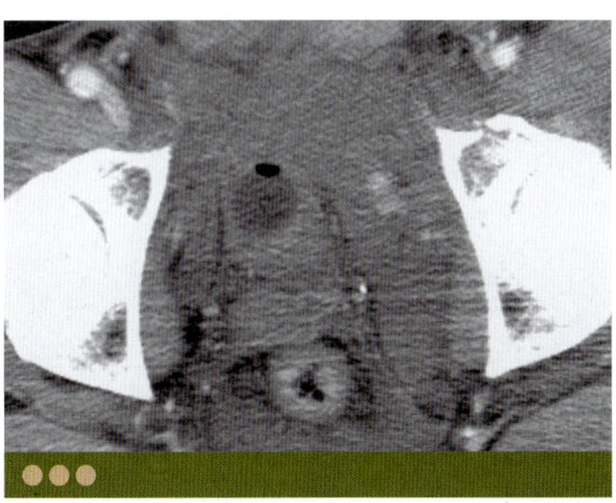

F. Pelvic hematoma: CECT from the same patient shows the bladder collapsed around a Foley catheter and surrounded by pelvic hemorrhage.

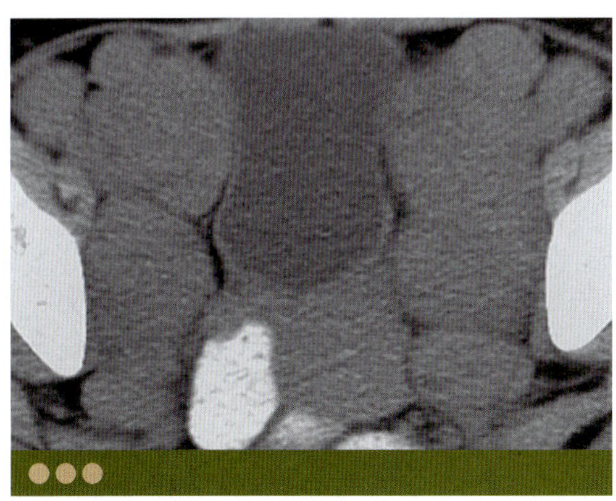

G. Lymphoma: CECT shows extensive lymphadenopathy causing bilateral and symmetric compression of the bladder.

IMAGE KEY

Common

Rare

Typical

Unusual

CHAPTER 9

URETHRA

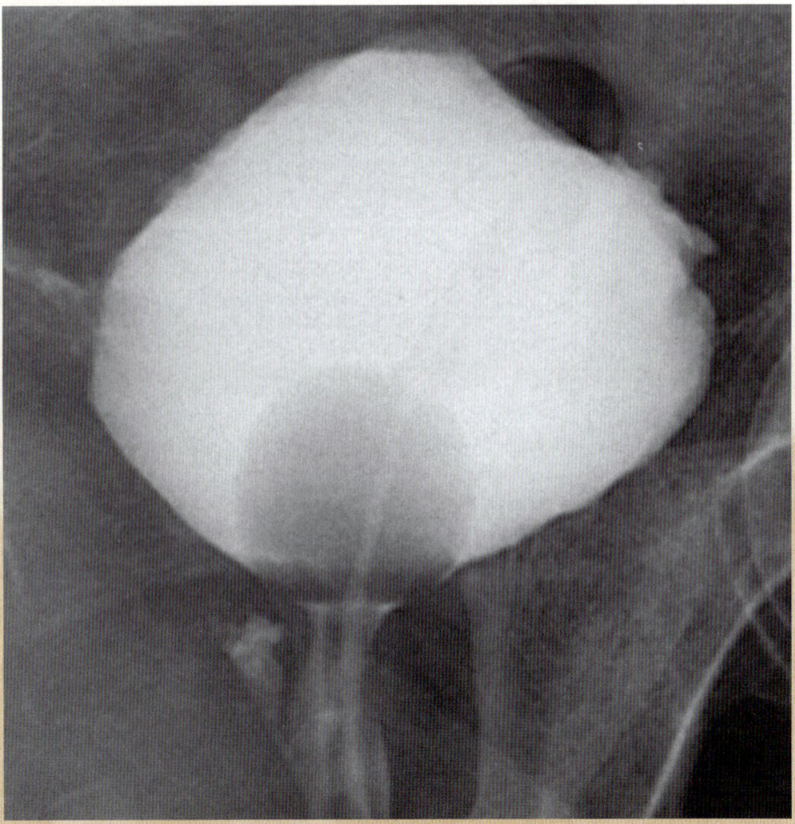

9–1 Normal Urethra

David D. Casalino

PRESENTATION

Dysuria.

FINDINGS

Cystogram shows a small lobulated collection of contrast extending cephalad from the right lateral aspect of the bulbous urethra.

DIFFERENTIAL DIAGNOSES

- *Anterior urethral injury*: May be iatrogenic or may be caused by blunt trauma or penetrating injury; clinical history usually includes mechanism of injury; blood at the meatus is the cardinal sign of anterior urethral injury.
- *Urethral fistula*: May result from infection, trauma, radiation injury, surgery, or, rarely, neoplasm; irregular tract that may be blind ending or communicate with a pelvic organ or another segment of urethra.
- *Urethral diverticulum*: Can be congenital or acquired; acquired diverticula may be caused by trauma, instrumentation, or infection and can involve any portion.

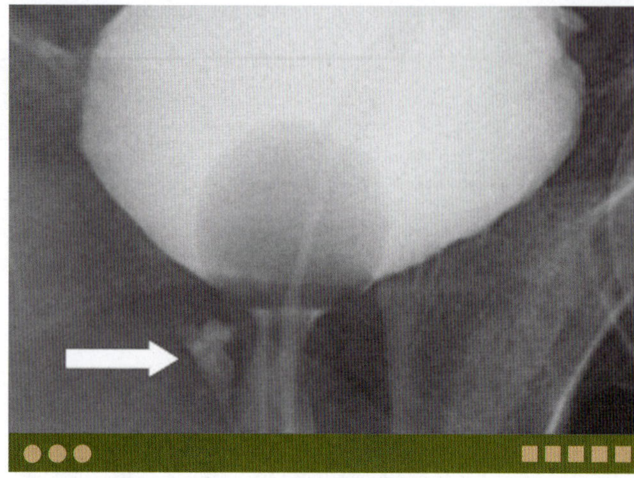

A. Cystogram shows a small lobulated collection of contrast extending cephalad via a smooth tract from the right lateral aspect of the bulbous urethra. The appearance is characteristic of a normal Cowper gland and duct.

COMMENTS

MALE URETHRA

The male urethra has a length of 17.5 to 20 cm and consists of anterior and posterior portions. The posterior urethra is divided into the prostatic and membranous urethras. The prostatic urethra is 3.5 cm long and extends from the internal sphincter at the bladder neck and terminates at the distal end of the verumontanum. The verumontanum is a 1-cm long oval protuberance at the posterior wall of the prostatic urethra. Two ejaculatory ducts and prostatic glands drain into the verumontanum. The membranous urethra is 1 to 1.5-cm long and extends from the distal end of the verumontanum to the external sphincter at the urogenital diaphragm. It is the narrowest portion of the urethra.

The anterior urethra is divided into the bulbous, or bulbar, and penile, or pendulous, portions. The bulbous urethra extends from the external sphincter to the penoscrotal junction, where there is slight angulation of the urethra by the suspensory ligament of the penis. The proximal bulbous urethra is dilated and has a conical shape at the bulbomembranous junction. Contraction of the constrictor nudae muscle may cause an anterior or circumferential indentation of the proximal bulbous urethra and should not be mistaken for a stricture. Cowper glands are paired glands that lie within the urogenital diaphragm and drain into either side of the dilated portion of the bulbous urethra via ducts that are 2 to 4 cm long. There are also periurethral glands of Littré that drain into the anterior urethra and are more numerous on the dorsal aspect. Contrast opacification of Cowper glands and ducts, glands of Littré, and prostatic ducts during urethrography is often associated with urethral inflammation or stricture, although not always. The penile urethra extends from the penoscrotal junction to the external meatus. The fossa navicularis is 1- to 1.5-cm long focal dilatation of the distal aspect of the penile urethra.

FEMALE URETHRA

The female urethra is 4 cm long and extends from the bladder neck obliquely in an anterior and inferior direction to the external orifice situated between the labia minora. The urethra is widest at its proximal aspect and tapers distally. Skene glands are groups of periurethral glands found distally and empty through two small ducts to either side of the external meatus.

PEARLS

- **The male urethra consists of anterior (prostatic and membranous) and posterior (bulbous and penile) portions.**
- **Contrast opacification of Cowper glands and ducts, glands of Littré, and prostatic ducts during imaging is often associated with urethral inflammation or stricture, but not always.**
- **The female urethra is widest at its proximal aspect and tapers distally.**

ADDITIONAL IMAGES (B-E)

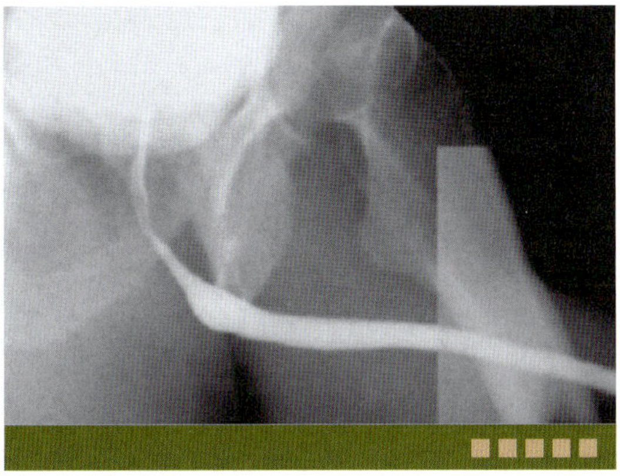

B. Retrograde urethrogram, a composite image, shows a normal urethra.

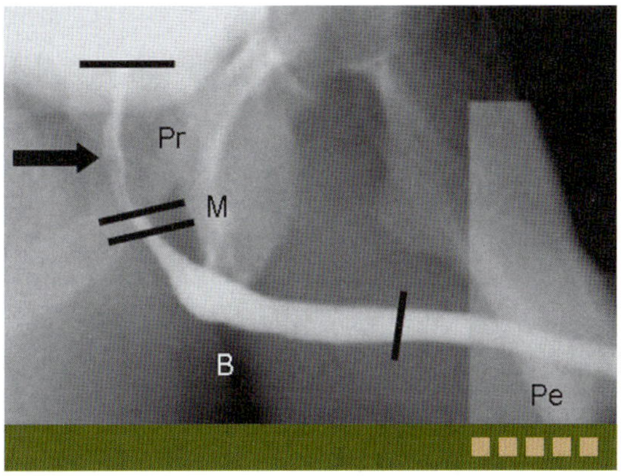

C. Retrograde urethrogram shows the verumontanum (arrow) and demarcation of prostatic (Pr), membranous (M), bulbar (B), and penile (Pe) portions of the urethra.

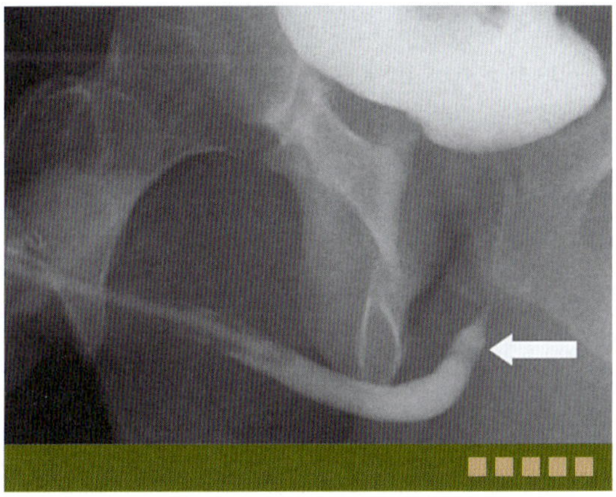

D. Retrograde urethrogram from a different male patient shows the normal conical shape of the proximal bulbar urethra with smooth focal indentation (arrow) caused by the constrictor nudae muscle.

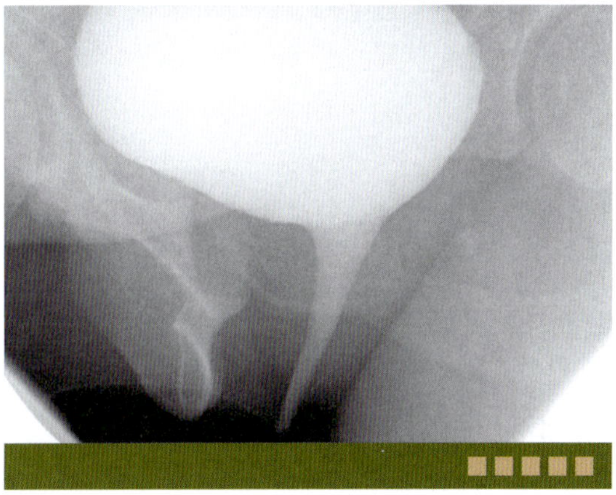

E. Voiding cystourethrogram shows a normal female urethra.

DIFFERENTIAL DIAGNOSES IMAGES (F-G)

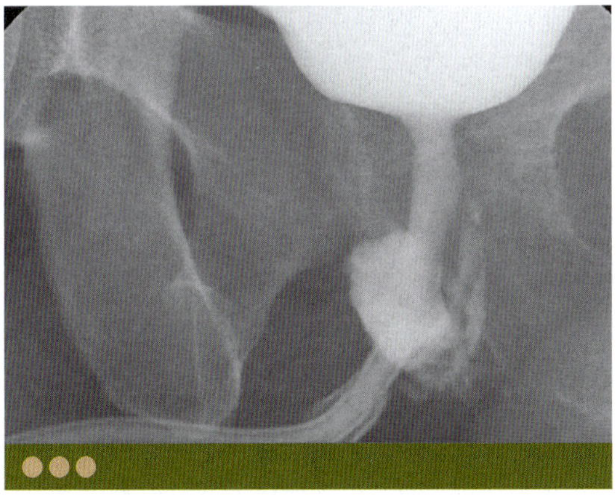

F. Iatrogenic anterior urethral injury: Retrograde urethrogram shows focal contrast leakage from the bulbous urethra after abdominoperineal resection.

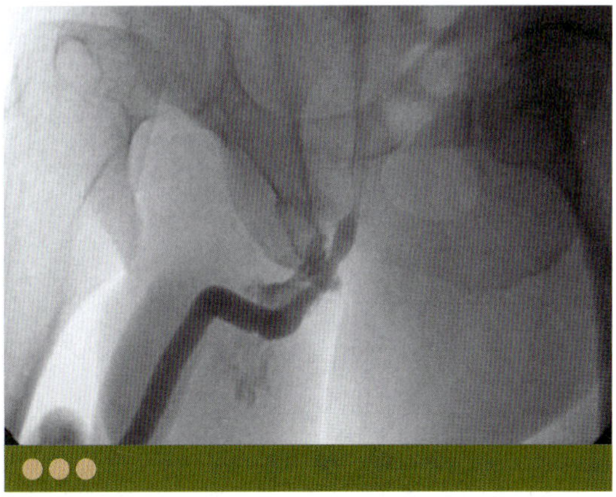

G. Traumatic anterior urethral injury: Retrograde urethrogram shows contrast leakage from the bulbous urethra with extension into the scrotum in a patient status post straddle injury.

IMAGE KEY

Common

Rare

Typical

Unusual

9–2 Female Urethral Carcinoma

David D. Casalino

PRESENTATION

Urethral mass associated with bleeding and dysuria.

FINDINGS

CT shows a slightly heterogeneous soft-tissue mass of the urethra.

DIFFERENTIAL DIAGNOSES

- *Other malignancy involving urethra*: Including bladder, gynecologic, and rectal cancers; may have clinical signs and symptoms specific for a particular tumor; imaging may not be able to differentiate; tissue diagnosis necessary.
- *Infectious process*: Including infected urethral diverticulum; signs and symptoms suggestive of infection.

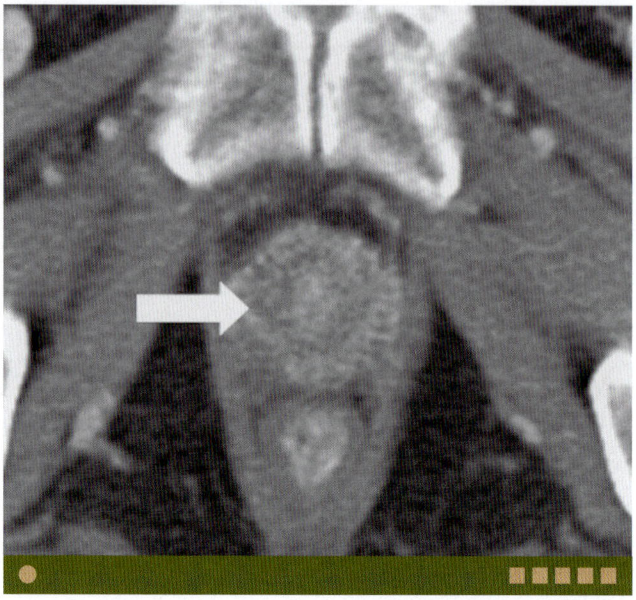

A. Axial CECT shows a slightly heterogeneous soft-tissue mass of the urethra (arrow).

COMMENTS

Carcinoma of the urethra accounts for less than 0.01% of all female malignancies. Most of the patients are white and 40 to 60 years old. Urethral carcinomas seem to develop in the setting of chronic irritation or urinary tract infections. Squamous cell carcinoma (SCC) is the most common histopathologic type, accounting for 60% to 75% of cases, followed by transitional cell carcinoma (TCC) (15%-20%) and adenocarcinoma. The distal third of the urethra is the most common site for SCC. Benign, synchronous lesions, such as caruncles, papillomas, and polyps of the urethra, are often present. Presenting symptoms may include urethral bleeding, frequency, dysuria, urethral obstruction, and urethral mass. The diagnosis is usually made by clinical examination.

Voiding cystourethrography (VCUG) may demonstrate irregular narrowing or a single or multiple irregular filling defects. CT and MR are helpful in assessing local invasion and nodal involvement. On CT, the tumor appears as a heterogeneous, soft-tissue attenuation mass. On MR, the tumor is typically hypointense on T1-weighted imaging, hyperintense on T2-weighted imaging, and enhances. Sagittal T2-weighted imaging is particularly useful for assessing tumor invasion of the bladder, vagina, and pelvic floor. Tumors of the distal third of the urethra, sometimes referred to as "anterior" urethral cancer, preferentially spread to the superficial and deep inguinal nodes. More proximal tumors, sometimes referred to as "entire" urethral cancer, spread to the internal and external iliac and obturator nodes and not uncommonly invade adjacent organs. While anterior lesions can usually be treated with local surgical excision, entire urethral lesions are often high-grade tumors, locally advanced, and may warrant a combination therapy that includes surgery, radiation therapy, and chemotherapy.

PEARLS

- **Urethral carcinoma is the only epithelial malignancy of the urinary tract that is more common in women with a 4:1 female-to-male ratio.**
- **SCC is the most common histopathologic type, followed by TCC and adenocarinoma.**
- **VCUG may demonstrate irregular narrowing or irregular filling defect(s).**
- **MR and CT are useful in the assessment of nodal disease and local invasion.**

ADDITIONAL IMAGE

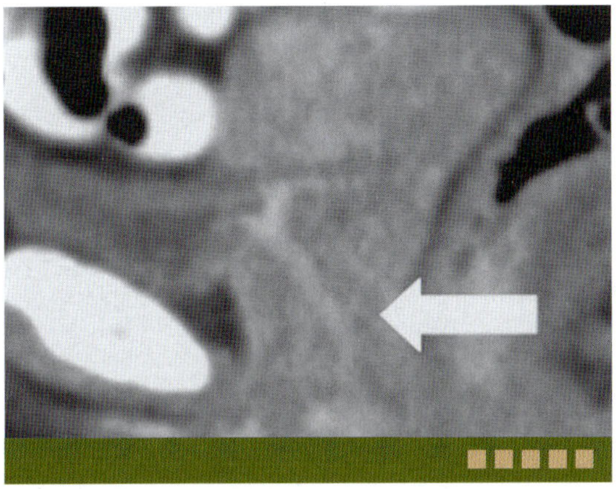

B. Sagittal CECT shows the urethral mass (arrow) without evidence of gross invasion into the surrounding structures. Biopsy and subsequent surgery diagnosed urethral SCC with extensive inflammatory change of the urethra.

DIFFERENTIAL DIAGNOSES IMAGES (C-E)

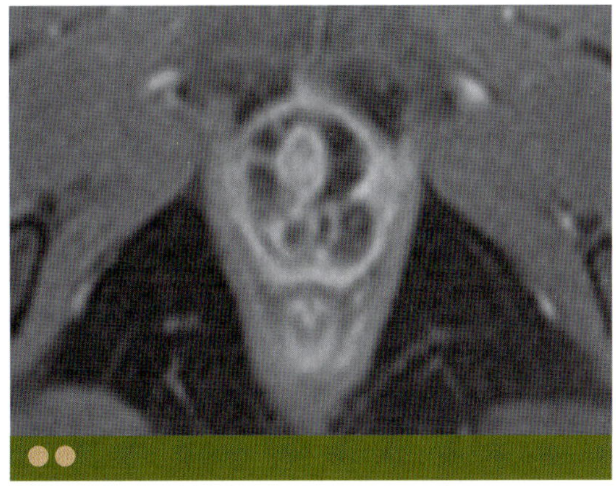

C. Urethral diverticulum, infected: Axial contrast-enhanced T1-WI shows a heterogeneous lesion surrounding the urethra. The mass is predominantly low-signal intensity with peripheral enhancement and septations.

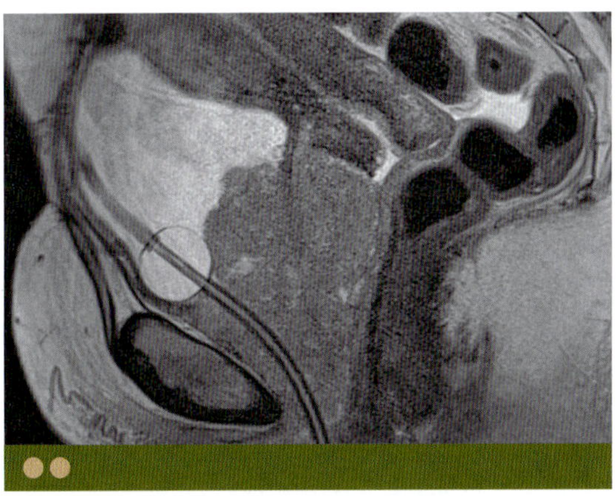

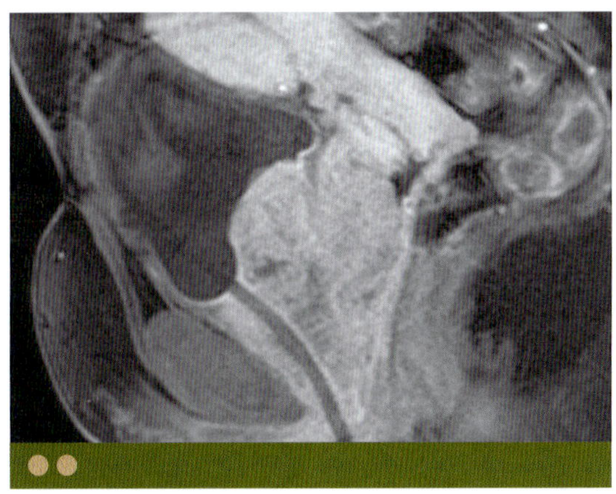

D. and **E. Vaginal SCC involving the urethra:** Sagittal T2-WI and contrast-enhanced T1-WI show a large, heterogeneously enhancing mass arising from the anterior vaginal wall and invading the urethra and bladder.

IMAGE KEY

Common

Rare

Typical

Unusual

9–3 Male Urethral Carcinoma

David D. Casalino

PRESENTATION

Hematuria, diminished urine stream, and palpable penile mass.

FINDINGS

MR shows a heterogeneous, enhancing mass involving the corpus spongiosum.

DIFFERENTIAL DIAGNOSES

- *Squamous cell carcinoma (SCC) of the penis*: Rare in the US, but accounts for 10% to 20% of all male malignancies in Asia, Africa, and South America; glans is involved in more than 50% of the cases; threefold increased risk in uncircumcised men.
- *Penile sarcoma*: Include epithelioid sarcoma, Kaposi, leiomyosarcoma, and rhabdomyosarcoma; rare, accounting for less than 5% of penile malignancies; those arising from a corpus tend to metastasize early.
- *Metastatic disease*: Often a known primary, such as bladder urothelial carcinoma or prostate adenocarcinoma.

COMMENTS

Primary urethral carcinoma is rare. SCC is most common, accounting for 80% of the cases, and most often arises in the bulbous or membranous urethra but can occur in the more distal urethra and, rarely, in the prostatic urethra. TCC is less common, accounting for 15% of cases, and usually occurs in the posterior urethra but can occur more distal. Adenocarcinoma is the least common and arises from Cowper glands or the glands of Littré. Urethral carcinoma usually occurs in men that are more than 50 years of age. Chronic irritation, gonococcal urethritis, and urethral stricture are considered risk factors for the development of urethral carcinoma. The most common presenting symptom is a palpable mass along the course of the urethra or in the perineum. Patients may also present with obstructive symptoms, hematuria, bloody discharge, pain, urethral fistula, or periurethral abscess.

Urethrography typically demonstrates segmental, irregular narrowing of the urethra. If there is a change in the appearance of a chronic stricture or if the margins of a stricture are irregular, carcinoma should be considered. Larger tumors may be seen as an infiltrative mass on CT or MR. On MR, the tumor is usually isointense to low-signal intensity relative to the surrounding corpus spongiosum on T1- and T2-weighted images. MR is useful in assessing tumor size and location and in local staging, which includes determination of invasion into the corpora and other adjacent structures. Urethral carcinoma may also spread to regional lymph nodes and hematogenously to more distant sites. Posterior urethral carcinomas are more often associated with extensive local spread, distant metastases, and a worse prognosis. Surgical excision is the most common treatment for urethral carcinoma.

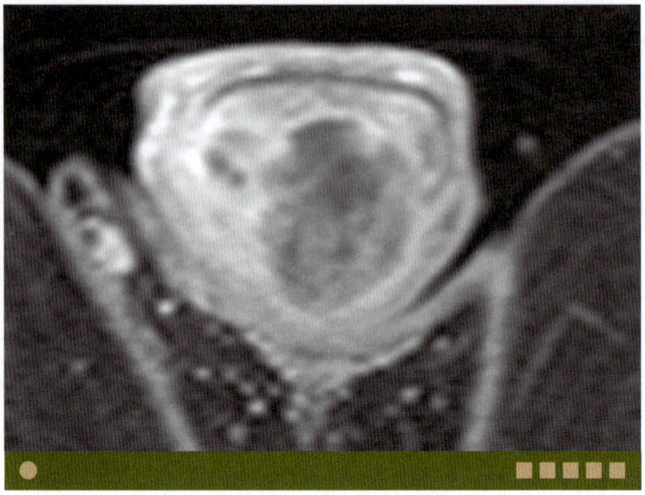

A. Axial contrast-enhanced T1-WI shows a heterogeneous, enhancing mass involving the corpus spongiosum, extending through its tunica into the intercavernous fascia.

PEARLS

- **Carcinomas of the urethra are SCC in 80% of the cases and most common in the bulbous and membranous portions.**
- **Patients with urethral carcinoma often have a history of urethral stricture and a palpable mass.**
- **Urethral carcinoma should be considered when urethrogram demonstrates a change in the appearance of a chronic stricture or if the margins of a stricture are irregular.**
- **MR is particularly helpful in local staging.**
- **Primary tumor stages are I: invades subepithelial connective tissue; II: invades corpus spongiosum prostate or periurethral muscle; III: invades corpus cavernosum beyond prostate capsule, anterior vagina, or bladder neck; and IV: invades other adjacent organs.**

ADDITIONAL IMAGES (B-D)

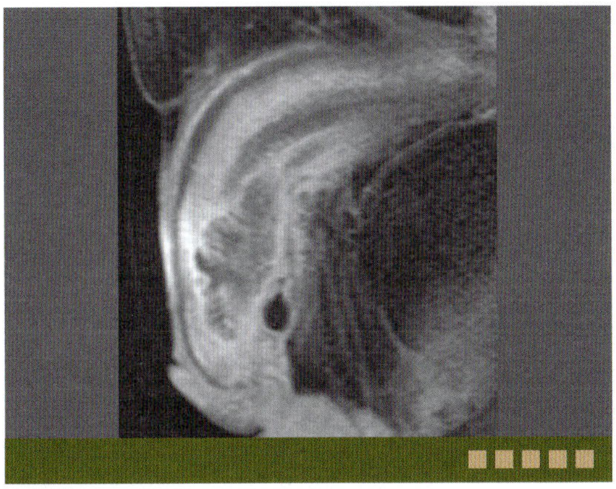

B. Sagittal contrast-enhanced T1-WI from the same patient shows the mass that involves the penile urethra. The glans penis is normal. Biopsy showed SCC of the urethra.

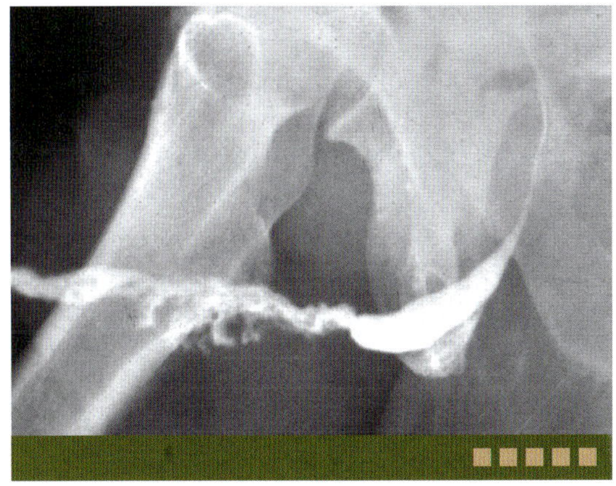

C. Retrograde urethrogram shows irregular narrowing of a long segment of anterior urethra caused by SCC.

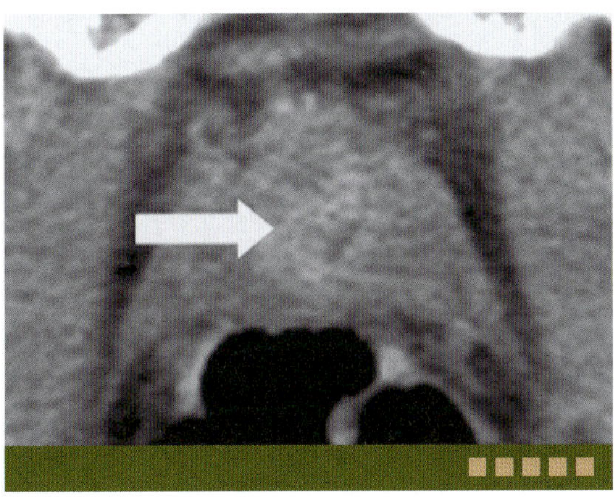

D. Axial CECT shows an enhancing mass (arrow) involving the central region of the prostate. Biopsy showed TCC of the prostatic urethra.

DIFFERENTIAL DIAGNOSES IMAGES (E-G)

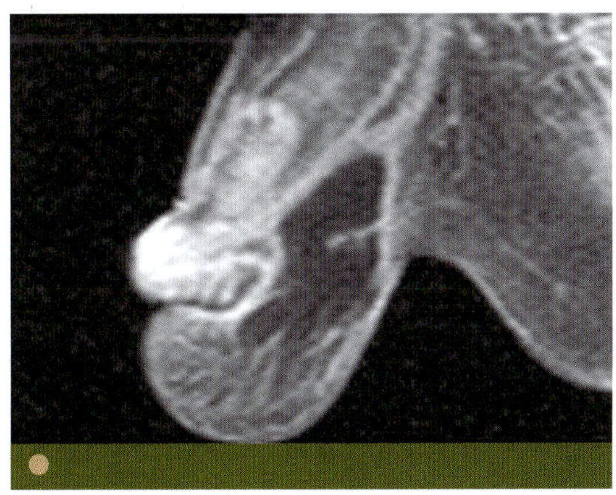

E. Squamous cell carcinoma of the penis: Sagittal contrast-enhanced T1-WI shows a large mass with central necrosis involving the glans penis as well as the ventral aspect of the corpus spongiosum and penile urethra.

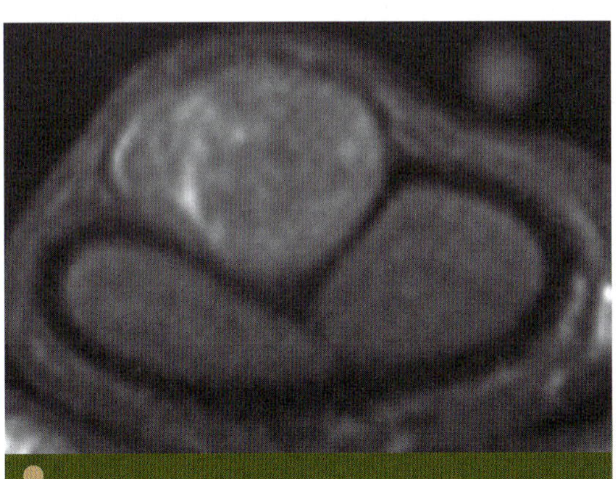

F. Penile leiomyosarcoma: Axial contrast-enhanced T1-WI shows a heterogeneous, enhancing mass arising from the corpus spongiosum with local invasion.

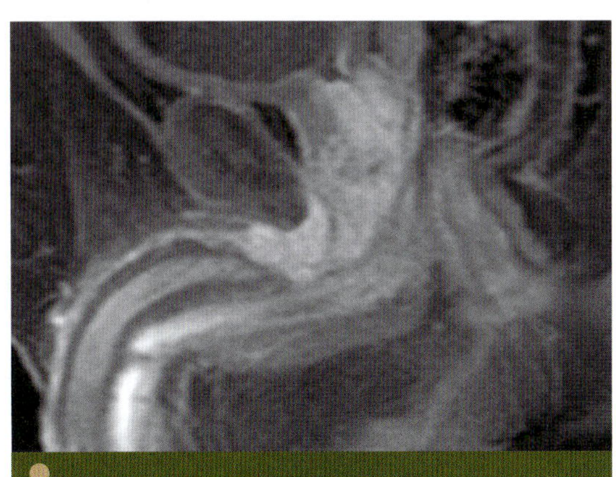

G. Metastatic disease: Sagittal contrast-enhanced T1-WI shows a heterogeneous, large enhancing mass involving the prostate, proximal urethra, and base of penis. Biopsy showed synovial sarcoma.

IMAGE KEY

Common

Rare

Typical

Unusual

9–4 Urethral Stricture

David D. Casalino

PRESENTATION

Decrease urine flow, hematuria, and dysuria.

FINDINGS

Urethrogram shows focal narrowing of the bulbous urethra.

DIFFERENTIAL DIAGNOSES

- *Iatrogenic stricture*: History of instrumentation, catheterization, or surgery.
- *Traumatic stricture*: History of trauma (blunt or penetrating); focal stricture; straddle injury typically involves the bulbous urethra.
- *Infectious or inflammatory stricture*: Relevant history of infection or inflammation; longer segment of urethra often involved; gonococcus most often involves the bulbous urethra.
- *Neoplasm*: Stricture is rarely only manifestation of neoplasm; elderly patient.

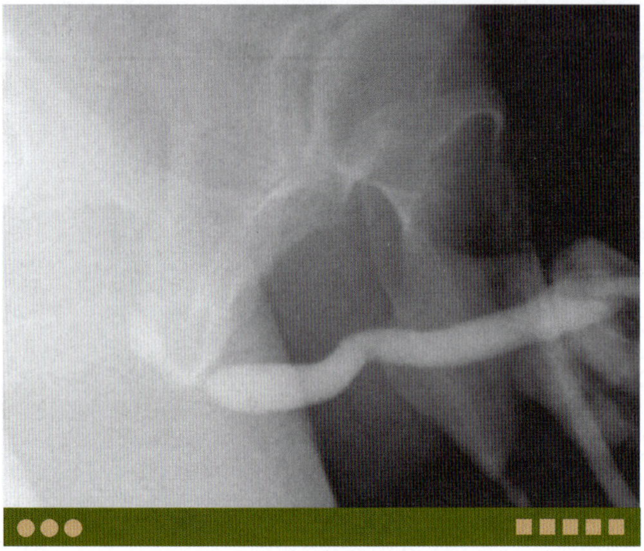

A. Retrograde urethrogram shows focal narrowing of the bulbous urethra because of a stricture related to prior straddle injury.

COMMENTS

A urethral stricture is an abnormal narrowing of any part of the urethra caused by fibrous scarring. Urethral strictures occur primarily in men. The most common causes of anterior urethral strictures are iatrogenic and traumatic, followed by infectious, inflammatory, and neoplastic. Congenital strictures are rare. Iatrogenic strictures may be because of instrumentation, catheterization, or surgery and usually occur in the bulbomembranous and penoscrotal junctions. They may be focal or long, solitary or multifocal. A straddle injury is the most common external trauma associated with anterior strictures. The bulbous urethra is usually involved focally. The most common infectious etiology is caused by *Neisseria gonorrhoeae*, which usually involves the bulbous urethra with multiple strictures. Strictures of the posterior urethra are usually the result of trauma or surgery, such as radical prostatectomy or transurethral resection of the prostate (TURP), causing urethral distraction or disruption. Patients with a urethral stricture may present with decreased urine flow, incomplete bladder emptying, dysuria, hematuria, or urinary tract infection.

The goals of imaging urethral strictures include assessment of the number, location, length, and severity of the strictures and detection of concomitant abnormalities, such as periurethral abscess, fistula, false passages between different portions of the urethra, and urine extravasation. This information is critical for determining appropriate treatment.

Retrograde urethrography is the primary imaging study for evaluating a urethral stricture. Proper patient positioning in a steep oblique orientation is necessary to avoid underestimating stricture length. Multiple projections may be complementary. Ultrasound and MR may be complementary in evaluating patients with strictures. Treatment options include dilatation, intraluminal stenting, cystoscopic urethrectomy, and open urethroplasty.

PEARLS

- **Urethral strictures occur primarily in men and are most often iatrogenic or traumatic.**
- **Infectious strictures are typically secondary to gonococcal urethritis.**
- **Retrograde urethrography is the primary imaging study for evaluating urethral strictures.**
- **Proper technique is critical in defining the extent and severity of strictures and should include steep oblique positioning of the patient and penis.**

ADDITIONAL IMAGE

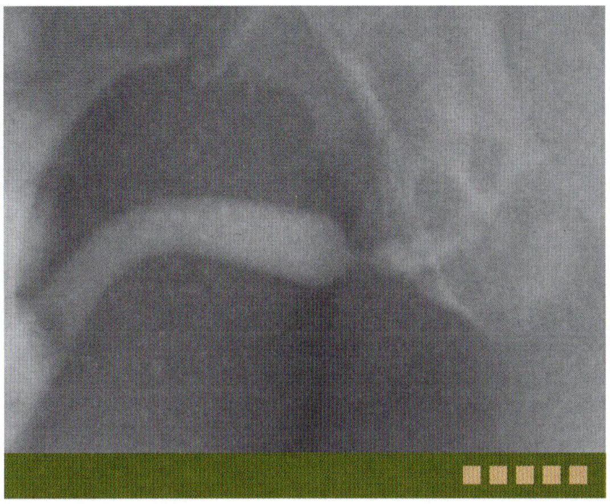

B. Retrograde urethrogram from a different patient shows a very focal and tight stricture also secondary to a straddle injury.

DIFFERENTIAL DIAGNOSES IMAGES (C-G)

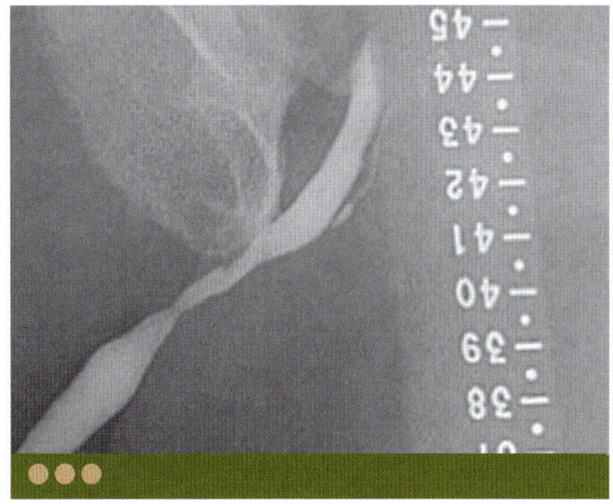

C. Iatrogenic stricture: Retrograde urethrogram shows a 3.5-cm-long stricture at the penoscrotal junction. The stricture was because of prior catheterizations. Contrast partially fills a Cowper duct.

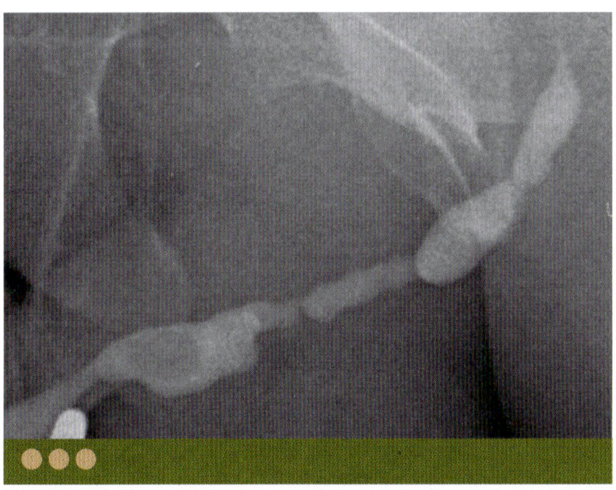

D. Iatrogenic stricture: Retrograde urethrogram shows irregularity with focal stricture involving the anterior urethra in a patient status post open urethral reconstruction using a buccal mucosal graft.

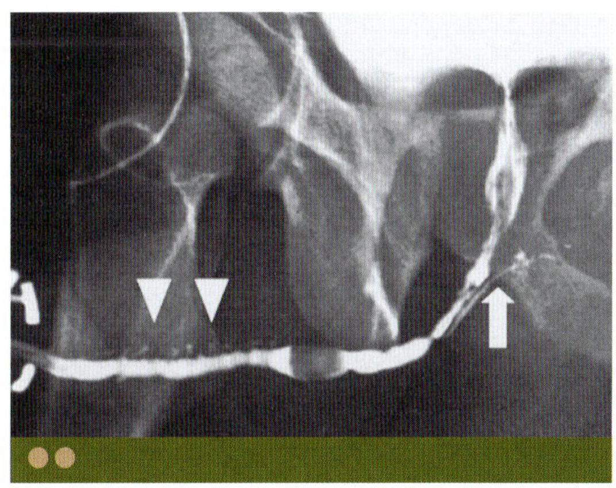

E. Infectious stricture: Retrograde urethrogram from a patient with gonococcal urethritis shows multiple strictures involving the bulbous urethra and penile urethra. There are glands of Littré abscesses (arrowheads) and involvement of Cowper ducts and glands (arrow). There is an air bubble at the penoscrotal junction.

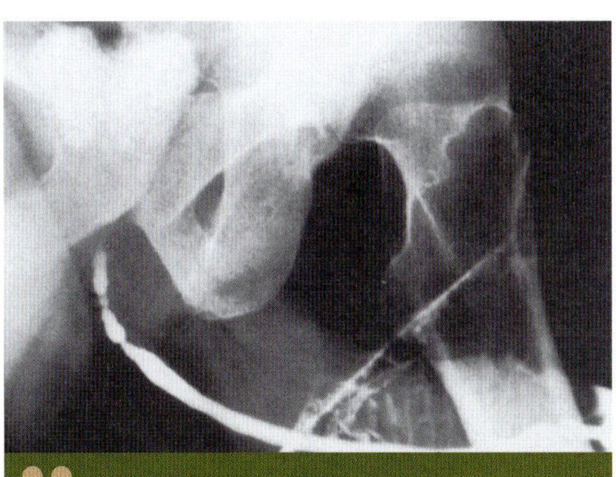

F. Infectious stricture: Retrograde urethrogram of a different patient with gonococcal urethritis shows a beaded stricture of the bulbous urethra.

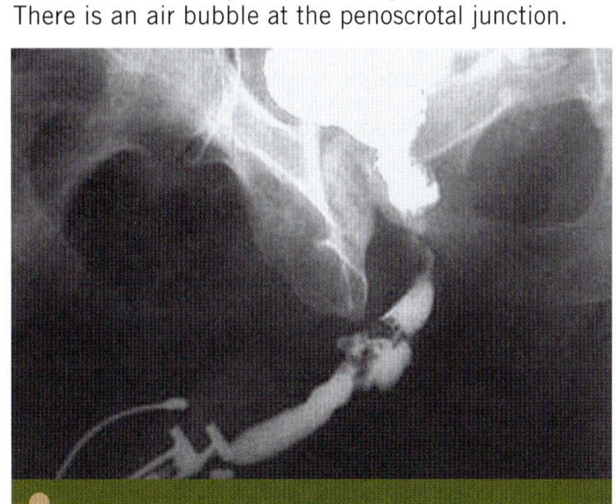

G.Neoplastic stricture: Retrograde urethrogram shows very irregular, focal narrowing of the bulbous urethra caused by SCC of the urethra. *(Figures E-G courtesy of Neil F. Wasserman, MD, Veterans Administration Medical Center, Minneapolis, MN.)*

IMAGE KEY

Common

Rare

Typical

Unusual

9–5 Gonococcal Urethritis

David D. Casalino

PRESENTATION

Decreased urine flow, incomplete bladder emptying, dysuria and history of antibiotic treatment for urethral discharge.

FINDINGS

Urethrogram shows focal narrowing of the bulbous urethra.

DIFFERENTIAL DIAGNOSES

- *Nongonococcal urethritis*: Urethral discharge usually scant; *Chlamydia trachomatis* accounts for up to 50% of the cases; complications, including stricture, are much less common; less than 5% develop a stricture.
- *Iatrogenic stricture*: History of instrumentation or surgery.
- *Trauma*: History of trauma (blunt or penetrating); focal stricture; straddle injury typically involves the bulbous urethra.
- *Neoplasm*: Stricture is rarely only manifestation of neoplasm; elderly patient.

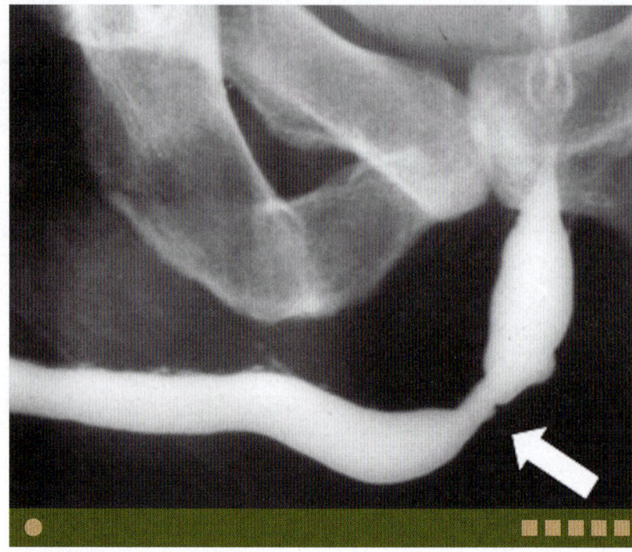

A. Retrograde urethrogram shows slightly irregular, focal narrowing (arrow) of the bulbous urethra and slight mucosal irregularity involving the penile urethra.

COMMENTS

Gonococcal urethritis is due to infection by *N gonorrhoeae*, a gram-negative diploccoccus, and is one of the most common causes of urethral stricture. The infection starts in the distal urethra and spreads proximally, though rarely proximal to the external sphincter. Fifteen percent of patients will develop a stricture in the late stages of infection. Patients with gonococcal urethritis usually present with a purulent discharge. Dysuria and painful or swollen testicles may also be present. Diagnosis is usually made on the basis of clinical and laboratory findings. Treatment involves antibiotics with coverage for *C trachomatis*, another common sexually transmitted disease often found in patients with gonorrhea.

No imaging is necessary for uncomplicated urethritis. Urethrography is usually performed to evaluate suspected complications that may include stricture, periurethral fistula, and periurethral abscess. Seventy percent of strictures involve the bulbous urethra, but they can involve the penile urethra. It is usually irregular or beaded and extends over several centimeters. Dilatation of Littré glands is not uncommonly seen on urethrography. Filling of Cowper ducts may also be seen proximal to the stricture. Mucosal hyperplasia may occur and create nodular filling defects in the urethra. Periurethral abscess is thought to arise from a Littré gland that has become obstructed and infected. These abscesses may be life-threatening if not diagnosed and treated quickly. The abscess may spread ventrally along the corpus spongiosum. On occasion, the Buck fascia may be penetrated and result in tissue necrosis and fistula formation between the urethra and perineum. "Watering can" or "watering pot" perineum refers to urination through urethroperineal fistulas, which are more commonly associated with tuberculosis of the urethra. Urethrography may demonstrate a periurethral abscess if it communicates with the urethra or fistula. Ultrasound may be helpful in the diagnosis of periurethral abscess. CT and MR imaging may demonstrate complications and the extent of the abscess. Treatment involves antibiotics, surgical debridement, and urinary drainage via suprapubic catheter.

PEARLS

- **Uncomplicated gonococcal urethritis is usually diagnosed on the basis of clinical and laboratory findings.**
- **Fifteen percent of the patients with gonococcal urethritis develop a stricture, which involves the proximal bulbous urethra in 70% of the cases.**
- **Periurethral abscesses and urethroperineal fistulas may complicate gonococcal urethritis.**

ADDITIONAL IMAGES (B-D)

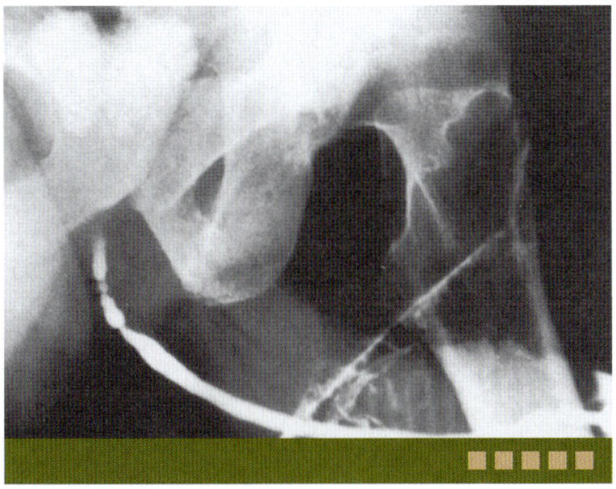

B. Retrograde urethrogram from a different patient with gonococcal urethritis shows a longer, beaded stricture of the bulbous urethra. *(Courtesy of Neil F. Wasserman, MD, Veterans Administration Medical Center, Minneapolis, MN.)*

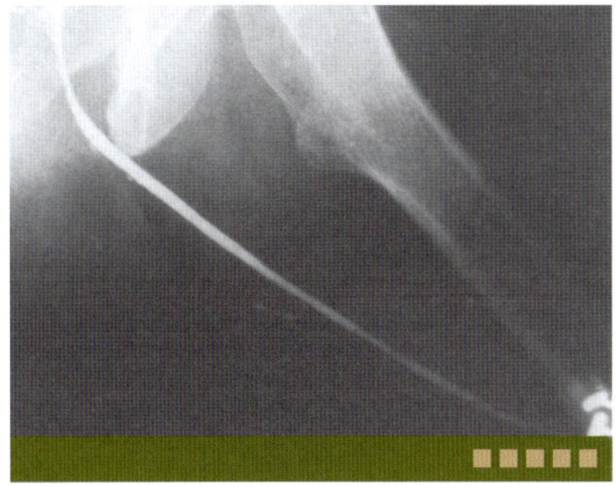

C. Retrograde urethrogram from a different patient shows a very long, smooth stricture of the bulbous and penile urethra. *(Courtesy of Neil F. Wasserman, MD, Veterans Administration Medical Center, Minneapolis, MN.)*

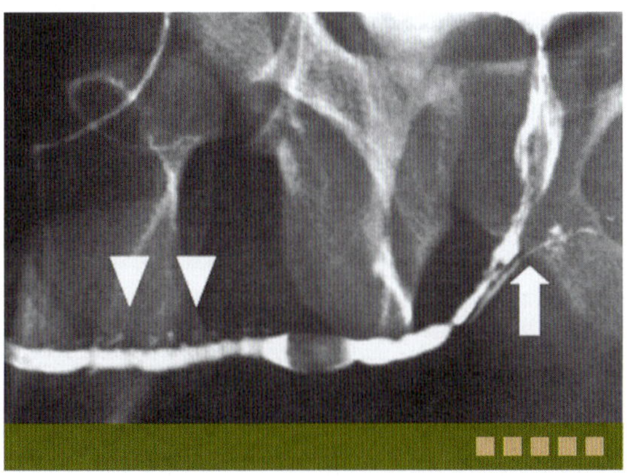

D. Retrograde urethrogram from a patient with gonococcal urethritis shows multiple strictures involving the bulbous urethra and penile urethra. There are glands of Littré abscesses (arrowheads) and involvement of Cowper ducts and glands (arrow). There is an air bubble at the penoscrotal junction. *(Courtesy of Neil F. Wasserman, MD, Veterans Administration Medical Center, Minneapolis, MN.)*

DIFFERENTIAL DIAGNOSES IMAGES (E-F)

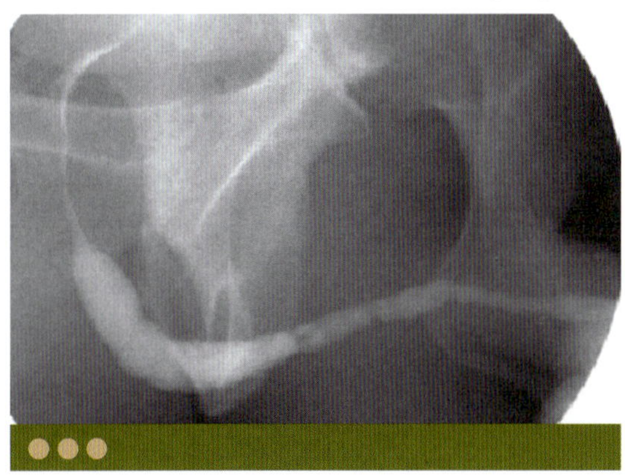

E. Iatrogenic stricture: Retrograde urethrogram shows beaded narrowing of a long segment of penile urethra and distal bulbous urethra. The stricture was presumably because of extended catheterization.

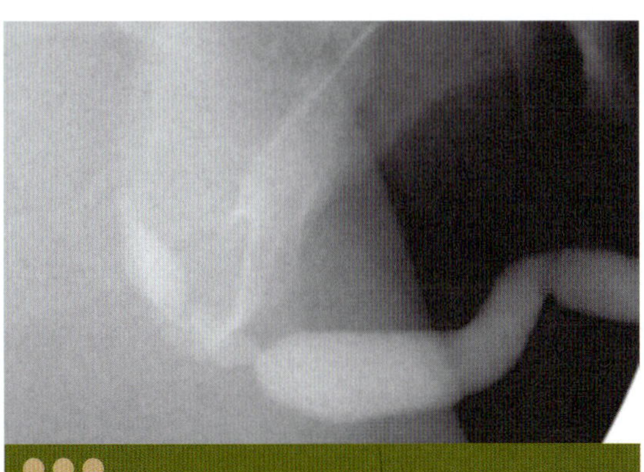

F. Traumatic stricture: Retrograde urethrogram shows a focal stricture of the bulbous urethra in a young adult who sustained a straddle injury when he was 9 years old.

IMAGE KEY

Common

Rare

Typical

Unusual

9–6 Balanitis Xerotica Obliterans, or Penile Lichen Sclerosus

David D. Casalino

PRESENTATION

Dysuria and weak urine stream in patients with atrophic white patches on the glans penis.

FINDINGS

Urethrogram shows smooth narrowing of the fossa navicularis and distal urethra.

DIFFERENTIAL DIAGNOSES

- *Infectious urethritis and stricture*: Much more common; relevant history of infection; discharge; more often multifocal; gonococcus most often involves the bulbous urethra.
- *Iatrogenic stricture*: History of instrumentation or surgery.
- *Trauma*: History of trauma (blunt or penetrating); focal stricture; straddle injury typically involves the bulbous urethra.
- *Neoplasm*: Stricture is rarely only manifestation of neoplasm; elderly patient.

COMMENTS

Balanitis xerotica obliterans (BXO) is a male genital variant of lichen sclerosus et atrophicus (LS), a skin disease of uncertain etiology that results in white, thickened plaques involving the prepuce, glans, and/or urethral meatus. BXO is a common cause of acquired phimosis and meatal stenosis in schoolboys. Urethral involvement is uncommon, starts at the meatus, and spreads proximally in a confluent manner. The involved segment typically shows smooth narrowing. In mild early BXO, patients may notice areas of grayish white coloration on the glans or inner layer of the foreskin. The involved areas may be itchy and are prone to fissuring and hemorrhagic blistering during intercourse. Fibrous phimosis may develop. When more aggressive, BXO may cause the surface of the glans and inner prepuce to ulcerate, producing a purulent discharge. BXO is considered premalignant and associated with SCC of the penis, which may develop long after the BXO has been treated.

Imaging is not necessary for the diagnosis of BXO, but urethrography may demonstrate urethral involvement, which typically appears as smooth narrowing of the fossa navicularis and distal urethra. Treatment of urethral involvement often includes meatotomy and urethroplasty.

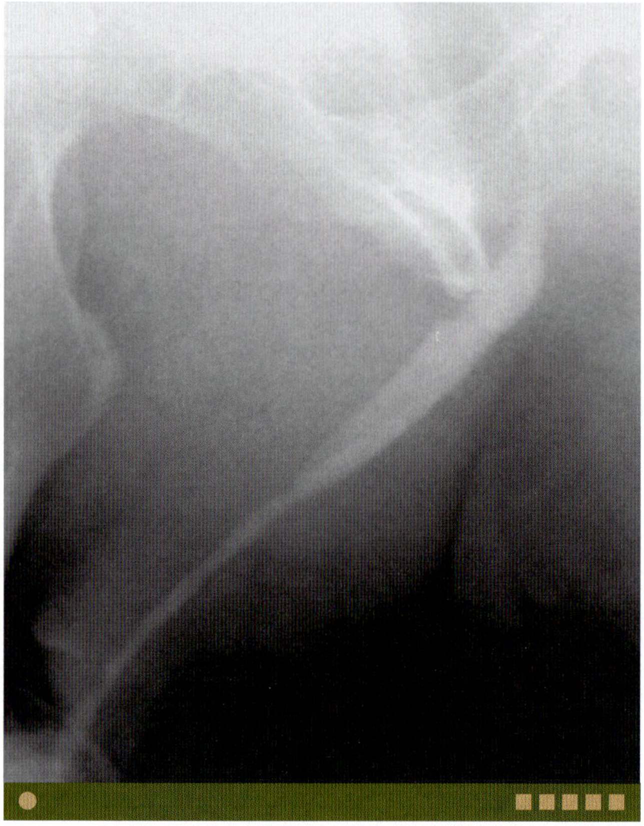

A Retrograde urethrogram shows smooth narrowing of the fossa navicularis and distal urethra.

PEARLS

- **BXO is synonymous with penile lichen sclerosus and male genital lichen sclerosus.**
- **BXO is associated with SCC of the penis.**
- **Urethral involvement is uncommon and spreads proximally in a confluent manner from the meatus.**
- **Urethral involvement results in smooth narrowing of the distal urethra.**

ADDITIONAL IMAGES (B-C)

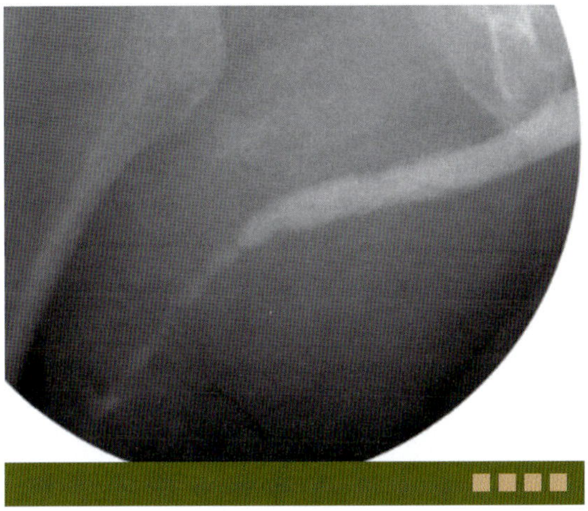

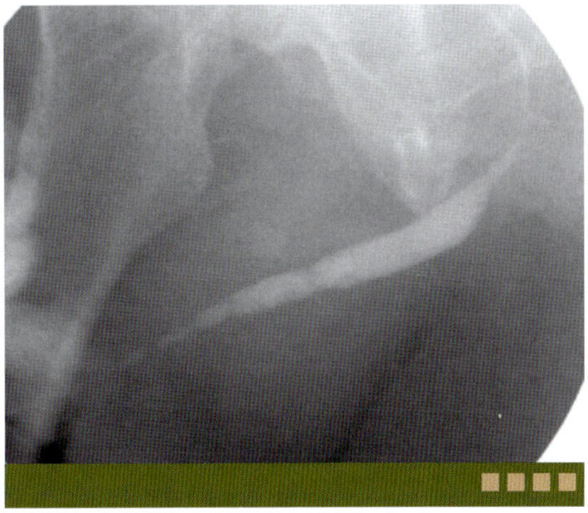

B. and **C.** Retrograde urethrogram from a different patient with BXO shows beaded narrowing of the distal urethra.

DIFFERENTIAL DIAGNOSES IMAGES (D-E)

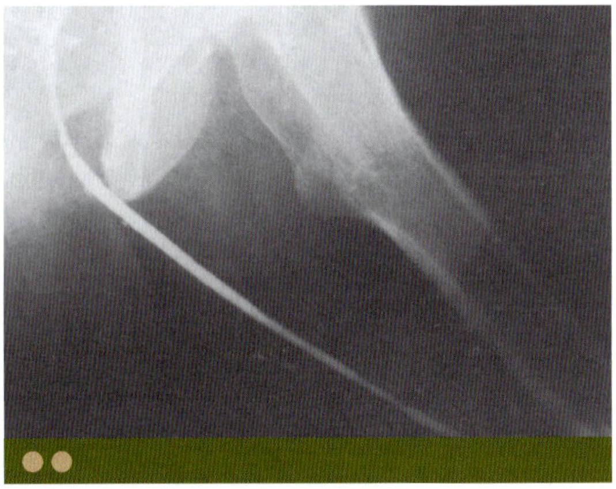

D. Infectious stricture: Retrograde urethrogram from patient with a history of gonococcus urethritis shows a very long, smooth stricture of the bulbous and penile urethra. *(Courtesy of Neil F. Wasserman, MD, Veterans Administration Medical Center, Minneapolis, MN.)*

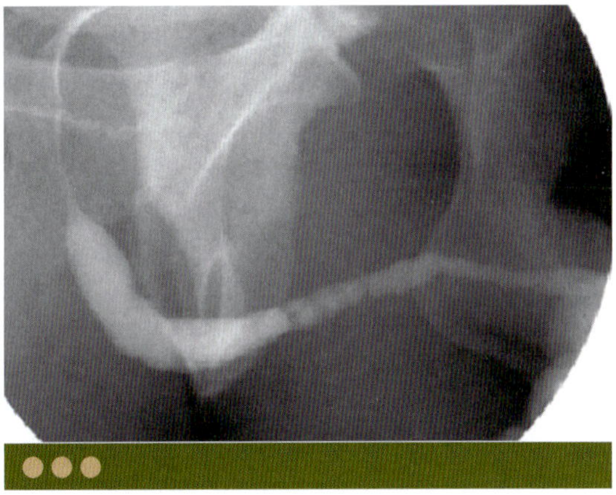

E. Iatrogenic stricture: Retrograde urethrogram shows beaded narrowing of a long segment of penile urethra and distal bulbous urethra. The stricture was presumably caused by extended catheterization.

IMAGE KEY

Common

Rare

Typical

Unusual

9-7 Urethral Fistula

David D. Casalino

PRESENTATION

Leakage of urine from the ventral surface of penis during micturition.

FINDINGS

Urethrogram shows a tract of contrast extending from the ventral aspect of the penile urethra to the skin surface.

DIFFERENTIAL DIAGNOSES

- *Acute anterior urethral injury*: May be iatrogenic or caused by blunt or penetrating injury; clinical history usually includes mechanism of injury; blood at the meatus is the cardinal sign of anterior urethral injury.
- *Urethral diverticulum*: Can be congenital or acquired; congenital diverticula usually involve the penile urethra; acquired diverticula may be caused by trauma, instrumentation, or infection and can involve any portion.
- *Cowper gland*: Paired glands that lie within the urogenital diaphragm and drain into either side of the dilated portion of the bulbous urethra via ducts that are 2 to 4 cm long.
- *Opacification of penile veins*: Typical anatomic distribution; transient; urethral obstruction may be present.
- *Ectopic insertion of ureter*: Above the urogenital diaphragm; continuity with rest of the ureter.

COMMENTS

A urethral fistula may be congenital or result from infection, trauma, radiation injury, surgery, or, rarely, neoplasm. Fistulas may communicate with the skin, a pelvic organ, such as bowel, vagina, or uterus, or another segment of urethra. A fistula may be blind ending. Posttraumatic fistulas may result if there is superinfection or a more distal obstruction causing increased pressures within the urethra. Urethroperineal fistulas are often the result of a periurethral abscess in men with urethral strictures but may also result from surgery to correct a stricture or repair hypospadias. Presenting signs and symptoms vary, depending on the point of termination; for example, urethrocutaneous fistulas to the perineum or scrotum may result in one or more openings that leak urine during micturition, so-called "watering pot" perineum.

Urethral fistulas are usually imaged with retrograde or voiding urethrography; although fistulography, fluoroscopic studies of the small bowel or colon/rectum, vaginography, or MR might be necessary for diagnosis. Imaging should attempt to determine the location, number and size of fistulas. During urethrography, lateral images of the lower pelvis are particularly important. A fistula typically appears as an irregular tract that may be blind ending or communicating to another structure. The size and shape can be widely variable. On MR, T2-WI in multiple planes is often helpful for assessment of fistulas, which are usually high-signal intensity and show enhancement.

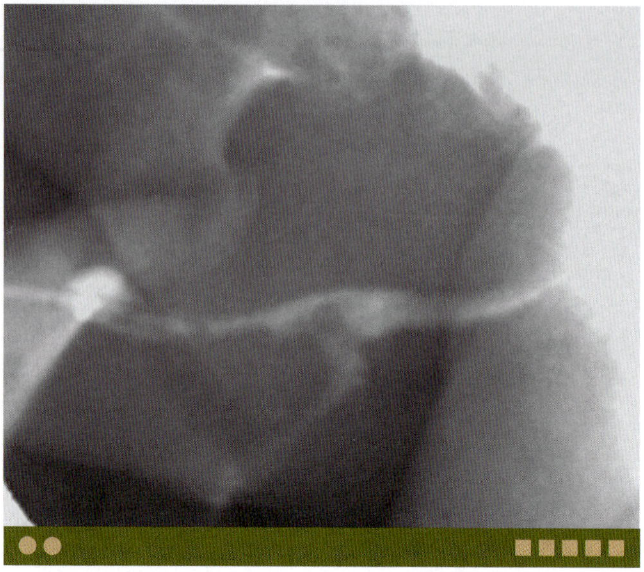

A. Retrograde urethrogram shows a fistula extending from the ventral aspect of the penile urethra to the skin surface.

PEARLS

- **Urethral fistulas may be blind ending or communicate with the skin, a pelvic organ, or another segment of urethra.**
- **Patient presentation depends on the point of termination.**
- **Imaging must be tailored to the type of fistula that is clinically suspected.**
- **Urethrography is usually the imaging study of choice.**
- **Multiplanar T2-WI may be very helpful as well.**

ADDITIONAL IMAGES (B-D)

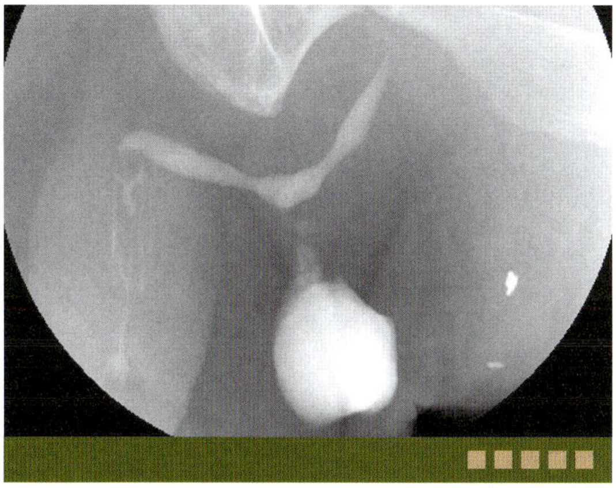

B. Retrograde urethrogram from a different patient shows an irregular tract of contrast extending from the ventral aspect of the penile urethra to a large round collection. The patient presented with postvoid dribbling and a history of prolonged catheterization.

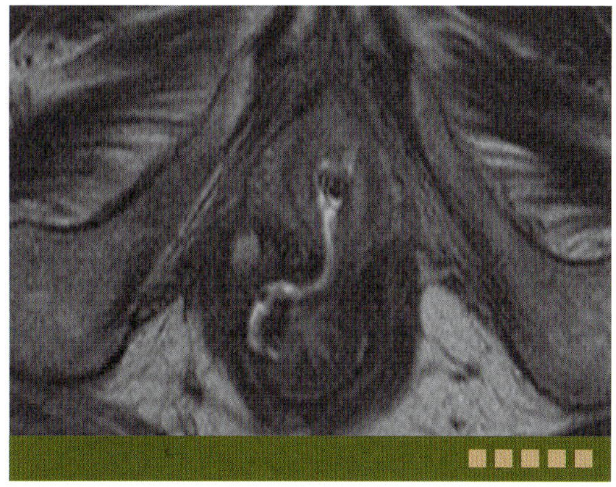

C. Axial T2-WI shows a thin hyperintense fistula between the right lateral wall of the anus and the urethra in a woman with Crohn disease.

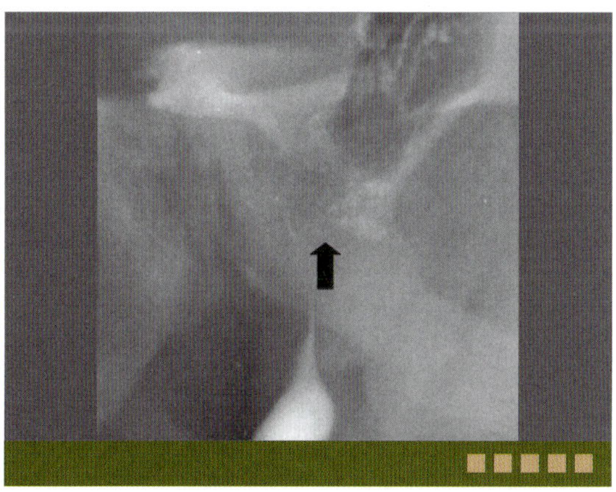

D. Retrograde urethrogram shows a small fistula (arrow) between the prostatic urethra and rectum in a young male with history of imperforate anus.

DIFFERENTIAL DIAGNOSES IMAGES (E-G)

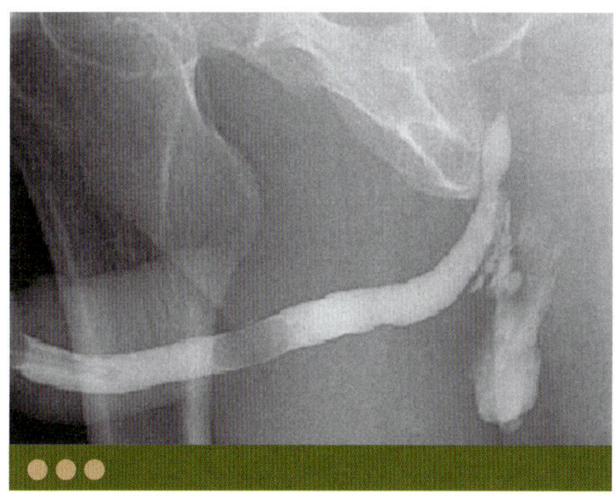

E. Anterior urethral injury: Retrograde urethrogram shows focal contrast leakage from the bulbous urethra with extension into the scrotum in a patient after straddle injury.

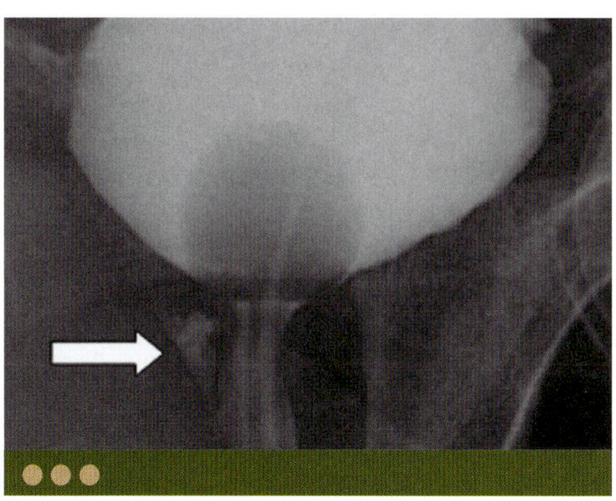

F. Cowper gland and duct: Cystogram shows a small collection of contrast (arrow) extending cephalad via a smooth tract from the right lateral aspect of the bulbous urethra. The appearance is characteristic of a normal Cowper gland and duct.

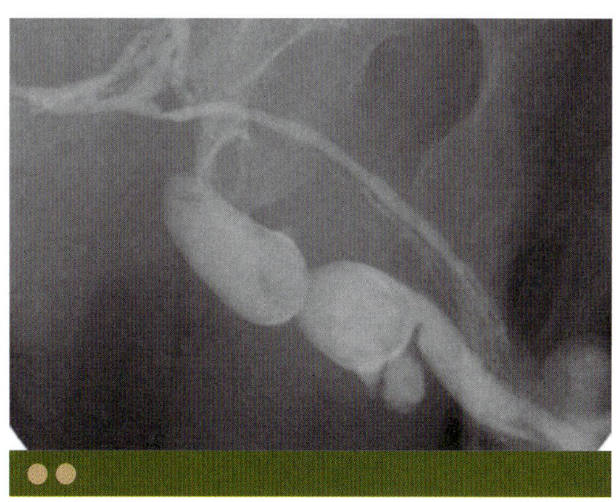

G. Penile veins: Retrograde urethrogram shows contrast opacification of multiple penile veins along the dorsal aspect of the penis in a patient with two large urethral diverticula filled with calculi and a high-grade proximal stricture.

IMAGE KEY

Common

Rare

Typical

Unusual

9–8 Urethral Diverticulum

Frank H. Miller

PRESENTATION

Lower urinary tract symptoms; urinary frequency, dysuria, recurrent UTI; dyspareunia.

FINDINGS

MR shows high-signal intensity lesion surrounding the urethra.

DIFFERENTIAL DIAGNOSES

- *Vaginal inclusion cyst*: May be difficult to distinguish, does not have connection to urethra; however, urethral diverticulum may not show connection on MR.
- *Endometrioma*: Generally different symptoms, seen as high-signal intensity on T1-WI and T2-WI from hemorrhage.
- *Ectopic ureterocele*: Connection to ureter.

COMMENTS

Urethra diverticula are saccular outpouchings from the urethra. They may be congenital or acquired. The majority is acquired and is a result of recurrent infection and obstruction or trauma to the periurethral glands. These dilated glands, then, rupture into the urethral lumen. They may also develop after urethral stricture. Urethral diverticula are more common in females than males. Congenital diverticula are rare, more common in males in the mid-penile urethra.

Diverticuli are often difficult to diagnose because of nonspecific symptoms and delay in diagnosis. Complications include infection, calculi, and rarely malignant degeneration. A tender periurethral mass may be palpated on physical examination.

The most common site of involvement is posterior or posterolateral wall of the mid-urethra. The diverticula may be unilocular or multilocular.

MR has advantages because of its lack of invasiveness, reproducibility, and ability to show surrounding anatomy with high spatial and contrast resolution. Urethral diverticula are typically seen as fluid signal intensity and as low-signal intensity on T1-weighted images and well seen based on their high-signal intensity on T2-weighted sequences. The multiplanar capability of MR helps localize the urethral diverticulum accurately. In women, the diverticula may wrap around the urethra referred to as "saddle-shaped" or "horseshoe-shaped" diverticula. Gadolinium-enhancement can be helpful to show the cystic nature and evaluate carcinoma. Complications including infection, calculi, or neoplasm can be detected on MR. Because of mass effect from the urethral diverticulum, the connection of a diverticulum to the urethra may not be seen. The distinction may require urethroscopy, biopsy, or surgical resection.

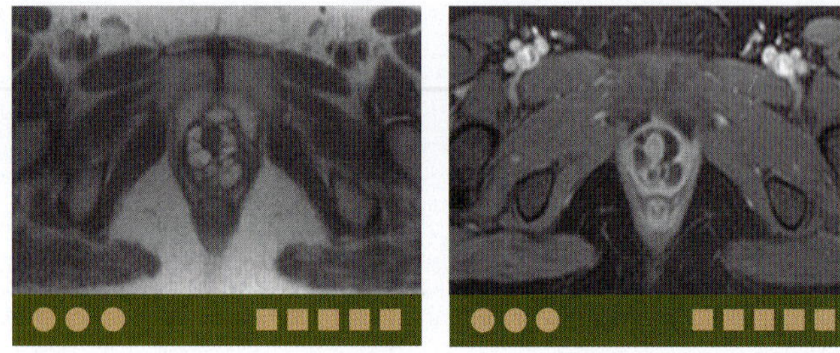

A. Axial T2-WI shows high-signal intensity mass surrounding the urethra.
B. Axial contrast-enhanced T1-WI shows the lesion is of fluid density and surrounds the urethra.

Urethroscopy may show the diverticulum and communication with the urethra but the connection may not always be seen. Voiding cystography may show the diverticulum, but it may be difficult to see as well as MR and have the patient void for the examination. Double-balloon catheter urethrography may show the diverticulum but is not performed everywhere and is more invasive and uncomfortable.

PEARLS

- **Urethral diverticula are often difficult to diagnose because of nonspecific symptoms and delay in diagnosis.**
- **Complications of urethral diverticula include infection, calculi, and rarely malignant degeneration.**
- **MR is least invasive method to show urethral diverticula.**

ADDITIONAL IMAGES (C-D)

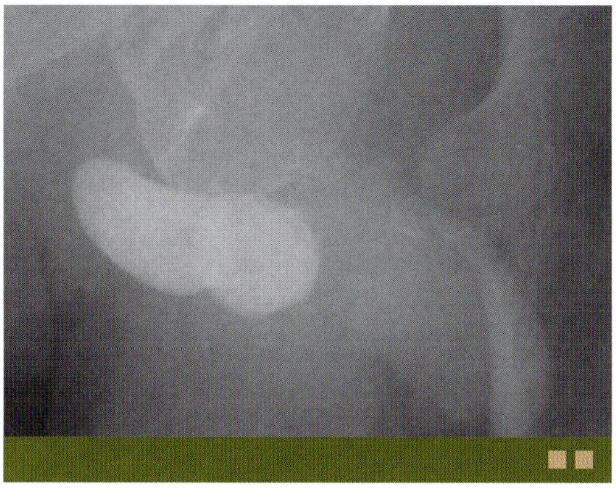

C. Scout image from urethrogram in elderly male with a firm nodule and weak urinary stream shows large calcifications projected over the urethra.

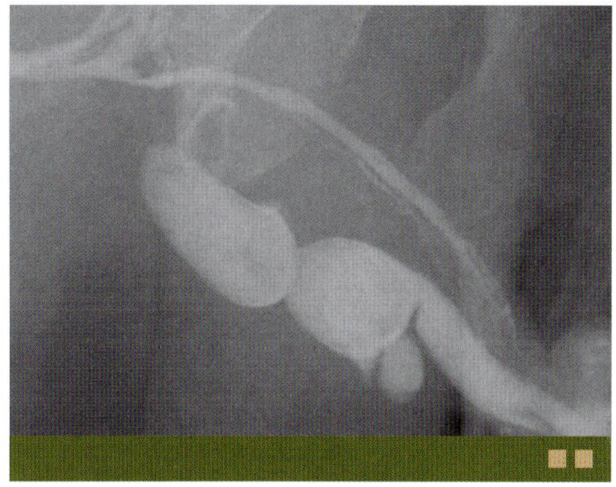

D. Retrograde urethrogram shows urethral diverticulum with calcifications in the urethra.

DIFFERENTIAL DIAGNOSES IMAGES (E-H)

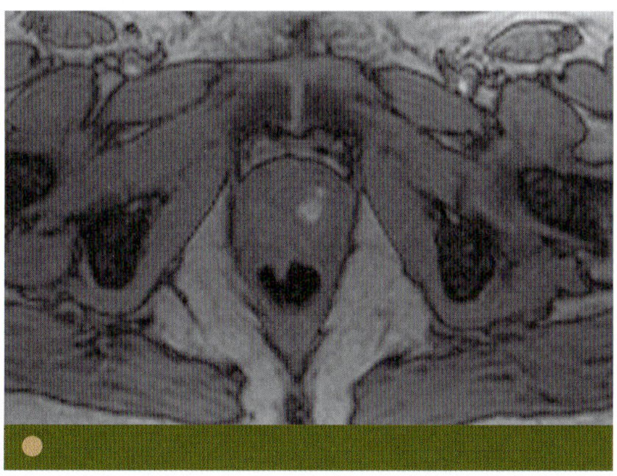

E. Endometriosis: Axial T1-WI shows high-signal intensity lesion from hemorrhage as a result of endometriosis mimicking urethral diverticulum. The patient had symptoms of endometriosis.

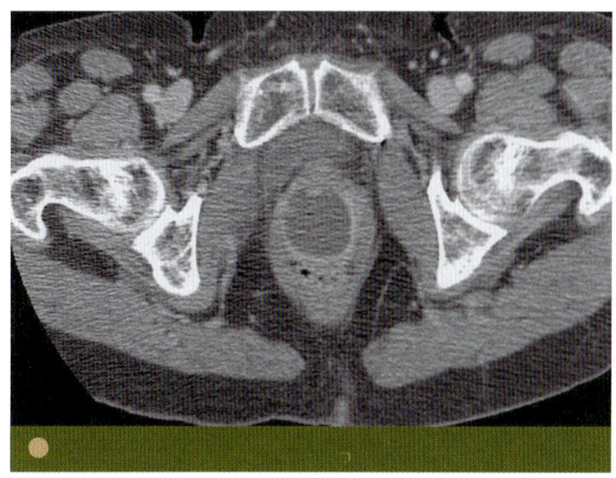

F. Vaginal inclusion cyst containing clear cell carcinoma: Axial CECT in a different patient shows mass near urethra and vagina.

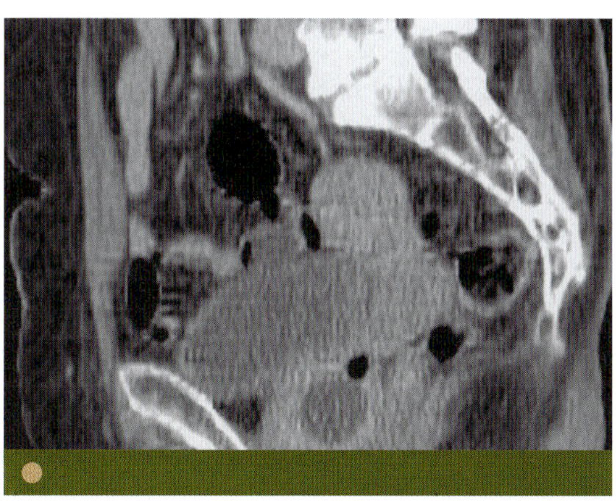

G. Vaginal inclusion cyst containing clear cell carcinoma: Sagittal CECT shows the mass is between the vagina and the urethra. It can be difficult to distinguish vaginal inclusion cysts from urethral diverticula.

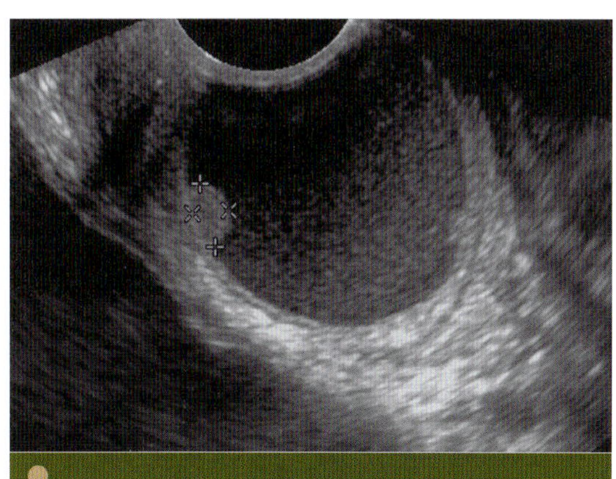

H. Vaginal inclusion cyst containing clear cell carcinoma: Longitudinal transvaginal sonogram shows the mass has an associated nodule which had flow. Surgical resection showed the lesion was a vaginal inclusion cyst containing clear cell carcinoma.

IMAGE KEY

Common

Rare

Typical

Unusual

CHAPTER 10

URINARY TRACT TRAUMA

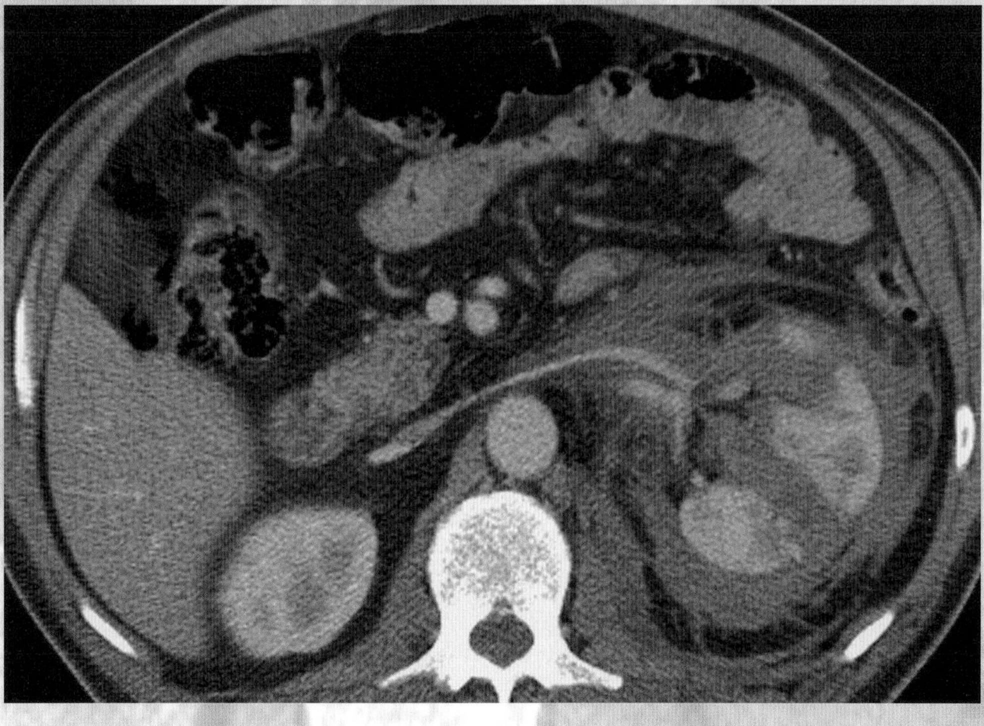

10–1 Subcapsular Hematoma

Nancy A. Hammond

PRESENTATION

Trauma.

FINDINGS

Crescentic hyperdense fluid collection with mass effect on the adjacent renal parenchyma.

DIFFERENTIAL DIAGNOSIS

- Subcapsular hematoma secondary to underlying mass lesion should be considered in the absence of significant trauma.

COMMENTS

Renal injuries are classified into five main categories by the American Association for the Surgery of Trauma (AAST) Grading System for Renal Injury. A Grade I injury is characterized as a parenychmal contusion and nonexpanding subcapsular hematoma without parenchymal laceration. These comprise the majority of renal trauma cases (75%-80%). Grade II injuries are defined as nonexpanding perirenal hematomas confined to the retroperitoneum and superficial lacerations (<1 cm in depth) in the renal cortex. Grade III injuries include lacerations involving less than 1 cm depth of the renal cortex without extension into the collecting system or urinary extravasation. Lacerations that extend through the renal cortex, medulla, and collecting system, injuries to the main renal artery or vein with contained hemorrhage, and thrombosis of the segmental renal artery without parenchymal lacerations are considered Grade IV injuries. Grade V injuries comprise lacerations that shatter the kidney, injuries to the renal hilum with devascularization of the kidney, and renal artery disruption or occlusion.

Subcapsular hematomas appear as crescentic collections between the renal capsule and renal parenchyma and are considered Grade I injuries. When small, there is minimal mass effect on the adjacent renal parenchyma but as they enlarge, there is compression of the adjacent renal parenchyma resulting in a biconvex collection. The attenuation values of these collections vary by the age of the clot. Acute hematomas are typically hyperattenuating (40-60 HU) relative to renal parenchyma on nonenhanced CTs (NECTs). On contrast-enhanced studies, subcapsular hematomas do not enhance. On MRI, the hematoma can have variable signal depending on the age.

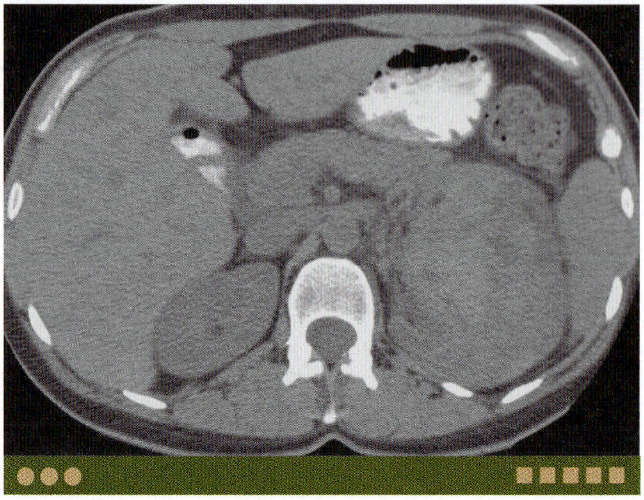

A. Axial NECT shows a large heterogeneous collection adjacent to the left kidney. Hyperdense regions are compatible with acute hemorrhage in this patient who sustained a motor vehicle collision.

On ultrasound, acute hematomas appear as echogenic collections in the subcapsular space. As the hematoma breaks down over time, the collection becomes more hypoechoic and may appear as a complex cystic structure with internal echoes and septations.

These injuries are treated conservatively. In the absence of significant trauma to account for the hematoma, follow-up imaging is warranted to exclude an underlying mass lesion as a source of the bleeding.

PEARLS

- **Grade I renal injuries account for the majority of renal injuries and are treated conservatively.**
- **Appear as subcapsular, crescentic fluid collections with mass effect on adjacent renal parenchyma dependent on the size of the hematoma.**
- **In the acute setting, subcapsular hematomas are hyperdense on NECT and do not enhance with contrast administration.**

ADDITIONAL IMAGES (B-D)

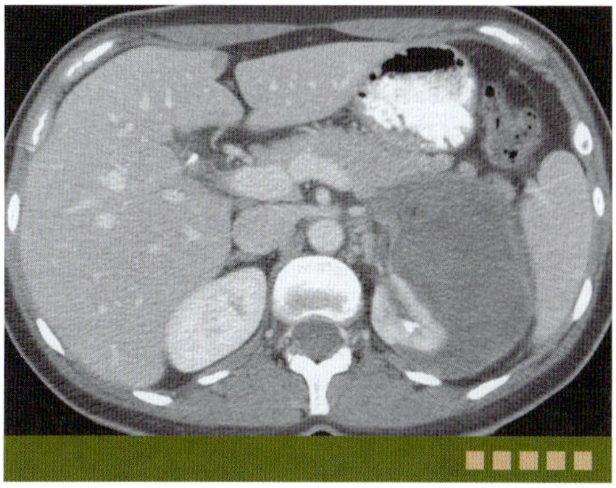

B. Axial CECT in the same patient shows the extent of the subcapsular hematoma and associated mass effect on the left kidney. There is delayed enhancement of the left kidney compared to the right as a result of the large hematoma.

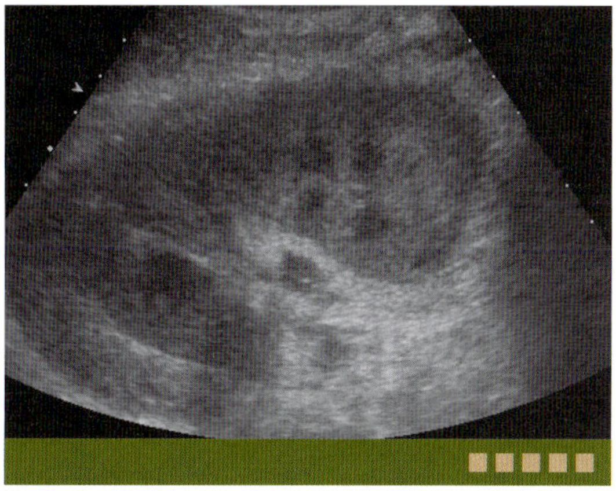

C. Longitudinal sonogram of a patient who recently underwent biopsy shows a crescentic, hyperechoic fluid collection at the upper pole of the transplanted kidney compatible with a subcapsular hematoma. No significant mass effect is present on this image.

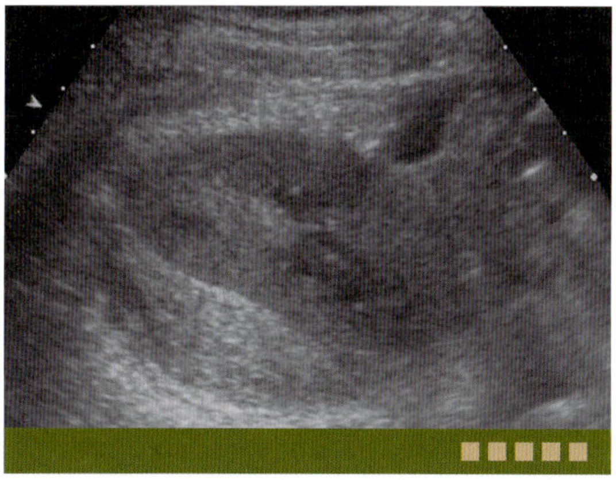

D. Transverse sonogram in the same patient as Figure C also shows the hyperechoic fluid collection in the subcapsular space. Mild mass effect on the adjacent renal parenchyma is better appreciated on this image.

DIFFERENTIAL DIAGNOSES IMAGES (E-F)

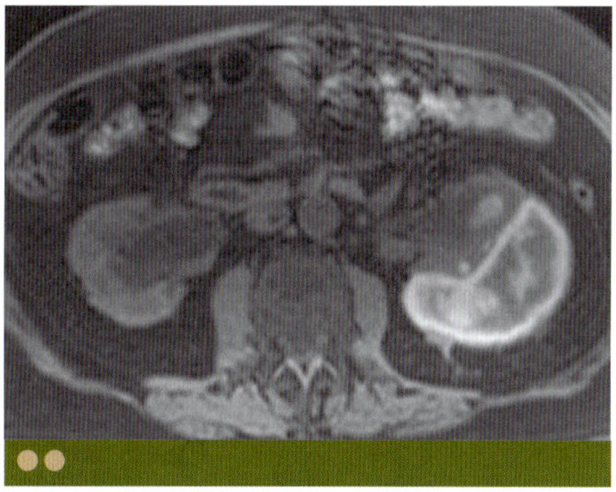

E. Hematoma secondary to underlying mass: Axial nonenhanced T1-WI shows a complex subcapsular hematoma in a patient without a history of trauma. The hematoma was found to be secondary to a hemorrhagic cyst.

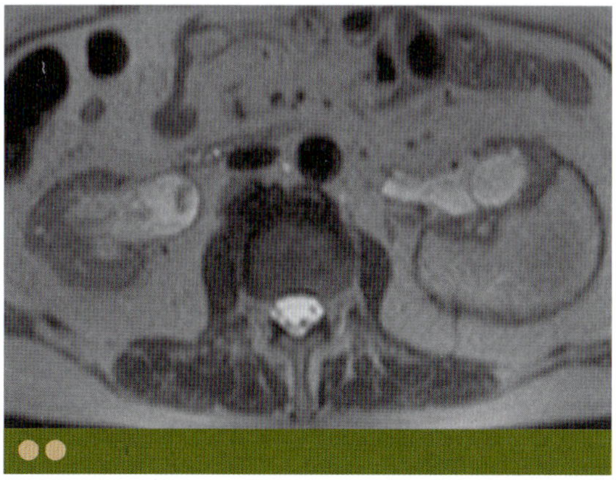

F. Hematoma secondary to underlying mass: Axial T2-WI shows the subcapsular hematoma to be hyperintense on T2-WI sequence. The adjacent renal parenchyma is better depicted on this sequence than on the T1-WI.

IMAGE KEY

Common

●●●●●
●●●●
●●●
●●
●

Rare

Typical

■■■■■
■■■■
■■■
■■
■

Unusual

10–2 Renal Contusion

Nancy A. Hammond

PRESENTATION

Status post fall with flank pain.

FINDINGS

Contrast-enhanced CT (CECT) demonstrates focal area of decreased enhancement.

DIFFERENTIAL DIAGNOSES

- *Focal pyelonephritis*: Similar CT findings. Diagnosis guided by clinical history.
- *Subsegmental infarction*: Appears as small, sharply demarcated, wedge-shaped areas of decreased enhancement. Renal contusions are typically less well defined than areas of infarction.

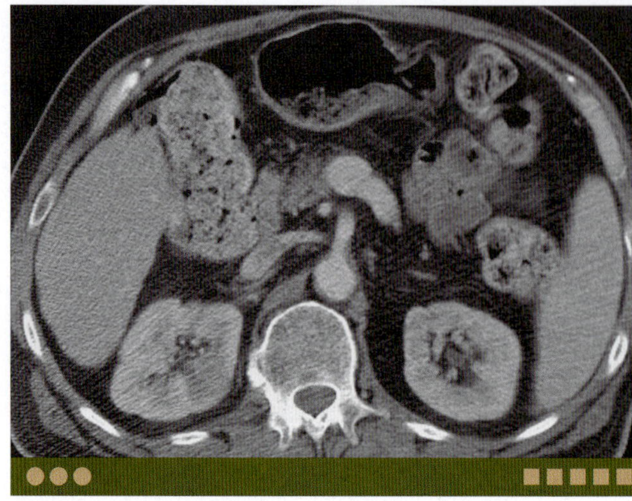

A. Axial CECT shows a subtle, ill-defined area of decreased attenuation in the posteromedial aspect of the right kidney in this patient presenting with right flank pain after trauma.

COMMENTS

Renal contusions are considered a Grade I injury based on the Renal Injury Scale for the AAST. A Grade I injury is characterized as a parenchymal contusion or nonexpanding subcapsular hematoma without parenchymal laceration and comprise the majority of renal trauma cases (75%-80%).

CT is the primary mode of imaging in the setting of trauma. On NECT, a renal contusion appears as a focal, hyperdense collection. This is because of focal interstitial edema and intraparenchymal extravasation of small amounts of bloody urine. On CECT, a renal contusion is an ill-defined, round hypoenhancing area. If delayed images are obtained, the contused parenchyma may show contrast staining.

MRI's use in the setting of trauma is limited by longer examination times, difficulties in monitoring patients during the examination, and general lack of availability. It is reserved as a trouble shooting modality with an inconclusive CT or in patients with a contraindication to CECT. In the uncommon instances that MRI is employed, a renal contusion appears also as an ill-defined area of hypoenhancement on postgadolinium sequences.

Renal contusions are treated conservatively.

PEARLS

- **Grade I injuries are the most common injuries in the setting of renal trauma and are treated conservatively.**
- **CT is the primary modality in evaluating patients with suspected renal trauma.**
- **Renal contusions are radiographically indistinguishable from focal pyelonephritis but can be distinguished based on clinical history.**

ADDITIONAL IMAGES (B-D)

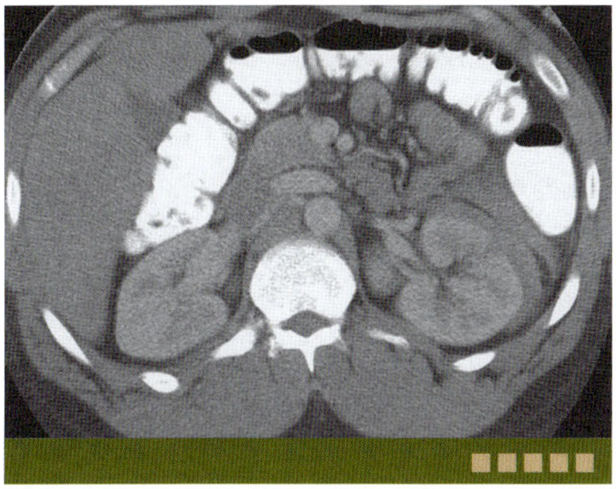

B. Axial CECT in a motor vehicular collision patient shows a subtle area of decreased attenuation at the periphery of the left kidney. A small amount of hyperdense fluid is noted adjacent to the left kidney compatible with a small perinephric hematoma.

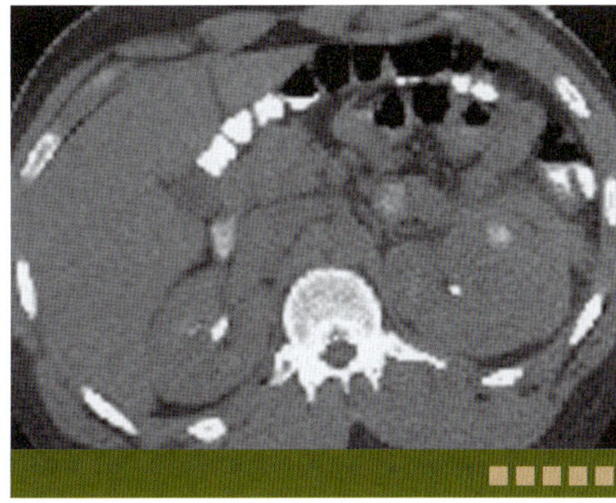

C. Axial delayed CECT delayed image in the same patient as Figure B at the same level shows retention of contrast material at a similar location as the previously noted decreased attenuation compatible with a small renal contusion.

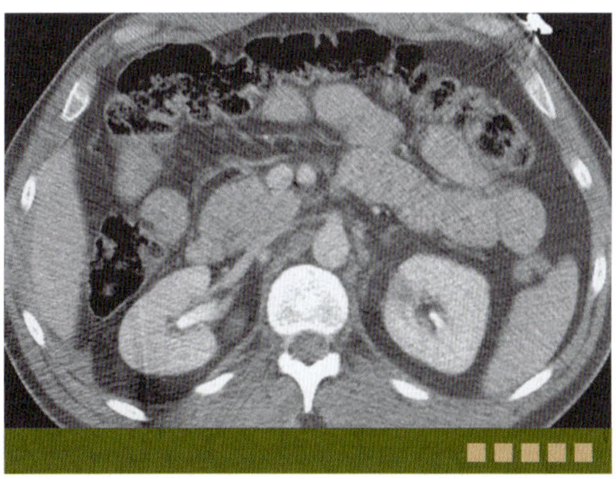

D. Axial CECT shows an ill-defined hypodense region in the anteromedial aspect of the left kidney. There is minimal stranding in the perinephric fat adjacent to the hypodense region. In the setting of trauma, findings are consistent with a small renal contusion.

DIFFERENTIAL DIAGNOSES IMAGES (E-F)

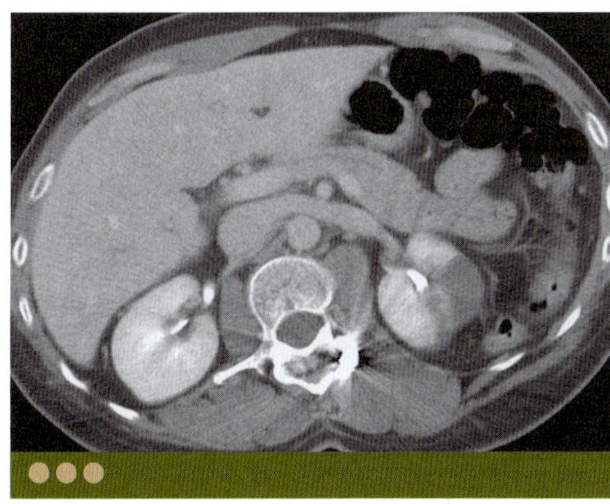

E. Renal infarction: Axial CECT shows decreased attenuation at the mid aspect of the left kidney. This region is more well defined than typically seen with renal contusion and compatible with acute renal infarction.

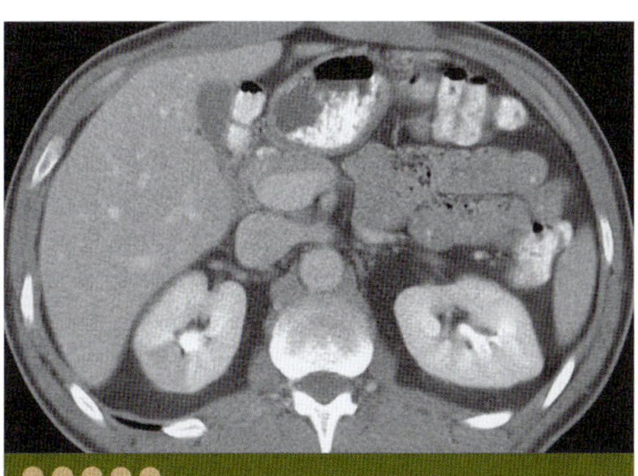

F. Pyelonephritis: Axial CECT shows a wedge-shaped area of decreased attenuation in the right kidney in a patient with clinically suspected pyelonephritis.

IMAGE KEY

Common

Rare

Typical

Unusual

10–3 Renal Laceration

Nancy A. Hammond

PRESENTATION

Blunt trauma.

FINDINGS

Linear low density extending from the renal cortex centrally; perinephric hematoma may or may not be present.

DIFFERENTIAL DIAGNOSIS

None

COMMENTS

AAST classifies renal trauma into five major grades. Approximately 90% of the renal trauma cases are as a result of blunt abdominal trauma, and the remaining 10% are attributed to penetrating trauma. Renal injuries present in 15% to 40% of patients with major blunt abdominal trauma. The majority of blunt trauma cases are considered Grade I injuries and can be treated conservatively. Conversely, the majority of renal injuries from penetrating trauma (66%) are significant. Grade I injuries include parenchymal contusions with or without a subcapsular hematoma. Grade II are characterized as superficial lacerations that involve less than 1 cm of the renal cortex with or without a perinephric hematoma. Grade III injuries are defined as lacerations that extend greater than 1 cm but do not involve the renal pelvis. Perinephric hematomas are likely present. Grade IV injuries include deep cortical lacerations which extend to the collecting system or vascular injuries without complete devascularization of the kidney. Grade V injuries comprise of lacerations that shatter the kidney or a devascularizing injury of the renal pedicle.

CECT is the first line modality in the setting of acute trauma. Excretory urography and MR are rarely used in the acute trauma setting. On contrast-enhanced CT, renal lacerations appear as linear hypodense areas extending from the renal cortex. If a perinephric hematoma is present, it appears as a hyperdense collection in the perirenal space. Unlike a subcapsular hematoma, mass effect on the adjacent renal parenchyma is not characteristically present.

Treatment of Grades I and II renal injuries is typically conservative. Nephrectomy rates have been shown to be higher in surgically explored patients (35%) versus observed patients (12%). Management of Grade III injuries depends on the clinical scenario. In cases of Grade IV injuries, treatment is conservative if less than 50% of the kidney is infarcted. In cases of thrombosis or avulsion of the main renal artery, rapid intervention is essential as permanent renal parenchymal loss and function can be incurred if treatment is delayed greater than 2 hours.

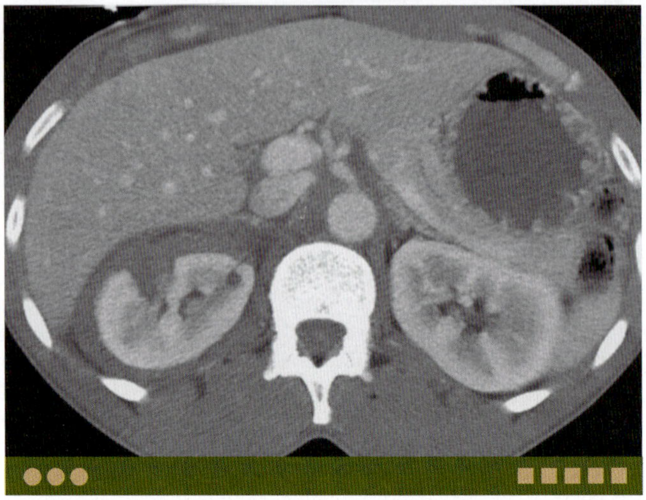

A. Axial CECT shows a linear area of nonenhancement involving the interpolar region of the right kidney. The laceration does not extend to the renal pelvis and is categorized as a deep cortical laceration or a Grade III injury. A small perinephric hematoma is also present.

PEARLS

- **Majority of blunt renal trauma injuries are Grade I or II and can be treated conservatively.**
- **Injuries caused by penetrating trauma are more likely to be significant and may require more aggressive management.**
- **Renal lacerations appear as linear hypodensities extending from the renal cortex. Evaluation of the depth of the laceration should be evaluated. Extension of the laceration into the renal pelvis is classified as a Grade IV injury.**

ADDITIONAL IMAGES (B-E)

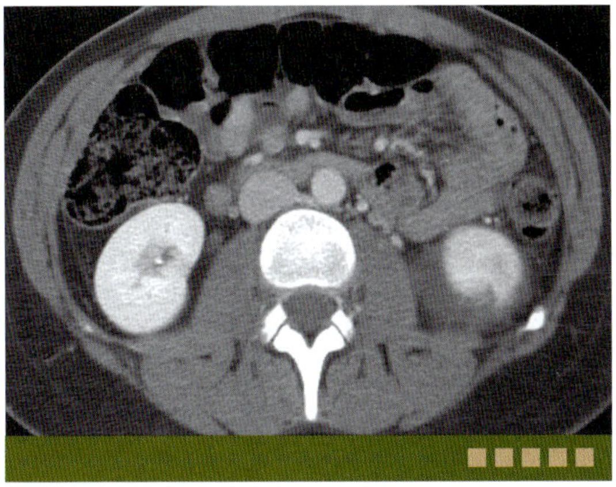

B. Axial CECT shows a small superficial laceration at the lower pole of the left kidney. The laceration involves less than 1 cm of the cortex consistent with a Grade II injury. A perinephric hematoma is also present.

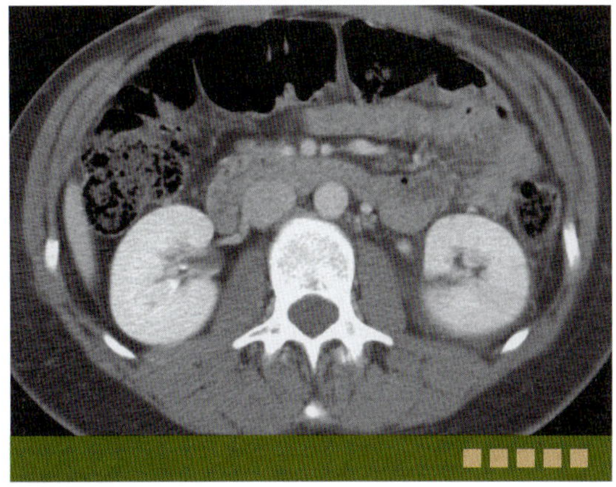

C. Axial CECT shows a deep laceration at the lower pole of the left kidney with a perinephric hematoma. It is unclear based on this image whether this laceration extends to the renal pelvis or not.

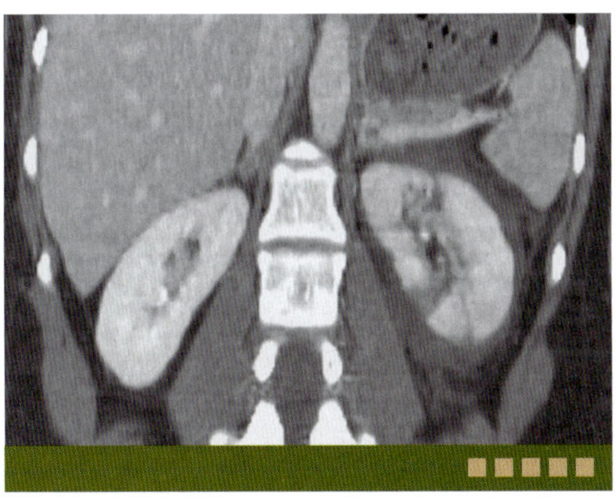

D. Coronal CECT in the same patient as Figure C confirms that the laceration does extend to the renal pelvis constituting a Grade IV injury.

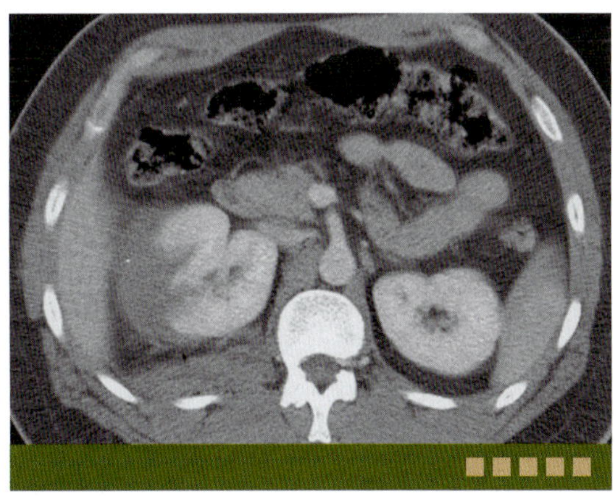

E. Axial CECT in a different patient shows a large laceration extending to the renal pelvis also consistent with a Grade IV injury. A perinephric hematoma is also present.

IMAGE KEY

Common

Rare

Typical

Unusual

10–4 Shattered Kidney

Nancy A. Hammond

PRESENTATION

Trauma.

FINDINGS

CECT shows multiple areas of parenchymal disruption and fragmentation of the kidney.

DIFFERENTIAL DIAGNOSIS

None

COMMENTS

The term "shattered kidney" refers to multiple renal lacerations resulting in fragmentation of the renal parenchyma. These are considered Grade V injuries and are usually associated with devitalized fragments, compromised excretion of contrast material, lacerations of the renal pelvis and collecting system, and active hemorrhage. CECT is the study of choice in the setting of trauma. Findings of shattered kidney include multiple linear densities extending to the central renal hilum with areas of parenchymal disruption. A perinephric hematoma is usually present. Examination for active extravasation is essential and evident by hyperdense foci similar in density to that of the enhanced vascular structures. Delayed images can be helpful in evaluating injury to the collecting system.

Conservative management is typically the treatment of choice for traumatic renal injuries with the exception of the most severe cases. The only absolute indication for operative management is life-threatening renal hemorrhage. Relative indications include (a) extensively devitalized tissue (>50%), (b) urinary extravasation not controlled by conservative means, and (c) arterial thrombosis. Angiography and embolization are important adjuncts in the stable patient with active bleeding.

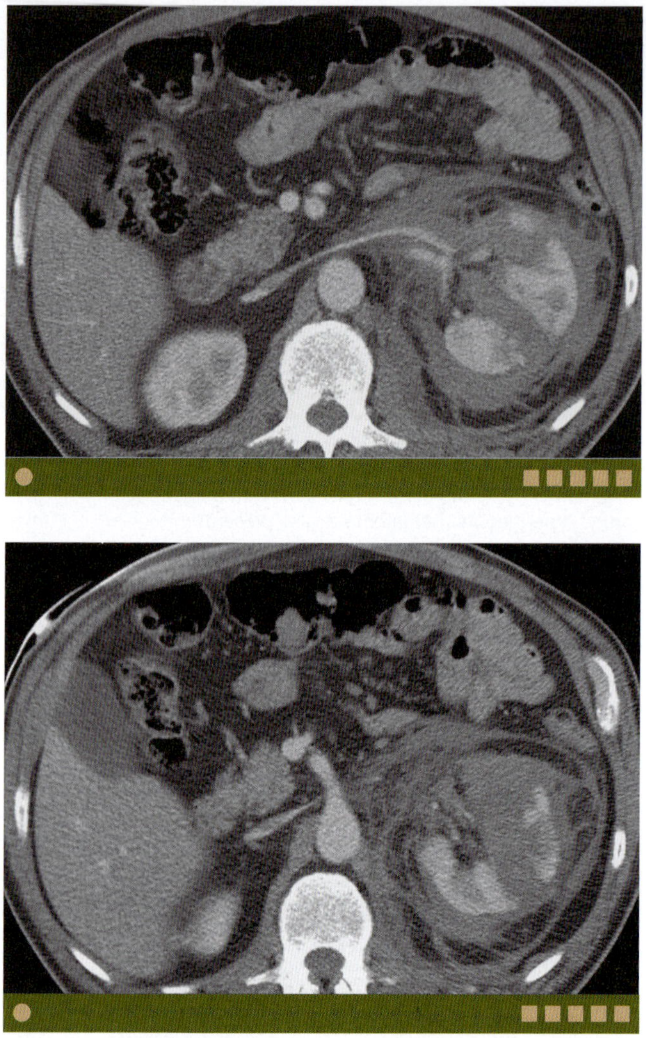

A. and **B.** Axial CECT shows multiple linear densities which extend to the renal sinus compatible with a shattered kidney. Additionally, a perinephric hematoma is present.

PEARLS

- **Shattered kidney refers to a Grade IV renal injury resulting in multiple renal lacerations and parenchymal disruption.**
- **Evaluation for active extravasation is essential as may require immediate intervention.**
- **Conservative management is the treatment of choice except in cases of life-threatening renal hemorrhage. Relative indications for surgical intervention are listed in the comments section.**

ADDITIONAL IMAGES (C-E)

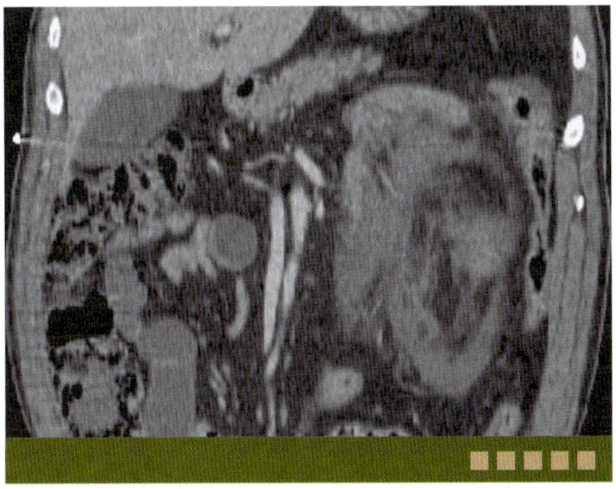

C. Coronal CECT in the same patient shows the extent of the perinephric hematoma.

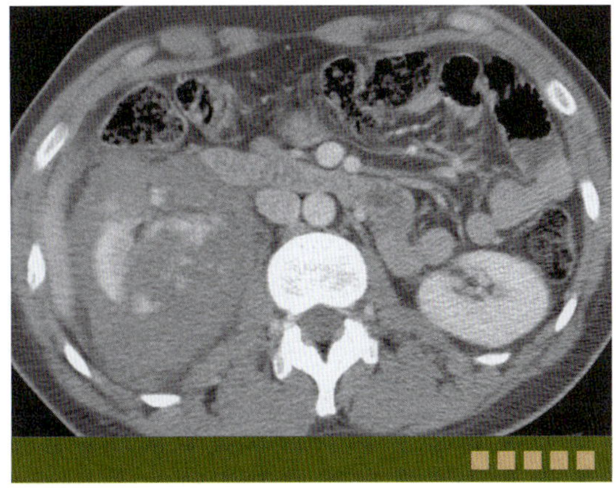

D. Axial CECT in a different patient also shows findings consistent with a shattered kidney and perineprhic hematoma involving the right kidney.

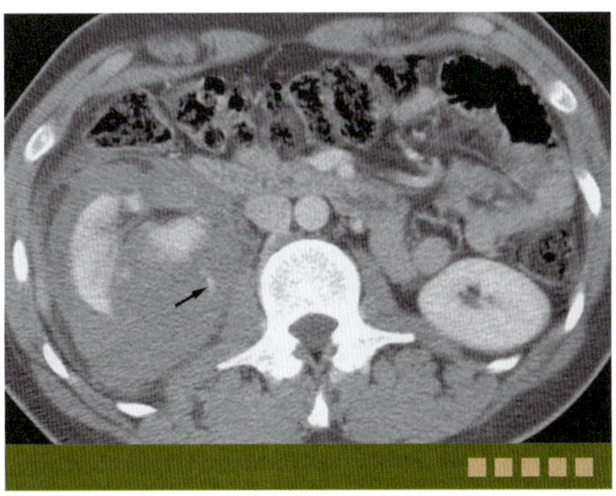

E. Axial CECT in the same patient as Figure D shows a curvilinear hyperdense at the medial aspect of the right kidney consistent with active extravasation of contrast material and acute hemorrhage (arrow).

IMAGE KEY

Common

Rare

Typical

Unusual

10–5 Vascular Pedicle Injury

Nancy A. Hammond

PRESENTATION

Blunt trauma.

FINDINGS

Nonenhancement of the involved kidney in the setting of abdominal trauma.

DIFFERENTIAL DIAGNOSIS

None

COMMENTS

Renal vascular injuries are characterized as either Grade IV or Grade V injuries by AAST. Grade IV renal injuries are described as vascular injuries without complete devascularization of the kidney and deep lacerations that extends to the renal pelvis. Grade V injuries include lacerations that shatter the kidney, injuries to the renal hilum/vascular pedicle with devascularization of the kidney, and renal artery disruption or occlusion. Grade V renal injuries make up only 3% to 4% of all blunt renal trauma injuries and are associated with significant abdominal or skeletal injuries elsewhere. Vascular pedicle injuries can result in either avulsion, intimal dissection, or traumatic occlusion of the renal artery or vein. The left kidney is more likely to suffer a pedicle injury than the right. The most common types of vascular pedicle injury are avulsion or laceration of the main renal artery and vein or thrombosis of the main renal artery. Patients may or may not (24%) have hematuria at presentation.

CT is the first line modality in the setting of acute trauma. Excretory urography does not adequately stage patients with extensive renal trauma. MR is rarely used in the setting of trauma because of time constraints and availability. Therefore, CECT should be performed in patients with suspected major trauma. On CECT, findings suggestive of a vascular injury include nonenhancement of the involved portion of the kidney. Acute thrombosis of the main renal artery results in infarction and an absent nephrogram of the affected kidney. Perinephric hematomas are typically small in this setting. The cortical rim sign or enhancement of the peripheral aspect of the kidney is usually absent in the immediate post-trauma period but develops by 1 week in most cases. Renal vein laceration or thrombosis is the least common type of vascular pedicle injury. CT typically demonstrates an enlarged kidney with a decreased early nephrogram, prolonged corticomedullary phase and absent to very little excretion of contrast. The renal vein may be enlarged, and a hyperdense clot may be identified on nonenhanced images. However, CT does not reliably detect venous injury and conventional venography may be necessary.

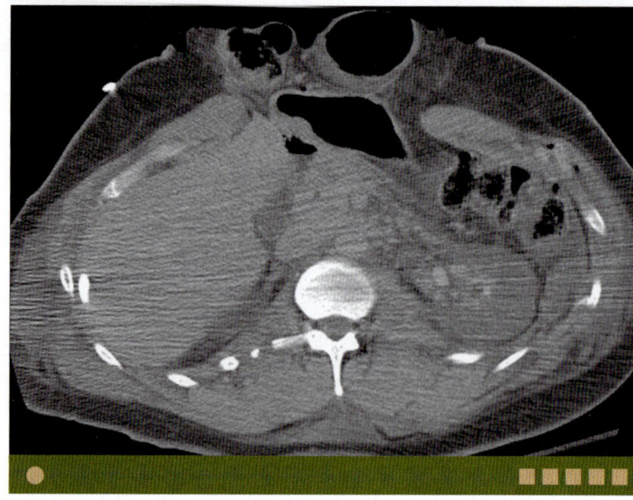

A. Axial CECT shows near complete lack of enhancement of the left kidney. An ischemic left kidney caused by vascular pedicle injury was found intraoperatively.

Clinically, Grade V injuries typically require surgical intervention. Angiography is useful in demonstrating intimal tears of the main renal artery, posttraumatic pseudoaneurysm and arteriovenous fistulae. If less than 50% of the renal parenchyma is involved, vascular injuries can be treated conservatively.

PEARLS

- **Grade V renal injuries comprise only 3% to 4% of blunt renal trauma injuries but are associated with significant skeletal or abdominal injuries elsewhere.**
- **Grade V renal injuries typically require surgical intervention.**
- **Vascular pedicle injuries demonstrate nonenhancement or decreased function of the involved kidney. A cortical rim sign is not present in the acute setting but usually develops within 1 week of the injury.**

ADDITIONAL IMAGES (B-F)

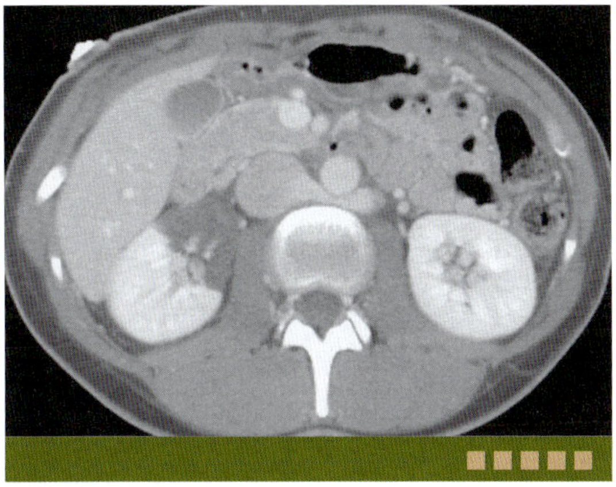

B. Axial CECT shows an area of nonenhancement involving the anteromedial aspect of the right kidney consistent with segmental infarction and a Grade IV injury. Less than 50% of the kidney was involved and the renal injury was treated conservatively.

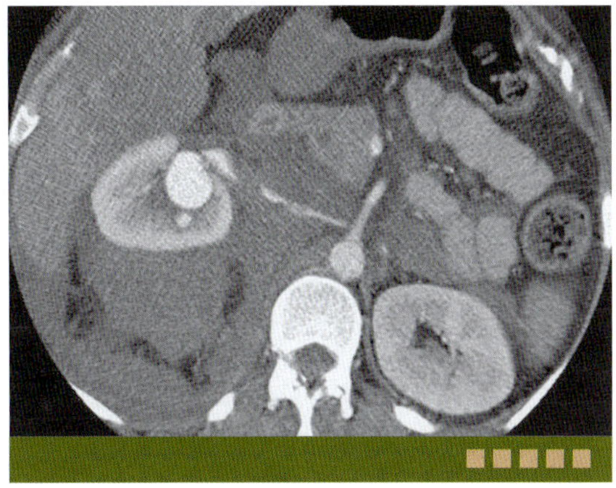

C. Axial CECT shows a round, focal hyperdense collection in the right renal pelvis consistent with a traumatic pseudoaneurysm. A large perinephric hematoma is also present displacing the kidney anteriorly.

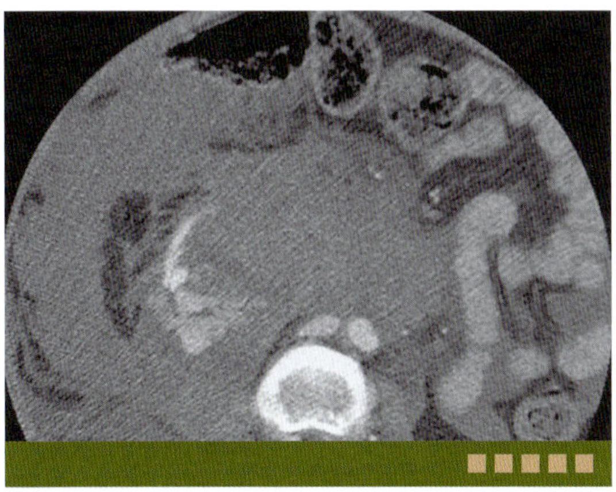

D. Axial CECT in the same patient as Figure C shows nonenhancement of the lower pole of the right kidney. A large retroperitoneal hematoma is present with curvilinear hyperdensity represent acute extravasation of contrast material.

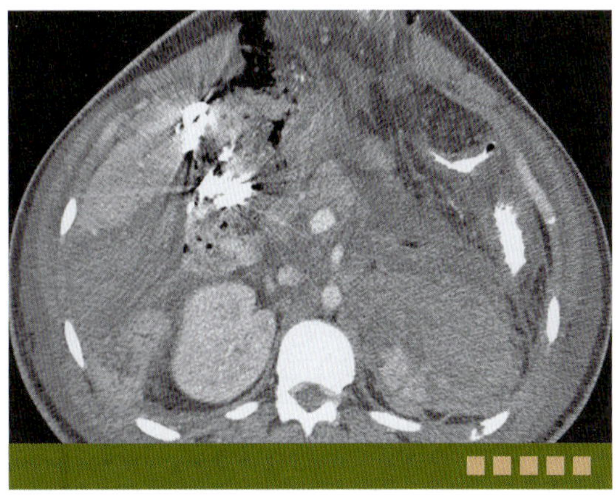

E. Axial CECT shows decreased enhancement of the enlarged, left kidney with minimal parenchymal enhancement noted posteriorly. A perinephric hematoma and open abdominal wound are also present. Venous injury was suspected and conventional venography was performed demonstrating laceration to the left renal vein.

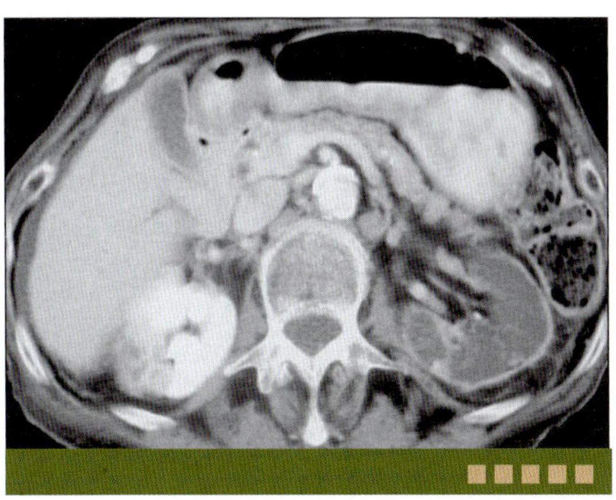

F. Axial CECT shows near complete nonenhancement of the left kidney with a thin peripheral rim of enhancement consistent with the cortical rim sign seen in subacute renal infarction.

IMAGE KEY

Common

Rare

Typical

Unusual

10–6 Traumatic Ureteropelvic Junction Injury

Nancy A. Hammond

PRESENTATION

Blunt abdominal trauma.

FINDINGS

CECT demonstrates extravasated contrast material at the level of the ureteropelvic junction (UPJ). Delayed images may be necessary to confirm extravasation. Additional signs of renal trauma are likely present.

DIFFERENTIAL DIAGNOSIS

None

COMMENTS

UPJ injuries are a rare consequence of blunt abdominal trauma. The mechanism of injury is sudden deceleration resulting in tension on the renal pedicle. Clinically, the diagnosis may be missed because of the absence of hematuria in approximately 30% of the patients. UPJ injuries are classified into two groups: complete avulsion and partial tear.

CECT is considered the first line imaging modality in the evaluation of trauma. In injury to the UPJ, CT demonstrates an intact intrarenal collecting system with medial perinephric urinary/contrast extravasation. As it can be difficult to distinguish a partial from a complete UPJ tear, the presence of contrast material in the distal ureter can help to differentiate a partial tear from a complete avulsion. Delayed contrast-enhanced images may be necessary to identify and characterize the extent of a UPJ injury. In equivocal cases, retrograde pyelography should be performed as the management differs. UPJ avulsions are treated with surgical repair. Lacerations can be treated conservatively or with stent placement.

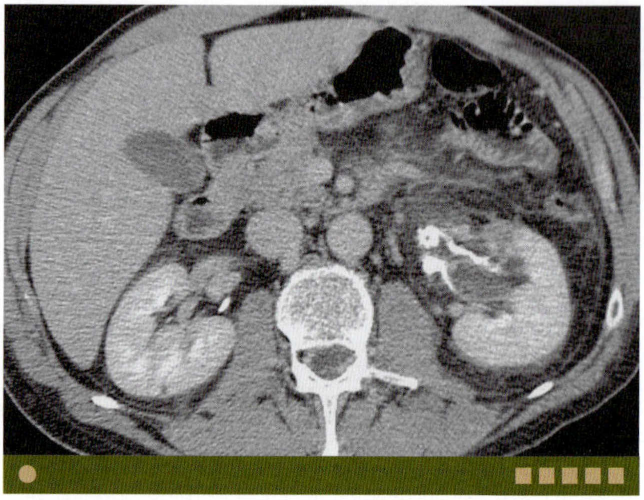

A. Axial CECT obtained in the excretory phase shows fluid in the left renal pelvis. Extravasated contrast material is present in the left renal pelvis.

PEARLS

- **Injury to the UPJ is an uncommon consequence of renal trauma and classified as either partial tears or complete avulsions.**
- **Stranding and fluid in the region of the UPJ should raise the suspicion of a UPJ injury. Delayed images can be obtained to confirm extravasation of contrast material.**
- **Partial tears are treated conservatively or with stent placement, whereas complete avulsions require surgical repair.**

ADDITIONAL IMAGES (B-F)

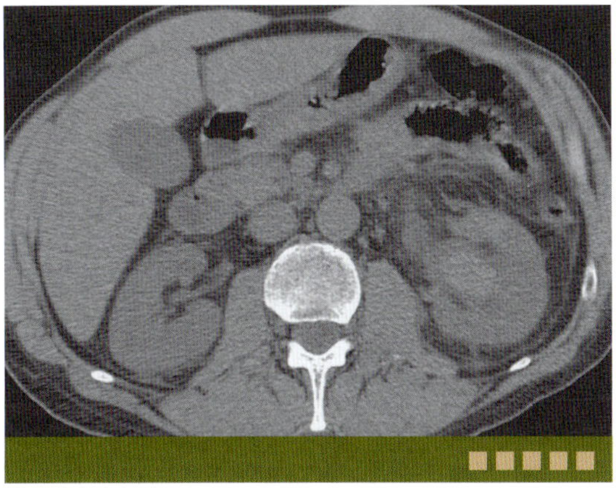

B. Axial NECT shows a hyperdense collection in the renal sinus consistent with a hematoma.

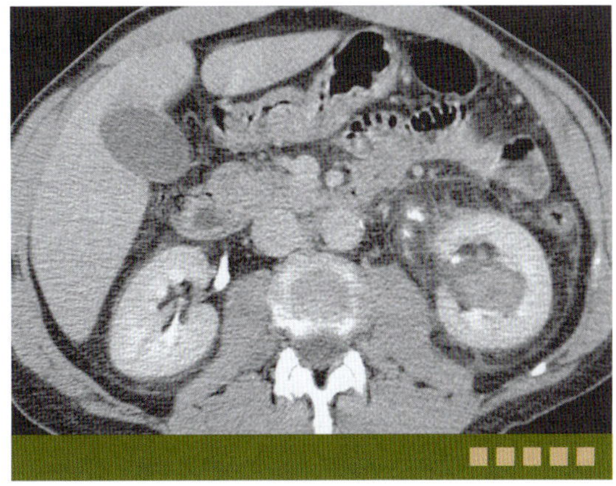

C. Axial-delayed CECT shows the renal sinus hematoma and extravasated contrast material exiting from the renal pelvis consistent with a UPJ injury.

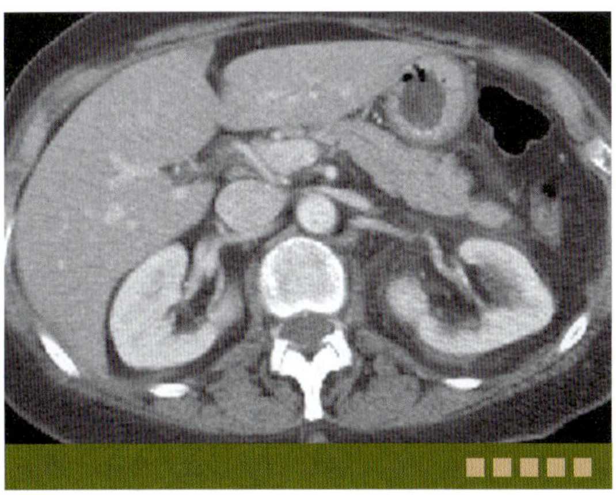

D. Axial CECT obtained in the nephrographic shows a small amount of perinephric fluid and fluid in the renal sinus raising suspicion for a UPJ injury. Delayed images are necessary to evaluate injury to the renal pelvis.

IMAGE KEY

Common

Rare

Typical

Unusual

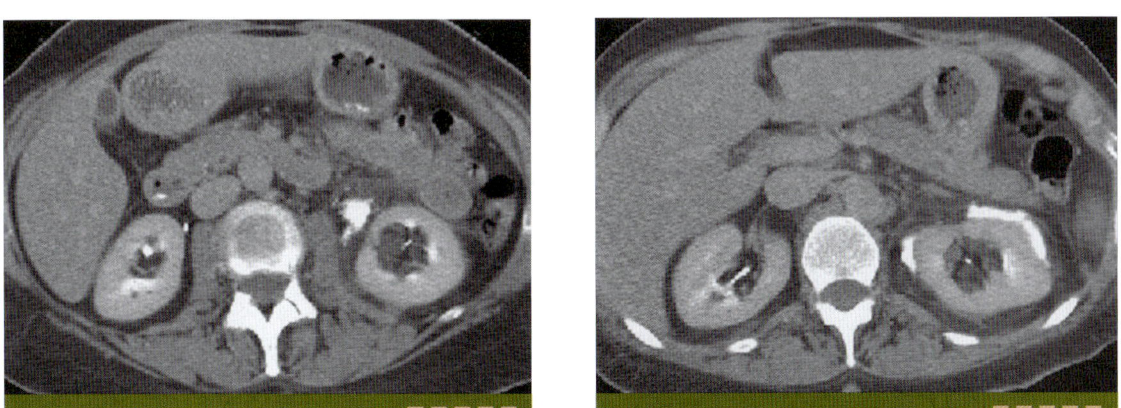

E. and **F.** Axial CECT in the same patient as Figure D show extravasated contrast material in a perinephric and periureteral location confirming a renal pelvis disruption.

10–7 Iatrogenic Ureteral Injury

Nancy A. Hammond

PRESENTATION

Surgically suspected ureteral injury.

FINDINGS

Extravasation of contrast material from ureter on delayed CECT.

DIFFERENTIAL DIAGNOSIS

None

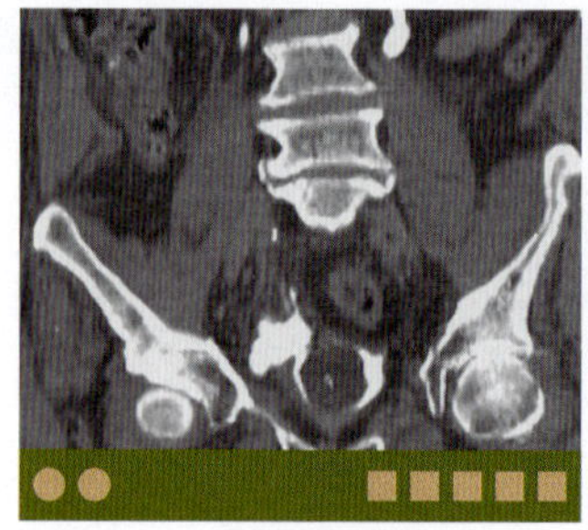

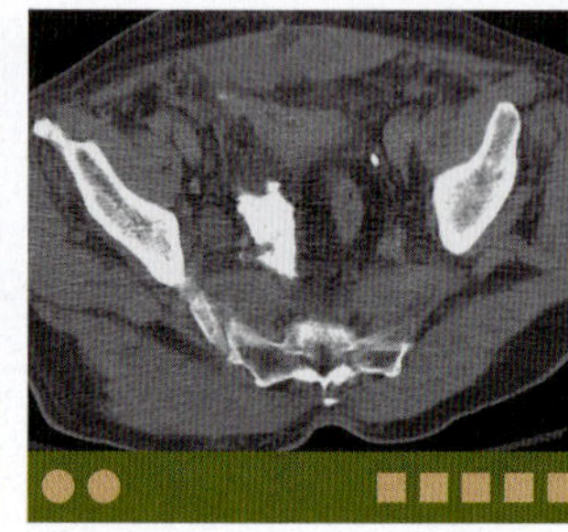

A. Delayed coronal CECT shows a focal collection of contrast material in the right hemipelvis arising from the distal right ureter consistent with distal right ureteral injury.
B. Delayed axial CECT in the same patient as Figure A also shows the extravasated contrast material.

COMMENTS

Injury to the ureter is typically secondary to iatrogenic causes and uncommonly associated with external trauma. Ureteric trauma is involved in less than 1% of all genitourinary injuries caused by external trauma. When ureteral injury is caused by external trauma, gunshot wounds account for 91% of the injuries. Iatrogenically, ureteral injuries occur during abdominopelvic surgery or ureteroscopy. Gynecologic surgeries account for the highest number of surgical injuries (75%) with colorectal surgeries being the second most common. The most common mechanisms of operative ureteral injury include crushing from misapplied clamp, ligation with suture, transsection, angulation of the ureter with secondary obstruction, ischemia from stripping or electrocoagulation, or resection of a segment of ureter.

The majority of iatrogenic ureteral injuries are diagnosed postoperatively. Patients can present with flank pain, fever and sepsis, fistula formation, urinoma, ileus, and renal failure.

CECT is a highly sensitive modality for evaluating for ureteral injury. Delayed images should be obtained to assess for extravasation of contrast material. Additionally, complications such as urinomas can be evaluated for. Urinomas appear as low density collections that fill with contrast material on delayed images. Intravenous urogram (IVU) can also be employed to evaluate for ureteral injury but is less sensitive than CT or retrograde studies. Findings on IVU suggesting injury to the ureter include delayed renal function, ureteral dilatation or deviation, extravasation of contrast and nonvisualization of the ureter. Retrograde pyelogram is the most sensitive study to evaluate for ureteral injury and can be utilized when injury is suspected intraoperatively.

Treatment of ureteral injuries depends on the extent, type, location, and time of presentation. Minor injuries can often be treated with ureteral stent placement while more serious injuries may require surgical management.

PEARLS

- **The majority of ureteral injuries are iatrogenic in origin and most commonly seen with abdominopelvic surgeries.**
- **Traumatic injury to the ureters is uncommon and typically seen in gunshot victims.**
- **CECT is a sensitive modality for evaluating ureteral injury but requires delayed imaging.**

ADDITIONAL IMAGES (C-F)

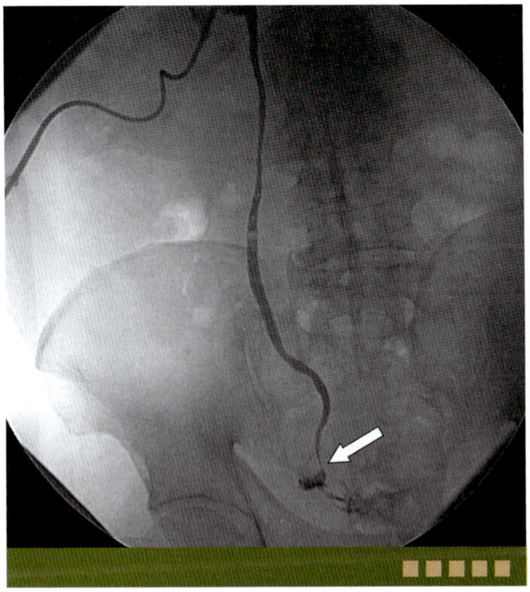

C. Injection via the patient's right percutaneous nephrostomy tube confirms the site of the leak to be the distal right ureter (arrow).

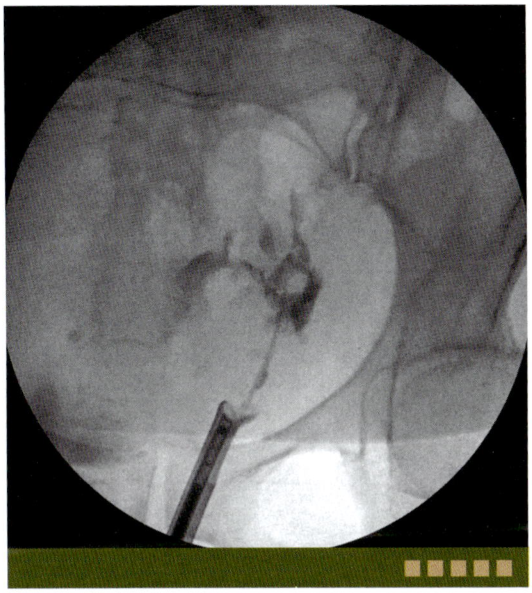

D. Retrograde left pyelogram shows extravasation of contrast material from the distal left ureter in this patient status post hysterectomy.

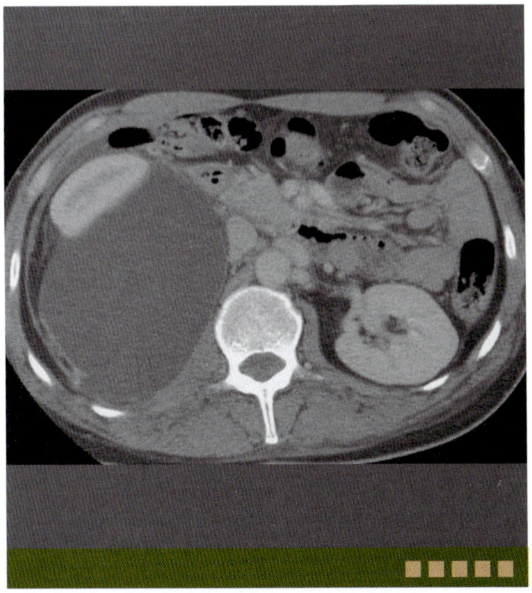

E. Axial CECT shows displacement of the right kidney anteriorly by a large fluid collection. There is a delayed nephrogram of the right kidney.

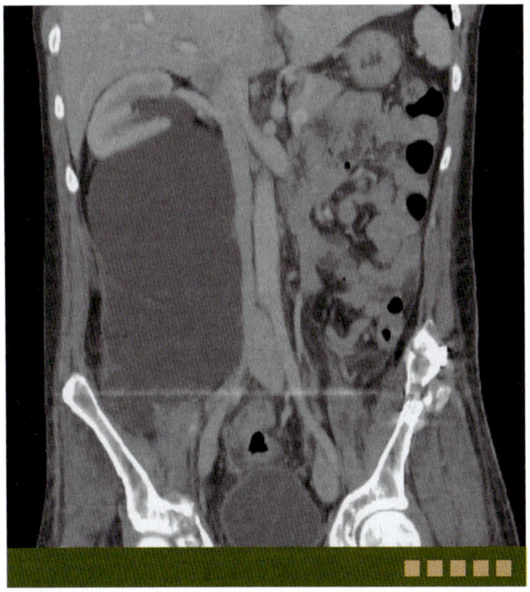

F. Coronal CECT in the same patient shows communication of the large retroperitoneal fluid collection with the proximal right ureter consistent with an urinoma.

IMAGE KEY

Common

Rare

Typical

Unusual

10-8 Anterior Urethral Injuries

David D. Casalino

PRESENTATION

Scrotal pain and blood at the urethral meatus after motor vehicle accident.

FINDINGS

Retrograde urethrogram shows contrast extravasation from the proximal bulbous urethra and opacification of the more proximal urethra and bladder; contrast also extends into the scrotum.

DIFFERENTIAL DIAGNOSES

- *Urethral fistula*: May result from infection, trauma, radiation injury, surgery, or, rarely, neoplasm; irregular tract that typically communicates with a pelvic organ or another segment of urethra but may be blind ending; communicating organ may determine clinical presentation.
- *Urethral diverticulum*: Can be congenital or acquired; congenital diverticula usually involve the penile urethra; acquired diverticula may result from trauma, instrumentation, or infection and can involve any portion; may be complicated by infection, calculi, and rarely malignancy.
- *Cowper gland*: Paired glands that lie within the urogenital diaphragm and drain into either side of the dilated portion of the bulbous urethra via ducts that are 2 to 4 cm long; opacification often associated with urethral inflammation or stricture, but not always.

COMMENTS

Anterior urethral injuries may be iatrogenic or caused by blunt trauma or penetrating injuries from gunshot or knife wounds. Iatrogenic causes include catheterization and instrumentation. The blunt trauma mechanism usually involves a straddle injury, or type V injury according to the Goldman et al expansion of the Calapinto and McCallum classification system. This type of injury involves a blunt force compressing the bulbous urethra and corpus spongiosum against the inferior aspect of the pubic bones. Pelvic fractures are typically not present. Blood at the meatus is the cardinal sign of anterior urethral injury. Patients may also have dysuria, hematuria, or an inability to void. Stricture and impotence may complicate anterior urethral injuries. Treatment usually involves urinary diversion and primary reconstruction, typically 3 to 6 months after the injury.

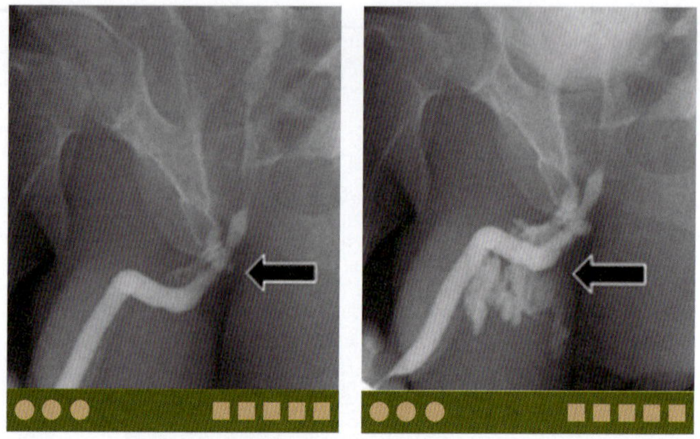

A. and **B.** Retrograde urethrogram shows contrast leakage from the bulbous urethra (arrows) with extension into the scrotum in a patient status post straddle injury.

Retrograde urethrography is the imaging study of choice for suspected urethral injury.

Anterior urethral injuries may be partial or complete tear or contusion with intact urethra.

A partial tear is diagnosed on retrograde urethrography when there is demonstration of contrast extravasation from the urethra and contrast opacification of the urethra proximal to the injury site. Extravasation from the injury site without more proximal urethral opacification is diagnostic of a compete tear. When a partial or complete tear is present, contrast may opacify the penile corpora and draining veins. Strictures may complicate anterior urethral injuries. The strictures are usually focal, well-defined, and involve the mid or proximal bulbous urethra.

PEARLS

- **A straddle injury typically involves a blunt force compressing the bulbous urethra and corpus spongiosum against the inferior aspect of the pubic bones.**
- **Blood at the meatus is the cardinal sign of anterior urethral injury.**
- **When a urethral injury is suspected, retrograde urethrography is the study of choice.**
- **When a stricture develops as a complication of anterior urethral injury, it is usually focal and well defined.**

ADDITIONAL IMAGES (C-D)

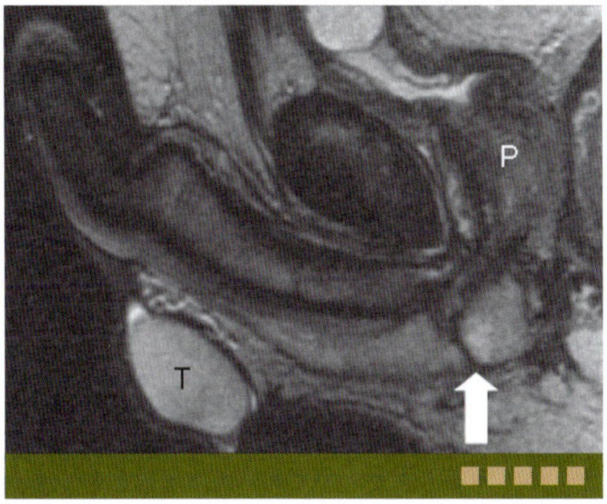

C. Sagittal T2-WI shows a hypointense fracture (arrow) through the corpus spongiosum and involving the bulbous urethra in a different patient status post straddle injury. P and T label the prostate and testis, respectively.

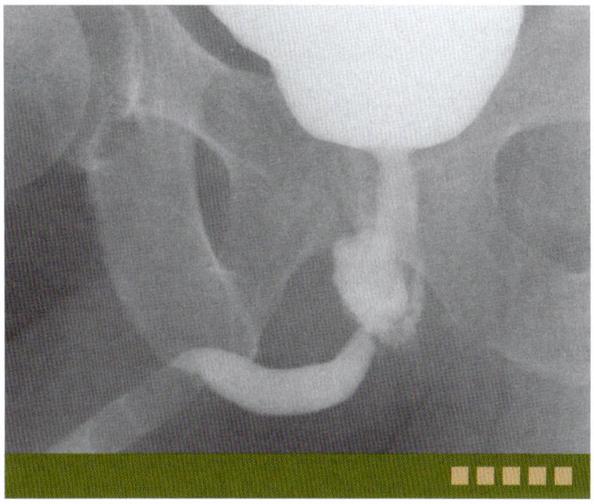

D. Retrograde urethrogram shows focal contrast leakage from the bulbous urethra after abdominoperineal resection.

DIFFERENTIAL DIAGNOSES IMAGES (E-G)

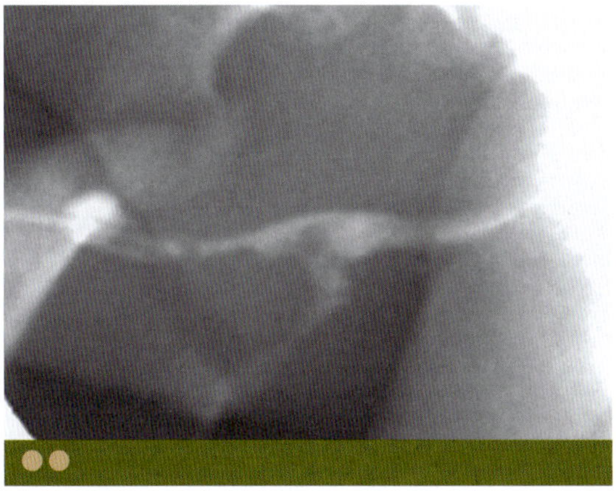

E. Urethral fistula: Retrograde urethrogram shows a fistula extending from the ventral aspect of the penile urethra to the skin surface.

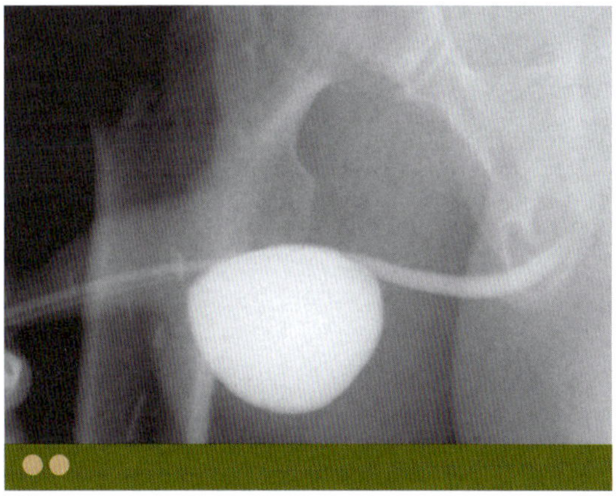

F. Urethral diverticulum: Retrograde urethrogram shows a large, smooth diverticulum arising from the penile urethra and the result of prolonged catheterization.

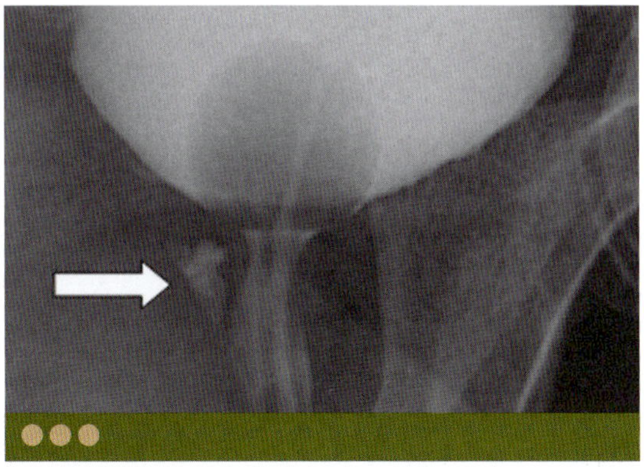

G. Cowper gland and duct: Cystogram shows a small collection of contrast (arrow) extending cephalad via a smooth tract from the right lateral aspect of the bulbous urethra.

IMAGE KEY

Common

Rare

Typical

Unusual

10–9 Posterior Urethral Trauma

Nancy A. Hammond

PRESENTATION

Trauma with blood at the meatus.

FINDINGS

Extravasation of contrast from the posterior urethra.

DIFFERENTIAL DIAGNOSES

- *Anterior urethra injury*: Involves the bulbous or penile urethra, typically isolated and associated with saddle injuries.
- *Bladder base injury*: Extraperitoneal bladder injury with contrast material extravasated around the base of bladder confined to the perivesical space. Bladder may have a tear-shaped morphology caused by surrounding hematoma.

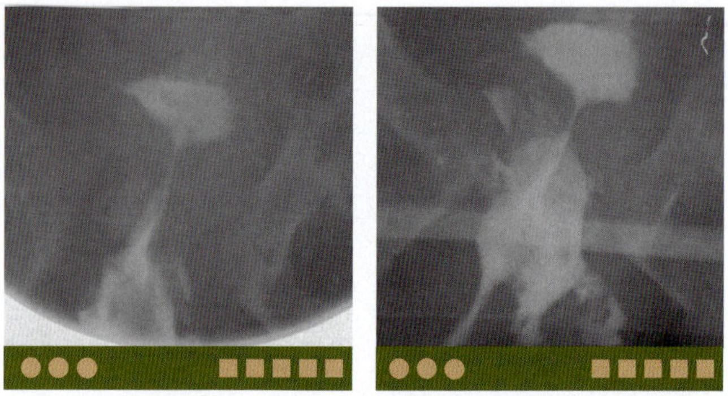

A. and **B.** Retrograde urethrogram shows extravasation of contrast material from the membranous portion of the posterior urethra into the extraperitoneal space. Contrast does not extend into the perineum consistent with an intact urogenital diaphragm. There is minimal filling of the urinary bladder suggesting that this represents a partial tear of the urethra. Diastasis of the pubic symphisis is also noted.

COMMENTS

The male urethra consists of two portions: the anterior and the posterior urethra. The anterior urethra extends from the external meatus to the inferior edge of the urogenital diaphragm and is further subdivided into the penile and bulbous urethra. The posterior urethra is divided into the membranous and prostatic urethra.

Traumatic urethral injury is four times more common in men than women because of the increased length of the male urethra. Urethral injury is typically seen in the setting of blunt abdominal trauma. Posterior urethral injury is associated with crush injuries with approximately 10% of the major pelvic ring fractures resulting in urethral injury. Associated bladder injury is seen 20% of the times in patients with pelvic fractures and urethral trauma. Trauma to the anterior urethra is seen secondary to saddle injuries and is usually isolated. Penetrating trauma to the urethra is uncommon, but when present, typically involves the anterior urethra. Blood at the meatus is seen in about 50% of significant urethral injuries.

When urethral injury is suspected, retrograde urethrogram should be performed. Posterior urethral injuries are classified based on findings on retrograde urethrography. With rupture of the puboprostatic ligaments, the prostatic urethra is stretched but the urethra remains intact on retrograde study. When the membranous urethra is torn above an intact urogenital diaphragm, retrograde study demonstrates extravasation of contrast from the torn urethra without extension into the perineum. In cases of a partial tear with an intact urogenital diaphragm, the prostatic urethra and bladder can be filled. When a complete tear occurs, no flow into the prostatic urethra or bladder is present. When there is concomitant disruption of the urogenital diaphragm, extravasated contrast is identified extending not only into the extraperitoneal space but also into the perineum. A superiorly positioned bladder can be seen with complete disruption of the membranous urethra. CECT may demonstrate extravasated contrast material on delayed imaging.

Treatment of urethral injuries consists of placement of a suprapubic catheter, endoscopic stent placement or delayed reconstruction procedure.

PEARLS

- **Traumatic injury to the urethra is four times more common in males than females and is typically seen in the setting of blunt abdominal trauma.**
- **Urethral trauma is divided into posterior and anterior urethral trauma with most cases of posterior urethral trauma associated with crush injuries.**
- **Clinically suspected urethra trauma should be evaluated with retrograde urethrogram.**

ADDITIONAL IMAGES (C-D)

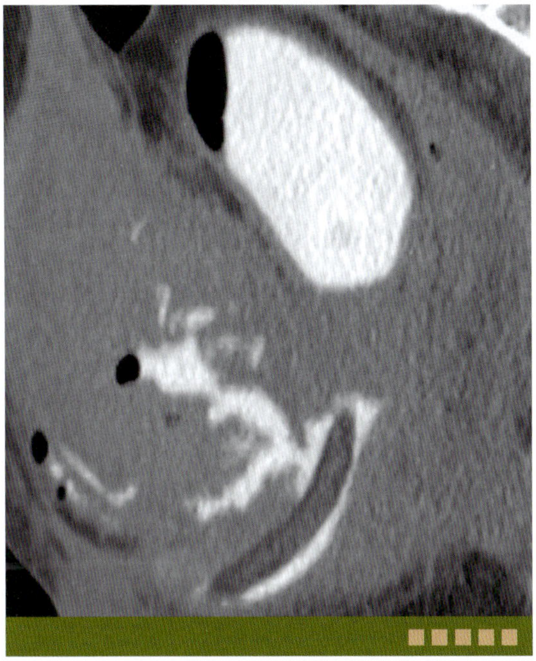

C. Sagittal CECT in the same patient shows extravasation of contrast material from the membranous urethra. Contrast extends anteriorly into the large extraperitoneal hematoma.

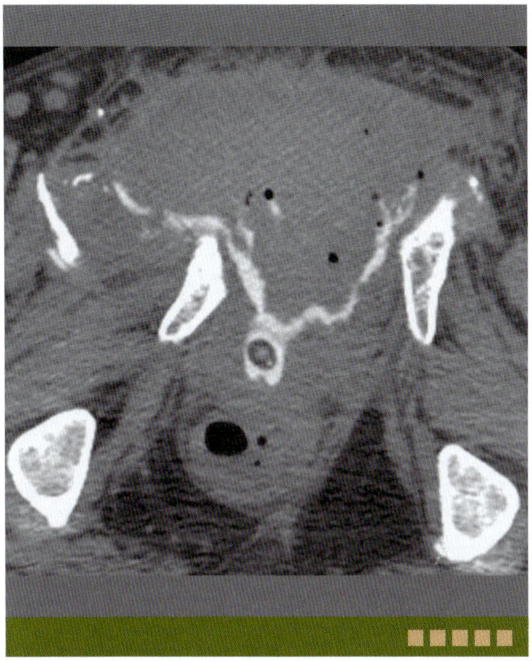

D. Axial CECT also shows the posterior urethral injury with contrast material extending into the prevesicular hematoma. The presence of air is likely associated with a recent procedure but may also imply superinfection.

DIFFERENTIAL DIAGNOSES IMAGES (E-F)

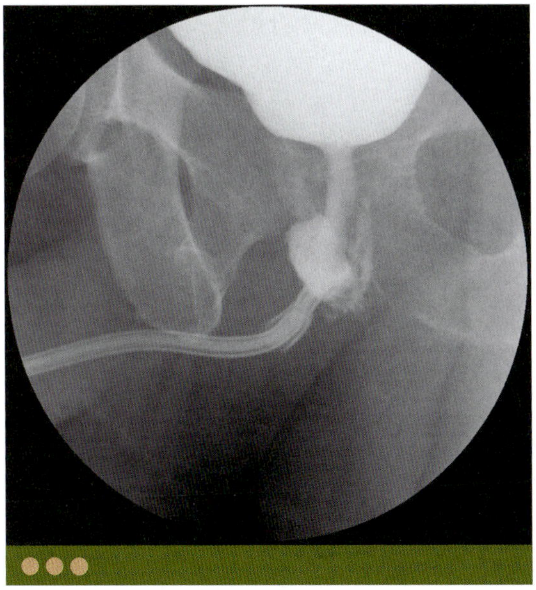

E. Anterior urethral injury: Retrograde urethrogram shows extravasation of contrast material from the proximal bulbar urethra.

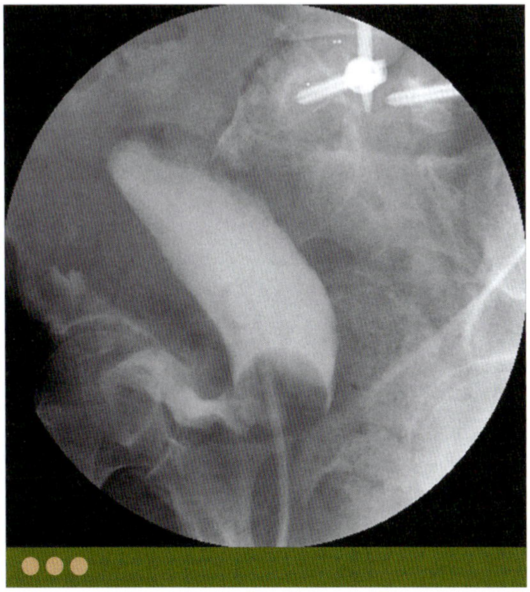

F. Bladder base injury: Spot image from a cystogram shows extravasation of contrast material from the base of the bladder.

IMAGE KEY

Common

Rare

Typical

Unusual

10–10 Extraperitoneal Bladder Rupture

David D. Casalino

PRESENTATION

Gross hematuria and pelvic pain post–motor vehicle accident.

FINDINGS

CT cystogram shows contrast distention of the bladder and hyperdense material in the anterior perivesical space.

DIFFERENTIAL DIAGNOSES

- *Intraperitoneal bladder rupture*: Contrast around bowel loops, in paracolic gutters, and in pouch of Douglas; less often associated with pelvic girdle fractures.
- *Urethral injury*: Typically present with blood in the urethral meatus, which should be evaluated with retrograde urethrography prior to bladder catheterization.
- *Pelvic bleeding*: Bleeding may be hyperdense and mimic contrast leakage from the bladder; often adjacent to fracture.
- *Bladder injury caused by penetrating or iatrogenic trauma*: Clinical setting will usually allow differentiation.

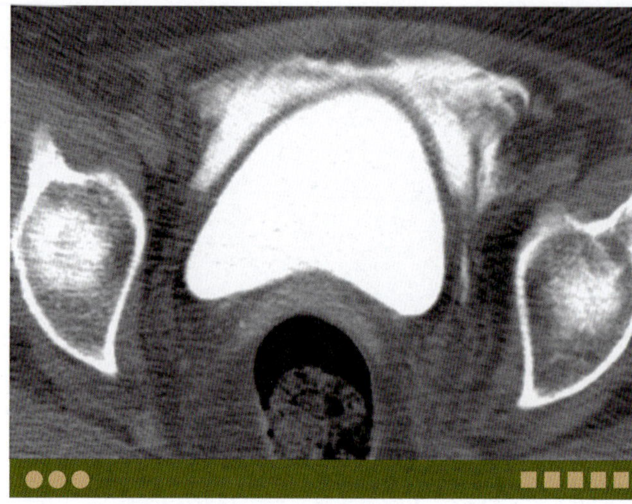

A. Axial NECT cystogram shows distention of the bladder and contrast extravasation into the anterior perivesical space.

COMMENTS

Bladder injury may result from penetrating, blunt, or iatrogenic trauma. Bladder rupture is the most common injury and may be classified as intraperitoneal or extraperitoneal. Bladder injuries are more likely to occur when the bladder is more distended. Sixty percent of all bladder ruptures are extraperitoneal. These injuries are almost always associated with pelvic girdle fractures, usually anterior pelvic arch fracture. The injury to the bladder may be caused by direct laceration by a bony fragment, a direct burst injury, or shearing force of the deforming pelvic ring. Bladder injuries commonly present with pelvic pain and hematuria. Patients may have difficulty voiding. Most extraperitoneal bladder ruptures can be managed with an indwelling bladder catheter.

Cystography has traditionally been the imaging study of choice for suspected bladder injury, but CT cystography is equally accurate and can be performed while the patient is being scanned for other injuries. One must always consider a urethral injury before attempting catheterization for cystography. Retrograde urethrogram may be warranted. Whether assessment of the bladder is performed by conventional or CT cystography, it is essential to obtain postvoid or postdrainage views, which may show delayed contrast leakage.

Contrast extravasation may be "flame-shaped" adjacent to the bladder. Contrast usually collects in the pelvic extraperitoneal space, including perivesical, space of Retzius (anterior prevesical) and retrorectal space, but may extend into scrotum, perineum, retroperitoneum, thigh, penis, or anterior abdominal wall. The bladder may assume a tear-drop shape as a result of compression by a pelvic hematoma.

PEARLS

- **Sixty percent of all bladder ruptures are extraperitoneal.**
- **Extraperitoneal rupture is almost always associated with pelvic girdle fractures.**
- **Most extraperitoneal ruptures can be managed with an indwelling bladder catheter.**
- **Extravasation may only be seen on postdrainage or postvoid views.**
- **Contrast usually collects in the pelvic extraperitoneal space.**

ADDITIONAL IMAGES (B-D)

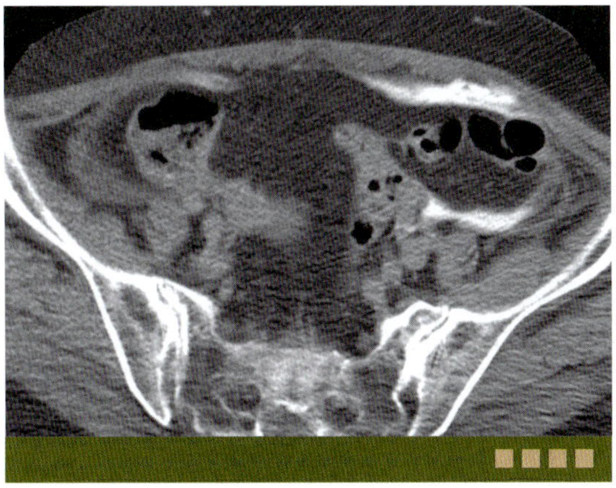

B. Axial NECT cystogram from the same patient shows cephalad contrast extension into the left anterior abdominal wall and retroperitoneum.

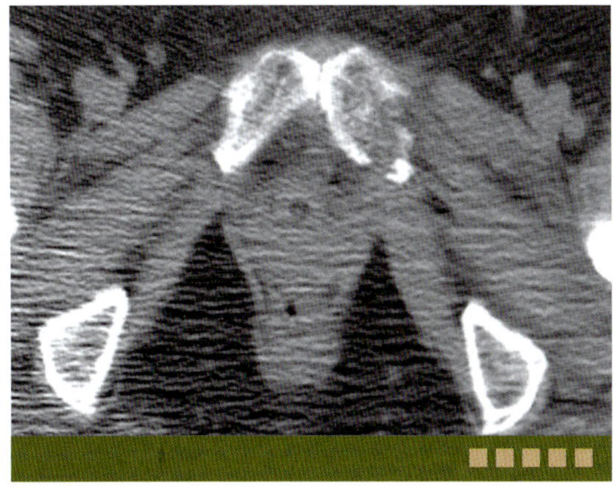

C. Axial NECT cystogram from the same patient shows a fracture through the left pubic bone.

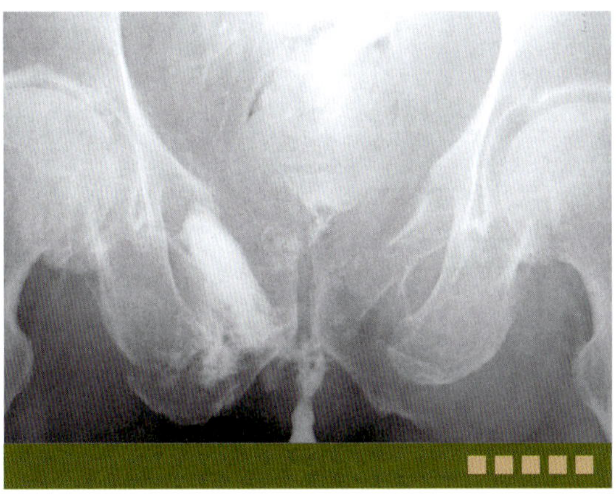

D. Cystogram from a different patient shows extraperitoneal contrast extravasation and numerous fractures of the pelvic girdle.

DIFFERENTIAL DIAGNOSES IMAGES (E-G)

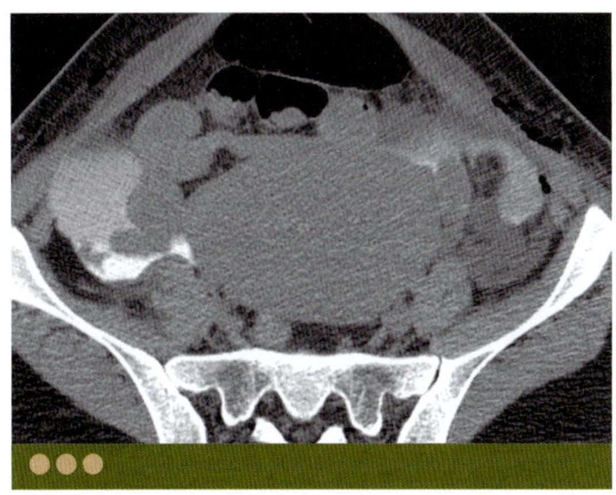

E. Intraperitoneal bladder rupture: Axial NECT cystogram shows contrast extravasation into the peritoneal cavity, around bowel loops.

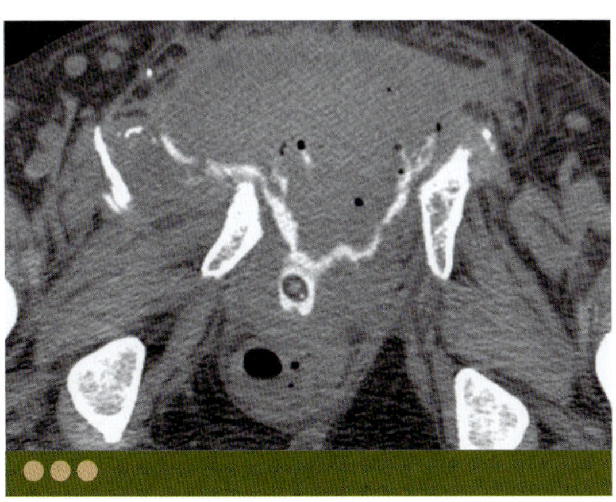

F. Urethral injury: Axial NECT cystogram shows contrast extravasation from the disrupted posterior urethra with large anterior pelvic hematoma and multiple pelvic fractures. A catheter is seen in the urethra.

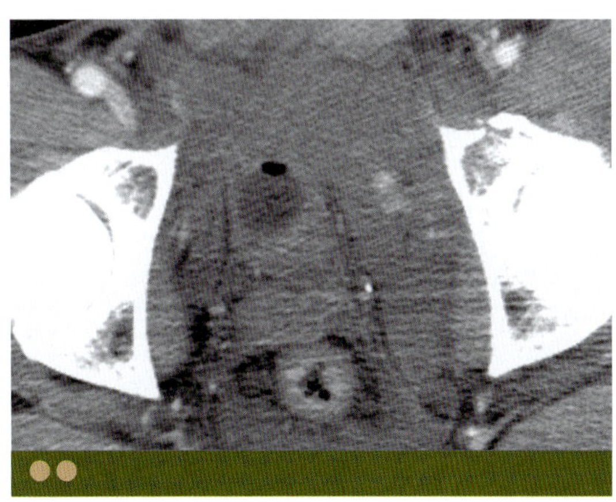

G. Pelvic bleeding: Axial CECT shows active bleeding into left pelvic musculature and an adjacent fracture. A Foley catheter is within the bladder, which is not contrast-filled.

IMAGE KEY

Common

Rare

Typical

Unusual

10–11 Intraperitoneal Bladder Rupture

David D. Casalino

PRESENTATION

Gross hematuria and pelvic pain post–motor vehicle accident.

FINDINGS

CT cystogram shows contrast distention of the bladder and intraperitoneal hyperdense material.

DIFFERENTIAL DIAGNOSES

- *Extraperitoneal bladder rupture*: Contrast usually collects in the pelvic extraperitoneal space, including perivesical, space of Retzius (anterior prevesical) and retrorectal space, and may extend into scrotum, perineum, retroperitoneum, thigh, penis, or anterior abdominal wall; more strongly associated with pelvic fractures.
- *Pelvic bleeding*: Bleeding may be hyperdense and mimic contrast leakage from the bladder; often adjacent to fracture.
- *Bowel perforation with intestinal contrast extravasation*: Usually denser contrast and pneumoperitoneum; often focal bowel abnormality, such as mural disruption.
- *Bladder injury caused by penetrating or iatrogenic trauma*: Clinical setting will usually allow differentiation.

COMMENTS

Bladder injury may result from penetrating, blunt, or iatrogenic trauma. Bladder rupture is the most common injury and may be classified at intraperitoneal or extraperitoneal.

Approximately 35% of bladder ruptures are intraperitoneal. Typically, this type of rupture occurs in the setting of blunt trauma to a distended bladder resulting in a sudden rise in intravesical pressure and disruption of the bladder dome. Children are prone to intraperitoneal ruptures because of the relative intra-abdominal position of the bladder. Adults in motor vehicle accidents are prone to this type of injury as a result of impact on a distended bladder, often by a seat belt or steering wheel. Twenty-five percent of the patients with intraperitoneal bladder rupture do not have associated pelvic fractures. Bladder injury commonly presents with pelvic pain and hematuria. Patients may have difficulty voiding because of blood clots. Intraperitoneal bladder rupture usually requires emergent surgical repair. Urine absorbed from the peritoneal cavity may result in electrolyte abnormalities, including hyperkalemia, hypernatremia, uremia, and acidosis.

Cystography has traditionally been the imaging study of choice for suspected bladder injury, but CT cystography is as accurate and can be performed while the patient is being scanned for other injuries. One must always consider a urethral injury before attempting catheterization for cystography. Retrograde urethrogram may be warranted. Whether assessment of the bladder is performed by conventional or CT cystography, it is essential to obtain postvoid or postdrainage views, which may show delayed contrast leakage.

The extravasated contrast may create a "cloudlike" appearance, outline loops of small bowel, collect in the rectovesical or rectouterine pouch, and extend into the paracolic gutters.

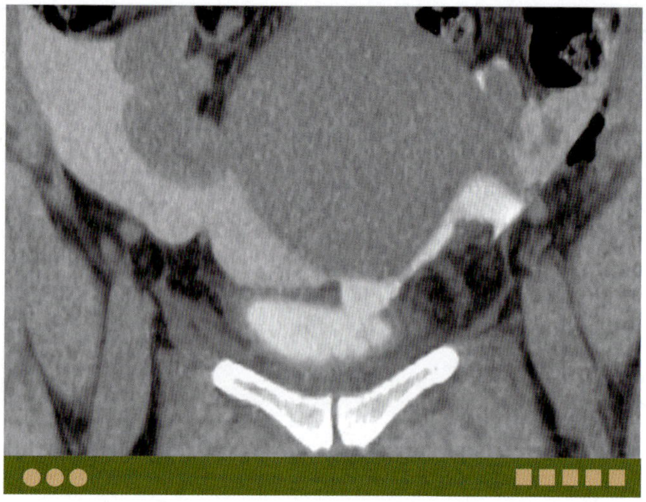

A. Coronal NECT cystogram shows contrast distention of the bladder with disruption of the bladder dome and intraperitoneal contrast extravasation.

PEARLS

- **35% of the bladder ruptures are intraperitoneal.**
- **25% of the patients with intraperitoneal bladder rupture do not have associated pelvic fractures.**
- **Intraperitoneal bladder rupture usually requires emergent surgical repair.**
- **Extravasation may only be seen on postdrainage or postvoid views.**
- **Contrast usually collects in the rectovesical or rectouterine pouch and may extend into the paracolic gutters and outline loops of bowel.**

ADDITIONAL IMAGES (B-D)

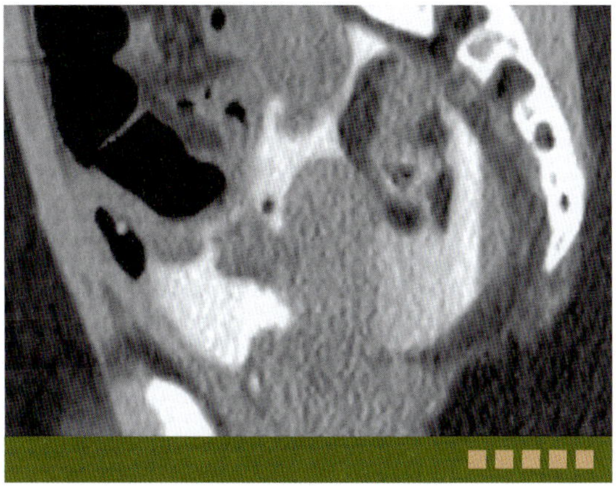

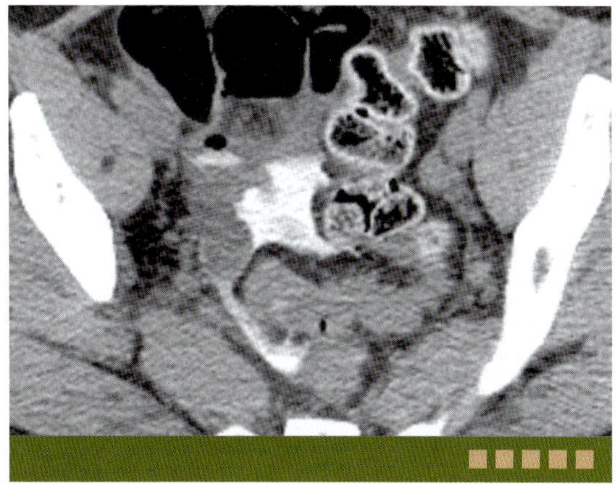

B. and **C.** Sagittal and axial NECT cystogram images from a different patient show disruption of the bladder dome with contrast collection in the rectouterine pouch and outlining bowel.

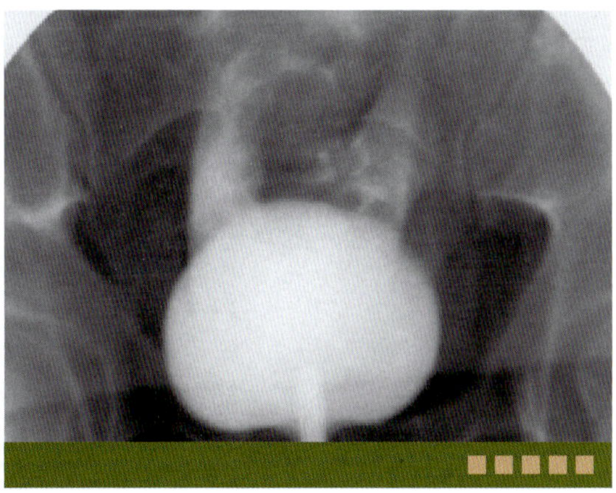

D. Intraoperative cystogram shows bladder dome disruption with intraperitoneal contrast extravasation.

DIFFERENTIAL DIAGNOSES IMAGES (E-G)

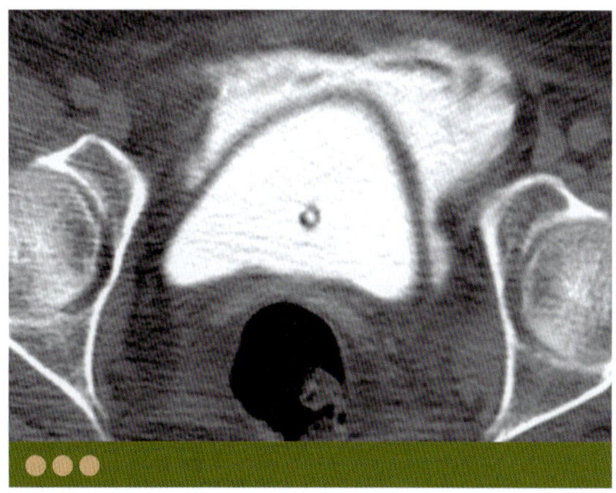

E. Extraperitoneal bladder rupture: Axial NECT cystogram shows distention of the bladder and contrast extravasation into the anterior perivesical space.

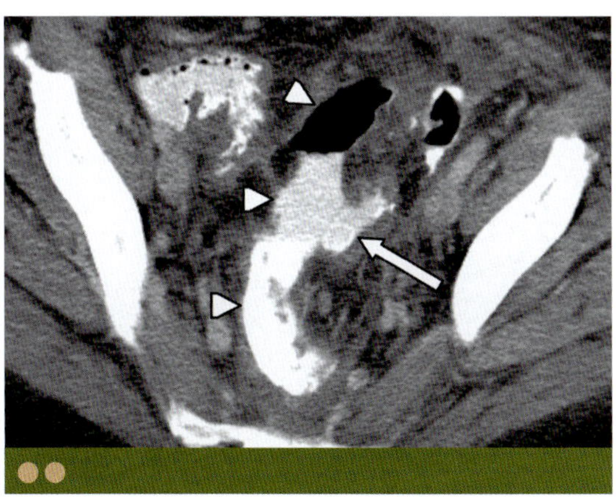

F. Bowel perforation: Axial CECT shows colonic contrast extravasation (arrowheads) from a disrupted sigmoid colonic anastomosis (arrow).

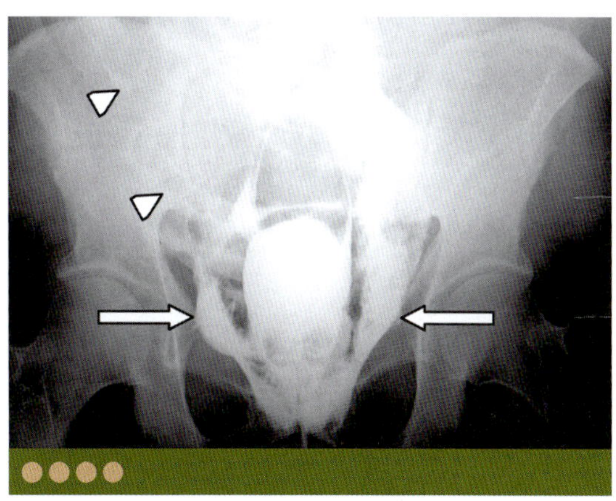

G. Iatrogenic bladder injury: Cystogram shows extraperitoneal (arrows) and intraperitoneal (arrowheads) contrast extravasation as a complication of prostatectomy.

IMAGE KEY

Common

Rare

Typical

Unusual

CHAPTER 11

NORMAL VARIANTS AND CONGENITAL ANOMALIES

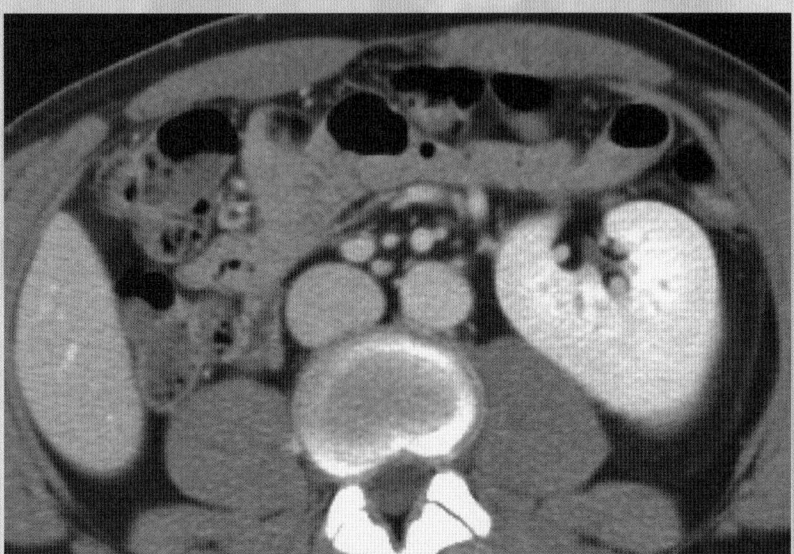

11–1 Renal Agenesis

Nancy A. Hammond

PRESENTATION

Incidental finding.

FINDINGS

Complete absence of the kidney.

DIFFERENTIAL DIAGNOSIS

- *Renal aplasia*: A small nonfunctioning kidney and a renal artery may be identified unlike renal agenesis.

COMMENTS

Renal agenesis is defined as complete congenital absence of renal tissue. It occurs as a result of *in utero* failure of formation of the ureteral bud or as a result of deficiency of the metanephric blastema in the fifth week of gestation. True renal agenesis also results in the absence of the bladder trigone and ureteral orifice. The ipsilateral renal artery is absent. These findings are in distinction to renal aplasia. Agenesis is usually an isolated sporadic anomaly but is also seen with chromosomal abnormalities and in association with genetic syndromes or developmental defects (VACTERL).

Bilateral renal agenesis is extremely rare and incompatible with life. Males are more commonly affected than females. Infants with bilateral renal agenesis have characteristic features of Potter facies including low set ears and prominent palpebral folds.

Unilateral agenesis is seen in 1 in 1000 to 2000 births, is asymptomatic, and is typically found incidentally. It is associated with a variety of genital abnormalities. In males, these include ipsilateral seminal vesicle cysts, ipsilateral absence of the vas deferens, hypoplasia or agenesis of the testicle, and hypospadias. In females, genital abnormalities include Müllerian duct anomalies including unicornuate or bicornuate uterus, absence or hypoplasia of the uterus, and absence or aplasia of the vagina (Rokitansky-Kuster-Hauser syndrome). Unilateral renal agenesis affects both kidneys equally.

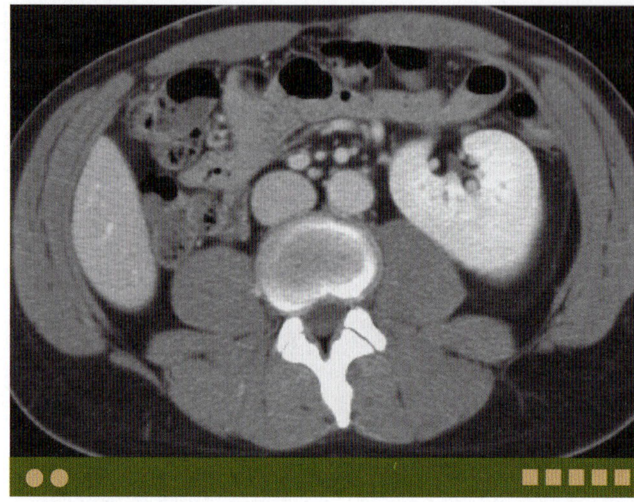

A. Axial CECT shows complete absence of the right kidney. A right renal artery was not identified.

Conventional radiographs may demonstrate colon occupying the affected renal fossa. Cross-sectional imaging and sonography demonstrates the absence of renal parenchyma, ispilateral ureter, and ipsilateral renal artery. In 8% to 10% of the cases, the ipsilateral adrenal gland will be absent. Compensatory hypertrophy of the contralateral kidney is typically present.

PEARLS

- **Bilateral renal agenesis incompatible with life and extremely rare.**
- **Unilateral renal agenesis is uncommon, usually found incidentally, and associated with genital abnormalities.**
- **Imaging demonstrates complete absence of renal parenchyma, ipsilateral ureter, and ipsilateral renal artery.**

ADDITIONAL IMAGES (B-D)

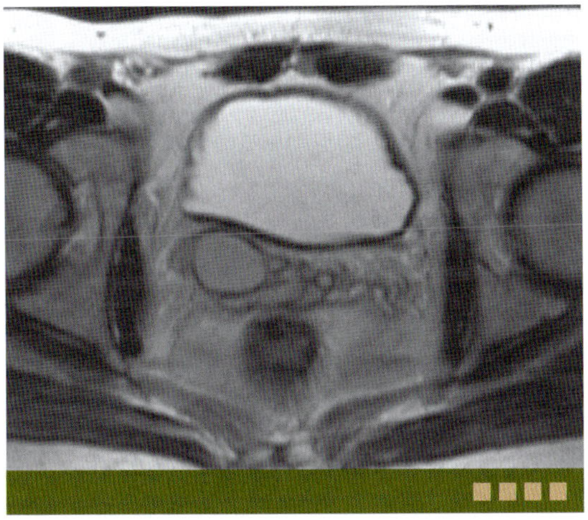

B. Axial T2-WI in the same patient shows a hyperintense lesion in the right seminal vesicles. Contrast-enhanced T1-WI showed nonenhancement of this structure (not shown). Findings are compatible with a seminal vesicle cyst.

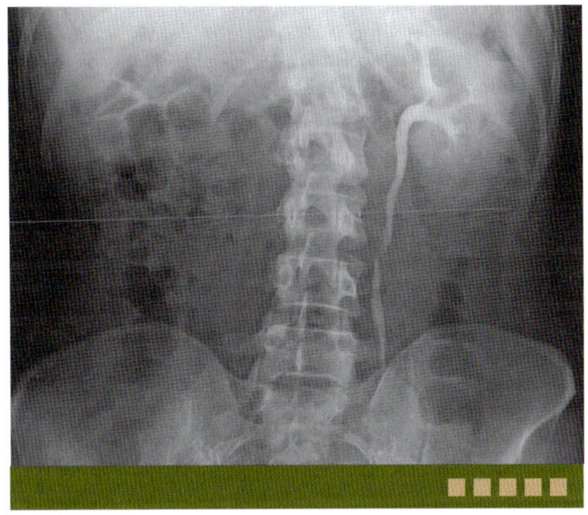

C. Fifteen minute radiograph from an intravenous urogram (IVU) shows nonvisualization of the right kidney. The left kidney measured 13.2 cm compatible with compensatory hypertrophy. This patient was being evaluated for infertility and found to have a uterine anomaly on hysterosalpingogram (HSG).

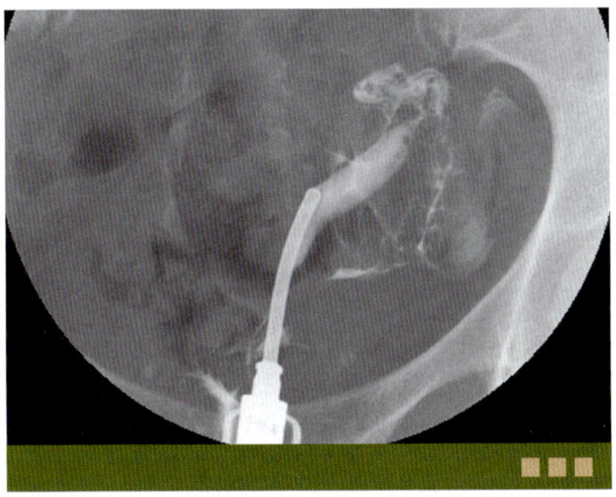

D. HSG in the same patient as Figure C shows filling of a single horn of the uterus compatible with unicornuate uterus.

DIFFERENTIAL DIAGNOSIS IMAGES (E-F)

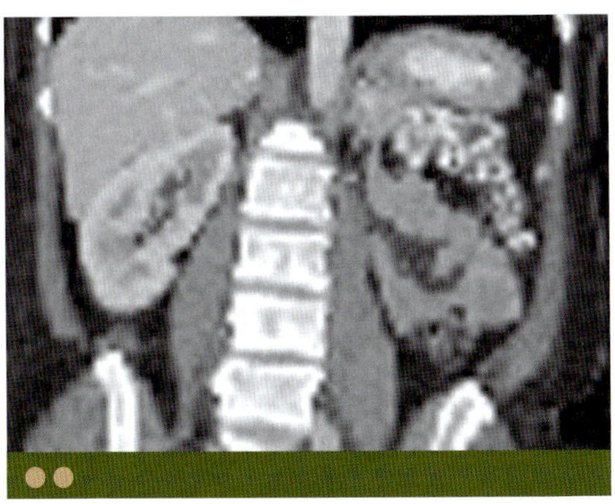

E. Renal aplasia: Coronal CECT in a different patient shows nonvisualization of the left kidney.

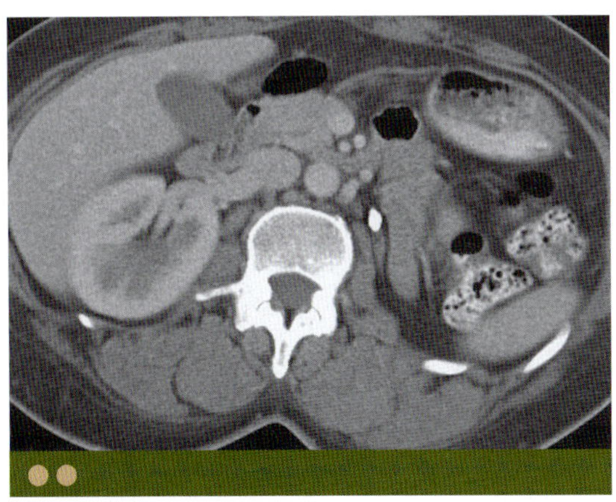

F. Renal aplasia: Axial CECT in the same patient as Figure E shows a small calcification in the left renal fossa compatible with anaplastic kidney rather than renal agenesis.

IMAGE KEY

Common

Rare

Typical

Unusual

11–2 Persistent Fetal Lobation

Nancy A. Hammond

PRESENTATION

Incidental finding on imaging.

FINDINGS

Smooth, regular indentations of the renal cortex without cortical loss.

DIFFERENTIAL DIAGNOSES

- *Cortical scar:* Associated parenchymal loss; Usually occurs in the cortex overlying the calyx.
- *Neoplasm*: Cross-sectional imaging demonstrates a true lesion with different signal, density, or echogenicity than adjacent renal parenchyma.
- *Multiple renal infarcts*: Usually seen in patients with small vessel disease; associated cortical atrophy is present.

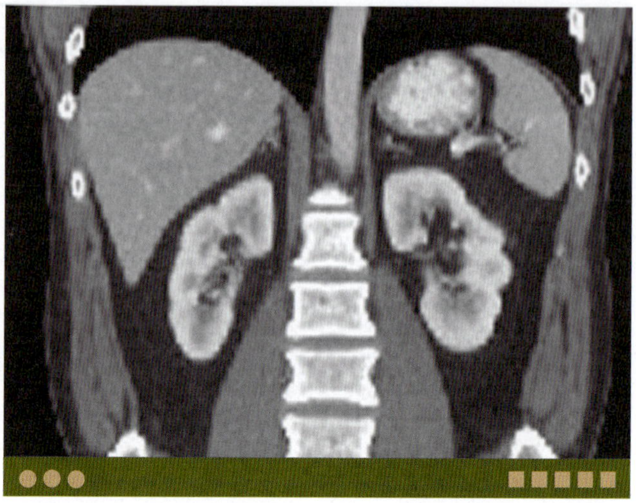

A. Coronal CECT shows smooth regular indentations of the renal cortex most marked involving the left kidney. The indentations occur between the renal pyramids, and there is no associated cortical loss or renal atrophy.

COMMENTS

Persistent fetal lobation can be identified in approximately 5% of the adults undergoing renal imaging. It is of no clinical significance but can be mistaken for an underlying mass or areas of cortical scarring. Embryologically, the kidney is composed of several lobules that eventually fuse to form the kidney. Typically, the renal surface becomes smooth and the interlobar grooves become invisible during the third trimester. However, incomplete fusion of the lobules resulting in small residual clefts can persist postnatally and into adulthood causing persistent fetal lobation of the kidney.

On intravenous urography, CT, MR, or sonography, persistent fetal lobations appear as smooth, regular indentations in the renal contour. There is no associated parenhcymal thinning or abnormalities of the underlying calyx. The renal indentations should be smooth and regular. They overlie the space between the pyramids. This is in distinction to cortical scarring which typically involves the cortex overlying the calyx. Radiographically, persistent fetal lobation can be confirmed by the presence of a renal pyramid in the bulge bounded by septa of Bertin on either side.

PEARLS

- **Persistent fetal lobation seen in about 5% of the adults undergoing imaging studies.**
- **Fetal lobation is of no clinical significance.**
- **Imaging studies demonstrate smooth regular indentations of the renal contour without parenchymal loss. In distinction to cortical scarring, the indentation occurs between the renal calyces/pyramids.**

ADDITIONAL IMAGE

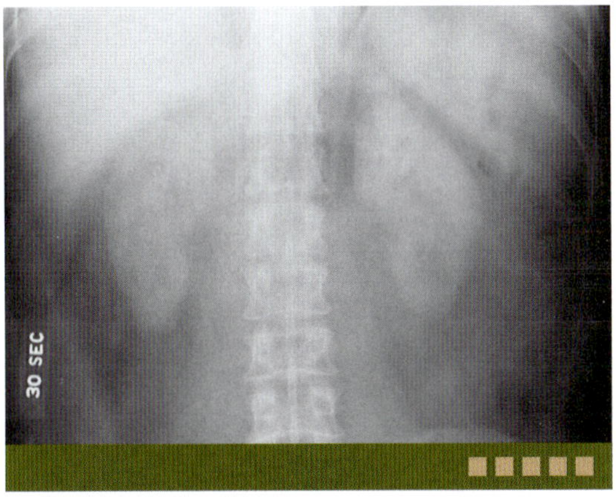

B. Tomogram from an IVU after injection of contrast shows mild undulation of the renal contour slightly more prominent on the right than on the left.

DIFFERENTIAL DIAGNOSES IMAGES (C-F)

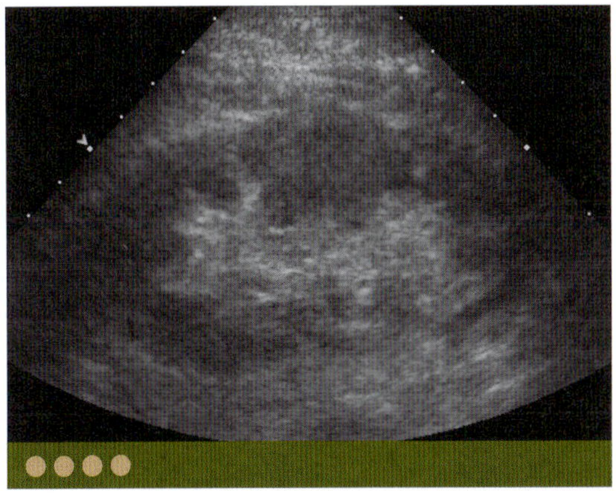

C. Renal cell carcinoma: Longitudinal sonogram shows mild contour bulge of the mid aspect of the left kidney with bulging of the inner margin of the renal cortex raising the possibility of an underlying mass.

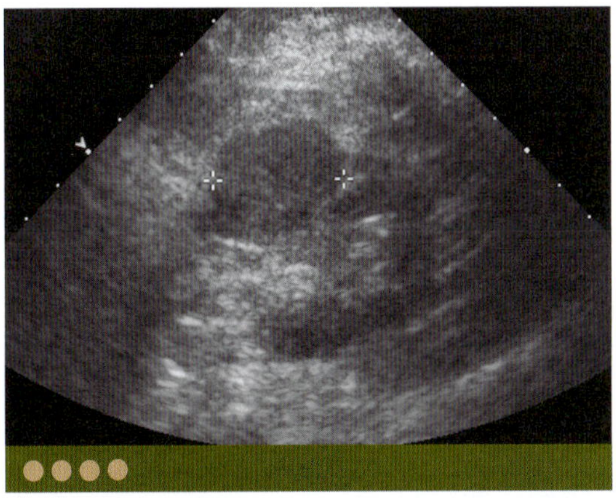

D. Renal cell carcinoma: Transverse sonogram in the same patient confirms the presence of a solid renal mass.

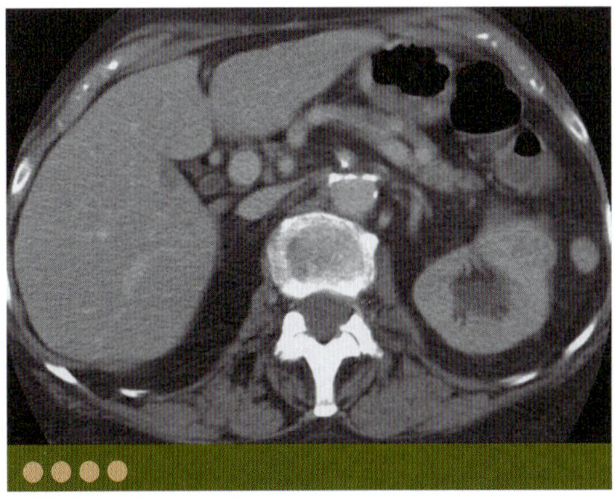

E. Renal cell carcinoma: Axial CECT in the same patient further shows the solid, enhancing mass in the left kidney subsequently found to represent a renal cell carcinoma.

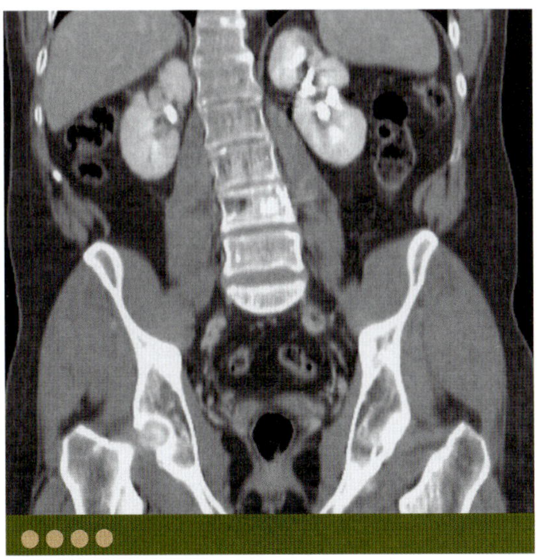

F. Cortical scarring: Coronal CECT shows a focal indentation of the renal cortex involving the mid aspect of the left kidney with associated cortical loss. The focal indentation on the left overlies a calyx and is characteristic of scarring.

IMAGE KEY

Common

Rare

Typical

Unusual

11–3 Dromedary Hump

Nancy A. Hammond

PRESENTATION

Incidental finding on renal imaging.

FINDINGS

Cortical hump at the mid to upper aspect of the left kidney.

DIFFERENTIAL DIAGNOSIS

- *Focal renal mass*: A discrete mass is identified on contrast-enhanced images.

COMMENTS

The term dromedary hump refers to an apparent pseudomass at the lateral aspect of the left kidney. This is felt to be created by molding of the renal tissue by the adjacent spleen during fetal development resulting in a prominent cortical hump at the interpolar region. A dromedary hump should have the appearance of normal renal parenchyma regardless of the imaging modality with uniform thickness of renal parenchyma between the bulge and the underlying renal calyces. The area should be subtended by a normal collecting system element and a normal interpapillary line should be present.

IVU demonstrates a prominent cortical hump in the characteristic location with elongation of the calyx. Sonogram also demonstrates a prominent cortical hump that maintains uniform thickness and is isoechoic to the remainder of the renal cortex. On nonenhanced cross-sectional studies, the region should be isointense or isodense to the remaining renal parenchyma. Contrast-enhanced studies should demonstrate normal parenchymal enhancement of the region. It is important to be aware of the typical location and appearance of this finding to avoid unnecessary imaging to evaluate for a presumed renal mass.

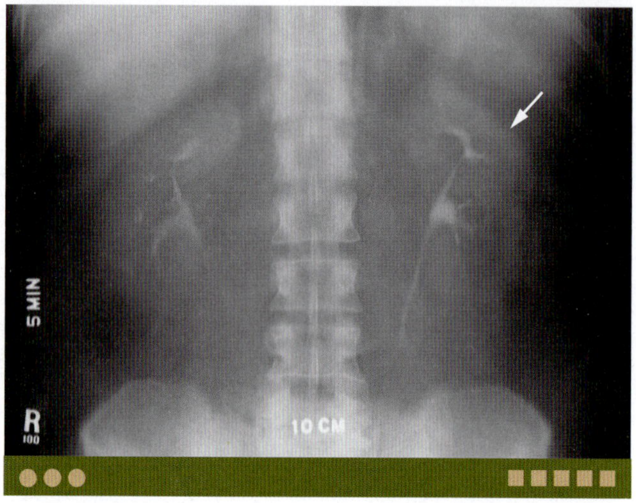

A. Tomogram from an IVU obtained at 5 minutes shows the characteristic cortical bump along the lateral margin of the mid aspect of the left kidney.

PEARLS

- **Normal anatomic variant secondary to molding of the renal tissue by the adjacent spleen during fetal development.**
- **It is important to be aware of characteristic location and appearance involving the mid to upper aspect of the left kidney.**
- **A cortical hump is seen at the lateral aspect of the left kidney with preservation of normal cortical thickness. On cross-sectional imaging, this region remains isodense, isoechoic, or isointense to the remainder of the renal cortex.**

CHAPTER 11
Normal Variants and Congenital Anomalies

CASE
Dromedary Hump

ADDITIONAL IMAGES (B-C)

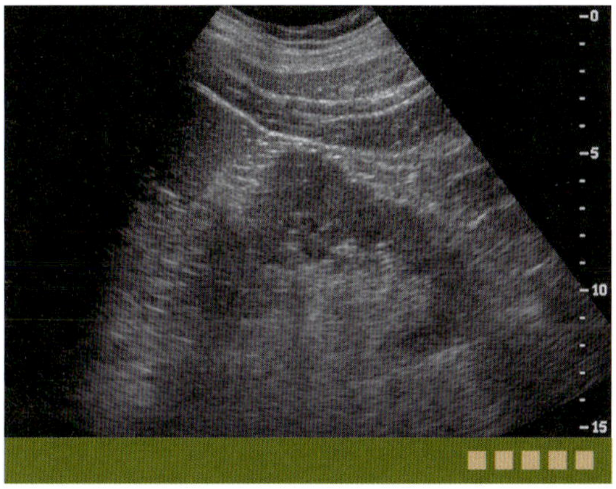

B. Longitudinal sonogram shows a prominent bulge of the outer cortical margin at the mid aspect of the left kidney. Note uniform cortical thickness throughout the left kidney despite the cortical hump

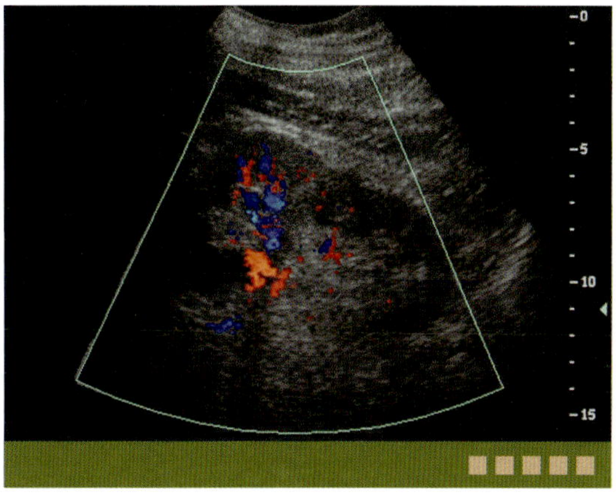

C. Longitudinal color sonogram in the same patient as Figure B shows normal blood flow to this region confirming that this finding relates to a dromedary hump rather than an underlying mass.

DIFFERENTIAL DIAGNOSIS IMAGES (D-E)

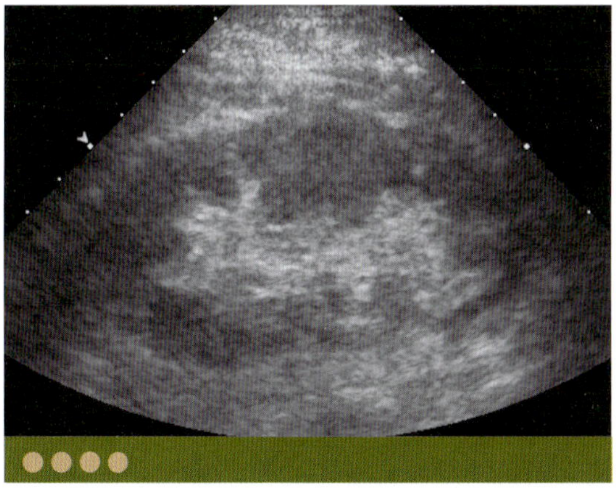

D. Renal mass: Longitudinal sonogram also shows a cortical bump at the mid aspect of the left kidney. However, the cortex is thickened at this level and slightly more echogenic than the more inferior and superior renal cortex.

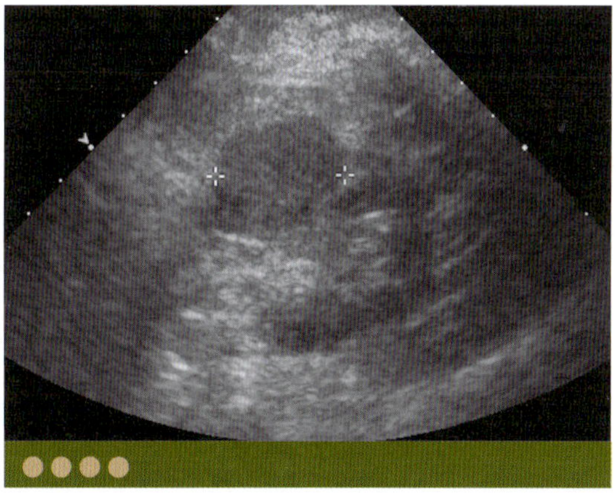

E. Renal mass: Transverse sonogram in the same patient as Figure D confirms the presence of an echogenic, solid renal mass.

IMAGE KEY

Common

Rare

Typical

Unusual

11–4 Hypertrophied Column of Bertin

Nancy A. Hammond

PRESENTATION

Renal ultrasound performed for hematuria.

FINDINGS

Mass-like protuberance into the renal sinus at the junction of the mid and upper pole of the kidney.

DIFFERENTIAL DIAGNOSIS

- *Renal mass*: Characteristic location and appearance of hypertrophied column of Bertin distinguishes from a true mass.

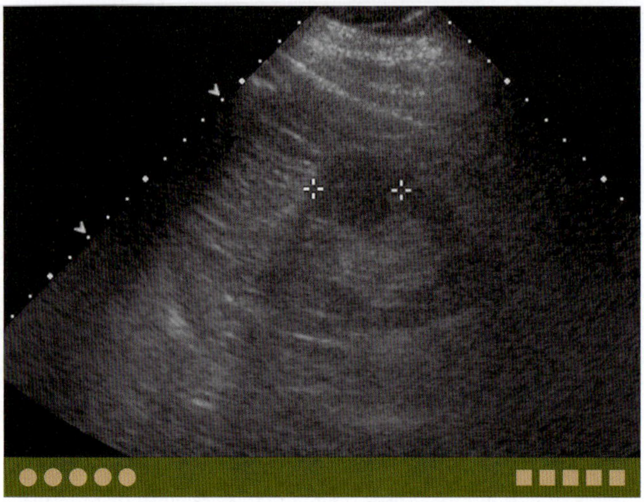

A. Transverse sonogram shows a hypoechoic mass-like protusion in the interpolar region of the left kidney. The mass is near isoechoic to adjacent renal cortex.

COMMENTS

A prominent or hypertrophied column of Bertin is a normal anatomic variant resulting from hypertrophied cortical tissue located between the pyramids that project into the renal sinus. In the 1740s, the prominent column of Bertin was described by a French anatomist, Exupere Joseph Bertin, as a thickened aggregate of cortical tissue. Bertin's original studies noted that some of these projections were more prominent than others; however, it was not until the 1960s that radiologist became aware of the characteristic findings of a hypertrophied column of Bertin distinguishing them from a mass lesion. Until this time, a number of unnecessary nephrectomies were performed for presumed neoplasms. A prominent column of Bertin is the most common cause of a renal pseudotumor on cross-sectional imaging.

They most typically occur at the junction of the upper and middle thirds of the kidney and are seen in both kidneys but more common on the left than on the right. The column of Bertin forms from the fusion of two layers of septal cortex of two adjacent lobes or renunculi. In some cases, this fusion of normal cortex may be more prominent and project into the renal sinus resulting in a pseudomass.

Sonographically, a prominent column of Bertin appears as a projection of renal cortex into the renal sinus engulfed by renal sinus fat. The echogenicity is identical to that of the adjacent renal cortex. A small hypoechoic focus that represents an engulfed papilla can be seen in the center of the hypertrophied column has also been described on IVU as a small central lucency. Color or power Doppler ultrasound may demonstrate blood vessels coursing through the region. Unlike cases of true renal masses that distort the renal contour, a normal contour is seen with a hypertrophied column. CT and MRI confirm the presence of normal renal parenchyma with a prominent column of Bertin being isodense/isointense to adjacent renal parenchyma.

PEARLS

- **Prominent column of Bertin is a normal anatomic variant secondary to hypertrophied cortical tissue and usually seen at the junction of the upper and middle pole of the kidney.**
- **Most common cause of a renal pseudotumor.**
- **Imaging studies demonstrate a normal renal contour. The prominent column demonstrates the same echogenicity, density, or signal intensity of adjacent renal cortex.**

ADDITIONAL IMAGES (B-C)

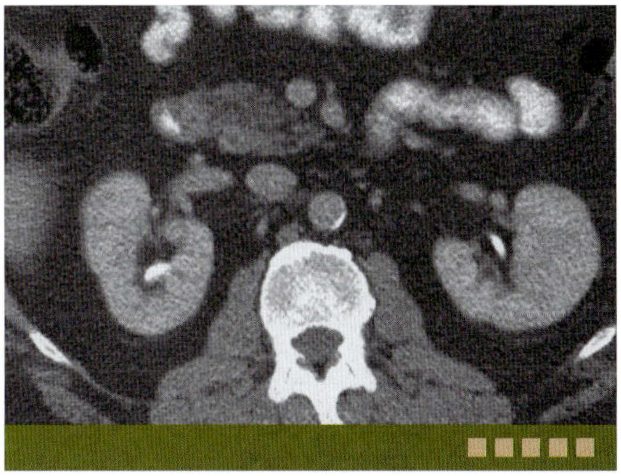

B. Axial CECT in the same patient as Figure A shows the pseudomass projecting into the renal sinus to be isodense to renal cortex.

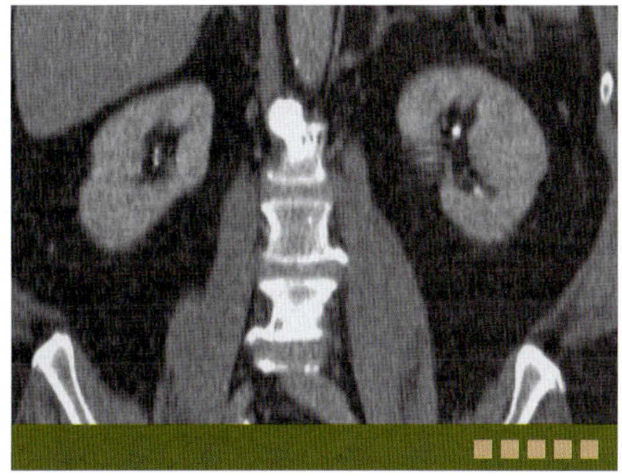

C. Coronal CECT further shows the prominent column of Bertin projecting into the renal sinus.

DIFFERENTIAL DIAGNOSIS IMAGES (D-F)

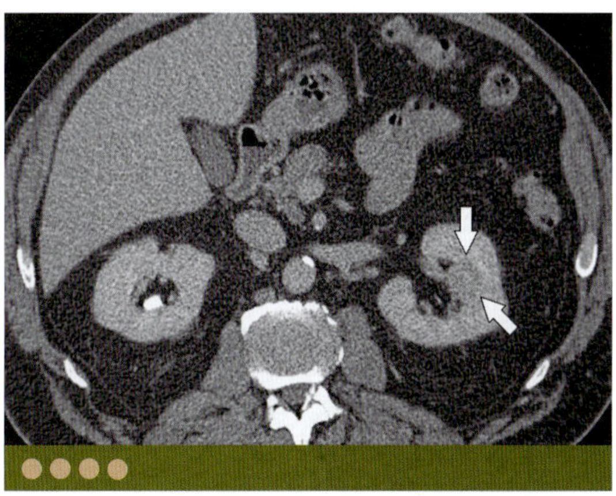

D. Renal cell carcinoma: Axial CECT shows a subtle hypodense region in the renal cortex of the left kidney in the typical location of a hypertrophied column of Bertin. However, given that this region was slightly less dense than adjacent renal cortex, the possibility of a renal mass was raised and MRI was recommended.

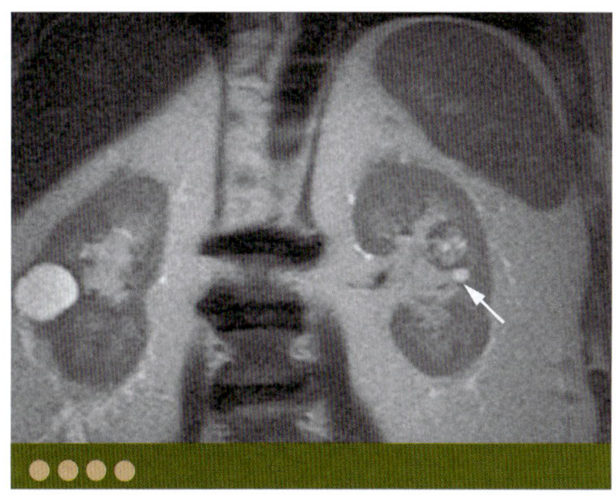

E. Coronal T2-WI in the same patient as Figure E confirms the presence of a solid mass in the interpolar region of the left kidney. The mass shows heterogeneous signal intensity and is slightly hyperintense to normal renal cortex (arrow).

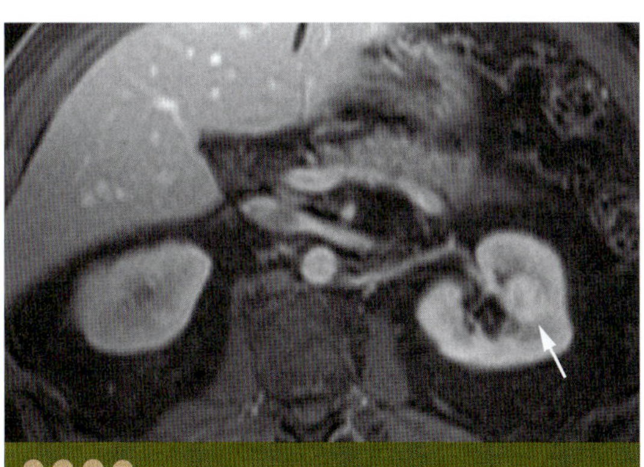

F. Axial contrast-enhanced T1-WI shows the mass to enhance mildly heterogeneously (arrow).

IMAGE KEY

Common

Rare

Typical

Unusual

11–5 Renal Lobar Dysmorphism

Paul Nikolaidis

PRESENTATION

Incidentally discovered renal mass on CT.

FINDINGS

Triple phase CT shows a smoothly marginated central mass projecting into the renal sinus. It enhances to the same degree as normal renal parenchyma on all phases of the examination.

DIFFERENTIAL DIAGNOSIS

- *Renal neoplasms*: Neoplastic lesions should not enhance in the exact same fashion as the normal renal parenchyma on all phases of the CT or MR examination. Areas of heterogeneity, hemorrhage, or altered enhancement are typically seen.

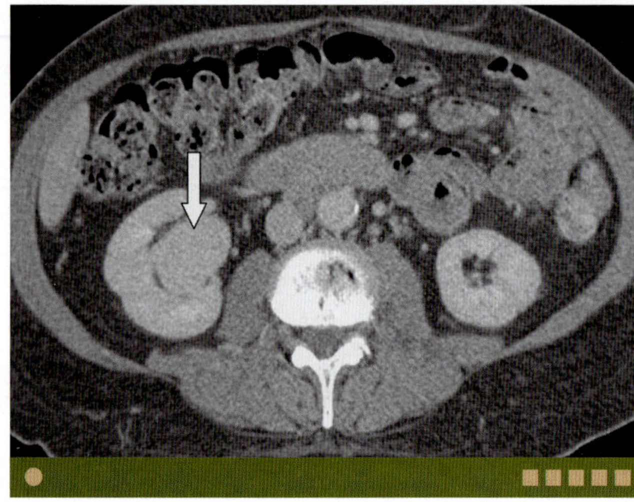

A. Axial CECT obtained during the nephrographic phase of imaging shows an enhancing mass arising, extending into the renal sinus at the mid to lower aspect of the right kidney**.**

COMMENTS

Renal pseudotumors are histologically composed of normal renal tissue but can mimic a neoplasm on cross-sectional imaging or urography. One common pseudotumor is renal lobar dysmorphism, which is a developmental malposition of a renal lobe. It is caused by abnormal embryological development of the kidney (abnormal fusion), resulting in a condition where a complete renal lobe is located deep within the renal substance. This anomaly has been reported to represent "junctional parenchyma". The presence of a complete lobe is suggested by the presence of a calyx centrally within the mass, which is a diagnostic feature.

Lobar dysmorphism is one of a number of normal anatomic variants that may simulate mass lesions on imaging studies. Most are located between the upper and middle thirds of the kidney, near the renal sinus, while a minority are located in the lower third of the kidney.

On sonography, a lobar dysmorphism is usually isoechoic to renal parenchyma, and may project into the renal sinus fat. Lobar dysmorphism can be correctly diagnosed on triple phase CT, when its typical medullary and cortical structures are confirmed during the corticomedullary and nephrographic phases of contrast enhancement. CT should demonstrate a smoothly marginated mass deep in the interpolar parenchyma, usually projecting into the renal sinus. Lesions should enhance to the same degree as the normal renal parenchyma on all phases of the examination. On the nephrographic phase, the majority of the mass should enhance to the same degree as the renal cortex. In the pyelographic phase, a dense medullary blush should be seen; the presence of a small calyx is diagnostic.

PEARLS

- **Renal pseudotumors can mimic neoplasms on imaging, but are histologically composed of normal renal tissue.**
- **Lobar dysmorphism is one of several normal anatomic variants that may simulate a renal neoplasm.**
- **On CT, a smoothly marginated mass which enhances to the same degree as the normal renal parenchyma is seen deep in the interpolar parenchyma.**
- **The presence of a small calyx is diagnostic.**

ADDITIONAL IMAGES (B-C)

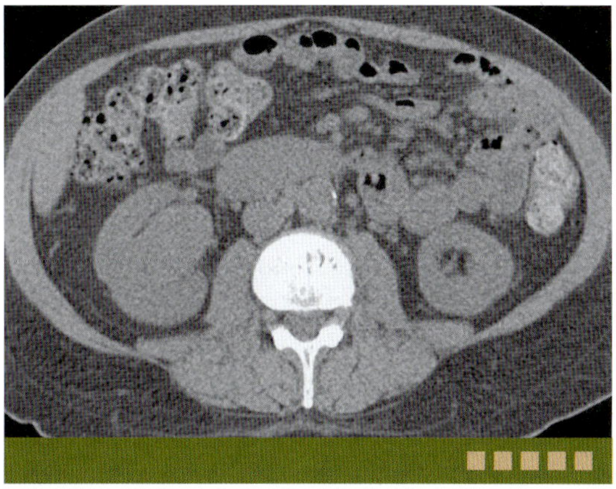

B. Corresponding axial NECT shows the mass to be isodense to renal parenchyma.

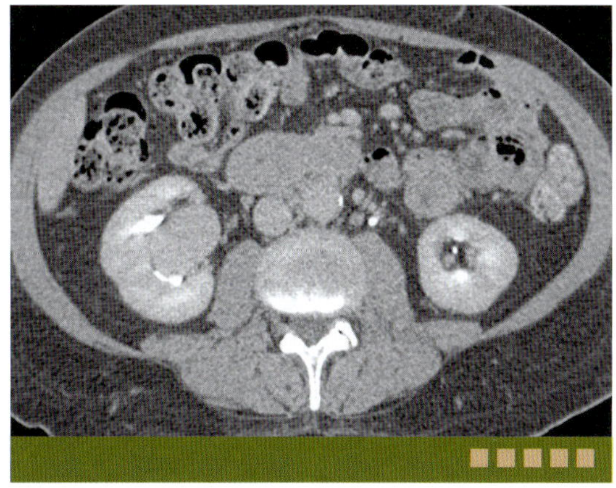

C. Corresponding axial CECT obtained during the excretory phase of imaging shows that the mass enhances similar to the normal renal parenchyma.

DIFFERENTIAL DIAGNOSIS IMAGES (D-F)

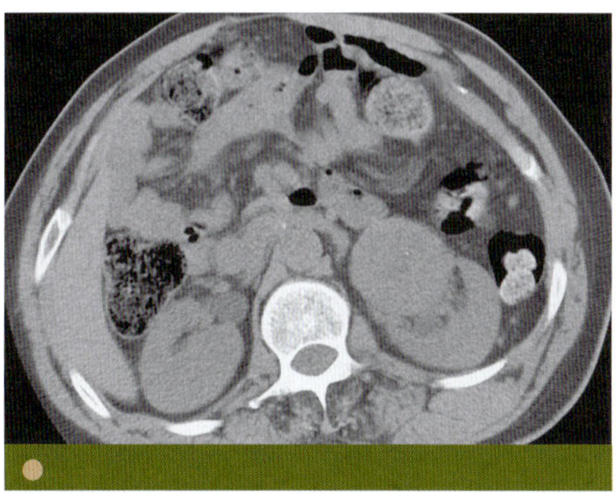

D. Leiomyosarcoma of the kidney: Axial NECT shows a large centrally located mass extending anteriorly in the mid to lower aspect of the right kidney.

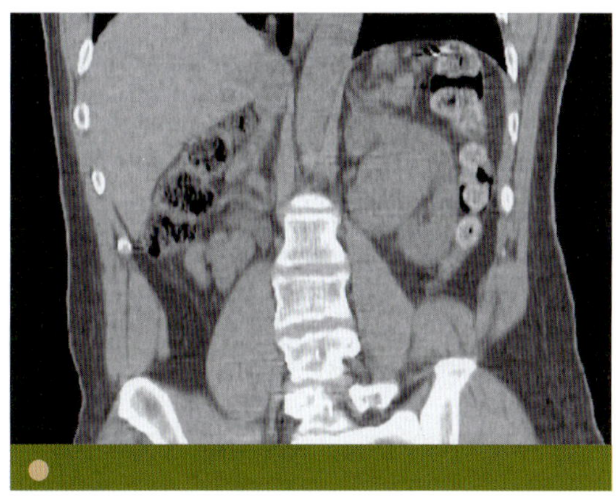

E. Leiomyosarcoma of the kidney: Corresponding coronal NECT reformation shows the mass to be approximately isodense to renal parenchyma.

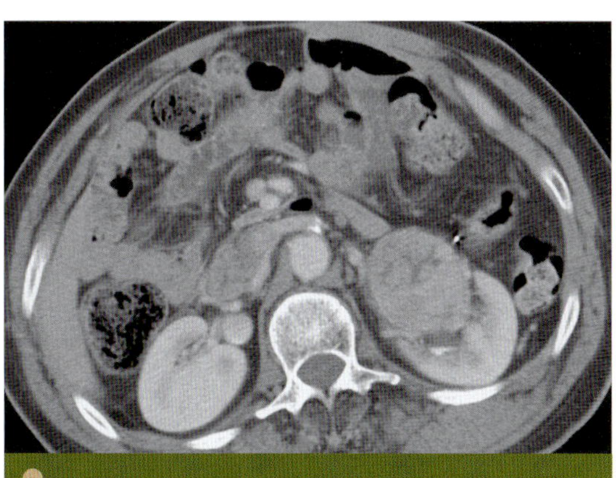

F. Leiomyosarcoma of the kidney: Corresponding axial CECT obtained during the excretory phase of imaging shows that the mass is quite heterogeneous and does not enhance in a similar pattern as the normal renal parenchyma.

IMAGE KEY

Common

Rare

Typical

Unusual

11–6 Junctional Parenchymal Defect

Nancy A. Hammond

PRESENTATION

Incidental finding on imaging.

FINDINGS

Triangular hyperechoic focus at the anteriosuperior aspect of the right kidney.

DIFFERENTIAL DIAGNOSES

- *Cortical scar*: Demonstrates associated cortical loss.
- *Neoplasm (AML or RCC)*: Mass-like configuration; may have enhancing component.

COMMENTS

Junctional parenchymal defects (JPD) are a normal anatomic variant and seen in approximately 30% of the population. Most commonly, these are found incidentally in examinations performed for the evaluation of other suspected pathology. JPDs form as a result of extension of the renal sinus at the junction of the renal poles because of incomplete fusion of the two embryonic parenchymatous masses called renunculi. It is most commonly seen in the right kidney but has been described in the left kidney sometimes.

Sonographically, JPDs appear as triangular, hyperechoic focus at the anterosuperior or posteroinferior aspect of the kidney on sagittal imaging. The hyperechoic structure can typically be traced to the renal sinus when followed medially. Intravenous pyelogram may demonstrate a radiolucent triangular defect in a typical location for JPD which is best appreciated on tomograms. As JPD can be mistaken for a mass, knowledge of its characteristic location and shape is essential to make the diagnosis. CT and MR demonstrate fat attenuation signal that is continguous with the perinephric fat and extends to the renal sinus at the site of the defect.

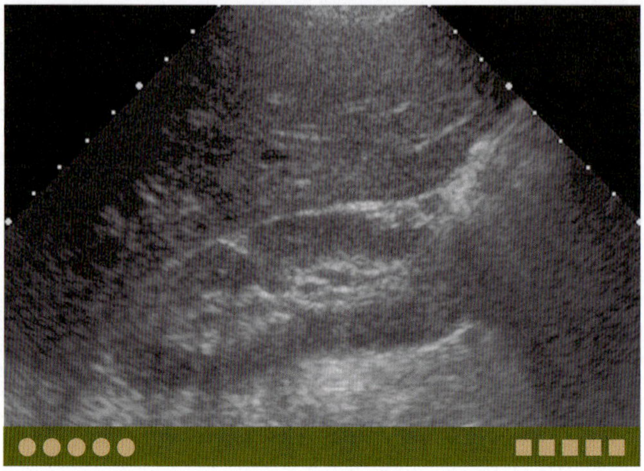

A. Longitudinal sonogram of the right kidney shows a triangular hyperechoic focus at the anterosuperior aspect of the kidney.

PEARLS

- **JPD is a common anatomic variant seen in approximately 30% of the population.**
- **JPD results from incomplete fusion of two renunculi in the embryo.**
- **A characteristic hyerechoic, triangular focus is present at the anterosuperior or posteroinferior aspect of the kidney and is seen most commonly in the right kidney but can involve the left kidney.**
- **JPD can be distinguished from a pathologic condition by its characteristic location and shape.**

ADDITIONAL IMAGES (B-D)

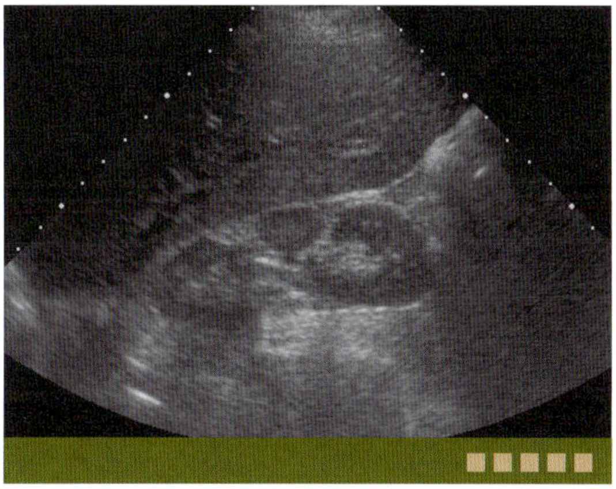

B. Longitudinal sonogram in the same patient further shows the hyperechoic lesion clearly extending to the renal sinus and confirming the diagnosis of a junctional parenchymal defect.

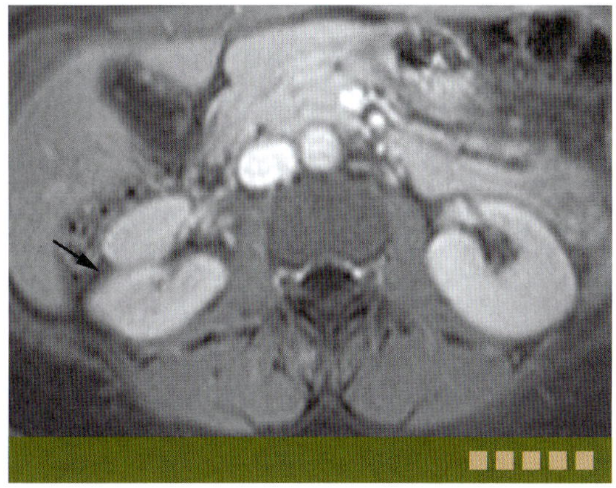

C. Axial contrast-enhanced T1-WI in a different patient shows a triangular defect in the right kidney with extension to the renal sinus (arrow). The cortical defect follows the signal of fat on all sequences.

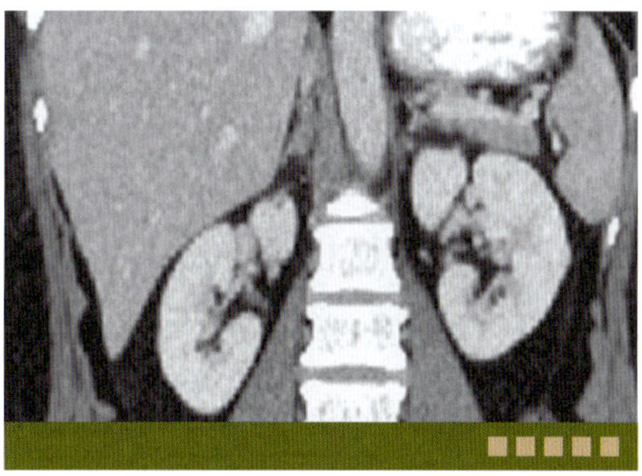

D. Coronal CECT shows bilateral fat density defects involving the upper poles of the kidneys compatible with bilateral JPDs.

DIFFERENTIAL DIAGNOSES IMAGES (E-F)

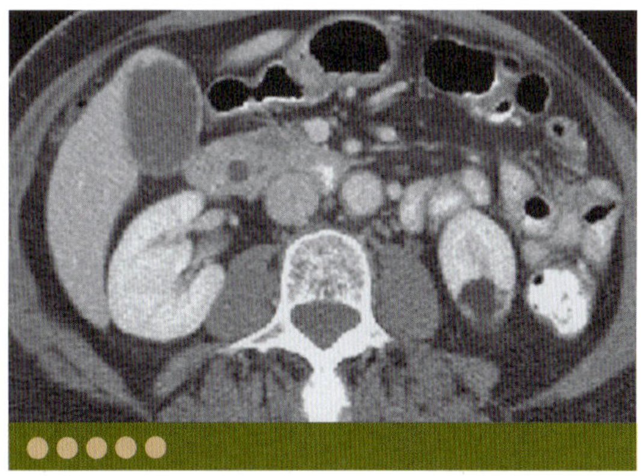

E. Angiomyolipoma: Axial CECT shows a fat density mass at the peripheral aspect of the left kidney consistent with an angiomyolipoma. In distinction to JPD, this has a mass-like configuration, does not extend to the renal pelvis, and is in an atypical location for a JPD.

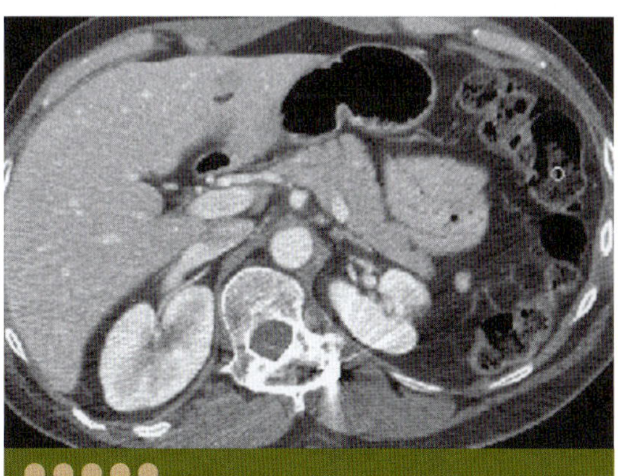

F. Cortical scar: Axial CECT shows a defect in the mid portion of the left kidney with associated cortical loss compatible with cortical scar in this patient with a history of renal infarct.

IMAGE KEY

Common

Rare

Typical

Unusual

11–7 Ureter Herniation with Ligation in Patient with Crossed Fused Renal Ectopia

Frank H. Miller

PRESENTATION

- *Ureteral hernia*: Groin mass.
- *Crossed fused ectopia*: Abdominal or flank pain, palpable mass, nonspecific symptoms; often incidentally detected.

FINDINGS

Crossed fused ectopic better shown on CT with abnormal excretion of lateral moiety resulting from ligation of a ureteral hernia during surgery.

DIFFERENTIAL DIAGNOSIS

None

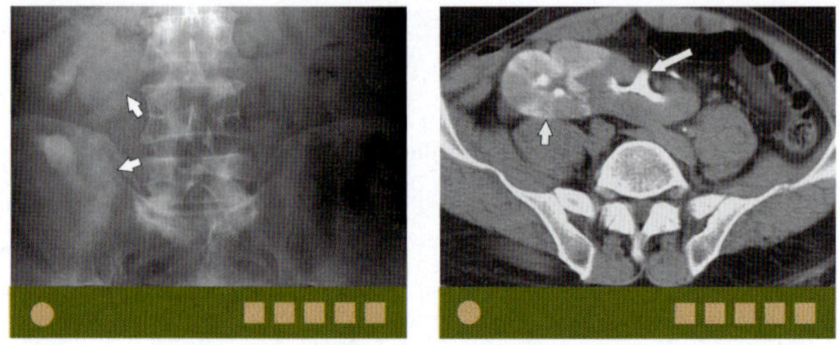

A. IVU film obtained 15 minutes after contrast shows delayed nephrogram and excretion from the ureter of the more lateral moiety (arrows). Crossed fused ectopia and ureteroinguinal hernia diagnosed after ureter was ligated during hernia repair.
B. Axial CT (with residual contrast from the IVU performed shortly before CT) better shows the presence of fused kidneys. Note the striated appearance of the more lateral moiety (short white arrow). The medial portion showed normal excretion into the ureter (long white arrow).

COMMENTS

Ureter herniations are rare with less than 200 reported cases. Reported sites of ureteral herniation include the scrotum (inguinal), groin (inguinal or femoral), buttock (sciatic), and chest (foramen of Bochdalek). Ureteroinguinal hernia is the most common form of ureteral herniation. The ureter is pulled into the inguinal canal and scrotum. These hernias most commonly present as groin masses usually in the fourth or fifth decade of life. Urinary and obstructive bowel symptoms are common. As in this patient, they are associated with crossed fused ectopia although crossed fused ectopia is not always seen. CT and other imaging studies show the ureter extending into the inguinal canal because of ureteroinguinal hernia. An IVU of ureteral hernias may show the characteristic "loop the loop" or "curlicue ureter." This finding represents the superimposition of the afferent and efferent ureter limbs as they cross the hernia sac and is best seen with the patient supine.

Crossed fused ectopia is a rare abnormality of the urinary tract. The ectopic kidney crosses over the midline and joins the other kidney (usually caudal to it) while retaining the normal ureteral insertion into the bladder. Crossed renal ectopia can be divided into four subtypes: crossed ectopia with fusion (90%), crossed ectopia without fusion, solitary crossed renal ectopia, and bilaterally crossed ectopia. This patient had crossed ectopia with fusion. Imaging examinations will show empty renal fossa on one side and fusion of the kidneys on the other side.

This case shows accidental ureteral ligation during an inguinal hernia repair with unsuspected ureteroinguinal hernia and associated crossed fused renal ectopia. The ureteral hernia and crossed fused ectopia were not diagnosed prior to hernia repair and CT was useful in identifying the significant findings and the need for immediate repair. With the increasing use of CT, radiologists need to be aware of the appearance of ureteroinguinal hernia and its association with crossed fused ectopia.

PEARLS

- **Imaging findings of crossed fused renal ectopia include fused kidneys with two collecting systems.**
- **Ureteroinguinal hernias are rare but most common type of ureter hernia.**
- **Ureteroinguinal hernias are important to identify to avoid iatrogenic injury to the ureter.**

ADDITIONAL IMAGES (C-G)

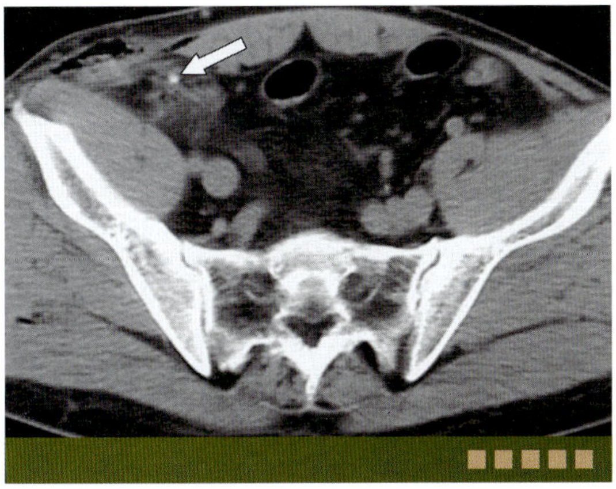

C. More distal CT in same patient shows the right ureter has opacified to the level of the groin where the surgery was performed (arrow).

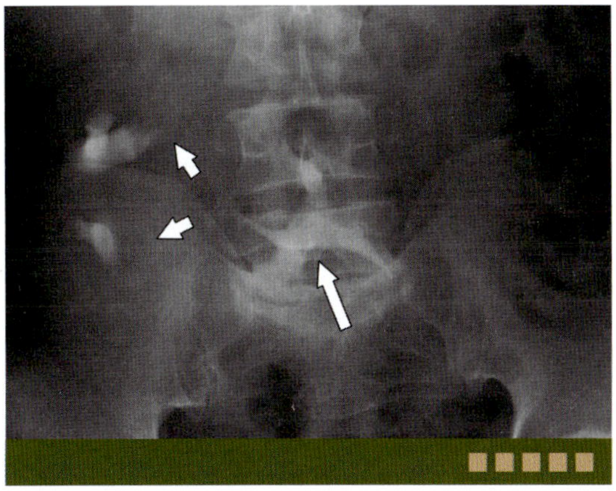

D. Follow-up IVU 2 months after surgery shows normal function of both renal moieties (lateral=short arrows, medial=long arrow).

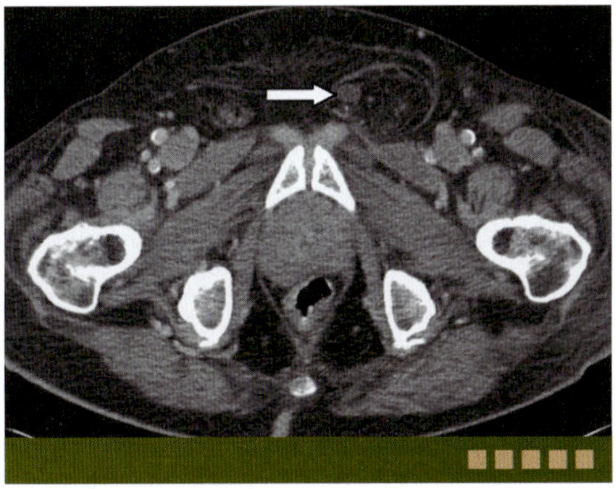

E. Ureteroinguinal hernia: Axial CECT shows left inguinal hernia containing tubular structure that is the ureter (arrow) in hernia.

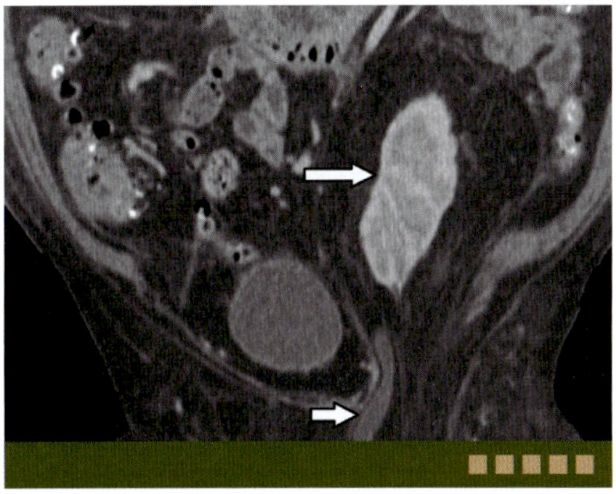

F. Coronal reformatted CECT shows the left ureteroinguinal hernia (short arrow) with ptotic left kidney (long arrow). The patient has hemorrhagic pancreatitis.

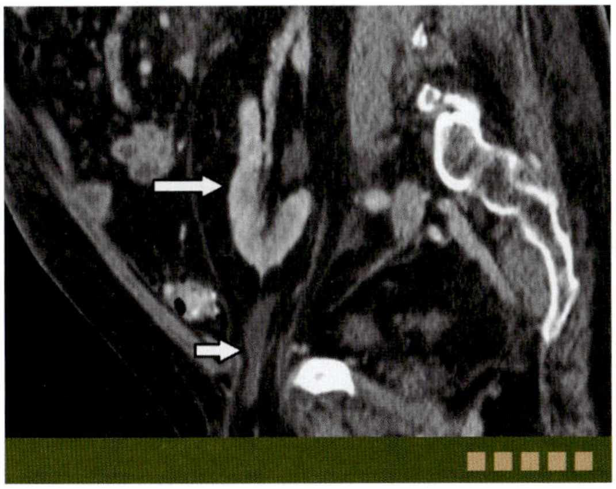

G. Sagittal reformatted CECT shows ptotic kidney (long arrow) and left ureteroinguinal hernia (short arrow).

IMAGE KEY

Common

Rare

Typical

Unusual

11–8 Renal Cell Carcinoma in Patient with Horseshoe Kidney

Frank H. Miller

PRESENTATION

Asymptomatic; hematuria.

FINDINGS

MR shows horseshoe kidney with enhancing renal cell carcinoma.

DIFFERENTIAL DIAGNOSIS

None

COMMENTS

Horseshoe kidney is the most common renal fusion anomaly seen in approximately 1 in 400 people. There is fusion of two distinct kidneys each with its own ureter and renal pelvis. Unlike crossed fused ectopia, horseshoe kidney refers to a situation when each kidney lies on one side of the spine. Most commonly in more than 90% of the cases, the lower poles of the kidney are fused with a fibrous or renal parenchymal band across the midline. The kidneys are malrotated with the renal pelvis directed more anteriorly. The lower poles are directed medially. The inferior mesenteric artery hinders renal ascent in development with the isthmus of the kidney trapped under it. The horseshoe kidney lies more caudal than normal.

Reported complications include increased likelihood of traumatic injury and urinary stasis leading to hydronephrosis, reflux, stones, and infection. Ureteropelvic junction (UPJ) obstruction is a common complication. There is an increased risk of injury of the isthmus based on its position anterior to the spine. Many with horseshoe kidney are asymptomatic with the findings detected incidentally on imaging studies.

The diagnosis of horseshoe kidney can be made using excretory urography, ultrasound, CT, or MR. Excretory urography often has difficulty in identifying the isthmus and distinguishing fibrous from parenchymal isthmus. The diagnosis by ultrasound may be difficult and requires a high index of suspicion based on the abnormal appearance of the kidney. The renal arteries are often multiple and ectopic. The ureters extend anteriorly.

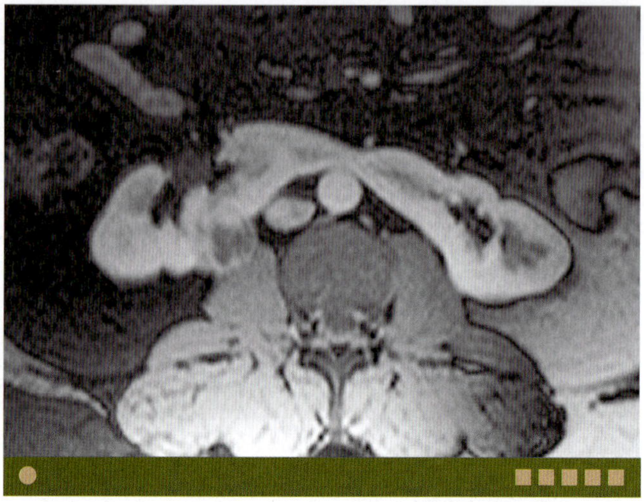

A. Axial contrast-enhanced T1-WI shows fused kidneys with parenchymal isthmus at the lower poles. Note enhancing renal mass from renal cell carcinoma.

The isthmus can be supplied by the renal artery or arise directly from the aorta above or below the isthmus. The blood supply can less commonly arise from the common iliac, external iliac, or inferior mesenteric arteries.

PEARLS

- **Horseshoe kidney is the most common renal anomaly seen in approximately 1 in 400 births.**
- **Kidneys are connected by isthmus that may be parenchymal or fibrous.**
- **Many patients are asymptomatic with increased likelihood of obstruction, infection, stones, and injury by blunt trauma.**
- **Diagnosis of horseshoe kidney is best made by CT or MR.**

ADDITIONAL IMAGES (B-G)

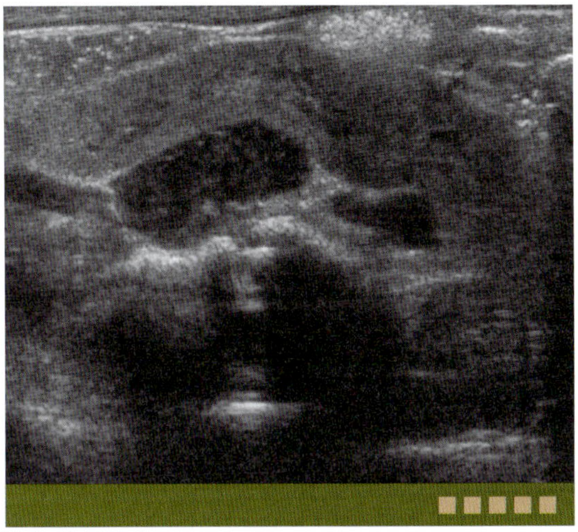

B. Longitudinal sonogram shows horseshoe kidney in a newborn boy. Band consists of parenchymal tissue seen anterior to the aorta and inferior vena cava.

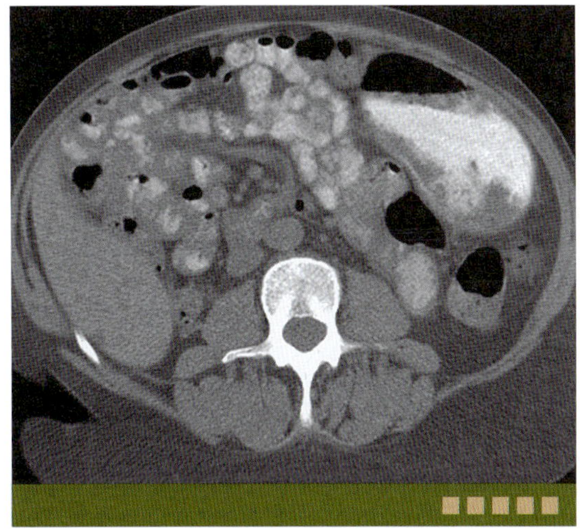

C. Axial NECT shows kidneys not seen in their normal position.

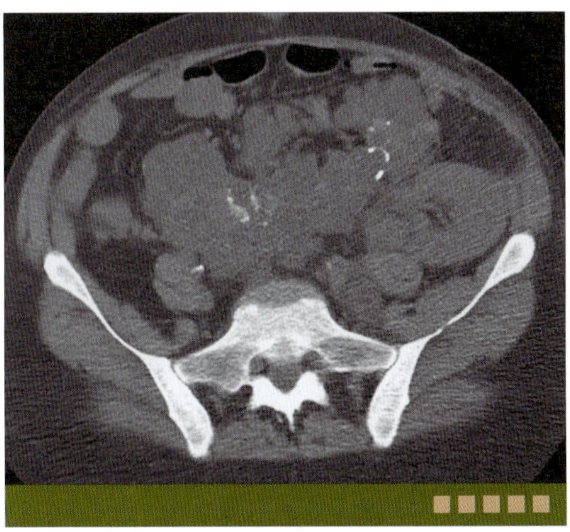

D. Axial NECT in the same patient as Figure C shows polycystic kidney disease involving horseshoe kidney with left renal transplant.

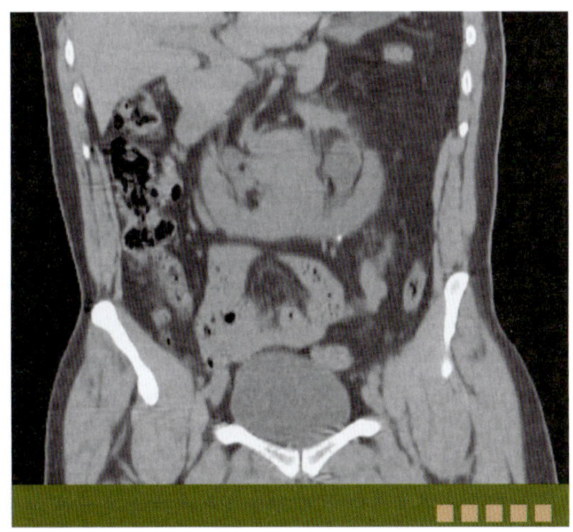

E. Coronal NECT shows horseshoe kidney with left ureteral stone.

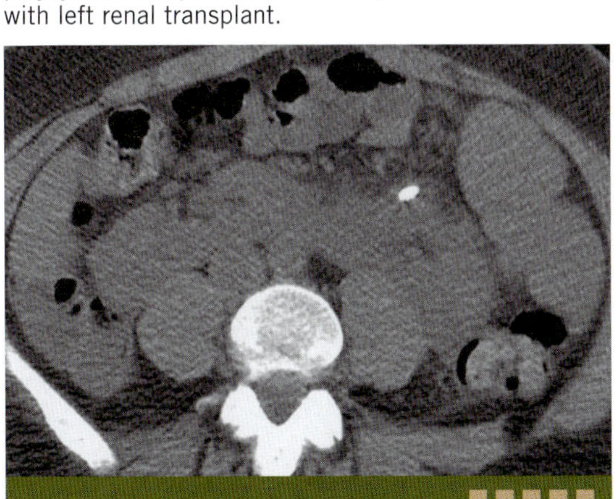

F. Axial NECT shows left ureteral stone.

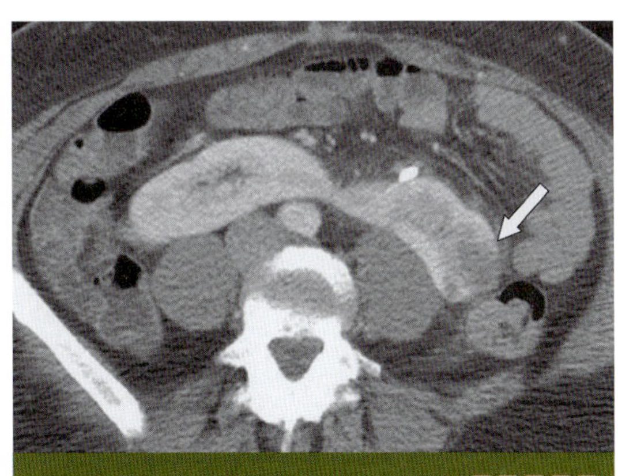

G. Axial CECT in the same patient as Figure E shows left renal lesion from acute pyelonephritis (arrow).

Figures C and D are the same patient.
Figures F and G are the same patient, but different from Figure E.

IMAGE KEY

Common

Rare

Typical

Unusual

11–9 Nephroptosis

David D. Casalino

PRESENTATION

Asymptomatic; IVU performed to map ureters prior to gynecologic surgery.

FINDINGS

IVU, erect film, shows a lower position of right kidney compared to the left kidney and angulation of the proximal right ureter.

DIFFERENTIAL DIAGNOSES

- *Ectopic kidney*: Displacement of the kidney is permanent, not positional; ureter is short and arterial blood supply is usually ectopic as well.
- *Displacement of kidney*: Most often resulting from hepatomegaly and not positional.

COMMENTS

Nephroptosis refers to greater than normal excursion of a kidney with change in the patient position. An excursion of up to two vertebral bodies is considered to be within the range of normal. The ureter is normal length in nephroptosis. Ptosis commonly produces kinks or angulations of the ureter; however, ptosis, even when severe, rarely produces symptoms. On rare occasions, it may be associated with obstruction. Dietl crisis refers to painful nephroptosis caused by position-dependent renal arterial compromise or acute intermittent hydronephrosis.

On IVU, an erect film provides the best view for demonstrating renal ptosis. Ptotic kidneys have normal length ureters, and their arteries usually arise from normal sites.

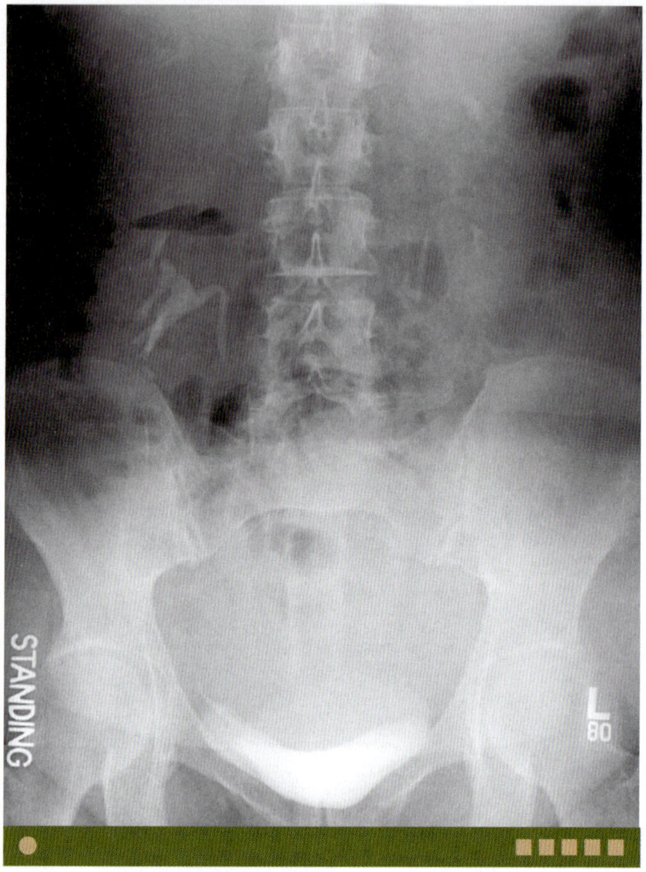

A. IVU, erect film, shows the right kidney to be rotated and in a lower position than the left kidney. The superior aspect of the right kidney is at the L2-3 level, and there is angulation of its ureter proximally.

PEARLS

- **Nephroptosis is renal excursion of greater than two vertebral bodies.**
- **Nephroptosis is usually asymptomatic.**
- **An erect image from an IVU is best for the diagnosis of renal ptosis.**
- **Ureteral length and renal artery origin are typically normal.**

ADDITIONAL IMAGE

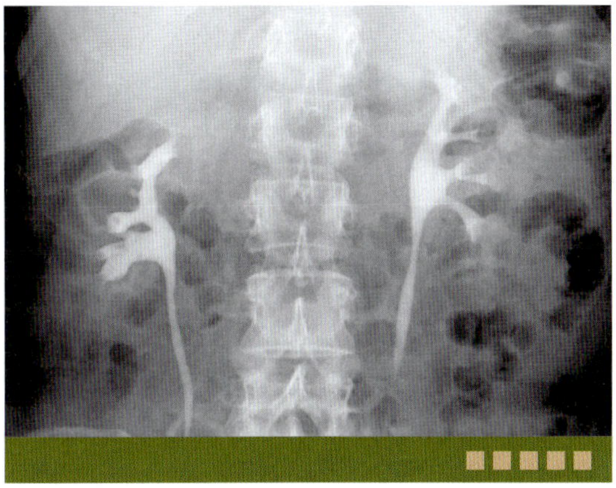

B. IVU, supine film in the same patient, shows the right kidney to have its superior aspect at the T12-L1 level. The right ureter is normal in length and without proximal angulation.

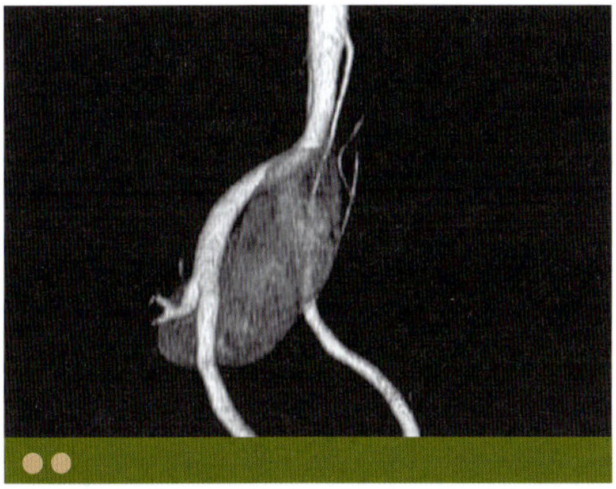

D. Ectopic kidney: Oblique 3-D computed tomography angiogram (CTA) shows the right renal artery to be ectopic, arising from the aorta just above the level of the bifurcation.

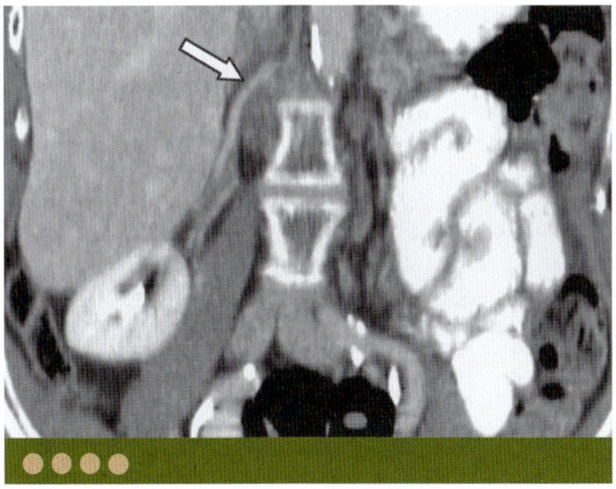

F. Displaced kidney: Coronal CECT, in the same patient, shows downward displacement of the right kidney by an enlarged liver. The right renal artery (arrow) is not ectopic.

DIFFERENTIAL DIAGNOSES IMAGES (C-F)

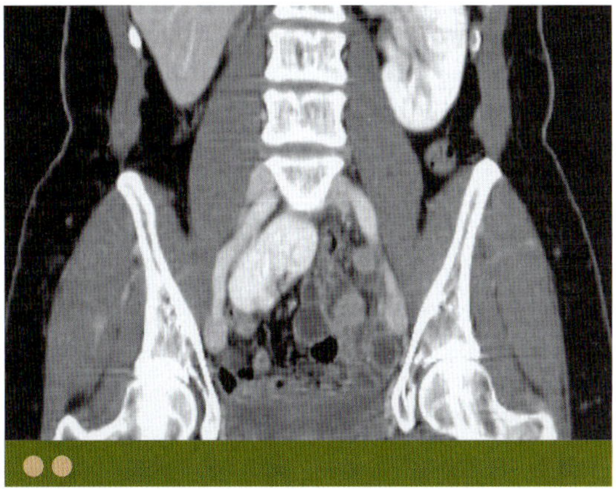

C. Ectopic kidney: Coronal CECT shows right kidney at level of common iliac vessels. The ureter was shown on other images to be short compared to the left ureter.

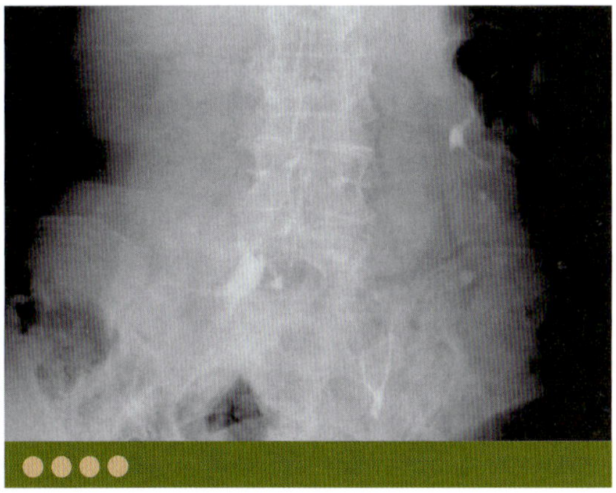

E. Displaced kidney: IVU, supine film, shows the rotated right kidney at the level of the upper sacrum. The right ureter is slightly redundant. The kidney position did not change on the erect film (not shown).

IMAGE KEY

Common

Rare

Typical

Unusual

11–10 Ureteropelvic Junction Obstruction

David D. Casalino

PRESENTATION

Hematuria and intermittent flank pain, particularly when drinking a few beers.

FINDINGS

CT image shows moderate dilatation of the left pelvocalyceal system. An artery and vein (arrow) are seen crossing the UPJ. The left ureter was normal in caliber (not shown).

DIFFERENTIAL DIAGNOSES

- *Mechanical obstruction of the proximal ureter*: Can be caused by stone, stricture, or tumor; stone or tumor may be apparent; usually symptomatic.
- *Peripelvic cysts*: Usually asymptomatic and bilateral; excretory phase imaging is most helpful in making the diagnosis.

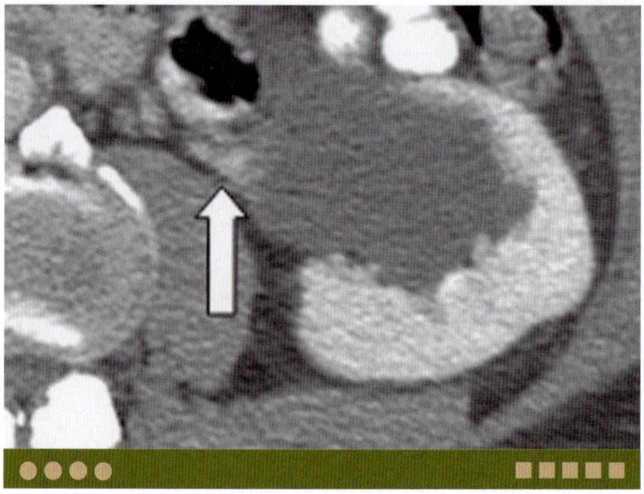

A. Axial CECT shows moderate dilatation of the left pelvocalyceal system. An artery and vein (arrow) are seen crossing the UPJ. The left ureter was normal in caliber (not shown).

COMMENTS

Congenital obstruction of the urinary tract occurs most commonly at the UPJ. The etiology of UPJ obstruction is uncertain, but it is a functional obstruction involving the proximal ureter. The age at which a patient is diagnosed depends in part on the severity of the obstruction. It may be diagnosed *in utero* during obstetrical ultrasonography. UPJ obstruction may present as an abdominal mass in a neonate. It may be diagnosed in later adulthood or remain asymptomatic. Symptoms in adults may include hematuria, urinary tract infection, and pain that is intermittent and precipitated by high urine flow rates. Twenty percent of cases are bilateral. The left kidney in males is more commonly involved. Associated anomalies include contralateral renal agenesis or multicystic dysplastic kidney, vesicoureteral reflux, and ureteral duplication.

On imaging, the pelvocalyceal system is usually dilated with focal narrowing at the UPJ. If the functional obstruction is severe, there may be massive hydronephrosis with renal enlargement, delayed renal enhancement and excretion, and cortical thinning. The ipsilateral ureter is normal in caliber. In some cases, radionuclide diuresis renography or Whitaker test may be necessary to make the diagnosis.

Surgical pyeloplasty has been considered the treatment choice, yet endoscopic pyeloplasty may be effective for treating UPJ obstruction. Imaging with CT or MR angiography prior to endoscopic pyeloplasty is helpful in identifying vessels that may be crossing the site of obstruction.

PEARLS

- **UPJ obstruction is a congenital, functional obstruction involving the proximal ureter.**
- **UPJ obstruction may be diagnosed prenatally through late adulthood or remain asymptomatic, depending upon the severity of the obstruction.**
- **The pelvocalyceal system is usually dilated with focal narrowing at the UPJ and a normal caliber ipsilateral ureter.**
- **Imaging may be helpful in identifying vessels crossing the UPJ obstruction prior to endoscopic pyeloplasty.**

ADDITIONAL IMAGES (B-D)

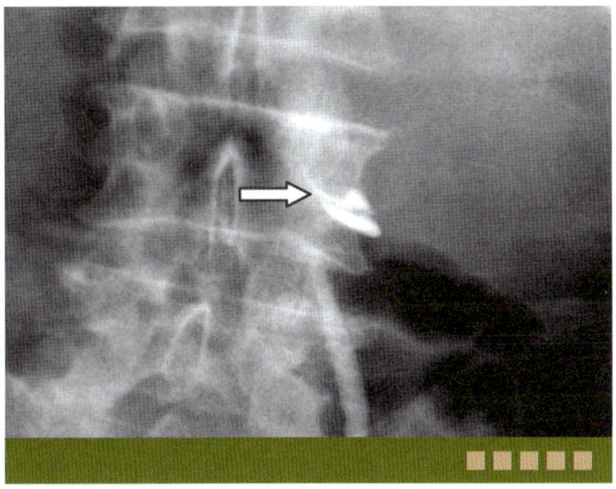

B. Retrograde urogram from the same patient shows focal narrowing and sharp angulation of the proximal left ureter (arrow).

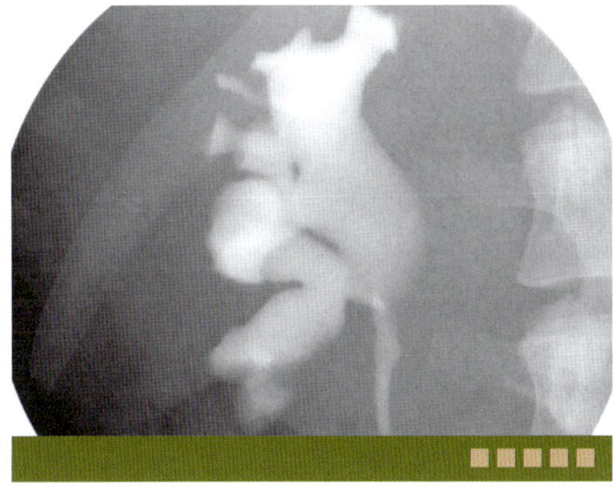

C. Retrograde urogram from a different patient shows focal narrowing of the proximal left ureter and moderate pelvocalyceal dilatation.

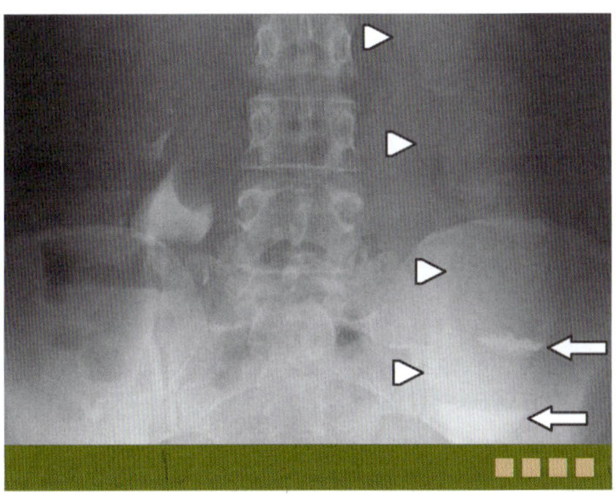

D. IVU upright image shows massive left pelvocalyceal system dilatation (arrowheads) with faint contrast opacification and numerous small layering stones (arrows).

DIFFERENTIAL DIAGNOSES IMAGES (E-G)

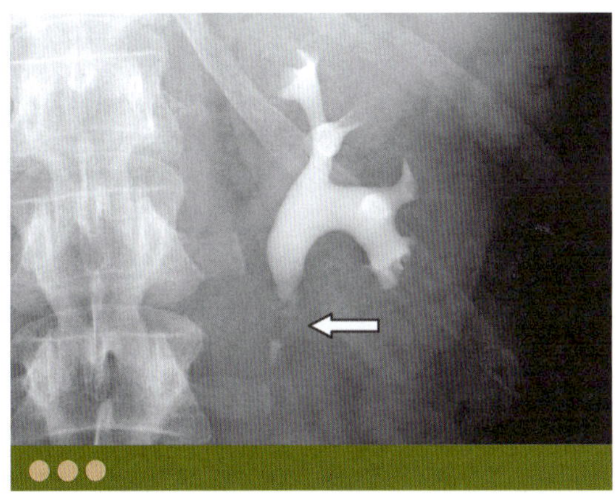

E. Transitional cell carcinoma: IVU shows mild to moderate pelvocalyceal system dilatation and an irregular, noncalcified filling defect (arrow) at the left UPJ. Goblet sign is seen involving the ureter at the inferior margin of the mass.

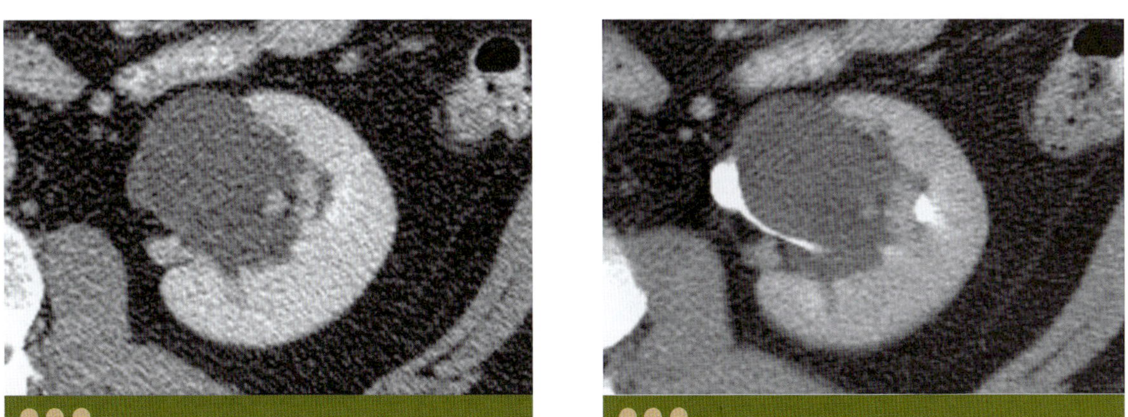

F. and G. Peripelvic cysts: Axial CECT, nephrographic phase, shows fluid attenuation filling the renal sinus. Axial CECT, excretory phase, shows contrast-filled collecting system being stretched and attenuated by the peripelvic cysts.

IMAGE KEY

Common

Rare

Typical

Unusual

11–11 Duplication of the Collecting System

David D. Casalino

PRESENTATION

Intermittent right flank pain, hematuria.

FINDINGS

CT shows two dense, round structures in the right retroperitoneum on excretory phase imaging.

DIFFERENTIAL DIAGNOSES

- *Blind-ending ureteral duplication*: Only one limb extends to the renal collecting system.
- *Calcification adjacent to contrast-filled ureter*: Calcification most often within a lymph node, vein, or artery; will not be in continuity with the ipsilateral collecting system.

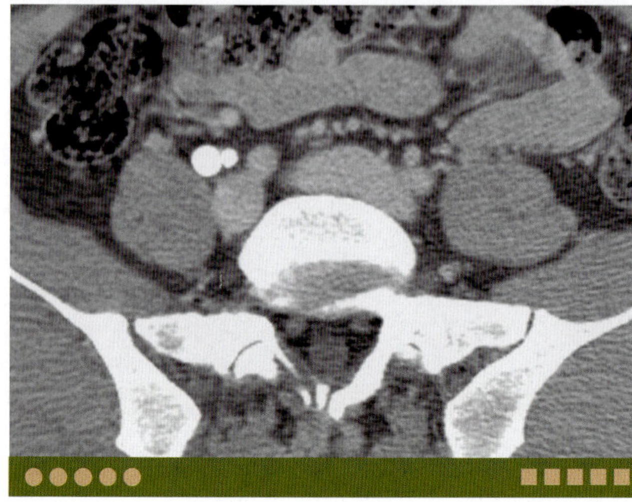

A. Axial CECT during excretory phase shows two dense, round structures in the right retroperitoneum.

COMMENTS

Duplication anomalies are the most common of the urinary tract and occur in 4% of the population. There is a spectrum of duplication anomalies that include bifid renal pelvis, incomplete, or partial, duplication, and complete duplication.

A bifid renal pelvis or incomplete duplication is usually an incidental finding on imaging; although a partial duplication with "yo-yo" reflux, that is peristalsis down one ureteral limb driving urine up the other relaxed limb, may be associated with flank pain and urinary tract infection.

Patients with a complete duplication more often have imaging finds reflecting clinically significant abnormality. In complete duplication, the lower moiety ureter typically inserts into the trigone and may be associated with vesicoureteral reflux. This reflux may result in extensive scarring of the renal lower pole. The upper moiety ureter is ectopic and usually inserts caudal and medial to the normal insertion site (Weigert-Meyer rule). This ectopic ureter may have an ureterocele and/or extravesical insertion. An ectopic ureterocele is a focal dilatation of the distal ureter that is usually associated with obstruction of the ectopic ureter and may, if large enough, also obstruct the ipsilateral lower moiety ureter or bladder outlet resulting in bilateral hydronephrosis. Ectopic ureteroceles are more common in female patients. A "drooping lily" configuration on IVU is the result of obstruction of the ectopic ureter causing severe upper pole hydronephrosis and enlargement that compresses the lower pole. An extravesical insertion in females may be below the urogenital diaphragm and associated with urinary incontinence. An example is insertion into the vagina. Sites of ectopic insertion in males are always above the urogenital diaphragm.

PEARLS

- **Duplication anomalies occur in 4% of the population.**
- **In complete duplication, lower moiety ureter usually inserts into the trigone and may be associated with vesicoureteral reflux.**
- **Upper moiety ureter is ectopic, usually with more caudal and medial insertion site, and may have an ureterocele and/or extravesical insertion.**
- **Ectopic ureteroceles are more common in females with a female:male ratio of 4:1.**

ADDITIONAL IMAGES (B-E)

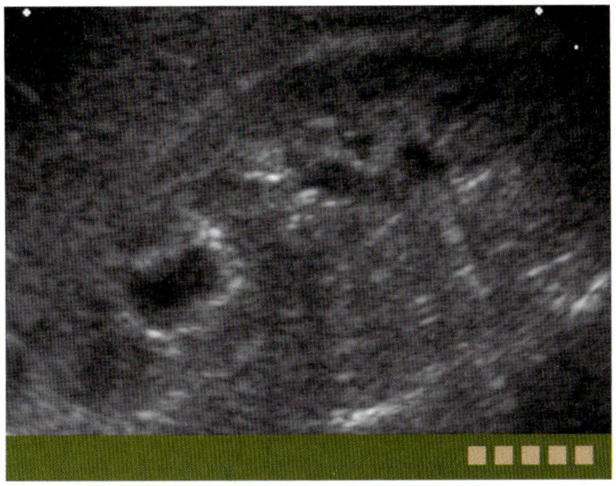

B. Longitudinal sonogram of the right kidney in the same patient shows a duplicated collecting system with dilated upper pole collecting system and a band of renal parenchyma crossing the central echo complex.

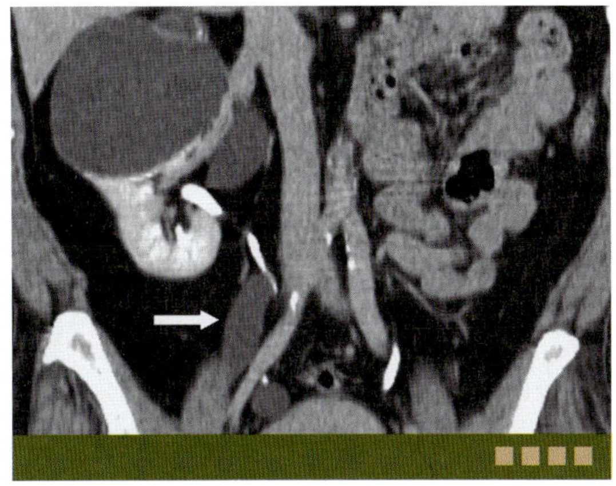

C. Coronal CECT during excretory phase shows complete duplication on the right with the lower moiety ureter contrast filled and the upper pole collecting system markedly dilated with absence of excretion and dilated ureter (arrow).

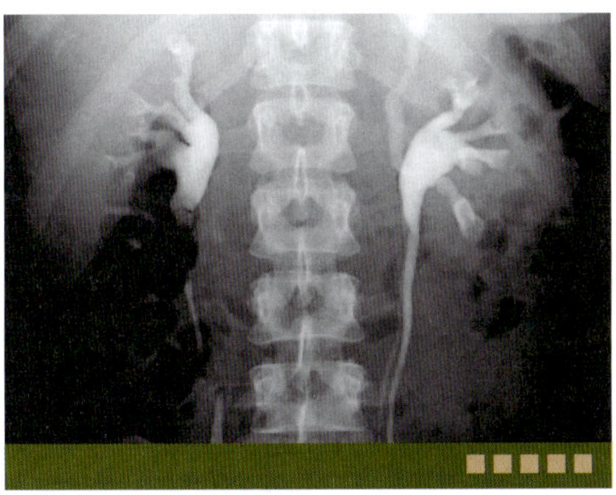

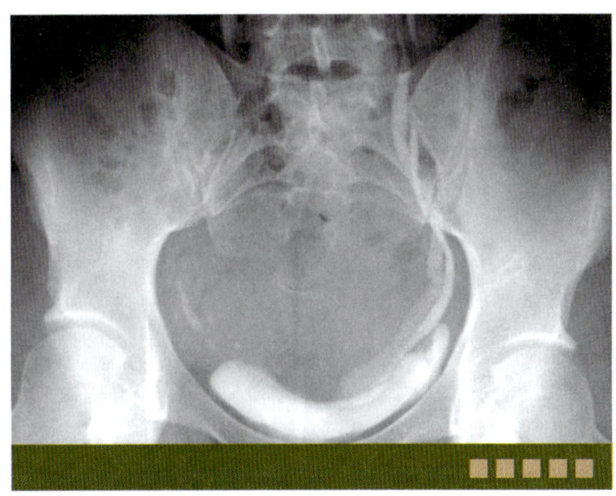

D. and E. IVU show complete duplication on the left with the upper moiety ureter having a more inferomedial insertion site and an ureterocele.

DIFFERENTIAL DIAGNOSES IMAGES (F-G)

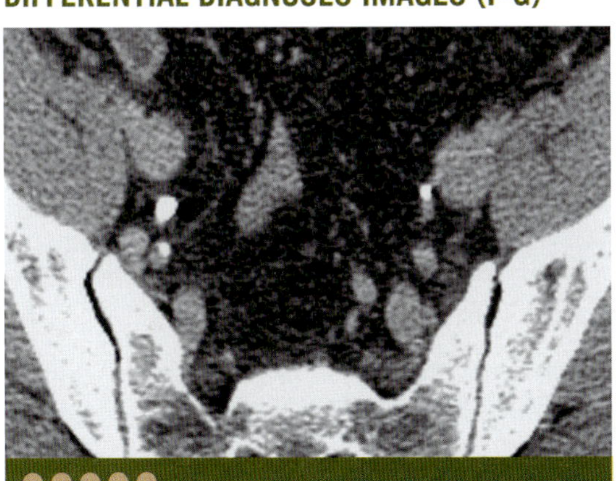

F. Atherosclerotic calcification: Axial CECT shows bilateral, contrast-filled ureters and a focal calcification associated with the right internal iliac artery.

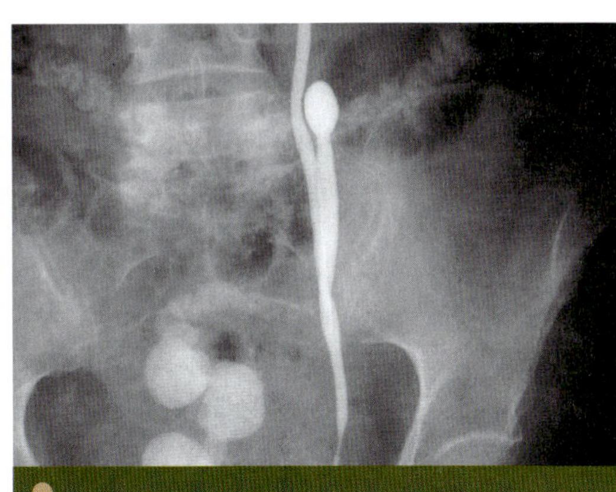

G. Blind-ending ureteral duplication: Retrograde urogram shows a blind-ending ureteral bud arising from the left ureter. The left renal collecting system was normal (not shown).

IMAGE KEY

Common

Rare

Typical

Unusual

11–12 Blind-Ending Ureteral Duplication

David D. Casalino

PRESENTATION

Hematuria.

FINDINGS

Retrograde urogram shows bifurcation of the distal left ureter with one branch extending to the renal pelvis and the other having a bulbous blind end.

DIFFERENTIAL DIAGNOSES

- *Ureteral leak*: Usually in the setting of trauma or surgery; the collecting system above the site of injury may be dilated.
- *Partial duplication of collecting system*: Involves two proximal ureters in communication with a duplicated renal collecting system, unless one ureter is obstructed.

COMMENTS

Blind-ending ureteral duplication is an unusual ureteral duplication anomaly. This anomaly is also referred to as blind-ending ureteral bud or blind-ending branch of a bifid ureter. It likely develops from a duplicated ureteric bud when one of the limbs fails to induce the metanephrogenic blastema or fails to become associated with it.

This anomaly may be first detected at any age and is twice as common in females. Patients are usually asymptomatic; although symptoms, such as dysuria, pain, or hematuria, may result if there is associated urinary stasis or reflux with infection or stone formation. Transitional cell carcinoma in a blind-ending bud has been reported. There is a reported association with abnormalities of the contralateral upper tract, in particular partial and complete duplication.

On imaging, the blind-ending ureter almost invariably connects to an otherwise normal ureter and has its blind end directed cranially. A blind-ending ureter can arise from any part of the ureter. Rarely, two blind-ending ureters can arise from a single ureter. The blind-ending branch may be cylindrical or saccular. A long ureteral bud may extend cranially to the base of the renal pelvis or higher. An IVU usually demonstrates the blind-ending ureteral bud via ureteroureteral reflux. Retrograde urography may be helpful in equivocal cases or to evaluate possible intraureteral abnormality. CT axial images may be confusing with demonstration of a single ureter more proximally and two ureters more distally. Coronal reformatted images may simplify making the diagnosis.

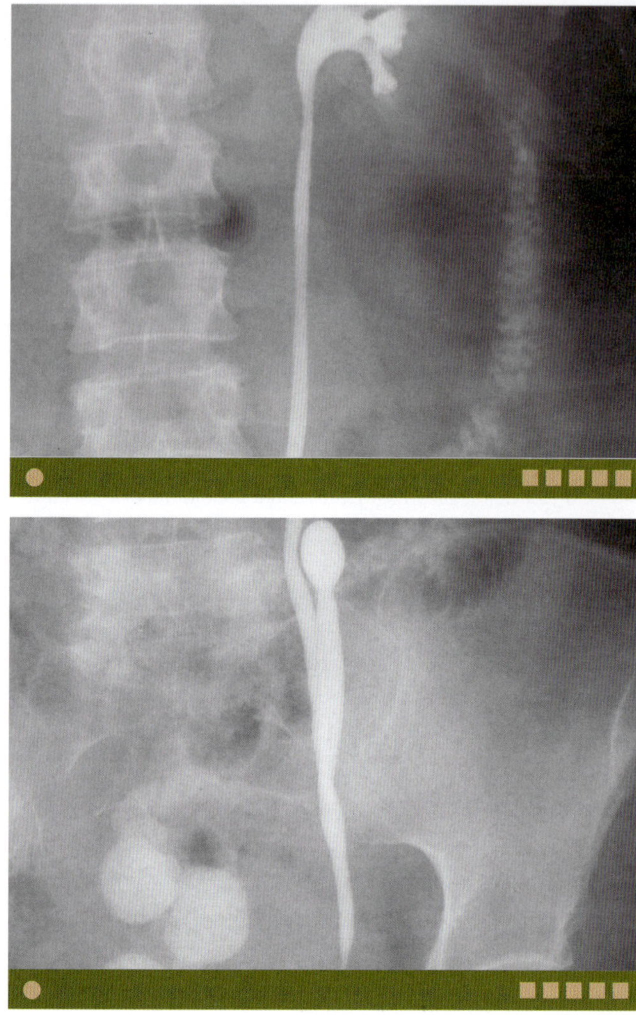

A. and B. Retrograde urogram shows a blind-ending ureteral bud arising from the left ureter. The left renal collecting system appears normal.

PEARLS

- **Blind-ending ureteral duplication is usually an incidental finding but may be complicated by infection, stone formation, or neoplasm.**
- **A blind-ending ureter may not be well visualized on IVU if there is little or no ureteroureteral reflux.**
- **Retrograde urography is the study of choice for diagnosis and evaluation of intraureteral abnormalities.**

ADDITIONAL IMAGES (C-D)

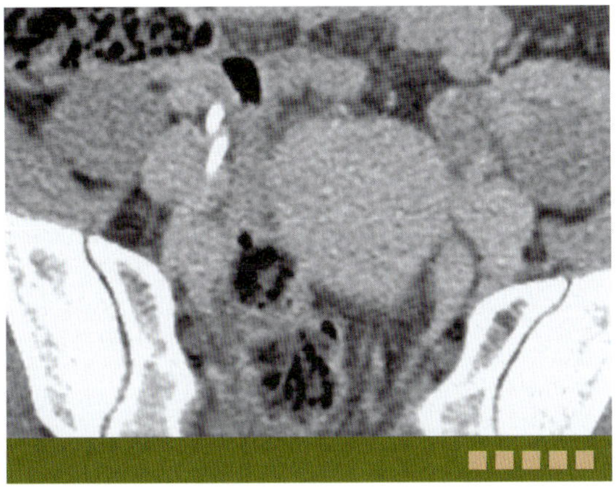

C. Axial CECT, excretory phase, from a different patient shows two contrast-filled ureters on the right.

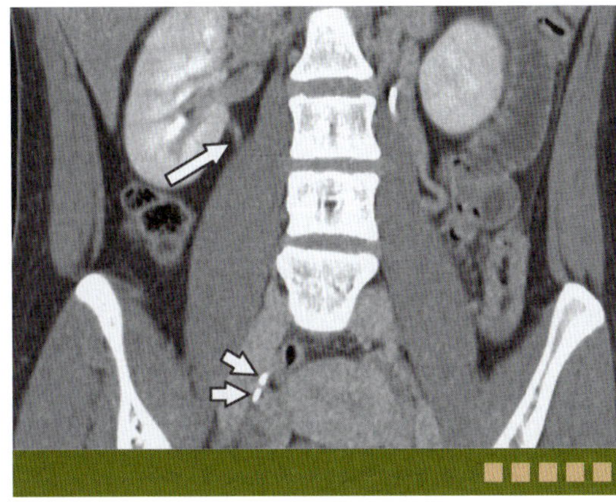

D. Coronal CECT, from the same patient in the prior figure, shows a single proximal ureter (long arrow) and two more distal ureters (short arrows), one normal and one blind-ending.

DIFFERENTIAL DIAGNOSES IMAGES (E-G)

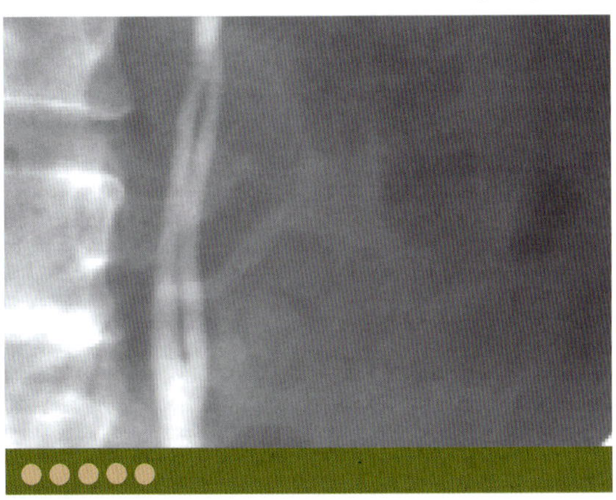

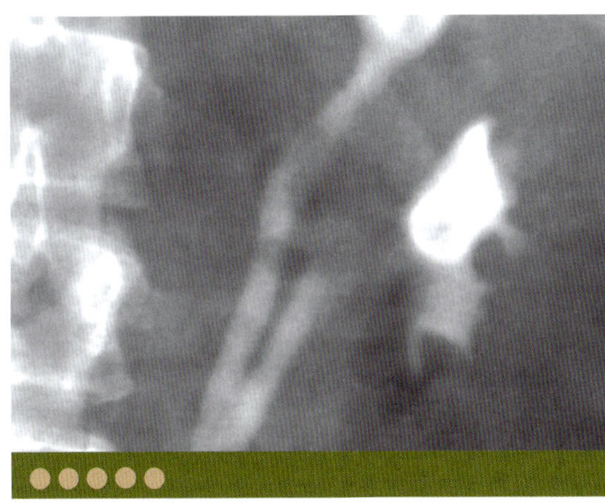

E. and **F. Partial duplication:** Retrograde urogram shows branching of a single ureter distally into two ureters, which extend cranially and communicate with the duplicated renal collecting system.

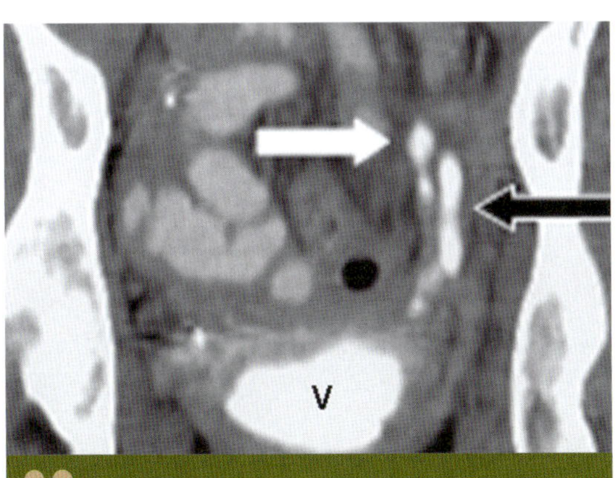

G. Ureteral leak: Coronal CECT, excretory phase, shows a linear contrast leak (black arrow) extending cranially from the site of injury to the left ureter (white arrow). There is also an uretero-vaginal fistula, accounting for the vagina (V) being contrast-filled.

IMAGE KEY

Common

Rare

Typical

Unusual

11-13 Retrocaval, or Circumcaval, Ureter

David D. Casalino

PRESENTATION

Currently asymptomatic with a history of kidney stones and occasional right flank pain.

FINDINGS

IVU shows medial deviation of the proximal right ureter at the L3 level. The ureter then gradually extends laterally to a more normal position.

DIFFERENTIAL DIAGNOSES

- *Retroperitoneal fibrosis*: Usually involves both ureters, but may be unilateral; usually at the L3 to L5 level; often hydronephrosis and ureteral narrowing.
- *Renal tumor or lateral retroperitoneal mass*: Mass may be palpable.
- *Postoperative*: Example, retroperitoneal lymph node dissection; maybe bilateral; surgical history and surgical sutures and/or clips usually present.

COMMENTS

A retrocaval ureter is a developmental anomaly of the inferior vena cava (IVC) that is caused by the persistence of the posterior cardinal vein. Two types of retrocaval ureter have been described. Type I (low loop) is much more common and involves the right ureter coursing inferomedially behind the IVC and then crossing laterally over the anterior aspect of the IVC. The right ureter typically has a reversed J appearance, and the medial-most portion is medial to the adjacent vertebral pedicle. When obstruction is present, it usually occurs proximally, 1 to 2 cm past the lateral IVC margin. Type II (high loop) involves the ureter coursing behind the IVC at or just above the level of the UPJ. This second variety may mimic a UPJ obstruction.

Most cases of a retrocaval ureter are asymptomatic, but patients may present with back or flank pain that is related to ureteral obstruction or hydronephrosis. A retrocaval ureter is more common in males with a male to female ratio of 3:1. Most symptomatic patients present in the third or fourth decade of life. Obstruction may be complicated by infection or stone formation.

The appearance on IVU is usually diagnostic but can be confirmed by CT. The anomaly almost always involves the right ureter except in patients with a left IVC or situs inversus. If there is obstruction because of the retrocaval course of the ureter, surgery can be performed and involves resection of the narrowed portion of ureter and reanastomosis anterior to the IVC.

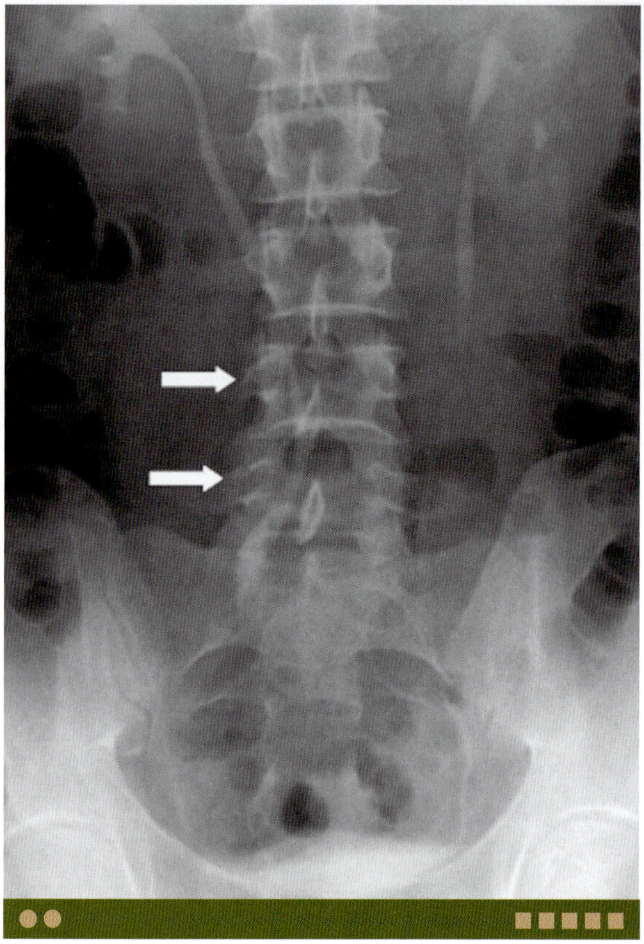

A. IVU shows medial deviation of the proximal right ureter such that its medial-most portion is medial to the adjacent vertebral pedicles (arrows). The ureter, then, gradually extends laterally to a more normal position. The course of the left ureter is normal.

PEARLS

- **The appearance of a retrocaval ureter on IVU is usually diagnostic.**
- **The right ureter is involved in a vast majority of cases.**
- **Most cases are asymptomatic, but obstruction can occur and be associated with pain, infection, and stone formation.**

ADDITIONAL IMAGES (B-D)

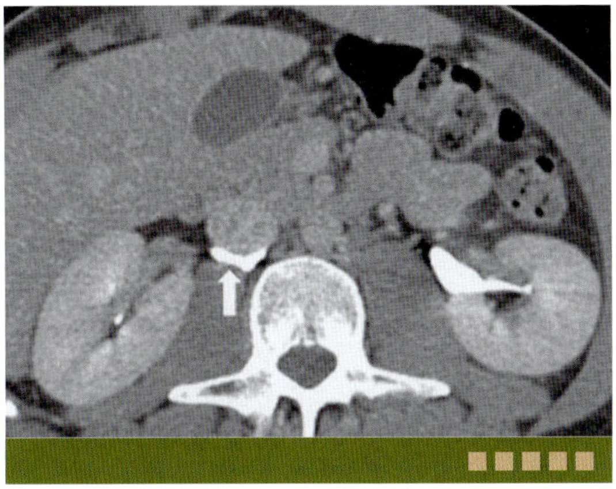

B. Axial CECT from a different patient shows the proximal portion of the right ureter (arrow) coursing behind the IVC.

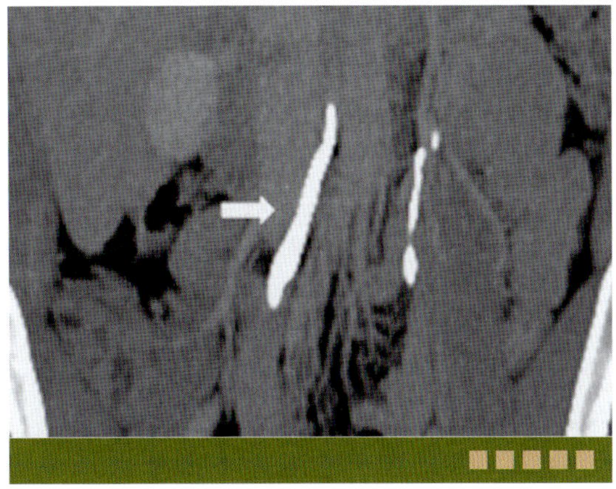

C. Coronal CECT shows the more distal portion of the right ureter (arrow) coursing laterally over the anterior aspect of the IVC.

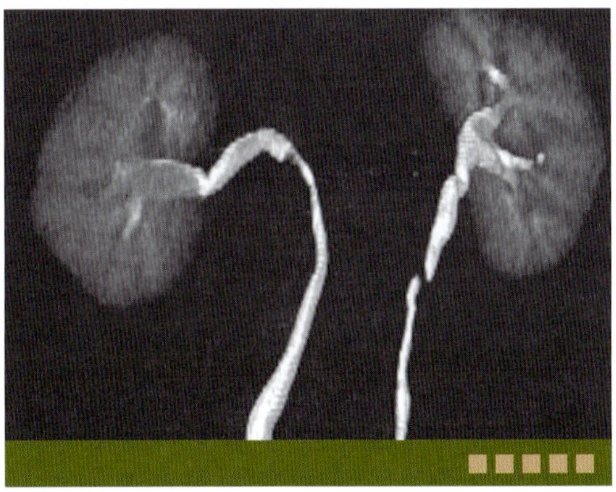

D. Coronal CECT with 3-D post processing shows the course of the retrocaval right ureter with abrupt medial deviation of the proximal segment creating a reversed J, or fishhook, appearance.

DIFFERENTIAL DIAGNOSES IMAGES (E-G)

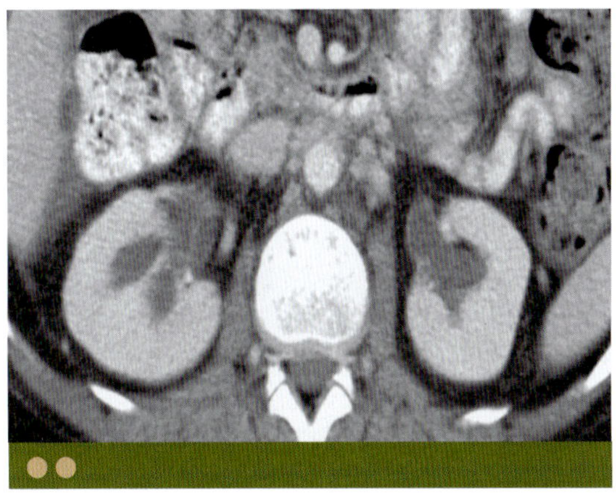

E. Retroperitoneal fibrosis: Axial CECT shows bilateral hydronephrosis and abnormal retroperitoneal soft tissue confirmed to be fibrosis in patient status post radiation therapy for lumbar spine metastases.

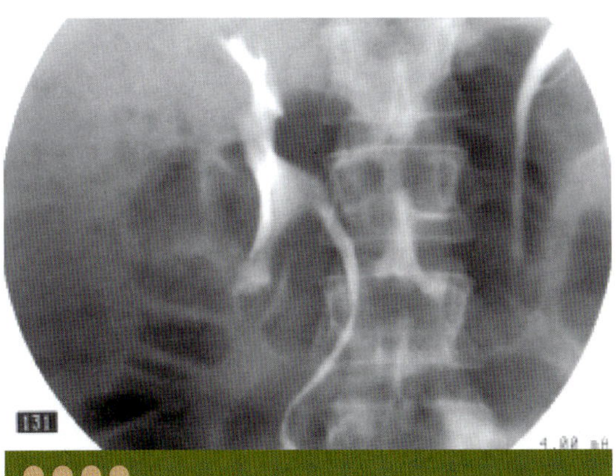

F. Renal tumor: Retrograde urogram shows medial deviation of the proximal right ureter and renal collecting system, which is also splayed.

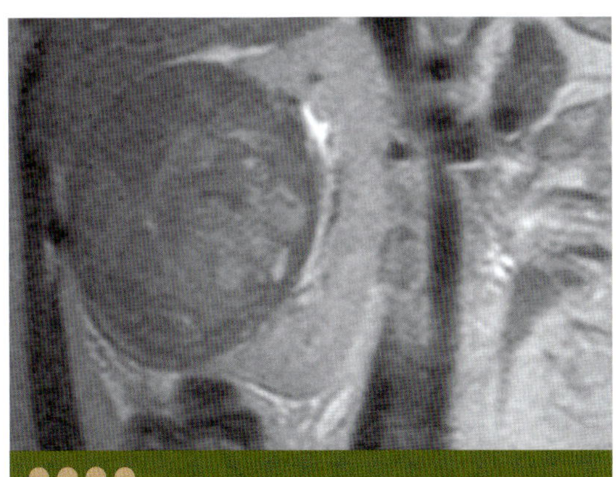

G. Renal tumor: Coronal T2-WI from the same patient shows a large hypointense mass arising from the lateral cortex of the right kidney. The mass effect accounts for the retrograde urogram findings.

IMAGE KEY

Common

Rare

Typical

Unusual

11–14 Primary Megaureter

David D. Casalino

PRESENTATION

Pain, hematuria, and clinical features of urinary tract infection.

FINDINGS

IVU shows marked dilatation of the lower third of the left ureter with a short segment of distal tapering and less extensive dilatation of the more proximal collecting system.

DIFFERENTIAL DIAGNOSES

- *Distal obstruction*: Etiology, such as stone, tumor, or ectopic ureterocele, may be seen on imaging; usually symptomatic; usually diffuse ureteral dilatation and pelvicaliectasis.
- *Vesicoureteral reflux*: Distal tapering not a feature; usually diagnosed in infants and children and associated with urinary tract infection and cortical scarring; extent of dilatation varies and is graded with voiding cystourethrography (VCUG) or radionuclide cystography.
- *Increased urine volume (eg, diabetes insipidus or polydipsia)*: Usually bilateral; clinical information often helpful.

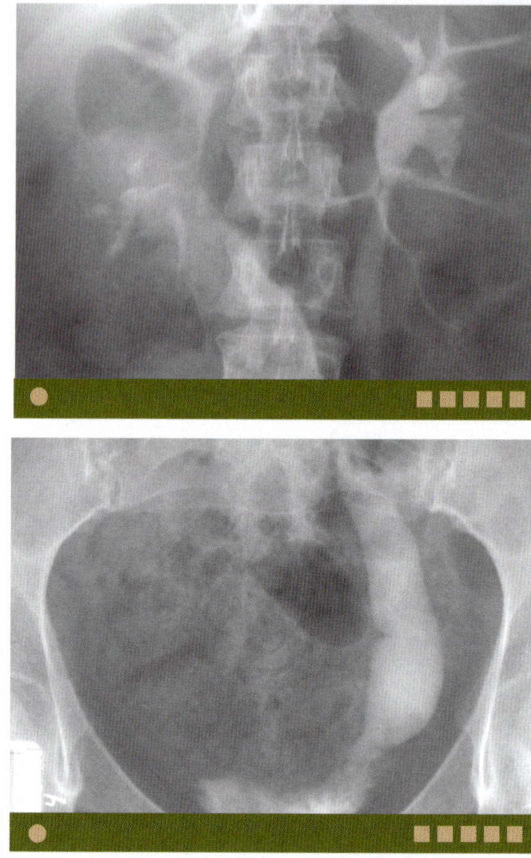

A. and B. IVU shows marked dilatation of the lower third of the left ureter with a short segment of distal tapering, mild to moderate dilatation of the more proximal ureter, and nondilated calyces.

COMMENTS

Primary megaureter is an idiopathic congenital abnormality that causes abnormal ureteral dilatation. It results from an abnormality of the musculature that causes a functional impairment of peristalsis in the distal ureter. Primary megaureter may present at any age and often incidentally, although severe cases are usually diagnosed in infancy and childhood. It is more common in male patients, unilateral in 75% of the cases, and more often involving the left ureter. When symptomatic, patients may present with pain, hematuria, abdominal mass, or signs and symptoms of urinary tract infection or stone formation.

Primary megaureter may be associated with other anomalies in up to 40% of the cases. These include ipsilateral ureteropelvic junction obstruction, contralateral or ipsilateral vesicoureteral reflux, contralateral agenesis, ipsilateral megacalicosis, and others. The coexistence of primary megaureter and megacalicosis may mimic a chronic mechanical obstruction. Megacalicosis results in an increased number of calyces that are squared or laminated in shape.

The severity of primary megaureter is variable and will affect the imaging findings. It is most commonly mild and inconsequential with fusiform dilatation, perhaps up to 3 cm in diameter, of the distal ureter proximal to a tapered distal segment that may be up to 4 cm in length. With greater severity, there is more extensive ureteral dilatation without significant dilatation of the calyces. In the rare, severe cases there may also be blunting of the calyces, an obstructive pattern in dynamic imaging studies, and impaired renal function. VCUG can be helpful in differentiating primary megaureter from vesicoureteral reflux.

PEARLS

- **Rare and attributed to a functional impairment of peristalsis in the distal ureter.**
- **Variable severity and resulting clinical signs and symptoms.**
- **Most often mild with asymptomatic dilatation of the distal ureter, proximal to a tapered segment.**

DIFFERENTIAL DIAGNOSES IMAGES (C-H)

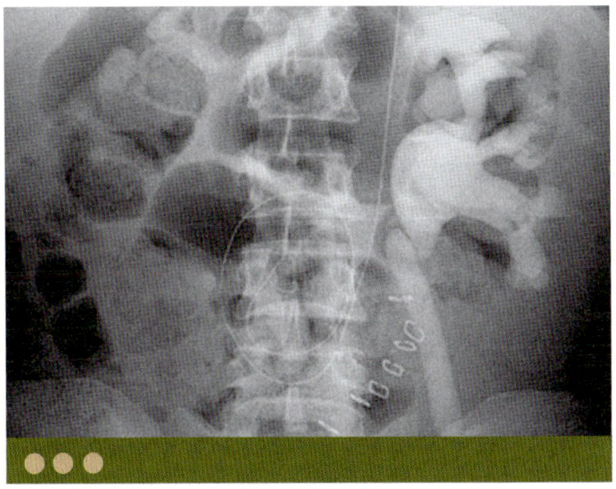

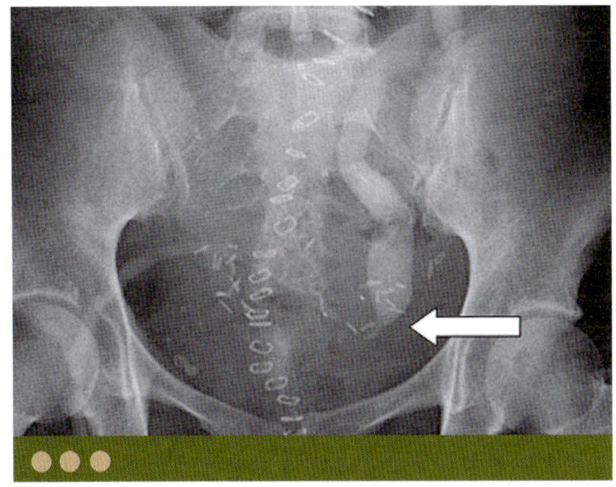

C. and **D. Distal ureteral obstruction (iatrogenic):** IVU shows marked dilatation of the left ureter and renal collecting system because of accidental clipping of the distal ureter (arrow) at the time of emergent cesarean section. The patient had increasing left flank pain.

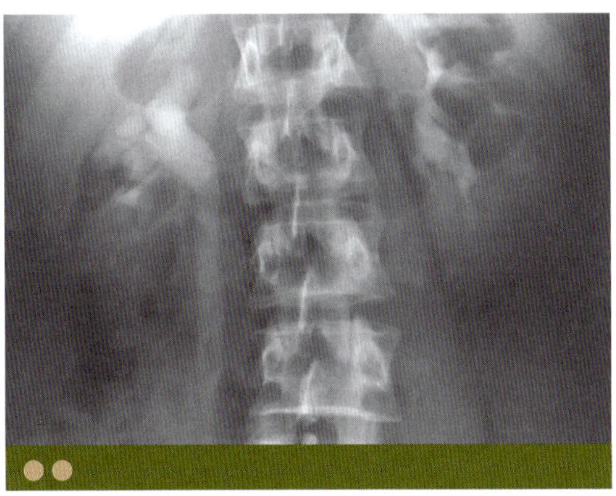

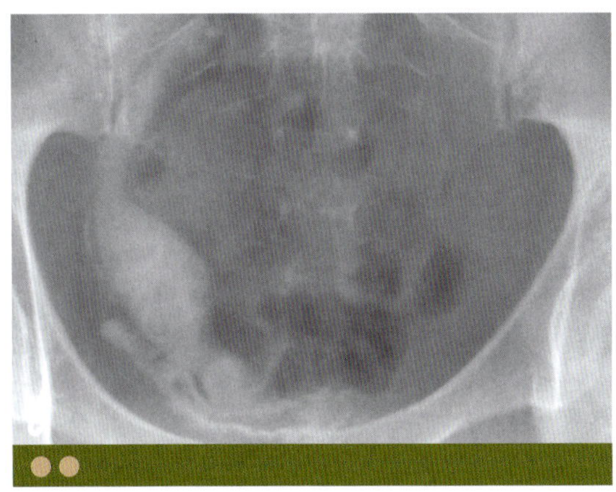

E. and **F. Distal ureteral obstruction (ectopic ureterocele):** IVU postvoid image shows persistent marked dilatation of the right kidney upper moiety and associated ureter of a duplicated collecting system. The obstruction is caused by an ectopic ureterocele.

IMAGE KEY

Common

Rare

Typical

Unusual

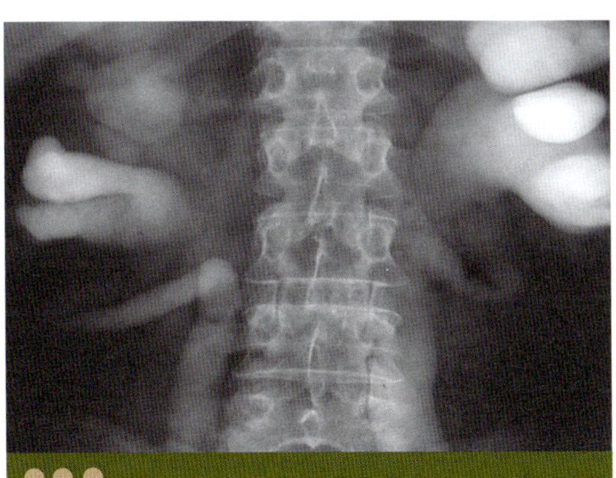

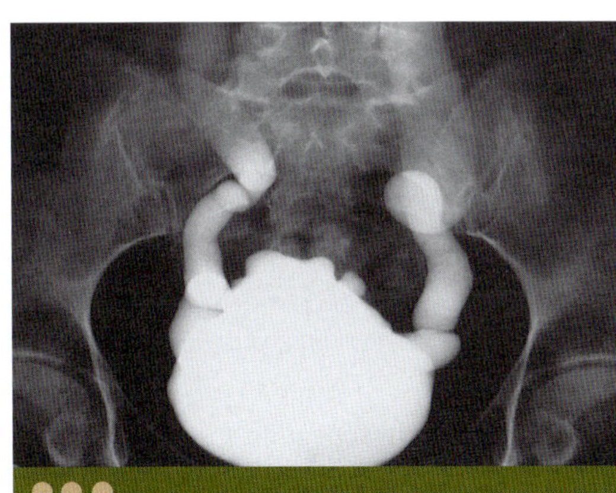

G. and **H. Vesicoureteral reflux:** Cystogram shows bilateral high-grade reflux with marked tortuosity and dilatation of the ureters and calyces.

11–15 Calyceal Diverticulum

David D. Casalino

PRESENTATION

Usually asymptomatic, but may present with pain, hematuria, or symptoms of infection.

FINDINGS

IVU tomogram shows a focal, oval collection of contrast superimposed over the medial cortex of the interpolar region of the right kidney.

DIFFERENTIAL DIAGNOSES

- *Focal caliectasis caused by infundibular narrowing*: More central; may visualize infundibular tumor or filling defect.
- *Papillary necrosis*: Smaller contrast cavities extending from the fornix or in the center of papilla; often flame shaped or clubbed calyx; usually multiple; history may be helpful.
- *Rupture of cyst or abscess into a calyx*: Usually does not communicate with fornix; history may be helpful.
- *Ruptured calyceal fornices in hydronephrosis*: More irregular than a diverticulum; typically symptomatic with pelvicaliectasis.

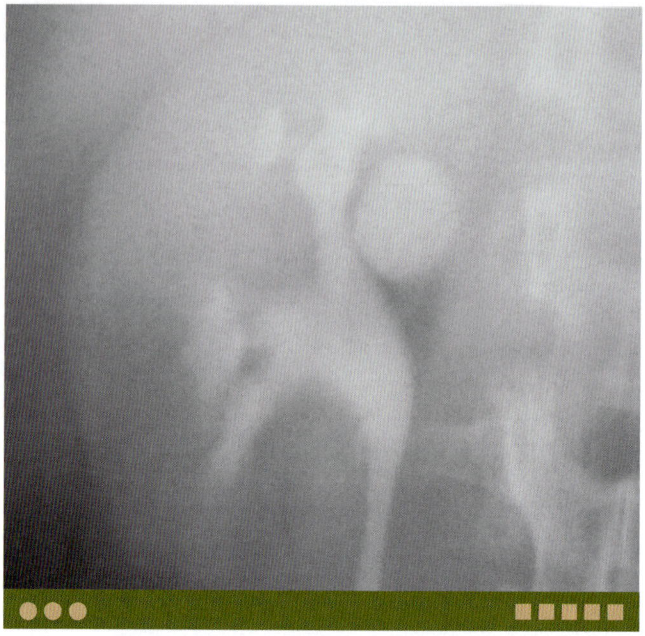

A. IVU tomogram shows a smooth-walled, contrast-filled diverticulum superimposed over the medial cortex of the interpolar region of the right kidney. The patient presented with recurrent hematuria.

COMMENTS

A calyceal diverticulum, or pyelocalyceal diverticulum, is an urothelium-lined cavity that extends from the pelvocalyceal system into the adjacent renal parenchyma. Calyceal diverticula are thought to be congenital. Three types of calyceal diverticulum have been described. Type I is most common and arises from a minor calyx. Type II arises from an infundibulum in communication with a major calyx. Type III is least common and arises from the renal pelvis.

Calyceal diverticula may be seen at any age and are found with equal frequency in both sexes. They are usually asymptomatic; but stone formation or infection may lead to presentation with hematuria, pain, or sign and symptoms of urinary tract infection. Ten to fifty percent of calyceal diverticula contain calculi. Transitional cell carcinoma can develop in a diverticulum.

On imaging, calyceal diverticula usually appear as solitary, round, smooth-walled outpouchings from the collecting system. On IVU and excretory-phase CT and MR, they will usually fill with contrast material. Diverticula vary in size from 0.5 to 5 cm and usually involves the upper pole of the kidney. A calyceal diverticulum may mimic a cortical cyst on ultrasonography or CT and MR imaging performed without contrast or prior to contrast excretion. A single stone or a cluster of small stones in the periphery of the kidney suggests a calyceal diverticulum. Layering milk of calcium may be seen in a diverticulum.

No treatment is needed for asymptomatic diverticula, yet surgical intervention may be necessary in patients with recurrent or persistent urinary tract infection, hematuria, or intractable pain.

PEARLS

- **Stone formation within a calyceal diverticulum is not uncommon and may result in pain and hematuria.**
- **The diverticulum may mimic a cortical cyst.**
- **The diverticulum will typically fill with excreted contrast.**
- **A filling defect within a diverticulum may be a stone, clot, or neoplasm and warrants further evaluation.**

ADDITIONAL IMAGES (B-D)

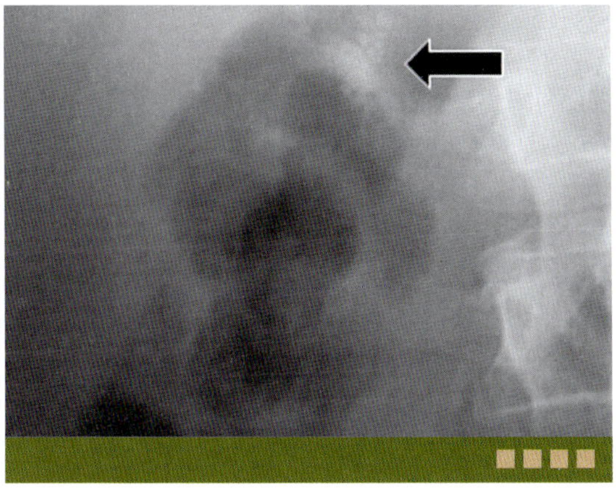

B. IVU scout radiograph from the same patient shows a cluster of small calculi (arrow) in the location of the diverticulum.

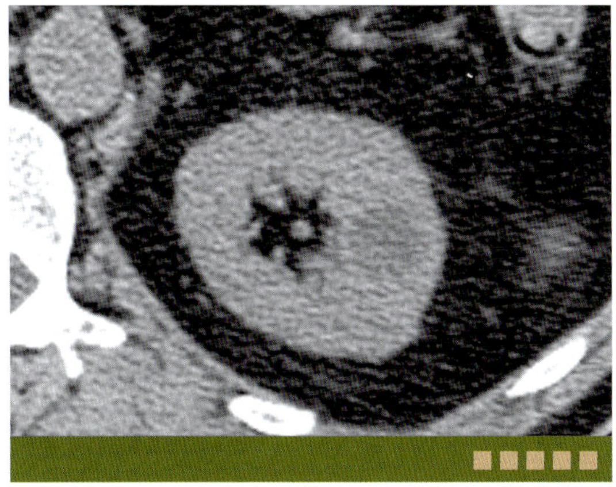

C. Axial NECT from a different patient shows a 1.5-cm cystic mass in the lateral cortex of the left kidney.

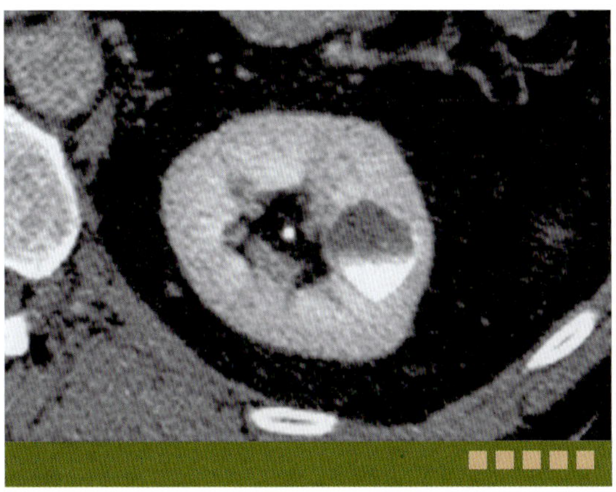

D. Axial CECT from the same patient and during the excretory phase shows contrast filling of the cystic mass, characteristic of a calyceal diverticulum.

DIFFERENTIAL DIAGNOSES IMAGES (E-G)

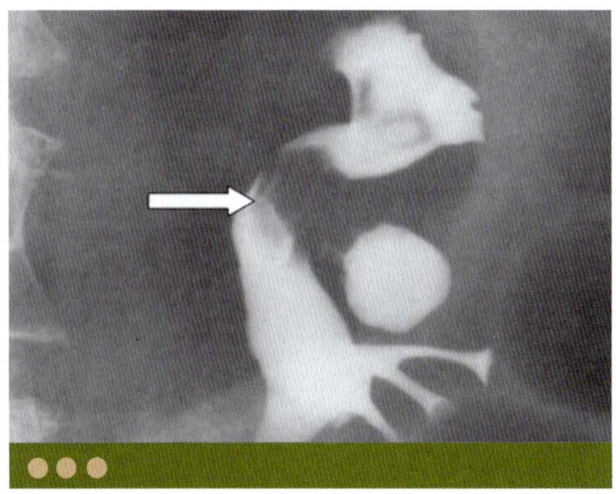

E. Focal caliectasis caused by TCC: Retrograde urogram shows an irregular filling defect (arrow) involving the infundibula of the upper pole and interpolar region collecting system and resulting in caliectasis.

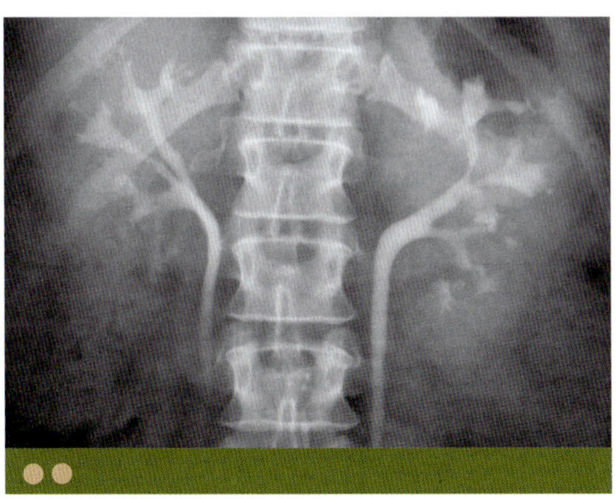

F. Papillary necrosis: IVU from patient with S – hemoglobinopathy shows elongated contrast-filled cavities situated eccentrically in multiple papillae.

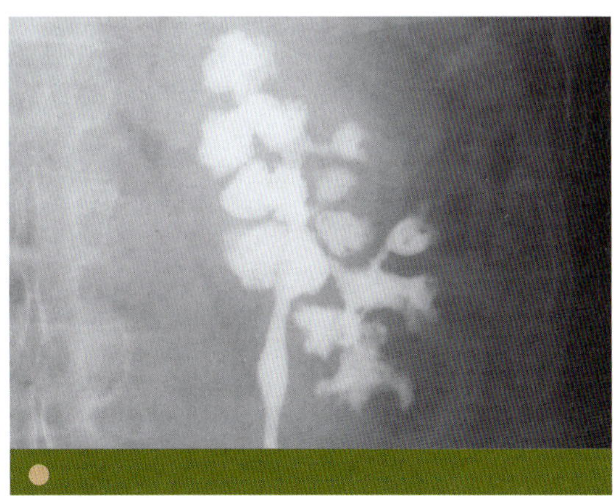

G. Tuberculosis: Retrograde urogram shows multiple irregular calyces and irregular parenchymal cavities, due to cavitation of granulomatous masses and erosion into the collecting system.

IMAGE KEY

Common

Rare

Typical

Unusual

CHAPTER 12

PROSTATE AND PENIS

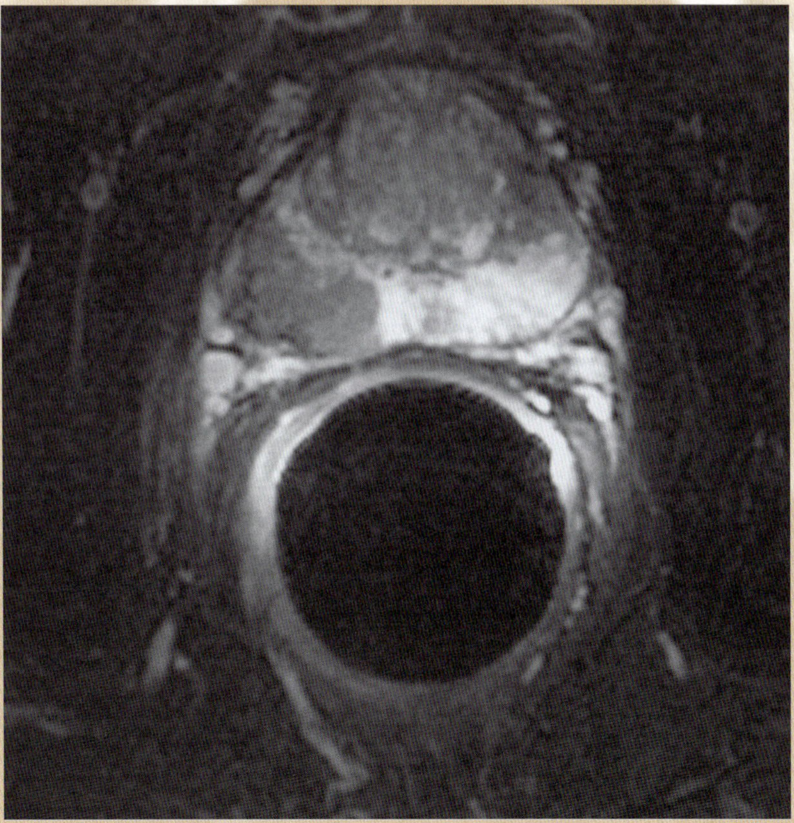

12–1 Prostate Carcinoma

Nancy A. Hammond

PRESENTATION

Elevated PSA.

FINDINGS

T2-weighted MR shows enlargement of the prostate with a hypointense abnormality in the right peripheral zone.

DIFFERENTIAL DIAGNOSES

- *Benign prostate hypertrophy (BPH)*: Typically involves the central gland but may involve the peripheral zone.
- *Focal prostatitis*: Imaging features similar to prostate cancer; clinical signs and symptoms may be helpful.

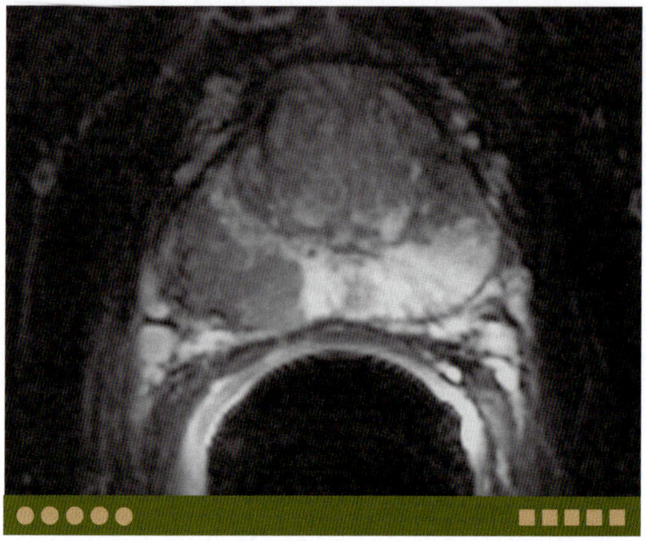

A. Axial T2-WI of the prostate gland performed with an endorectal coil shows a hypointense mass in the right aspect of the peripheral zone without extracapsular extension. Normal appearing T2 hyperintense peripheral zone is seen on the left.

COMMENTS

Prostate cancer is the most commonly diagnosed noncutaneous malignancy in American men. It is rare in men younger than 50 years of age but increases significantly with age thereafter. Histologically, more than 95% of prostate cancers are adenocarcinomas. Less common prostate malignancies include squamous cell carcinomas, endometrioid carcinomas, and mesenchymal neoplasms.

Transrectal ultrasound (TRUS) is utilized to evaluate and biopsy the prostate gland. Biopsies are taken of any focal abnormality in the peripheral zone as well as six random biopsies. The Gleason system is used to grade prostate cancer. A grade ranging from 1 to 5 (1 = well differentiated, 5 = poorly differentiated) is assigned to the two most prevalent patterns of cell differentiation seen at biopsy. The Gleason score is the sum of the two grades. A Gleason score of less than 4 is not likely to have metastasized while a score greater than 8 suggests a high likelihood of metastases.

On TRUS, prostate cancer appears as a hypoechoic lesion in the peripheral zone. This appearance can also occur with benign conditions including atypical hyperplasia, focal prostatitis, and prostatic cysts. However, approximately 30% of prostate cancers are isoechoic to normal prostate gland on TRUS. Focal abnormal vascularity on color Doppler US may aid in identifying cancers when gray scale abnormalities are not present.

CT is useful in evaluating for advanced disease. Detection of prostate cancer with MRI is limited to those occupying the peripheral zone. Those involving the transitional zone are difficult to distinguish from BPH. Utilizing an endorectal coil, MR can evaluate for extracapsular extension. Prostate cancer is typically isointense to normal prostate tissue on T1-WI sequences. On T2-WI sequences, prostate cancer demonstrates decreased signal relative to the hyperintense peripheral zone. If the patient has undergone a recent biopsy, increased T1 signal may be present as a result of hemorrhage. Most cancers are resistant to intratumoral hemorrhage, so the presence of increased signal on T1-WI sequences can help determine where the cancer is not present. Data suggests MR specificity and sensitivity can be improved by using MR spectroscopy, analysis of dynamic enhancement, and diffusion imaging. MR spectroscopy of the prostate detects indicator lines of citrate, choline, and creatine. Normal prostate tissue shows high levels of citrate and low levels of choline. Prostate cancer uses citrate for energy metabolism and shows high levels of choline. Therefore, the ratio of (choline + creatine)/citrate can be used to distinguish healthy from cancerous prostate tissue.

PEARLS

- **Prostate cancer is the most commonly diagnosed malignancy and the second leading cause of cancer deaths in males in the United States.**
- **When occurring in the peripheral zone, MR demonstrates a T2 hypointense mass relative to the normal hyperintense peripheral zone.**
- **TRUS is the initial modality utilized for biopsies in patients with suspected prostate cancer. Lesions typically are hypoechoic but 30% of prostate cancers are isoechoic to normal prostate gland on TRUS.**

ADDITIONAL IMAGES (B-E)

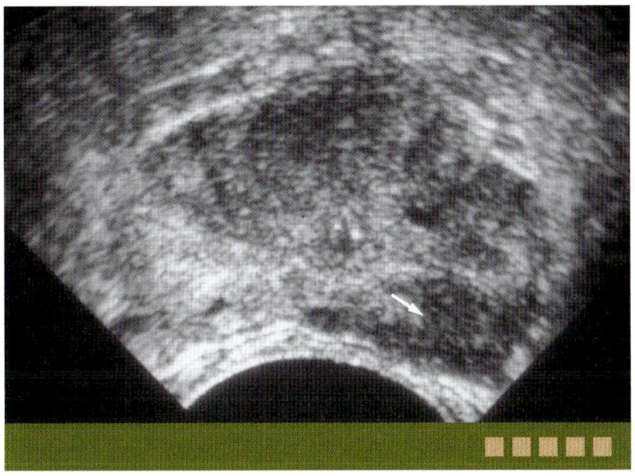

B. Transverse TRUS shows a hypoechoic mass in the left peripheral zone (arrow).

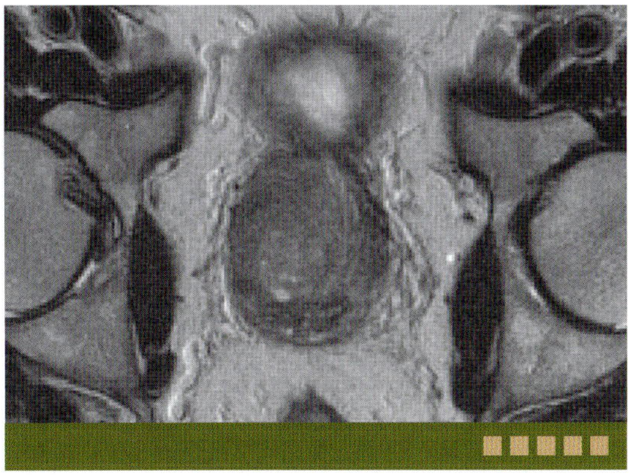

C. Axial T2-WI in a different patient shows a mildly hyperintense mass, occupying the central zone and right peripheral zone compatible with prostate cancer.

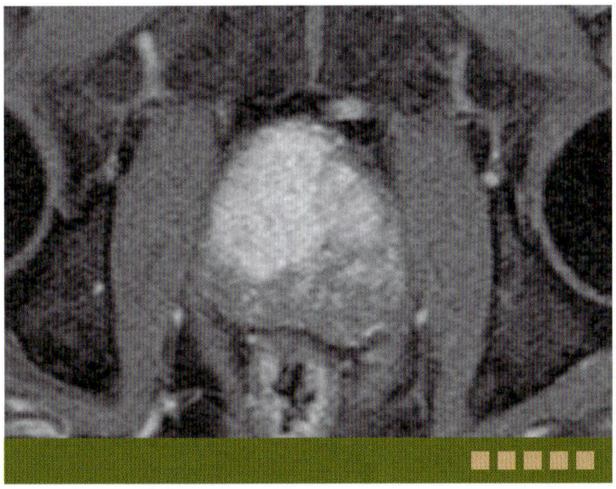

D. Axial contrast-enhanced T1-WI in the same patient as Figure C shows heterogeneous enhancement of the prostatic mass.

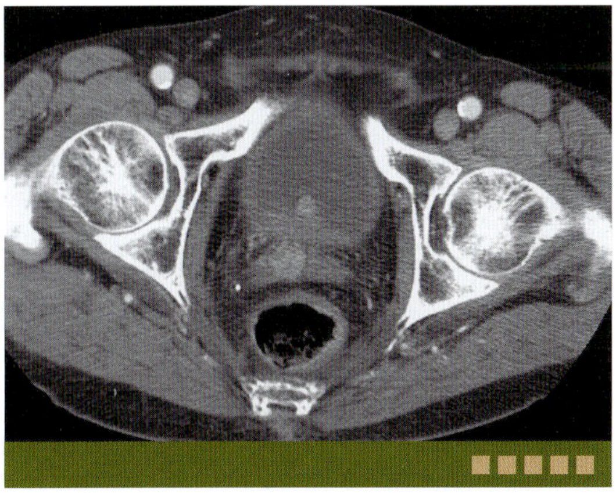

E. Axial CECT in a patient with prostate cancer shows a focal area of enhancement in the right seminal vesicle compatible with extension of disease.

IMAGE KEY

Common

Rare

Typical

Unusual

12–2 Metastatic Prostate Carcinoma

Nancy A. Hammond

PRESENTATION

Known prostate cancer with rising PSA level.

FINDINGS

Prostatic mass with extracapsular extension and seminal vesicle involvement.

DIFFERENTIAL DIAGNOSIS

None

COMMENTS

Prostate cancer is the most commonly diagnosed malignancy and the second leading cause of cancer deaths in American males. It is considered a tumor of older men with the median age of diagnosis being 72 years. Prostate cancer is often responsive to treatment when widespread and can be cured when localized. As tumor growth varies from slow to moderately rapid, patients can have prolonged survival even when metastases have occurred. Survival of the patient is related to the extent and behavior of the tumor. When disease is confined to the prostate gland, the 5-year survival rate is high. Locally advanced disease is considered not curable and a substantial portion of these patients will die from prostate cancer. If distant metastases are present, the median survival is typically 1 to 3 years. However, even in advanced disease, there are indolent clinical courses with longer survival times.

While CT is not accurate in assessing for early extracapsular extension of the disease, it can evaluate for advanced disease by demonstrating pathologic lymphadenopathy and distant metastases. Distant metastases are most commonly found in the bones and lymph nodes. Bony metastases are typically sclerotic and can also be detected with nuclear medicine bone scan.

MRI with an endorectal coil is useful in evaluating for extracapsular extension. Signs of extracapsular extension on MRI include focal contour abnormalities, large tumor volume, an apical location, broad margins with the prostate capsule, and infiltration of the periprostatic fat. Signs of neurovascular bundle invasion include direct tumor extension posterolaterally into the neurovascular bundle, decreased signal intensity obliterating the rectoprostatic angle, and focal contour abnormalities within the posterolateral aspect of the gland on axial T2-WI. Seminal vesicle invasion is characterized by low T1 and T2 signal within the lobules of the seminal vesicles and an adjacent prostate cancer. Like CT, MRI can be useful in evaluating for pelvic lymphadenopathy and osseous metastases.

The treatment approach to prostate cancer is influenced by the stage of the disease, patient age and coexisting medical problems. Two systems are used for the staging of prostate cancer. The Jewett system utilizes an A through D nomenclature; Stage A represents clinically undetectable tumor confined to the prostate gland, Stage B represents tumor confined to the prostate gland, Stage C is tumor clinically localized to the periprostatic area but extending through the prostatic capsule with or without seminal vesicle involvement, and Stage D includes disease with distant metastases. The American Joint Committee on Cancer (AJCC) utilizes a tumor, nodes, metastasis (TNM) system that employs the same broad T stage categories as the Jewett system but includes subcategories of T stage. This TNM system is clinically useful and more precisely stratifies newly diagnosed patients. Treatment options include surgery, radiation therapy, cryotherapy, and hormonal therapy. Surgery is utilized in patients with tumors confined to the prostate gland (Stages I and II) and who are in good health.

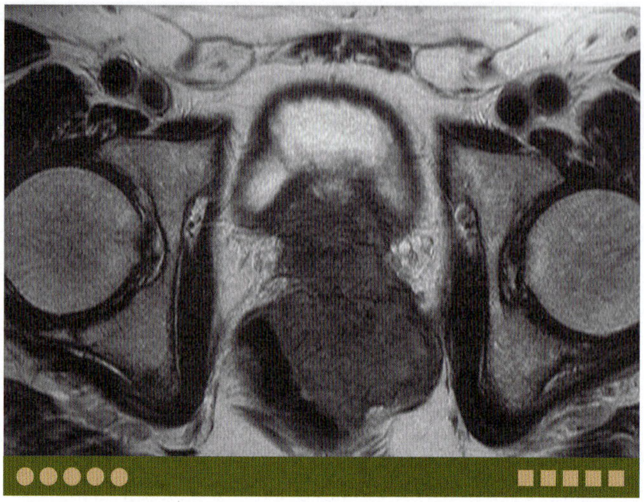

A. Axial T2-WI shows a mildly hyperintense mass occupying the expected location of the prostate gland. Extracapsular extension is present with loss of the normal fat plane between the urinary bladder anteriorly and the rectum posteriorly.

PEARLS

- **While the tumor is commonly latent, disease progression depends on the histologic grade/stage and tumor volume.**
- **CT and MR are both useful in evaluating for distant metastases but only MR is helpful in detecting extracapsular extension.**
- **Pelvic lymphadenopathy usually precedes distant metastases.**

ADDITIONAL IMAGES (B-E)

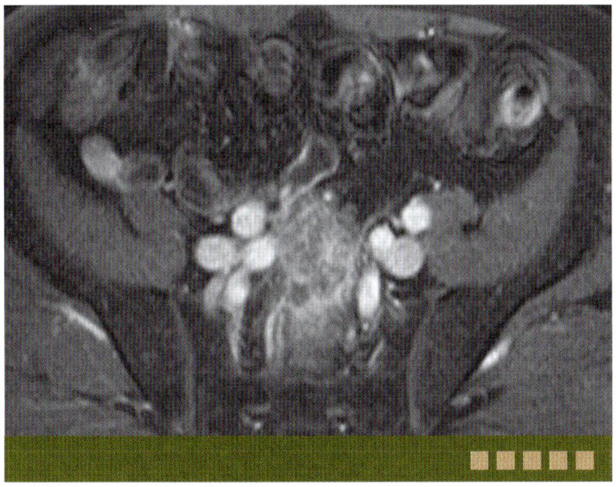

B. Axial contrast-enhanced T1-WI in the same patient shows a heterogeneously enhancing mass just inferior to the aortic bifurcation compatible with metastatic disease.

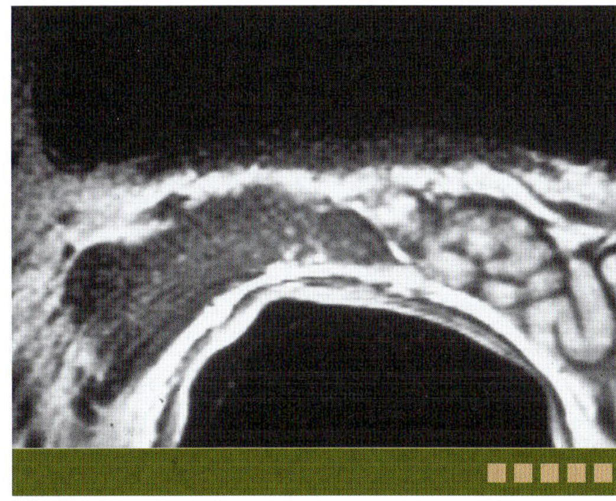

C. Axial T2-WI utilizing an endorectal coil obtained at the level of the seminal vesicles in a patient with known prostate cancer shows T2 hyperintensity replacing the right seminal vesicle consistent with tumor extension from the prostate gland.

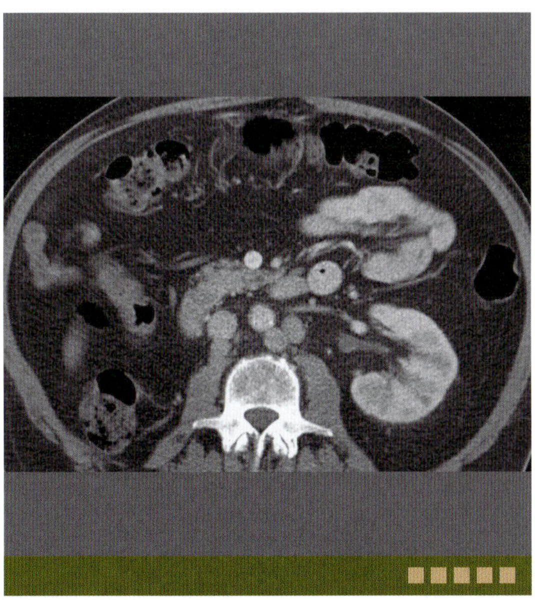

D. Axial CECT in a patient with known prostate cancer and rising PSA shows retroperitoneal lymphadenopathy along the left para-aortic chain compatible with metastatic disease.

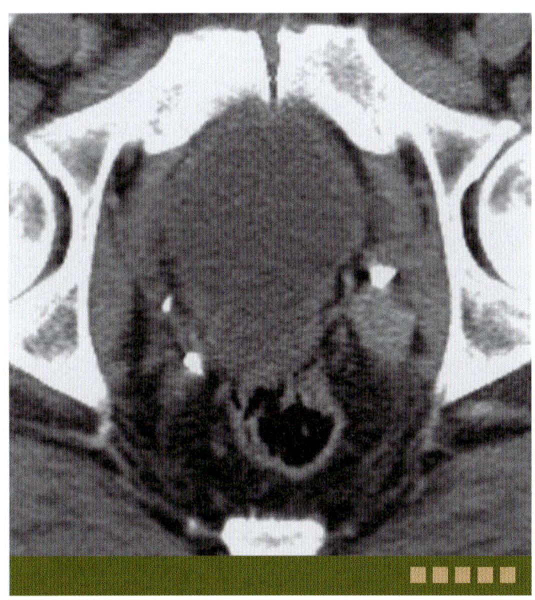

E. Axial CECT in a patient that is status postprostatectomy for prostate cancer with rising PSA shows an enhancing soft tissue nodule in the left ischiorectal fossa just posterior to a surgical clip consistent with recurrent prostate cancer.

IMAGE KEY

Common

Rare

Typical

Unusual

12–3 Benign Prostatic Hypertrophy

Nancy A. Hammond

PRESENTATION

Obstructive/irritative voiding symptoms.

FINDINGS

Enlarged prostate gland.

DIFFERENTIAL DIAGNOSIS

- *Prostate cancer*: More commonly involves the peripheral zone than central gland.

COMMENTS

Benign prostatic hypertrophy (BPH) is a common condition affecting greater than 50% of males 50 years or older in age. It is characterized by hyperplasia of prostatic adenomatous tissue. Tissue hypertrophy occurs in the periurethral transitional zone. Symptoms relate more to the pattern of hypertrophy than to the absolute volume of enlargement. "Median-lobe hypertrophy" of the periurethral tissues at the bladder base is responsible for symptoms including urinary hesitancy, frequent urination, increased risk of urinary tract infections and urinary retention. Prostate specific antigen (PSA) can be elevated in patients with BPH because of increased organ volume and inflammation secondary to urinary tract infections.

Radiographically, intravenous urogram (IVU) demonstrates a smooth mass-like impression on the base of the urinary bladder caused by prostatic enlargement. Findings of bladder outlet obstruction may be evident, including poor bladder emptying, bladder wall trabeculations, and bladder diverticula. As a result of the elevation of the interureteric ridge, "hooking" of the distal ureters may be present. If obstruction is longstanding, there may be dilatation of the upper urinary tracts, delayed excretion of contrast, and impaired renal function.

TRUS demonstrates prostatic enlargement with adenomata involving the transitional zone and periurethral glandular tissue but is usually only indicated when prostate cancer is suspected. The ultrasound diagnosis of BPH is based on an enlarged prostate gland (>40 g). The involved transitional zone or inner gland is heterogeneously hypoechoic with coarsened echotexture. Calcifications may be present. Multiple nodules may be present that are usually hyperechoic but can be hypoechoic or isoechoic. Cystic changes can occur because of degeneration of hyperplasic nodules.

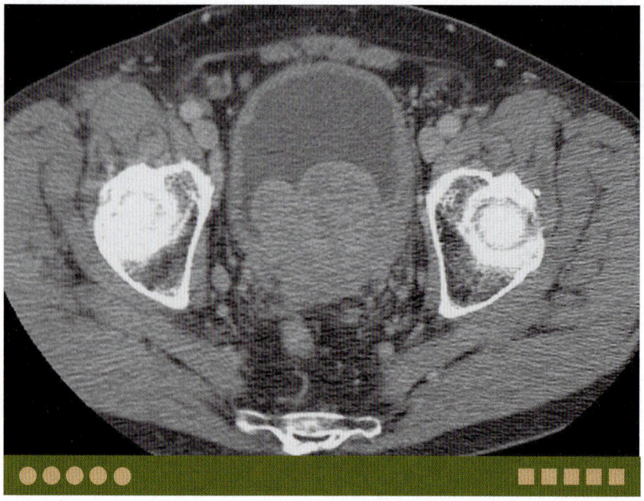

A. Axial CECT shows an enlarged, nodular prostate gland extending into the base of the bladder. There is mild diffuse bladder wall thickening present in this image.

CT demonstrates enlargement of the prostate gland. In some cases of BPH, CECT demonstrates the posterior peripheral zone to be lower attenuation than the centrally located adenoma. Underlying prostate cancer cannot be excluded based on CT.

MRI also demonstrates an enlarged gland with multiple nodules of varying signal on T2-weighted sequences. Low-signal nodules are predominantly stoma-rich foci of BPH and higher signal nodules are glandular-rich nodules.

Treatment of BPH depends on the severity of systems ranging from medical to surgical management.

PEARLS

- **BPH affects greater than 50% of males over the age of 50.**
- **Imaging demonstrates enlargement of the gland. Frequent changes of bladder outlet obstruction are present.**
- **Underlying prostate cancer cannot be excluded based on imaging studies.**

ADDITIONAL IMAGES (B-F)

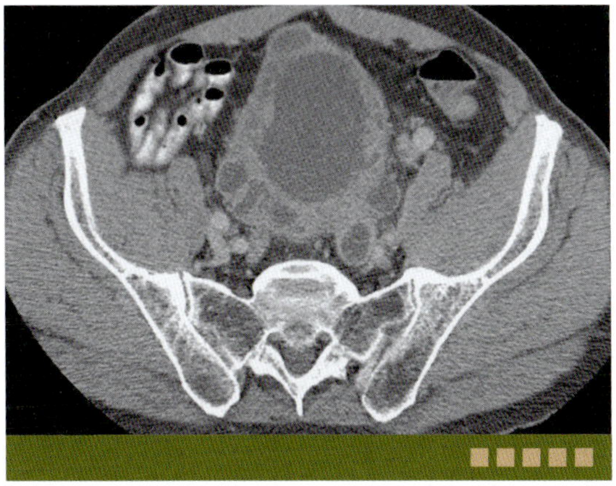

B. Axial CECT in the same patient shows multiple bladder diverticula, trabeculation to the bladder wall, and bladder wall thickening consistent with bladder outlet obstruction caused by BPH.

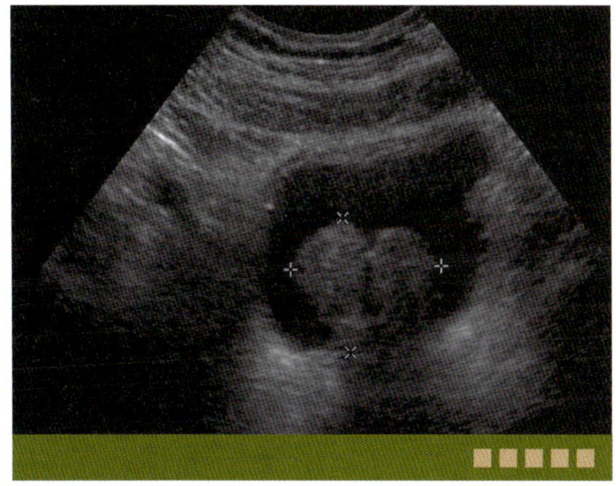

C. Transverse sonogram through the urinary bladder shows a nodular soft tissue mass projecting into the base of the bladder. This most likely arises from the prostate.

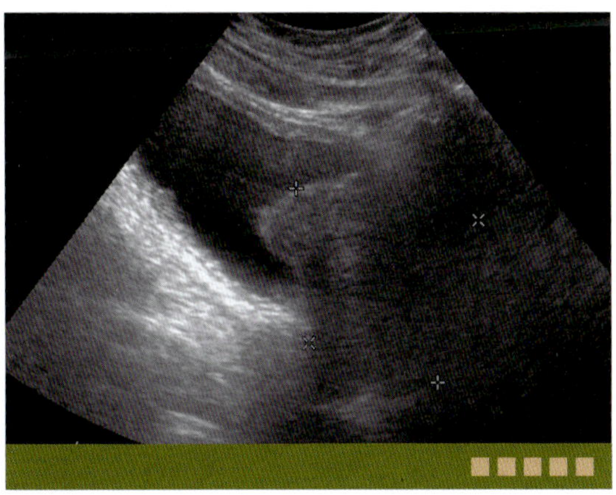

D. Longitudinal sonogram in the same patient confirms that the mass is related to the enlarged nodular prostate gland consistent with BPH. An underlying prostate cancer cannot be excluded based on this study. Correlation with PSA levels is warranted.

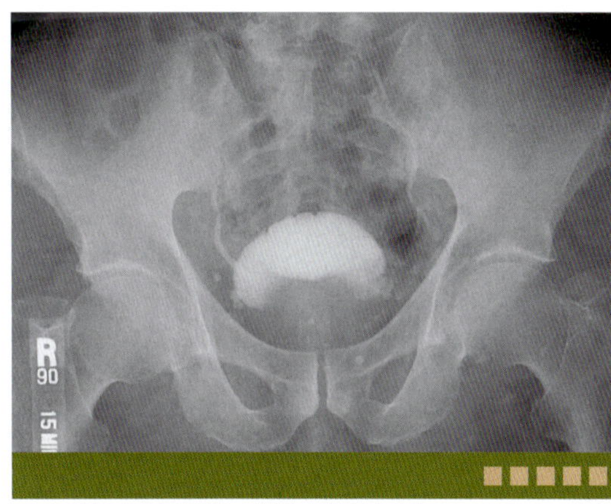

E. Contrast-enhanced IVU shows mass effect on the base of the bladder resulting from the enlargement of the prostate gland. Bladder wall trabeculation secondary to bladder outlet obstruction is present. This was confirmed with the postvoid image (not shown) which showed significant retention of contrast in the urinary bladder.

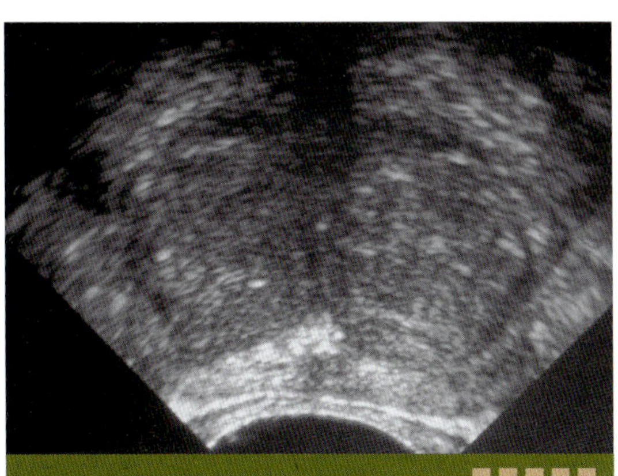

F. Transverse TRUS shows an enlarged prostate gland. The transitional zone is heterogeneously hypoechoic with a coarsened architecture.

DIFFERENTIAL DIAGNOSIS IMAGE

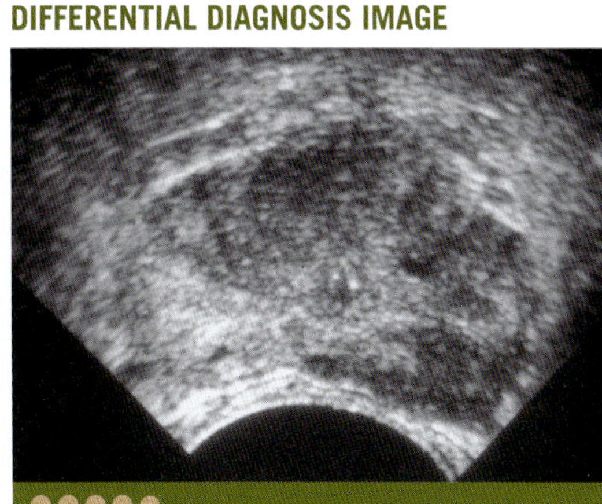

G. Prostate cancer: Transverse TRUS shows an enlarged prostate gland. A hypoechoic mass in the left peripheral zone was found on biopsy to represent adenocarcinoma of the prostate gland.

IMAGE KEY

Common

Rare

Typical

Unusual

12-4 Prostatitis

Nancy A. Hammond

PRESENTATION

Fever and dysuria.

FINDINGS

CT shows a heterogeneous prostate gland with low density in the peripheral zone. Mild stranding around the prostate gland may be present.

DIFFERENTIAL DIAGNOSIS

- *Prostate cancer*: Typically appears as focal low T2 signal in the peripheral zone. Chronic prostatitis may also have this appearance but is usually more diffuse with prostatitis than malignancy. Clinical presentation may help in distinguishing the two, but biopsy may be necessary.

COMMENTS

Acute prostatitis is typically caused by a retrograde bacterial infection with *Escherichia coli* accounting for more than 80% of the infections. It usually presents as a urinary tract infection with symptoms including frequency, dysuria, fever, perineal pain, and urethral discharge. Acute prostatitis is usually associated with predisposing risk factors, including bladder outlet obstruction secondary to BPH or an immunosuppressed state. It is much less common than chronic prostatitis but is easier to diagnose because of its more uniform clinical presentation. Chronic prostatitis often occurs without an acute episode and can be bacterial, inflammatory, or without an identifiable pathologic lesion. Like prostate cancer, prostatitis tends to involve the peripheral zone.

Conventional radiographs and IVU have a limited role in evaluating prostatitis. Transabdominal ultrasound, CT, and MRI are usually not necessary in evaluating acute prostatitis but can help in finding complications of acute prostatitis, including abscess formation. CT of acute prostatitis may demonstrate enlargement of the gland with periprostatic stranding. MRI shows an enlarged gland with decreased signal on T1-WI sequences and increased signal on T2-WI. Areas of inflammation enhance on contrast-enhanced sequences. Stranding in the adjacent fat and involvement of the seminal vesicles may be present. Chronic prostatitis can appear similar to prostate cancer as both demonstrate low signal on T2-weighted sequences. In distinction to prostate cancer, chronic prostatitis is more likely to demonstrate diffuse low T2 signal in the peripheral zone without a focal mass.

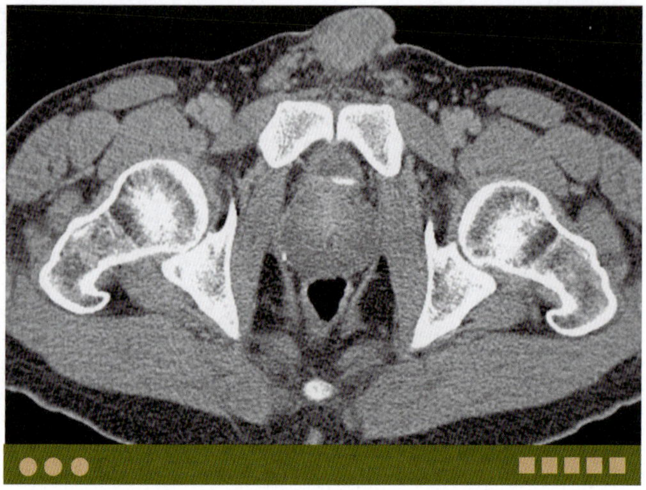

A. Axial CECT shows mild enlargement of the prostate gland. There is greater than typically seen low attenuation noted in the peripheral zone. The patient reported fever and dysuria and was found to be tender over the prostate gland on digital rectal examination (DRE).

TRUS demonstrates varying areas of altered echogenicity in the prostate gland. When located in the peripheral zone, this finding can be difficult to distinguish from cancer. Other features that have been described on TRUS include capsular thickening, prostatic calculi, a hypoechoic halo in the periurethral region, and enlargement and thickening of the septa of the seminal vesicles.

Treatment of uncomplicated acute prostatitis includes antibiotic therapy. In cases of chronic prostatitis in which inflammation is felt to be present, a 4-week trial of antibiotics is recommended. Otherwise, supportive measures including analgesics, alpha-blocking agents, hydration, stool softeners, and sitz baths are often used.

PEARLS

- **Acute prostatitis is much more common than the chronic form and usually presents as a urinary tract infection.**
- **Imaging may be helpful in diagnosing complications, such as abscess formation.**
- **Prostatitis and prostate cancer may have indistinguishable imaging features.**

ADDITIONAL IMAGES (B-D)

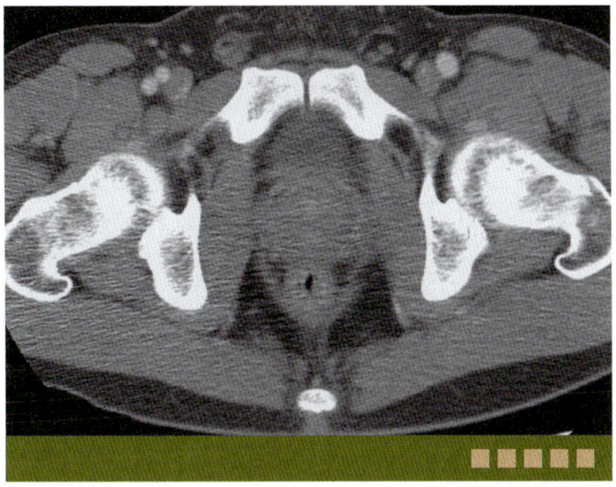

B. Axial CECT in a different patient shows heterogeneity to the prostate gland with haziness to the prostatic margins and mild periprostatic stranding. The patient was clinically suspected of having prostatitis.

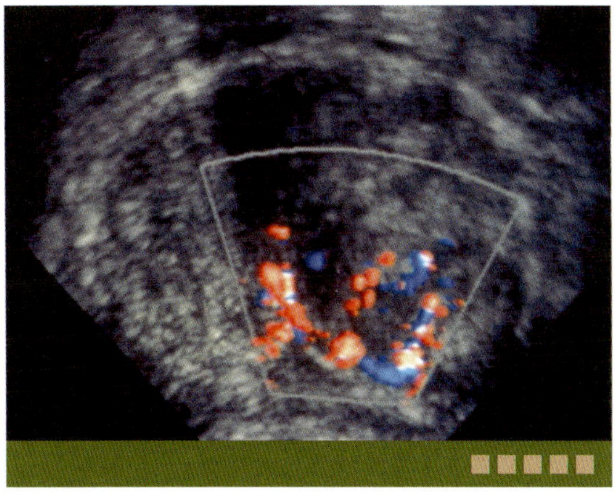

C. Color Doppler TRUS shows a heterogeneous appearance to the prostate gland with increased flow to the peripheral zone.

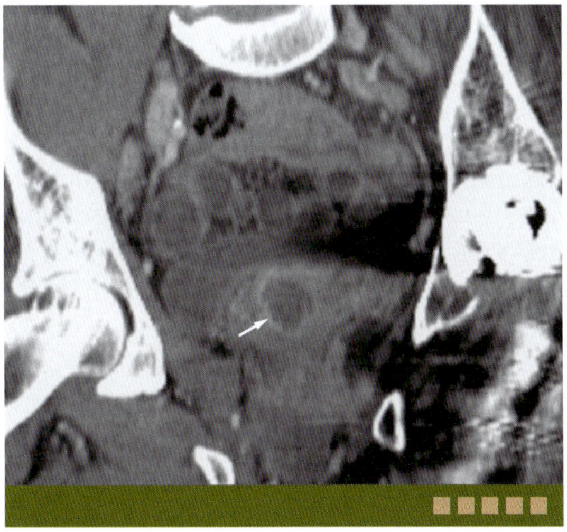

D. Coronal CECT in a patient with known prostatitis shows a rim enhancing fluid collection consistent with a prostatic abscess (arrow).

DIFFERENTIAL DIAGNOSIS IMAGE

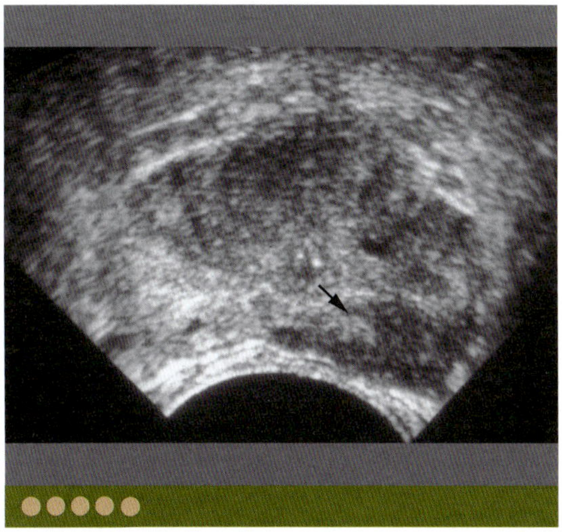

E. Prostate cancer: TRUS shows a focal, hypoechoic mass in the left peripheral zone (arrow).

IMAGE KEY

Common
●●●●●
●●●●
●●●
●●
●
Rare

Typical
■■■■■
■■■■
■■■
■■
■
Unusual

12–5 Prostatic Abscess

Nancy A. Hammond

PRESENTATION

Fever and dysuria.

FINDINGS

CT images show a complex fluid collection in the prostate gland.

DIFFERENTIAL DIAGNOSES

- *Utricle cyst*: Midline cystic structure without rim enhancement; clinical presentation different from abscess; wall enhancement may be present if superinfected.
- *TURP defect*: Midline location with communication to the urinary bladder; no peripheral enhancement.

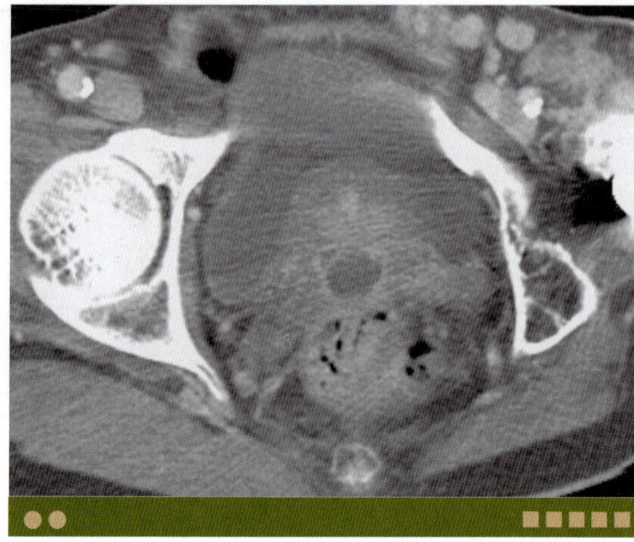

A. Axial CECT shows a rim-enhancing low-density fluid collection in the prostate gland.

COMMENTS

Prostatic abscesses are a rare complication of either acute or chronic bacterial prostatitis. Less commonly, they can be secondary to hematogeneous spread of infection. Abscess formation as a complication of prostatitis has significantly decreased with the advent of antibiotic therapy. The clinical diagnosis of a prostatic abscess can be difficult to make as symptoms are non-specific. The diagnosis should be suspected when symptoms of prostatitis do not resolve despite appropriate antibiotic therapy. Prostatic abscesses are most common in diabetic and immunocompromised patients and in patients with indwelling urinary catheters. They are usually caused by *E coli, Staphylococcus* and gram-negative colon bacteria.

IVU and conventional radiographs are noncontributory in the diagnosis of prostatic abscesses. TRUS demonstrates a loculated fluid collection within the prostate gland. The abscess may demonstrate ill-defined borders, irregular walls, occasionally septations and a hypoechoic halo surrounding the collection. The fluid is homogeneously hypoechoic or heterogeneous because of the presence of debris. If gas is present, ring-down or comet tail artifact may be detected. Color flow typically shows periabscess hypervascularity. CT demonstrates a focal low-density collection with rim enhancement often within an enlarged gland. MRI demonstrates a complex cystic fluid collection that is hyperintense on T2-WI sequences and demonstrates rim enhancement on contrast-enhanced T1-WI sequences. Prostatic abscesses are seen most commonly in the transitional and central zones of the prostate gland. It is important to image through the urogenital diaphragm as the abscess can extend inferiorly and involve the base of the penis.

Treatment includes appropriate antibiotic therapy, drainage, or surgical treatment when necessary.

PEARLS

- **Incidence of prostatic abscesses has decreased since the advent of antibiotics in treating prostatitis.**
- **Seen most commonly in diabetic and immunocompromised patients or patients with indwelling Foley catheters.**
- **Appear as rim-enhancing fluid collection on CECT and MR.**

ADDITIONAL IMAGES (B-C)

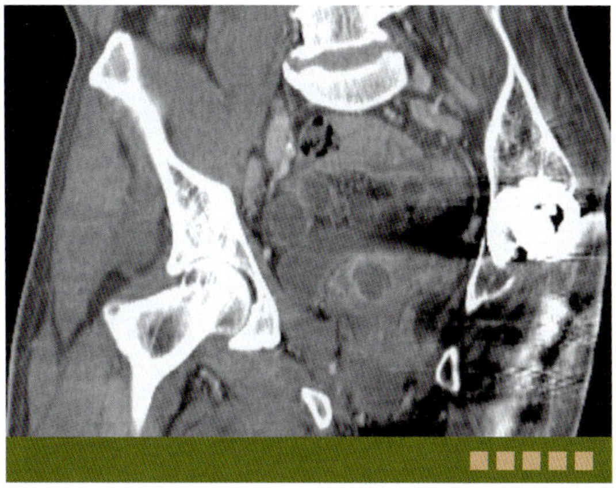

B. Coronal CECT in the same patient as Figure A further shows the prostatic abscess.

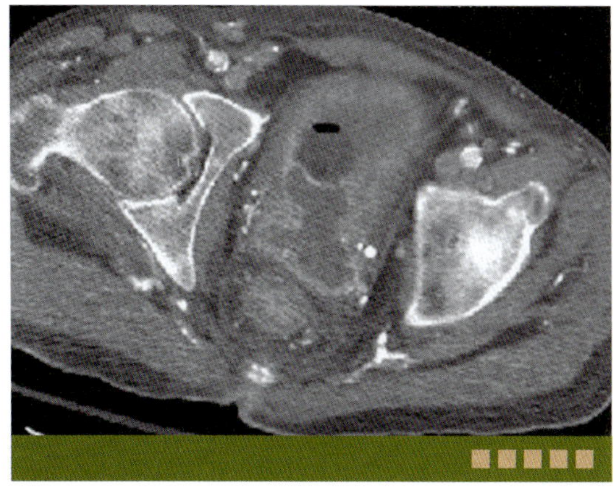

C. Axial CECT in a different patient shows an irregular fluid collection within the prostate gland. This collection also shows rim enhancement. Additionally, a Foley catheter is present.

DIFFERENTIAL DIAGNOSES IMAGES (D-G)

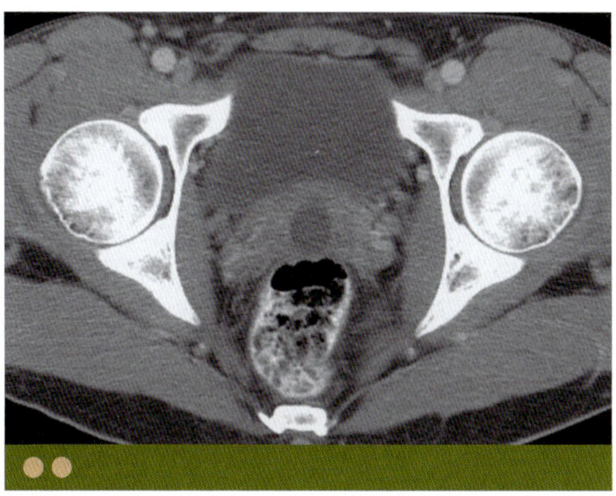

D. Utricle cyst: Axial CECT in an asymptomatic patient shows a midline low density, round fluid collection in the prostate gland. No wall enhancement is present.

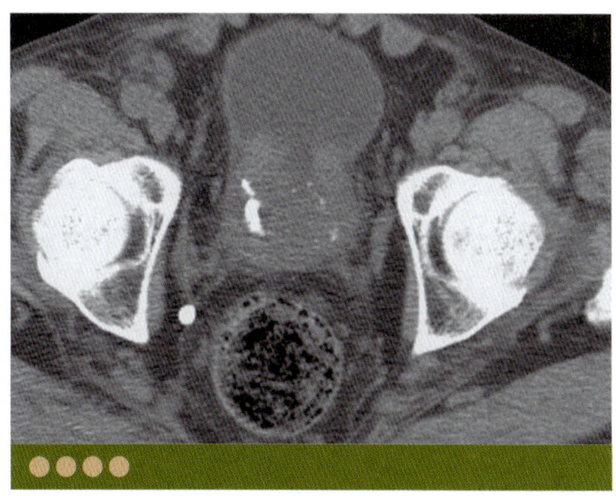

E. TURP defect: Axial NECT in a patient with BPH shows a low-density structure at the anterior superior aspect of the prostate gland which is contiguous with the urinary bladder. There is no rim enhancement.

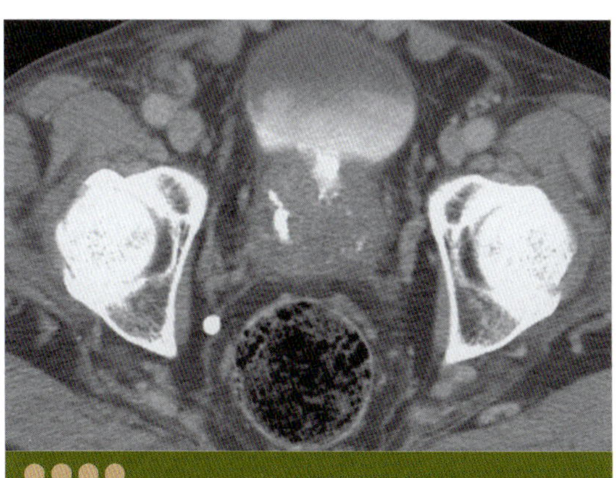

F. TURP defect: Axial delayed CECT in the same patient as Figure E shows filling of the structure with excreted contrast material compatible with a TURP defect.

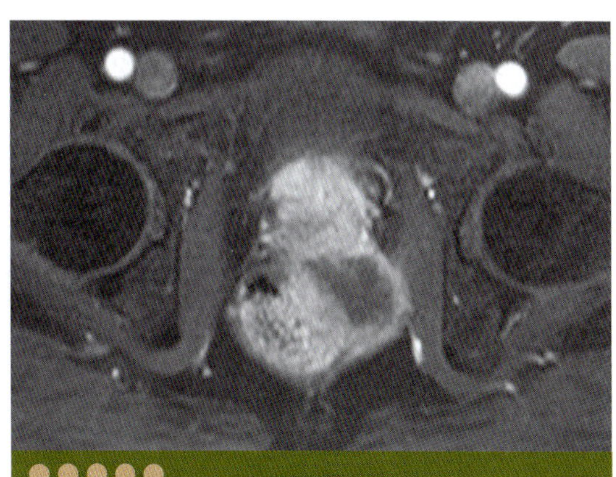

G. Prostate cancer with necrosis: Axial contrast-enhanced T1-WI shows a region of decreased enhancement in the left peripheral zone of the prostate gland inferiorly. An enhancing mass consistent with prostate cancer is present more superiorly (not shown).

IMAGE KEY

Common

Rare

Typical

Unusual

12–6 Prostatic Cystic Mass

David D. Casalino

PRESENTATION

Urinary frequency and hesitancy and weak urine stream.

FINDINGS

MR shows the prostate to have an enlarged heterogeneous transition zone with cystic focus just right of midline.

DIFFERENTIAL DIAGNOSES

- *Müllerian duct cyst and prostatic utricle cyst*: May cause urinary obstructive symptoms; both in the region of verumontanum and at the midline.
- *Ejaculatory duct cyst*: Rare, usually small; lateral to the midline in the central zone of the prostate; when large, may extend above the prostate.
- *Cysts associated with tumors*: Malignant tumors include adenocarcinoma, papillary cystadenocarcinoma, and liposarcoma; benign tumors include multilocular prostatic cystadenoma and leiomyoma.
- *Prostate abscess*: Clinical signs and symptoms of infection.
- *Ectopic ureter*: Continuity with the rest of the ureter.

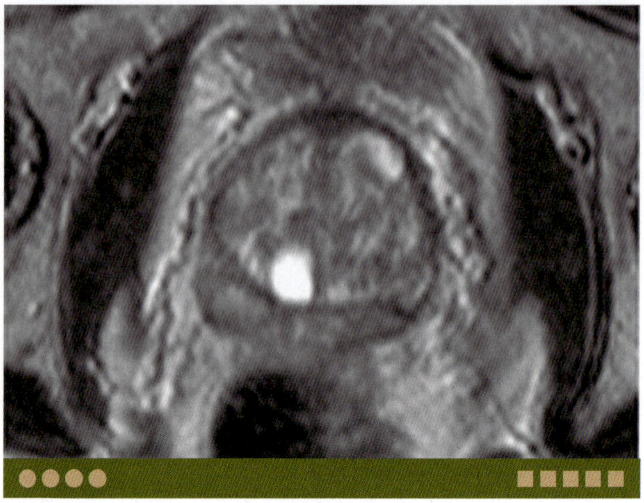

A. Axial T2-WI shows the prostate to have an enlarged, heterogeneously hypointense transition zone, characteristic of BPH, with area of cystic degeneration just right of midline.

COMMENTS

Prostatic cystic masses are uncommon but occasionally identified on imaging. Cyst location, associated imaging findings, and clinical features may allow a specific diagnosis or reduce the number of possible etiologies. Most prostatic cysts represent cystic degeneration of benign prostatic hypertrophy (BPH). These cysts are typically in the transition zone of the prostate, not uncommonly multiple, and of various sizes. BPH may cause obstructive symptoms. Müllerian duct cysts and prostatic utricle cysts may be impossible to differentiate on the basis of imaging. Both are usually midline in the region of the verumontanum, may cause urinary obstructive symptoms and rarely ejaculatory duct obstruction, and may be complicated by infection and stone formation. Müllerian duct cysts usually extend above the prostate, may be slightly lateral to the midline, and do not communicate with the urethra. Prostatic utricle cysts arise from the verumontanum, are always midline, and communicate with the urethra. As a result, prostatic utricle cysts may be associated with postvoid dribbling and contain spermatozoa. These cysts may also be associated with unilateral renal agenesis, cryptorchidism, and hypospadia. Ejaculatory duct cysts are rare and result from duct obstruction. Presenting symptoms may include hematospermia, dysuria, and infertility. Typically, they are just lateral to the midline in the central zone of the prostate, but when large may extend above the prostate and appear central. Ejaculatory duct cysts often contain calculi and may be complicated by infection. Malignant prostatic tumors, including adenocarcinoma, which most often arises from the peripheral zone and elevates serum PSA, papillary cystadenocarcinoma, and liposarcoma, and benign prostatic tumors, including multilocular cystadenoma and leiomyoma, may show cystic components. Prostate abscesses usually result from an acute bacterial infection. Patients typically present with clinical signs and symptoms of infection. On imaging, prostate abscesses typically show thick walls and heterogeneous contents.

PEARLS

- **Most prostatic cysts occur in nodules of BPH.**
- **Müllerian duct cysts and prostatic utricle cysts are typically midline in the region of the verumontanum and may be impossible to differentiate on imaging.**
- **Ejaculatory duct cysts are rare, just lateral to the midline, and often contain calculi.**
- **Prostatic tumors may have cystic components, almost always in combination with solid components.**

DIFFERENTIAL DIAGNOSES IMAGES (B-G)

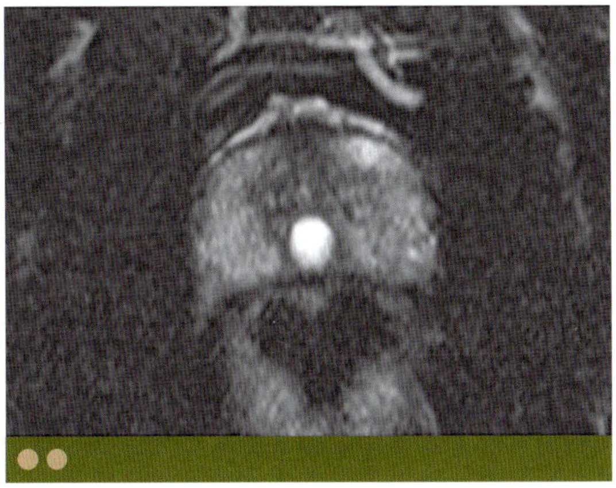

B. Utricle cyst: Axial T2-WI shows a small, midline cyst in the region of the verumontanum.

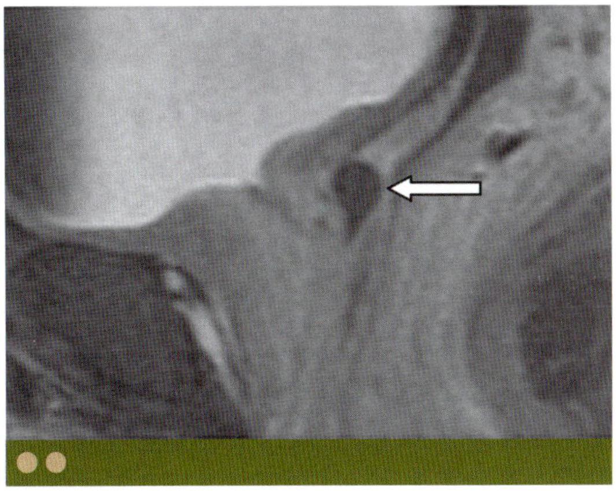

C. Müllerian duct cyst: Sagittal contrast-enhanced T1-WI shows a hypointense, nonenhancing cystic mass (arrow) at the midline and extending above the prostate.

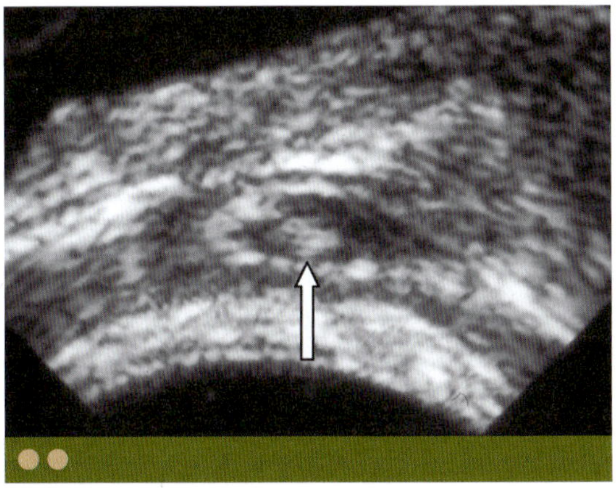

D. Ejaculatory duct cyst: Longitudinal sonogram shows a right of midline cyst that contains a small echogenic stone (arrow). The patient presented with hematospermia.

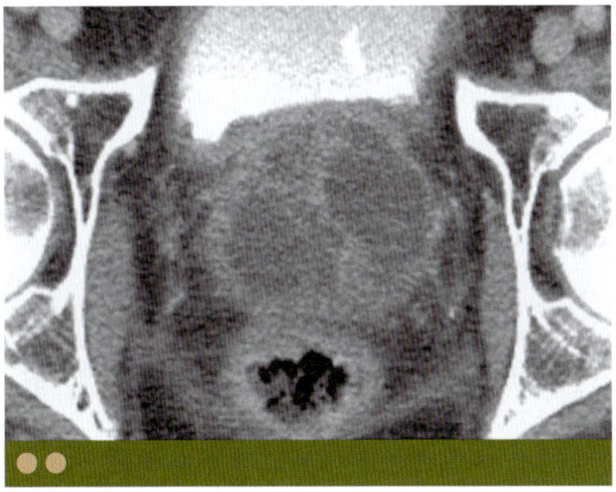

E. Cystic necrosis within prostatic adenocarcinoma: Axial CECT shows the prostate to be diffusely heterogeneous with prominent cystic areas intermixed with solid areas in a patient with elevated serum PSA.

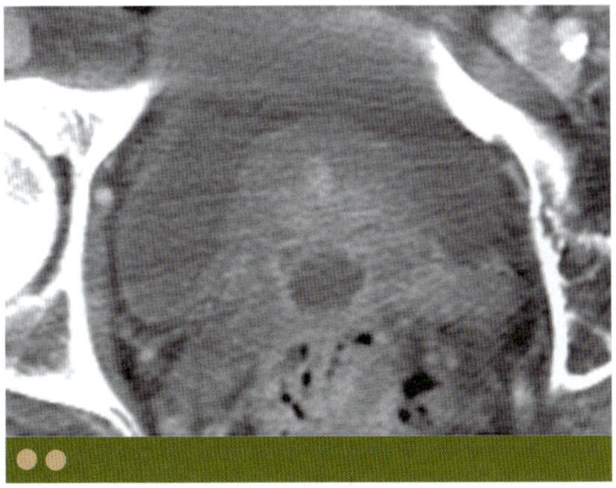

F. Prostate abscess: Axial CECT shows a near midline cystic mass with a thick, enhancing wall. Patient had pain, fevers, and history of prostatitis.

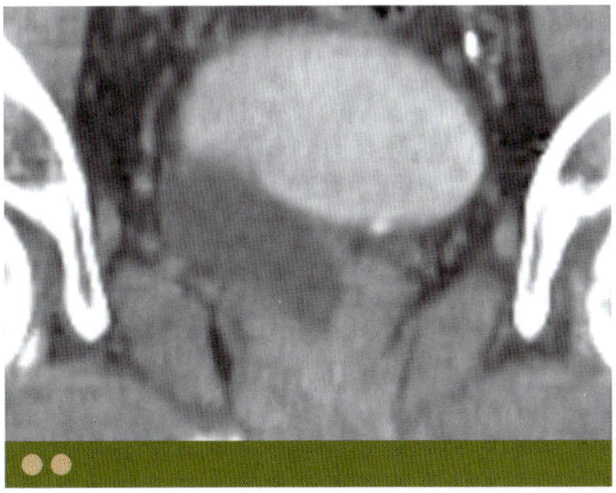

G. Ectopic ureter: Coronal CECT shows a large cystic abnormality involving the right side of the prostate. This abnormality was shown to be dilated, ectopic ureter from a duplicated right collecting system.

IMAGE KEY

Common

Rare

Typical

Unusual

12–7 Seminal Vesicle Cyst and Renal Agenesis

Frank H. Miller

PRESENTATION

Asymptomatic or present in early adulthood with perineal pain on ejaculation or defecation, dysuria, urinary frequency or pelvic mass on physical examination.

FINDINGS

Cyst in the right seminal vesicle.

DIFFERENTIAL DIAGNOSES

- *Prostatic cysts, cystic cancer and abscesses*: Different location.
- *Utricle cyst*: Tends to be midline.
- *Ejaculatory duct cysts*: Midline in location.
- *Ectopic ureterocele*: Distinguished based on relationship to ureter.
- These conditions are not associated with renal agenesis.

COMMENTS

Seminal vesicle cysts can be congenital or acquired. Congenital cysts are usually unilateral and associated with anomalies of the kidneys or mesonephric ducts. It most commonly is associated with renal agenesis as seen in this patient. Unilateral renal agenesis occurs in 1 out of 1000 births. The cysts result from maldevelopment of the distal mesonephric duct with failure of development of the ureteric bud and atresia of the ejaculatory duct; this leads to obstruction of the seminal vesicle and cyst formation. Acquired cysts are often bilateral and occur as a result of inflammatory disorders including prostatitis, inflammation of the seminal vesicle, and prostatic surgery due to obstruction of the ejaculatory duct.

Seminal vesicle cysts are usually smaller than 5 cm and asymptomatic, discovered as a palpable abdominal mass, or on DRE as a fluctuant mass. They may be seen incidentally on imaging studies. They may present with symptoms from bladder irritation. Symptoms include abdominal, perineal and pelvic pain, pain on ejaculation, urinary frequency or dysuria, hematuria, and urinary tract infections. Other reported symptoms include infertility and hematospermia. When larger than 12 cm, they are referred to as giant cysts and can cause bladder and colonic obstruction.

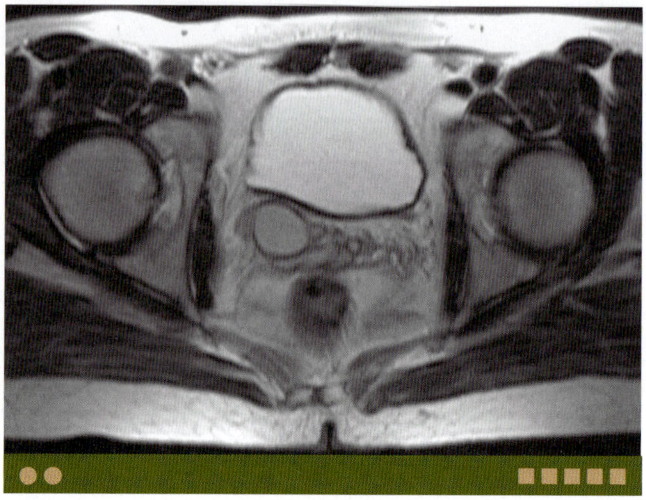

A. Axial T2-WI shows high-signal intensity cyst in the right seminal vesicle.

Sonography may show the cystic nature of the mass and its location. The masses are generally anechoic but may contain a thick wall and internal debris from prior bleeding or infection. CT findings vary from fluid density to increased density fluid from hemorrhage, protein, or infection. Diagnostic findings include a normal seminal vesicle and the contralateral absent seminal vesicle associated with a thick-walled cyst. On MR, the cyst when composed of simple fluid is low-signal intensity on T1-WI and high-signal intensity on T2-WI. When complex, they may be high-signal intensity on T1-WI and T2-WI because of hemorrhagic or proteinaceous material.

When symptomatic, the seminal vesicle cysts can be treated endoscopically or via laparoscopic cystectomy.

PEARLS

- **Seminal vesicle cysts are usually asymptomatic.**
- **Seminal vesicle cysts are usually smaller than 5 cm.**
- **Seminal vesicle cysts may be diagnosed with ultrasound, CT, or MR.**
- **Seminal vesicle cysts are associated with renal agenesis.**

ADDITIONAL IMAGES (B-C)

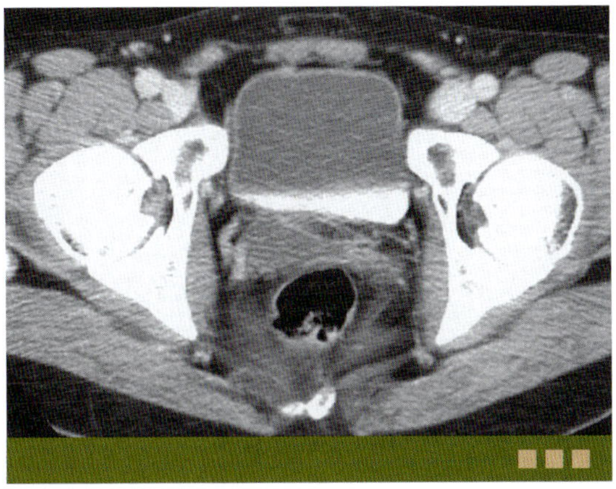

B. Axial CECT shows a cystic area in the right seminal vesicle. The diagnosis is easier on MR than on CT.

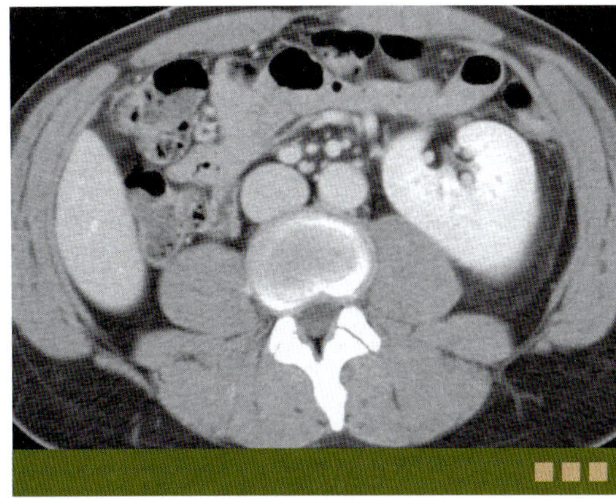

C. More superior axial CECT shows right renal agenesis with normal left kidney. This helps confirm diagnosis of seminal vesicle cyst.

DIFFERENTIAL DIAGNOSES IMAGES (D-F)

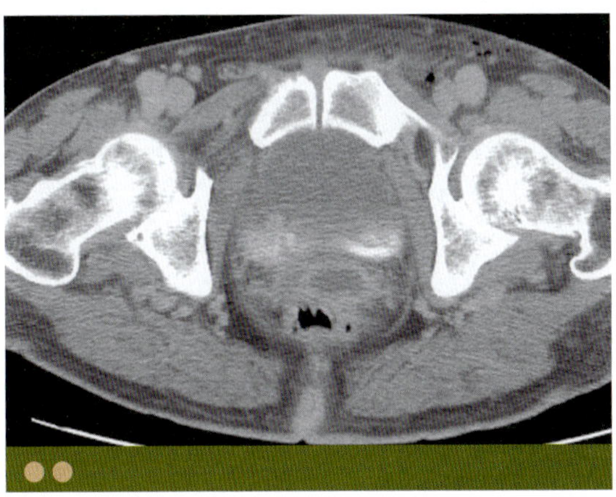

D. Prostate abscess: Axial CECT shows a peripherally enhancing cystic collection caused by prostate abscess. The location and patient's symptoms help distinguish it from a seminal vesicle cyst.

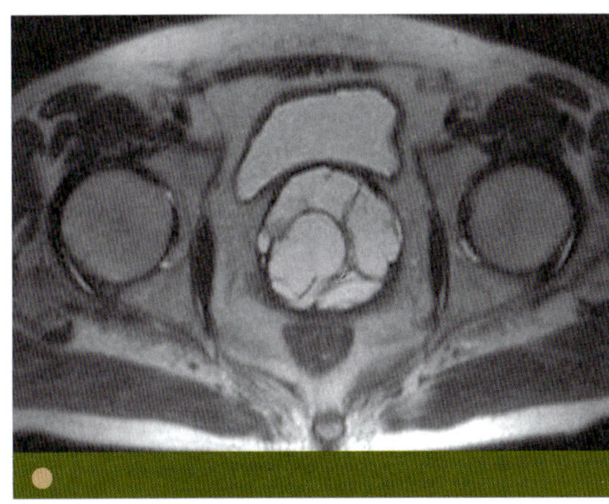

E. Multicystic prostatic cancer: Axial T2-WI shows a multi-septated cystic mass replacing the prostate because of cancer. The location helps distinguish the lesion from a seminal vesicle cyst.

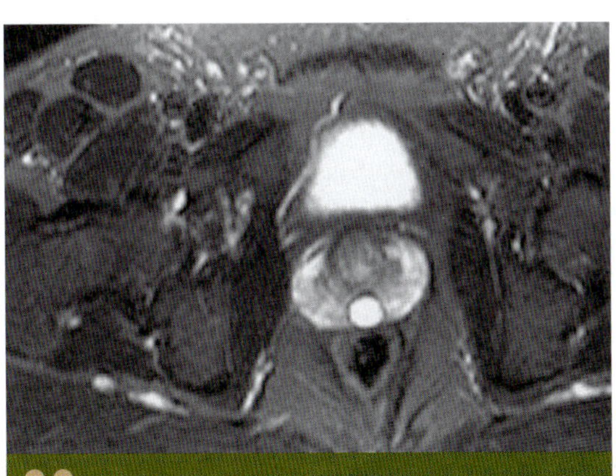

F. Prostatic utricle cyst: Axial T2-WI shows a midline cystic mass caused by utricle cyst. The midline location helps distinguish the lesion from a seminal vesicle cyst.

IMAGE KEY

Common

Rare

Typical

Unusual

12–8 Penile Cancer

Frank H. Miller

PRESENTATION

Firm mass in the tip of the penis; generally not painful.

FINDINGS

Enhancing penile mass.

DIFFERENTIAL DIAGNOSES

- *Metastases to the penis*: Generally known primary malignancy; may be multiple.
- *Peyronie disease*: Seen as enhancing plaques.
- *Penile trauma*: Not seen as enhancing mass; can usually distinguish based on history.

COMMENTS

Primary penile cancer is rare in the US accounting for less than 1% of genitourinary tumors in males. The most common tumor involving the penis is squamous cell carcinoma (SCC) seen in more than 95%. Penile cancer is most common in the sixth and seventh decade of life. Being uncircumcised is associated with penile cancer. Patients generally present with a firm mass but may delay seeking attention because of the lack of symptoms delaying the diagnosis.

Penile cancer most often arises in the skin of the glans penis. MR is the most sensitive examination to show depth of invasion. T2-weighted and gadolinium-enhanced fat suppressed T1-WI are useful to delineate the primary tumor and show invasion into the tunica albuginea, corpora, and urethra. Tumor tends to be hypointense to the corpora cavernosa on T1 and T2-WI and hypoenhances relative to the corpora. MRI helps show the draining inguinal lymph nodes for which the coronal images are quite helpful. To image the penis, the scrotum and penis should be elevated on towels to the anterior abdominal wall with the tip extending cephalad. A small surface coil should be used for higher resolution images. A pelvic phased array coil is used to evaluate the pelvic lymph nodes.

Using the TNM staging classification of penile cancer, T1 is seen as invasion of the subepithelial connective tissue, T2 as invasion of the corpus spongiosum or cavernosum, T3 as invasion of the urethra or prostate and T4 as invasion of other adjacent structures. N1 refers to metastasis in a single superficial inguinal node, N2 for metastasis in multiple or bilateral superficial inguinal nodes, and N3 for metastasis in deep inguinal or pelvic lymph nodes. M1 refers to distant metastases. The Jackson classification includes Stage 1 as confined to the glans or prepuce or both, Stage 2 as extending onto the penile shaft, Stage 3 as inguinal lymph node involvement, and Stage 4 for deep pelvic lymph nodes or distant metastases. Treatment usually requires surgical radical or partial penectomy.

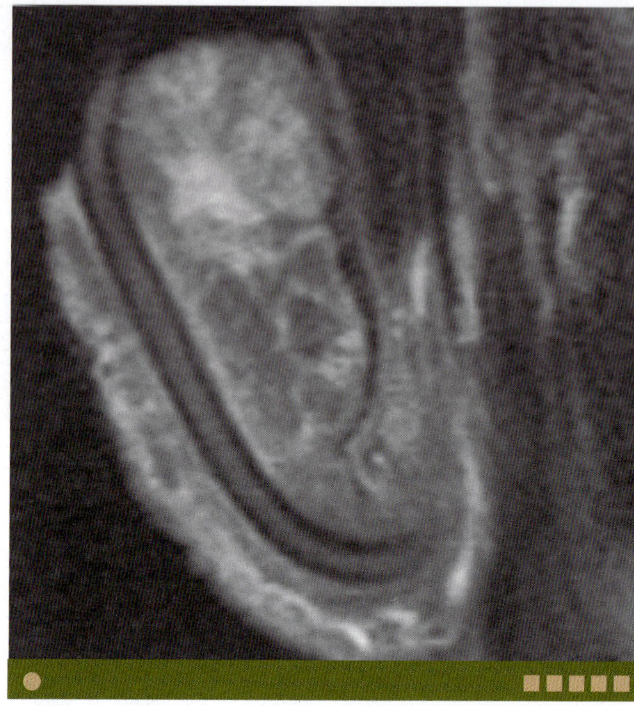

A. Sagittal contrast-enhanced T1-FS MR shows mass with heterogeneous signal intensity involving the glans penis and the corpora cavernosa.

PEARLS

- **Primary penile cancer is rare and is most often resulting from SCC.**
- **Penile cancer is most common in the sixth and seventh decade of life.**
- **Penile cancer involves the glans of the penis.**
- **Penile cancer is often hypointense on T1 and T2-WI and hypoenhances relative to the corpora.**
- **A small surface coil should be used to evaluate the penis with a pelvic or body coil for imaging regional lymph nodes.**

ADDITIONAL IMAGES (B-D)

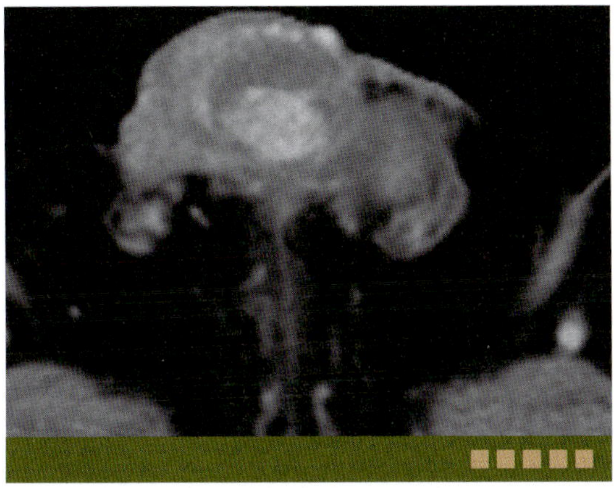

B. Axial CECT in different patient shows a heterogeneous enhancing mass resulting from penile cancer.

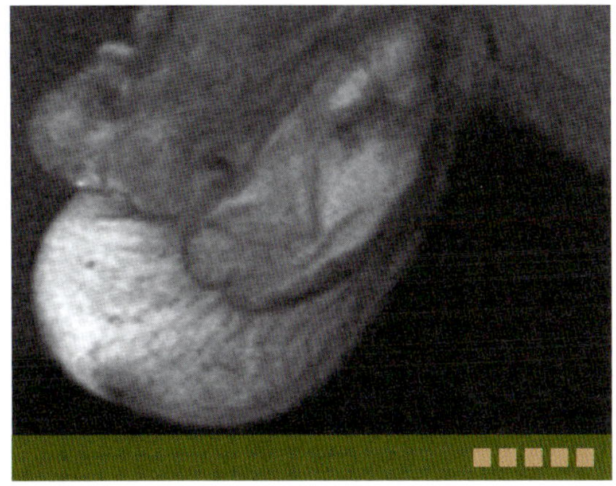

C. In a different patient, sagittal T2-WI shows a heterogeneous predominately hyperintense mass extending from distal penile shaft and glans as a result of squamous penile cancer.

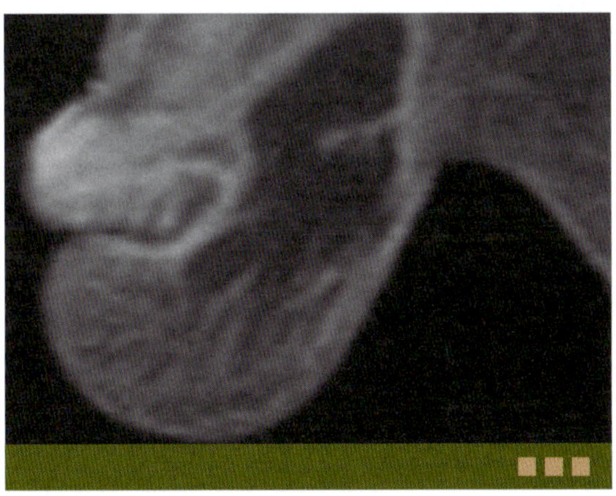

D. Sagittal contrast-enhanced T1-FS MR show the mass enhances heterogeneously and has large area of necrosis.

DIFFERENTIAL DIAGNOSES IMAGES (E-G)

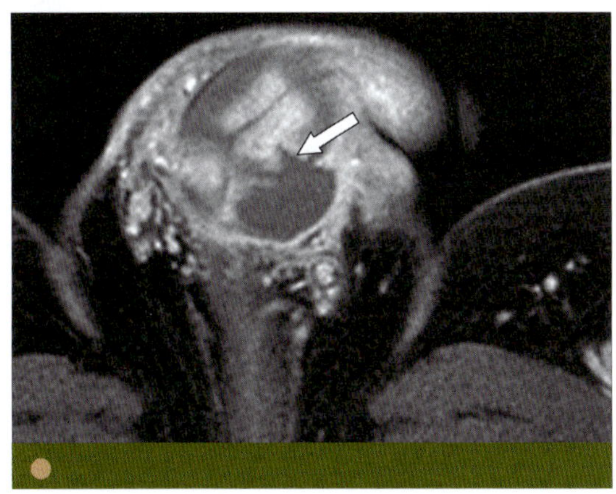

E. Penile fracture: Axial contrast-enhanced T1-WI shows a fracture of the tunica albuginea of the corpus cavernosum (arrow) as discontinuity of the tunica albuginea.

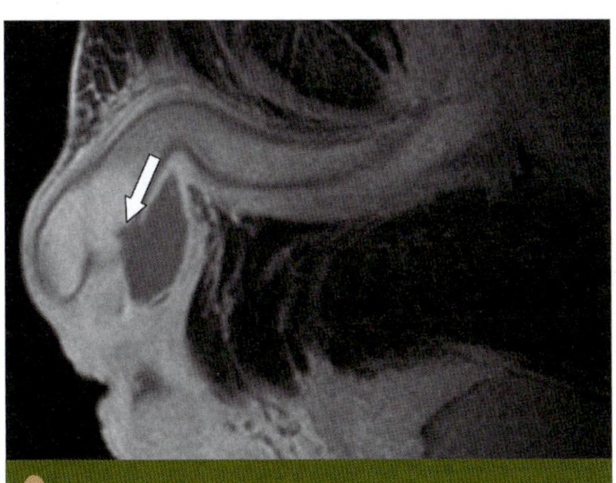

F. Penile fracture: Sagittal contrast-enhanced T1-WI shows linear disruption of the tunica albuginea (arrow) with adjacent hematoma.

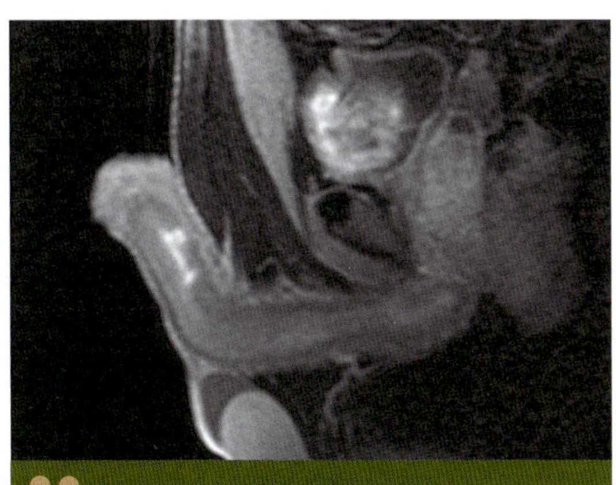

G. Peyronie disease: Sagittal contrast-enhanced T1-WI shows linear enhancement of fibrous plaque because of active disease. The abnormality involves the tunica and is not an enhancing mass unlike penile cancer.

IMAGE KEY

Common

Rare

Typical

Unusual

12–9 Penile Fracture

Frank H. Miller

PRESENTATION

"Crack" during sexual intercourse with marked penile swelling and erythema; sudden pain and instantaneous loss of erection; hematuria and dysuria may occur if there is associated urethral injury.

FINDINGS

Fracture of the tunica albuginea of the corpus cavernosum seen as discontinuity of the tunica albuginea.

DIFFERENTIAL DIAGNOSES

- *Peyronie disease*: Different history and imaging findings (plaques on ultrasound and MR).
- *Penile cancer*: Different history and imaging findings (solid mass and not history of trauma).

COMMENTS

Penile fracture consists of rupture of the corpus cavernosum and tunica albuginea and sometimes of the corpus spongiosum and urethra. It is usually caused by trauma to the erect penis during sexual intercourse or masturbation. An audible crack, sudden onset of pain, swelling, and loss of erection and deviation of the penis toward the side opposite the injury are characteristic clinical findings. Penile fracture is a urologic emergency that requires prompt surgical treatment to avoid complications such as penile curvature, fibrosis and erectile dysfunction.

MRI is the best imaging study to evaluate penile fracture. MR has excellent soft tissue contrast and the advantage of multi-planar imaging. It is helpful to identify the site and severity of the lesion for surgical planning and to assess urethral injury. MRI shows discontinuity of the hypointense T2-weighted tunica albuginea and Buck fascia. The tear is generally in the ventral portion of the corpus cavernosum. There may be associated hematoma. Gadolinium-enhanced MR may delineate the tunica tear. A tear in the tunica albuginea or disruption of the urethra may require surgical repair. Urethral injuries may be seen on MR but are better evaluated on retrograde urethrogram. Corpus cavernosum and/or extra-tunical hematomas as well as subcutaneous edema are also usually present but generally do not require surgery. Ultrasound may be performed for the diagnosis but may be difficult because of severe pain and is not as reliable as MR.

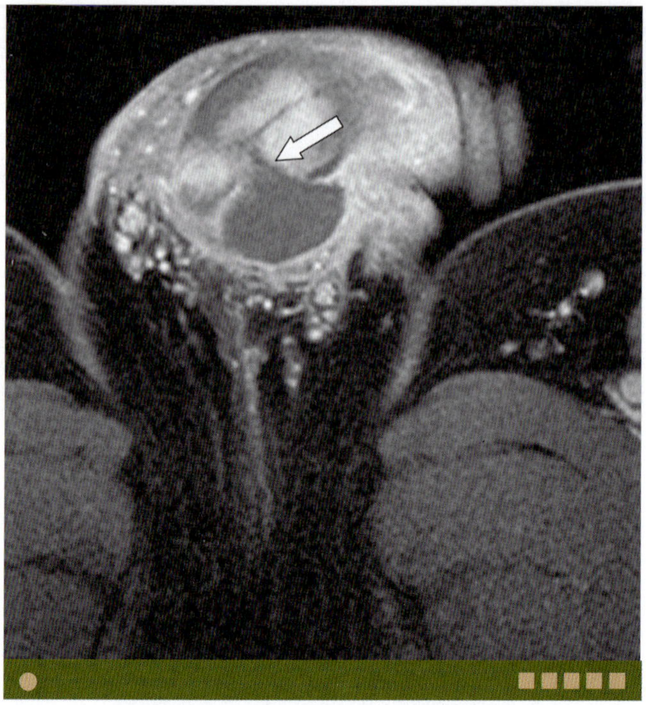

A. Fracture of the tunica albuginea in patients with pain following vigorous sexual intercourse. Axial contrast-enhanced T1-WI shows a fracture of the tunica albuginea of the corpus cavernosum as discontinuity of the tunica albuginea.

PEARLS

- **Penile fracture is a urologic emergency that requires prompt surgical treatment.**
- **MR is the best method to evaluate for penile fractures.**
- **Penile fractures are seen as discontinuity of the hypointense tunica albuginea.**
- **MR can be helpful to show which patients have disruption of the tunica albuginea and require surgery.**
- **Tears are generally seen in the ventral portion of the corpus cavernosum.**

ADDITIONAL IMAGES (B-E)

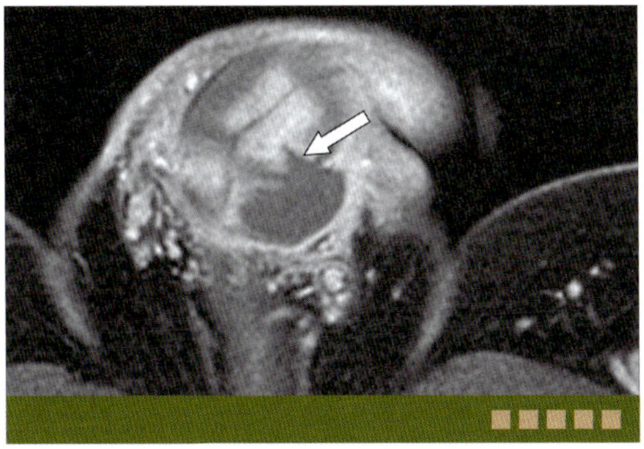

B. Axial contrast-enhanced T1-WI shows a discontinuity of the hypointense tunica albuginea (arrow) because of tear with adjacent fluid collection.

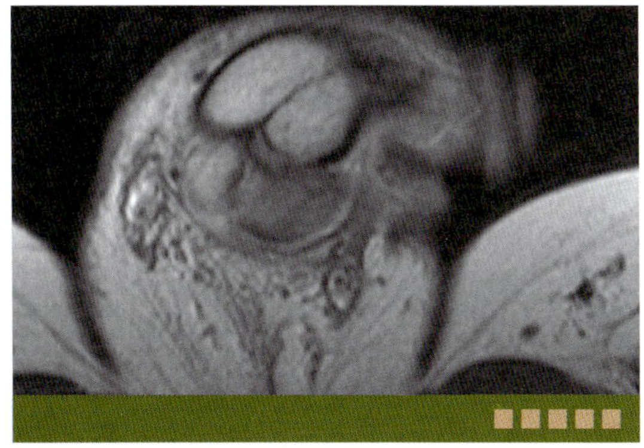

C. Axial T2-WI shows the adjacent hematoma that measures approximately 3 cm.

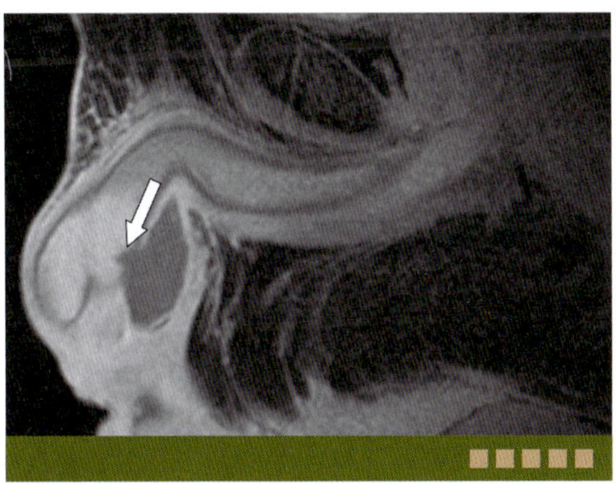

D. Sagittal contrast-enhanced T1-WI shows linear disruption of the tunica albuginea (arrow) with adjacent hematoma.

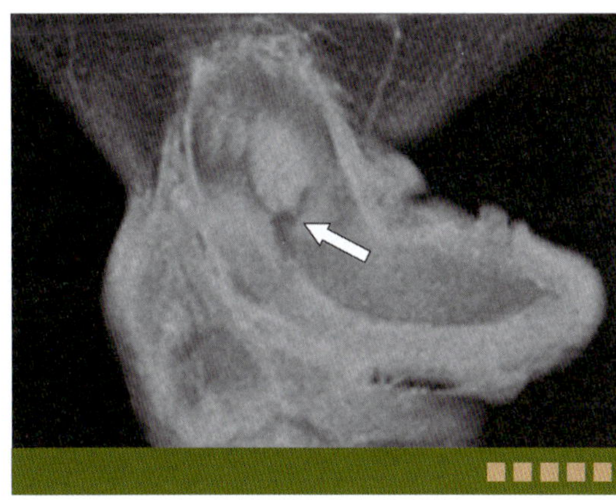

E. Coronal contrast-enhanced T1-WI shows a jagged line caused by fracture (arrow). The penis is deviated to the left.

DIFFERENTIAL DIAGNOSES IMAGES (F-G)

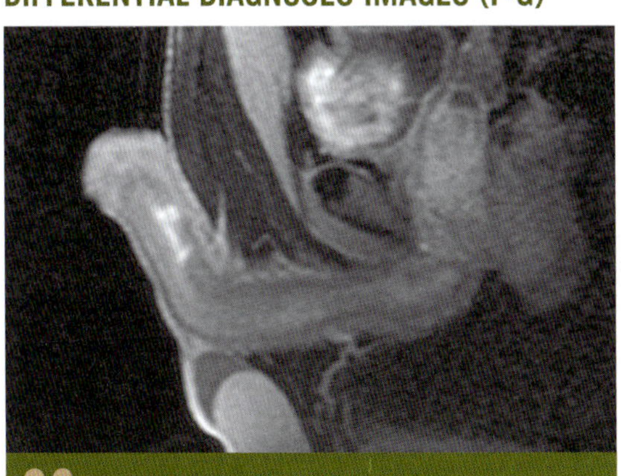

F. Peyronie disease: Sagittal contrast-enhanced T1-WI shows linear enhancement of fibrous plaque caused by active disease. No fracture is seen.

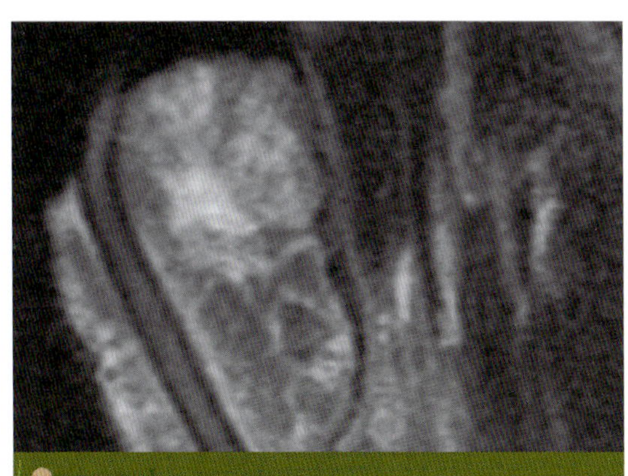

G. Penile cancer: Sagittal contrast-enhanced T1-WI shows a large enhancing heterogeneous mass from penile cancer.

IMAGE KEY

Common

Rare

Typical

Unusual

12–10 Peyronie Disease

Frank H. Miller

PRESENTATION

Penile pain, penile curvature, and erectile dysfunction.

FINDINGS

Echogenic foci with shadowing because of calcifications related to Peyronie disease.

DIFFERENTIAL DIAGNOSES

- Localized penile fibrosis from trauma or cavernous injections.
- *Penile fracture*: Associated history of trauma or injury and associated findings of trauma on imaging studies.
- *Penile tumor*: Mass seen on imaging studies.

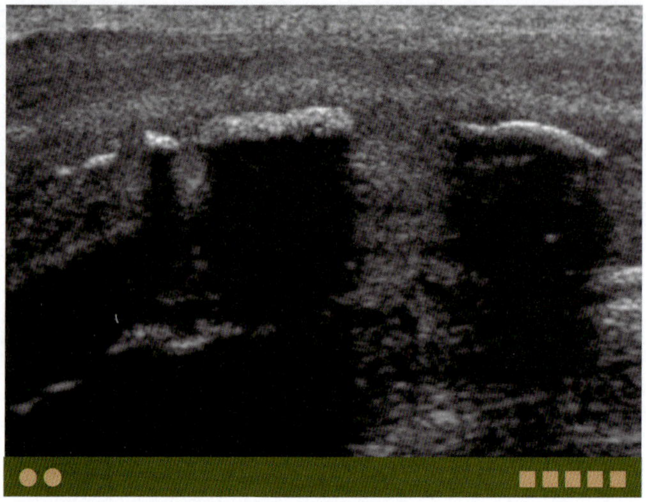

A. Longitudinal sonogram shows hyperechoic plaques because of calcifications with posterior shadowing.

COMMENTS

Peyronie disease is an acquired inflammatory disorder of the tunica albuginea leading to the formation of fibrotic plaques, which may or may not be calcified. The plaques can be associated with penile curvature, erectile dysfunction and pain on erection. The early stages of Peyronie disease include inflammation beneath the tunica albuginea with fibroblast proliferation creating a thickened plaque of fibrous tissue in the tunica albuginea and leading to calcifications.

Penile plaques in Peyronie disease are usually identified by palpation and do not require imaging; however, those located at the penile base may not be palpable and may require MRI for diagnosis. Ultrasound is generally the preferred method for detection of plaques and shows calcifications which is not seen on MR. Ultrasound is readily available and allows examining the patient at the time of the examination. Ultrasound confirms that the palpable abnormality correlates with the imaging findings which are generally seen as calcifications and not as a mass. The ultrasound examination should be performed with a high resolution linear transducer. Because the calcifications are seen as low signal intensity on MR, they may not be seen on T1 and T2-WI easily. The administration of IV gadolinium helps identify enhancement, which is felt to relate to peri-plaque enhancement from "inflammatory" foci of Peyronie. Enhancing plaques have been suggested to show active inflammation, which is a potential advantage of MR although not always of clinical relevance in affecting therapy.

PEARLS

- **The plaques of Peyronie disease can be associated with penile curvature, erectile dysfunction and painful erection.**
- **The diagnosis of Peyronie disease is generally made by palpation.**
- **High-resolution ultrasound is the best method to show calcifications associated with the fibrotic plaques.**
- **MR shows the plaques as enhancing lesions which suggest active inflammation.**

ADDITIONAL IMAGES (B-D)

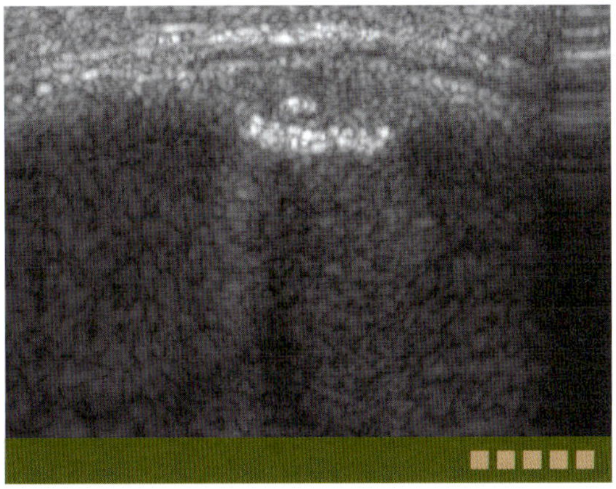

B. Transverse sonogram shows hyperechoic plaques involving tunica albuginea because of calcifications with posterior shadowing.

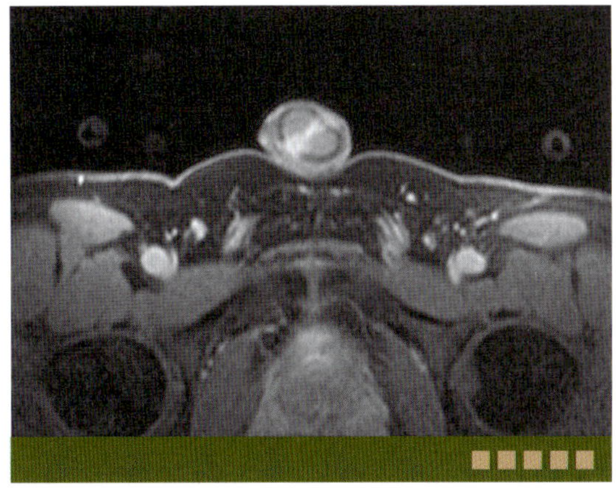

C. Axial contrast-enhanced T1-WI shows enhancement of the plaques from Peyronie disease.

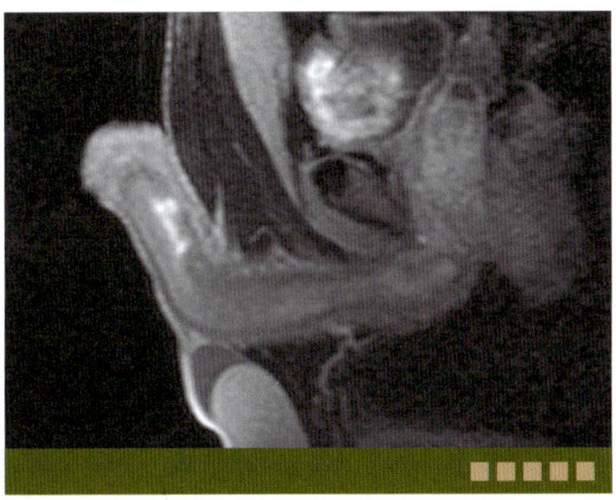

D. Sagittal contrast-enhanced T1-WI shows linear enhancement of fibrous plaque from active disease.

DIFFERENTIAL DIAGNOSES IMAGES (E-G)

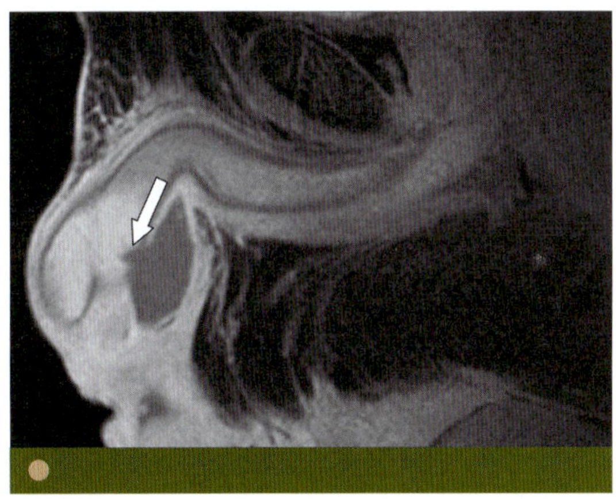

E. Penile fracture: Sagittal contrast-enhanced T1-WI shows a penile fracture (arrow) with adjacent hematoma in patient with trauma.

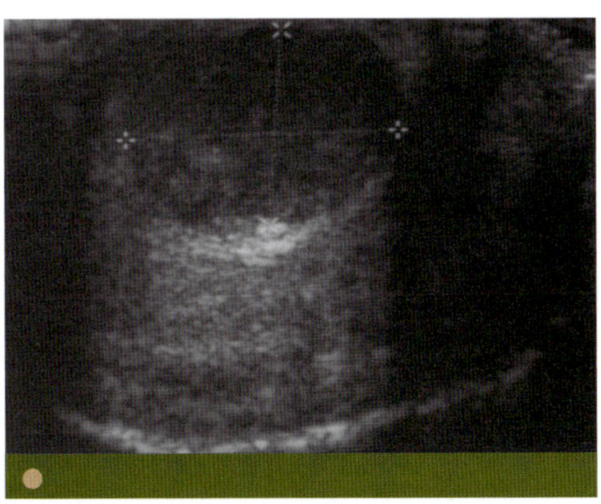

F. Penile leiomyosarcoma: Longitudinal sonogram shows a mass involving the corporus spongiosum.

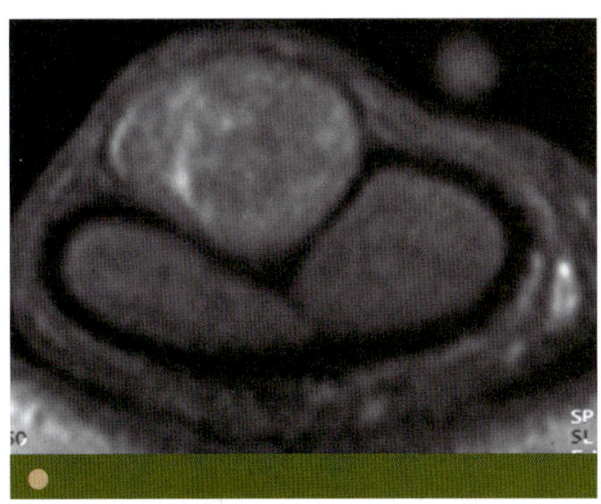

G. Penile leiomyosarcoma: Axial contrast-enhanced T1-WI shows the enhancing mass involving the corporus spongiosum.

IMAGE KEY

Common

Rare

Typical

Unusual

CHAPTER 13

SCROTUM

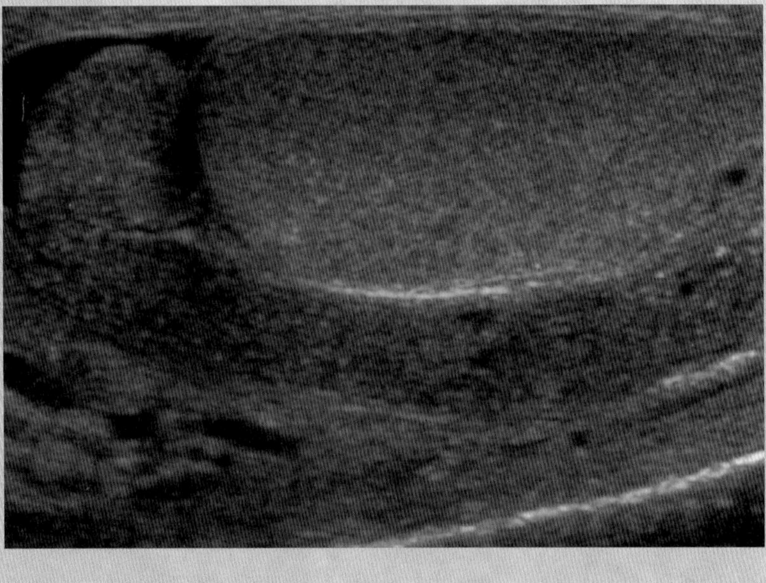

13–1 Epididymitis

Frank H. Miller

PRESENTATION

Acute scrotal pain in adolescent and adults; may be associated fever, dysuria, or pyuria.

FINDINGS

Enlarged, hypoechoic epididymis with increased flow.

DIFFERENTIAL DIAGNOSES

- *Spermatoceles*: Generally asymptomic unlike epididymitis; cysts of epididymal head.
- *Adenomatoid tumor*: Generally asymptomatic unlike epididymitis; solid extratesticular lesion.
- *Varicocele*: Different symptoms; serpigenous vessels adjacent to testis.

COMMENTS

Epididymitis is the most common cause of intrascrotal inflammation in postpubertal men. Descending infection, most often by urinary tract organisms from the bladder or prostate most often causes acute epididymitis. It most commonly is associated with *Escherichia coli*, *Pseudomonas*, *Proteus mirabilis*, *Chlamydia trachomatis* and *Neisseria gonorrhoeae*. Epididymitis involves the adjacent testes in 20% to 40% of patients and can be focal or diffuse. Patients with epididymitis present with fever, scrotal pain, and swelling. There is often dysuria and pyuria.

Ultrasound is the best method to evaluate the scrotum and testes in the setting of acute pain. Sonographic findings include enlarged and heterogeneous, mainly hypoechoic, epididymis and spermatic cord, reactive hydrocele, and scrotal skin thickening. Epididymitis is often associated with orchitis. Color and power Doppler show hyperemia resulting from inflammation as increased blood flow to the epididymis and testis, which helps distinguish it from complete torsion where there is absence of flow. Involvement may be seen in the entire epididymis or only a portion because of epididymitis. Focal hypoechoic or anechoic areas may develop as a result of abscesses. When chronic, the epididymis may become hyperechoic and develop calcifications. When treated early with antibiotics, patients have an excellent outcome. When severe, epididymo-orchitis may lead to ischemia and testicular infarction because of compression of the testicular vessels from epididymal inflammation.

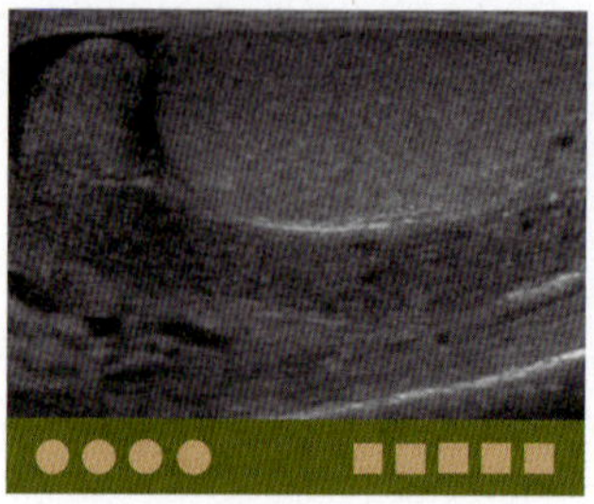

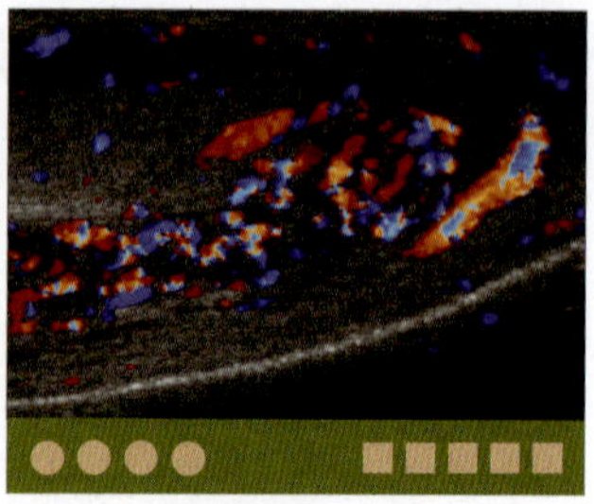

A. Epididymitis. Longitudinal sonogram shows enlarged hypoechoic epididymis.
B. Epididymitis. Color Doppler sonogram in the same patient shows increased flow from hyperemia and inflammation.

PEARLS

- **Epididymitis is the most common cause of intrascrotal inflammation.**
- **Gray scale ultrasound shows an enlarged epididymis, which generally is hypoechoic.**
- **Color Doppler is helpful to show hyperemia as increased flow in the involved epididymis.**
- **Can distinguish from torsion which on color Doppler is generally seen as absent flow.**

ADDITIONAL IMAGES (C-D)

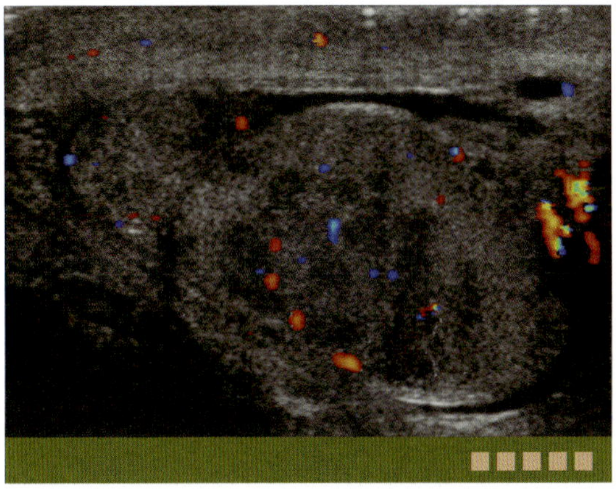

C. Left epididymo-orchitis. Longitudinal sonogram in different patient shows enlarged and hypoechoic epididymis with focal area of hypoechogenicity in the testes as a result of orchitis. The involvement of the testis may mimic a cancer.

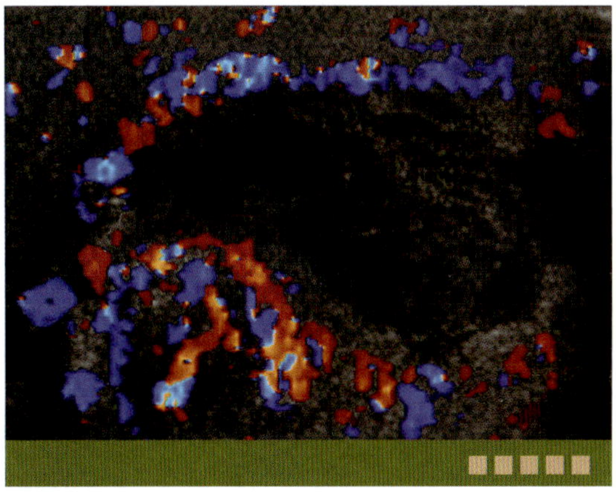

D. Epididymitis with developing abscess. Longitudinal sonogram in different patient shows enlarged epididymis with increased flow and hypoechoic area caused by developing abscess.

DIFFERENTIAL DIAGNOSES IMAGES (E-F)

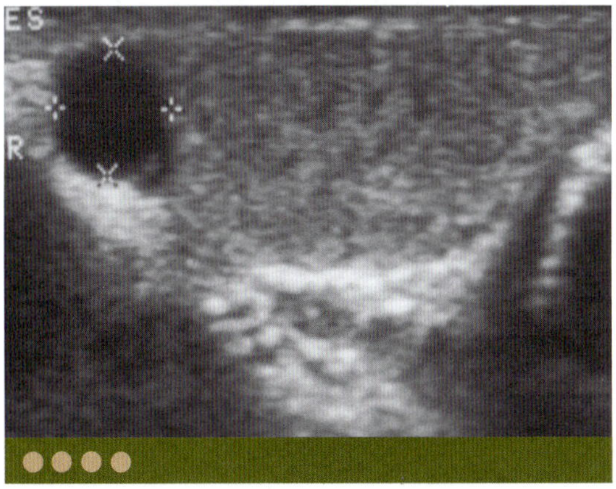

E. Spermatocele: Transverse sonogram shows anechoic fluid collection that is extratesticular as a result of spermatocele in epididymal head. Spermatocele tend to be asymptomatic.

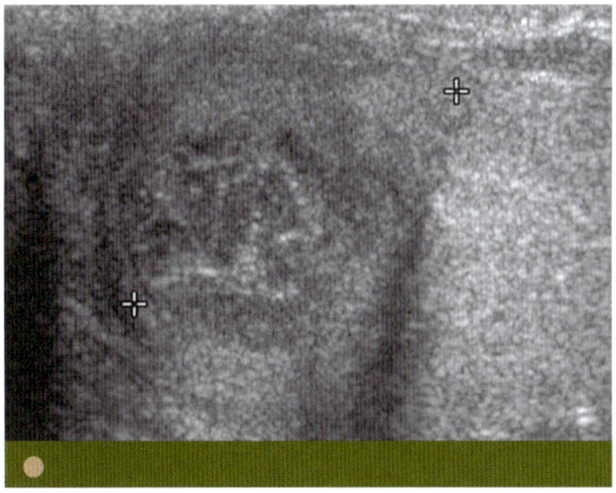

F. Adenomatoid tumor: Transverse sonogram shows solid lesion in the right epididymis which differs from epididymitis. They also have different clinical presentations.

IMAGE KEY

Common

Rare

Typical

Unusual

13–2 Epididymal Abscess

Paul Nikolaidis

PRESENTATION

Unresolved or persistent severe epididymitis, fever, and palpable scrotal mass.

FINDINGS

Sonogram shows a small hypoechoic, avascular epididymal lesion in the background of an enlarged heterogeneous epididymis with marked increase in vascularity.

DIFFERENTIAL DIAGNOSES

- *Epididymal neoplasms (ie, adenomatoid tumor)*: No significant hyperemia should be seen in the surrounding epididymis; usually painless, palpable lesions.
- *Epididymal cyst*: Very common and generally anechoic; there should be no clinical signs of infection. The surrounding normal epididymis should not be hyperemic.
- *Epididymal hematoma*: A rare entity usually with a classic reticular pattern and internal linear echoes; there should be no secondary signs of infection. Often there is a history of trauma.

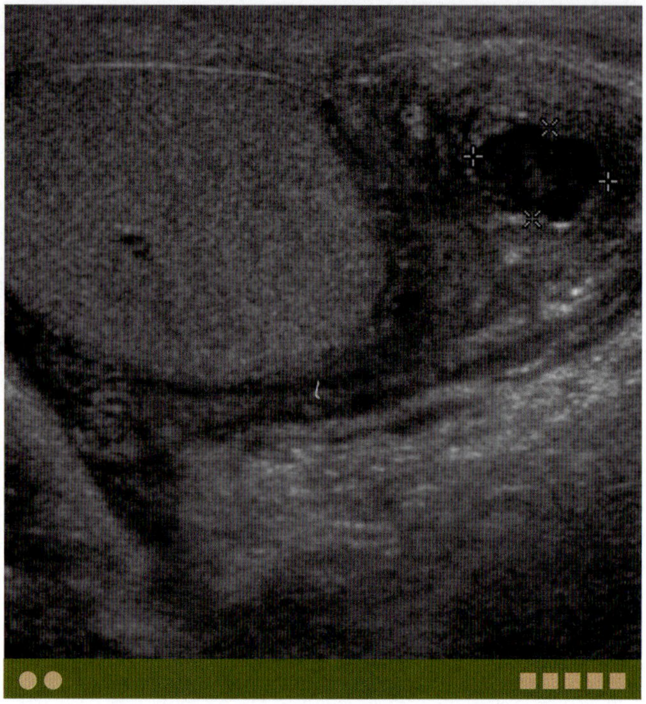

A. Longitudinal sonogram shows a central hypoechoic lesion within the epididymis (calipers). The surrounding epididymis is enlarged and heterogeneous.

COMMENTS

Epididymal abscesses are an uncommon complication of epididymitis, and may occur in cases of severe or untreated epididymitis. Usual causative organisms are *C trachomatis* and *N gonorrhoeae* in younger men and *E coli* or *P mirabilis* in patients over 35. Patients typically present with signs and symptoms of infection. The scrotum is usually erythematous, inflamed, and tender. Epididymal abscesses should be considered in patients not improving on antibiotics.

On sonography, they appear as either well-circumscribed or ill-defined anechoic or hypoechoic areas that may mimic a neoplasm or an area of infarction. However, color flow and Doppler imaging should show a marked increase in vascularity around the lesion, indicative of its inflammatory nature. Concomitant sonographic findings usually include an enlarged and heterogeneous epididymis with focal areas of decreased or mixed echogenicity. In addition, scrotal wall thickening, testicular heterogeneity or increased vascularity caused by a superimposed orchitis, a hydrocele, or pyocele may be present.

Complications include rupture, in addition to ischemia or infarction. Surgical drainage is often the treatment of choice.

PEARLS

- **Usually occurs in cases of severe or untreated epididymitis.**
- **On gray-scale sonography, they are anechoic or hypoechoic and may mimic a neoplasm, infarction, or hematoma.**
- **Color Doppler imaging helps make the diagnosis by showing a marked increase in vascularity surrounding the lesion.**
- **Complications include rupture and testicular ischemia or infarction.**

ADDITIONAL IMAGES (B-D)

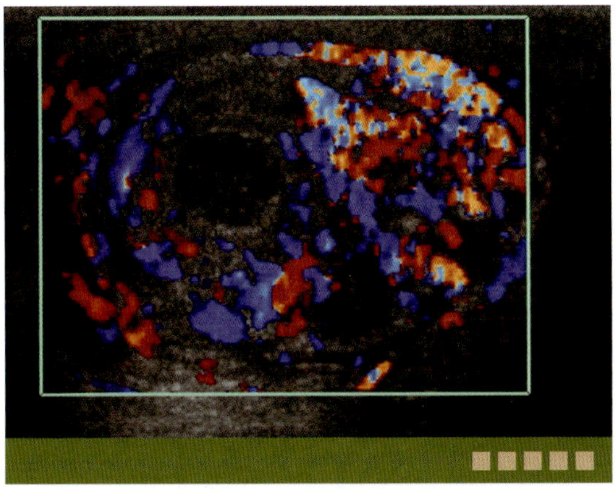

B. Transverse sonogram with color Doppler shows the small epididymal abscess to be avascular. The surrounding epididymis is markedly hypervascular.

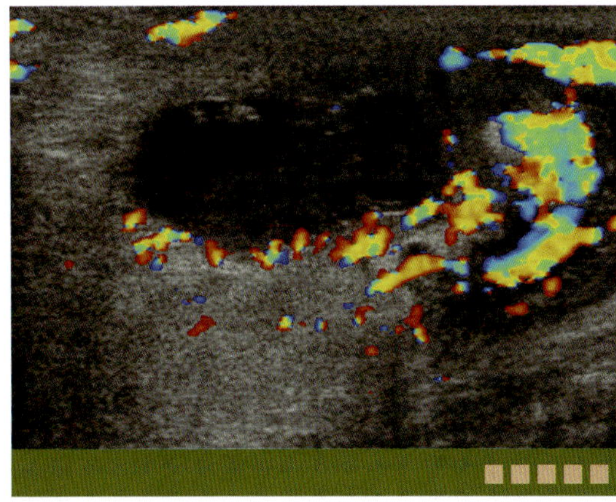

C. Longitudinal sonogram with color Doppler on a different patient shows a hypoechoic, avascular lesion in the tail of the epididymis. The surrounding tissue is hyperemic.

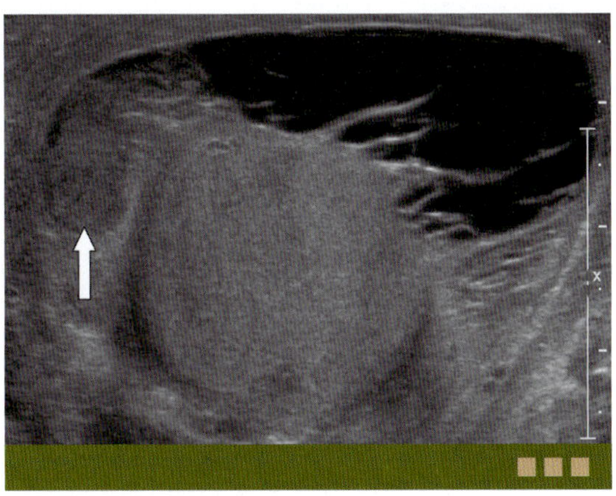

D. Transverse sonogram in another patient shows a mildly hypoechoic lesion within the epididymis (arrow). The patient also had a complex hydrocele and a concomitant orchitis. This subsequently developed into an epididymal abscess.

DIFFERENTIAL DIAGNOSES IMAGES (E-G)

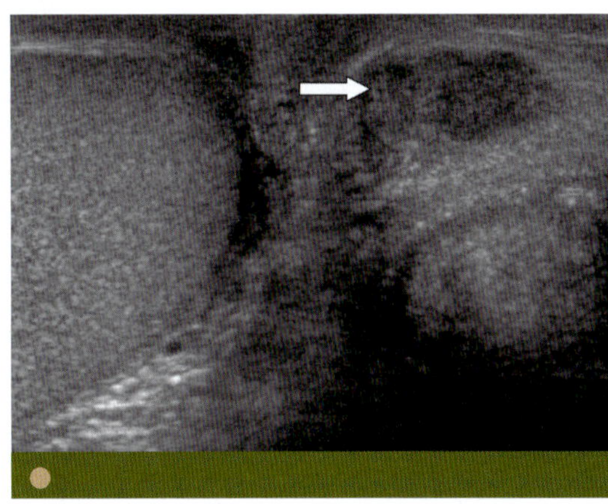

E. Adenomatoid tumor: Transverse sonogram in a patient with a palpable abnormality shows a solid, hypoechoic epididymal lesion (arrow). Note the absence of surrounding inflammatory changes.

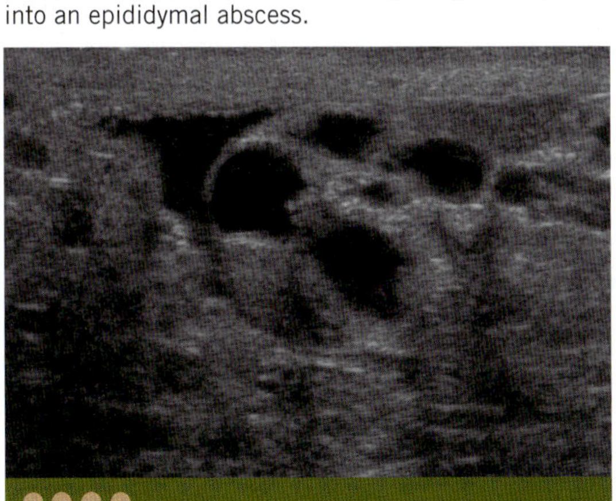

F. Epididymal cysts: Transverse sonogram in a patient with a palpable lump shows multiple anechoic epididymal lesions. The patient was asymptomatic. These have classic features of simple cysts.

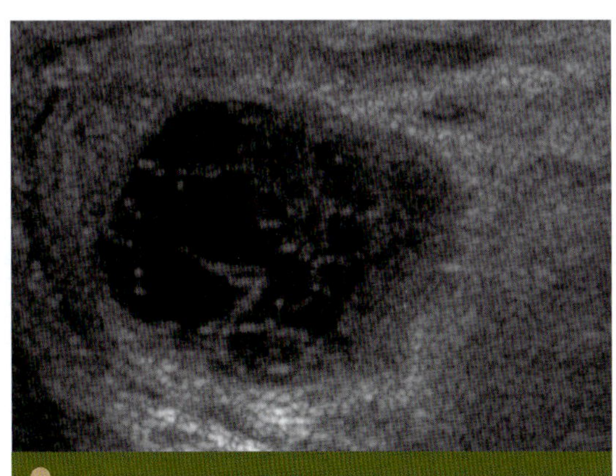

G. Epididymal hematoma: Transverse sonogram in a patient with history of testicular injury shows a hypoechoic lesion in the head of the epididymis. It shows a reticular pattern and internal linear echoes, features compatible with a hematoma. Follow-up sonogram in three months confirmed resolution.

IMAGE KEY

Common

●●●●●
●●●●
●●●
●●
●

Rare

Typical

■■■■■
■■■■
■■■
■■
■

Unusual

13-3 Orchitis

Frank H. Miller

PRESENTATION

Acute scrotal pain; may be associated nausea and fever.

FINDINGS

Enlarged, hypoechoic testes with increased flow.

DIFFERENTIAL DIAGNOSES

- *Torsion*: Can have similar symptoms, can be usually distinguished on the basis of imaging as absent flow, although intermittent or incomplete torsion can have flow and severe epididymo-orchitis can lead to infarction.
- *Tumor*: Less common cause of pain, can be distinguished on ultrasound as focal masses.
- *Leukemia and lymphoma*: Rare mimicker, usually bilateral, while infection is often unilateral. Lymphoma can look similar on imaging but is generally painless and will not resolve with antibiotic therapy.
- *Trauma*: Can distinguish generally based on history and clinical findings.

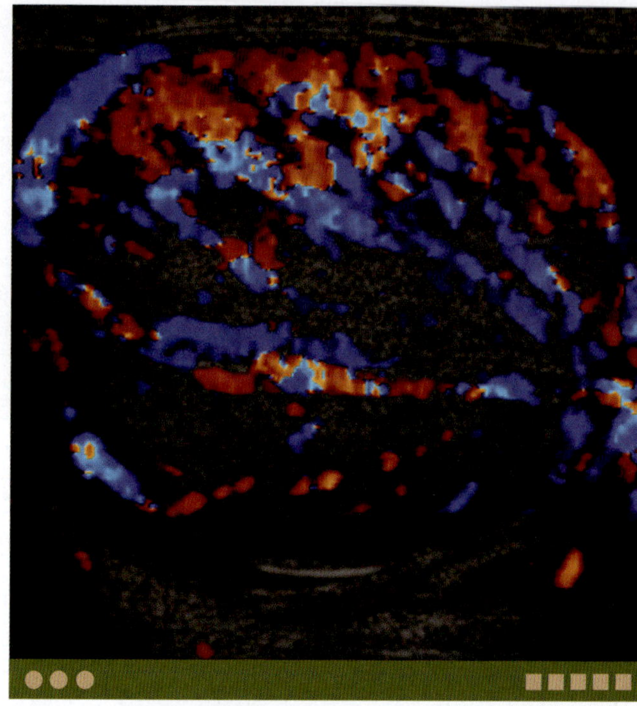

A. Transverse color Doppler sonogram shows increased flow within the testis because of orchitis.

COMMENTS

Orchitis is the most common cause of acute scrotum in adolescents and adult males. Descending infection, most often by urinary tract organisms, usually causes acute epididymitis. In older patients and children, it is often caused by infections that lead to bacteriuria, *E coli* and *P mirabilis*. In sexually active men, epididimo-orchitis is often caused by sexually transmitted organisms such as *C trachomatis* and *N gonorrhoeae*. Orchitis is generally preceded by and associated with epididymitis. Isolated orchitis is uncommon and generally caused by viruses. Mumps orchitis caused by paramyxovirus may be seen as orchitis without epididymitis and may be bilateral. Granulomatous disease including tuberculosis, brucellosis, and sarcoidosis are less common causes of orchitis especially in the United States.

Ultrasound is the best method to evaluate the scrotum in the setting of acute pain. Sonographic findings include enlarged and heterogeneous mainly hypoechoic testes, reactive hydrocele, and scrotal skin thickening. Color Doppler show hyperemia caused by inflammation as increased blood flow to the testis, which helps distinguish it from complete torsion where there is absence of flow. An enlarged, hypoechoic ipsilateral epididymis with increased flow is often associated with orchitis and may help distinguish it from tumor. Gray scale sonography can be normal in orchitis while the color Doppler is abnormal emphasizing the importance of Doppler. It is helpful to compare the suspected abnormal testis with the normal testis to detect subtle cases. Spectral Doppler showing decreased vascular resistance is useful for diagnosis. Multiple hypoechoic areas may be seen in the testicular parenchyma, mimicking tumor. Focal hypoechoic areas may develop because of abscesses. Follow-up sonography to demonstrate resolution of the findings and confirm infection may be required when it is difficult to distinguish from tumor. Symptoms usually resolve with antibiotics when bacterial in origin. When severe, epididymo-orchitis may lead to ischemia and testicular infarction. Following resolution of inflammation, the testis may atrophy.

PEARLS

- **Orchitis is the most common cause of acute scrotum in adolescent and young men.**
- **Gray scale ultrasound shows an enlarged testis that generally is hypoechoic.**
- **Color Doppler is helpful to show hyperemia as increased flow in the involved testis.**
- **Can distinguish from torsion that on color Doppler is generally seen as absent flow.**
- **Focal orchitis may be difficult to distinguish on imaging from neoplasm.**
- **The epididymis often has associated involvement with orchitis.**

ADDITIONAL IMAGES (B-C)

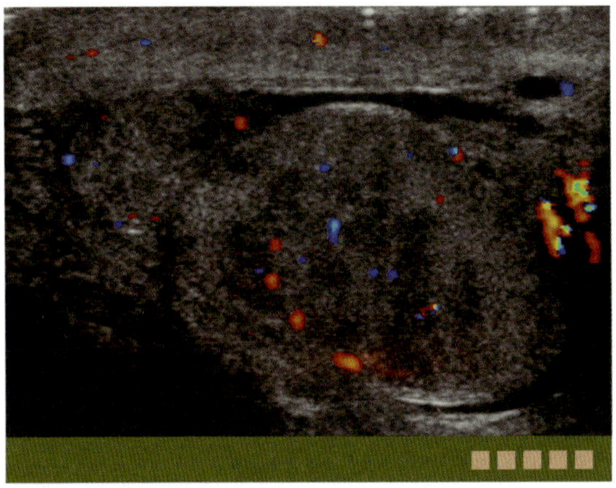

B. Left epididymo-orchitis: Longitudinal sonogram in different patient shows enlarged and hypoechoic epididymis with focal area of hypoechogenicity in the testes caused by orchitis. The involvement of the testis may mimic a cancer.

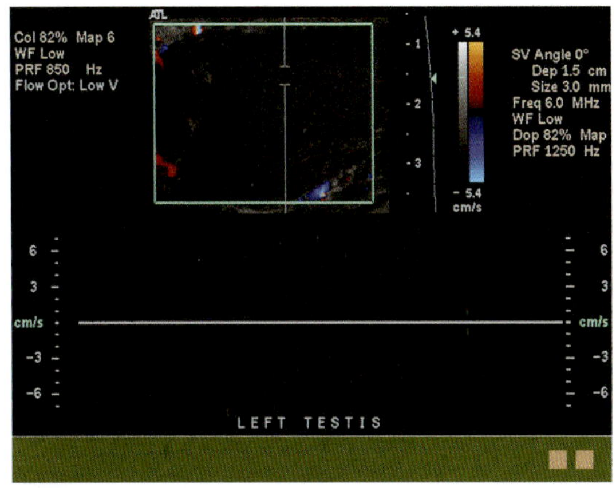

C. Ischemia caused by orchitis: Sagittal color Doppler image of the left testis shows absence of flow in this patient with the clinical diagnosis of severe orchitis.

DIFFERENTIAL DIAGNOSES IMAGES (D-F)

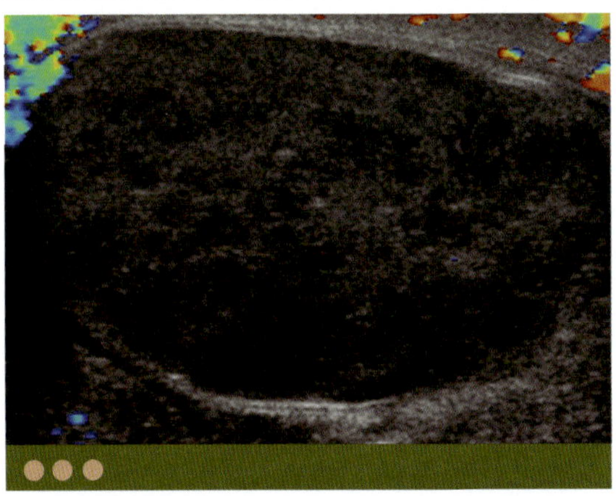

D. Testicular ischemia caused by torsion: Color Doppler image of the right testis shows heterogeneous hypoechoic appearance with lack of flow because of torsion.

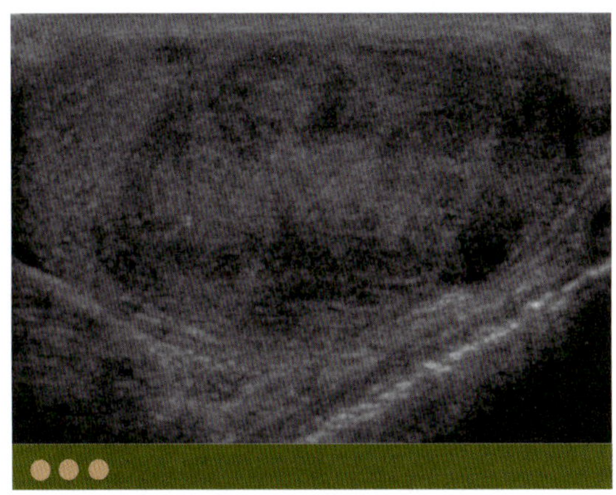

E. Seminoma: Longitudinal sonogram shows large hypoechoic mass, which replaces large part of the testis.

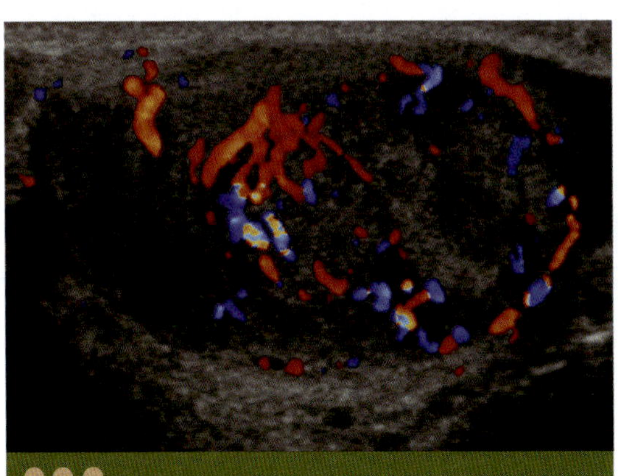

F. Seminoma: Color Doppler image in the same patient shows increased flow within the seminoma. Tumors tend to be more focal masses. If unable to distinguish tumor from focal orchitis, then short interval follow-up sonogram may be considered.

IMAGE KEY

Common

Rare

Typical

Unusual

13–4 Tuberculous Epididymitis and Orchitis

Paul Nikolaidis

PRESENTATION

Scrotal swelling and pain, fever, night sweats.

FINDINGS

Sonography shows an enlarged and hypoechoic epididymis, with increased vascularity.

DIFFERENTIAL DIAGNOSES

- *Pyogenic epididymo-orchitis*: Lack of response to conventional antibiotics may aid in diagnosis of TB. A combination of markedly heterogeneous echotexture, scrotal skin thickening, abscess formation, extratesticular calcifications, and scrotal sinus tracts suggest tuberculous over pyogenic epididymo-orchitis.
- *Lymphoma*: A rare mimic; may differentiate by clinical history, sometimes biopsy is necessary.
- *Testicular neoplasms*: Involvement with TB of only the testicle is extremely rare, but in those instances, it may be difficult to differentiate from tumor.

COMMENTS

Tuberculous epididymo-orchitis is uncommon. The GU tract is the most frequent site of extrapulmonary involvement with TB. The kidneys are typically the first organ affected in the genitourinary system. Epididymal and testicular involvement occur after retrograde seeding of the epididymis (initially the tail) from the prostate or seminal vesicles. Tuberculous involvement of the testicle is almost always secondary to spread from the epididymis. Primary involvement of only the testicle is exceedingly rare and would be difficult to differentiate from a testicular tumor. Involvement of both the epididymis and testicle suggests infection as the cause, except for lymphoma in rare occasions where the epididymis is also involved.

Sonographically, the affected epididymis, or portion thereof, appears enlarged. Echogenicity and echotexture have been described as having several patterns: diffusely heterogeneous, nodular heterogeneous, and less commonly diffusely homogeneous and hypoechoic. The marked sonographic heterogeneity in tuberculous epididymitis is because of the variety of underlying pathologic components, including caseation necrosis, fibrosis, granuloma formation, and fibrosis.

Other possible sonographic findings of tuberculous epididymitis include scrotal wall thickening, abscess formation, and the presence of a hydrocele. It has been reported that

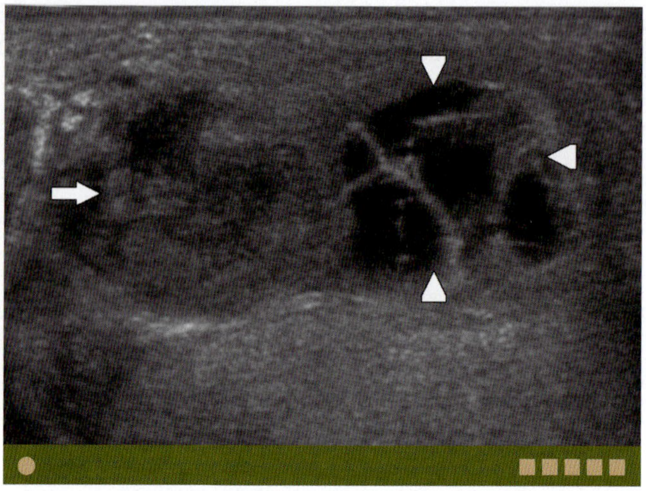

A. Longitudinal sonogram of the scrotum shows an enlarged, heterogeneous epididymis (arrow). In addition, there is an adjacent complex septated collection representing a small abscess (arrowheads). There was no significant associated heterogeneity in the testicular echotexture.

tuberculous epididymitis preferentially involves the tail of the epididymis. When the testicle is also involved, it is usually enlarged and hypoechoic with ill-defined hypoechoic foci or focal masses. Intrascrotal extratesticular calcifications and scrotal sinus tracts to the skin can also be seen.

The lack of a rapid response to treatment with conventional antibiotics should suggest TB, especially if there is a history of tuberculous infection in other organs.

PEARLS

- **Epididymal involvement in TB occurs after retrograde seeding of the epididymis (initially the tail) from the prostate or seminal vesicles.**
- **The affected epididymis is enlarged and quite heterogeneous.**
- **The testes are usually not involved, particularly in the absence of epididymal involvement.**
- **There may be scrotal skin thickening, abscess formation, extratesticular calcifications and scrotal sinus tracts in TB of the scrotum.**
- **A lack of any response to conventional antibiotics should suggest TB.**

ADDITIONAL IMAGES (B-D)

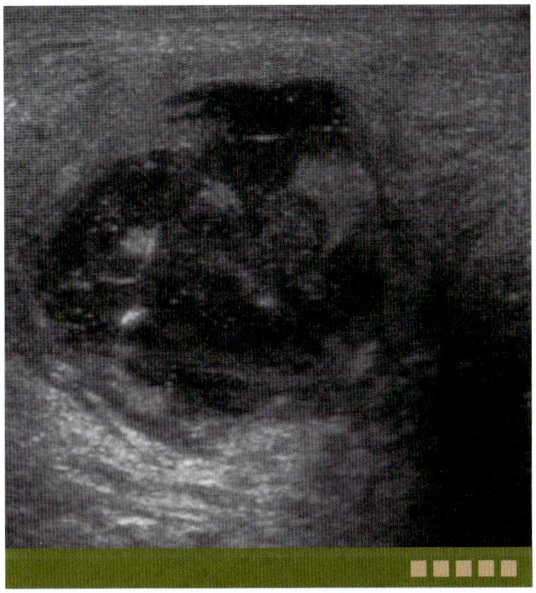

B. Transverse sonogram on the same patient shows an additional scrotal wall abscess. Scrotal wall thickening, abscess formation, and sinus tracts are often seen in tuberculous infection.

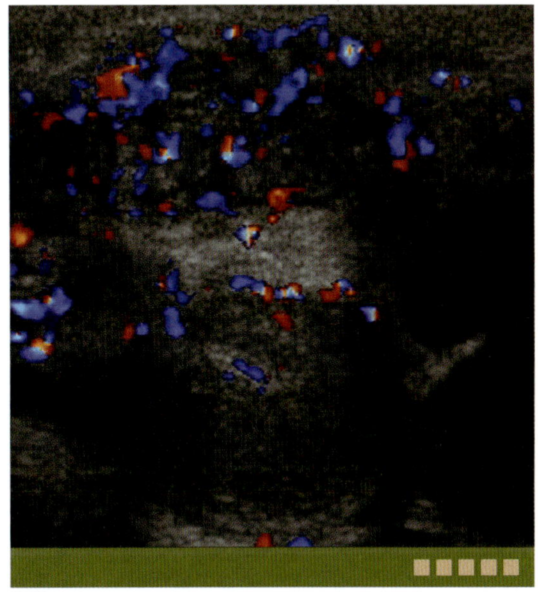

C. Longitudinal color Doppler sonogram in another patient shows an enlarged and hypoechoic left epididymis. There is also increased vascularity. This did not respond to several courses of conventional antibiotics.

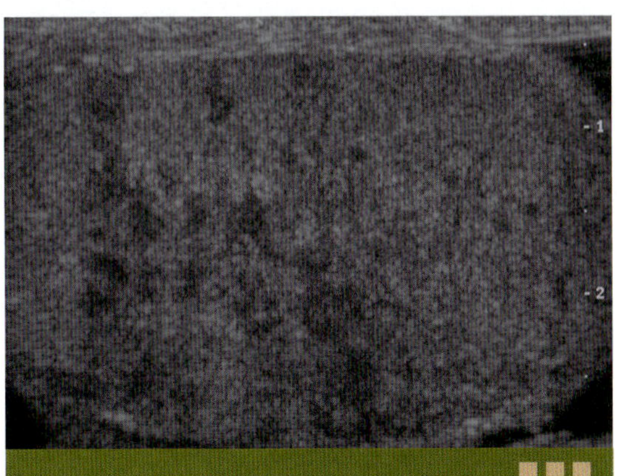

D. Transverse sonogram of the left testicle in the same patient shows marked heterogeneity and multiple small focal hypoechoic nodules. Tuberculous infection spread from the epididymis to the testicle in this patient.

DIFFERENTIAL DIAGNOSES IMAGE

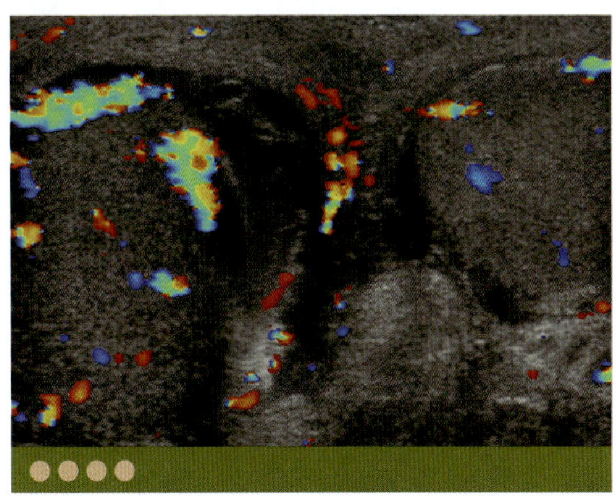

E. Acute bacterial (nontuberculous) epididymo-orchitis: Transverse sonogram with color Doppler shows enlargement and heterogeneity of the right epididymis and testis. Gonococcal infection was identified as the cause. The patient improved on antibiotics.

IMAGE KEY

Common
●●●●●
●●●●
●●●
●●
●
Rare

Typical
■■■■■
■■■■
■■■
■■
■
Unusual

13–5 Testicular Infarction Caused by Acute Infection

Paul Nikolaidis

PRESENTATION

Scrotal pain, erythema, or swelling.

FINDINGS

Color Doppler sonogram shows complete absence of flow within an abnormal-appearing right testicle.

DIFFERENTIAL DIAGNOSIS

- *Testicular torsion*: Even though patients with torsion typically present with acute onset of pain and swelling and no preceding signs of infection, differentiation may be difficult.

COMMENTS

Testicular infarction is rare but may occur in sickle cell disease, polycythemia vera, trauma, vasculitis, or in the acute phase of testicular infection or inflammation. When severe, epididymitis and/or epididymo-orchitis may cause compression of the testicular vasculature and can compromise blood flow to the testis.

Testicular infarction, which may be focal or global, is typically hypoechoic on sonography, with absence of color Doppler flow. Focal intratesticular infarction may mimic a tumor or an abscess. In addition to absence of intratesticular color Doppler flow, increased flow is often seen in the paratesticular tissues. A surrounding hyperechoic or hypoechoic rind may be seen encircling the affected testis. Differentiating testicular infarction secondary to acute epididymitis or epididymo-orchitis from subacute testicular torsion may not be possible unless a patient has clinical and/or sonographic findings typical of acute inflammation prior to developing infarction. In both entities, there is absence of intratesticular color Doppler flow often with increased flow in the paratesticular tissues.

Early diagnosis of vascular compromise and prompt epididymotomy may be necessary to prevent infarction.

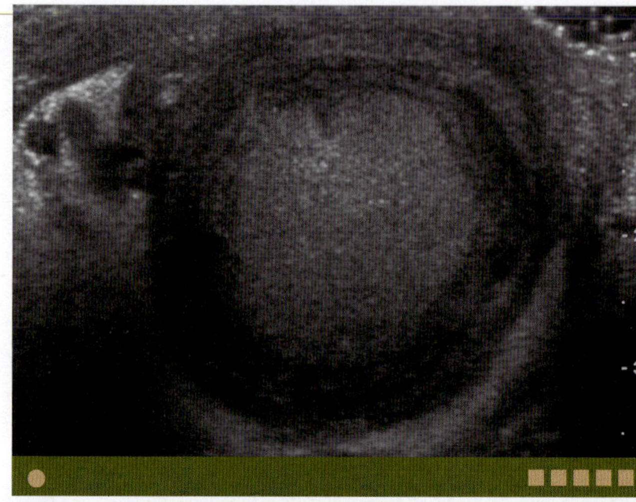

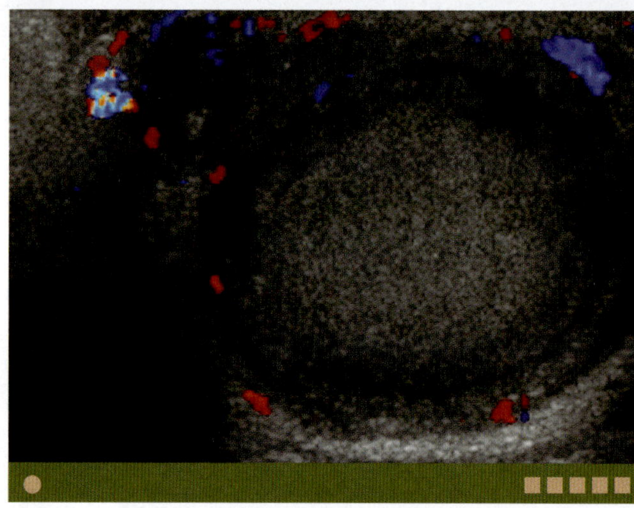

A. Transverse gray-scale sonogram of the right testicle shows a thick, relatively hypoechoic rind surrounding the right testicle. The testicle is slightly heterogeneous in echogenicity.
B. Corresponding transverse color Doppler sonogram shows complete absence of flow within the right testicle. Note that there is mildly increased flow in the tissues immediately surrounding the right testicle. In addition, the right epididymis is enlarged, slightly heterogeneous and hyperemic in this patient with acute epididymo- orchitis.

PEARLS

- **Severe epididymitis or epididymo-orchitis may result in testicular infarction caused by compression of the testicular vasculature.**
- **Testicular infarction may also occur in sickle cell disease, polycythemia vera, trauma, and vasculitis.**
- **On sonography, it may be difficult to distinguish from torsion unless there is clinical history of preceding infection.**
- **The affected area is usually hypoechoic with absent intratesticular color Doppler flow, which may be accompanied by hyperemia of the surrounding tissues.**

ADDITIONAL IMAGES (C-D)

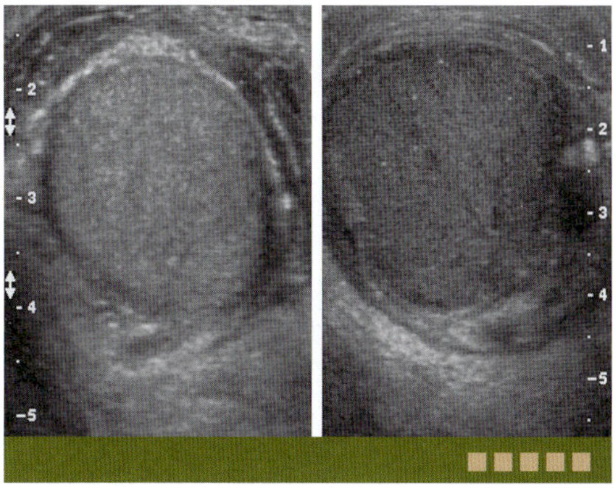

C. Transverse sonogram of both testicles in another patient show relative enlargement of the left testicle. The left testicle is also relatively hypoechoic and is surrounded by a thin hyperechoic rind. On color Doppler examination, there was no flow within the left testicle.

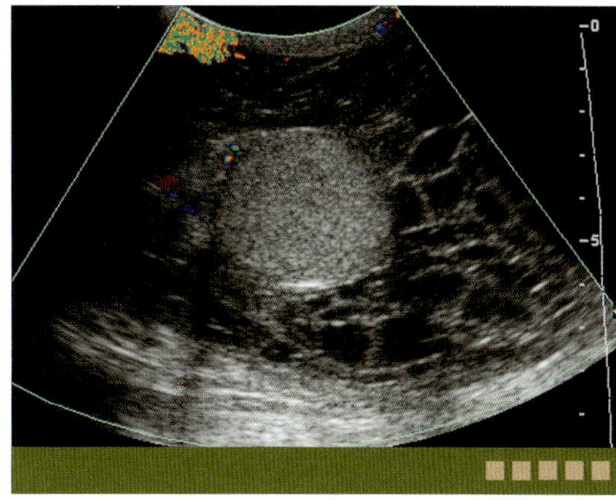

D. Transverse color Doppler sonogram of the right testicle in another patient with clinical signs of infection. The right testicle is relatively hyperechoic and is surrounded by a large, complex pyocele. There was complete absence of blood flow in the right testicle.

DIFFERENTIAL DIAGNOSIS IMAGES (E-F)

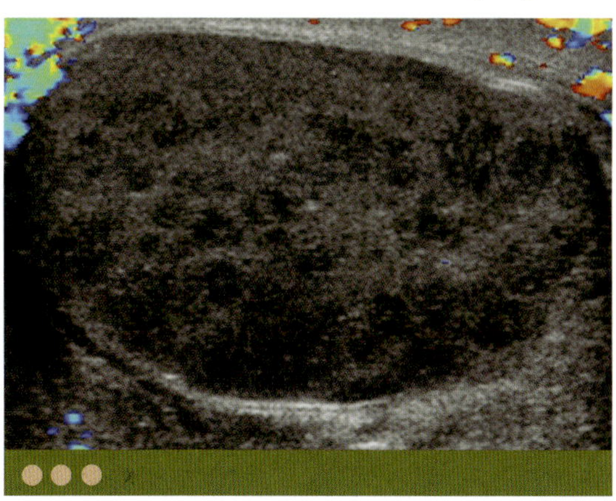

E. Testicular torsion: Longitudinal sonogram on a patient with acute onset right scrotal pain shows complete absence of flow within the right testicle. The right testicle is also markedly heterogeneous.

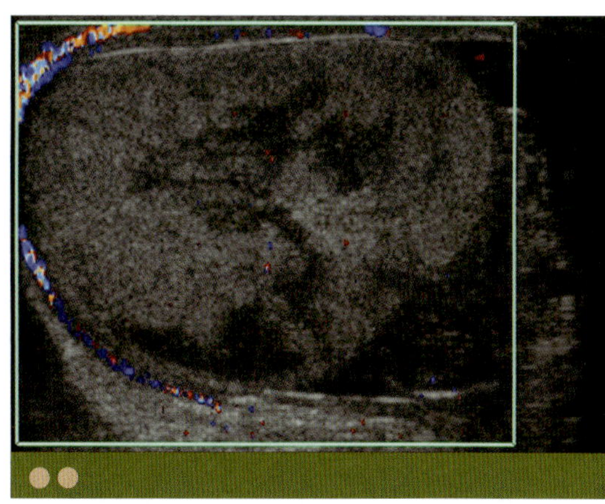

F. Testicular torsion with hemorrhagic infarction: Transverse color Doppler sonogram in another patient with a one-day history of severe left testicular pain shows near complete absence of flow within the left testicle. Note multiple linear and stellate hypoechoic areas, which on surgical pathology were shown to represent areas of hemorrhagic infarction.

IMAGE KEY

Common

●●●●●
●●●●
●●●
●●
●

Rare

Typical

■■■■■
■■■■
■■■
■■
■

Unusual

13–6 Xanthogranulomatous Orchitis

David D. Casalino

PRESENTATION

Hard, nontender left testis.

FINDINGS

T2-weighted MR image shows the left testis to have abnormally high-signal intensity with a central linear area of intermediate signal intensity and a rim of low-signal intensity.

DIFFERENTIAL DIAGNOSES

- *Testicular neoplasms*: More common; vascularity or enhancement often seen within the mass; necrosis may occur; imaging feature may not allow differentiation.
- *Chronic infectious or inflammatory process, including tuberculous (TB) orchitis and testicular malakoplakia*: Uncommon; often lack of response to conventional antibiotics; scrotal skin thickening, abscess formation, and sinus tracts more common than in pyogenic orchitis. Other organs commonly involved by the process include pulmonary TB and bladder malakoplakia.
- *Acute pyogenic orchitis*: Usually a typical clinical history, including intense testicular pain, and expected response to conventional antibiotics.
- *Intratesticular hematoma or contusion*: Painful; almost always a history of testicular trauma; follow-up sonography may be helpful; MR may demonstrate blood products.

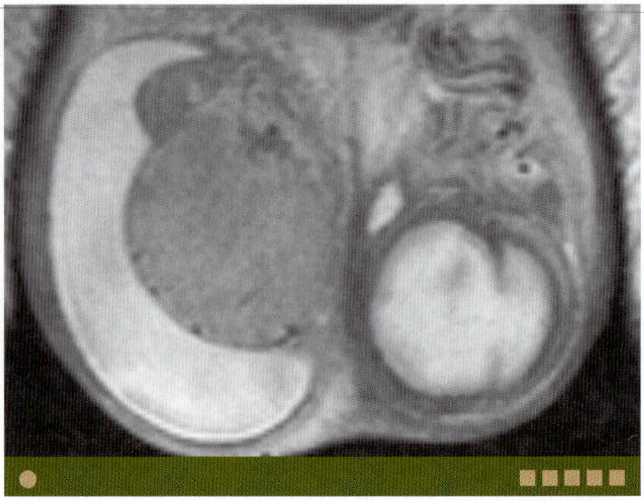

A. Coronal T2-WI shows the left testis to have abnormally high-signal intensity with a central linear area of intermediate signal intensity and a rim of low-signal intensity. The right testis and epididymis show signal intensity abnormalities consistent with mild epididymo-orchitis.

COMMENTS

Xanthogranulomatous inflammation is an uncommon destructive process marked by the presence of lipid laden macrophages (also referred to as xanthoma cells or foamy macrophages) and lymphocytes. It is predominantly seen in the kidneys but has also been described in multiple other organs, including the gallbladder, testicles, epididymides, ovaries, urinary bladder, appendix, vagina, and bones. The exact etiology of the xanthogranulomatous inflammation is unknown; however, it is often seen in association with long standing or recurrent infection.

At least 19 cases of xanthogranulomatous inflammation involving the testicles and epididymides have been described in the literature. While a microbial organism is often not identified, xanthogranulomatous orchitis (XGO) has been described in association with *E coli, Pseudomonas aeruginosa and actinomyces*. Obstruction of the spermatic tract has also been implicated as a possible etiology of XGO. Diabetes, neuropathic bladder, benign prostatic hypertrophy and repeated genitourinary tract infection may be risk factors for XGO.

Because of the destructive nature of the process and the difficulty of excluding the possibility of testicular neoplasm, removal of the involved testicle is often performed, particularly in cases refractory to antibiotic therapy.

Imaging findings are nonspecific. The most common sonographic finding described is a heterogeneous, hypoechoic testicular mass. Associated scrotal swelling, hyperemia, and fistulas have also been reported. MRI findings in the presented case include a T2 hyperintense and T1 hypointense cavity which is surrounded by a wall which is T2 hypointense and T1 hyperintense.

PEARLS

- **XGO is a very rare inflammatory process characterized by the infiltration of lipid-laden macrophages and parenchymal destruction.**
- **The etiology is unknown, but XGO is typically seen in association with long standing or recurrent infection.**
- **On imaging, it often has features of a complex cystic mass that is difficult to distinguish from a necrotic neoplasm.**
- **Treatment is usually orchiectomy.**

ADDITIONAL IMAGES (B-C)

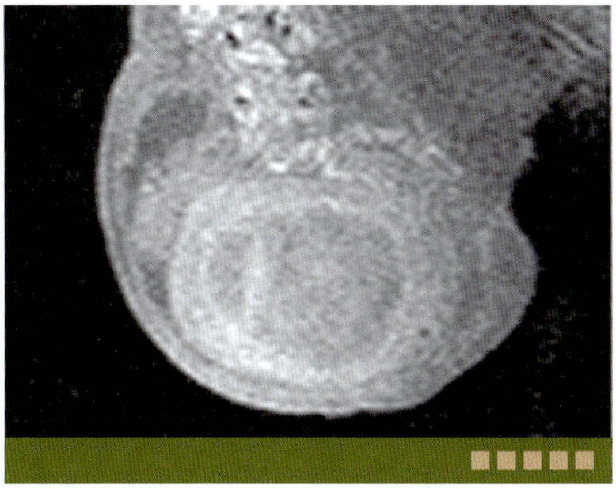

B. Sagittal T1-WI of the left testicle shows the lesion to be low T1-signal intensity and have a thin rim of higher signal intensity. The patient refused intravenous contrast.

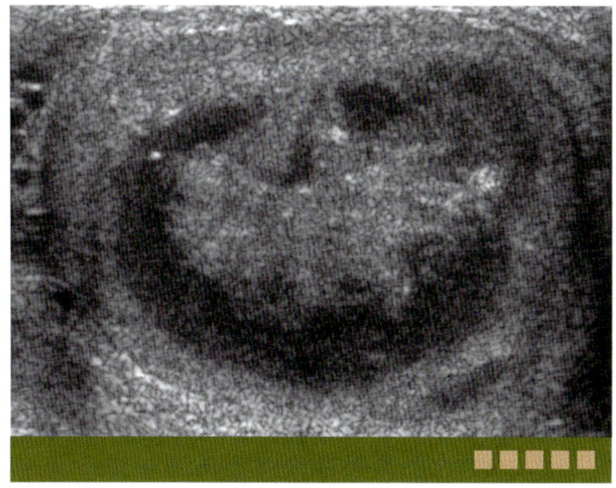

C. Longitudinal sonogram of the left testicle in the same patient shows a heterogeneous, hypoechoic lesion with posterior acoustic enhancement and absence of internal color Doppler flow.

DIFFERENTIAL DIAGNOSES IMAGES (D-G)

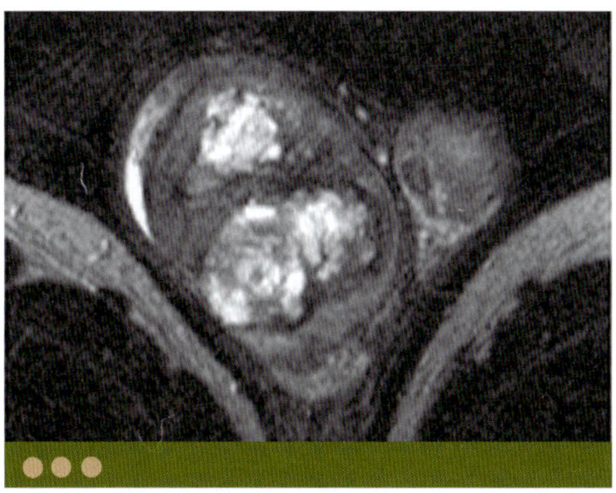

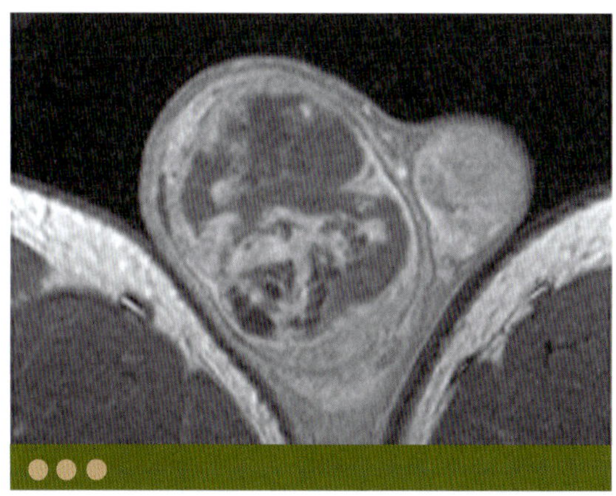

D. and **E. Mixed germ cell cancer:** Axial T2-WI and contrast-enhanced T1-WI show a large, heterogeneous mass of the right testis. The tumor has areas of T2 hyperintense necrosis intermixed with irregular areas of enhancement.

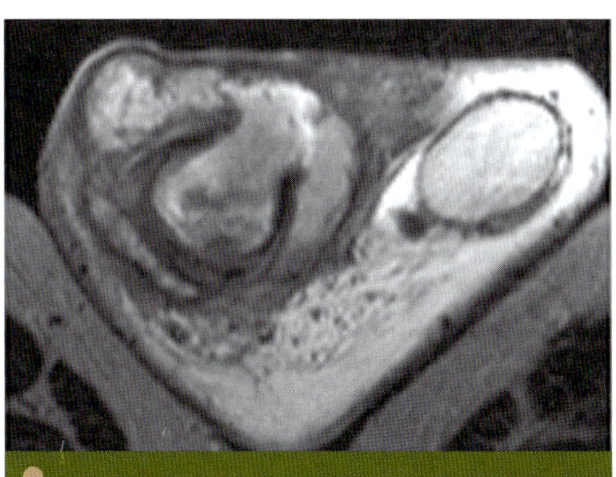

F. Malakoplakia: Axial T2-WI shows extensive necrosis and disruption of the right testis associated with anterior hyperintense scrotal abscess and scrotal wall inflammation.

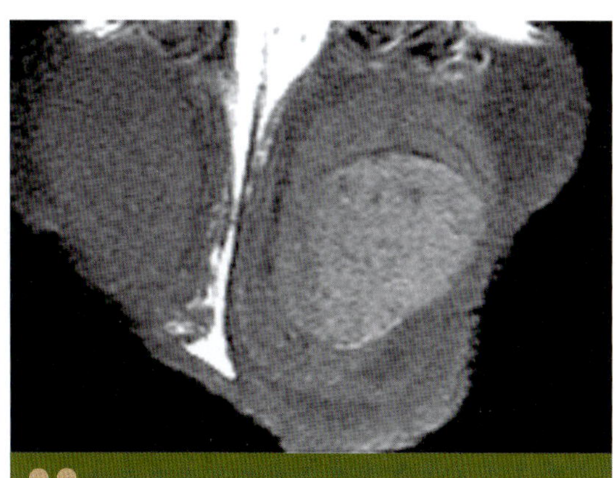

G. Intratesticular hematoma: Coronal T1-WI shows a hyperintense hematoma involving the left testis in a patient who received a kick to the scrotum.

IMAGE KEY

Common

Rare

Typical

Unusual

13–7 Fournier Gangrene

Frank H. Miller

PRESENTATION

Genital pain, tenderness, and crepitus.

FINDINGS

CT shows air and fluid dissecting into scrotum and perineum.

DIFFERENTIAL DIAGNOSES

- *Postoperative gas*: Distinguished based on history.
- *Penetrating injury*: Distinguished based on history.
- *Gas-forming scrotal abscess*: Distinguish based on imaging.
- *Emphysema from barotrauma from mechanical ventilation*: Distinguished based on clinical findings.

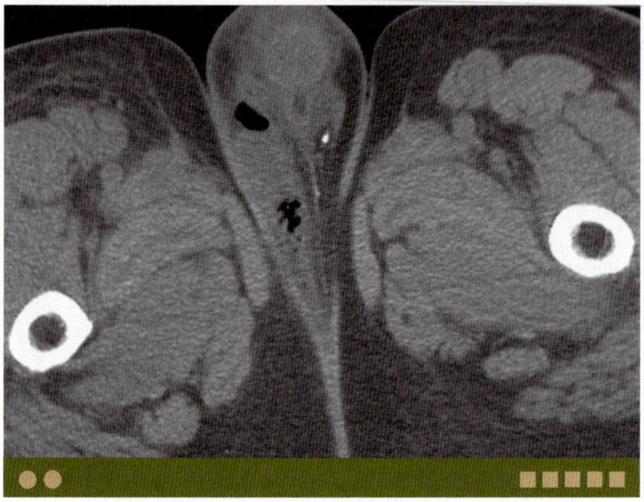

A. Axial NECT shows air and fluid extending into groin and scrotum caused by Fournier gangrene.

COMMENTS

Fournier gangrene is a potentially fatal, necrotizing infection of the perineal, genital, or perirectal area. If untreated, the infection can rapidly spread to the buttocks and abdominal wall. Patients often have a history of diabetes, HIV, or other immunosuppressive condition. The etiology is because of an infectious source. Infections are often polymicrobial and most often isolated organisms include *Klebsiella, E coli, Proteus, Streptococcus, and Staphlococcus.* Air is seen in the soft tissues from anerobic infections. Patients often present with scrotal swelling and pain. Crepitus as a result of subcutaneous air is highly suggestive.

Imaging studies help confirm the diagnosis. Radiographs show air in the soft tissues of the scrotum and perineum. Sonography may be performed if orchitis or epididymitis is suspected. Sonography may show gas in the scrotal wall and perineum. CT is the best imaging modality for the diagnosis. CT scans show skin and facial thickening and fat stranding and associated fluid collections. CT is more sensitive for smaller amounts of gas than plain films and can show the extent of disease and presence of abscesses. CT can show an underlying cause. MRI examinations, while they show the soft tissue involvement better than CT, do not show the presence of gas as well. In addition, MR is often less readily available in the emergency setting.

Fournier gangrene is a surgical emergency requiring surgical debridement of the necrotic tissue and broad-spectrum intravenous antibiotics. A high index of suspicion is required, and the radiologist may be the first to suggest the diagnosis and recommend surgical consultation.

PEARLS

- **Fournier gangrene is surgical emergency often requiring debridement of necrotic tissue and antibiotics.**
- **Radiologist may be the first person to suggest the diagnosis of Fournier gangrene.**
- **CT is the most sensitive test to show associated air and abscesses.**
- **The lack of history of surgery or penetrating injury makes the diagnosis of Fournier gangrene most likely.**

ADDITIONAL IMAGE

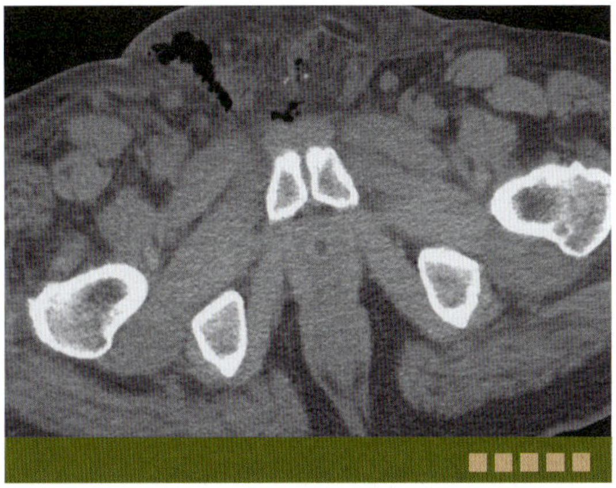

B. Axial NECT shows air involving the perineum along the anterior aspect of the pelvis. The patient required surgical debridement of the necrotic tissue.

IMAGE KEY

Common

Rare

Typical

Unusual

13–8 Testicular Torsion

Nancy A. Hammond

PRESENTATION

Acute scrotal pain and swelling.

FINDINGS

Absence of flow to the involved testicle.

DIFFERENTIAL DIAGNOSIS

- *Ischemia from severe infection*: Can be difficult to distinguish on the basis of imaging; clinical scenario may help.

COMMENTS

Testicular torsion most commonly occurs in peripubertal boys or young adult males under the age of 30 with a reported peak age of 14. Patients usually present with scrotal pain and swelling. The pain may radiate to the groin and lower abdomen and is often associated with nausea and vomiting. Marked scrotal tenderness is present on physical examination. Testicular torsion is a urologic emergency requiring immediate surgery. There is 100% salvage rate of the involved testicle in patients who undergo detorsion within 6 hours of the onset of pain. Salvage rates decrease to 70% if surgery is performed within 6 to 12 hours of onset of symptoms and only 20% when surgery is delayed more than 12 hours.

Torsion occurs in patients where the normal attachment of the testis to the posterior scrotal wall is congenitally absent, the "bell clapper" deformity. This results in the testis being suspended in the scrotal sac via its vascular pedicle. When present, the bell clapper deformity is bilateral 50% to 80% of the time.

Sonography is the first line modality in evaluating the patient with scrotal pain. On gray-scale images, the torsed testis can appear normal in its early stage. The presence of a normal appearing testicle suggests viability in the setting of torsion. A heterogeneous or hypoechoic testicle suggests non-viability. A twisted cord or "torsion knot" may or may not be seen on gray scale images and can be confused with an enlarged epididymal head. Color Doppler imaging is essential in the diagnosis of torsion and demonstrates absent or asymmetrically decreased testicular vascularity. Scanning of the testicular parenchyma should be performed utilizing low-flow detection Doppler settings (low pulse repetition frequency, low wall filter, and high Doppler gain). It is important to remember that severe infection can also cause decreased or absent flow to the testis. The clinical scenario is helpful in distinguishing the two entities. False-negative Doppler findings can occur when torsion is intermittent, low grade, or resolves spontaneously.

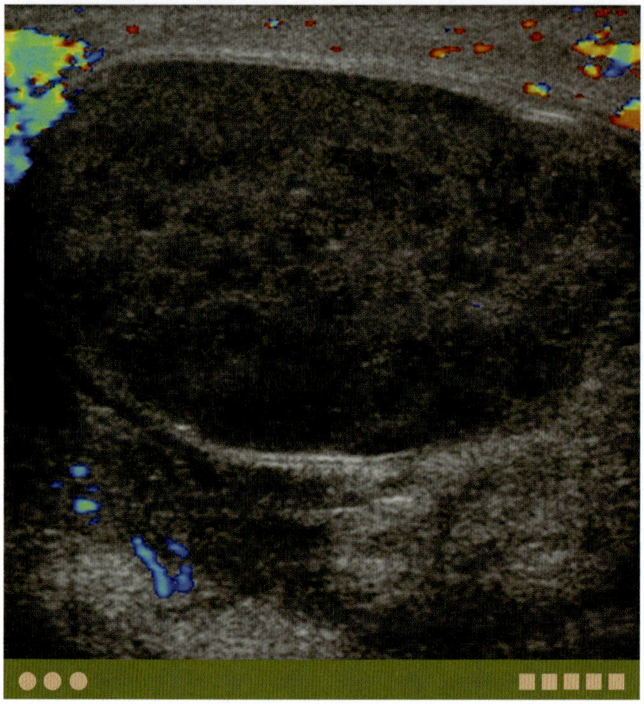

A. Color Doppler sonogram of the right testicle shows absence of flow. The testicle appears heterogeneous and hypoechoic.

Although less commonly utilized, radionuclide scans of the testes can also be used to evaluate for testicular torsion. In patients with torsion, the scan will show decreased uptake in the involved testis. Color Doppler is more sensitive for showing decreased testicular flow in complete torsion than nuclear scintigraphy.

PEARLS

- **Occurs most commonly in peripubertal or young adult males.**
- **Occurs as a result of bell clapper deformity with color doppler.**
- **Sonography is first line modality in diagnosis.**
- **Gray scale may be normal in early torsion; color Doppler is essential.**

ADDITIONAL IMAGE

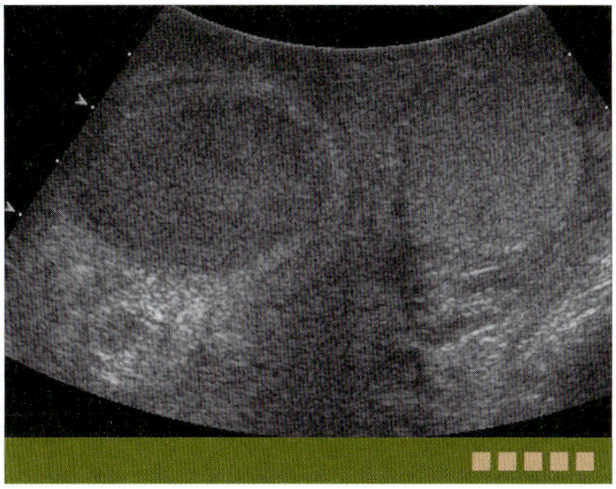

B. Gray-scale sonogram of both testicles in the same patient shows decreased echogenicity of the right testis compared to the left suggesting non-viability. The testis was found to be ischemic operatively.

DIFFERENTIAL DIAGNOSIS IMAGES (C-E)

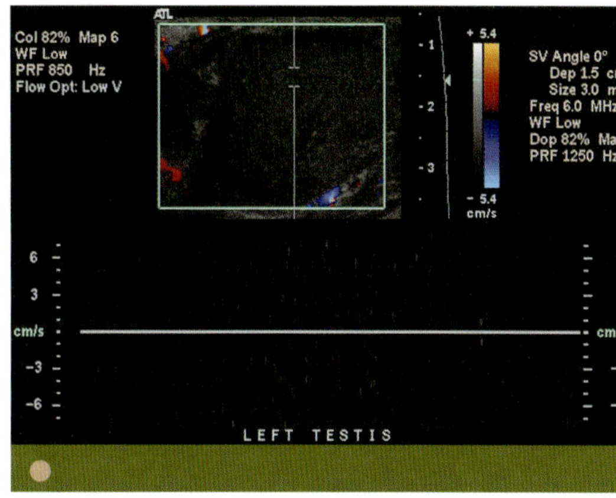

C. Ischemia caused by orchitis: Transverse gray-scale sonogram of both testes shows enlargement of and decreased echogenicity to the left testis. Edema to the surrounding soft tissues is present.

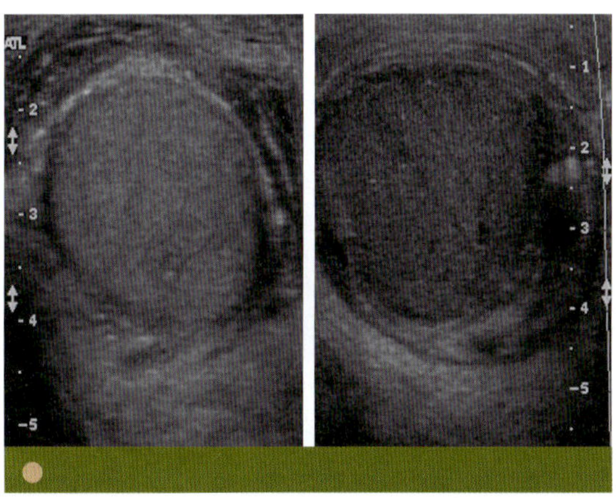

D. Ischemia caused by orchitis: Transverse gray-scale sonogram of both testes in the same patient shows decreased echogenicity of the left testis compatible with nonviability. Surgically, the left testis was found to be ischemic.

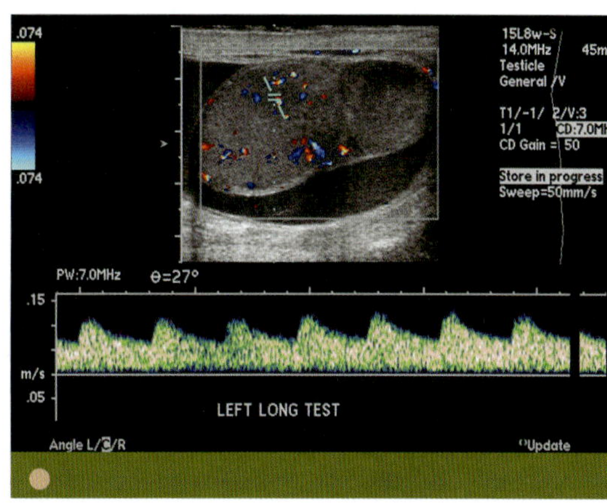

E. Ischemia caused by trauma: Sagittal color Doppler sonogram of the left testis in a different patient who sustained blunt trauma to the scrotum while playing basketball shows a region of no flow at the inferior aspect of the left testis. A complex hydrocele compatible with a hematocele is present.

IMAGE KEY

Common

Rare

Typical

Unusual

13–9 Torsion of the Epididymal Appendix

Paul Nikolaidis

PRESENTATION

Acute onset scrotal pain.

FINDINGS

Sonography shows a hypoechoic nodule adjacent to the testis without color Doppler flow and a surrounding small hydrocele. The patient experienced significant pain when scanning over this area.

DIFFERENTIAL DIAGNOSES

- *Normal epididymal appendix*: Mere visualization of an appendix without discernible flow is not sufficient to make the diagnosis, unless supported by the clinical history and physical examination.
- *Acute epididymo-orchitis*: In epididymal and/or testicular infection, increased flow throughout the testis and/or epididymis may be seen; there may be epididymal or testicular enlargement.
- *Testicular torsion*: Absence of flow is seen in the entire testis.

COMMENTS

The appendix epididymidis is a remnant of the mesonephric duct that is attached to the epididymal head. This structure is present in approximately 20% of younger patients. The appendix epididymidis is commonly stalked (in almost 80%), which makes it more prone to torsion. The normal epididymal appendices usually measure between 3 and 8 mm. They appear as a long stalked structure projecting from the head of the epididymis and are also isoechoic to it.

Torsion of either the testicular appendix or the appendix epididymis can clinically mimic testicular torsion which is managed differently as it has a high-morbidity rate. Almost 80% of cases occur between the ages of 7 and 14; almost half the cases of acute scrotum in children are caused by torsion of the appendix testis. Torsion of an appendix may occasionally occur in adult patients, however. On physical examination a tender, firm, mobile, pea-size nodule is palpated in the appropriate location, anterosuperior to the testis.

On sonography, a round or oval lesion often with an echogenic peripheral rim and central hypoechogenicity has been described. It can also appear as an ill-defined hypoechoic or echogenic nodule. There should be no internal flow on color Doppler. Secondary signs include a thickened scrotal wall, a reactive hydrocele, epididymal or testicular enlargement, and increased blood flow to the ipsilateral testis or adjacent epididymis. The appendix epididymis should be located posterolateral to the head of the epididymis, and may measure up to 9 to16 mm.

Routine surgical exploration of a torsed appendix testis is usually not necessary. Unlike testicular torsion, treatment is usually conservative and includes rest, ice, and anti-inflammatory medications.

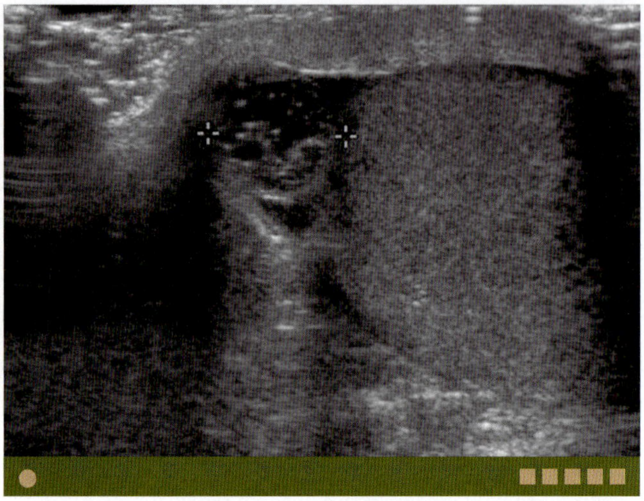

A. Transverse sonogram shows a heterogeneous 12-mm structure posterolateral to the epididymis (outlined by calipers). The patient experienced significant tenderness over the site. (*Image courtesy of Dr Carrie Donaldson, Evanston Hospital, Northwestern University, Evanston, Illinois.*)

PEARLS

- **The appendix epididymidis is a remnant of the mesonephric duct and is attached to the epididymal head, usually by a long stalk.**
- **A painful, firm, mobile, pea-size nodule is palpated anterosuperior to the testis.**
- **A tender nodule without color Doppler flow is seen on ultrasound.**
- **A thickened scrotal wall, reactive hydrocele, epididymal, or testicular enlargement or hyperemia may be seen.**

ADDITIONAL IMAGES (B-C)

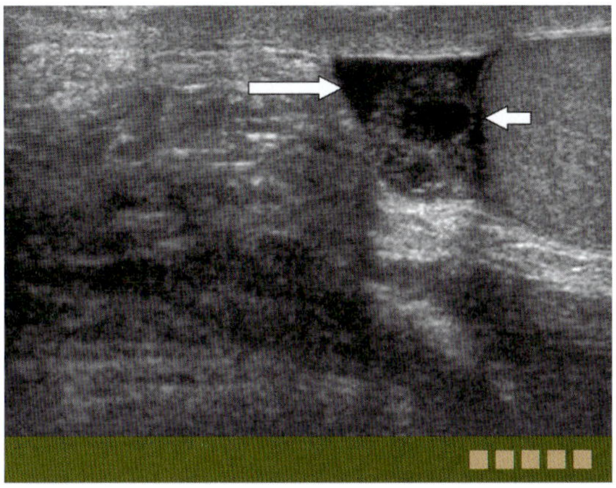

B. Additional high resolution ultrasound of the area shows the structure has anechoic components. It is surrounded by a small amount of fluid. Often a torsed epididymal appendix will have an associated small reactive hydrocele. (*Image courtesy of Dr Carrie Donaldson, Evanston Hospital, Northwestern University, Evanston, Illinois.*)

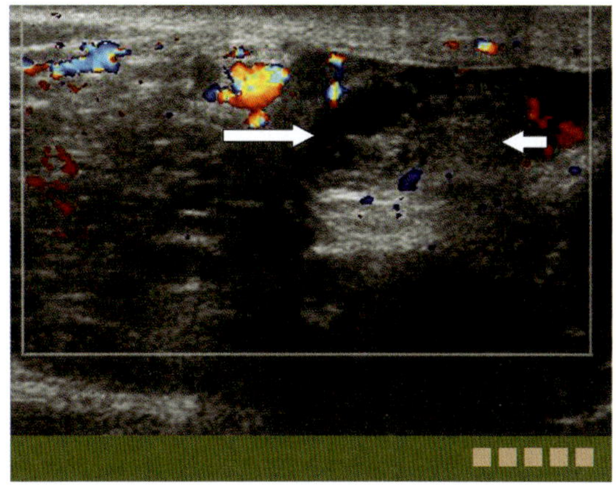

C. Transverse color Doppler sonogram on the same patient shows complete absence of flow within the abnormal heterogeneous structure representing a torsed epididymal appendix. (*Image courtesy of Dr Carrie Donaldson, Evanston Hospital, Northwestern University, Evanston, Illinois.*)

DIFFERENTIAL DIAGNOSES IMAGES (D-E)

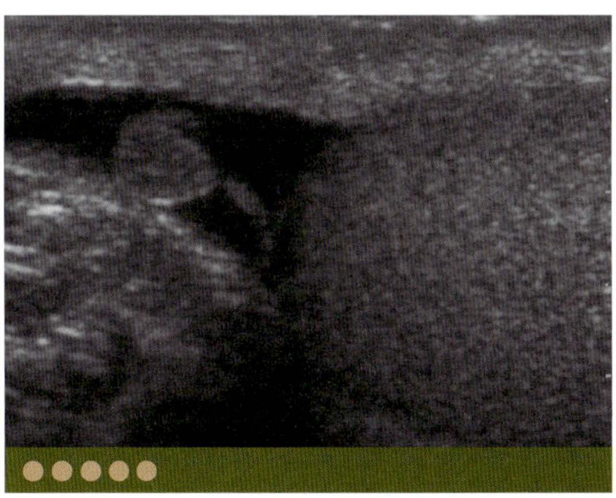

D. Normal epididymal appendix: Sagittal sonogram shows a long-stalked structure projecting from region of the epididymis. It is isoechoic to the epididymis. The patient was asymptomatic.

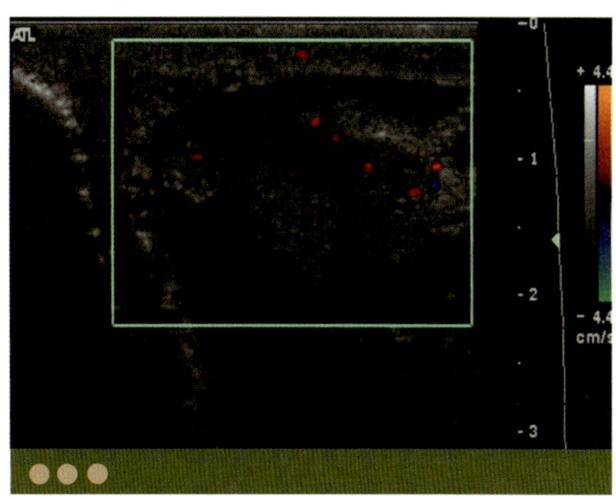

E. Normal epididymal appendix: Transverse color Doppler sonogram on another patient shows an appendix epididymis with discernible internal flow. It shows homogeneous echogenicity and measures approximately 7 mm. Trace physiologic fluid is seen surrounding it. The patient was asymptomatic.

IMAGE KEY

Common

Rare

Typical

Unusual

13–10 Scrotoliths

Frank H. Miller

PRESENTATION

Palpable mass.

FINDINGS

Extratesticular calcification.

DIFFERENTIAL DIAGNOSES

- *Cysts of the tunica albuginea*: Extratesticular lesion whose distinction is easily made with ultrasound as cyst and not calcification.
- *Microlithiasis*: Seen as multiple intratesticular calcifications.

COMMENTS

Calcifications in the scrotum may be intra- or extratesticular. When intratesticular, they may be a result of prior trauma or hematoma, burned out germ cell (Azzopardi) tumor, or associated with a tumor. Calcifications can involve the epididymis when associated with chronic epididymitis and injury. Scrotoliths also referred to as scrotal calculus or scrotal pearls are benign extratesticular calcifications that are mobile and arise from the tunica vaginalis. The scrotoliths may relate to prior injury or inflammation. They have been called scrotal pearls because of their macroscopic pearly white appearance. The reasons for their development include inflammation of the tunica vaginalis or torsion of the appendix testis or appendix epididymis that becomes calcified. Scrotoliths are separate from the epididymis. They tend to be less than 1 cm and often are associated with hydroceles and move. The patient or physician may palpate a hard mass and obtain an ultrasound to exclude a testicular mass. They are also often incidental findings on ultrasound and may be single or multiple. It is important to diagnose the abnormality as a scrotolith and not to confuse it with something more significant. No further work-up or follow-up examination is required.

A study by Frauscher in the journal *Radiology* describes the majority of extreme mountain bikers had scrotoliths felt as a result of trauma from the bike saddle during biking on rough terrain. These may be painful or asymptomatic.

Ultrasound of scrotoliths shows small calcifications with posterior acoustic shadows. They may be dependent in a hydrocele or free floating. It is important to not confuse these findings with significant pathology. No treatment is generally needed. Ultrasound examination is helpful if indicated to reassure the patient and referring doctor that a palpable mass is because of scrotoliths and not a neoplasm.

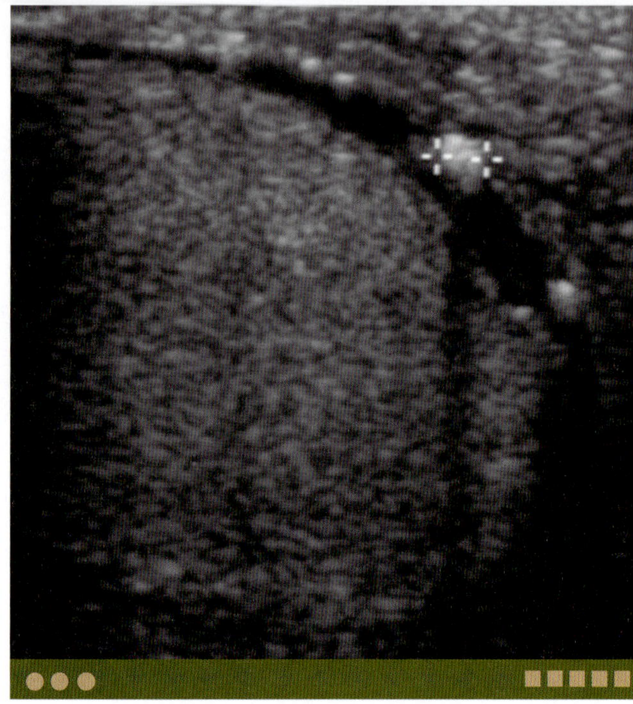

A. Transverse sonogram shows extratesticular echogenic focus with shadowing because of calcification attributed to scrotolith.

PEARLS

- **Scrotoliths are extratesticular calcifications that are benign. They do not require further evaluation.**
- **Scrotoliths are felt to result from prior trauma or inflammation.**
- **Ultrasound may be helpful in patients with palpable mass caused by scrotolith.**

DIFFERENTIAL DIAGNOSES IMAGES (B-C)

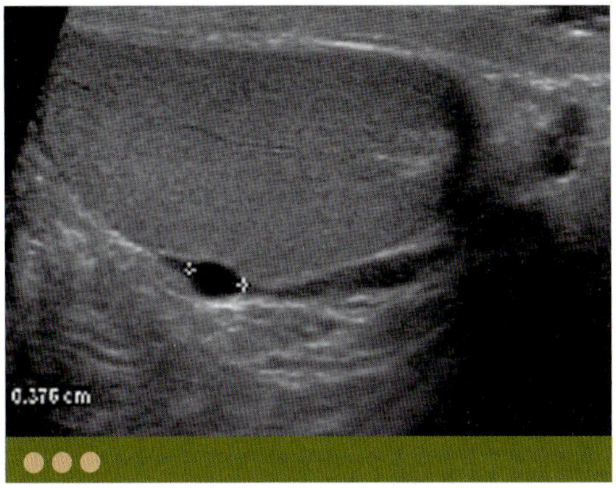

B. Cysts of the tunica albuginea: Sonogram shows tiny cystic 4-mm lesion involving the tunica albuginea without calcifications.

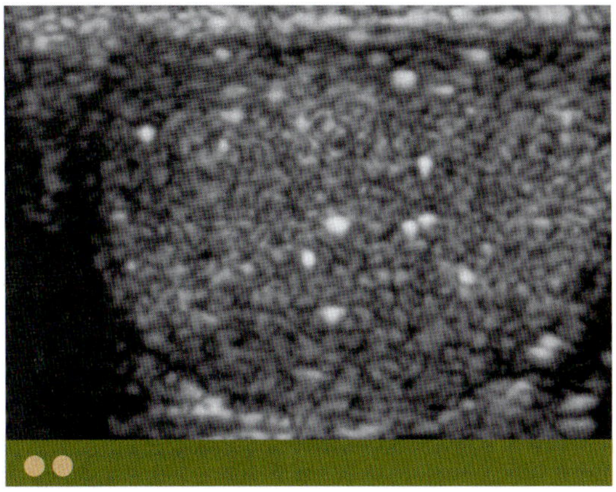

C. Microlithiasis: Longitudinal sonogram shows multiple echogenic foci from microlithiasis.

IMAGE KEY

Common

Rare

Typical

Unusual

13–11 Unilateral Striated Testicle from Fibrosis

Paul Nikolaidis

PRESENTATION

Often asymptomatic, but there may be a history of a prior insult (such as infection, trauma, or radiation to the testis).

FINDINGS

Multiple striations (linear hypoechoic bands) are seen emanating from the mediastinum in a testicle that is normal in size. There was no increased flow on color Doppler imaging.

DIFFERENTIAL DIAGNOSES

- *Infectious orchitis*: Orchitis can sometimes result in a striated pattern. Acute orchitis is typically associated with clinical signs of active infection, pain, epididymal enlargement, scrotal wall thickening, and increased vascularity.
- *Lymphoma*: In most reported cases of testicular lymphoma with a striated appearance, the involved testis was substantially enlarged with increased vascularity.

COMMENTS

A striated appearance of the testicle is defined as multiple hypoechoic bands radiating from the mediastinum testis. These striations have the same anatomic disposition as the interlobular septa, which are a component of the interstitium of the testis. Unilateral striated testicles are now more commonly encountered because of improvements in ultrasound equipment with higher resolution imaging. This finding is more often a result of fibrosis.

There are various patterns of fibrosis, including the striated pattern. Testicular fibrosis can have many etiologies including congenital disorders such as Klinefelter syndrome, alcoholism, aging, testicular trauma, inflammation, infection, radiation injury, and torsion. Other etiologies of a striated pattern include infectious orchitis and lymphoma, secondary to interstitial infiltration.

Sonographic findings in patients with a unilateral striated appearance secondary to fibrosis include a small- or normal-sized affected testicle. Vascularity on colorflow Doppler imaging should be normal or decreased. In the absence of clinical or sonographic findings to suggest malignancy or infection (such as testicular enlargement or hypervascularity), a striated pattern of a testis on sonography can be presumed to represent fibrosis. These patients should be followed clinically and/or sonographically and surgical exploration should be avoided.

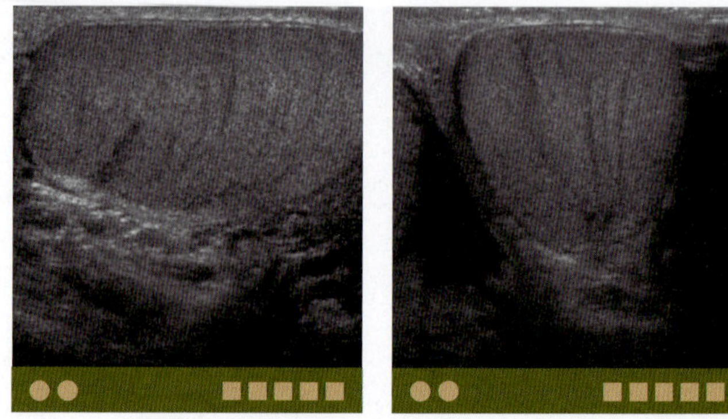

A. and **B.** Longitudinal (A) and transverse (B) sonograms of the testis show multiple linear hypoechoic bands emanating from the mediastinum testis. The testis was normal in size and did not demonstrate any increase in flow.

PEARLS

- **Multiple hypoechoic bands radiating from the mediastinum testis are seen.**
- **Testicular fibrosis is the most usual etiology.**
- **Fibrosis may be secondary to alcoholism, aging, prior trauma, inflammation, infection, radiation injury, or torsion.**
- **On sonography, the affected side is typically normal or small in size, and should demonstrate normal or decreased vascularity on color Doppler.**

ADDITIONAL IMAGES (C-D)

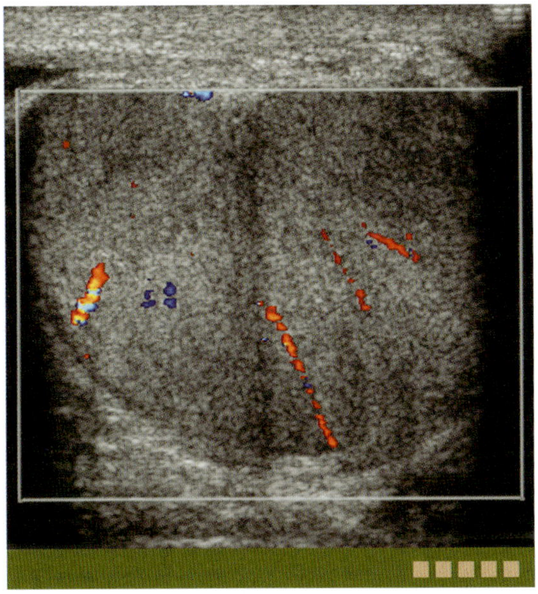

C. Color Doppler transverse sonogram of a striated testis in a different patient shows a normal pattern of flow.

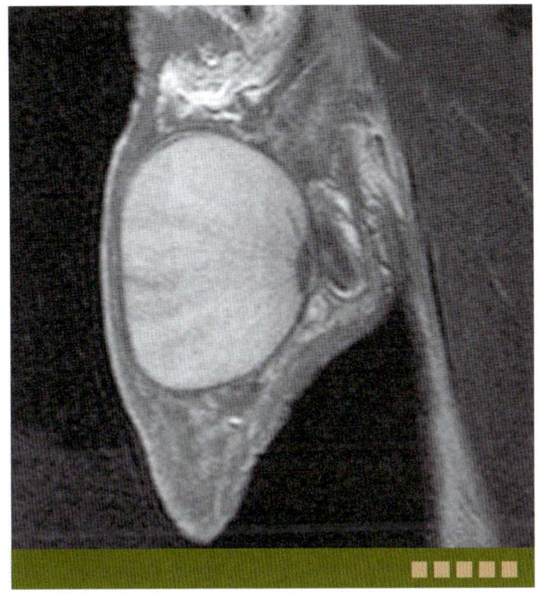

D. Sagittal contrast-enhanced T1-WI shows linear hypointense bands corresponding to the testicular striations seen on sonography.

DIFFERENTIAL DIAGNOSES IMAGES (E-F)

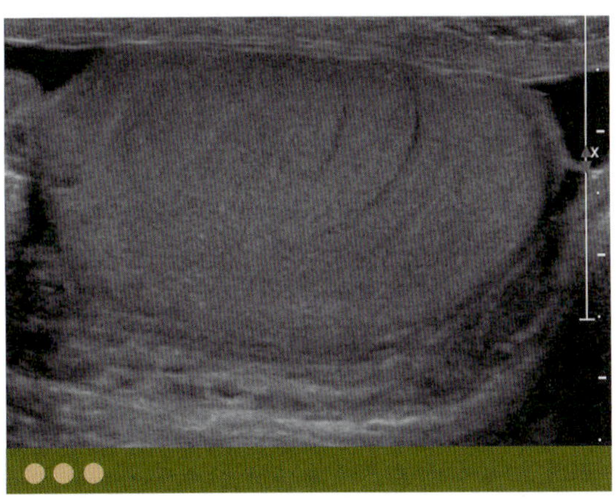

E. Acute infectious orchitis: Longitudinal sonogram on a patient with clinical signs of infection shows an enlarged, slightly heterogeneous right testis with linear hypoechoic striations.

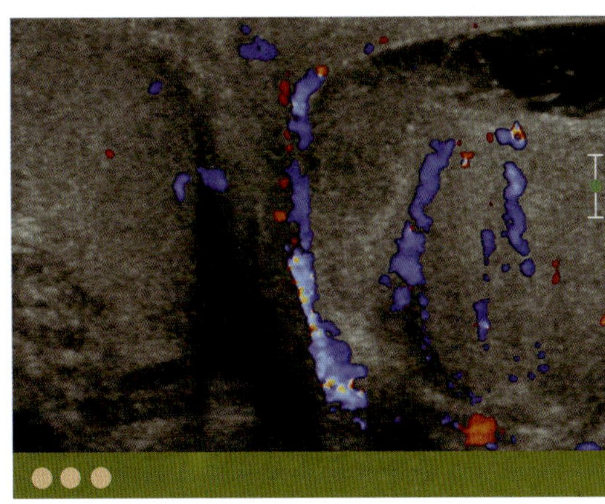

F. Acute infectious orchitis: Transverse color Doppler sonogram shows increased vascularity in the affected testis, also indicative of acute infection. A striated testis resulting from fibrosis would be expected to show normal or decreased flow.

IMAGE KEY

Common

●●●●●
●●●●
●●●
●●
●

Rare

Typical

■■■■■
■■■■
■■■
■■
■

Unusual

13–12 Testicular Rupture

Paul Nikolaidis

PRESENTATION

Testicular pain, scrotal swelling, and history of injury.

FINDINGS

Sonography shows an enlarged testicle with an abnormal overall shape, poorly defined margins, and heterogeneous echotexture. There are areas of discontinuity of the tunica albuginea.

DIFFERENTIAL DIAGNOSES

- *Intratesticular hematoma or contusion*: In cases of purely intratesticular injury, the tunica is not breached.
- *Extratesticular (scrotal) hematoma*: In an isolated extratesticular hematoma, the tunica is intact and the hematoma is localized outside the testicle.
- *Testicular neoplasm*: A large heterogeneous testicular mass may be seen in both instances; clinical history should help make the diagnosis, although in some cases, tumors are discovered following trauma.

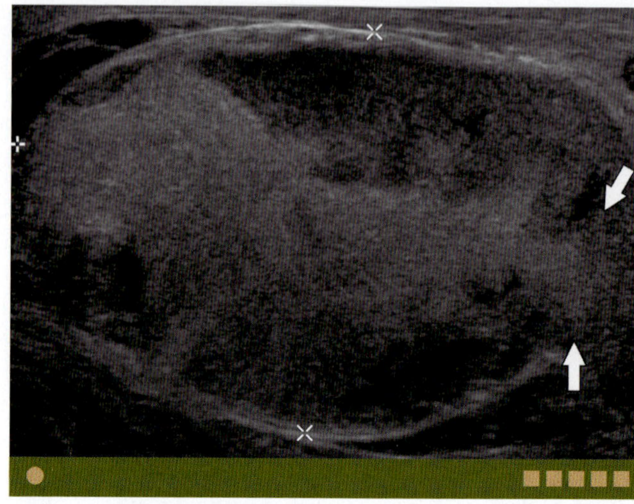

A. Longitudinal sonogram on a patient with direct injury to the scrotum shows a markedly heterogeneous right testicle. There is disruption of the tunica inferiorly with extrusion of testicular parenchyma (arrows).

COMMENTS

Scrotal injury, usually from athletic trauma, is not uncommon, and can result in contusion, hematoma, fracture, or rupture of the testicle. It is almost always the result of a direct blow. Of patients with scrotal trauma severe enough to seek medical attention, approximately 20% will have testicular rupture. Scrotal injury may also lead to the formation of a hematocele or hematoma elsewhere within the scrotum, with or without associated testicular abnormality.

Sonographic findings in testicular injury may include a scrotal wall hematoma, a hematocele, and an intratesticular hematoma, contusion, or testicular rupture. In cases of rupture, there is a break in the tunica with associated hemorrhage and extrusion of testicular contents into the scrotum. Discontinuity of the echogenic tunica, along with a poorly defined margin of the testicle, is highly suggestive of testicular rupture. Identification of the entire tunica albuginea with a high-frequency transducer is very important in evaluating for any areas of interruption, or testicular rupture may be missed. The testicular echotexture may be heterogeneous, with focal hyperechoic or hypoechoic areas because of underlying hemorrhage or infarction. Color and duplex Doppler images may show areas of decreased or absent flow.

Testicular rupture is a surgical emergency. More than 80% of the ruptured testes may be saved when surgically repaired within 72 hours. Simple intratesticular hematomas should resolve over time; no treatment is necessary.

PEARLS

- **Rupture is a surgical emergency with a salvage rate of over 80% if repaired within 72 hours.**
- **Sonographic findings pathognomonic for rupture are a break in the tunica albuginea with hemorrhage or spillage of the testicular contents.**
- **Color Doppler may show areas of decreased or absent flow.**

ADDITIONAL IMAGES (B-D)

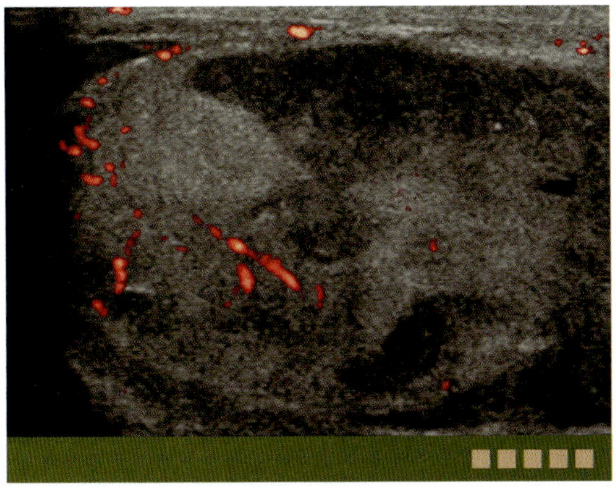

B. Corresponding longitudinal color Doppler sonogram shows absence of flow within a large portion of the injured right testicle.

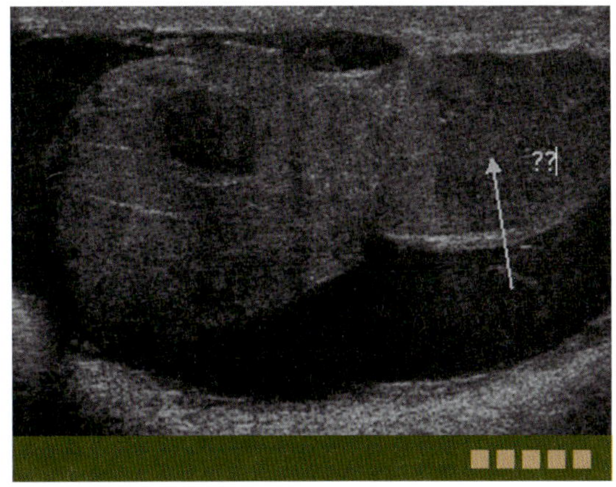

C. Longitudinal sonogram on another patient with acute injury to the scrotum shows an abnormal shape of the left testicle. There is disruption of the tunica inferiorly with extrusion of testicular parenchyma (arrow).

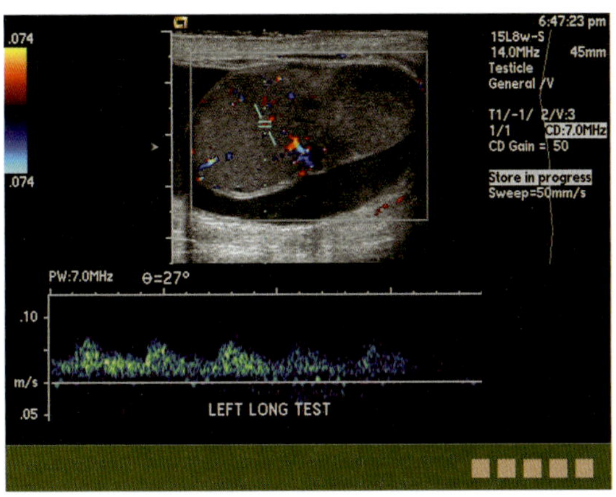

D. Corresponding longitudinal color Doppler sonogram shows complete absence of flow within the extruded portion of the left testicle.

DIFFERENTIAL DIAGNOSES IMAGES (E-G)

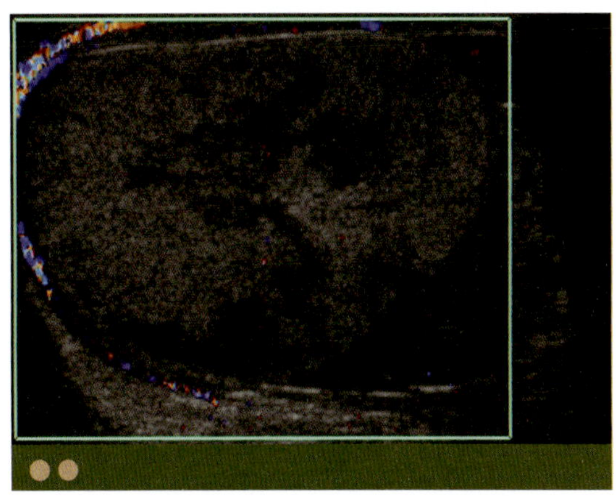

E. Testicular torsion with hemorrhagic infarction: Transverse color Doppler sonogram in a patient with a one-day history of severe left testicular pain shows near complete absence of flow within the left testicle. The testicle is markedly heterogeneous but the tunica appears intact.

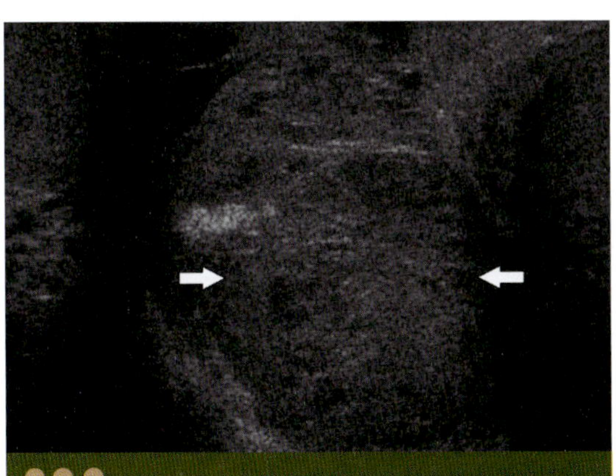

F. Extratesticular scrotal hematoma: Transverse sonogram in a patient with history of trauma shows a heterogeneous echogenic extratesticular lesion without flow on color Doppler located between the two testicles (arrows). Both testicles were normal.

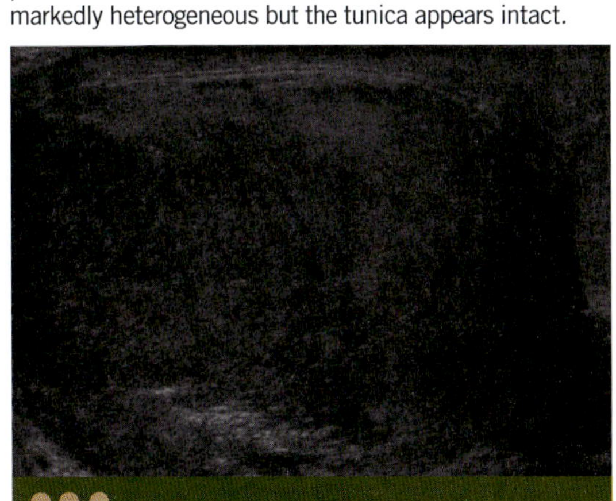

G. Testicular seminoma: Transverse sonogram in a patient with a large palpable scrotal mass shows a markedly heterogeneous right testicle. This mass demonstrated increased vascularity and also breached the tunica.

IMAGE KEY

Common

Rare

Typical

Unusual

13–13 Extratesticular Scrotal Hematoma

Paul Nikolaidis

PRESENTATION

Scrotal pain and/or scrotal swelling following trauma.

FINDINGS

Sonography shows an echogenic, heterogeneous, complex extratesticular lesion without any flow on color Doppler interrogation.

DIFFERENTIAL DIAGNOSES

- *Inguinal hernia*: They are generally larger and can be tracked to the internal inguinal ring; in some instances hernias may be reducible. Some hernias contain bowel loops that exhibit peristalsis on real-time sonography.
- *Spermatic cord lipoma or liposarcoma*: A lipomatous lesion of the spermatic cord should be centered in the inguinal canal; in addition the palpable abnormality usually develops over time, and there may be no history of trauma.
- *Abscess/Pyocele*: Typically a heterogeneous collection in a patient with clinical signs of infection. Usually, there is no history of traumatic injury.

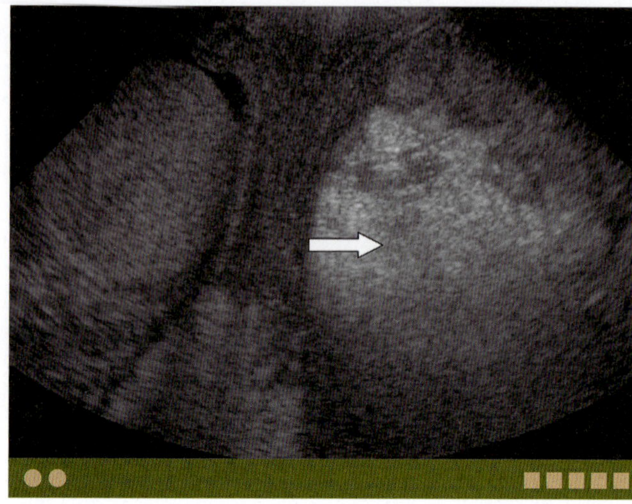

A. Transverse sonogram shows a hyperechoic focus medial to the right testicle (arrow) in a patient who sustained injury to the scrotum while playing soccer.

COMMENTS

Scrotal injury from direct trauma is not uncommon, and may result in contusion, hematoma, fracture, or rupture of the testicle. Scrotal injury may result in a hematocele or hematoma within the scrotum, with or without associated testicular injury. Concomitant severe testicular injury such as rupture should be excluded, as it is a surgical emergency.

Sonographic findings of an extratesticular scrotal hematoma include a heterogeneous, complex lesion without any flow on color Doppler interrogation. The classic sonographic reticulated appearance of a hematoma with linear fibrin strands may be present. The testes may be displaced by the hematoma. Careful sonographic examination of the testes to exclude the presence of a hematoma, fracture, rupture, or any compromise to blood flow is very important. If uncertain of this diagnosis, follow-up may be helpful, as a hematoma should regress over time and eventually resolve. Differential considerations of intrascrotal extratesticular and extra-epididymal lesions include lipomas and inguinal hernias. Clinical history and examination are very important in making the distinction.

Hematomas should resolve over time and treatment is usually not necessary.

PEARLS

- **Scrotal injury may result in a hematocele or hematoma within the scrotum, with or without associated testicular injury.**
- **Close scrutiny of the testicle for the presence of vascular compromise, intratesticular hematoma, or rupture is important.**
- **On sonography, hematomas are typically hyperechoic heterogeneous lesions.**
- **There should be no detectable flow on color Doppler.**

ADDITIONAL IMAGES (B-C)

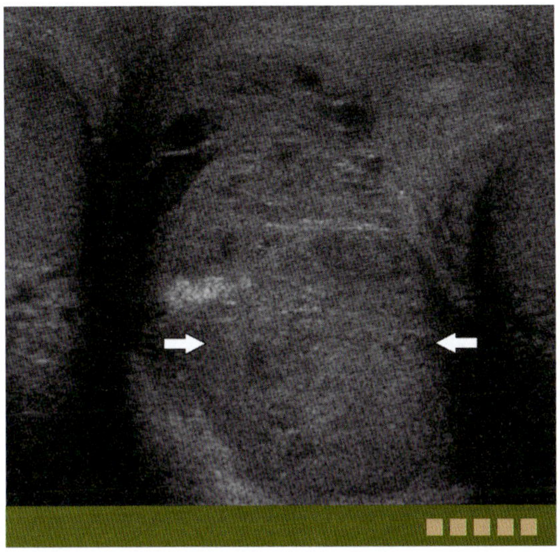

B. Transverse sonogram in a different patient shows a midline extratesticular hematoma situated between the two testicles (arrows).

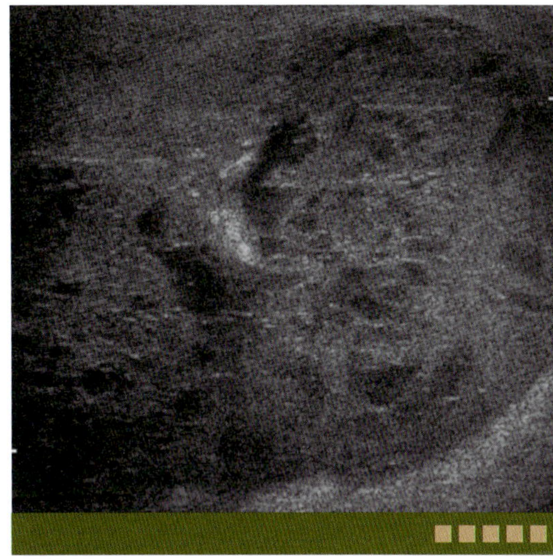

C. Corresponding longitudinal sonogram shows scattered linear hyperechoic strands and areas of reticulation, in addition to scattered hypoechoic foci.

DIFFERENTIAL DIAGNOSES IMAGES (D-G)

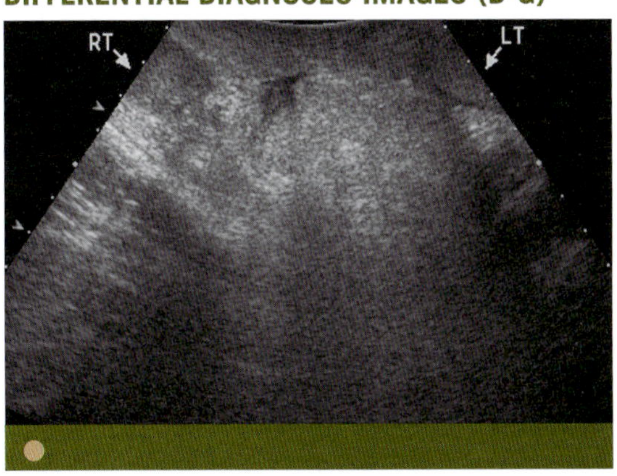

D. Lipoma of the spermatic cord: Transverse sonogram shows a large, predominantly hyperechoic lesion occupying a significant portion of the scrotum and displacing both testes laterally (arrows).

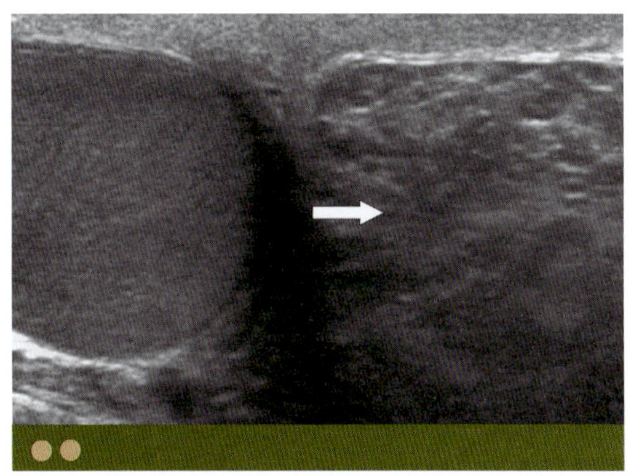

E. Fat containing inguinal hernia: Transverse sonogram shows a heterogeneous lesion adjacent to the right testicle (arrow). This was traced through the inguinal canal into the lower pelvis.

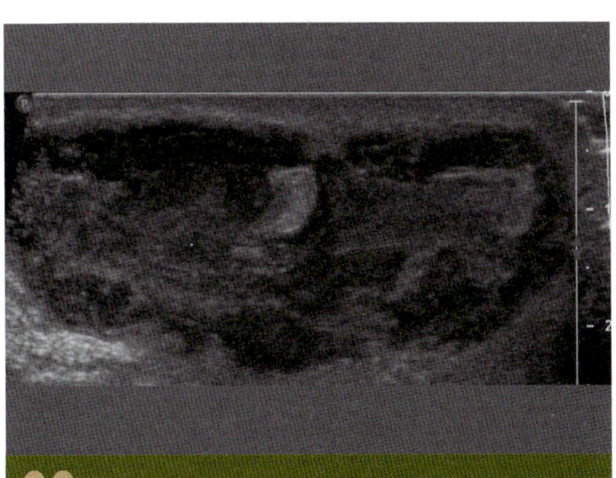

F. Abscess: Transverse sonogram in a patient with fever and tenderness shows a 5-cm heterogeneous lesion within the scrotum, separate from both testicles.

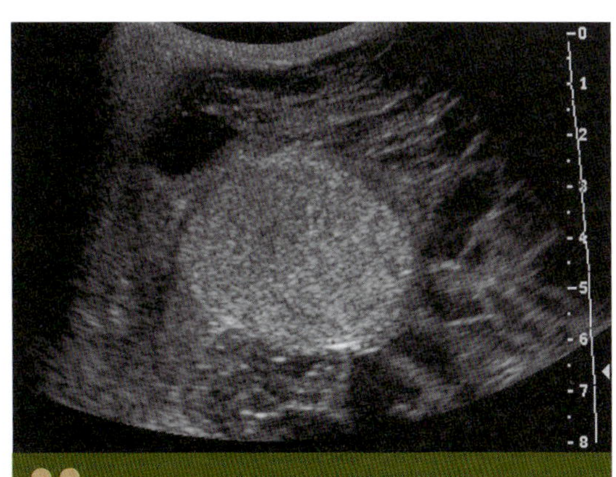

G. Pyocele: Transverse sonogram in another patient with clinical signs of infection shows a large, complex pyocele surrounding the right testicle.

IMAGE KEY

Common

Rare

Typical

Unusual

13–14 Germ Cell Tumor of the Testes

Frank H. Miller

PRESENTATION

Palpable testicular mass and testicular pain.

FINDINGS

Solid hypoechoic mass on ultrasound exam.

DIFFERENTIAL DIAGNOSES

- *Lymphoma and metastases*: Tend to be in older age group; often has a known history.
- *Leukemia*: Generally history of leukemia.
- *Epidermoid cyst*: Tends to have nearly pathognomonic target appearance with alternating areas of increased and decreased echogenicity.
- *Hematoma*: History of trauma; important to recognize that testicular cancer may be detected when reported history of trauma.
- *Leydig cell (and other nongerm cell tumors)*: Tend to be small and associated with hormone release such as estradiol; distinction often requires surgical pathology.
- *Orchitis*: Can look similar; clinical symptoms help distinguish; may need do follow-up imaging to exclude cancer.

COMMENTS

Primary testicular tumors represent 1% of all male cancers. Ninety-five percent of the testicular tumors are germ cell tumors, most often seen in the 25 to 35 years old age group. Germ cell tumors include seminoma (most common subtype), embryonal cell carcinoma, choriocarcinoma, and teratoma and mixture of types. Stromal tumors include leydig cell, Sertoli cell, granulosa cell, theca cell, and tumors of primitive gonadal stroma.

The most common germ cell tumor is seminoma seen in 40% to 50% of the cases. Two to five percent are bilateral. Fortunately, seminomas are the least aggressive and most sensitive to radiation and chemotherapy. There is increased incidence of tumors with cryptorchidism.

Patients generally present with testicular mass detected by patient or physician. Although masses seen in the setting of trauma may represent hematomas, it is important to recognize that patients with testicular tumors may present with history of trauma. The presence of flow within a mass should help suggest tumor. In addition, follow-up imaging of hematomas may be of value to exclude unsuspected neoplasm.

The diagnosis of germ cell tumor is best made with ultrasound having a sensitivity of nearly 100%. Ultrasound is

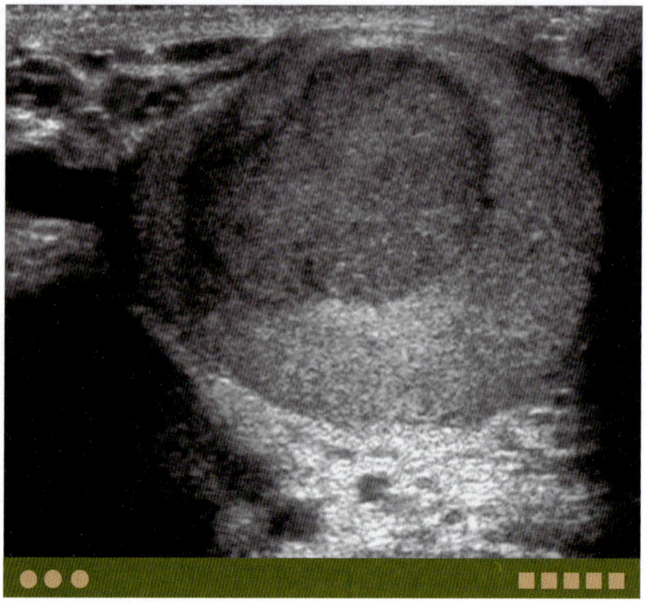

A. Longitudinal sonogram shows large hypoechoic mass caused by seminoma.

helpful in determining whether a mass is intratesticular or extratesticular. The majority of intratesticular masses are malignant.

On ultrasound, seminomas are most frequently seen as focal nodular or multinodular, homogeneous, and hypoechoic masses. They tend not to have calcifications. There is generally increased vascularity of the masses on Doppler sonography. Nonseminomatous tumors or mixed tumors tend to be more heterogeneous with cystic areas with necrosis and hemorrhage.

Treatment of testicular malignancies is orchiectomy with radiation or chemotherapy. CT scans of the abdomen and pelvis are helpful for staging purposes to assess for lymphadenopathy. Seminomas tend to be responsive to radiation and chemotherapy and have the best prognosis of the testicular neoplasms.

PEARLS

- **Germ cell tumors are most commonly seen between the age 25 and 35.**
- **The most common germ cell tumor is seminoma.**
- **The diagnosis of testicular tumors is best made with ultrasound.**
- **Seminomas tend to be homogeneous and well-defined and hypoechoic on ultrasound.**

ADDITIONAL IMAGE

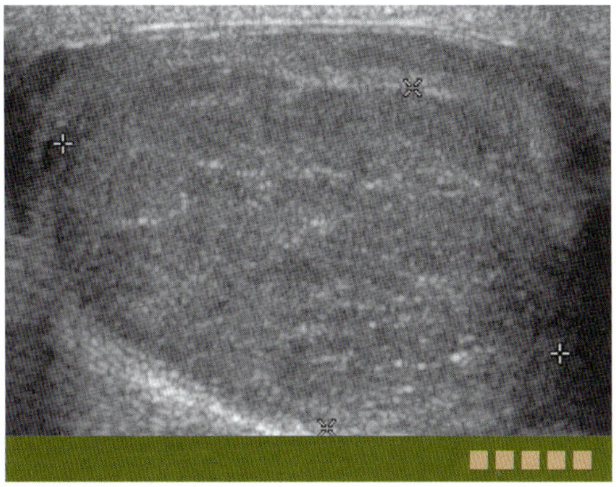

B. Transverse sonogram of testis in different patient shows large mass replacing the left testis.

DIFFERENTIAL DIAGNOSES IMAGES (C-G)

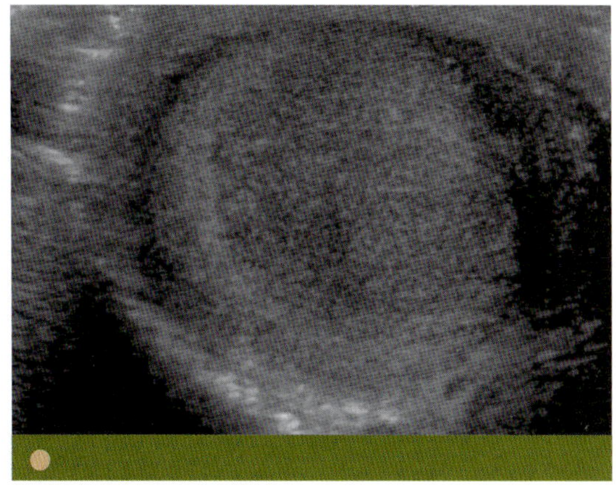

C. Myeloid sarcoma: The patient had a history of acute myeloid leukemia with recurrence as myeloid sarcoma in sinus and palpable testicle mass. The imaging appearance is identical to seminoma, but history makes it important to consider metastatic lesion.

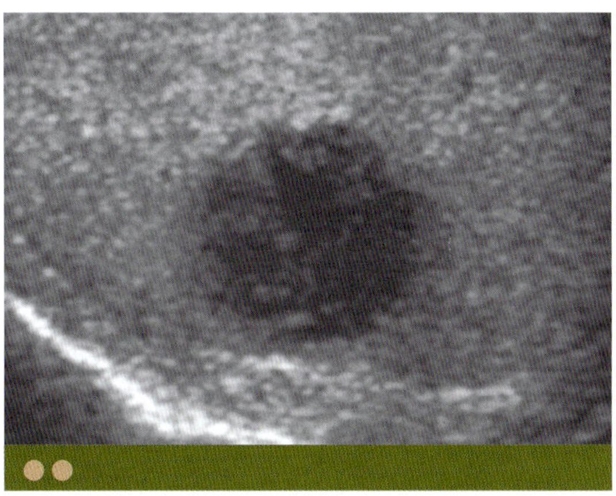

D. Testicular hematoma: Longitudinal sonogram in patient with a history of hockey puck injury shows hypoechoic intratesticular lesion from hematoma. The lesion did not have flow on color Doppler sonography. Follow-up imaging may be required to exclude underlying mass if the diagnosis is unclear.

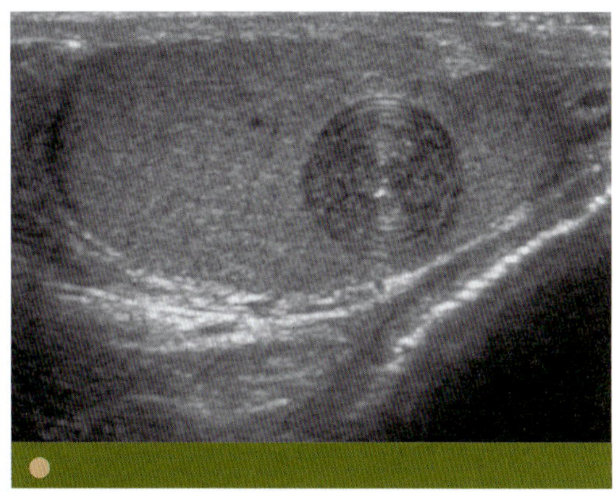

E. Epidermoid cyst: Longitudinal sonogram shows mass with "onion ring" appearance with alternating layers of increased and decreased echogenicity.

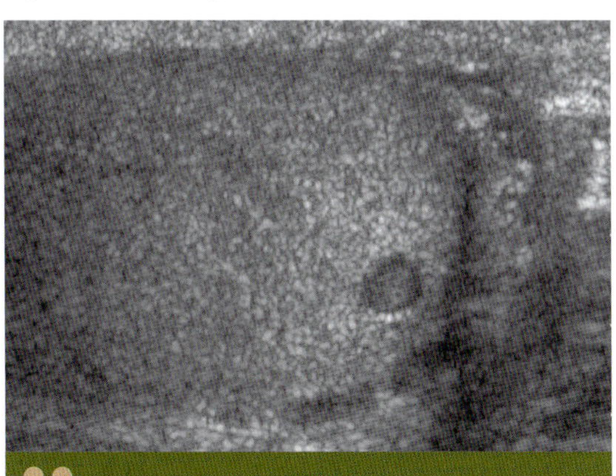

F. Leydig cell tumor: Longitudinal sonogram shows small hypoechoic intratesticular lesion. Leydig cell tumors tend to be smaller than seminomas and are associated with secretion of hormones like estradiol.

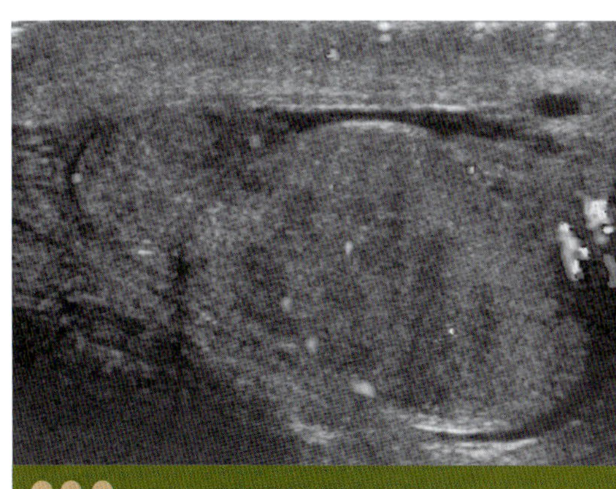

G. Orchitis and epididymitis: Longitudinal sonogram shows mass-like hypoechoic intratesticular lesion with increased flow having involvement of epididymis. Clinical symptoms were typical for the condition.

IMAGE KEY

Common

Rare

Typical

Unusual

13–15 Azzopardi Tumor

Frank H. Miller

PRESENTATION

35-year-old man with abdominal lymphadenopathy.

FINDINGS

Sonogram shows small focal echogenic foci in testis.

DIFFERENTIAL DIAGNOSES

- *Microlithiasis*: Seen as multiple small echogenic foci scattered throughout testis.
- *Microlithiasis with cancer*: Seen as associated mass with microlithiasis.
- *Trauma or hematomas or old infection*: Can generally be distinguished on the basis of clinical history and findings; would not generally have lymphadenopathy or evidence of malignancy.
- *Epidermoid with calcification*: Distinguished on the basis of classic imaging features.

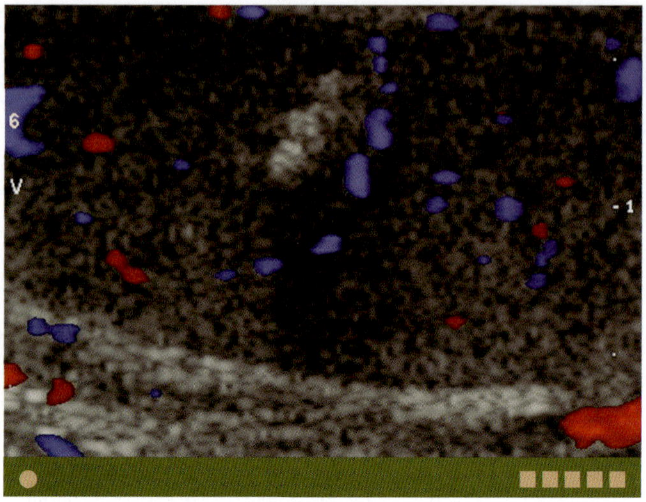

A. Longitudinal Color Doppler image shows echogenic foci caused by calcifications from burned-out testicular tumor.

COMMENTS

In 1961, Azzopardi described 17 patients who died from disseminated choriocarcinoma and other nonseminatous germ cell tumors. A primary neoplasm of the testes was not identified, but a fibrous scar was seen. These were felt to represent "burned-out" tumors or scar. The reason why they develop is felt to be a result of rapid tumor growth, outstripping its blood supply and later tumor regression.

Knowledge of the spread of testicular tumors is important to diagnose this condition. If lymph nodes are seen in the distribution of testicular tumor spread, then a sonogram of the testes should be performed to assess a neoplastic mass or much less commonly evidence of calcifications or scar to suggest a "burned-out" tumor. Most patients are suspected to have retroperitoneal germ cell tumors and not metastatic testicular tumor. Right testicular tumors tend to primarily involve aortocaval lymph nodes and lymph nodes adjacent to the aorta and inferior vena cava as well as right common and external iliac nodes. The left testicular tumors tend to spread near the left renal hilum in a paraortic or preaortic location but can also involve the left common and external iliac nodes less commonly. Hematogenous metastases can be seen typically via choriocarcinoma and embryonal carcinomas.

Sonography of the testes may not show a mass but can show these small burned out tumors as echogenic foci.

PEARLS

- **Azzopardi tumor is a result of spontaneous regression of a testicular tumor.**
- **Presence of typical distribution of metastases in a young male should suggest a testicular tumor.**
- **If a primary testicular tumor is not seen, a search for an Azzopardi occult tumor should be made.**
- **Occult tumors can present as scars or as echogenic linear bands and calcifications.**

ADDITIONAL IMAGES (B-C)

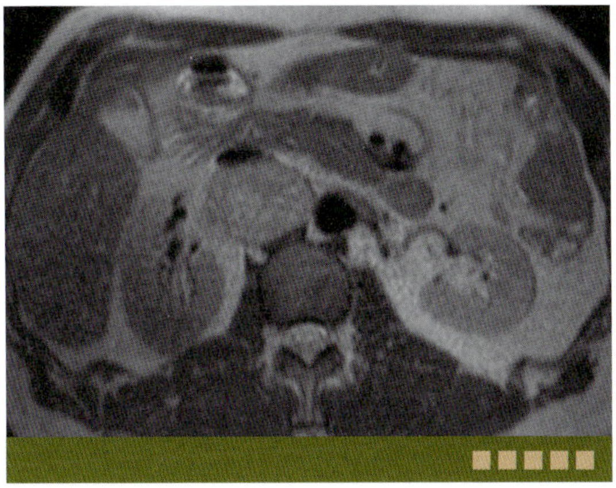

B. Axial T2-WI shows large right retroperitoneal lymph node mass.

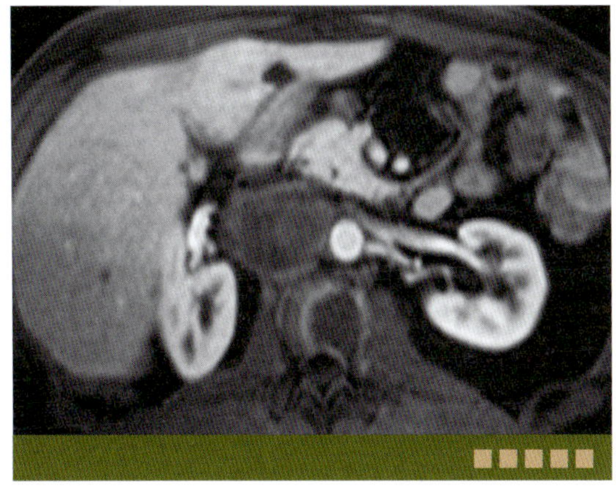

C. Axial contrast-enhanced T1-WI shows that mass is hypoenhancing.

DIFFERENTIAL DIAGNOSES IMAGES (D-F)

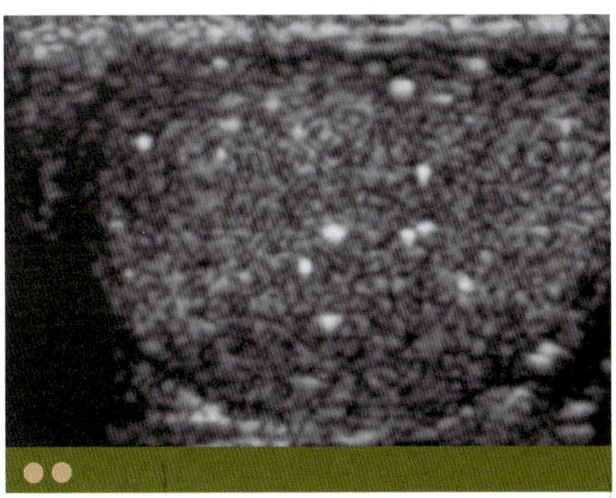

D. Microlithiasis: Longitudinal sonogram shows multiple echogenic foci from microlithiasis.

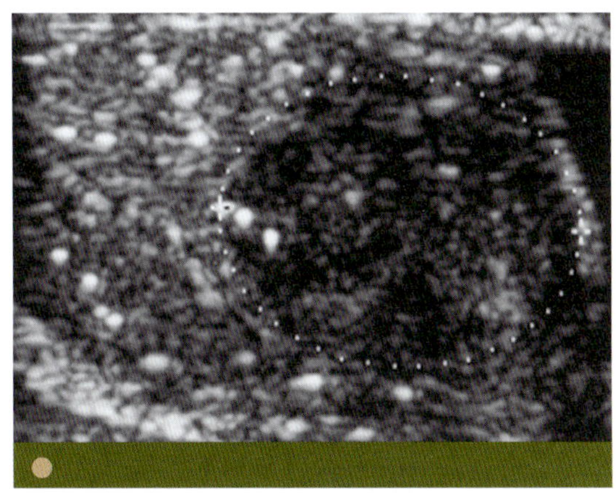

E. Microlithiasis with anaplastic seminoma: Longitudinal sonogram shows multiple shadowing echogenic foci from microlithiasis and hypoechoic mass that proved to be a seminoma.

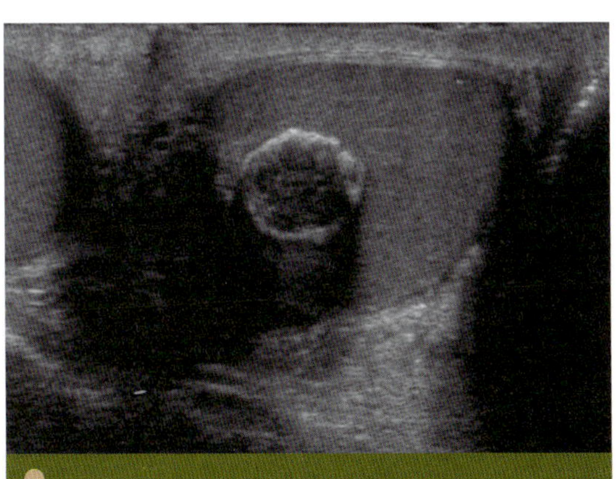

F. Epidermoid: Transverse sonogram shows round mass with peripheral calcifications that proved to be an epidermoid.

IMAGE KEY

Common

Rare

Typical

Unusual

13–16 Testicular Microlithiasis

Nancy A. Hammond

PRESENTATION

Incidental finding on scrotal ultrasound.

FINDINGS

Multiple, nonshadowing, hyperechoic foci (1 mm) scattered throughout both testicles.

DIFFERENTIAL DIAGNOSES

- *Macrocalcifications*: Larger calcifications that may have posterior shadowing.
- *Scrotolith*: Not intratesticular.

COMMENTS

Testicular microlithiasis is an uncommon condition in which multiple small calcifications are variably distributed within the testicular parenchyma. It is usually bilateral but can be unilateral. The condition can occur in normal males but has also been associated with a variety of conditions including germ cell neoplasms, Klinefelter syndrome, cryptorchidism, Down syndrome, male pseudohermaphroditism, pulmonary alveolar microlithiasis, previous radiotherapy, and subfertility states.

The exact cause of testicular microlithiasis remains unclear. Pathologically, the microliths are intratubular bodies with a central calcified core and surrounding concentric laminations composed of collagen fibers. The microliths are thought to result from defective phagocytosis of degenerate tubular cells by Sertoli cells.

The diagnosis of microlithiasis is made sonographically. It appears as multiple tiny (1-3 mm) hyperechoic foci scattered diffusely or clustered in the testicular parenchyma. The number of microliths required to diagnose testicular microlithiasis has been arbitrarily defined, but the current consensus is five foci on a single sonographic image. Posterior acoustic shadowing is rare and comet tail artifact can occasionally be seen. The presence of microlithiasis warrants a careful search for intratesticular masses. As an association with microlithiasis and testicular cancer has been demonstrated and tumors may develop subsequent to the discovery of microlithiasis, follow up ultrasound examinations are recommended to exclude developing neoplasms. A 6-month interval between examinations is a generally accepted time frame.

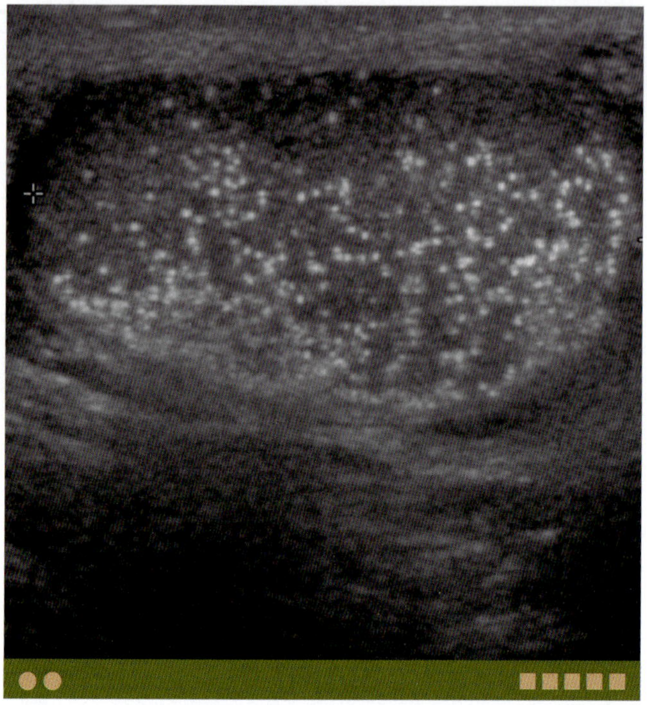

A. Longitudinal sonogram shows multiple punctate hyperechoic foci scattered throughout the left testicle compatible with microlithiasis. No associated posterior acoustic shadowing is present. No intratesticular mass lesions are present.

PEARLS

- **Microlithiasis is typically an incidental finding on testicular ultrasound performed for the evaluation for other pathology.**
- **Its association with germ cell neoplasms warrants a diligent search for coexisting neoplasm and continued follow-up with testicular ultrasound.**
- **Microlithiasis is considered to be present when >5 microcalcifications are seen on a single sonographic image.**

ADDITIONAL IMAGES (B-C)

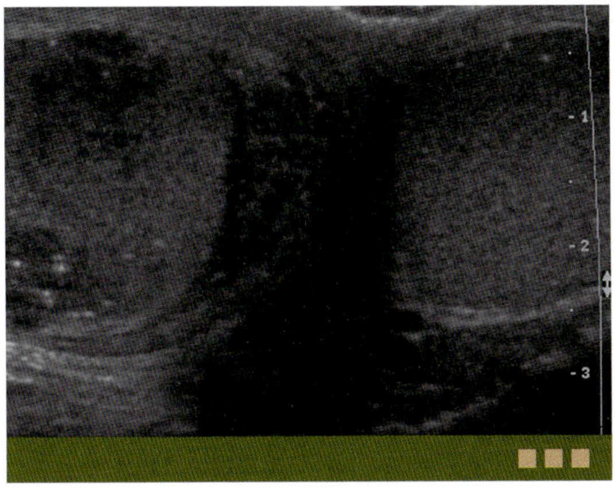

B. Transverse sonogram of both testicles shows bilateral hyperechoic foci compatible with microlithiasis. Additionally, an ill-defined hypoechoic mass is present in the right testicle.

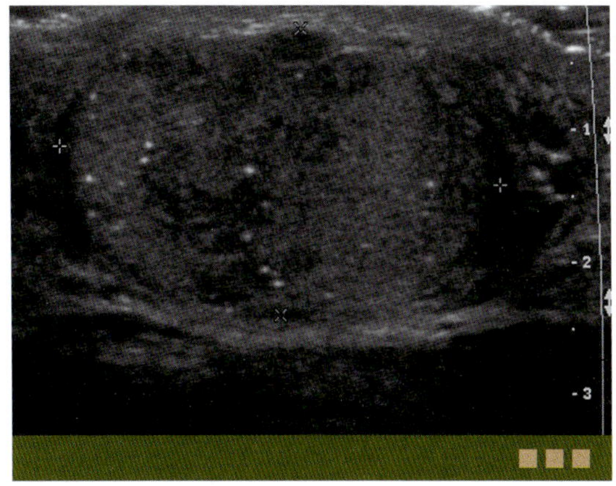

C. Transverse sonogram in the same patient as Figure B further shows intratesticular, hypoechoic mass that was subsequently proven to be a germ cell tumor.

DIFFERENTIAL DIAGNOSES IMAGES (D-E)

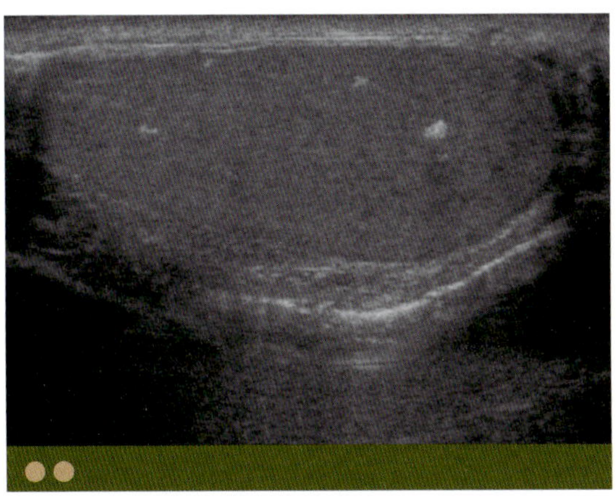

D. Macrocalcifications: Longitudinal sonogram of the left testicle shows a hyperechoic focus measuring approximately 6 mm in diameter compatible with macrocalcifications.

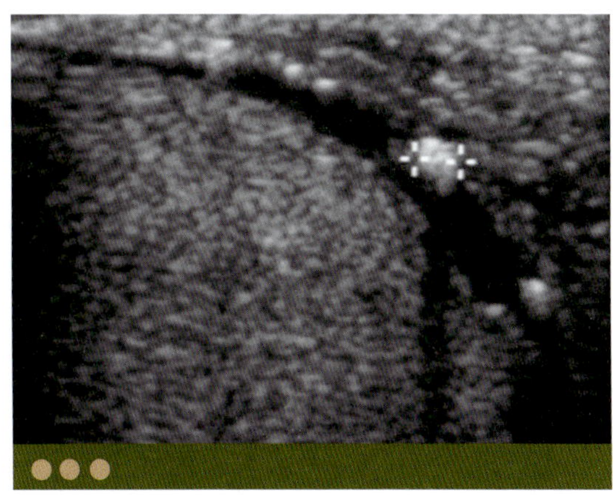

E. Scrotolith: Transverse sonogram shows an extratesticular hyperechoic focus with posterior acoustic shadowing compatible with a scrotolith.

IMAGE KEY

Common

Rare

Typical

Unusual

13–17 Testicular Lymphoma

Paul Nikolaidis

PRESENTATION

Painless testicular swelling, weight loss, fever, and night sweats.

FINDINGS

Sonography reveals diffuse involvement of the right testis with numerous ill-defined small hypoechoic foci in a background of diffuse heterogeneity.

DIFFERENTIAL DIAGNOSES

- *Testicular leukemia*: Usually with a similar sonographic appearance and often inseparable on imaging. They are similarly hypervascular on color Doppler sonography.
- *Infectious orchitis*: Infectious orchitis, especially severe, may have a similar appearance with testicular enlargement, hyperemia and loss of normal architectural features. Clinical symptomatology helps make the distinction.
- *Primary testicular neoplasms*: Primary (nonlymphomatous) testicular tumors may have a diffuse infiltrative appearance or may be multifocal, often with overlapping features (although most are solitary masses).
- *Testicular metastases*: Quite rare but may have overlapping features with lymphoma when multiple nodular foci of involvement are present.
- *Testicular rupture*: May present with testicular enlargement and loss of normal architectural features; the echogenic tunica albuginea should be disrupted. Clinical history should help differentiate.

COMMENTS

Primary testicular lymphoma accounts for approximately 5% of all testicular neoplasms and is the most common testicular malignancy in men over 60. However, testicular involvement is seen in less than 1% of the patients with lymphoma. Secondary lymphomatous involvement of the testis is more common.

Patients may present with painless testicular swelling that develops over weeks to months. On physical examination, a firm, nontender nodular testicle may be palpated.

Less commonly, patients have painful testicular swelling or may have a wide variety of constitutional symptoms including weight loss, fever, anorexia, and night sweats.

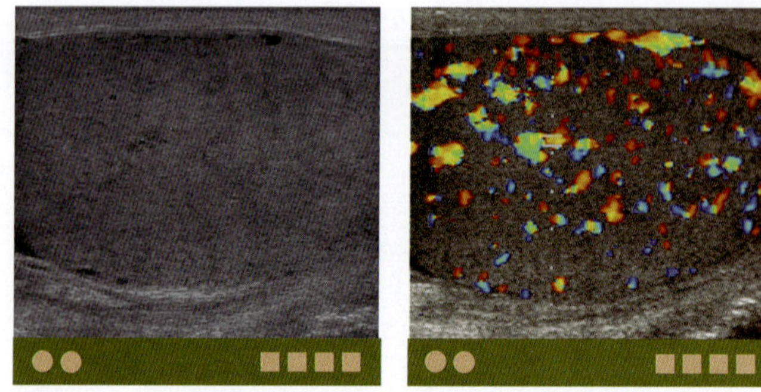

A. Longitudinal sonogram on a patient with a palpable scrotal mass shows an enlarged and heterogeneous right testicle. Vague areas of decreased echogenicity are seen throughout the testis. The epididymis was normal.
B. Corresponding longitudinal color Doppler sonogram shows multiple foci of markedly increased flow throughout the right testicle.

Sonographic findings include diffuse or focal involvement with areas of decreased echogenicity. Color Doppler sonography is very useful as lesions are frequently markedly hypervascular, even the smaller lesions. Involvement may be unilateral or bilateral. The epididymis may become involved in later stages, and will also be enlarged and hypoechoic. The testicular component is usually more extensive than the epididymal component.

The role of CT is generally confined to the identification of additional sites of involvement elsewhere in the body. MR can also detect testicular lesions and is also useful in evaluating extratesticular disease.

PEARLS

- **Most common testicular malignancy in men over 60.**
- **Secondary testicular lymphoma is more common than primary.**
- **On sonography, diffuse infiltration or multiple focal hypoechoic nodules are seen.**
- **Involved areas are almost always hypervascular on color Doppler.**

ADDITIONAL IMAGES (C-E)

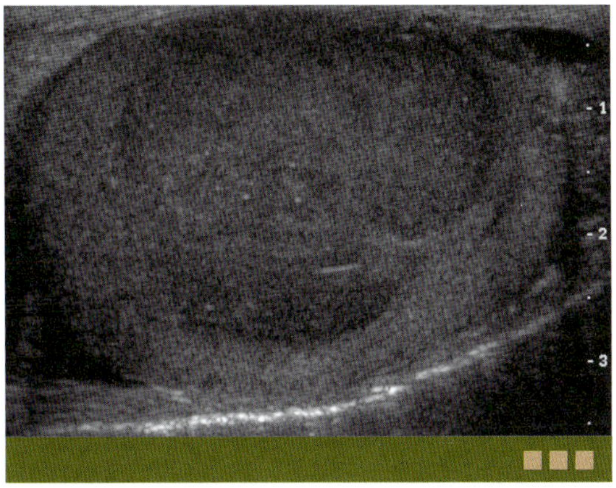

C. Longitudinal sonogram on another patient with testicular swelling shows a large infiltrative hypoechoic lesion in the right testicle.

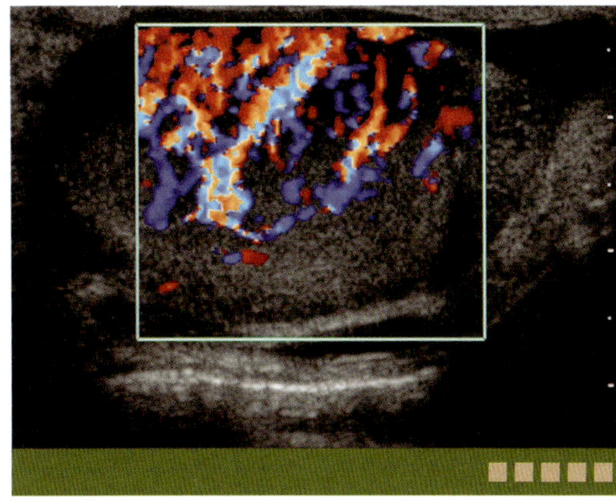

D. Corresponding longitudinal color Doppler sonogram shows markedly increased flow throughout the right testicular mass.

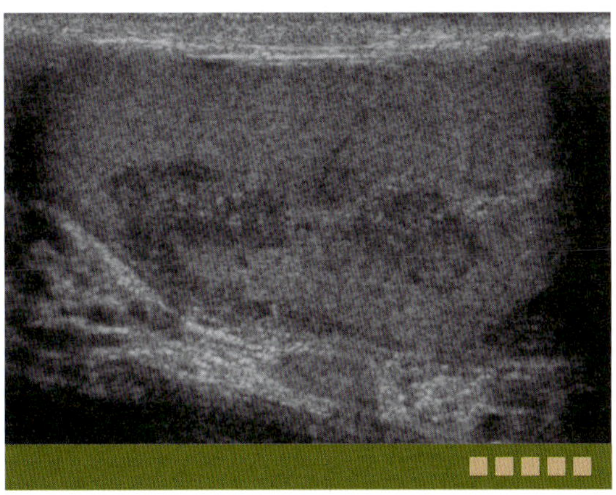

E. Longitudinal color Doppler sonogram of the right testicle in another patient with a history of lymphoma shows multiple areas of decreased echogenicity. Increased flow in the hypoechoic areas was seen on color Doppler images.

DIFFERENTIAL DIAGNOSES IMAGES (F-H)

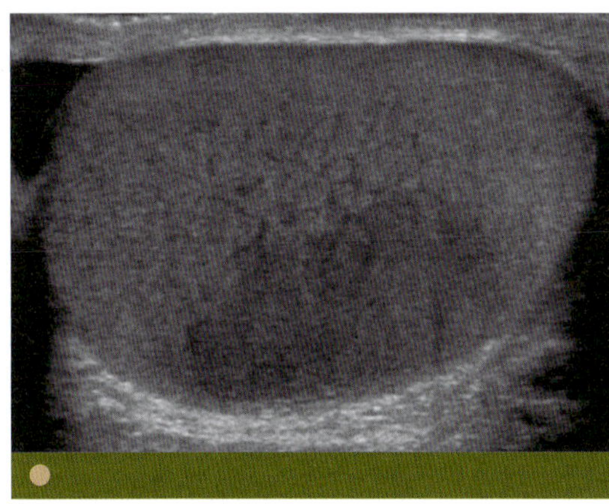

F. Testicular leukemia: Longitudinal sonogram on another patient with a history of leukemia shows a large peripheral hypoechoic lesion in the right testicle. This was also markedly hypervascular on color Doppler.

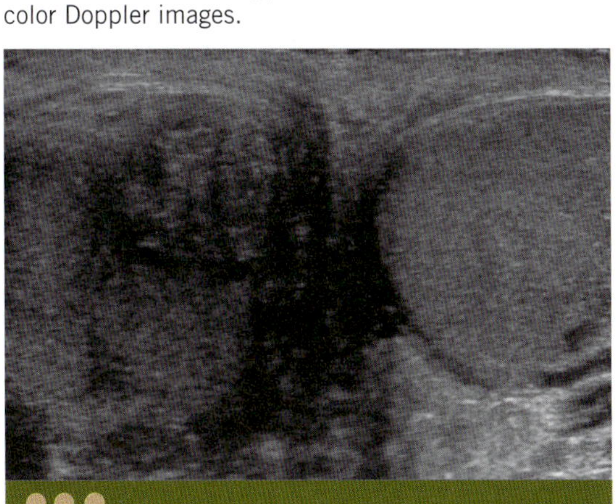

G. Acute infectious orchitis: Transverse sonogram on a patient with right-sided testicular pain and clinical signs of infection shows an enlarged, markedly heterogeneous right testis with several ill-defined hypoechoic areas. The left testicle is sonographically normal.

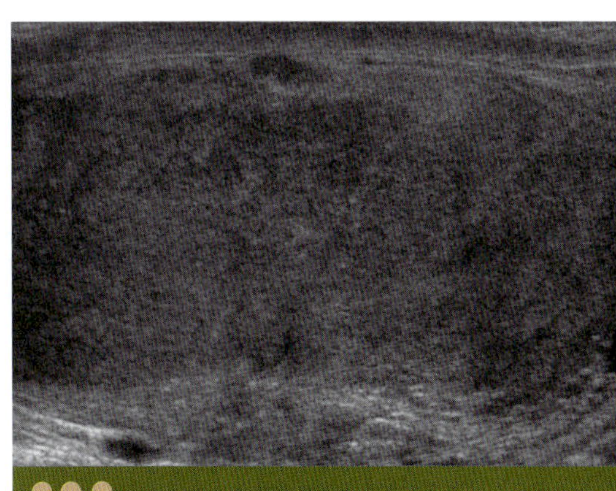

H. Testicular seminoma: Longitudinal sonogram in a patient with a palpable testicular mass shows a large heterogeneous mass occupying almost the entire right testicle. The mass demonstrated some areas of increased vascularity on color Doppler.

IMAGE KEY

Common

Rare

Typical

Unusual

13–18 Testicular Plasmacytoma (Plasma Cell Myeloma)

Paul Nikolaidis

PRESENTATION

Painless testicular swelling, weight loss, and back pain.

FINDINGS

Gray-scale sonogram in a patient with a history of multiple myeloma shows multiple hypoechoic, markedly hypervascular lesions within the testicle and in the scrotal wall.

DIFFERENTIAL DIAGNOSES

- *Testicular lymphoma*: Lesions may be more discrete in myeloma; but as increased vascularity on color flow imaging is seen in testicular leukemia and lymphoma, differentiation may be difficult.
- *Multifocal testicular seminoma*: Similarly may be impossible to differentiate. Lesions may show less vascularity.
- *Metastases*: Testicular metastases are rare. Patients usually have a known primary malignancy.
- *Sarcoid*: Scrotal lesions are typically multiple, small, and bilateral; although rarely, they can be solitary. Lesions are hypoechoic, with increased vascularity seen only in larger lesions on Doppler examination.

COMMENTS

Extramedullary plasmacytoma refers to a plasma cell myeloma arising in any organ outside the bone marrow. Ninety percent of these tumors develop in the head and neck; most commonly, they involve the upper respiratory tract. Rare sites of extraosseous myelomatoid involvement include the gastrointestinal tract, liver, spleen, pancreas, breast, vagina, testis, and skin. Most patients have previous or concurrent multiple myeloma or extramedullary plasmacytoma.

Sonographic appearances of testicular plasmacytoma that have been described include a solitary hypoechoic and markedly hypervascular lesion, as well as multiple hypoechoic lesions. An important sonographic feature is hyperemia on color flow and power Doppler images. Increased vascularity resembling inflammation on color flow imaging has also been described in testicular leukemia and lymphoma. Hyperechoic lesions have been reported less frequently. Lesions are usually homogeneous, but in some cases may be heterogeneous.

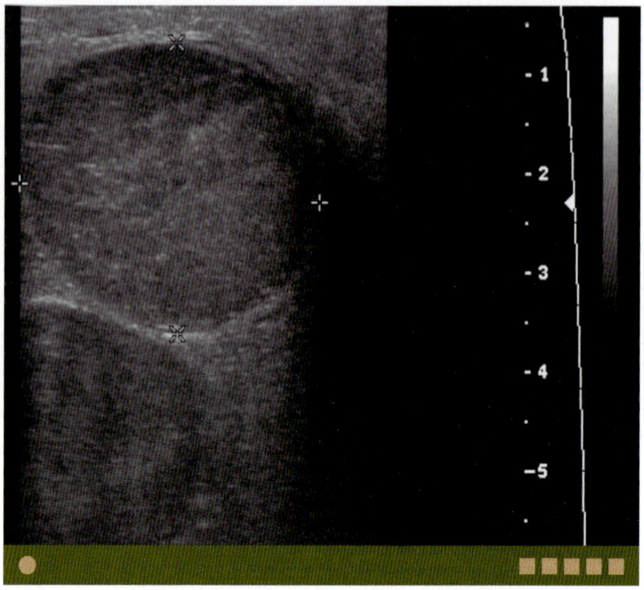

A. Longitudinal sonogram of the left testicle shows two intratesticular masses. The masses are slightly heterogeneous and predominantly hypoechoic.

The role of CT is generally confined to identification of additional sites of involvement elsewhere in the body. Multiplanar reformations may be helpful in better delineating the extent of osseous abnormalities. MR can also detect myelomatoid lesions in the testes and scrotum.

If there is no history of myeloma, biopsy is generally performed. If such lesions are identified in a patient with multiple myeloma, plasmacytoma should be considered.

PEARLS

- **The testis is a rare site of extraosseous involvement in multiple myeloma.**
- **Most patients have a history of multiple myeloma or extramedullary plasmacytoma.**
- **On sonography, diffuse or focal hypoechoic nodules are seen.**
- **Lesions are frequently hypervascular on color Doppler imaging.**

ADDITIONAL IMAGES (B-C)

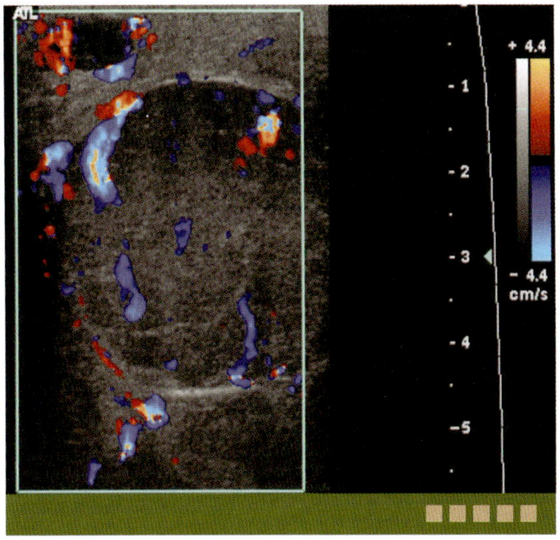

B. Longitudinal color Doppler sonogram on the same patient shows marked hypervascularity of one of the testicular masses.

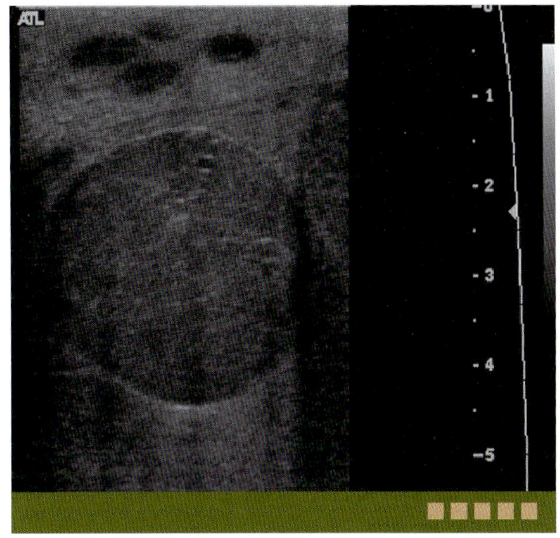

C. Transverse sonogram on the same patient shows four smaller hypoechoic scrotal wall lesions, in addition to the larger intratesticular mass.

DIFFERENTIAL DIAGNOSES IMAGES (D-F)

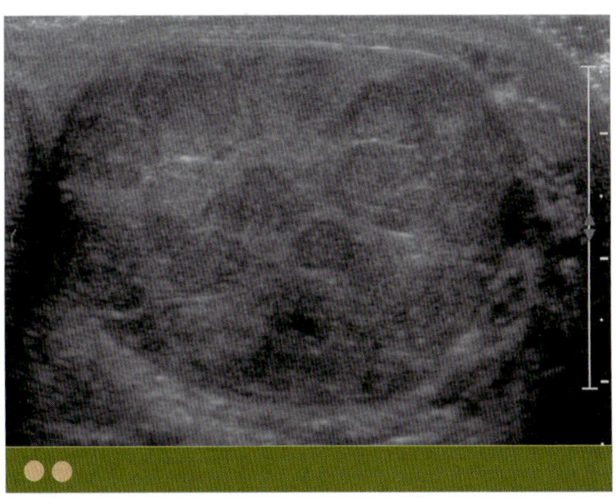

D. Multifocal seminoma: Longitudinal sonogram of the right testicle shows numerous hypoechoic intratesticular lesions. They were only moderately vascular on color flow imaging.

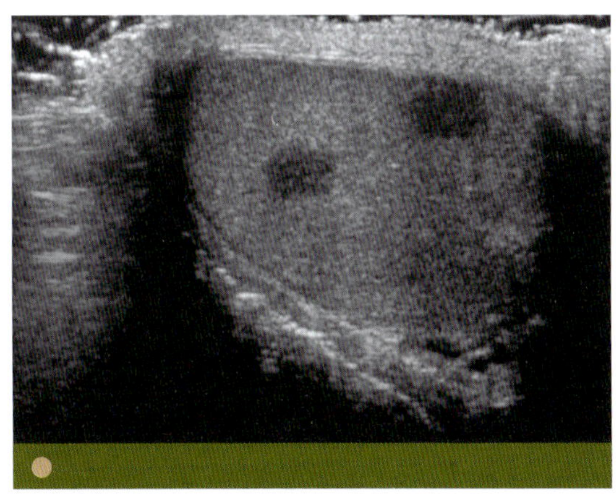

E. Sarcoid: Longitudinal sonogram of the left testicle shows a few small hypoechoic intratesticular lesions. On histopathologic analysis, these were shown to contain noncaseating granulomas. Subsequent chest CT demonstrated hilar and mediastinal lymphadenopathy.

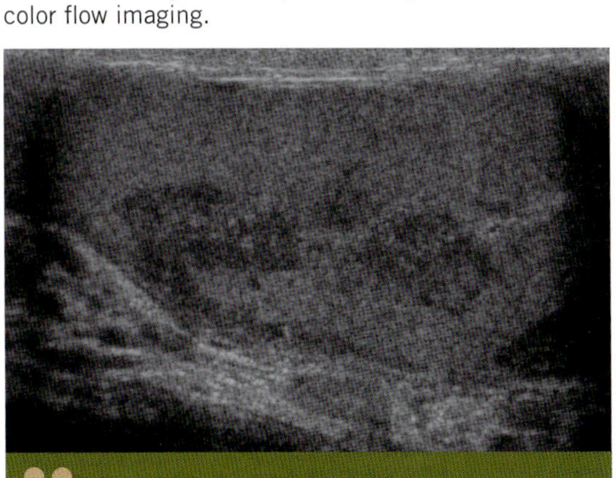

F. Lymphoma: Longitudinal sonogram of the right testicle shows a few ill-defined hypoechoic intratesticular lesions in a patient with a history of lymphoma.

IMAGE KEY

Common

Rare

Typical

Unusual

13–19 Leydig Cell Tumor

Paul Nikolaidis

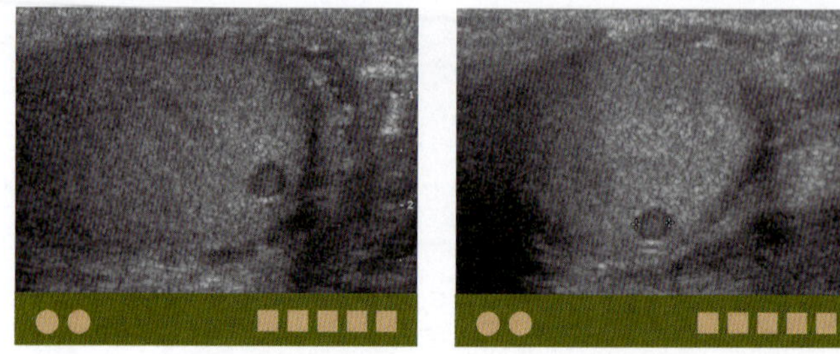

A. and B. Longitudinal (A) and transverse (B) sonogram of the right testis in a young male patient show a 4-mm solid hypoechoic intratesticular lesion.

PRESENTATION

Palpable testicular mass and gynecomastia.

FINDINGS

Sonography shows a single, well-defined small hypoechoic testicular lesion in a young patient.

DIFFERENTIAL DIAGNOSES

- *Seminoma and other testicular neoplasms*: Leydig cell tumors are usually solitary small hypoechoic lesions, sometimes hormonally active. They are often difficult to separate from a wide variety of testicular neoplasms.
- *Intratesticular hematoma or contusion*: An intratesticular hematoma may occur in the setting of testicular trauma. Necrosis and hemorrhage may be present in larger Leydig cell tumors. Clinical history and follow-up sonography may be important in making the distinction.

COMMENTS

Leydig cell tumors arise from the interstitial cells of Leydig, which are found adjacent to the seminiferous tubules. Together with Sertoli cells, they form the gonadal stroma of the testicle. Although Leydig cell tumors are the most common sex-cord stromal tumor, they account for only 1% to 3% of all testicular tumors. The sex-cord stromal tumors exhibit several histologic patterns, including Leydig, Sertoli, granulosa and theca cell, along with undifferentiated types. Mixed tumors are relatively common.

Leydig cell tumors can occur at almost any age, but there appear to be two peaks, the first in pediatric patients 5 to 10 years old and the second at 20 to 50 years. Approximately 10% to 20% of tumors in adults are malignant. They are very rarely malignant in children. Leydig cell tumors can secrete sex hormones such as estradiol and patients may present with gynecomastia. They can also secrete testosterone.

On sonography, they are typically small, solid and hypoechoic. In a young patient with a small intratesticular hypoechoic mass, Leydig cell tumor should always be considered in the differential. Benign tumors cannot be reliably distinguished from malignant ones on imaging. Malignant tumors are usually larger, often with an infiltrative margin, and may show spread beyond the testis. In approximately 25% of cases, foci of hemorrhage and necrosis may produce cystic spaces (particularly in larger lesions).

If a Leydig cell tumor is considered preoperatively, the patient can undergo excisional biopsy through an inguinal approach, with intraoperative sonography for localization of the mass. If the intraoperative frozen section diagnosis is benign, testicle-sparing resection can be performed.

PEARLS

- **Sex-cord stromal tumors include Leydig (most common), Sertoli, granulosa, and theca cell, along with undifferentiated and mixed types.**
- **Approximately 10% to 20% of Leydig cell tumors in adults are malignant; in children they are mostly benign. On sonography, they are typically small, solid, and hypoechoic.**
- **Sonography cannot reliably distinguish benign from malignant lesions.**
- **Larger tumors can have cystic spaces from necrosis and hemorrhage.**

ADDITIONAL IMAGES (C-D)

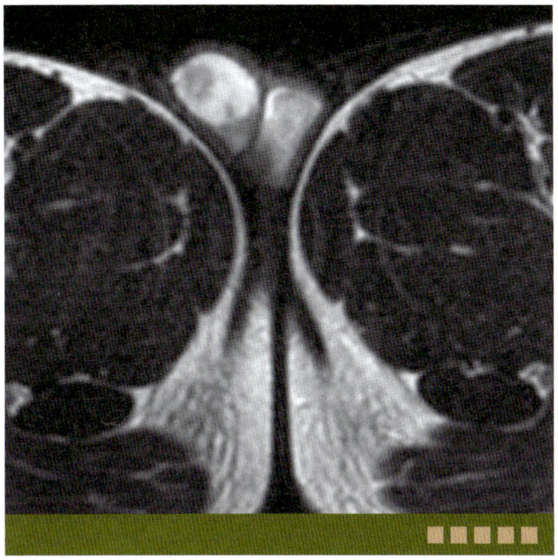

C. Axial non-contrast T1-WI of the right testis on a different patient shows a small hypointense intratesticular mass representing a Leydig cell tumor. (*Image courtesy of Dr Dana Weber, Dept. Ped. Radiology, University of Leipzig.*)

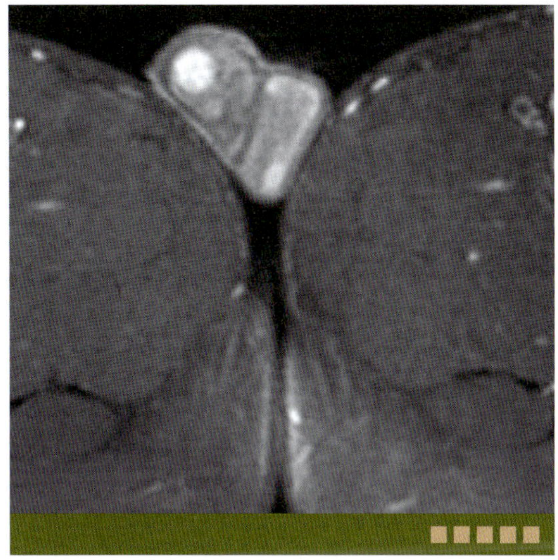

D. Axial contrast-enhanced T1-WI on the same patient shows that the tumor enhances avidly. (*Image courtesy of Dr Dana Weber, Dept. Ped. Radiology, University of Leipzig.*)

DIFFERENTIAL DIAGNOSES IMAGES (E-F)

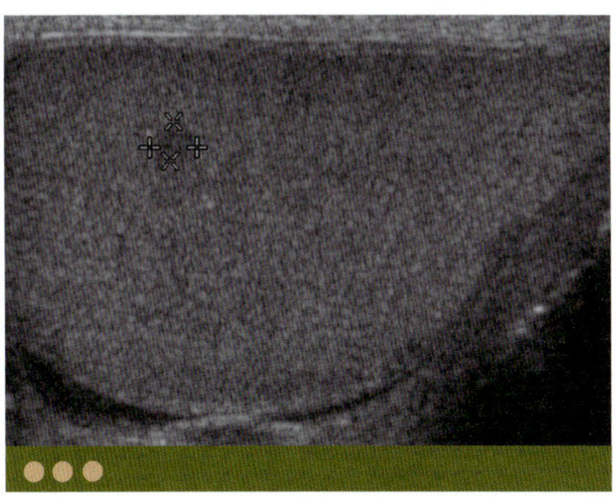

E. Seminoma: Longitudinal sonogram in a different patient shows a very small hypoechoic intratesticular lesion (outlined by the calipers). Surgical pathology confirmed a small seminoma.

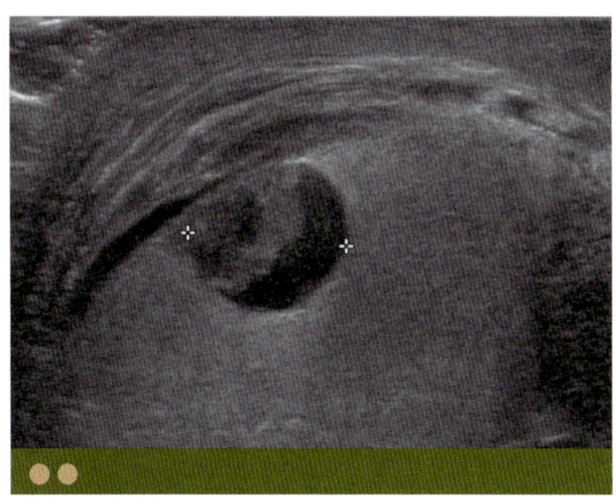

F. Intratesticular hematoma: Transverse sonogram in a patient with a history of trauma shows a peripheral intratesticular lesion of mixed echogenicity, but predominantly hypoechoic. Necrosis and hemorrhage may be present in larger Leydig cell tumors. This was presumed to represent a hematoma, and was followed with sonography. It subsequently resolved.

IMAGE KEY

Common

Rare

Typical

Unusual

13–20 Testicular Sarcoidosis

Frank H. Miller

PRESENTATION

Incidental lesions on ultrasound, history of respiratory symptoms.

FINDINGS

Irregular, hypoechoic solid masses in the testis.

DIFFERENTIAL DIAGNOSES

- *Neoplasm*: Less commonly multiple masses; often not involvement of both testes and epididymis; differentiated by clinical history or imaging findings of sarcoidosis.
- Lymphoma can involve both testis and epididymis, but testis is more often involved and patients are often older with known history of lymphoma. Biopsy often required for diagnosis.
- Inflammatory process such as tuberculosis or fungal infection; can have multiple masses in testes and epididymis; patients generally symptomatic.
- *Testicular infarcts*: Unusual appearance as multiple round masses; can be distinguished based on history and abnormal Doppler flow.

COMMENTS

Sarcoidosis is a systemic disease with noncaseous granulomas in affected organs. Nearly all organs have reportedly been involved with sarcoidosis, the most frequently involved organ is the lung. Genital involvement occurs in less than 1% of the patients with systemic sarcoidosis and may not be suspected or diagnosed prior to ultrasound exam.

Characteristically, sarcoidosis involving the testes is seen as irregular small hypoechoic solid masses involving the testes or epididymes. The lesions are typically multiple and small, and rarely are solitary. On sonography, the appearance may mimic inflammatory or neoplastic lesions. The lesions are generally painless. Patients may have acute or chronic epididymitis. Often the patient has symptoms related to sarcoidosis, but the diagnosis may not be known prior to the ultrasound examination. On further investigation, the patient often has respiratory symptoms and a chest X-ray or CT scan may show the characteristic hilar lymphadenopathy or pulmonary parenchymal disease of sarcoidosis. In other patients, the radiologist may not be aware of the diagnosis of sarcoidosis. Differential considerations include primary testicular tumor, metastatic disease, tuberculosis, fungal infections, and Wegener granulomatosis. Sarcoidosis may co-present with tuberculosis making the diagnosis more difficult. Surgery may be required for the diagnosis as the diagnosis may not be suspected; however, surgery may not be required for therapy as many cases of sarcoidosis may respond to steroids.

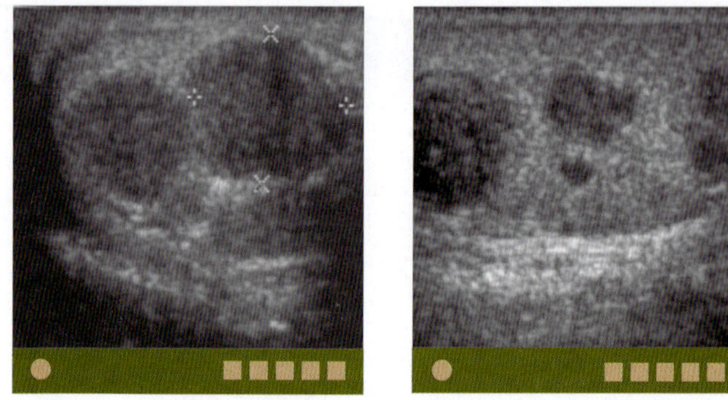

A. Ultrasound shows several hypoechoic lesions seen in the right testis.
B. Multiple lesions are also seen in the left testis.

PEARLS

- **Consider sarcoidosis when small hypoechoic epididymal and testicular lesions.**
- **To help diagnose sarcoidosis, a chest X-ray or CT scan may be helpful.**
- **Lesions from sarcoidosis are generally asymptomatic unlike those from infections or malignancy.**
- **Sarcoidosis responds to steroids.**

ADDITIONAL IMAGES (C-E)

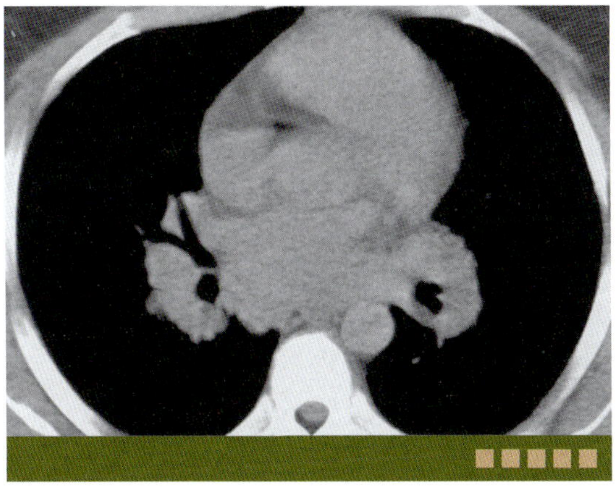

C. Axial NECT scan shows bilateral hilar adenopathy caused by sarcoidosis (arrows).

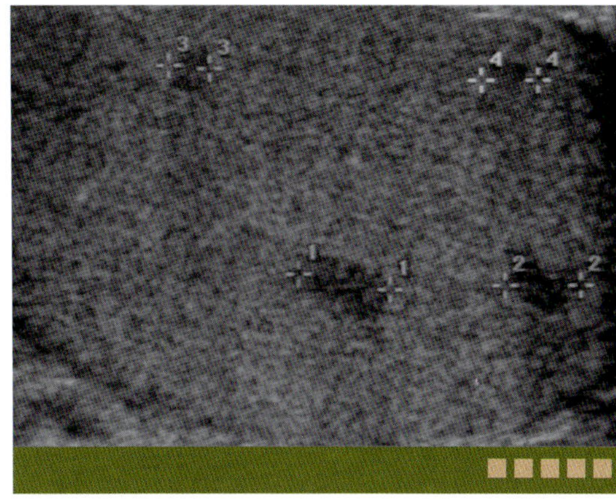

D. Sarcoidosis: In another patient, multiple small hypoechoic lesions are seen in the right testis.

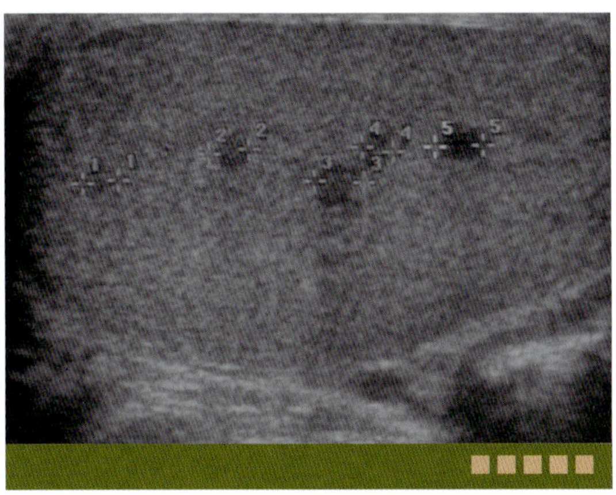

E. Multiple lesions are also seen in the left testis in same patient as in Figure D.

DIFFERENTIAL DIAGNOSES IMAGES (F-H)

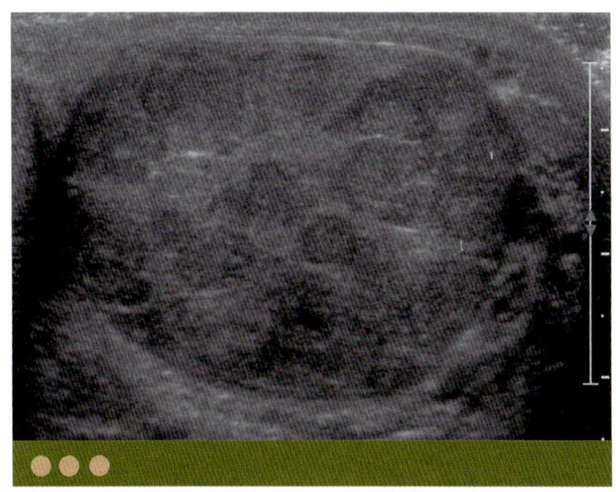

F. Multifocal seminoma: Longitudinal sonogram of the right testicle shows numerous hypoechoic intratesticular lesions.

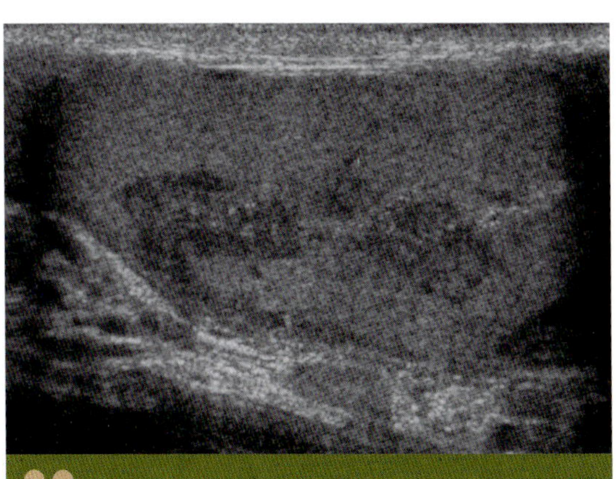

G. Lymphoma: Longitudinal sonogram of the right testicle shows a few ill-defined hypoechoic intratesticular lesions in a patient with history of non-Hodgkin lymphoma.

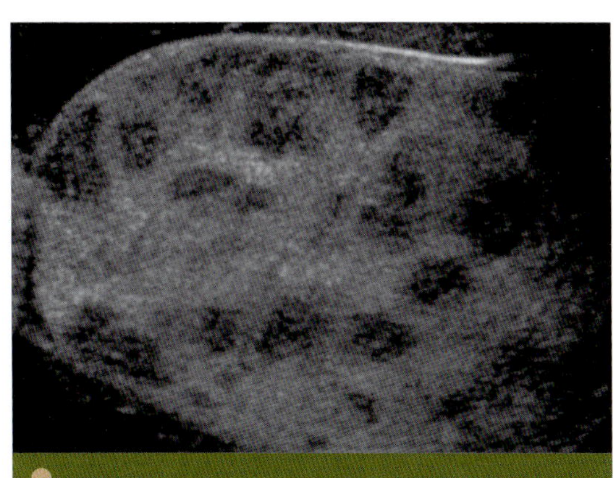

H. Infarct: Longitudinal sonogram shows multiple hypoechoic lesions in the testes with no flow seen in the testis caused by infarction.

IMAGE KEY

Common

Rare

Typical

Unusual

13–21 Inflammatory Pseudotumor of the Testis

Paul Nikolaidis

PRESENTATION

Painless testicular mass, often in immune-deficient patients.

FINDINGS

Sonography shows a solid peripheral hypoechoic testicular mass. There is some peripheral flow, with few penetrating vessels seen on color and power Doppler.

DIFFERENTIAL DIAGNOSES

- *Solid testicular neoplasms*: Inflammatory pseudotumor is a very rare lesion with a nonspecific sonographic appearance and differentiation from most neoplasms is usually not feasible. Patients with pseudotumors may be immune-deficient, as can patients with other testicular neoplasms however.
- *Intratesticular hematoma*: Rare, color flow should be absent. Clinical history very helpful.

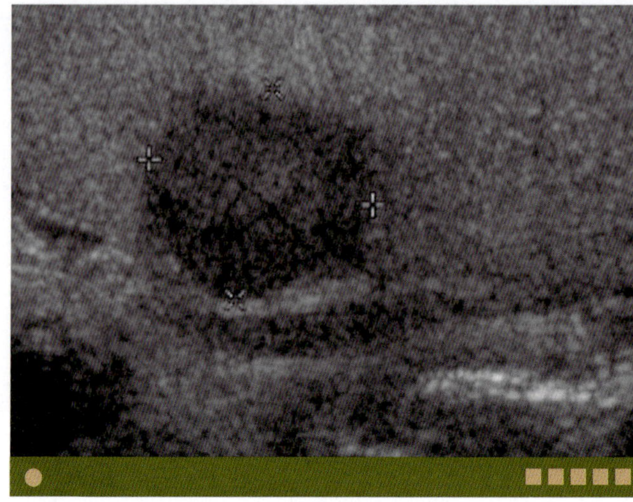

A. Longitudinal sonogram of the right testis shows a 1.2-cm peripherally located round hypoechoic mass.

COMMENTS

Inflammatory pseudotumor is a very rare entity that sonographically mimics a neoplasm. Inflammatory pseudotumors can occur anywhere and have been described in many organs, including the lung, spleen, and liver, but also rarely within the testicular stroma. Most of them are composed of a varying mixture of myofibroblasts, fibroblasts, lymphocytes, and plasma cells.

Testicular inflammatory pseudotumors are thought to represent a tissue reaction and may occur in the setting of previous trauma, surgery, infection, chemotherapy, radiation, or adjacent neoplasm.

Very few cases of inflammatory pseudotumor of the testis have been reported in the literature, and there are also a few reports of extratesticular scrotal pseudotumors. The few cases described have been solid, hypoechoic, and round. Some peripheral flow and a few penetrating vessels may be seen on color Doppler. Their sonographic appearance is highly nonspecific and differential considerations include primary and secondary testicular neoplasms.

Surgical resection is typically necessary to provide the definitive histologic diagnosis.

PEARLS

- **A rare entity that sonographically mimics a neoplasm.**
- **Rarely occurs in the scrotum, either within the stroma of the testes or in the extratesticular space.**
- **Thought to be tissue reaction to a previous insult (trauma, surgery, infection, chemotherapy, or radiation).**
- **Typically solid, homogeneous, and hypoechoic on sonography.**

ADDITIONAL IMAGES (B-C)

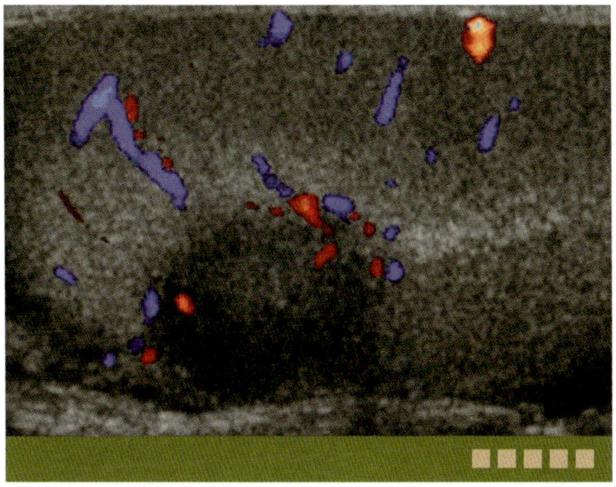

B. Corresponding longitudinal color Doppler sonogram of the right testicular lesion shows some peripheral flow. The lesion is otherwise predominantly hypovascular.

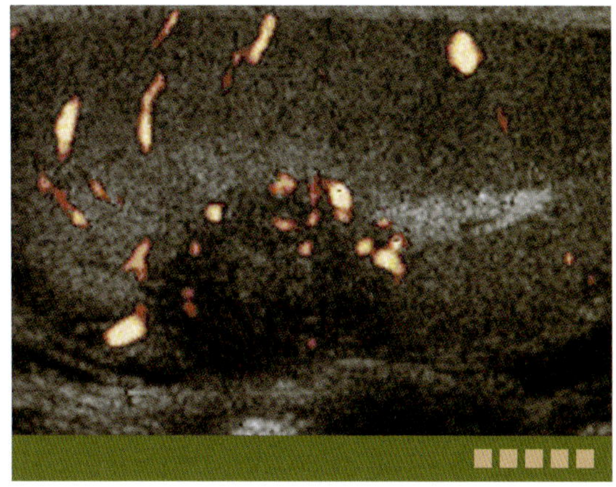

C. Corresponding longitudinal power Doppler sonogram of the right testis better shows the few penetrating vessels.

DIFFERENTIAL DIAGNOSES IMAGES (D-F)

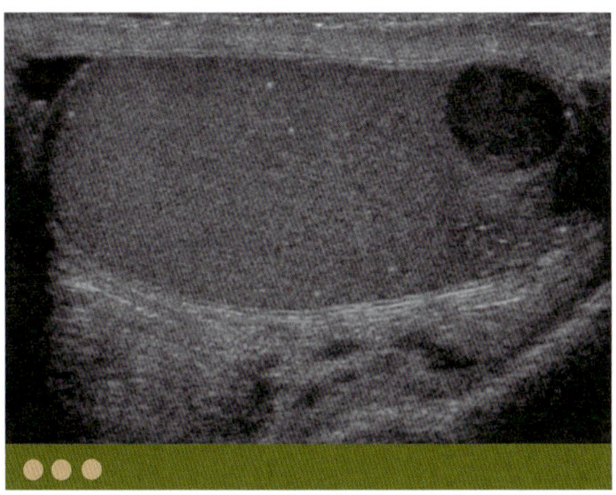

D. Seminoma: Longitudinal sonogram in a different patient shows an 8-mm peripheral hypoechoic, solid intratesticular lesion. Note the concomitant testicular microlithiasis.

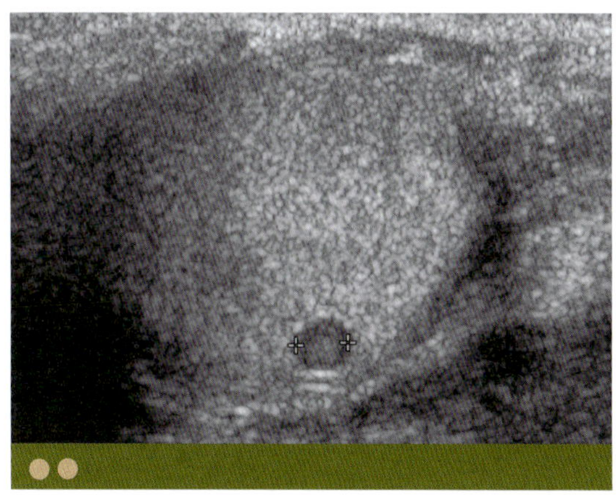

E. Leydig cell tumor: Transverse sonogram of the right testis in another patient shows a nonspecific, 4-mm, solid, hypoechoic intratesticular lesion.

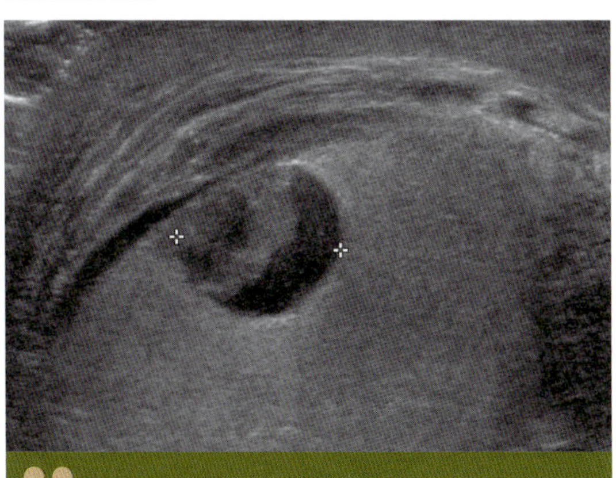

F. Intratesticular hematoma: Transverse sonogram in a patient with a history of trauma shows peripheral testicular lesion with mixed echogenicity (but predominately hypoechoic). There was no appreciable internal flow. This was presumed to represent a hematoma, and was sonographically followed to resolution.

IMAGE KEY

Common

Rare

Typical

Unusual

13–22 Epidermoid Cyst

Frank H. Miller

PRESENTATION

Palpable testicular mass; less often incidental on physical exam.

FINDINGS

Sonogram shows intratesticular mass with "onion ring" appearance with alternating areas of increased and decreased echogenicity.

DIFFERENTIAL DIAGNOSES

- *Teratoma*: Can have a similar imaging appearance on ultrasound, but they usually have positive tumor markers and Doppler vascularity, which are not seen in epidermoid cysts.
- *Seminoma*: Does not have the echogenic capsule or calcified rim.
- *Xanthogranulomatous orchitis*: Rare entity distinguish based on imaging appearance and history.

COMMENTS

Testicular epidermoid cyst is a rare benign lesion seen in 1% to 2% of resected testicular tumors. It is the most common benign tumor in the testis. Epidermoid cyst is a benign tumor of germ cell origin ranging in size from 1 to 3 cm. It is most commonly seen during the second to fourth decades of life. They are benign and have no malignant potential. They are treated with orchiectomy or enucleation.

The sonographic appearances of epidermoid cysts include: a well-defined, solid hypoechoic mass with an echogenic capsule or calcified rim; a halo with a central area of increased echogenicity—target appearance; and an "onion ring" appearance, with alternating layers of hyper and hypoechogenicity. The lesion is filled with flaky, cheesy-white keratin. It is important to recognize an epidermoid cyst at sonography, as it allows testis-sparing surgery. The lesions can be difficult to distinguish from rare teratoma requiring pathologic evaluation. MR findings include a high-signal intensity mass on T2-weighted images with or without low-signal intensity foci surrounded by a low signal intensity rim and lack of enhancement on contrast-enhanced T1-weighted images.

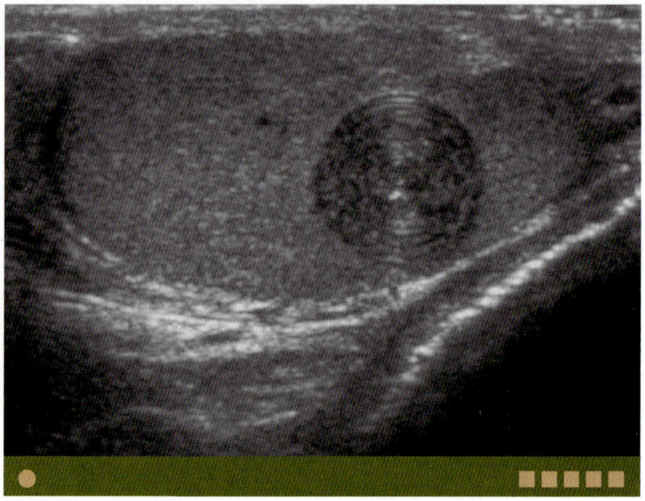

A. Longitudinal sonogram shows mass with "onion ring" appearance with alternating layers of increased and decreased echogenicity.

PEARLS

- **Testicular epidermoid is rare, seen in 1% to 2% of resected tumors.**
- **Epidermoid cysts are benign.**
- **Can have target or "onion ring" appearance.**
- **Important to identify as may perform testis sparing surgery.**

ADDITIONAL IMAGE

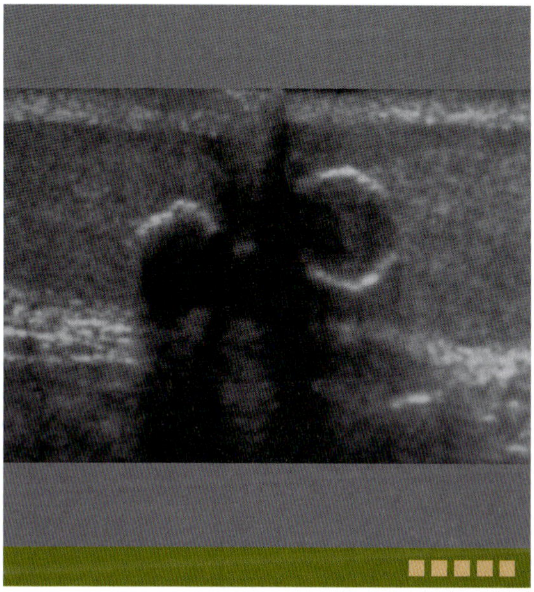

B. Longitudinal sonogram shows bilateral hypoechoic masses with echogenic rim characteristic of epidermoid. Bilateral involvement is rare.

DIFFERENTIAL DIAGNOSES IMAGE

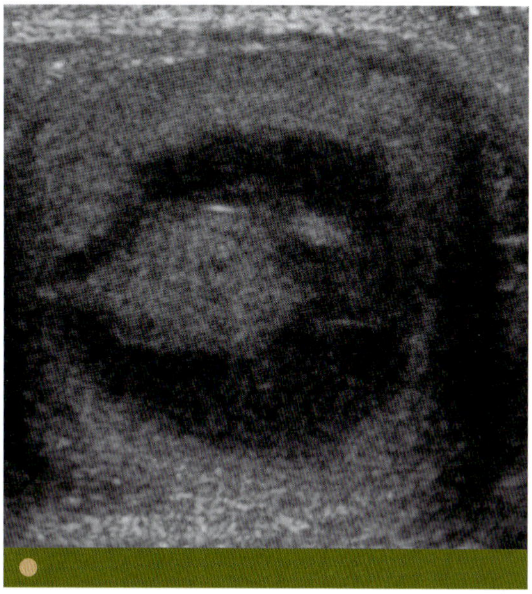

C. Xanthogranulomatous orchitis: Longitudinal sonogram shows complex mass with areas of increased and decreased echogenicity. The appearance is nonspecific and more heterogeneous than the epidermoid cysts. It was shown to be XGO following orchiectomy.

IMAGE KEY

Common

Rare

Typical

Unusual

13–23 Cysts of Tunica Albuginea

Frank H. Miller

PRESENTATION

Palpable mass.

FINDINGS

Sonogram shows extratesticular cyst measuring less than 1 cm with cystic appearance involving tunica albuginea.

DIFFERENTIAL DIAGNOSIS

None

COMMENTS

Cysts of the tunica albuginea can present with palpable mass and be confused clinically with neoplasms. (The tunica albuginea is the surrounding capsule of the testis.) The incidence of cysts of the tunica albuginea is about 0.3% of adult men. Patients with cyst of the tunica albuginea may have a mass which concerns patients or physicians for a testicular tumor. Often patients or physicians are concerned and the palpable mass prompts an ultrasound exam with suspicion of testicular tumor. Ultrasound is diagnostic in showing that it is not an intratesticular neoplasm. A cyst of the tunica albuginea is seen as an extratesticular cystic lesion typically in the upper anterior and lateral zone of the testis.

Testicular cysts are divided into intratesticular and extratesticular cysts. The extratesticular cysts include cysts of the tunica albuginea and those of the epididymis. Cysts of the tunica albuginea are most commonly seen in the 40- and 50-year-old males. They range in size from 2 to 5 mm and may be single or multiple. They may be larger and more complex. They may be initially triggered by prior infection or trauma.

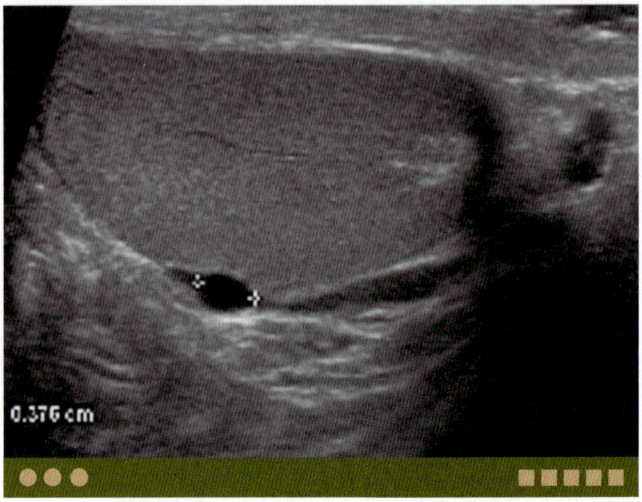

A. Longitudinal sonogram shows a 4-mm anechoic lesion caused by the cyst of the tunica albuginea.

PEARLS

- **Sonography is diagnostic in diagnosing cyst of the tunica albuginea.**
- **Extratesticular nodule smaller than 1 cm with cystic echogenicity and thin wall involving tunica albuginea is diagnostic of tunica albuginea.**
- **Cysts of tunica albuginea do not require surgery.**

IMAGE KEY

Common

Rare

Typical

Unusual

13–24 Cysts and Tubular Ectasia of the Rete Testis

Frank H. Miller

PRESENTATION

Asymptomatic middle-aged male.

FINDINGS

Sonogram shows cysts involving the rete testes and epididymal cysts.

DIFFERENTIAL DIAGNOSES

- *Cystic malignant testicular tumors such as teratoma*: Can occur anywhere in the testis and not only in the mediastinum. Different age group; positive tumor markers, tend to be in younger patients and palpable mass.
- *Rete testis cystadenoma*: Extremely rare; cystic lesion with multiple septations, large cystic components, and conglomeration of cysts.

COMMENTS

Tubular ectasia of the rete testis are dilatation of the tubules which transport sperm from the seminiferous tubules to the efferent tubules. They are often associated with ipsilateral spermatoceles and intratesticular cysts.

Unlike most intratesticular masses, cysts and tubular ectasia of the rete testes are benign. The diagnosis of tubular ectasia of the rete testis is important so that it should not be confused for testicular neoplasm. Unlike neoplasms, they tend to occur in middle-aged and elderly men. In addition, they typically are associated with the mediastinum testis and associated with spermatoceles. Unlike neoplasms, they are generally not palpable masses. Tubular ectasia of the rete testes is often bilateral and asymmetric. Neoplasms tend to be solid masses.

Sonography shows multiple small variable cystic lesions involving the mediastinum testis. On sonography, they have the appearance of cysts including anechoic lesions with increased through transmission and lack of flow. They tend to be in the superoposterior aspect of the testis involving the mediastinum. The cyst may range from a few millimeters to 15 mL. They may be surrounded by a hyperechoic rim.

Cystic tumors tend to occur in younger patients, have positive tumor markers, and do not meet all criteria of a simple cyst. Tubular ectasia is often bilateral unlike tumors.

Tubular ectasia of the rete testis is associated with epididymal obstruction secondary to inflammatory or traumatic lesions. There are variable-sized cystic lesions in the region of the mediastinum testis. They are frequently bilateral and associated with epididymal cysts.

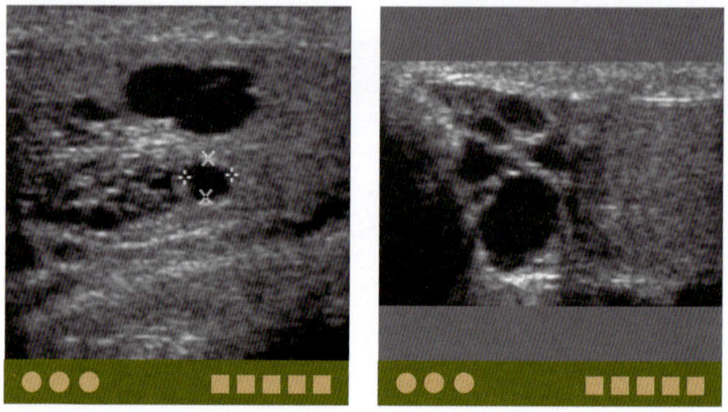

A. Longitudinal sonogram shows multiple different size cysts involving the mediastinum testes.
B. Longitudinal sonogram shows associated epididymal cysts.

PEARLS

- **Tubular ectasia of the rete testes tends to occur in middle-aged men.**
- **Cysts are seen in the region of the mediastinum testes.**
- **They are frequently seen involving both testes and associated with epididymal cysts.**

DIFFERENTIAL DIAGNOSES IMAGES (C-D)

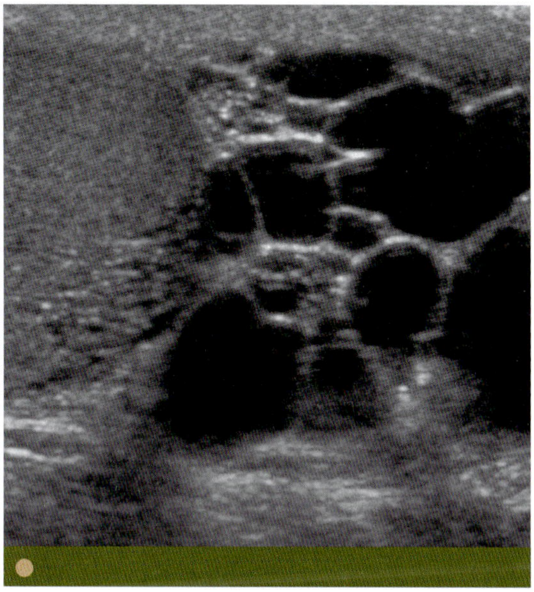

C. Cystadenoma of the rete testis: Transverse sonogram shows large complex cystic mass in right scrotum which is predominately extratesticular. The mass is seen adjacent to the rete testes.

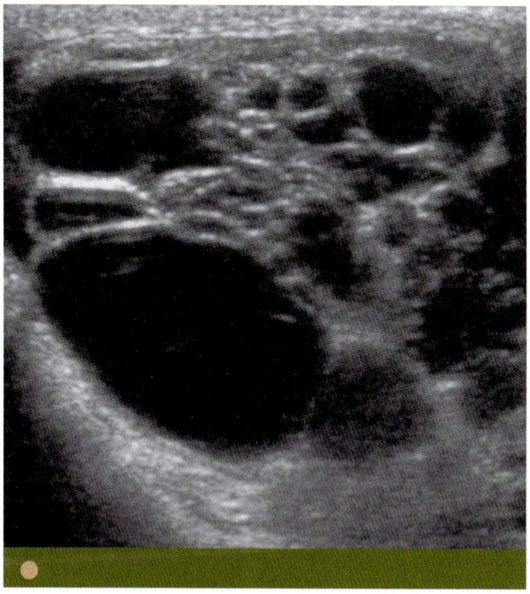

D. Cystadenoma of the rete testis: In the same patient, the mass is shown to have large cystic components and large conglomeration of cysts on sonography.

IMAGE KEY

Common
Rare

Typical
Unusual

13–25 Cystadenoma of the Rete Testis

Paul Nikolaidis

PRESENTATION

Painless mass on examination, scrotal swelling.

FINDINGS

Sonography reveals a large multicystic, septated lesion of the left testicle, with significant extratesticular extension.

DIFFERENTIAL DIAGNOSES

- *Cystic ectasia of the rete testis*: With minimal dilatation, cystic ectasia presents as subtle linear echoes around very small cystic spaces in the mediastinum testis. With increasing dilatation, the tubules have a more cystic appearance.
- *Epididymal cysts*: Rete cystadenomas may become large and grow predominantly into the extratesticular space. However, the multitude of septations, extensive cystic components, and focal conglomeration should help distinguish them from epididymal cysts.
- *Cystadenocarcinoma of the rete testis*: Cystadenocarcinoma is indistinguishable from rete testes cystadenoma. Histologic diagnosis is always required.

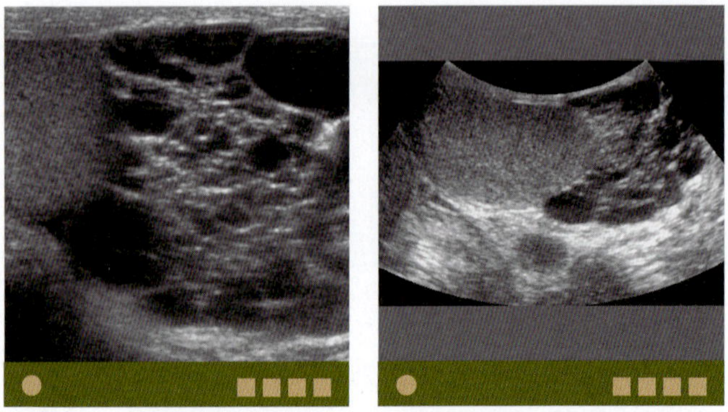

A. and B. Transverse smaller field of view (A) and larger field of view (B) sonogram shows a large predominantly extratesticular complex cystic mass in the right scrotum containing numerous septations.

COMMENTS

The rete testis is an anastomotic network of ducts that is often a site of benign cystic change. Cystic ectasia, also termed cystic dilatation of the rete testis, is the most common abnormality of the rete testis. Its appearance depends on the extent of tubular dilatation. With minimal dilatation, cystic ectasia appears as subtle linear echoes posterior to small cystic spaces in the region of the mediastinum. With increasing dilatation, the tubules take on a more cystic appearance. Rarely, neoplasms of the rete testis may occur, including benign cystadenomas and malignant cystadenocarcinoma. Other processes that may involve the rete testis include hyperplasia, cysts, hamartomas, and other neoplasms.

Sonographically, cystadenomas appear as multiseptated or multiloculated lesions with or without associated nodularity. Although the rete testis is mainly located within the testicle, these lesions can become quite large and grow mostly into the extratesticular space. Features which distinguish a cystadenoma from other scrotal cystic lesions such as epididymal cysts are the multitude of septations and cystic components as well as the focal conglomeration of the cysts.

Treatment of cystadenomas is usually surgical excision and clinical follow up. If not removed in their entirety, they can recur. Patients should be followed clinically and with ultrasound after surgery. If removed completely, the prognosis is excellent, in contrast to cystadenocarcinomas.

PEARLS

- **Neoplasms of the rete testis, including benign cystadenomas and malignant cystadenocarcinoma, are rare.**
- **On sonography, they are typically multiseptated or multiloculated lesions, in some cases with significant associated nodularity.**
- **The closest benign sonographic mimics are cystic ectasia of the rete testis, along with cysts and hamartomas which are rare.**
- **Treatment is surgical excision with close follow-up as they can recur if not removed in their entirety.**

ADDITIONAL IMAGES (C-D)

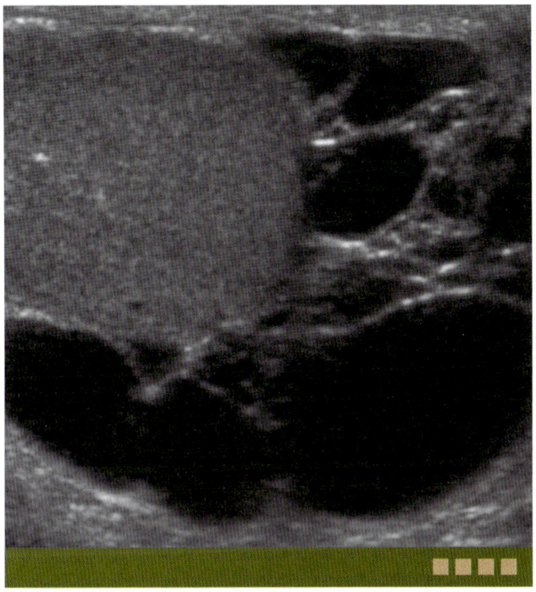

C. Longitudinal sonogram on the same patient shows larger cystic components that are part of this extensive lesion. Note that while the mass originates from the rete testis, it is predominantly extratesticular.

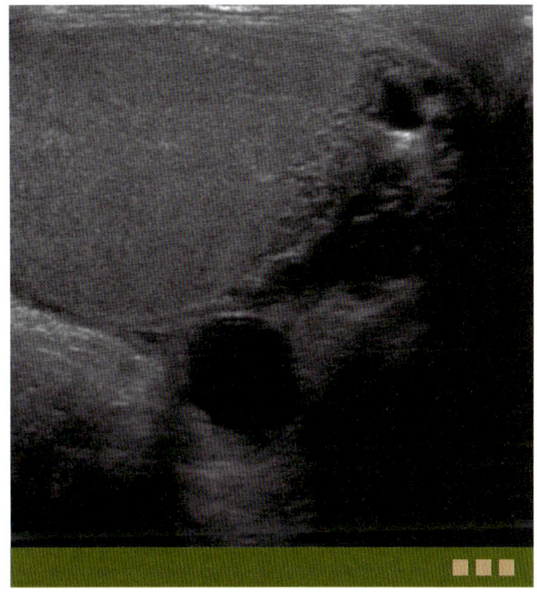

D. Transverse sonogram on the same patient obtained 2 years after surgical resection of the rete testis cystadenoma shows recurrence of the lesion. Note that it has similar sonographic features.

DIFFERENTIAL DIAGNOSES IMAGES (E-F)

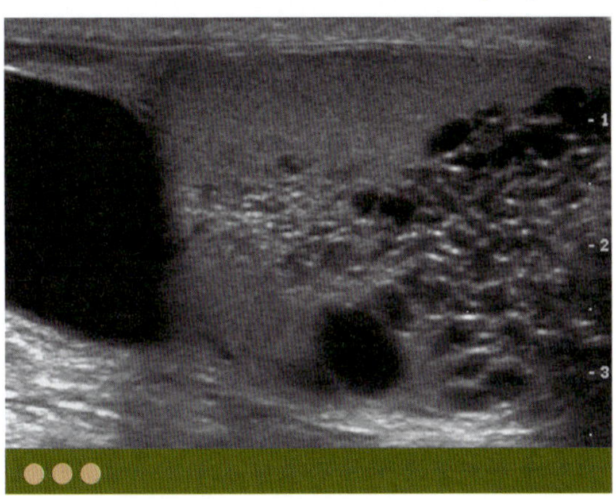

E. Cystic ectasia of the rete testis: Longitudinal sonogram of the right testis shows numerous small cysts extending along the mediastinum testis, some with a more tubular appearance. Findings are pathognomic for extensive ectasia of the rete testis.

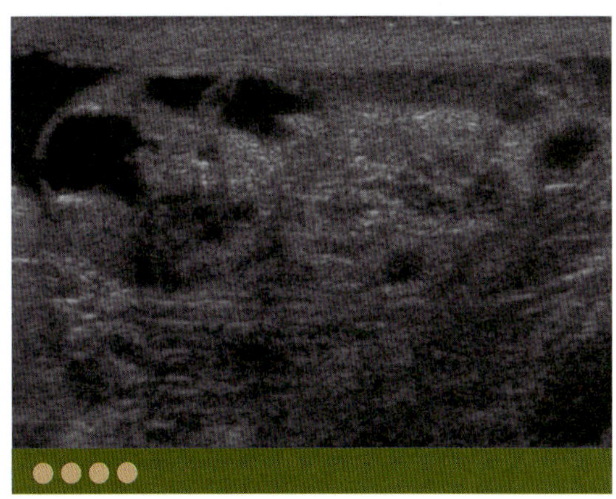

F. Epididymal cysts: Longitudinal sonogram of the left epididymis shows several discrete anechoic lesions compatible with simple cysts.

IMAGE KEY

Common

Rare

Typical

Unusual

13–26 Intratesticular Varicocele

Paul Nikolaidis

PRESENTATION

Asymptomatic, testicular pain, or infertility.

FINDINGS

Sonography reveals an anechoic tubular intratesticular lesion, which fills on color flow imaging.

DIFFERENTIAL DIAGNOSES

- *Extratesticular varicocele*: In a purely extratesticular varicocele, prominent vessels are located along the course of the spermatic cord and peritesticular region, but not within the testicle.
- *Cystic ectasia of the rete testis*: Cystic spaces are seen in the mediastinum testis, without any venous flow.
- *Cystadenoma of the rete testis*: Larger multiseptated or multiloculated lesions often with associated nodularity, and without any internal venous flow.

COMMENTS

An extratesticular varicocele (ETV) is a common entity that occurs in approximately 8% to 20% of males. ETVs occur secondary to increased dilatation of the veins of the spermatic cord, primarily caused by incompetent valves with impaired drainage into the internal spermatic vein. Less commonly, ETV is a result of venous compression. Sonography shows multiple dilated veins, exceeding 2 mm in diameter, located along the course of the spermatic cord or in the paratesticular region. ETV is more commonly left-sided (85%). Color or pulsed Doppler sonography shows a normal venous flow pattern at rest and increased velocities and retrograde filling during Valsalva manoeuvre.

An intratesticular varicocele (ITV) may occur in patients with an ETV. It is described as dilated veins radiating from the mediastinum testis into the testicular parenchyma. While it may be associated with testicular pain, ITV is usually an incidental finding on sonography. It is an unusual entity, with an incidence between 0.1% and 2% in patients undergoing scrotal ultrasound. They are most frequently found in the left testis. Some studies have suggested that an ITV may be bilateral in up to 40%.

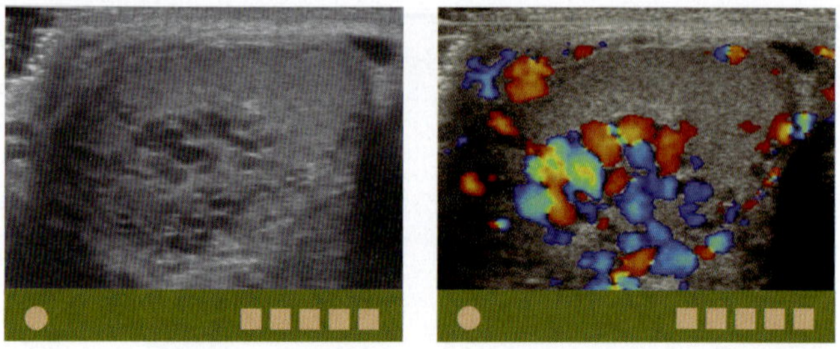

A. and **B.** Transverse gray-scale (A) and color flow (B) sonogram of the left testis shows a large serpentine anechoic intratesticular structure that fills in on color flow imaging.

Color Doppler sonography is diagnostic for ITV. Straight or serpentine hypoechoic structures will be seen within the mediastinum testis radiating into the testicular parenchyma. Color flow and duplex Doppler should demonstrate the presence of (retrograde) venous flow that increases on Valsalva. It has been reported that the Valsalva manoeuvre plays a very important role in the diagnosis of ITV because in most cases the retrograde flow will not show up spontaneously.

The clinical significance of ITVs is not certain. Treatment options are similar to ETV. Percutaneous sclerotherapy and catheterization of the spermatic vein for embolization of the lesion have also been reported with successful results. Some authors suggest that all symptomatic or infertile patients with ITV must be treated, even if an ETV is not present.

PEARLS

- **ITV refers to intratesticular dilated veins radiating from the mediastinum testis.**
- **An uncommon entity, usually asymptomatic.**
- **Color Doppler should demonstrate the presence of retrograde venous flow that increases on Valsalva.**
- **Treatment options are similar to ETV and include percutaneous sclerotherapy.**

ADDITIONAL IMAGES (C-E)

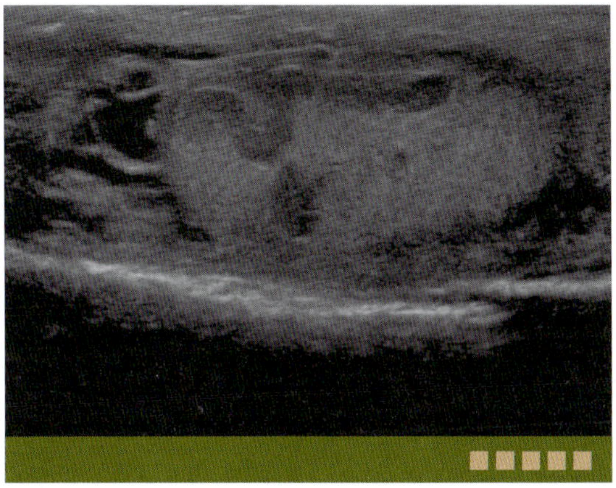

C. Longitudinal sonogram of the right testis in a different patient shows a large anechoic tubular structure traversing the testicular parenchyma.

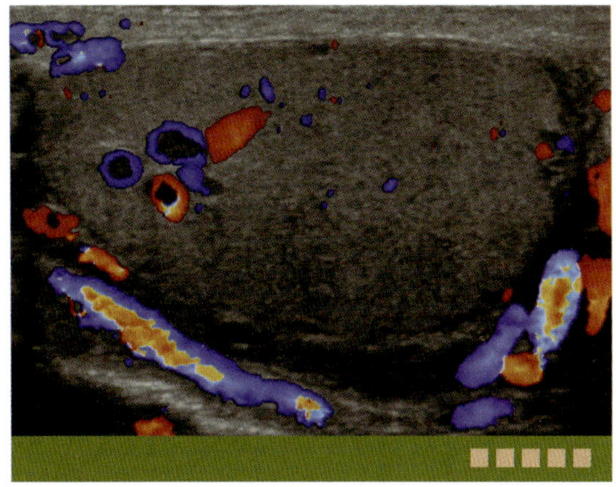

D. Corresponding longitudinal color Doppler image of the right testis shows the presence of retrograde venous flow, which increases on Valsalva.

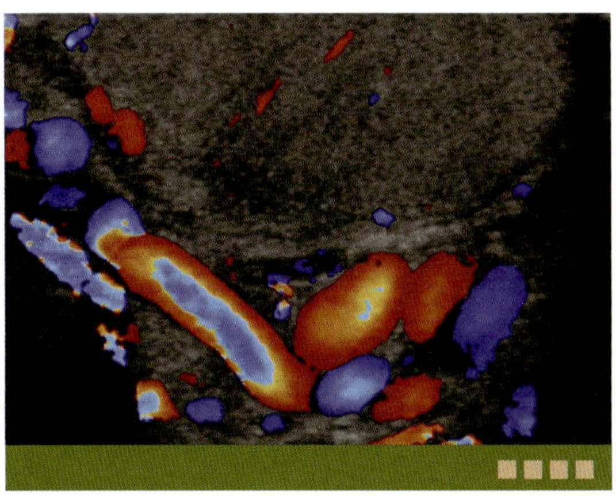

E. Longitudinal color Doppler image of the left testis in the same patient shows that the patient also has a left-sided ETV.

DIFFERENTIAL DIAGNOSES IMAGES (F-H)

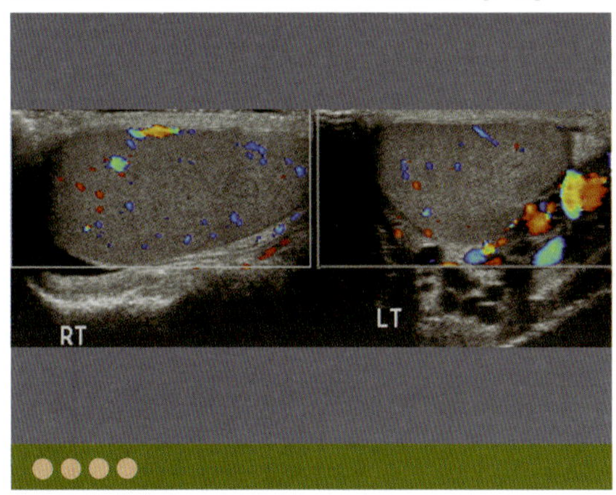

F. Extratesticular varicocele: Longitudinal sonograms of both testes show a left sided ETV. There was no accompanying ITV on either side.

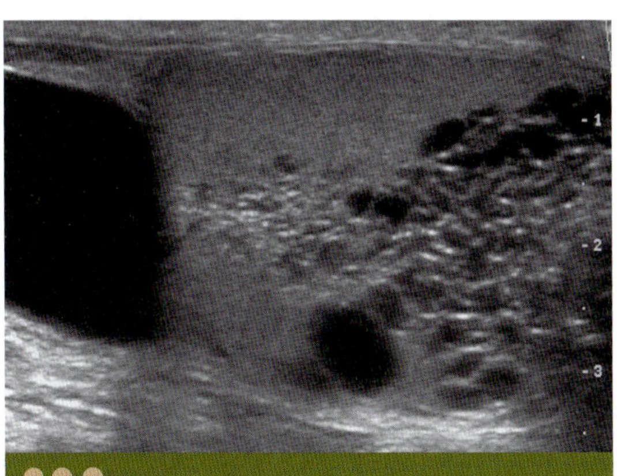

G. Cystic ectasia of the rete testis: Longitudinal sonogram of the right testis shows numerous small cysts extending along the mediastinum testis, some with a more tubular appearance. There was no flow on color Doppler imaging. Findings are pathognomic for cystic ectasia of the rete testis.

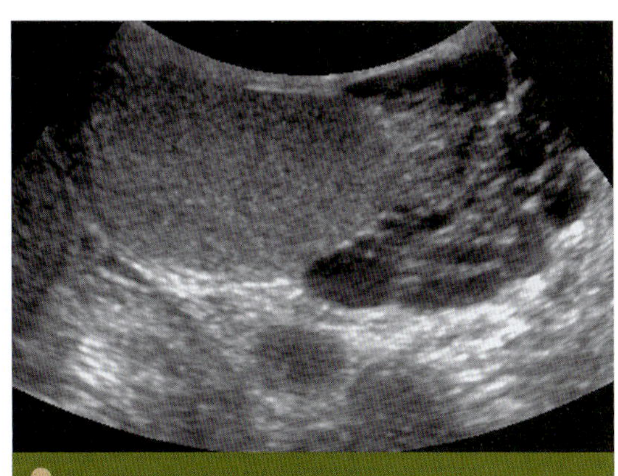

H. Cystadenoma of the rete testis: Longitudinal sonogram of the testis shows a large intra- and extratesticular complex cystic mass in the right scrotum containing numerous septations. There was no internal venous flow on color flow imaging.

IMAGE KEY

Common

Rare

Typical

Unusual

13–27 Polyorchidism

Paul Nikolaidis

PRESENTATION

Palpable scrotal mass/lump.

FINDINGS

Sonography demonstrates a third uniformly homogeneous echogenic structure within the scrotum with echogenicity identical to the normal testes.

DIFFERENTIAL DIAGNOSES

- *Other extratesticular, intrascrotal lesions*: The supernumerary testis may also be confused with other extratesticular intrascrotal lesions, including epididymal tumors. Careful attention to the sonographic appearance and exact location of the lesion should lead to the correct diagnosis.
- *Extratesticular hematoma*: Usually a more heterogeneous, ill-defined complex lesion without flow on color Doppler. Patients typically have a history of preceding trauma.

COMMENTS

Polyorchidism (testicular duplication) is a rare congenital anomaly of the genitourinary tract. The most common form is triorchidism. Patients may present in infancy or in late adulthood. Patients usually present with a painless palpable mass. Most commonly it represents a bifid or duplicated testis, with a single epididymis or vas deferens. Complete duplication of the testis, epididymis, and vas deferens is less common.

Sonography demonstrates a uniformly homogeneous structure with echogenicity identical to a normal testis. The supernumerary testicle is usually located superior and lateral to the normal testis. In three out of four cases, it is located on the left. An association with varicoceles, epididymitis, and infertility has been reported. MRI can also demonstrate the duplicated testis which should have identical signal characteristics as the normal testes.

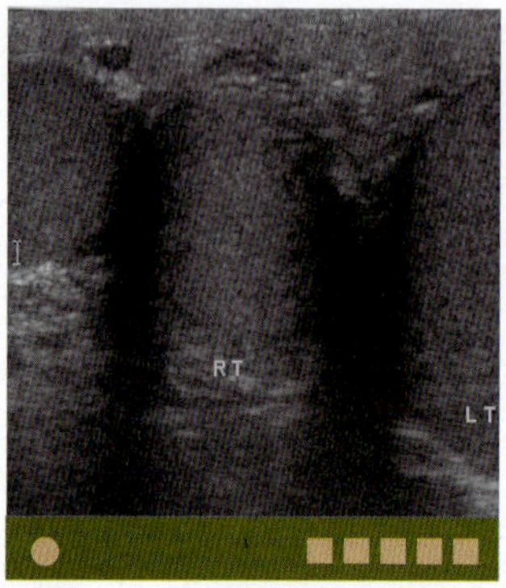

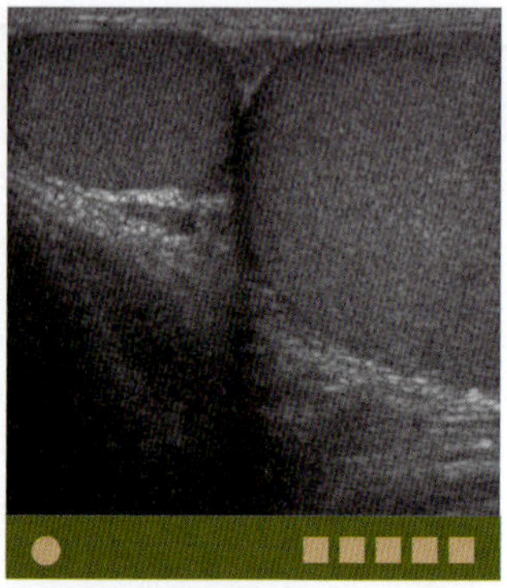

A. Transverse sonogram shows three isoechoic oval structures representing three separate testicles within the scrotum.
B. Longitudinal sonogram on the same patient shows the supernumerary testis, located lateral and superior to the right testis. Note that both structures have identical echogenicity and echotexture.

In planning management, the exact location of the supernumerary testis (intrascrotal, ectopic in the inguinal canal, or intra-abdominal), along with its size, reproductive potential, and age of the patient should be taken into account. Surgical intervention is generally not required in asymptomatic patients. Torsion is the most frequent complication of polyorchidism.

PEARLS

- **The most common form of polyorchidism is triorchidism.**
- **On sonography, they are typically homogeneous and isoechoic to the normal testis, located superior and lateral to it.**
- **Associated with varicoceles, epididymitis, and infertility.**
- **Torsion is the most frequent complication.**

ADDITIONAL IMAGES (C-D)

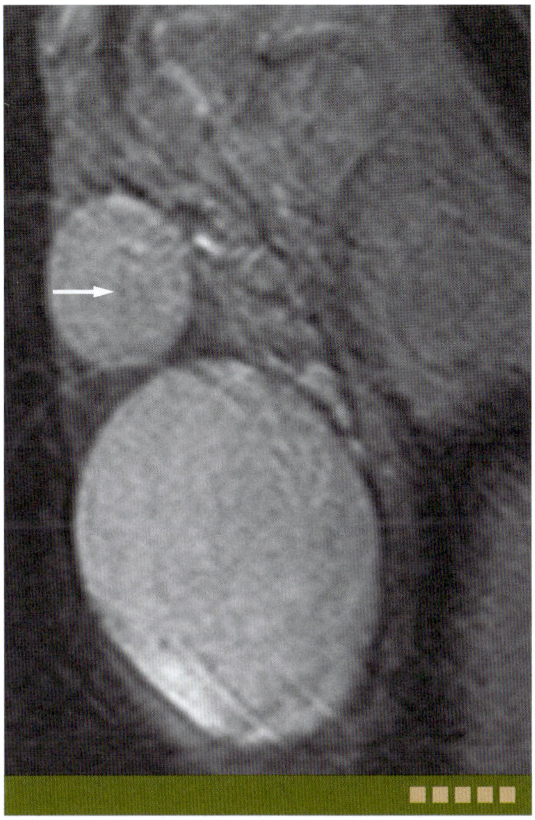

C. Sagittal T2-WI on the same patient shows the smaller supernumerary testis, which is located lateral and superior to the right testis, but with identical signal characteristics (arrow).

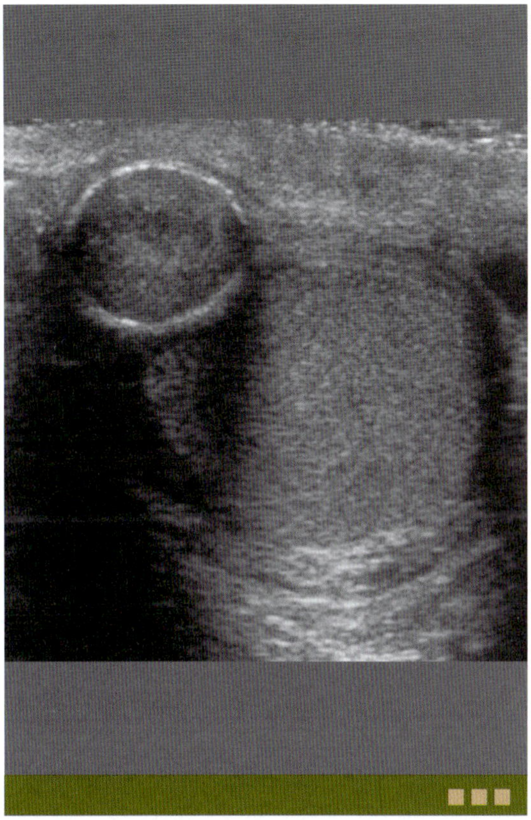

D. Transverse sonogram on a different patient shows a supernumerary testis with peripheral calcification. Note that the testicular parenchyma is slightly heterogeneous. This appearance is because of prior torsion and infarction.

DIFFERENTIAL DIAGNOSES IMAGES (E-F)

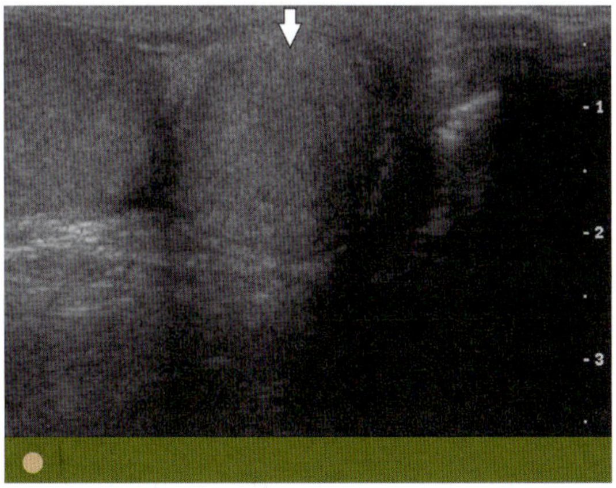

E. Paratesticular fibroma: Longitudinal sonogram on a patient with a palpable testicular lump shows an additional intrascrotal lesion, which is almost isoechoic to the right testis (arrow).

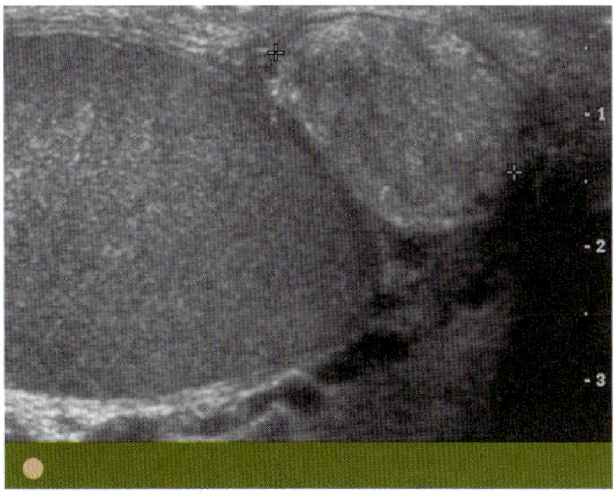

F. Paratesticular fibroma: More detailed, high-resolution longitudinal sonogram of the scrotum in the same patient, shows the lesion to be slightly hyperechoic and heterogeneous.

IMAGE KEY

Common

Rare

Typical

Unusual

13–28 Cryptorchid Testis

Frank H. Miller

PRESENTATION

Absence of testis in the scrotum.

FINDINGS

Sonogram shows undescended testis in inguinal canal.

DIFFERENTIAL DIAGNOSIS

None

COMMENTS

Cryptorchid testis refers to complete or partial failure of the intra-abdominal testes to descend into the scrotal sac. The undescended testes may be abnormally located anywhere along the normal path. Most frequently they are seen in the inguinal canal, but they may be seen in the abdomen, internal inguinal ring, external ring, or between the external ring and the scrotum.

Sonography is the initial test to assess for the absent testis and is helpful for inguinal testes but limited for pelvic or abdominal testes unless associated with malignancy. On ultrasound, the undescended testis is smaller and slightly less echogenic than the normal testes. The shape tends to be oval and homogeneous. A bright echogenic band representing the mediastinum testes may be helpful in identifying the tissue as testis. If ultrasound is not able to detect the testes, MR or CT may be helpful. In prior studies, CT and MR had sensitivities and specificities in the 80% to 100% range but did not include high abdominal testes. The use of oral and rectal contrast can be helpful when using CT to delineate the bowel. On MR, the testes are seen as having high-signal intensity on T2-weighted imaging. MR can be helpful in the diagnosis based on the lack of radiation in these young patients, multiplanar capability, and high contrast resolution.

Complications of cryptorchidism include increased risk of malignancy, torsion, and infertility. Orchiopexy of cryptorchid testes will not change the risk of malignancy but does help in surveillance. The highest incidence for the development of neoplasm is in those that have intra-abdominal location.

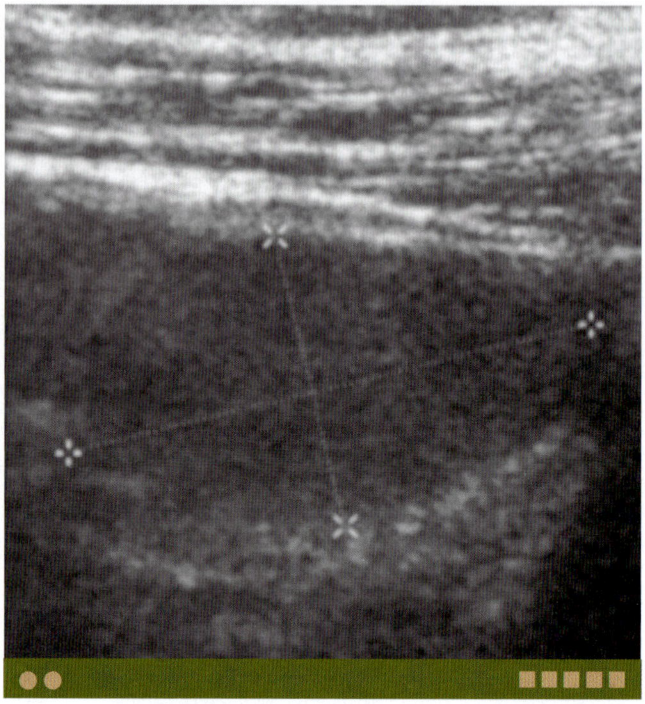

A. Longitudinal sonogram shows oval-shaped hypoechoic testis found in the inguinal canal in patients with undescended testes.

PEARLS

- **Sonography is initial test for undescended testes and is over 90% accurate when near inguinal canal but less accurate when intra-abdominal.**
- **CT and MR can be helpful when ultrasound does not show the undescended testes.**
- **Complications of cryptorchidism include increased risk of malignancy, torsion, and infertility.**

ADDITIONAL IMAGES (B-G)

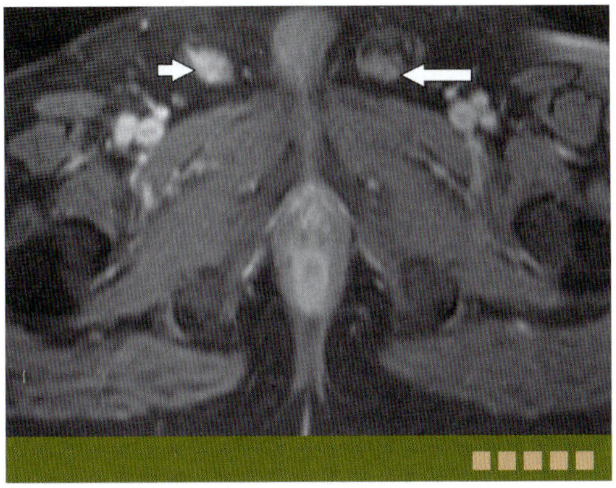

B. Axial contrast-enhanced T1-WI in a different patient shows enhancing testis (arrows) along inguinal canal which look similar to lymph nodes. The exam was performed to identify the undescended testes.

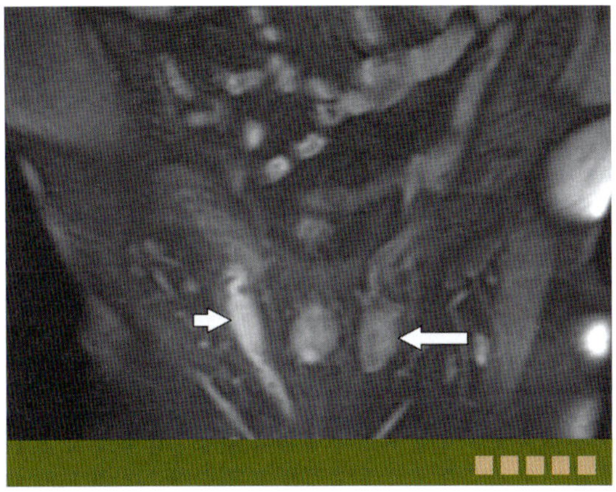

C. Coronal contrast-enhanced T1-WI in the same patient helps to show the enhancing testis (arrows) along the path of descent of the testes.

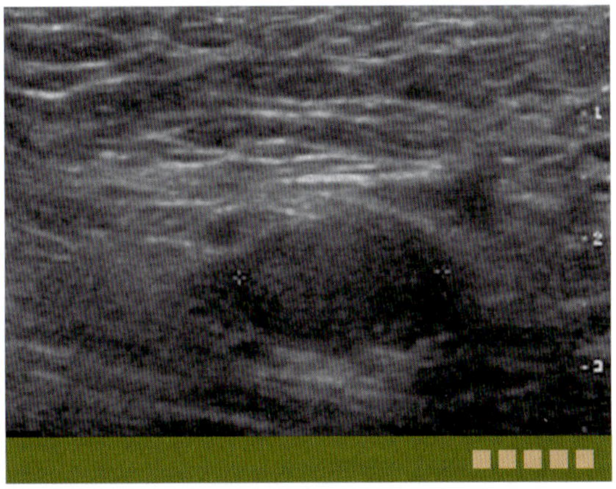

D. Longitudinal sonogram in the same patient shows the undescended testis.

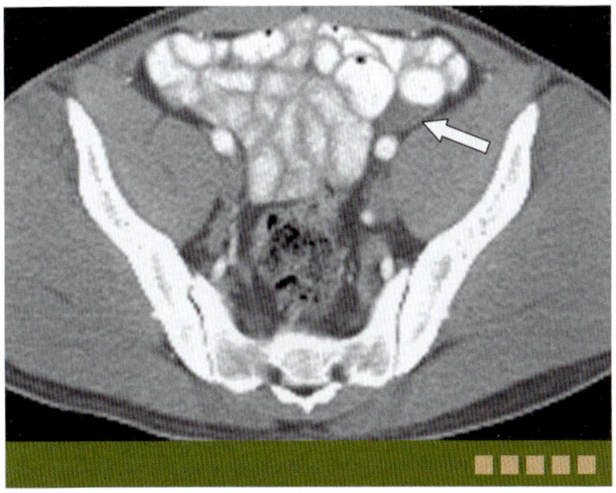

E. Different patient. Axial CECT shows the undescended testis (arrow) near the external iliac vessels.

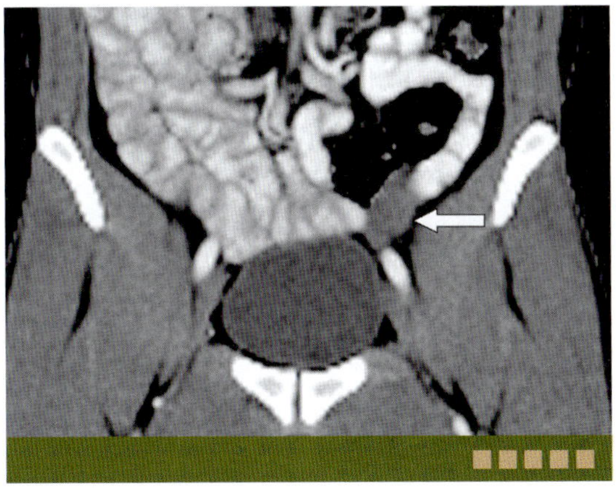

F. Coronal reformatted CECT in the same patient shows the ovoid undescended testis (arrow) that is slightly hypodense to muscle.

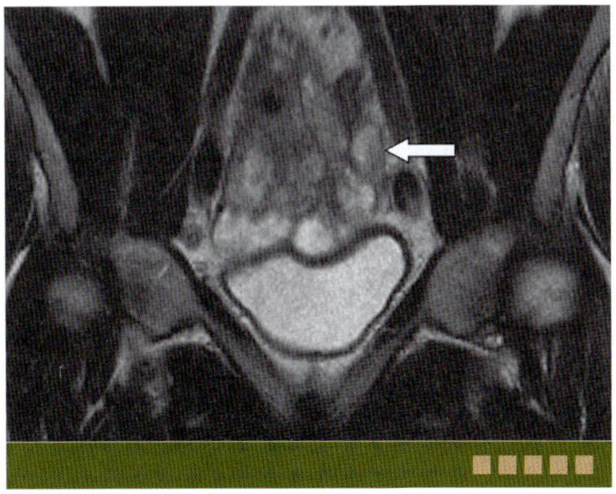

G. Coronal T2-WI shows the lesion is increased signal intensity (arrow).

IMAGE KEY

Common

Rare

Typical

Unusual

13–29 Seminoma in Undescended Testes

Frank H. Miller

PRESENTATION

Asymptomatic incidentally discovered mass in patients with cryptorchid testis.

FINDINGS

Solid mass in the pelvis of patients with undescended testis.

DIFFERENTIAL DIAGNOSIS

- *Other neoplasm, including lymphoma and sarcomas*: May have similar appearance, differentiated on the basis of clinical history of cryptorchidism and laboratory findings; tissue diagnosis, that is, biopsy or resection, necessary.

COMMENTS

Undescended testes are 5 to 48 times more likely to develop cancer than scrotal testes. The risk of cancer increases as the testes is more cephalad. A small percentage of testes (10%) are intra-abdominal, and these have as much as a 200-fold increased risk of cancer. The peak age for cancer in undescended testes is in the third and the fourth decade of life similar to scrotal testes. Seminoma is the most common type.

The diagnosis is often difficult at imaging studies as the radiologist may not be aware that the patient had a history of cryptorchid testis. In addition, patients may have had reported surgery for cryptorchidism in childhood and not know that orchiectomy did not occur as the testis may not have been found. Undescended testes can have other significant complications including infertility and ischemia with torsion.

Physicians may be aware of the increased risk of cancer in patients with undescended testes; however, the diagnosis may not be suspected. Even when malignant, patients may not be seen by physicians early as they are often asymptomatic. The patients may present with symptoms from mass effect. Symptoms may mimic appendicitis, urinary symptoms from mass effect on the bladder, or acute abdominal symptoms from torsion.

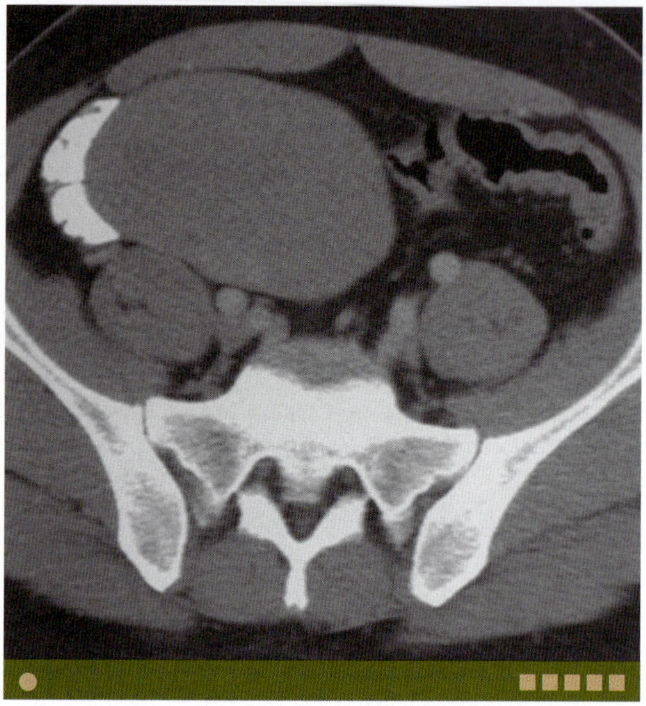

A. Axial CECT shows a mass in the pelvis because of undescended testis developing seminoma. The patient had a history of inguinal hernia repair.

Ultrasound is initially advocated to identify undescended testes with CT and MR helpful in difficult cases, especially those that are intra-abdominal and not identified on ultrasound.

PEARLS

- **Undescended testes are more likely to develop cancer.**
- **The diagnosis is often difficult at imaging studies as the history of a cryptorchid testis is often not known.**
- **A small percentage of testes are intra-abdominal which have significantly increased risk of cancer.**
- **Ultrasound, CT, or MR may be helpful in the diagnosis of undescended testes.**

(*Images reproduced with permission from Miller FH, Whitney WS, Fitzgerald SW, Miller EI. Seminomas complicating undescended intra-abdominal testes in patients with prior negative surgical exploration.* AJR *1999; 172:425-428.*)

ADDITIONAL IMAGES (B-F)

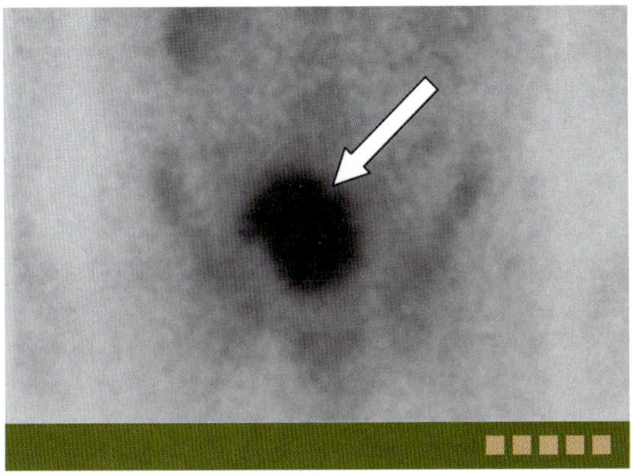

B. Gallium scan shows uptake in the mass in the pelvis (arrow). The patient had gallium scan for pulmonary evaluation for night sweats and persistent cough. As a result, the CT scan was performed. The patient had prior hernia repair and scrotal exploration. The testis was not identified but no further workup had been done 12 years prior to the exam.

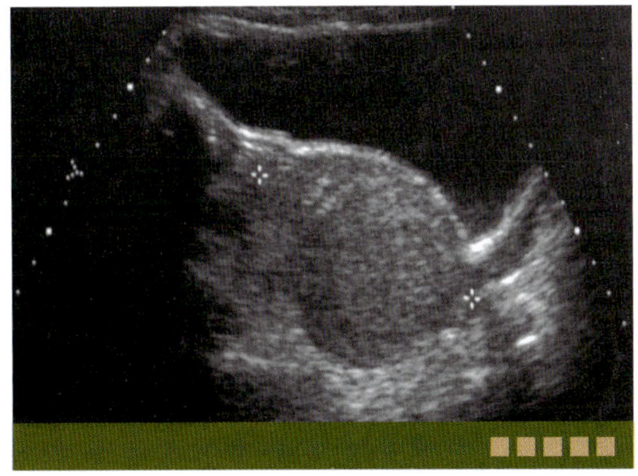

C. Longitudinal sonogram shows ovoid mass in the pelvis that is nonspecific in appearance but in patients with undescended testis is suspicious for cancer. The patient was suspected to have appendicitis clinically and thought he had a prior orchiectomy for undescended testes as child.

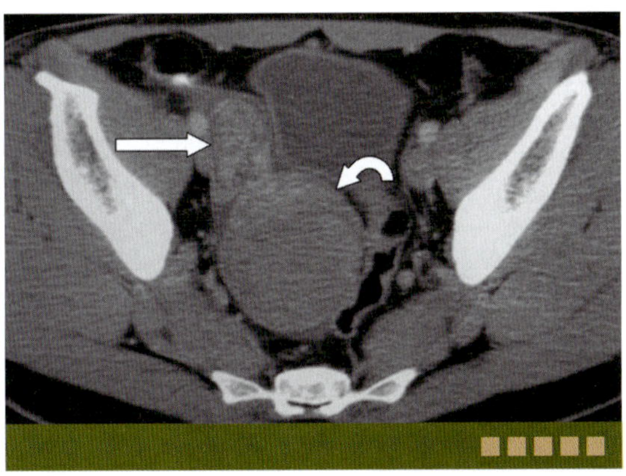

D. CECT shows heterogeneous mass (curved arrow) in the pelvis with dilated pedicle (straight arrow) because of torsion of seminoma demonstrated at surgery.

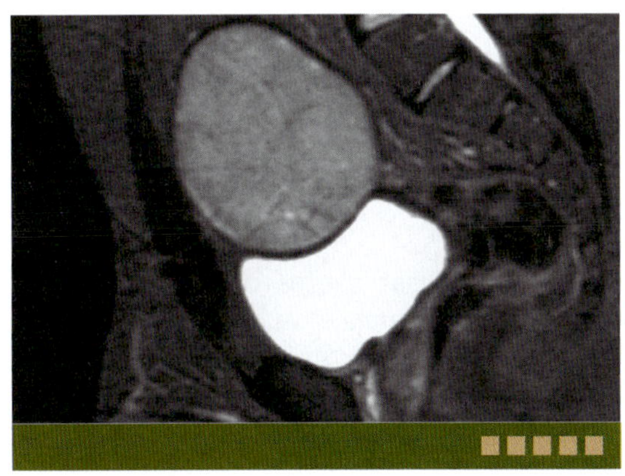

E. Sagittal short inversion time recovery image shows mass as hyperintense to muscle.

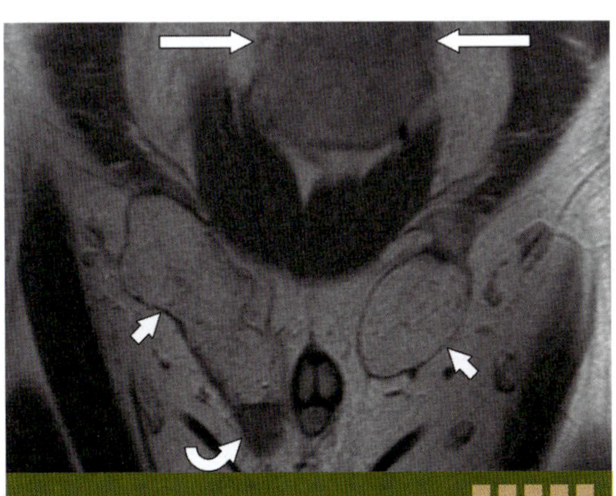

F. Coronal T1-WI shows mass as isointense to muscle (straight long arrows). Left testis is absent from scrotum. Right testis is seen just distal to the external ring (curved arrow). Bilateral fat-containing inguinal hernias are seen (small straight arrows).

DIFFERENTIAL DIAGNOSIS IMAGE

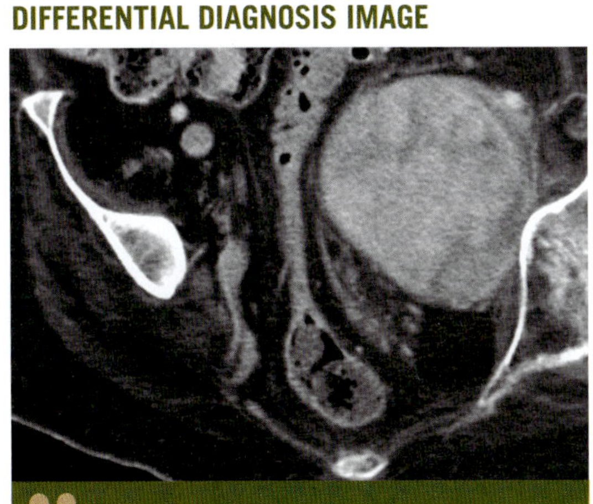

G. Pelvic leiomyosarcoma: Axial CECT shows a large, heterogeneously enhancing mass in the pelvis. Patient did not have cryptorchidism.

C and D are the same patient.
E and F are the same patient.

IMAGE KEY

Common

Rare

Typical

Unusual

13–30 Spermatocele

Frank H. Miller

PRESENTATION

Usually asymptomatic; freely movable mass superior and posterior to the testis on physical examination.

FINDINGS

Extratesticular fluid-containing mass attributed to spermatocele.

DIFFERENTIAL DIAGNOSES

- *Epididymal cysts*: May occur throughout the epididymis, while spermatoceles usually occur in the epididymal head.
- *Adenomatoid tumor*: Solid extratesticular lesion.
- *Cysts of the tunica albuginea*: Extratesticular lesion whose distinction is easily made with ultrasound.
- *Varicocele*: Serpigenous vessels adjacent to testis.
- *Hernia*: May see bowel or fat within the scrotum.

COMMENTS

Spermatoceles are one of the main causes of scrotal masses. Ultrasound can help differentiate intratesticular from extratesticular masses. Most extratesticular masses are benign while intratesticular masses are generally malignant. Spermatoceles consist of sperm-containing cystic dilatations of obstructed efferent ductules most commonly in the head of the epididymis. Spermatoceles contain spermatozoa unlike epididymal cysts that contain clear serous fluid. Both lesions are usually asymptomatic unless they rarely cause mass effect and can be managed conservatively. Most spermatoceles are small (1-2 cm in size), but they can sometimes be larger. Sonography shows a unilocular or multilocular well-defined hypoechoic lesion with posterior acoustic enhancement. These lesions may contain low-level echoes and septations from proteinaceous fluid or sperm that may suggest spermatocele instead of epididymal cyst, although the distinction is not critical. They may displace the testis inferiorly.

Spermatoceles are usually an incidental finding in patients in the fourth and the fifth decades of life. Spermatoceles are associated with tubular ectasia of the testes.

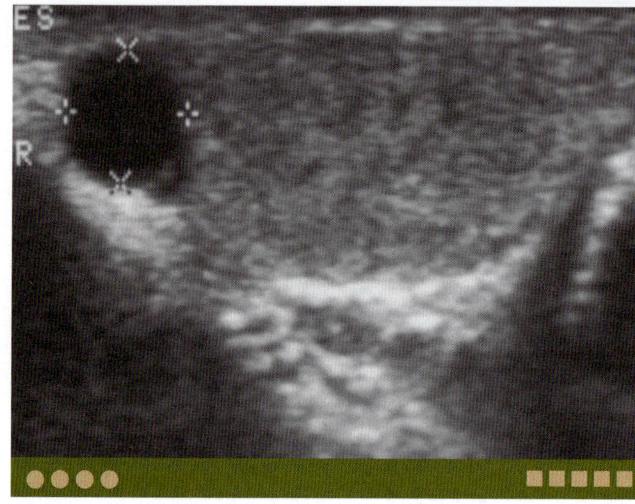

A. Sonogram shows anechoic fluid collection that is extratesticular as a result of spermatocele in epididymal head.

Spermatoceles can easily be differentiated from varicoceles using color Doppler sonography. Spermatoceles do not have flow unlike varicoceles. When a cyst is seen involving the epididymis, a spermatocele cannot be differentiated from an epididymal cyst. The distinction most likely is not critical. It is more important to distinguish spermatoceles from especially intratesticular tumors using ultrasound if it cannot be made on physical examination.

PEARLS

- **Spermatoceles are one of the most common causes of scrotal masses.**
- **Ultrasound helps distinguish spermatoceles from intratesticular masses if required.**
- **Spermatoceles are often associated with tubular ectasia of the testes.**
- **Spermatoceles are usually asymptomatic.**

DIFFERENTIAL DIAGNOSES IMAGES (B-F)

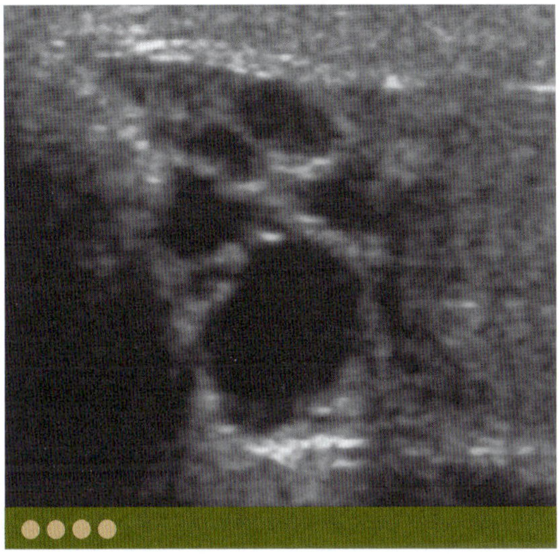

B. Epididymal cysts and cysts of the rete testes: Transverse sonogram shows epididymal cysts.

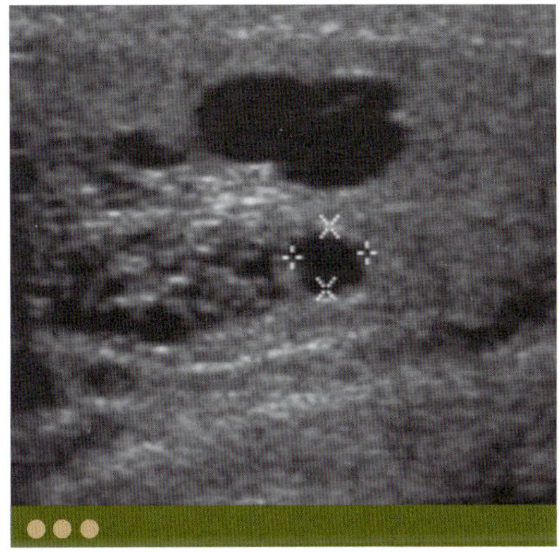

C. Epididymal cysts and cysts of the rete testes: Sonogram shows cysts of the rete testes that are associated with the epididymal cysts in the same patient as B.

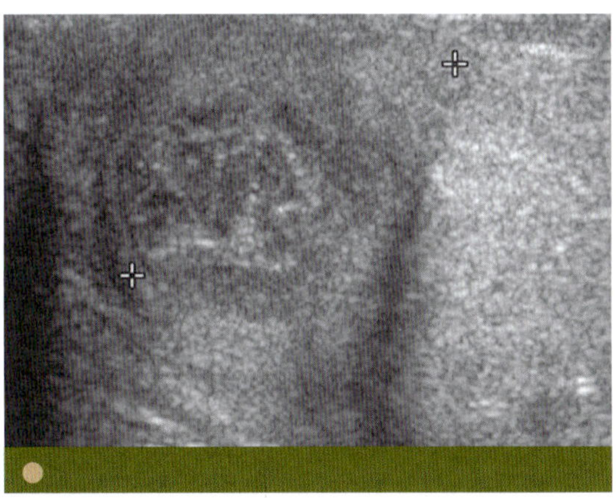

D. Adenomatoid tumor: Transverse sonogram shows solid lesion in the right epididymis that differs from the predominately cystic lesions seen with spermatoceles.

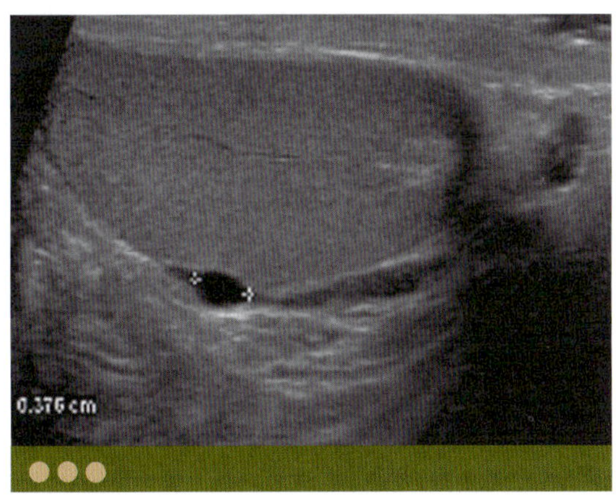

E. Cysts of the tunica albuginea: Sonogram shows tiny 4-mm lesion involving the tunica albuginea unlike spermatoceles.

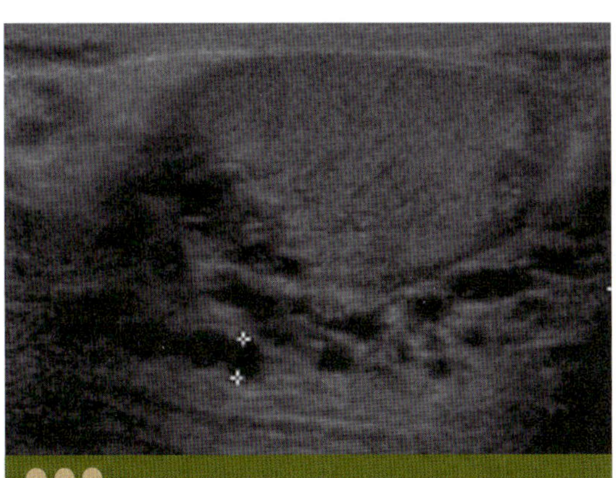

F. Varicocele: Sonogram easily makes distinction from spermatocele by showing serpigenous vessels adjacent to testis.

IMAGE KEY

Common

Rare

Typical

Unusual

13–31 Adenomatoid Tumors

Frank H. Miller

PRESENTATION

Incidental painless firm scrotal mass; may present with pain; slow growing.

FINDINGS

Ultrasound shows solid hypoechoic mass of the epididymis.

DIFFERENTIAL DIAGNOSES

- *Other benign tumors including lipoma, leiomyoma, neurofibroma, hemangioma, and granular cell tumor*: Can look similar, although lipoma may be able to be diagnosed because of fat.
- *Malignant tumors including sarcoma, metastases, and adenocarcinoma*: Tend to be large heterogeneous masses in older patients.
- *Epididymal cyst*: Would be cystic not solid extratesticular lesion.
- *Polyorchidism*: Rare entity with more than two testes; the extra testis is similar echogenicity to the testes and similar signal intensity on MR. Doppler ultrasound shows flow similar to testes.
- *Papillary cystadenoma*: Strong association with von Hippel Lindau disease (seen in up to 25% patients with von Hippel Lindau).

COMMENTS

Adenomatoid tumor is the most common epididymal tumor and accounts for approximately 30% of tumors of the paratesticular tissue. Adenomatoid tumors are uncommon masses. They are referred to as nonpapillary benign mesothelioma. They can occur in any age group but are most commonly present between the third and the fourth decades. Most adenomatoid tumors involve the epididymis, most often in the tail. They can occur in the testicular tunica albuginea and spermatic cord as well. They tend to be asymptomatic and slow-growing masses but may present with pain. They are benign.

Ultrasound is helpful to show the masses are extratesticular and not caused by testicular cancer. The intratesticular form cannot be distinguished from primary germ cell tumors. The treatment is surgical removal. These extratesticular tumors are solid and well defined on sonographic examination unlike the more common epididymal cysts or spermatoceles, which neither tends to be solid nor have flow in them. Adenomatoid tumors have variable echogenic patterns including hypoechoic, hyperechoic, or isoechoic relative to adjacent tissues. Adenomatoid tumors can look similar to other benign tumors including leiomyoma, neurofibroma, and granular cell tumors. Neoplasms involving the epididymis are rare. Malignant lesions are usually fibrosarcoma, malignant fibrous histiocytoma, or lymphosarcoma and often are larger and more heterogeneous and do not arise from the epididymis. Metastases to the epididymis are rare and may arise from cancers of the stomach, kidney, prostate, colon and rectum.

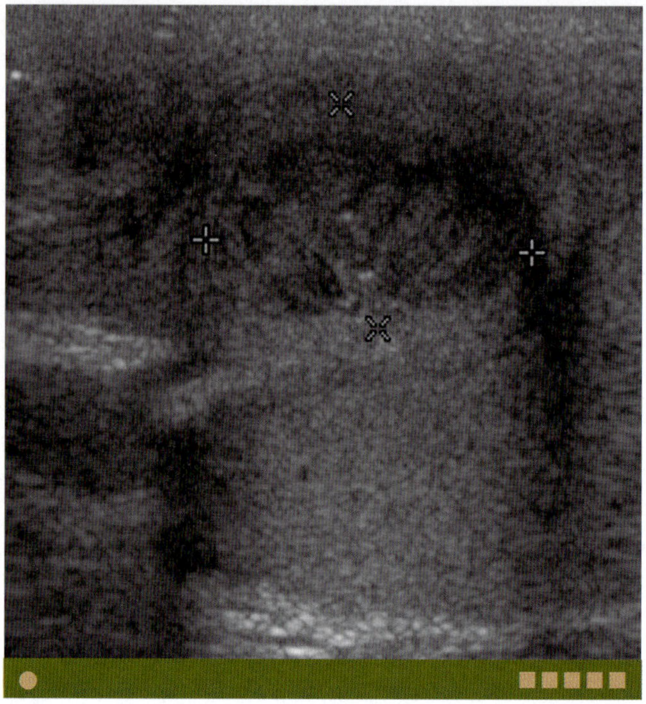

A. Transverse sonogram shows a round, solid hypoechoic mass of epididymis. Color Doppler images (not shown) showed increased flow in the mass.

PEARLS

- **Adenomatoid tumor is the most common extratesticular tumor.**
- **Ultrasound can be helpful to show mass is extratesticular.**
- **Adenomatoid tumors are solid lesions which have flow and can have variable echogenicity.**
- **Treatment of adenomatoid tumors is surgical removal.**

ADDITIONAL IMAGES (B-C)

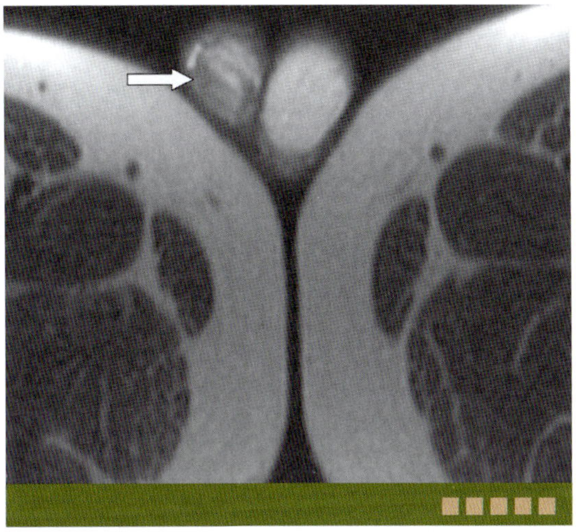

B. Axial T1-WI shows hypointense lesion from adenomatoid tumor (arrow).

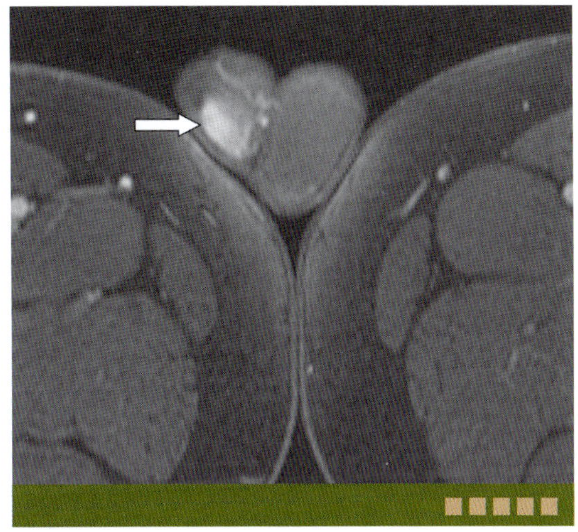

C. Axial T1-WI enhanced shows lesion enhancing.

DIFFERENTIAL DIAGNOSES IMAGES (D-G)

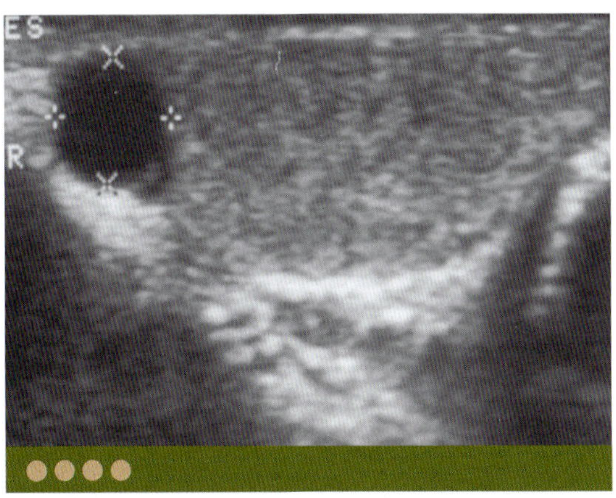

D. Epididymal cyst: Transverse sonogram shows anechoic fluid collection that is extratesticular because of spermatocele in epididymal head unlike solid lesion of adenomatoid tumor.

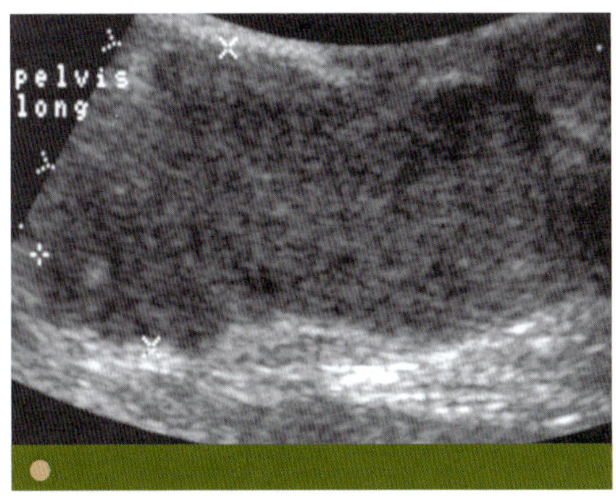

E. Extratesticular malignancy: Longitudinal sonogram shows large heterogeneous mass, which was separate from the testes and epididymis. Unlike adenomatoid tumor, the lesions tend to be large and heterogeneous. The lesion was removed and was caused by malignant fibrous histiocytoma.

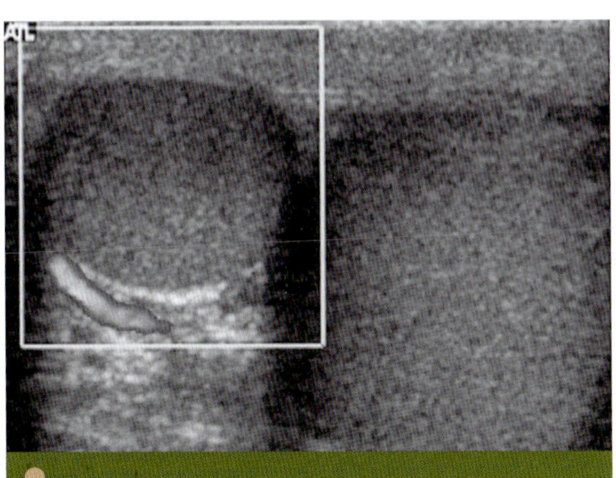

F. Polyorchydism: Longitudinal sonogram shows smaller right extratesticular lesion with similar echogenicity and flow to the normal testes.

F and G are the same patient.

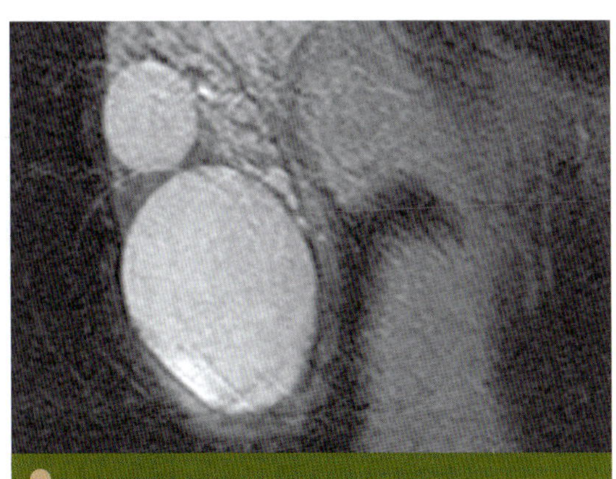

G. Polyorchidism: Sagittal T2-WI shows extratesticular lesion is similar MR signal intensity as the testis. The lesion was similar to the normal testes in signal intensity and enhancement on all sequences.

IMAGE KEY

Common

Rare

Typical

Unusual

13–32 Extratesticular Malignant Fibrous Histiocytoma

Frank H. Miller

PRESENTATION

Large complex mass of spermatic cord in older patient.

FINDINGS

Ultrasound shows large solid heterogeneous extratesticular mass displacing the testis; mass was separate from the epididymis.

DIFFERENTIAL DIAGNOSES

- *Hernia*: May be difficult to distinguish, helpful if can confirm bowel loops; may need an additional imaging.
- *Thick left spermatic cord from testicular detorsion*: Can usually be distinguished on the basis of history and associated imaging findings.
- *Hydrocele*: Usually fluid and not solid.

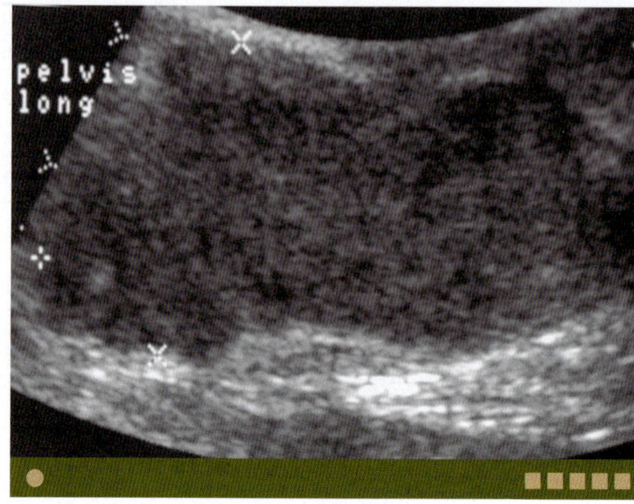

A. Longitudinal ultrasound shows large heterogeneous mass that was separate from the testes and epididymis.

COMMENTS

Although most extratesticular masses are benign, they can be malignant. Lipomas are the most common extratesticular neoplasm and are benign. Most malignant tumors of the spermatic cord are mesenchymal sarcomas, mainly rhabdomyosarcoma (in children) and liposarcoma (in adults). Liposarcomas can be diagnosed on the basis of the presence of fat. Other malignant tumors that can involve the spermatic cord include malignant fibrous histiocytomas, leiomyosarcomas, fibrosarcomas, and undifferentiated sarcomas. These are distinguished only at the time of pathologic analysis as they can appear similar on imaging studies. They are seen in older patients most frequently. Most patients present with a slowly enlarging painless mass in the inguinal canal or scrotum.

Imaging features include a large, complex solid mass. The diagnosis is difficult to make on the basis of clinical findings. Differential diagnosis based on clinical findings includes hernia, hydrocele, spermatocele, testicular tumors, epididymal infections, and tumors. Ultrasound is invaluable in distinguishing intratesticular from extratesticular masses. It is important to exclude hernias based on physical examination and ultrasound as they may appear as complex masses from omental fat and vessels. Peristalsis to suggest bowel contents may not be seen in all hernias. At times, MR examination may be helpful to demonstrate a solid mass and distinguish it from a hernia. MR also is helpful to identify blood products in characterizing hematomas or hemorrhagic masses which can be difficult to characterize with ultrasound.

PEARLS

- **Most extratesticular masses are benign, but they may be rarely malignant.**
- **Ultrasound helps distinguish intratesticular from extratesticular masses.**
- **Large complex masses that are not caused by hernias may represent tumors.**
- **Malignant fibrous histiocystoma is diagnosed based on pathology and is generally seen in older patients with slowly growing mass.**

DIFFERENTIAL DIAGNOSES IMAGES (B-D)

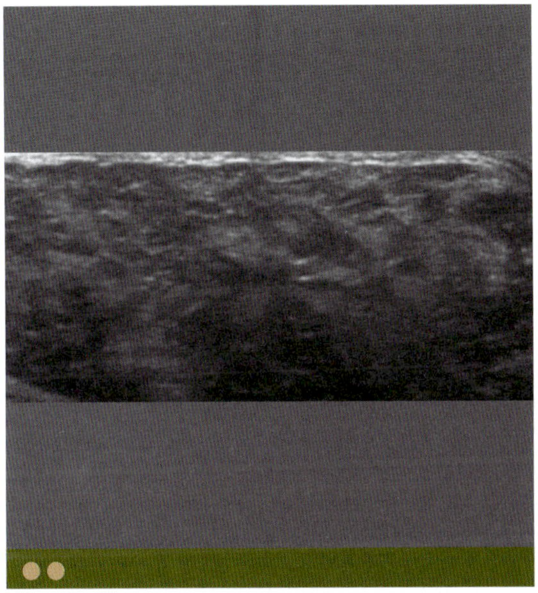

B. Hernia: Longitudinal ultrasound shows a large, complex mass from hernia which has nonspecific appearance on ultrasound.

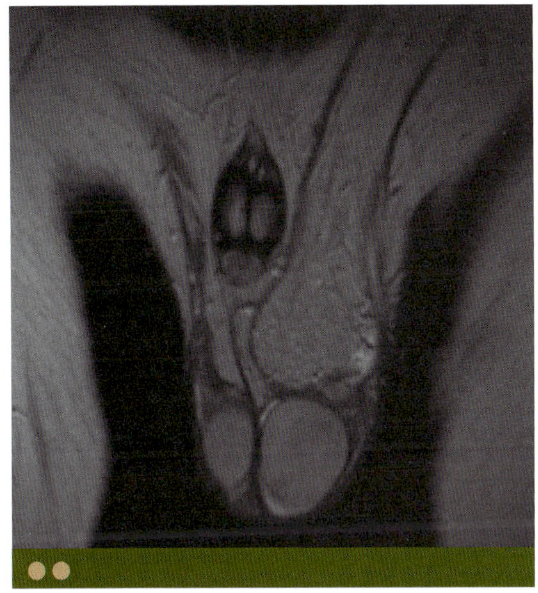

C. Hernia: Coronal T2-WI is helpful to show left inguinal hernia that is composed of high-signal intensity fat and extends from the pelvis into the scrotum.

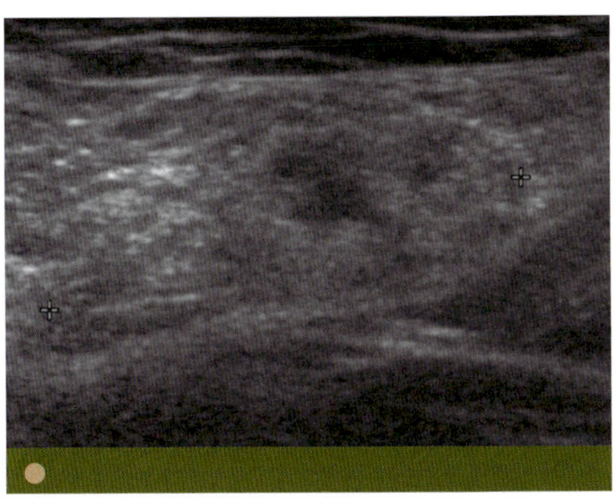

D. Testicular detorsion: Longitudinal sonogram shows thick left spermatic cord from testicular detorsion.

IMAGE KEY

Common

Rare

Typical

Unusual

Figures B and C are the same patient.
Figure D is a different patient.

13–33 Spermatic Cord Lipoma

Paul Nikolaidis

PRESENTATION

Palpable inguinal or scrotal mass.

FINDINGS

Sonography of the scrotum shows a large hyperechoic mass displacing the right testicle medially.

DIFFERENTIAL DIAGNOSES

- *Liposarcoma*: This is usually a more heterogeneous mass with increased nodularity and larger soft tissue components; however may be difficult to distinguish on imaging, particularly on ultrasound.
- *Inguinal hernia*: They are generally larger and may contain bowel loops exhibiting peristalsis. They also may be reducible on physical examination.
- *Hematoma*: Usually distinguished by a history of direct trauma; rarely patients on anticoagulation may get hematomas without known trauma.
- *Other intrascrotal, extratesticular lesions*: These may arise from the testicle, epididymis, or may be caused by infection (abscesses). They should not extend into the inguinal canal.

COMMENTS

Lipomas are the most common benign spermatic cord neoplasm. The spermatic cord consists of a group of structures that course through the inguinal canal to the testis. These include the vas deferens, testicular artery, testicular venous plexus, lymphatic vessels, and the genital branch of the genitofemoral nerve. The spermatic cord also contains fat and connective tissue. Spermatic cord lipomas usually present as an incidental, palpable nontender mass. There is no age predilection. There is significant variation in their size.

On sonography, they typically demonstrate a relatively homogeneous hyperechoic appearance. However, they may be difficult to distinguish from a liposarcoma. The sonographic findings of a liposarcoma are variable and nonspecific; sometimes, they are hypoechoic and heterogeneous, but they may be more homogeneous and hyperechoic. Lipomas should also be differentiated from omental fat in an inguinal hernia. This distinction is sometimes difficult. Lipomas are usually smaller and more homogeneous, whereas a hernia is a large elongated mass that can often be traced back to the internal inguinal ring.

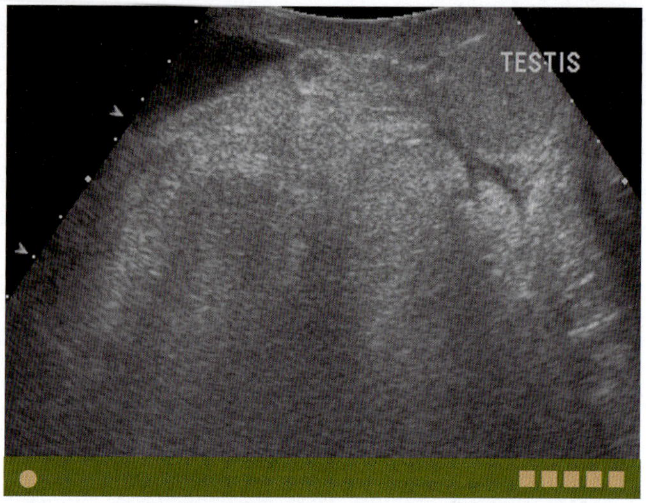

A. Transverse sonogram of the scrotum shows a large hyperechoic mass adjacent to the right testicle.

CT and MR may be performed for confirmation. Lipomas should be of uniform low attenuation at CT; however, atypical lipomas may have small solid elements or nodularity. On MR, simple lipomas are homogenous masses that are hyperintense on T1- and T2-WI, and show uniform decreased signal on sequences utilizing fat suppression.

The pathologic distinction between lipomas and the surrounding fat is based on the observation of slight variation in the size and shape of the fat cells; they are generally larger than the surrounding mature fat cells. If symptomatic, patients may benefit from surgical excision.

PEARLS

- **Benign neoplasms of the spermatic cord include lipomas, epidermoid cysts, leiomyomas, and lymphangiomas.**
- **On sonography, spermatic cord lipomas are typically homogeneous and hyperechoic.**
- **The closest sonographic mimics are liposarcoma and omental fat in an inguinal hernia.**
- **They should also be distinguished from other extratesticular, purely intrascrotal lesions such as hematomas, supernumerary testes, and epididymal lesions.**

ADDITIONAL IMAGES (B-C)

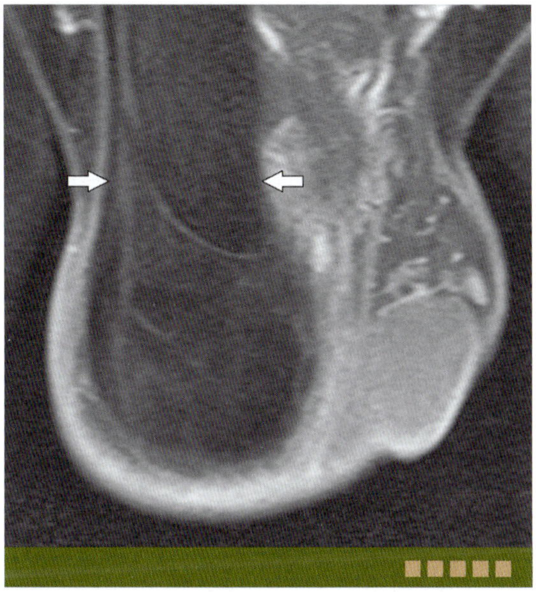

B. Coronal contrast-enhanced T1-WI on the same patient as in Figure A shows a fatty mass extending from the inguinal canal into the scrotum (arrows).

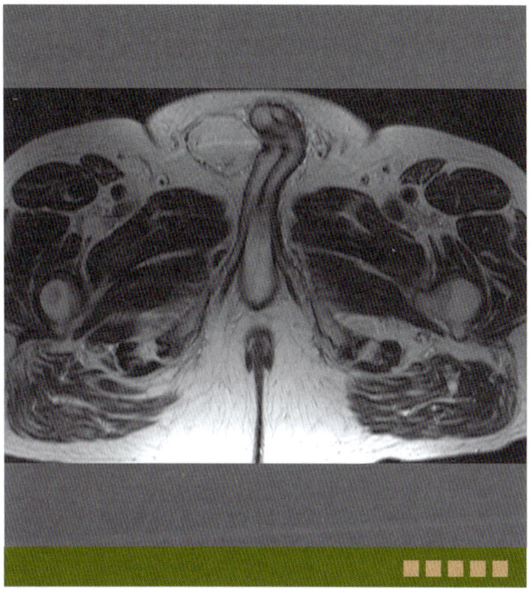

C. Corresponding axial T2-WI shows the fatty mass within the inguinal canal.

DIFFERENTIAL DIAGNOSES IMAGES (D-E)

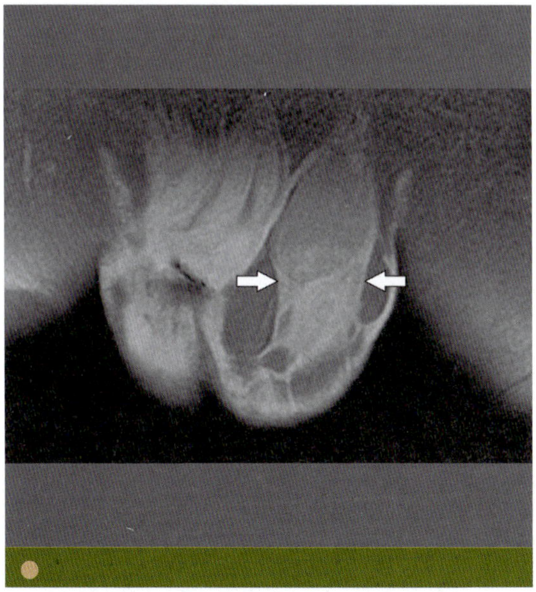

D. Liposarcoma of the spermatic cord: Coronal contrast-enhanced T1-WI shows a large fatty mass with solid enhancing components (arrows) extending through the left inguinal canal into the scrotum.

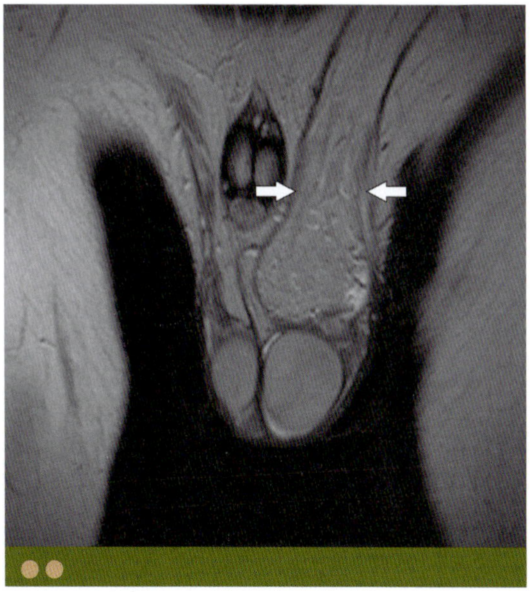

E. Inguinal hernia: Coronal T2-WI shows a fatty mass extending from the lower abdominal cavity through the inguinal canal into the scrotum (arrows). This was a hernia containing only fat.

IMAGE KEY

Common

Rare

Typical

Unusual

13–34 Spermatic Cord Liposarcoma

Paul Nikolaidis

PRESENTATION

Palpable inguinal mass, progressive scrotal swelling, enlarging scrotal mass.

FINDINGS

MR shows a heterogeneous solid lesion with fatty elements in the left inguinal canal.

DIFFERENTIAL DIAGNOSES

- *Inguinal hernia*: Hernias should be tracked through the internal inguinal ring, although large liposarcomas may occasionally extend through it into the abdominal cavity. Hernias may contain bowel loops exhibiting peristalsis and may be reducible on physical examination.
- *Lipoma of the spermatic cord*: Often indistinguishable; lipomas are usually smaller and more homogeneous without nodularity or large non-fatty soft tissue components.

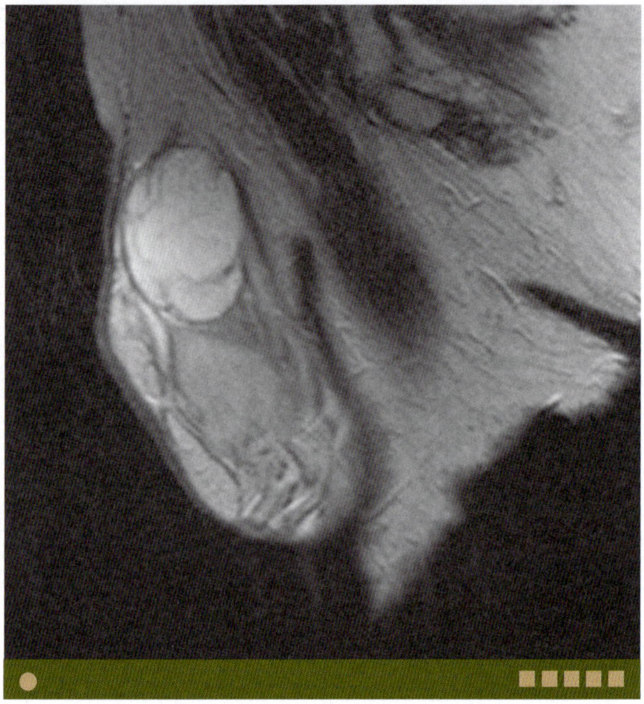

A. Sagittal non-enhanced T1-WI shows a heterogeneous partially fatty mass with solid elements extending through the left inguinal canal into the scrotum.

COMMENT

Spermatic cord liposarcomas (SCL) are rare malignant spermatic cord neoplasms, with only few hundred cases reported in the literature. Liposarcomas comprise approximately 7% of paratesticular sarcomas. They usually present with painless scrotal swelling progressing slowly during a period ranging from months to years. Occasionally, a previously stable mass can rapidly increase in size. They may become quite large by the time of diagnosis. Often they are clinically suspected to represent inguinal hernias. SCL should be suspected in patients experiencing recurrent hernias of the inguinal region. Average patient age at presentation is 55 years.

The sonographic findings of a SCL are variable and nonspecific; sometimes they are hypoechoic and heterogeneous, but they may be more homogeneous and hyperechoic. They should be differentiated from omental fat in an inguinal hernia. This distinction is sometimes difficult. A hernia should appear as an elongated mass that can often be traced back to the internal inguinal ring.

CT or MR is usually performed for confirmation and for evaluation of any additional sites of involvement. SCLs usually have solid elements or nodularity in addition to heterogeneous or homogeneous fatty elements.

Treatment should consist of radical orchiectomy with wide local excision. The need for regional and retroperitoneal lymphadenectomy and the usefulness of adjuvant radiotherapy or chemotherapy are not yet established. Although most cases of SCL are low in grade and stage, they have a high propensity for local recurrence. Close clinical and imaging follow-up is required.

PEARLS

- **Liposarcomas are rare malignant spermatic cord neoplasms.**
- **On sonography they have a nonspecific appearance, but are usually heterogeneous.**
- **MR or CT should be obtained preoperatively.**
- **Treatment consists of radical orchiectomy with wide local excision; patients should be followed closely.**

ADDITIONAL IMAGES (B-C)

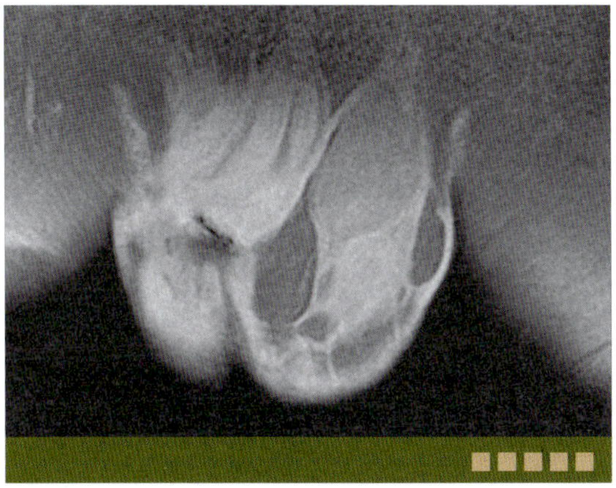

B. Corresponding coronal contrast-enhanced T1-WI shows numerous solid enhancing components within the fatty mass that extends into the scrotum.

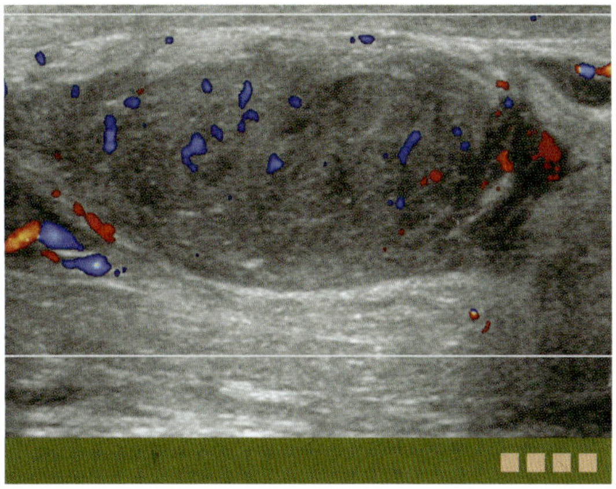

C. Transverse color Doppler sonogram on the same patient shows a large heterogeneous mass within the scrotum. It shows increased vascularity.

IMAGE KEY

Common

Rare

Typical

Unusual

DIFFERENTIAL DIAGNOSES IMAGES (D-E)

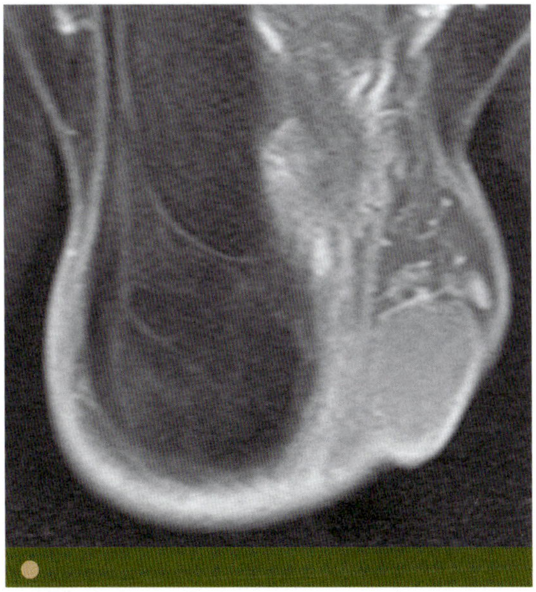

D. Spermatic cord lipoma: Coronal contrast-enhanced T1-WI shows a fatty mass extending from the right inguinal canal into the scrotum. It contains only few linear striations, but no areas of nodularity or significant soft tissue components.

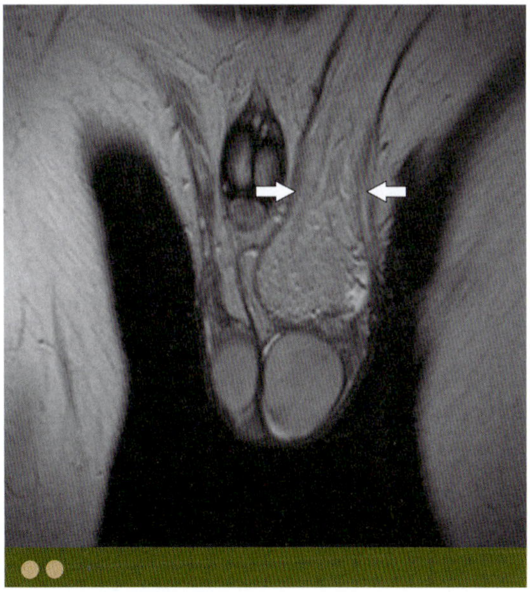

E. Inguinal hernia: Coronal T2-WI shows a fatty mass extending from the lower abdominal cavity through the inguinal canal into the scrotum (arrows). This represented a hernia containing only fat and no bowel.

13–35 Varicocele

Frank H. Miller

PRESENTATION

Infertility, scrotal mass—"bag of worms".

FINDINGS

Hypoechoic serpiginous vessels adjacent to the testis that show flow.

DIFFERENTIAL DIAGNOSIS

None

COMMENTS

Varicocele is the most common mass of the spermatic cord. A varicocele is a dilatation of the pampiniform venous plexus and internal spermatic vein. It is present in 15% to 20% of men. Patients may be asymptomatic or have dull, aching scrotal discomfort, more prominent when standing and relieved when laying down. Varicoceles represent the most common surgically correctable cause of male infertility. Most varicoceles occur on the left side or are bilateral. The diagnosis often is made clinically based on palpation of a "bag of worms" in the scrotum. They may be idiopathic or develop secondary to an abdominal mass that compresses the renal vein or inferior vena cava. Idiopathic varicoceles usually occur in 15 to 25 years old patients. Secondary varicoceles occur in older patients, usually over 40 years of age. Idiopathic varicoceles more often are seen on the left likely because of the longer course and perpendicular path of the left testicular vein into the left renal vein with "nutcracker" compression of the left renal vein between the superior mesenteric artery and aorta. This increased pressure may lead to incompetent valves and development of varicocele. The right testicular vein has a more direct and shorter course directly into the inferior vena cava. When the vessels are noncompressible or there is an isolated right varicocele, it is important to exclude an underlying retroperitoneal mass or inferior vena cava thrombus because of right renal tumor.

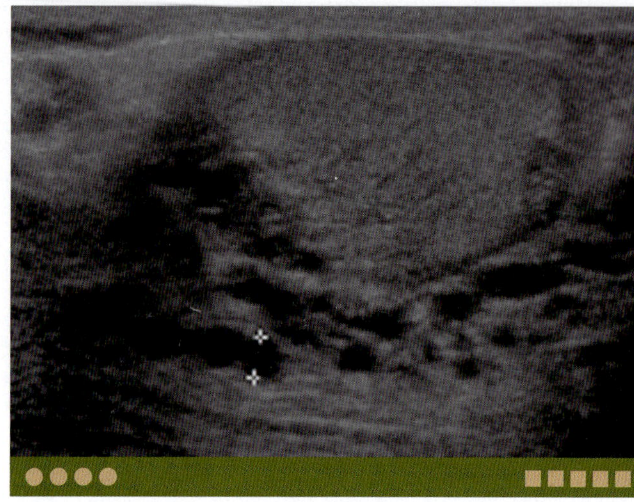

A. Transverse sonogram shows serpiginous structures because of varicocele seen outside the left testis.

Sonography shows hypoechoic serpiginous structures larger than 2 mm in diameter supero-lateral to the testis that increase in size and augmented flow with Valsalva. Color Doppler and duplex Doppler sonography show the venous flow pattern to confirm the diagnosis. Examination should be performed in both supine and standing position with Valsalva. The sensitivity and specificity of sonography for varicoceles is extremely high, near 100%.

PEARLS

- **Varicoceles are best diagnosed by sonogram.**
- **Color Doppler sonography helps show low flow velocity from venous flow.**
- **Multiple tubular structures larger than 2 mm in diameter are seen.**

ADDITIONAL IMAGES (B-D)

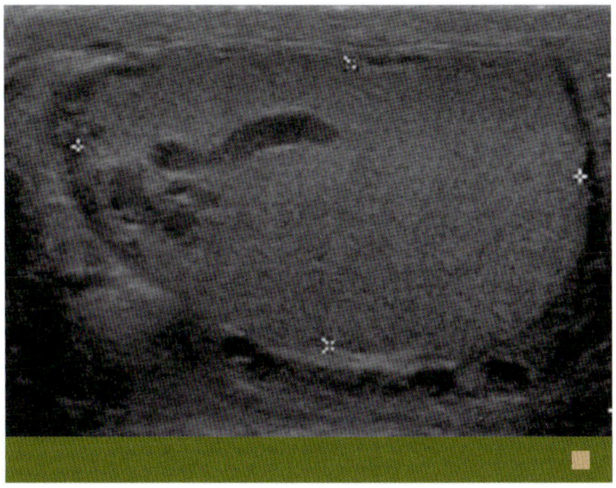

B. Transverse sonogram shows serpiginous structures within the testis because of varicocele with intratesticular component.

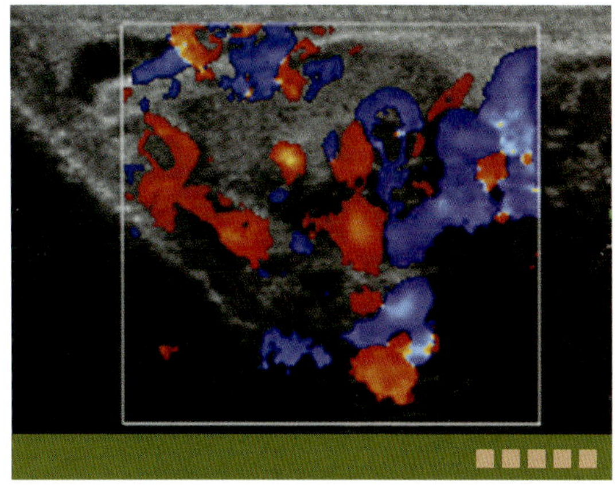

C. Transverse Color Doppler image shows flow within the varicoceles which augment with Valsalva.

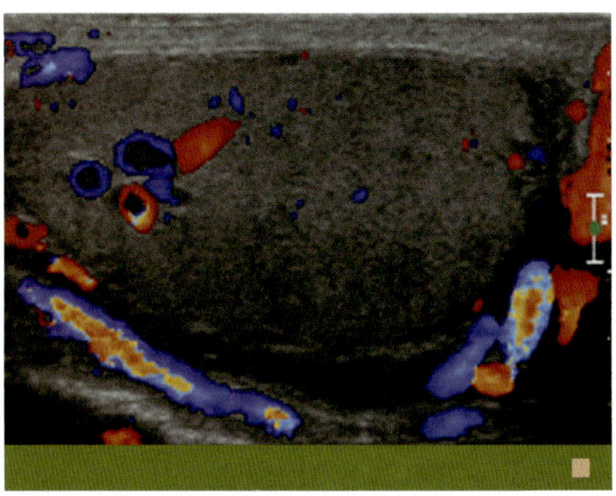

D. Longitudinal Color Doppler image shows flow within the intratesticular varicocele.

IMAGE KEY

Common

●●●●●
●●●●
●●●
●●
●

Rare

Typical

■■■■■
■■■■
■■■
■■
■

Unusual

CHAPTER 14

ADRENAL GLAND

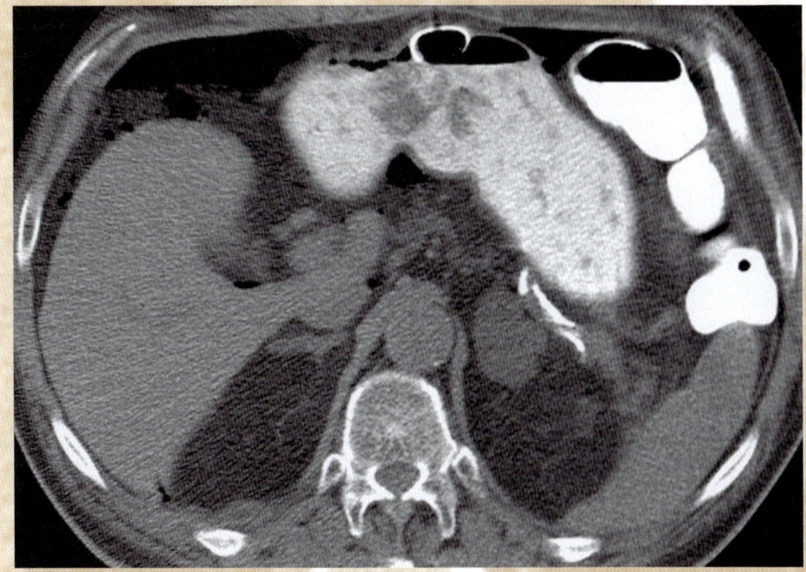

14–1 Adrenal Adenoma on Unenhanced CT

Frank H. Miller

PRESENTATION

May be incidental finding on imaging studies; may be hyperfunctioning and associated with hyperaldostonism (Conn syndrome) or hypercortisolism (Cushing syndrome) or hyperandrogenism from overproduction of androgens.

FINDINGS

Low-density lesion of adrenal gland.

DIFFERENTIAL DIAGNOSES

- *Adrenal metastases*: Often history of malignancy; may be indistinguishable on CECT; higher density on NECT.
- *Adrenal myelolipoma*: Has macroscopic fat; so typically lower (fat) density.
- *Adrenal pheochromocytoma*: Distinguish based on history of hypertension and elevated catecholamines, can be of lower density when cystic.
- *Adrenal cyst*: Tends to be fluid density.
- *Adrenal hemorrhage*: Seen as increased density.
- *Adrenal cell carcinoma*: Tends to be large, heterogeneous, may invade vessels, higher density on NECT.

COMMENTS

Imaging plays a critical role in the detection and characterization of adrenal masses. As patients are being imaged more frequently, adrenal masses are being detected more frequently. Incidental adrenal lesions are detected in about 5% of the population. The vast majority of these in patients without malignancy are benign. It is important to distinguish the benign from malignant lesions. Adenomas, more commonly, are small and have smooth margins with homogenous density. In contrast, features that suggest malignancy include larger size (>3 cm), heterogeneous and irregular margins. These findings are not specific.

Adrenal adenomas often can be distinguished from other benign and malignant lesions based on their imaging appearance. Adrenal adenomas unlike other lesions have high percentage of intracytoplasmic lipid. Those that are "lipid-rich" which may represent as many as 80% of adenomas have low Hounsfield units (HU) on unenhanced CT. On routine CT studies, which often are obtained following IV contrast, the appearance is often nonspecific.

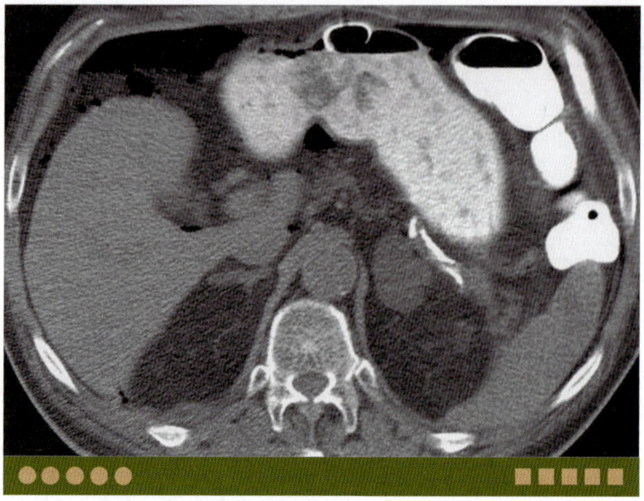

A. Axial NECT in patients without malignancy shows left adrenal mass which measured 3.8 × 2.9 cm and measured 5 HU. Lesion has smooth margins and is well defined. Findings are characteristic of adrenal adenoma.

Various threshold levels on unenhanced CT to characterize an adrenal lesion as adenomas have various sensitivities and specificities. A threshold of 2 HU is nearly 100% specific for an adrenal adenoma as almost all masses with this low density are adenomas; however, it has a relatively low sensitivity of approximately 50%. As a result, many adenomas may be considered indeterminate and may undergo unnecessary biopsy or be suspicious for malignancy. With a small false-negative rate, the use of a threshold of 10 HU will give a very high specificity of 98% and acceptable sensitivity of 71%. It is important to use a region of interest over the adrenal gland that includes the majority of the lesion without including periadrenal fat. The use of a high specificity is most likely more important than high sensitivity to ensure that the diagnosis of a false-positive test does not lead to incorrect treatment.

PEARLS

- **Adrenal adenomas usually contain lipid.**
- **An adrenal lesion that is less than 10 HU on NECT is usually caused by an adenoma.**
- **Metastases tend to be high density, greater than 20 HU on NECT.**

ADDITIONAL IMAGE

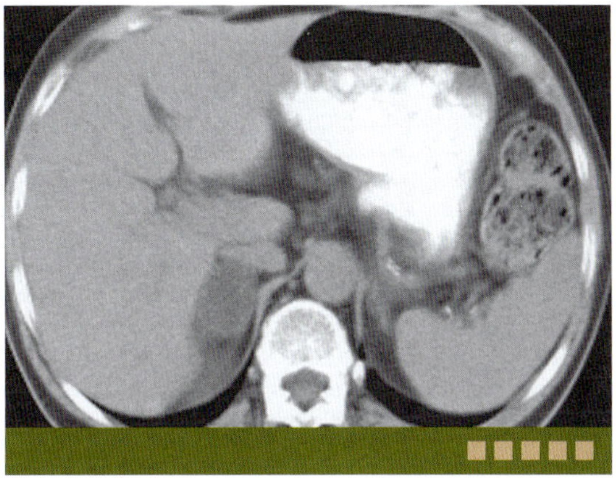

B. Axial NECT scan shows right adrenal lesion which was hypodense, well-defined, and with smooth margins from adrenal adenoma.

DIFFERENTIAL DIAGNOSES IMAGES (C-G)

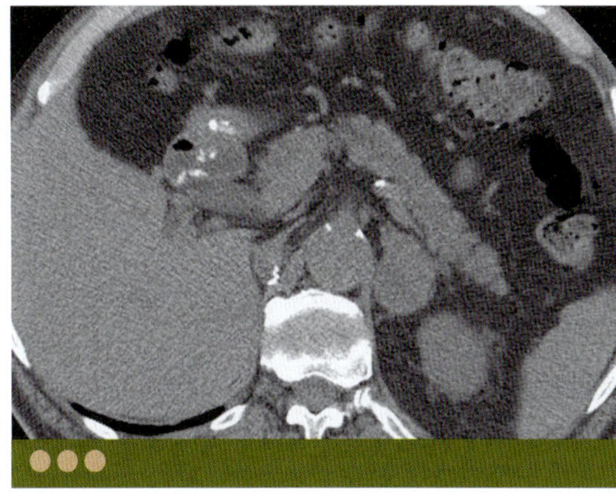

C. Adrenal metastasis from lung cancer: Axial NECT shows increased density left adrenal lesion that measures higher density than an adrenal adenoma.

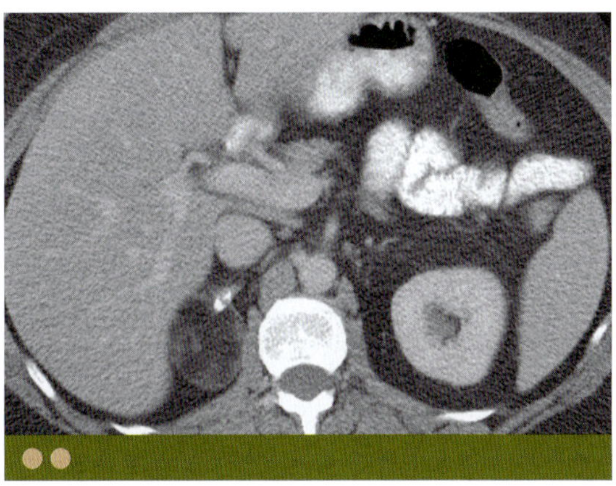

D. Adrenal myelolipoma: Axial CECT shows right adrenal mass that is predominately fat-containing and has associated calcification.

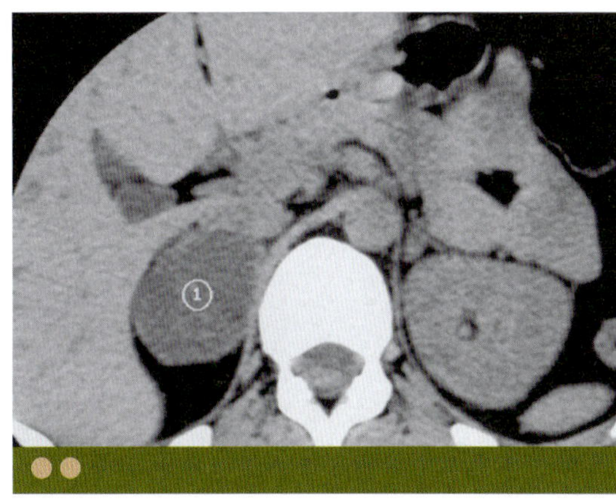

E. Cystic pheochromocytoma: Axial NECT shows a low-density 3-cm right adrenal mass in patients with history of hypertension. Lesion measured 14 HU. This history should prompt consideration of pheochromocytoma and functional adenoma. The patient had biochemical evidence of pheochromocytoma.

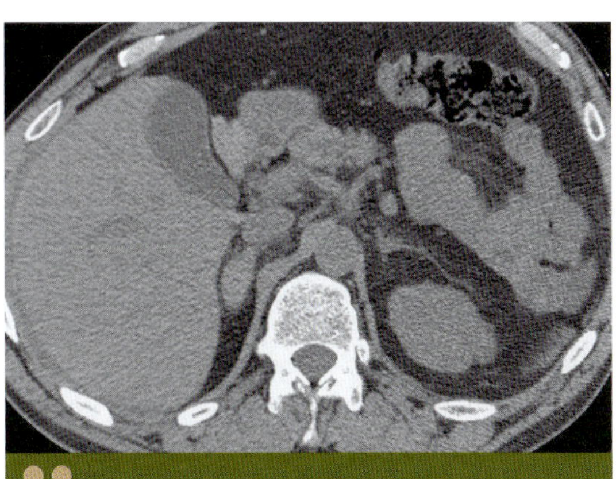

F. Adrenal hemorrhage: Axial NECT shows high-density right adrenal mass from adrenal hemorrhage. Density is higher than uncomplicated lipid-rich adenoma.

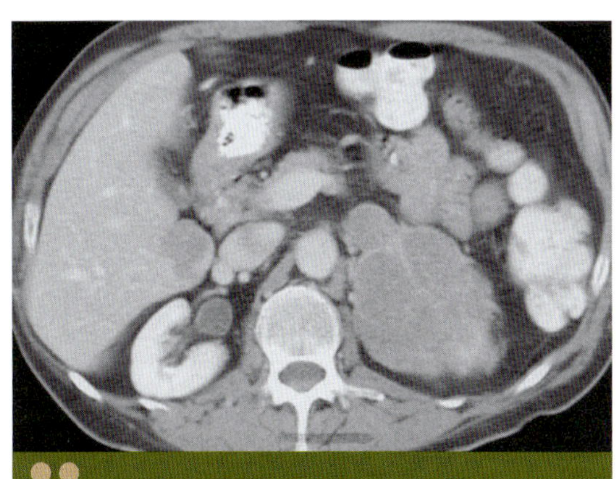

G. Adrenal cell carcinoma: Axial CECT shows large heterogeneous mass in the left adrenal gland and liver metastasis. The adrenal mass is larger and more heterogeneous than adrenal adenomas.

IMAGE KEY

Common

Rare

Typical

Unusual

14–2 Adrenal Adenoma Washout

Frank H. Miller

PRESENTATION

Incidental finding on imaging studies.

FINDINGS

Adrenal lesion with rapid washout of contrast material.

DIFFERENTIAL DIAGNOSES

- *Adrenal metastases*: Often history of malignancy; can be indistinguishable on routine CT from lipid-poor adenoma but differ based on washout.
- *Adrenal cell carcinoma*: Tends to be large, heterogeneous; may invade vessels and may have hemorrhage and necrosis.
- *Adrenal pheochromocytoma*: Distinguished on the basis of clinical history and laboratory findings, case reports have described abnormal washout similar to adenomas.
- *Adrenal myelolipoma*: Has macroscopic fat; so typically of lower density but does not show rapid washout.
- *Adrenal cyst*: Tends to be of fluid density but does not enhance.

COMMENTS

Unenhanced CT scans to characterize adrenal lesions as adenomas can be useful but have limitations. Approximately 20% to 30% of all adenomas are lipid-poor, and as a result, unenhanced CT may not be able to diagnose and characterize them. In addition, the majority of CT scans where lesions are detected incidentally especially in oncology patients are intravenous contrast-enhanced CT scans where the Hounsfield levels are not reliable unlike unenhanced CT scans. Chemical shift MR can be helpful to characterize adrenal lesions.

Another imaging parameter besides unenhanced CT to evaluate the adrenal gland relates to enhancement or perfusion. In patients where adrenal mass is greater than 10 HU and those who do not have an unenhanced scan, the use of adrenal washout on CT may be helpful. An adrenal protocol includes an unenhanced and venous CT obtained 60 seconds after the start of the injection and 10 or 15 minute delayed CT.

Adenomas tend to have rapid enhancement and washout of contrast material relative to nonadenomas. Rapid washout of contrast is seen in lipid-rich and lipid-poor adenomas. In contrast, malignancies tend to have abnormal vasculature and high endothelial permeability and as a result may show rapid enhancement, but contrast tends to accumulate and stay longer. Unlike unenhanced CT, an absolute attenuation value cannot be used as it varies based on the contrast dose, concentration, injection rate, and cardiac output. The percentage washout reflects the percentage of contrast enhancement values that is washed out on delayed scans.

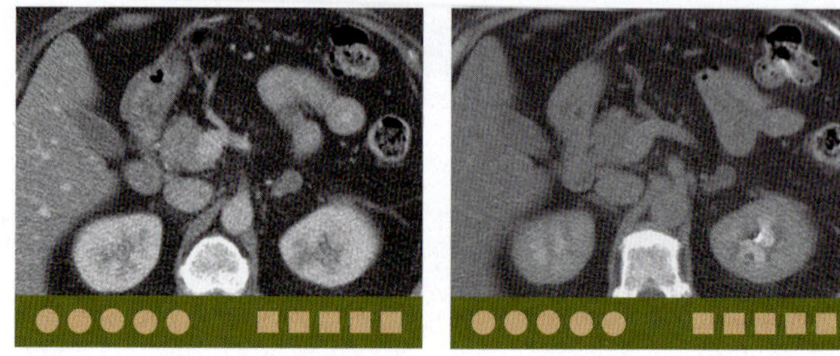

A. Axial CECT during venous phase shows 1-cm left adrenal lesion that measures 50 HU.
B. Axial CECT after 10-minute delay shows the adrenal mass measures 17 HU. The relative percentage change in washout is (50-17)/50 or 66%. The findings are consistent with an adrenal adenoma.

The absolute percentage washout is calculated on the basis of the equation (E-D/E-U) × 100 where E = early, D = delayed enhancement, and U = unenhanced value). Using a threshold of 60% yielded a sensitivity of 88% and specificity of 96%. In some patients, where the patient had a CT scan showing an adrenal mass, they can be reexamined using delayed images without returning for unenhanced CT. If unenhanced CT is not obtained, the relative washout is obtained with the equation of [(E-D)/E] × 100. A relative washout of 40% results in sensitivity of 96% and specificity of 100% for adenoma.

PEARLS

- **Adrenal adenomas are lipid poor in 20% to 30% of patients.**
- **Lipid-poor adenomas on NECT have HU greater than 10.**
- **Adrenal adenomas show rapid washout of contrast on CT.**
- **Rapid washout of contrast is seen in lipid-rich and lipid-poor adenomas.**
- **Metastases show slow washout of contrast.**

ADDITIONAL IMAGES (C-E)

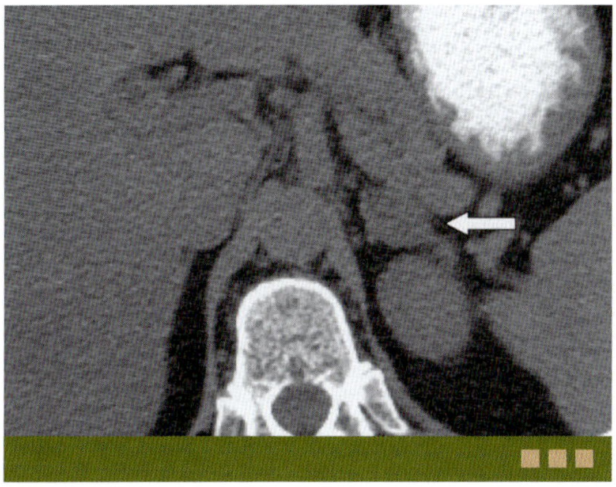

C. Lipid-poor adrenal adenoma. Axial NECT shows left adrenal mass, which measured 20 HU.

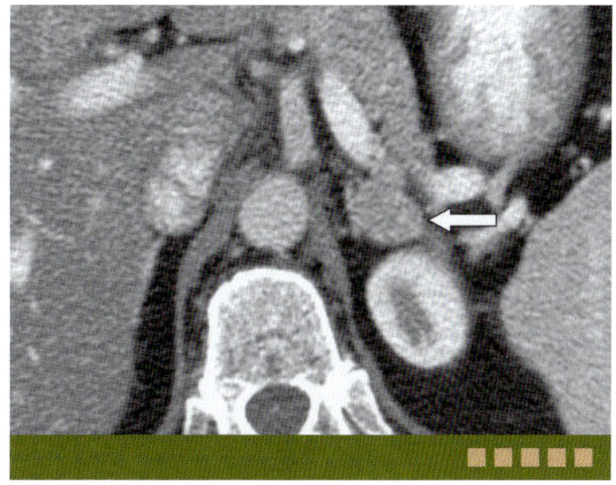

D. Axial CECT during venous phase shows enhancement of the lesion measuring 86 HU.

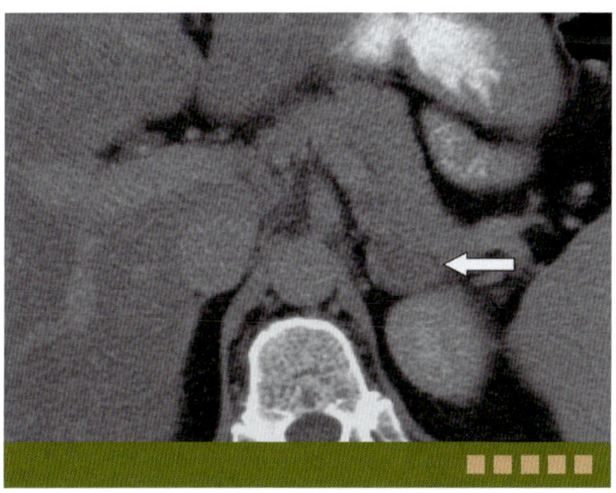

E. Axial CECT after 10-minute delay shows lesion measures 32 HU. The relative percentage washout is (86-20)/86 or 77%. The findings are consistent with adrenal adenoma.

DIFFERENTIAL DIAGNOSES IMAGES (F-G)

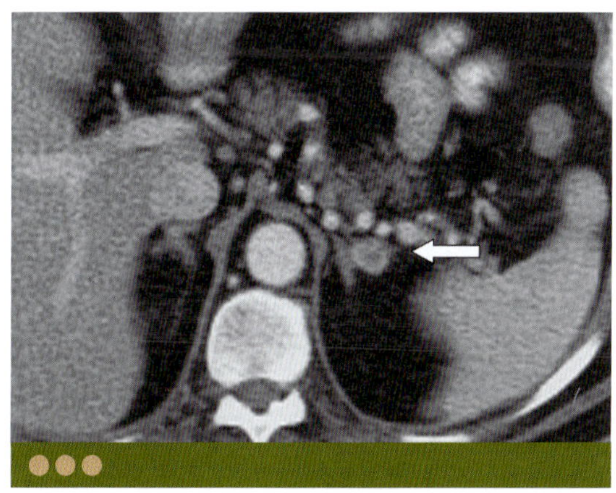

F. Renal cell carcinoma metastases to adrenal gland: Axial CECT shows left adrenal gland mass that measured 75 HU in patients with renal mass suspicious for renal cell carcinoma.

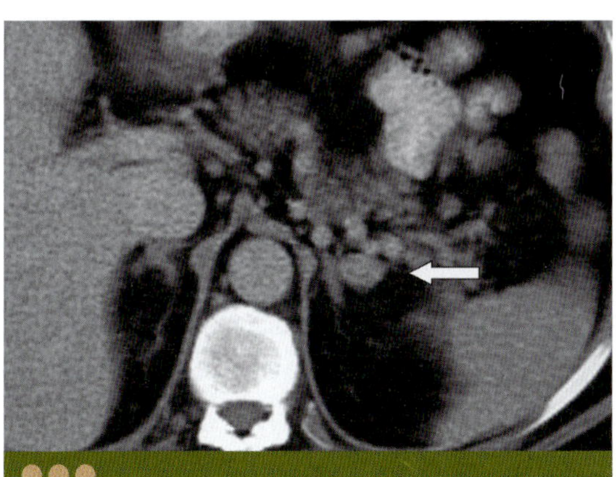

G. Axial CECT after 10 minutes delay shows the adrenal mass measured 66 HU. There was no significant washout to suggest that the lesion was an adrenal adenoma. This was a metastasis confirmed at surgery.

Figures C, D, and E are of the same patient.
Figures F and G are of the same patient.

IMAGE KEY

Common

Rare

Typical

Unusual

14–3 Adrenal Adenoma on MR

Frank H. Miller

PRESENTATION

Mass incidentally detected on ultrasound; nonspecific in appearance.

FINDINGS

Adrenal lesion loses signal intensity on opposed-phase MR images.

DIFFERENTIAL DIAGNOSES

- *Metastasis*: Usually associated with history of malignancy, vast majority do not contain lipid (do not drop in signal on opposed-phase imaging).
- *Adrenal cell carcinoma*: Rare tumor, generally large and heterogeneous in signal intensity from hemorrhage and necrosis; does not generally drop in signal on opposed-phase imaging.
- *Myelolipoma*: Uncommon masses; often heterogeneous with generally "macroscopic" fat.

COMMENTS

Adrenal lesions occur in 4% to 8% of autopsy series populations and are seen by radiologists on a routine basis when imaging patients. Adrenal lesions are frequently incidental lesions that are nonspecific on routine contrast-enhanced imaging. The distinction between adrenal adenomas and other lesions such as metastases can be critical, especially in patients with known malignancies. The presence of fat in adrenal adenomas, which is generally not seen in other adrenal lesions, helps differentiate adenomas from the other lesions. Unenhanced CT and chemical shift (in- and opposed-phase) MR imaging can be used to identify the presence of abundant intracytoplasmic lipid within the adrenal lesions to suggest that they represent adenomas.

The use of chemical shift MR imaging is based on fat and water protons precessing differently. On in-phase imaging, the water and fat signal are additive. On opposed-phase images, the fat and water are out of phase and cancel each other and appear dark. Therefore, adenomas are dark on opposed-phase imaging.

At 1.5 Tesla, the in-phase images are obtained at echo times (TE) values of 4.2 ms and multiples of 4.2 while the opposed-phase images are obtained at TE values of 2.1 ms and odd multiples of 2.1. When obtaining images using chemical shift imaging, it is important to keep all the parameters including TR, slice thickness and position, and flip angle the same. It is best to obtain these images as part of

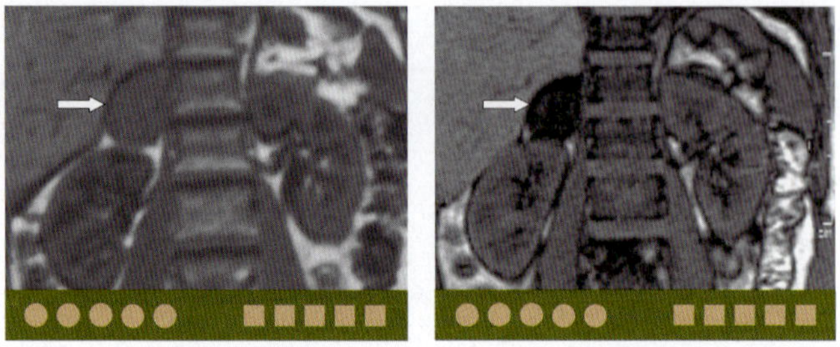

A. The patient had a 3-cm nonspecific right adrenal lesion incidentally detected on ultrasound. Coronal in-phase MR image shows the adrenal lesion was iso-intense with the muscle and liver on in-phase imaging.
B. Coronal opposed-phase MR image shows the lesion has signal loss relative to the liver and spleen. It can be identified as opposed-phase image as the organs are etched in black. These findings are consistent with a lipid-rich adrenal adenoma.

a single dual echo acquisition where the only parameter that varies is the TE. T2-weighted images (T2-WI) are not helpful in distinguishing adrenal lesions such as adenomas as the signal intensity on T2-WI is quite variable.

Suppression of signal on opposed-phase images can be determined subjectively or objectively. In general, the spleen is used as an internal reference as it does not generally change in signal intensity on in- and opposed-phase imaging. The liver is generally not used as it can have fatty infiltration accounting for a drop in signal on opposed-phase images. If it is not clear whether an adrenal lesion is suppressing on the opposed-phase imaging, then subtraction imaging can be used where the opposed-phase images are subtracted from the in-phase images.

PEARLS

- **Important to characterize adenomas accurately and not confuse them as metastases and prevent curative therapy when metastasis to adrenal.**
- **Chemical shift MR is excellent method to characterize adrenal lesions as adenomas.**
- **It is important to keep all parameters on MR the same with the exception of TE.**
- **On the opposed-phase imaging, adrenal adenomas lose signal when lipid-rich.**

ADDITIONAL IMAGES (C-F)

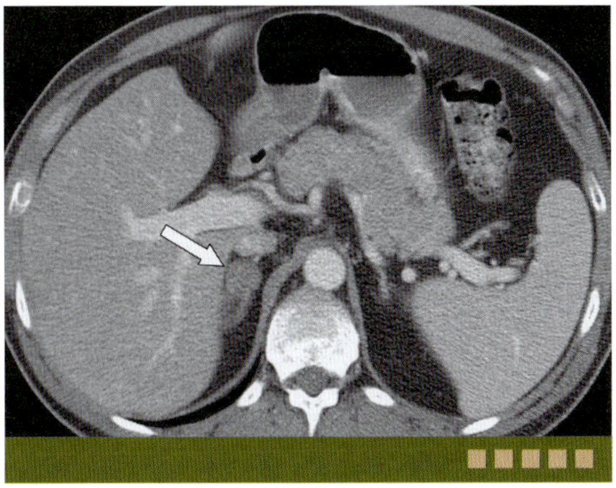

C. Axial CECT scan shows a nonspecific enhancing right adrenal lesion. If better characterization of the lesion is required, unenhanced CT or MR would be required.

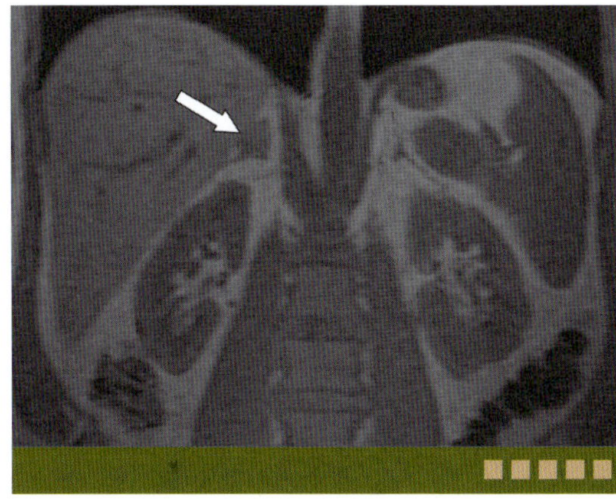

D. Coronal in-phase MR images show the lesion is similar in signal intensity to the spleen.

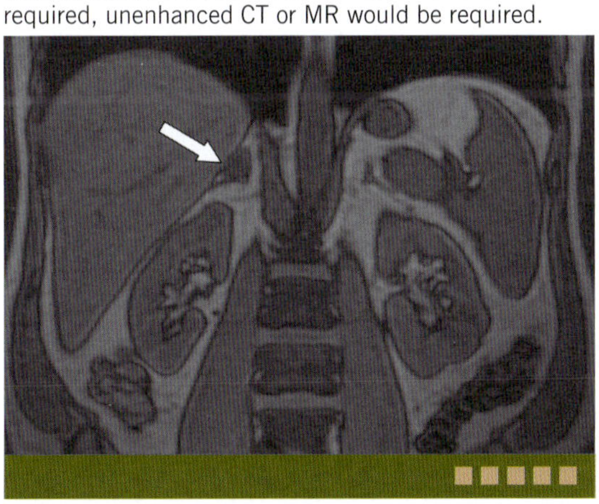

E. Coronal opposed-phase MR image shows the difficulty in this patient in determining if the lesion drops in signal intensity. It is similar signal intensity to the liver on in- and opposed-phase images. Regions of interest to measure signal intensity can be used or subtraction images.

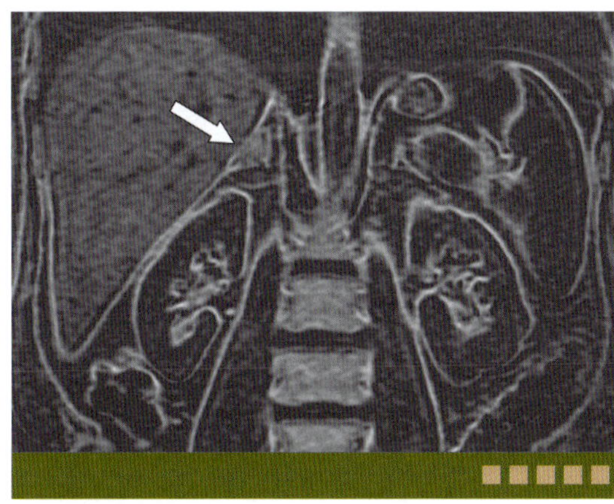

F. Subtraction image where the opposed-phase image is subtracted from the in-phase image shows that the adrenal gland is bright (arrow) as a result of the drop in signal from fat. This confirms the adrenal lesion is an adenoma. Note the liver is also bright because of fatty infiltration. This shows why the spleen is used as the standard and not the liver as the liver may also lose signal from fatty infiltration.

DIFFERENTIAL DIAGNOSES IMAGES (G-H)

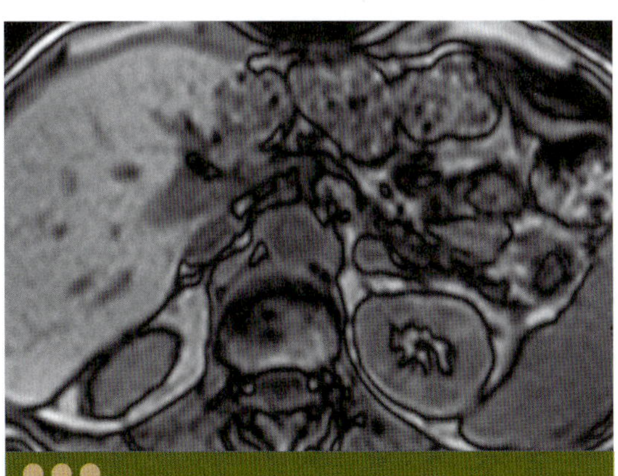

G. Adrenal metastasis from esophageal cancer: Opposed-phase image shows the lesion does not drop in signal intensity relative to the spleen. In-phase image is not shown.

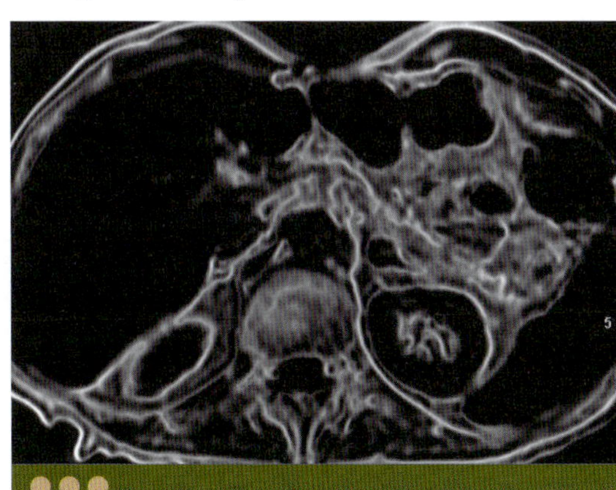

H. Subtraction image in the same patient created by subtracting the opposed-phase images from the in-phase images shows the adrenal lesion is not high-signal intensity to suggest the presence of fat. Lesion was proven to be metastasis from esophageal cancer.

Figures C, D, E, and F are of the same patient. Figures G and H are of the same patient.

IMAGE KEY

Common

Rare

Typical

Unusual

14–4 Atypical Adrenal Adenoma on MR

Frank H. Miller

PRESENTATION

Asymptomatic; hypercortisolism, and depressed adrenocorticotropic hormone (ACTH).

FINDINGS

Heterogeneous appearance of adrenal gland with areas that drop in signal with areas that do not drop in signal on opposed-phase MR imaging.

DIFFERENTIAL DIAGNOSES

- *Collision tumors*: Rare lesions generally result of two coexisting lesions such as adenoma and metastasis which may have different features, that is, adenoma shows signal drop and metastasis does not show signal drop on opposed imaging.
- *Adrenal cell carcinoma*: Generally very large heterogeneous mass unlike adenoma; may rarely have small focus of fat.
- *Typical adrenal adenoma*: Shows homogeneous suppression.
- *Metastases*: Generally do not suppress on opposed-phase images unless few types such as some renal cell carcinomas and hepatocellular carcinomas.

COMMENTS

Adrenal lesions are commonly seen in 4% to 8% of population on the basis of autopsy series and are routinely seen by radiologists on imaging studies. It is critical to distinguish benign adrenal adenomas from malignancies including metastases.

Chemical shift MR imaging is helpful in characterizing adrenal adenomas. The basis of distinction of adenomas from other lesions is the presence of abundant intra-cytoplasmic lipid in adenomas. The MR criterion for adenoma typically is complete suppression.

Gabriel et al. observed that some lesions demonstrate heterogeneous, incomplete suppression and the appearance is not typical for adenomas or for metastases.[1] In a study of 242 patients with adrenal lesions on MR, heterogeneous suppression was commonly seen in 34 patients (14%). All patients with heterogeneous suppression had a combination of interwoven lipid-rich cells and compact lipid-poor cells. The amount and distribution of the cell types correlated with the MR findings. In this small series with heterogeneous suppression, they all had a benign lesion. Their

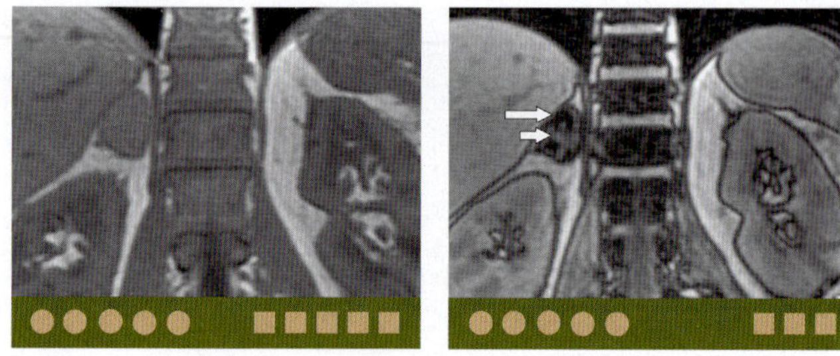

A. Coronal in-phase image (TE = 4.2 ms) shows 3-cm lesion which is similar in signal intensity to the liver.
B. Coronal opposed-phase image (TE = 2.1 ms) shows speckled pattern of heterogeneous suppression of the adrenal nodule with foci of suppression (long arrow) and nonsuppression (short arrow).

conclusion was that in the appropriate clinical setting, follow-up of these patients may be considered especially in patients without known malignancy.

Although rare, another cause for heterogeneous suppression is the presence of an adrenal collision tumor. Collision tumors refer to two different types of adrenal lesions that coexist, such as a metastasis and an adenoma. The imaging appearance is a combination of the two lesions. As a result, an adrenal adenoma with a metastatic focus may have a focus on nonsuppression on opposed-phase images. If a lesion grows, changes in appearance, or is somewhat large or heterogeneous, a collision tumor should be considered. In addition, case reports have described adrenal cortical carcinomas that contain fat, resulting in potentially heterogeneous suppression. These tumors, which are rare usually, present as very large masses and may contain necrosis and calcifications on CT unlike adenomas.[1]

PEARLS

- **Homogeneous suppression of adrenal lesions on opposed-phase MR images is typical for adrenal adenomas.**
- **Heterogeneous suppression on opposed-phase images is not rare.**
- **Heterogeneous suppression on opposed-phase images is most suggestive of atypical adrenal adenomas especially in patients without known malignancy.**
- **Heterogeneous suppression is a result of lipid-rich and lipid-poor cells in adrenal adenomas.**

[1]Gabriel H, Pizzitola V, McComb EN, Wiley, E, Miller FH. Adrenal lesions with heterogeneous suppression on chemical shift imaging: clinical implications. *JMRI* 2004; 19:308-316.

ADDITIONAL IMAGE

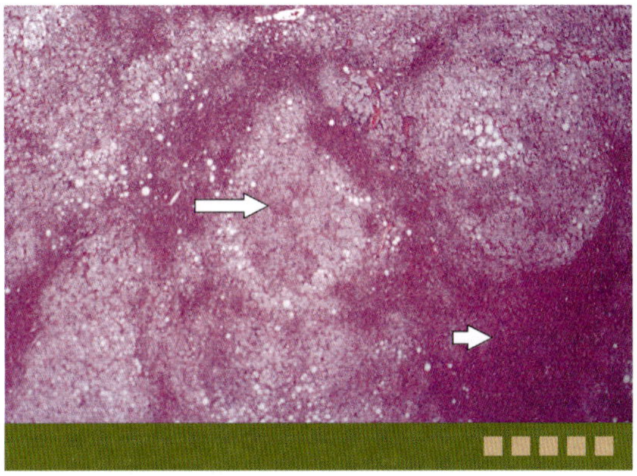

C. The corresponding pathology specimen reveals a mixture of vacuolated lipid-rich cells (long arrow) and lipid-poor cells (short arrow) within one high power field. This distribution of lipid-rich and lipid-poor cells account for the MR appearance of regions of signal drop-off on opposed-phase images resulting from lipid-rich cells and lack of signal drop-off caused by lipid-poor cells.

DIFFERENTIAL DIAGNOSES IMAGES (D-H)

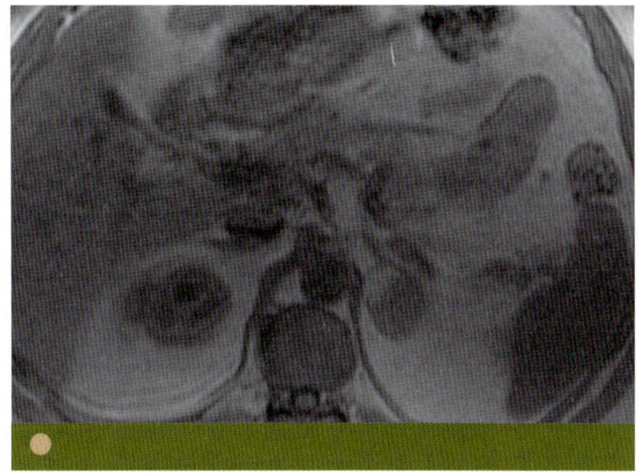

D. Collision tumor: In-phase image shows complex left adrenal lesion with the more anteromedial component is high-signal intensity.

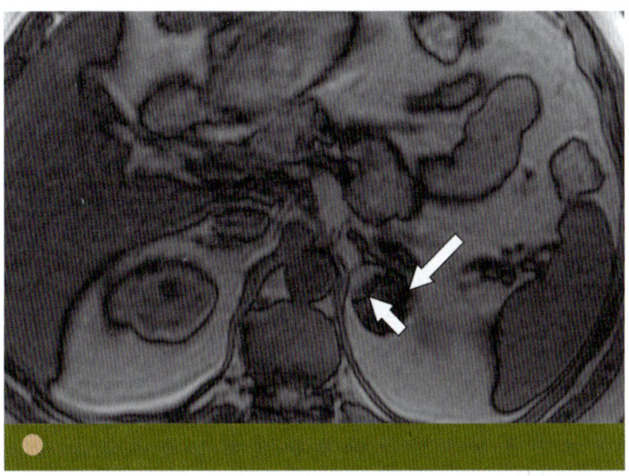

E. Opposed-phase image in the same patient shows that the lesion has area of signal drop-off (large arrow) because of microscopic fat with more medial portion not dropping in signal intensity (short arrow). Chemical shift or India ink artifact is seen between the more anterior macroscopic fat signal intensity area and the more lateral aspect of the adrenal gland.

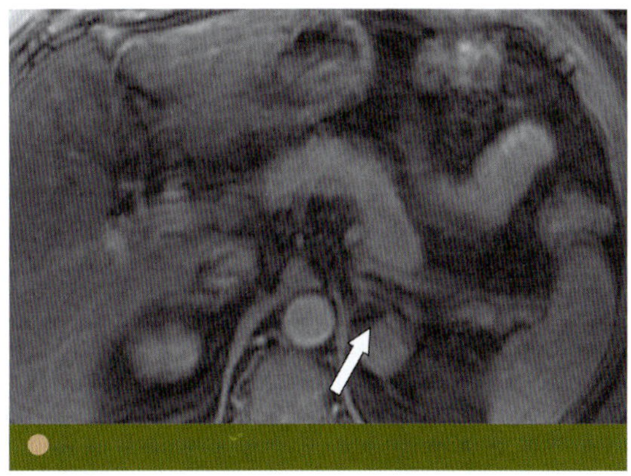

F. Axial frequency selective fat-suppressed image shows signal drop in the more medial portion (arrow) of the adrenal gland relative to the in-phase image. The drop in signal intensity is caused by macroscopic fat which is suggestive of adrenal myelolipoma. The lesion may represent a collision tumor with myelolipoma (seen as more anterior fat signal intensity) and adenoma (seen as the more lateral area which drops in signal intensity). It may also relate to a myelolipoma with areas that are lipid-rich and lipid-poor.

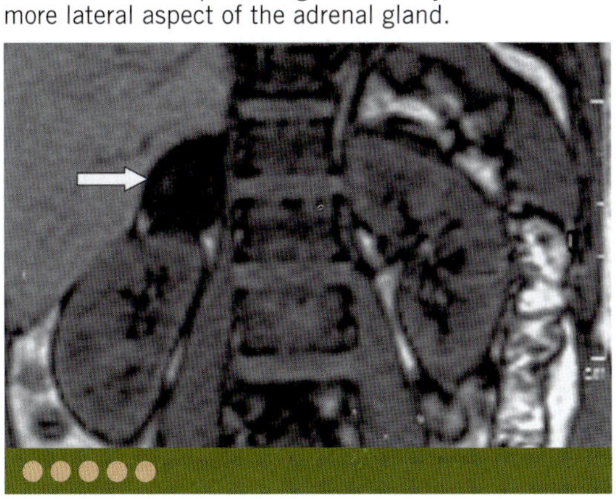

G. Typical adrenal adenoma: Coronal opposed-phase image shows drop in signal relative to in-phase image (not shown) because of right adrenal adenoma (arrow).

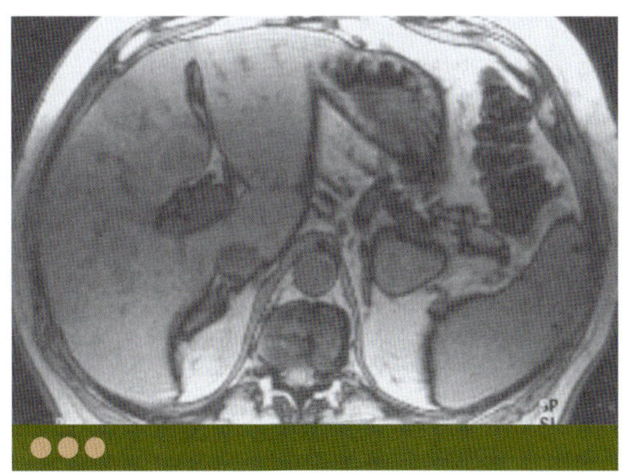

H. Adrenal metastases from duodenal cancer: Axial opposed-phase image shows left adrenal metastases that do not drop in signal intensity relative to in-phase image (not shown). Multiple liver metastases are also seen.

Figures D. to F. are of the same patient.

IMAGE KEY

Common

Rare

Typical

Unusual

14–5 Adrenal Metastasis

Frank H. Miller

PRESENTATION

Generally asymptomatic; patients with known malignancy elsewhere; may have evidence of adrenal insufficiency.

FINDINGS

Adrenal lesion of higher density on unenhanced CT than adenomas; heterogeneous enhancement following contrast.

DIFFERENTIAL DIAGNOSES

- *Adrenal adenoma*: Can distinguish if lipid-rich adenoma as tend to be lower density on CT.
- *Adrenal cortical carcinoma*: Tend to be rare and large and heterogeneous.
- *Pheochromocytoma*: Often hyperintense on T2 MR and hypervascular but can be nonspecific on imaging studies; history of hypertension and clinical findings help distinguish.

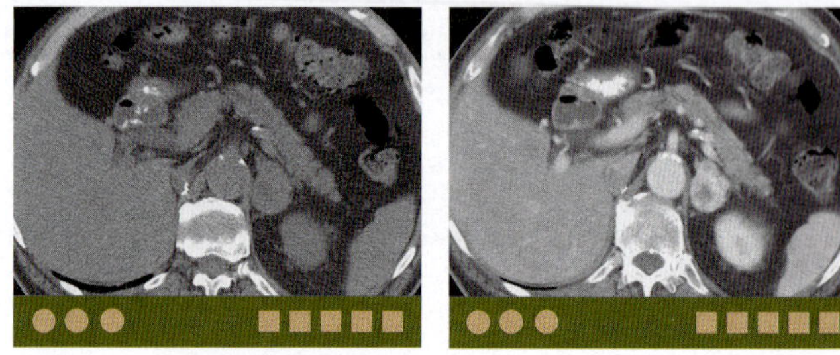

A. Adrenal metastasis from lung cancer. Unenhanced CT shows increased density left adrenal lesion that measures higher density than an adrenal adenoma.
B. Axial CECT scan in the same patient shows heterogeneous enhancing mass of the left adrenal gland with peripheral enhancement.

COMMENTS

Adrenal metastases are the most common malignant lesions of the adrenal glands. Adrenal metastases are often associated with primary cancers arising from the breast, lung, kidney, skin (melanoma), and colon. It is critical to be able to differentiate adrenal metastases from adenomas as the distinction may affect therapy in patients with a known malignancy.

The distinction of adrenal adenomas from metastases can generally be made with MR or CT based on the detection of lipid. Lipid is generally seen in adenomas and not in metastases. Exceptions do exist including some types of renal cell carcinoma and hepatomas that can contain lipid. Using CT, the density of metastases on unenhanced CT is generally higher than adenomas. Metastases on MR do not generally lose signal on opposed-phase images. The appearance of adrenal metastases can be variable. They may be small or large, unilateral or bilateral. When large, they tend to show findings suggestive of malignancy, including heterogeneous density or signal intensity and heterogeneous enhancement. They do not tend to show signal drop on opposed-phase images. Following contrast administration, metastases often have heterogeneous enhancement; however, when smaller, they are often homogenous and more difficult to distinguish from benign etiologies.

Benign adrenal lesions cannot always be distinguished from malignant adrenal lesions. At times, biopsy, PET scans, or follow-up imaging can be useful. Features that raise suspicion for malignancy include larger size (>5 cm), irregular shape, and ill-defined margins, heterogeneity, and lack of fat on CT or chemical shift MR. On follow-up examinations, metastases generally grow in size unless treatment for the cancer has been administered.

PEARLS

- **In patients with known malignancy, the possibility of adrenal metastases needs to be considered.**
- **Adrenal metastases can generally be distinguished from adrenal adenomas on the basis of the lack of lipid in metastases.**
- **Features that suggest malignancy include larger size (>5 cm), irregular shape, and ill-defined margins, heterogeneity, and lack of fat on CT or chemical shift MR.**
- **On follow-up examinations, metastases generally grow in size unless treatment for the cancer has been administered.**

ADDITIONAL IMAGES (C-F)

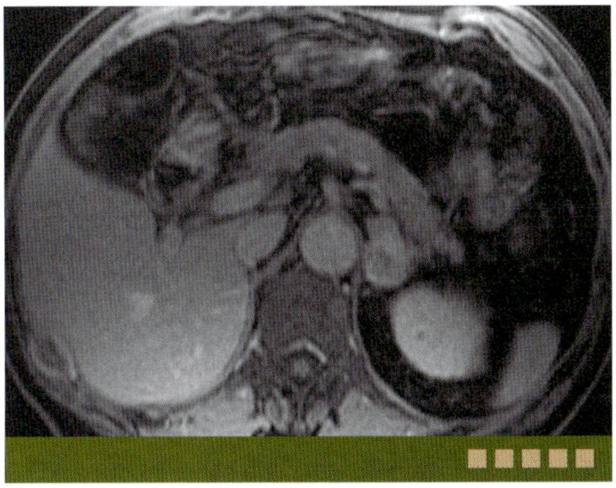

C. Axial contrast-enhanced MR shows heterogeneously enhancing left adrenal metastasis as well as right rib metastasis.

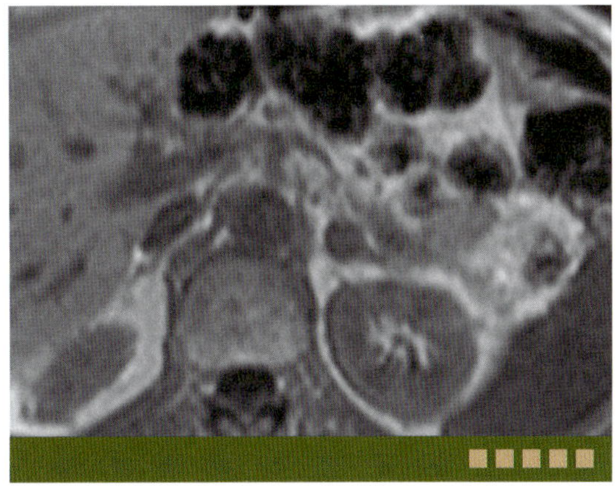

D. Adrenal metastasis from esophageal cancer. In-phase image shows left adrenal lesion which is similar signal intensity to the spleen.

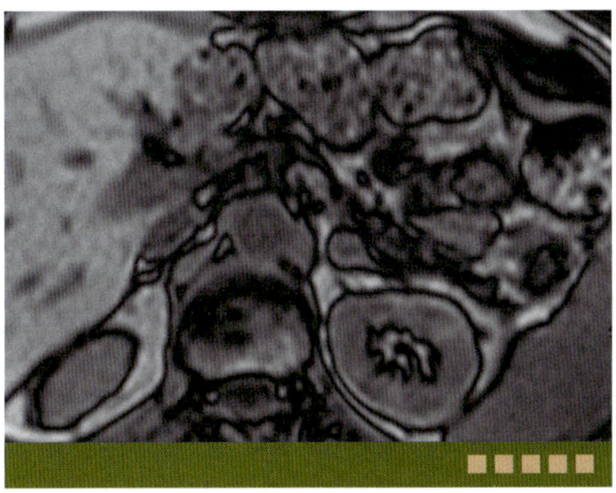

E. Opposed-phase image in the same patient shows the lesion does not drop in signal intensity relative to the spleen.

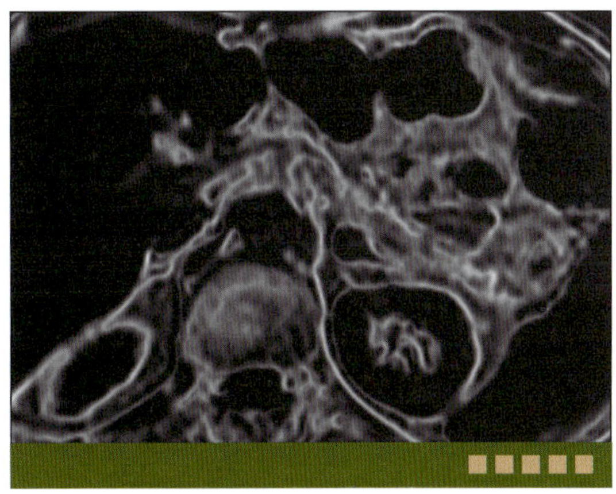

F. Subtraction image in the same patient created by subtracting the opposed-phase images from the in-phase images shows the adrenal lesion is not high-signal intensity to suggest presence of fat.

DIFFERENTIAL DIAGNOSES IMAGES (G-H)

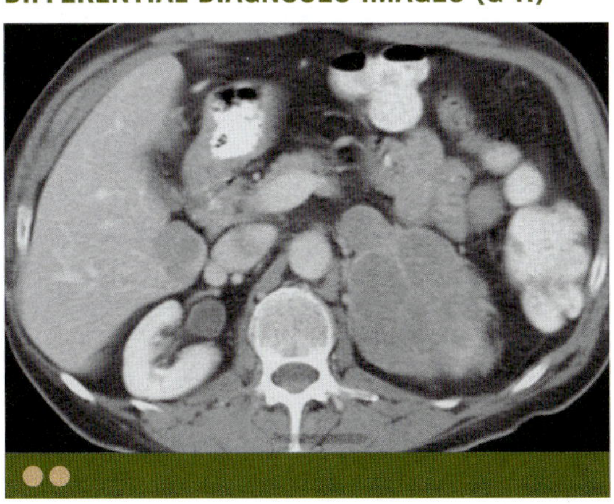

G. Adrenal cell carcinoma with liver metastasis: Axial CECT scan shows large heterogeneous lesion involving the left adrenal gland. Adrenal cell carcinoma is significantly less common than metastasis to the adrenal gland. Biopsy is required to make the distinction.

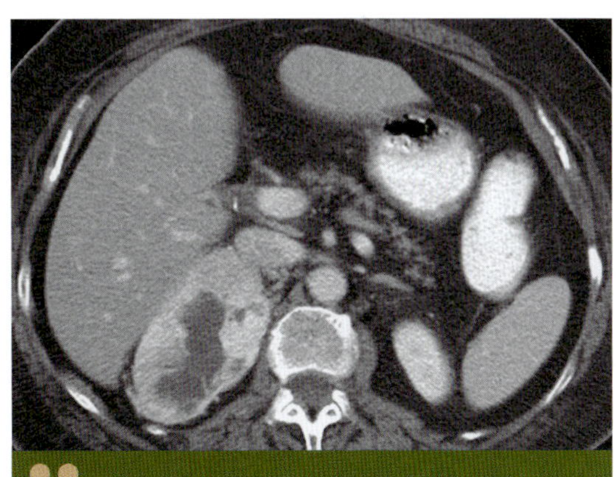

H. Pheochromocytoma: Axial CECT shows a large heterogeneous mass of the right adrenal gland. Pheochromocytomas are imaging chameleons mimicking other lesions. The history of hypertension and abnormal laboratory findings allow the distinction from other lesions.

IMAGE KEY

Common

Rare

Typical

Unusual

14–6 Adrenal Metastasis from Renal Cell Carcinoma Mimicking Adenoma

Frank H. Miller

PRESENTATION

Adrenal lesion; history of resected renal cell carcinoma.

FINDINGS

Adrenal lesion drops in signal intensity on opposed-phase MR images.

DIFFERENTIAL DIAGNOSES

- *Adrenal adenoma*: Looks same; generally does not increase in size; consider metastasis from renal cell cancer on the basis of the history of renal cell carcinoma or lesion suggestive of renal cell carcinoma.
- *Adrenal metastases from other lesions*: Metastases besides renal cell carcinoma or hepatocellular carcinoma generally do not drop in signal intensity.
- *Adrenal cell carcinoma*: Generally does not drop in signal intensity on opposed-phase images or only small portion of lesion which contains fat may drop in signal intensity.

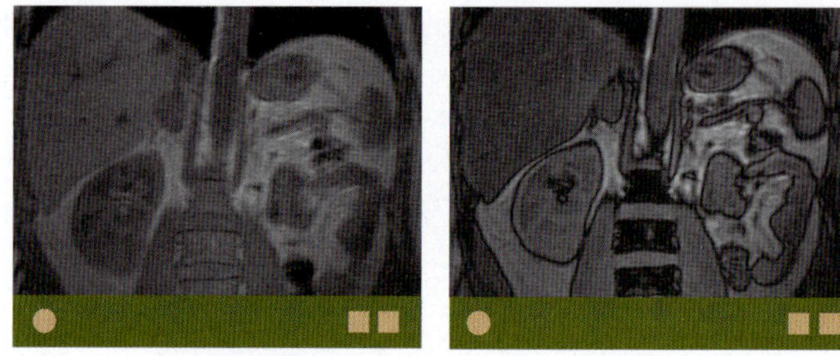

A. Coronal in-phase MR image shows right adrenal lesion that is similar signal intensity to the liver.
B. Coronal opposed-phase MR image shows the lesion drops in signal intensity but remains similar in signal intensity to the liver. Follow-up images showed growth of lesion, and biopsy showed metastatic renal cell carcinoma.

COMMENTS

Adrenal adenomas have microscopic lipid, and the presence of fat generally allows their diagnosis and their differentiation from other adrenal lesions. The use of MR, and specifically chemical shift imaging, is used to diagnose adrenal adenomas and differentiate these benign lesions from other lesions. The diagnosis of adrenal adenoma using MR is extremely specific and is made on the basis of the drop in signal intensity of the adrenal lesion on the opposed-phase images relative to the in-phase images.

Renal cell carcinoma, especially the clear cell subtype, and less often, the granular cell subtype, can have microscopic fat and mimic adenoma. Hepatocellular carcinoma can also have fat and metastasize to the adrenal gland. As a result of this fat, the lesion may drop in signal intensity on opposed-phase imaging. Renal cell carcinoma can metastasize to the adrenal gland and can have microscopic fat and mimic an adrenal adenoma as seen in this patient. As a result, in patients with neoplasms such as renal cell carcinoma that contain microscopic fat, it is important for radiologists to recognize that adrenal lesions that have microscopic fat may not represent adrenal adenomas but may represent metastases. Follow-up imaging, PET scan, or biopsy may be required. In the general population, the presence of an adrenal lesion that drops in signal intensity on opposed-phase images represents an adrenal adenoma. In this patient, the adrenal lesion was suspected to be an adrenal adenoma, but it grew on follow-up imaging. The history of renal cell carcinoma attributed to clear cell subtype made the lesion suspicious for a metastatic lesion that was confirmed on fine needle aspiration.

PEARLS

- **The vast majority of adrenal lesions that drop in signal intensity on opposed-phase images represent an adrenal adenoma.**
- **Renal cell carcinomas especially clear cell subtype can have microscopic fat.**
- **Adrenal lesions that drop in signal on opposed-phase images in setting of renal cell carcinoma may represent metastases.**
- **PET scan, follow-up imaging, or biopsy may be required to diagnose metastasis and distinguish from adenoma.**

ADDITIONAL IMAGE

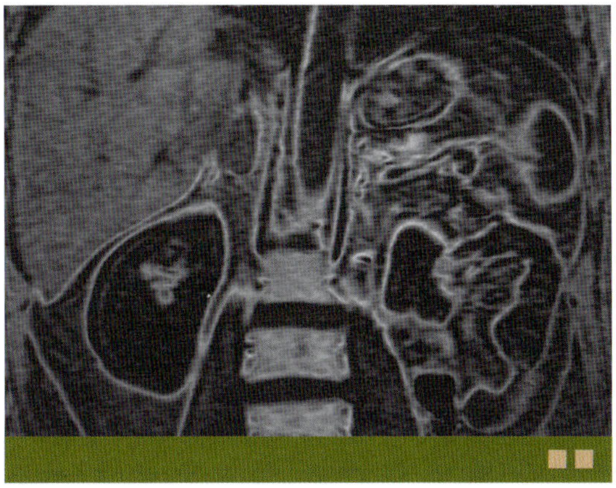

C. Subtraction image, where opposed-phase image is subtracted from in-phase image, shows that the right adrenal gland and the liver are increased signal from fat. This suggests adrenal adenoma; however, the history of clear cell renal cell carcinoma that has fat is one of the few examples where an adrenal lesion can lose signal because of metastatic lesion.

DIFFERENTIAL DIAGNOSES IMAGES (D-H)

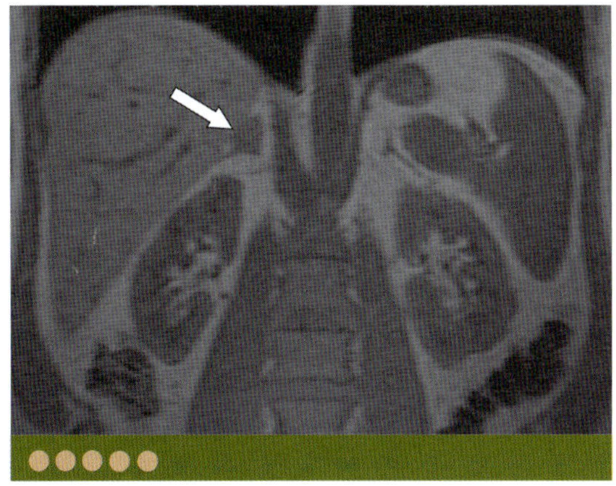

D. Adrenal adenoma: Coronal in-phase MR shows the adrenal lesion (arrow) is similar in signal intensity to the liver.

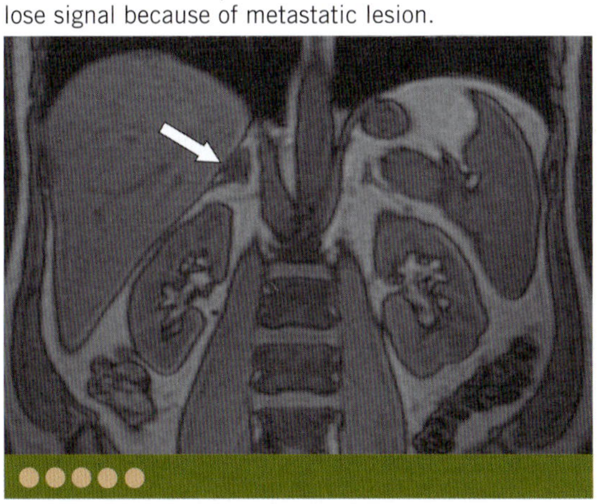

E. Coronal opposed-phase MR image in the same patient shows drop in signal intensity of adrenal (arrow) which is difficult to appreciate visually.

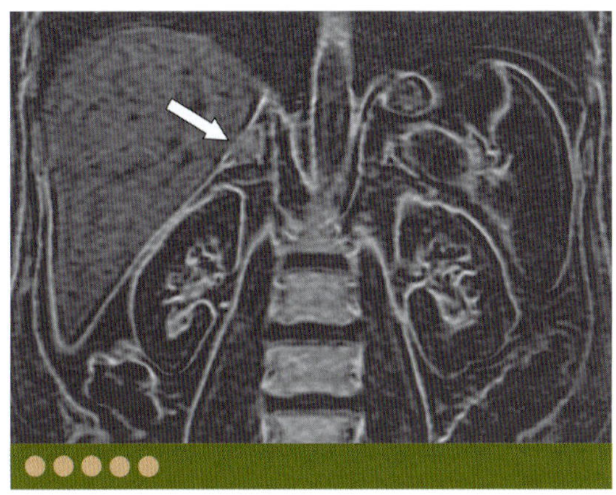

F. Coronal subtraction image (inopposed-phase image) shows drop in signal intensity of the liver and right adrenal lesion (arrow). The appearance is associated with adrenal adenoma. The patient did not have a history or findings of renal cell carcinoma to suggest metastases.

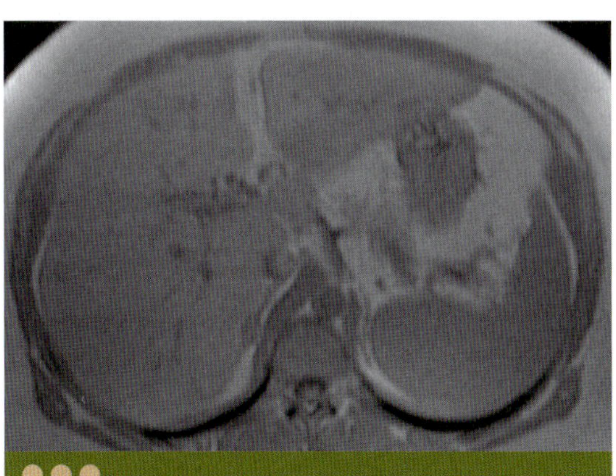

G. Renal cell metastasis to contralateral adrenal: In-phase MR image shows right adrenal lesion that has similar signal intensity as the liver and spleen.

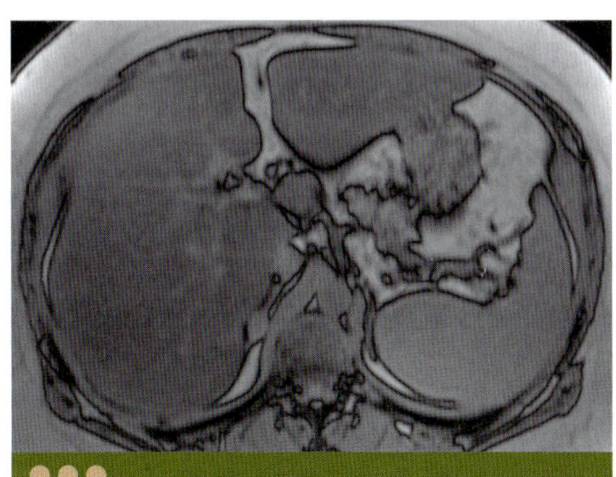

H. Opposed-phase MR image shows the right adrenal lesion has the same signal intensity as the spleen and does not drop in signal intensity because of metastasis which did not contain fat.

Figures D to F are the same patient.
Figures G and H are the same patient.

IMAGE KEY

Common

Rare

Typical

Unusual

14–7 Adrenal Collision Tumor

Frank H. Miller

PRESENTATION

History of lung cancer and adrenal mass.

FINDINGS

Complex adrenal lesion with imaging features that are a combination of the two lesions.

DIFFERENTIAL DIAGNOSES

- *Myelolipoma*: Can appear as a complex lesion but typically has macroscopic fat.
- *Atypical adrenal adenoma*: Can have lipid-rich and lipid-poor regions leading to heterogeneous appearance.
- *Pheochromocytoma*: Can have a variety of appearances, but clinical history and laboratory findings usually can help distinguish.
- *Adrenal metastases*: Can appear complex; generally does not have microscopic fat unless some type of renal cell carcinoma or hepatoma.
- *Adrenal cell carcinoma*: Tend to be large infiltrative masses which can have small foci of fat as well as hemorrhagic and necrotic material.

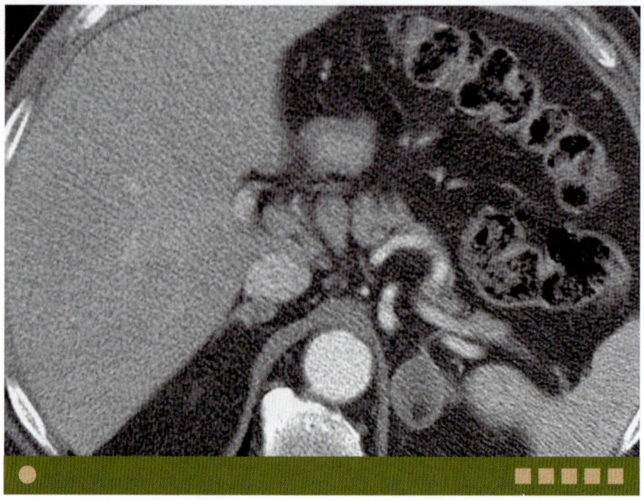

A. Axial CECT shows 3-cm left adrenal mass that is mainly soft tissue density with focal area of decreased density. Biopsy showed metastatic nonsmall cell carcinoma with cluster of adrenal cells consistent with adenoma.

COMMENTS

Collision tumors are extremely rare and the prevalence is unknown. Collision tumors refer to two different types of adrenal lesions that coexist: often a metastasis and an adenoma, but both lesions may be metastases or benign lesions.

The imaging appearance of collision tumors is a combination of the two lesions. As a result, an adrenal adenoma with a metastatic focus may have an area on suppression on opposed-phase MR images because of an adrenal adenoma and a focus of nonsuppression on opposed-phase images from the metastatic focus. Adrenal collision tumors may mimic an atypical adrenal adenoma that has areas of lipid-rich and lipid-poor regions. Collision tumors on unenhanced CT may be seen as a low-density area from a lipid-rich adenoma and higher-density area from a metastasis or nonadenoma. In addition, collision tumors may comprise a myelolipoma and adenoma making the distinction difficult. Collision tumors should be suspected in patients that have a known malignancy that have heterogeneous adrenal masses suspected to be an atypical adenoma and grows, changes in appearance, or have an adrenal lesion that becomes more heterogeneous or is somewhat large. Rarely, adrenal cortical carcinomas contain fat, resulting in potentially heterogeneous suppression suggestive of a collision tumor. These tumors, which are very rare, usually present as very large masses and may contain necrosis and calcifications on CT unlike that of adenomas. The diagnosis of collision tumors is best made by biopsy or surgical resection.

PEARLS

- **Collision tumors refer to two types of adrenal lesions that coexist.**
- **Collision tumors may be a result from metastasis and adenoma but can also be two benign or malignant lesions.**
- **Imaging features of collision tumors are a combination of the two coexisting lesions.**
- **Suspect collision tumor in patients that have a known malignancy that have heterogeneous adrenal masses suspected to be an atypical adenoma and grows, changes in appearance, or have an adrenal lesion or becomes more heterogeneous or is somewhat large.**
- **Diagnosis is confirmed by biopsy.**

ADDITIONAL IMAGES (B-C)

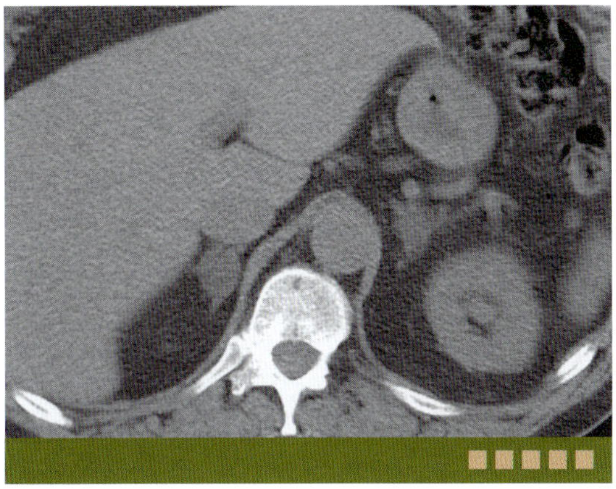

B. Axial CECT shows right adrenal lesion that measured 2 HU from adrenal adenoma. The patient also had left adrenal adenoma.

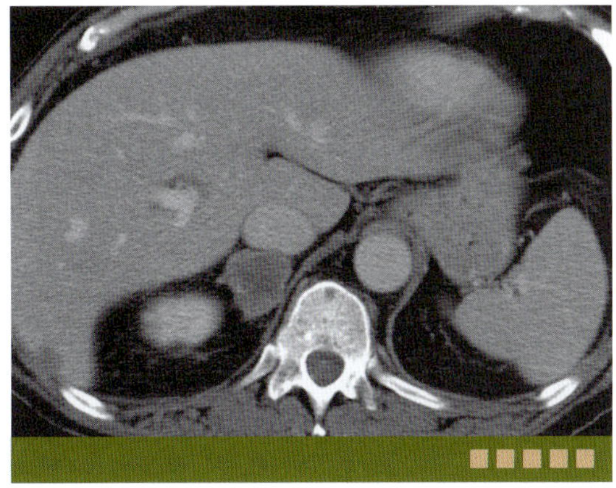

C. Axial CECT performed 2 1/2 years later showed lung mass as a result of cancer and new liver metastases. The right adrenal mass has increased in size to 3 cm and has increased in density. Patient was felt to develop metastatic lesion to an adrenal adenoma, a type of collision tumor. Small liver metastasis is seen.

DIFFERENTIAL DIAGNOSES IMAGES (D-G)

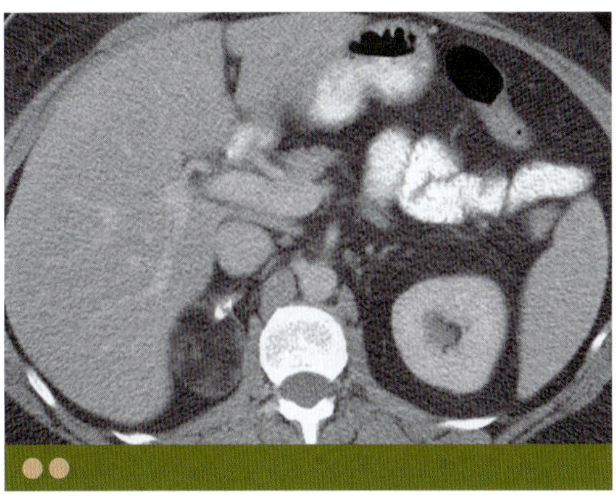

D. Adrenal myelolipoma: Axial CECT shows right adrenal lesion that is heterogeneous and has areas of fat density and areas of increased density and calcifications.

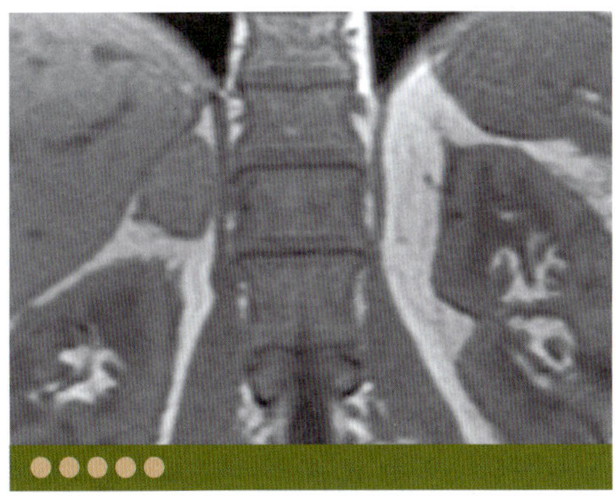

E. Atypical adrenal adenoma: Coronal in-phase image shows that lesion is similar signal intensity to the liver.

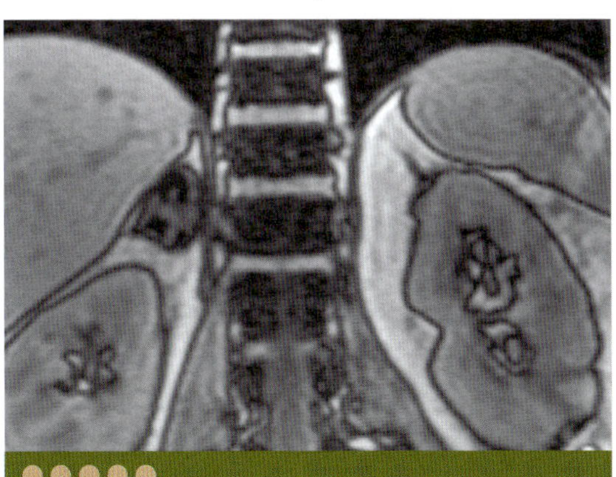

F. Atypical adrenal adenoma: Coronal opposed-phase image shows areas that drop in signal and areas that do not drop in signal with a speckled pattern. The appearance is a result of atypical adenoma.

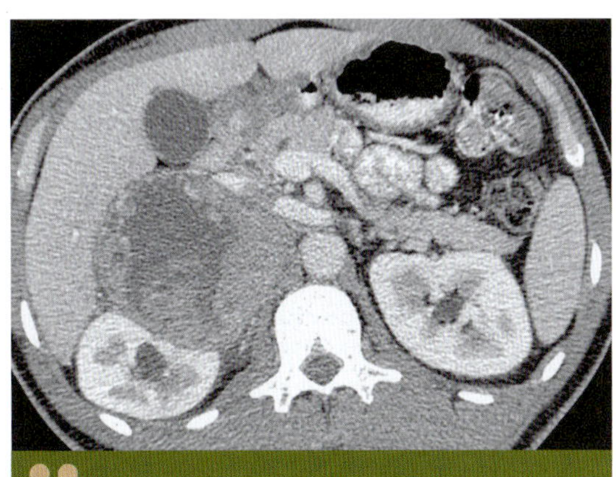

G. Adrenal cell carcinoma: Axial CECT shows large complex mass involving the right adrenal gland from hemorrhage and necrosis that is typical of adrenal cell carcinoma.

Figures B and C are the same patient.
Figures E and F are the same patient.

IMAGE KEY

Common

Rare

Typical

Unusual

14-8 Cystic Pheochromocytoma, Low-Density Mass on CT

Frank H. Miller

PRESENTATION

Headache, palpitations, diaphoresis, and hypertension.

FINDINGS

On the unenhanced CT, the mass had a density of 14 HU. Some may suggest that this lesion is an adenoma on the basis of the density of the lesion on unenhanced CT.

DIFFERENTIAL DIAGNOSES

- *Adrenal cyst*: High SI on T2-WI but does not enhance after contrast; no history of hypertension.
- *Adrenal lymphangioma*: Also high-signal intensity on T2; does not enhance after contrast; no history of hypertension.
- *Adrenal adenoma*: History of hypertension makes it imperative to exclude pheochromocytoma.
- *Adrenal metastasis*: Usually history of malignancy; lesion is not typical appearance for malignancy as it is of low density.

COMMENTS

Pheochromocytomas are functionally active tumors that arise from the chromaffin cells of the adrenal medulla. They secrete epinephrine and norepinephrine. They are also known as the "10% tumor": approximately 10% are bilateral, 10% are extra-adrenal, 10% occur in children, 10% are malignant, and 10% are inherited. The diagnosis is generally made on the basis of clinical findings with elevated urinary metaneprhine or vanillylmandelic acid seen in 90% of the patients. Imaging studies are important to preoperatively localize the tumors and guide surgery. In addition, imaging studies can determine if there is bilateral or multifocal involvement. In addition, these studies can determine malignant behavior, including metastases and local invasion as pathologic distinction of malignancy is difficult.

Pheochromocytomas, typically, are large tumors measuring larger than 3 cm. On unenhanced CT, they generally have densities similar to the liver and show marked enhancement as a result of their hypervascularity. Larger tumors can undergo cystic degeneration secondary to necrosis and hemorrhage. MR is helpful in the diagnosis with the signal intensity similar or lower than liver, kidney, or muscle on T1-weighted images (T1-WI). They may be higher if associated with hemorrhage. Similar to CT, the lesions following contrast show rapid enhancement. Unlike adrenal adenomas, pheochromocytomas typically do not show phase cancellation on out-of-phase sequences in comparison to in-phase sequences. On T2-weighted sequences, pheochromocytomas classically demonstrate longer T2 relaxation times with marked hyperintensity (described as "light bulb" bright). Several studies, and our experience, confirm that a large percentage of lesions are not the characteristic high signal intensity with many showing heterogeneous and moderate hyperintensity.

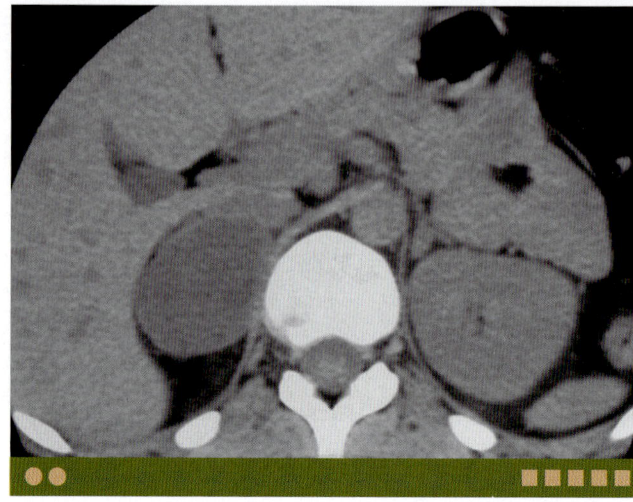

A. Axial NECT shows a low-density, 3-cm right adrenal mass in patients with history of hypertension. This history should prompt consideration of pheochromocytoma and functional adenoma.

PEARLS

- **Low-density adrenal lesions on CT may be seen with pheochromocytomas and not only adrenal adenomas.**
- **Not all low-density lesions of the adrenal gland on CT are from adrenal adenomas.**
- **Pheochromocytoma must also be considered especially in patients with hypertension.**
- **CT and MR often show hypervascular masses.**
- **High-signal intensity on T2-WI is commonly seen and used to be considered characteristic of pheochromocytoma but is often not seen.**
- **Imaging studies are helpful for localization purposes.**

ADDITIONAL IMAGES (B-D)

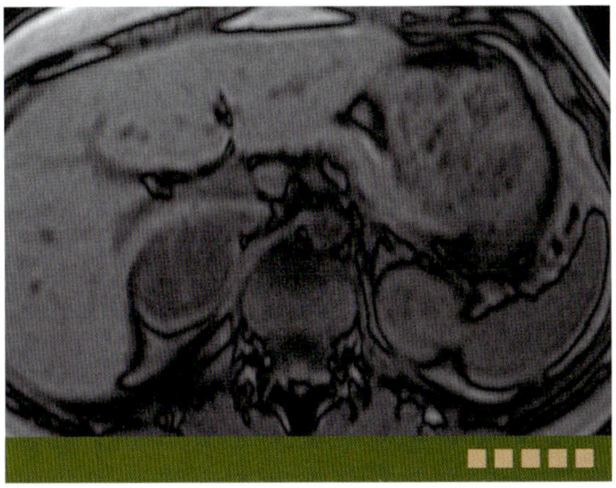

B. Axial opposed-phase MR image shows that the adrenal mass does not drop in signal intensity as would be expected for an adrenal adenoma relative to the in-phase images (not shown).

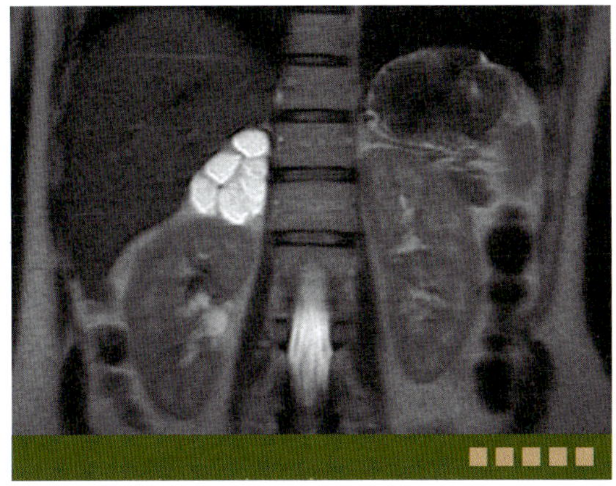

C. On coronal T2-WI, the right adrenal mass is high-signal intensity with septations.

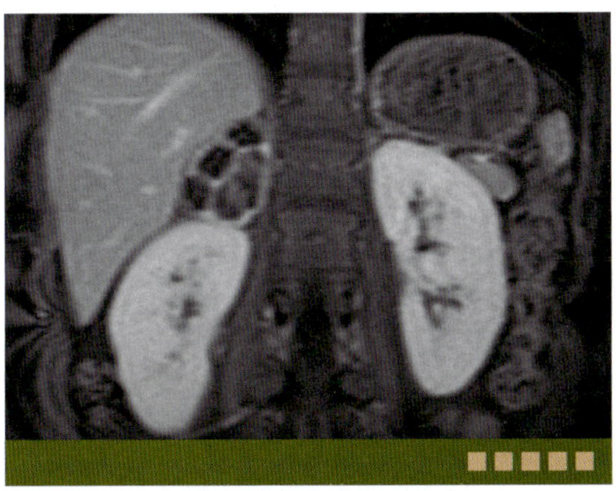

D. Coronal contrast-enhanced T1-WI shows the mass appears cystic with multiple septations.

DIFFERENTIAL DIAGNOSES IMAGES (E-G)

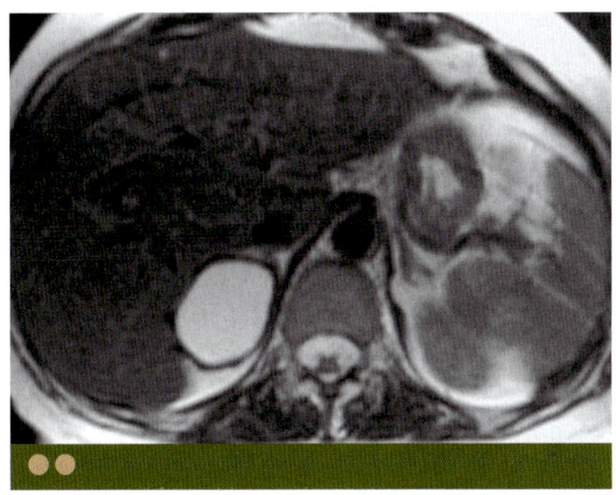

E. Adrenal cyst: Axial T2-WI shows lesion that is high signal.

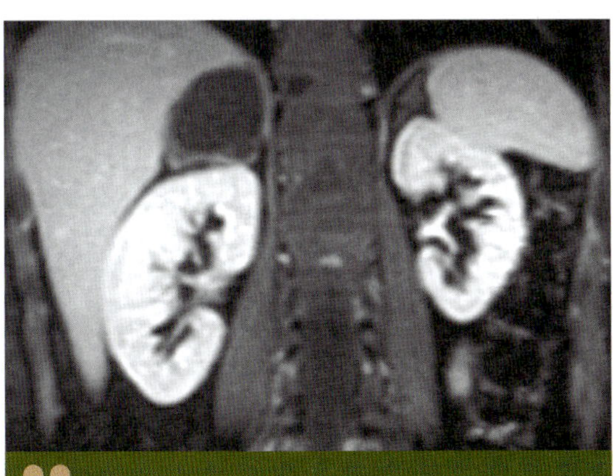

F. Adrenal cyst: Coronal contrast-enhanced T1-WI in the same patient as in Figure E shows nonenhancing fluid-containing right adrenal cyst. The patient had no history of hypertension to suggest pheochromocytoma, and the lesion is not as complex as the cystic pheochromocytoma.

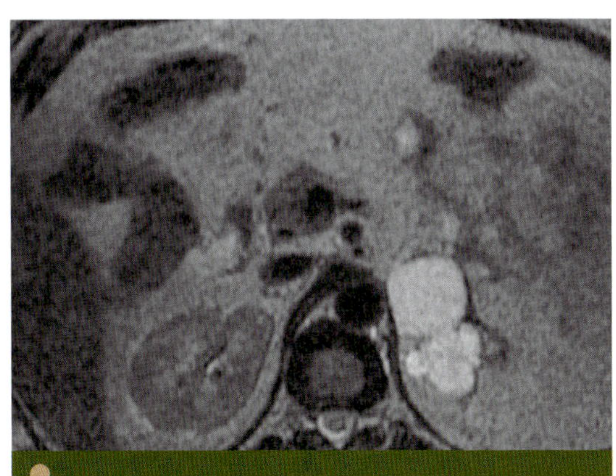

G. Lymphangioma: Axial T2 shows multilobulated fluid-containing lesion. The patient did not have any history of hypertension or trauma.

Figures A to D are the same patient.
Figures E and F are the same patient.

IMAGE KEY

Common

Rare

Typical

Unusual

14–9 Adrenal Pheochromocytoma with Hemorrhage

Frank H. Miller

PRESENTATION

Abdominal pain and hypertension.

FINDINGS

Left adrenal mass with high signal on T1- and T2-WI with low-signal rim on T2-WI from hemorrhage.

DIFFERENTIAL DIAGNOSES

- Adrenal hemorrhage from anticoagulation.
- Adrenal hemorrhage from other benign and malignant lesions.
- Adrenal hemorrhage from trauma.

COMMENTS

Adrenal hemorrhage may be a result of trauma, anticoagulation, sepsis, or stress as a result of surgery. Trauma accounts for 80% of the cases of adrenal hemorrhage. Adrenal hemorrhage on CT is seen as a lesion of increased density. On MR, hemorrhage is often seen as high-signal intensity on T1-WI from methemoglobin and has a dark rim on T2-WI because of hemosiderin. The MR appearance of hemorrhage may vary depending on the age of the hemorrhage.

The presence of adrenal hemorrhage warrants determination of the cause. In the absence of trauma and anticoagulation or sepsis, an underlying mass needs to be excluded. Even patients undergoing anticoagulation may have an underlying adrenal mass that bled. In this patient, there was a history of hypertension. The patient had laboratory evidence of pheochromocytoma. The diagnosis was confirmed at surgical resection. This case emphasizes the importance of determining the etiology of hemorrhagic masses of the adrenal gland and to consider pheochromocytoma.

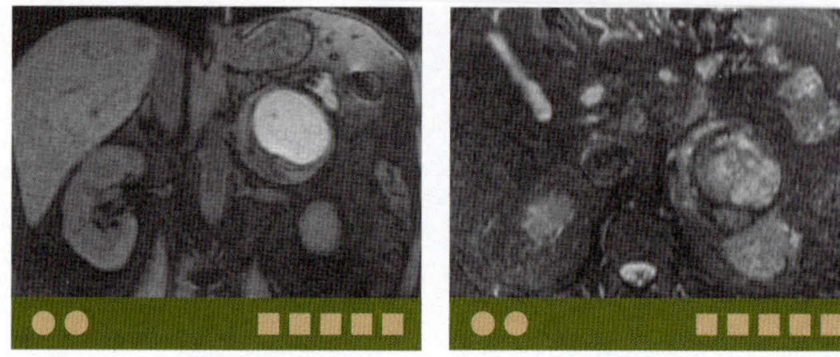

A. Coronal T1-WI shows 7-cm adrenal lesion that is of high-signal intensity.
B. Axial T2-WI shows mass is of high-signal intensity with low-signal intensity rim from the hemosiderin rim.

The classic dogma for pheochromocytomas used to be that pheochromocytomas are light bulb bright on T2-WI on MR from intracellular water; however, many pheochromocytomas are not bright on T2-WI. As illustrated, the MR appearance of pheochromocytoma is often nonspecific. Suggestive features of pheochromocytoma include a very hyperintense signal on T2-WI and hypervascular enhancement following gadolinium. The diagnosis, however, should be based on clinical and laboratory findings. MR is mainly performed for localization purposes.

PEARLS

- **Adrenal hemorrhage may be a result of trauma, anticoagulation, sepsis, or stress as a result of surgery.**
- **The etiology of adrenal hemorrhage needs to be determined.**
- **Pheochromocytomas are nonspecific in appearance and often not of high-signal intensity ("light bulb bright") on T2-WI.**

ADDITIONAL IMAGE

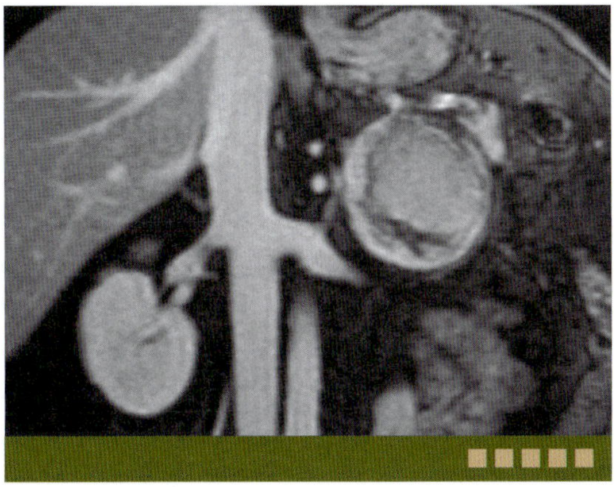

C. Coronal contrast-enhanced T1-WI shows enhancement of the periphery of the mass and lack of central enhancement. The patient had a history of hypertension and was shown to have a pheochromocytoma.

DIFFERENTIAL DIAGNOSES IMAGES (D-G)

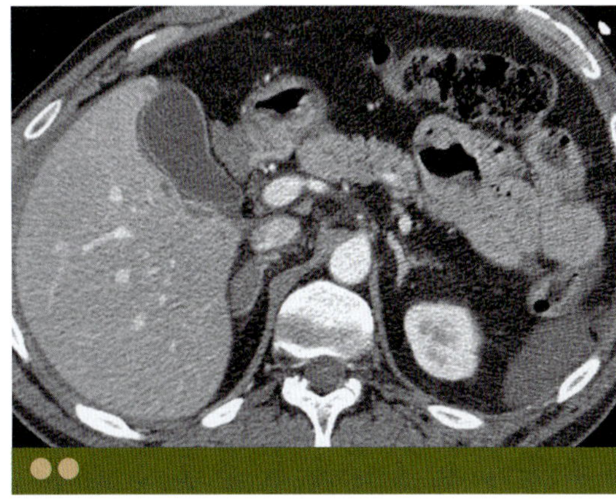

D. Adrenal hemorrhage from trauma: Axial CECT shows nonspecific right adrenal mass.

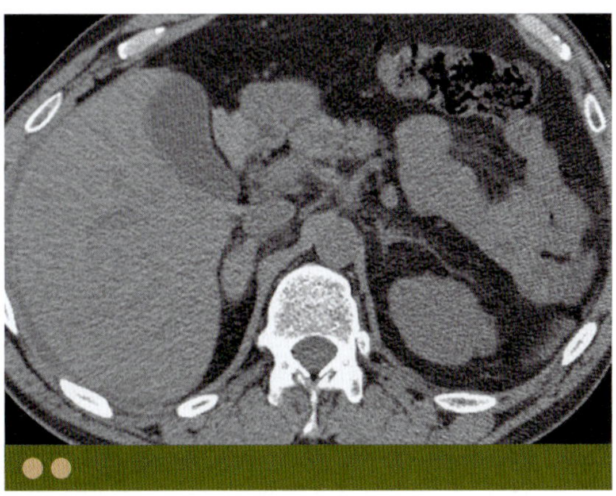

E. Adrenal hemorrhage from trauma: Axial NECT in the same patient as Figure D shows that the mass is of high density from hemorrhage.

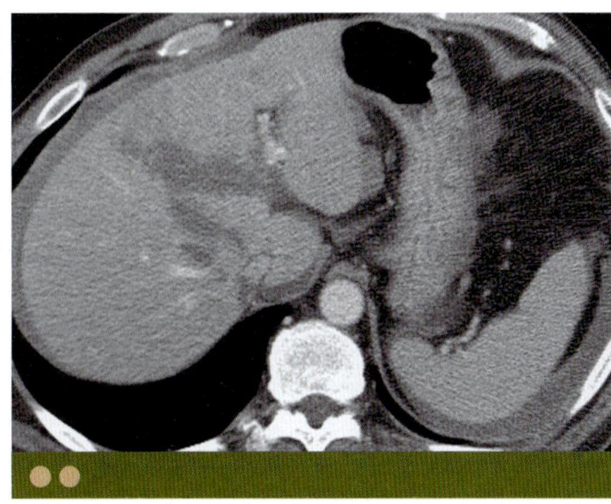

F. Adrenal hemorrhage from trauma: Axial CECT shows liver laceration with blood surrounding the liver and spleen. The patient had motor vehicle accident accounting for liver laceration and adrenal hemorrhage.

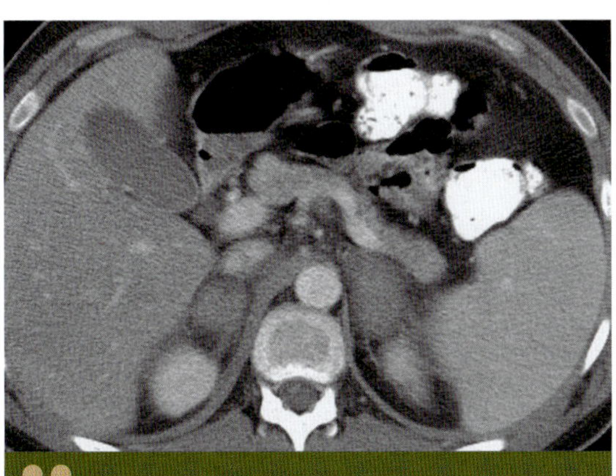

G. Bilateral adrenal hemorrhage: Axial CECT shows bilateral adrenal hemorrhage from anticoagulation.

Figures A to C are the same patient.
Figures D to F are the same patient.

IMAGE KEY

Common

Rare

Typical

Unusual

14–10 Paraganglioma of Organ of Zuckerkandl

Frank H. Miller

PRESENTATION

Hypertension, headache, sweating, and palpitations.

FINDINGS

Left para-aortic enhancing mass.

DIFFERENTIAL DIAGNOSES

- *Lymphoma*: Generally associated with multiple lymph nodes; may be distinguished on the basis of history.
- *Metastatic disease*: Generally known malignancy; additional metastases; different history and clinical findings.
- *Retroperitoneal sarcoma*: May look similar but often can be distinguished on the basis of clinical history; often larger heterogeneous masses.

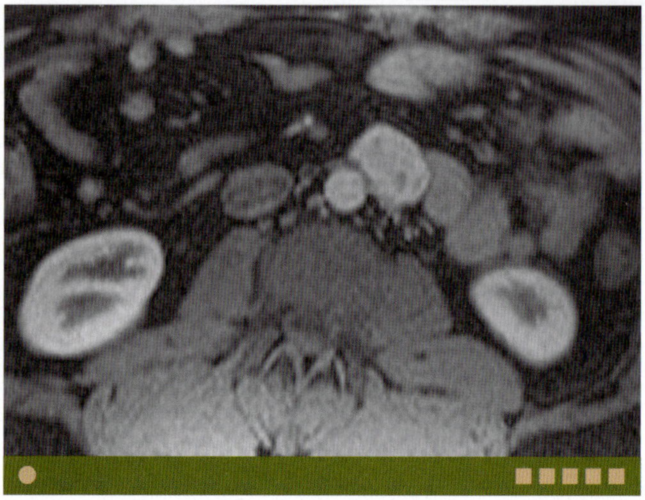

A. Axial contrast-enhanced T1-WI shows enhancing para-aortic mass along the organ of Zuckerkandl proven to be paraganglioma.

COMMENTS

Pheochromocytomas occur most commonly in adults and are associated with catecholamine release, including headache, sweating, hypertension, and palpitations. In patients with elevated catecholamines and normal adrenal glands, the sympathetic chain should be evaluated for extra-adrenal pheochromocytomas seen in approximately 10% of the cases. These lesions are referred to as paragangliomas as illustrated by this MR image of a paraganglioma at the organ of Zuckerkandl, near the bifurcation of the aorta. Other sites of extra-adrenal involvement include the sympathetic chain, including para-aortic region, skull base, and neck and near the bladder. The organ of Zuckerkandl is para-aortic extending from a level of the superior mesenteric artery or renal arteries to below the level of the aortic bifurcation with the highest concentration generally near the origin of the inferior mesenteric artery. The extra-adrenal paragangliomas are more likely multifocal compared to adrenal pheochromocytomas.

Pheochromocytomas are said to follow the "rule of ten": 10% are extra-adrenal, 10% are malignant, 10% are silent, 10% are bilateral, 10% are familial, and 10% occur in children. On CT, there are no specific features, but they often are hypervascular. On MR, they classically are relatively hyperintense on T2-WI and have intense enhancement. Many pheochromocytomas, however, are not specific. Metaiodobenzylguanidine (MIBG) scans or Octreoscan can be used to identify multiple lesions, metastases, and lesions not seen on CT and MR. Before biopsy of an indeterminate adrenal or retroperitoneal mass, correlation with biochemical markers should be performed to exclude pheochromocytoma or paraganglioma. If present, catecholamine blockade is recommended prior to biopsy or surgical resection.

The treatment is surgical excision. Approximately 10% to 40% of extra-adrenal paragangliomas are malignant. The diagnosis of malignancy can reliably be made only by the detection of metastatic involvement at imaging or recurrence following surgical resection.

PEARLS

- **Extra-adrenal pheochromocytomas are referred to as paragangliomas.**
- **Extra-adrenal pheochromocytomas are seen in 10% of pheochromocytomas.**
- **Paragangliomas of the organs of Zuckerkandl occur in a para-aortic location.**
- **Paragangliomas are more often malignant than intra-adrenal pheochromocytomas.**

ADDITIONAL IMAGES (B-F)

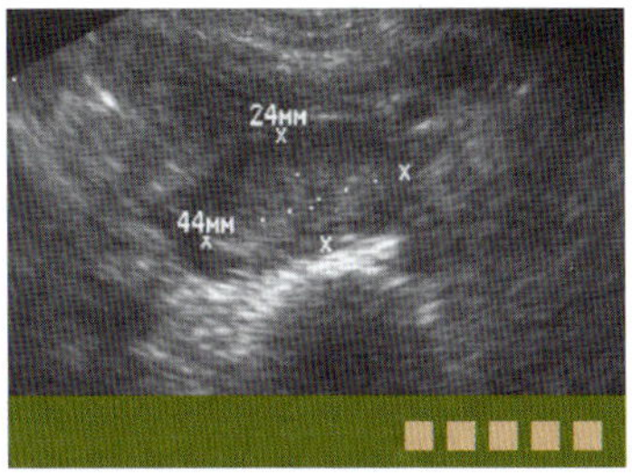

B. Transverse sonogram shows 4.4-cm mass anterior to the spine in a different patient.

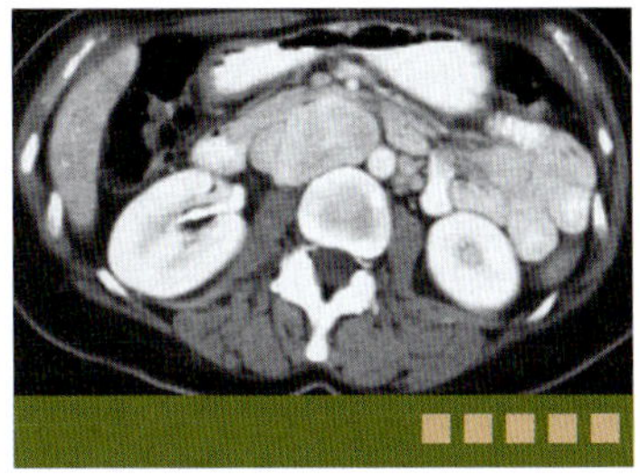

C. Axial CECT in the same patient as Figure B. shows enhancing aorta-caval mass proven to be paraganglioma.

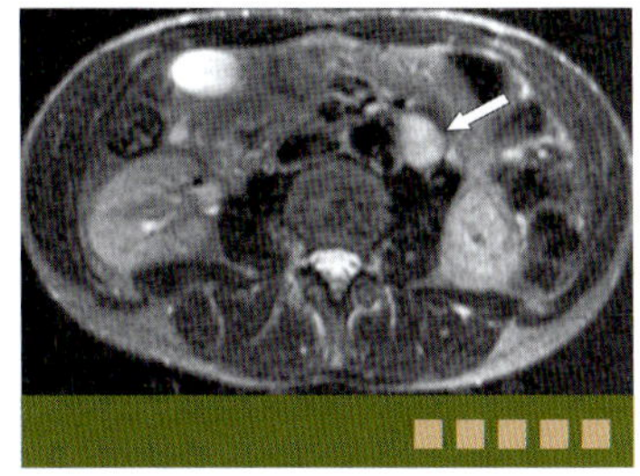

D. T2-WI in a different patient shows high-signal intensity left para-aortic mass (arrow) caused by paraganglioma of the organ of Zuckerkandl.

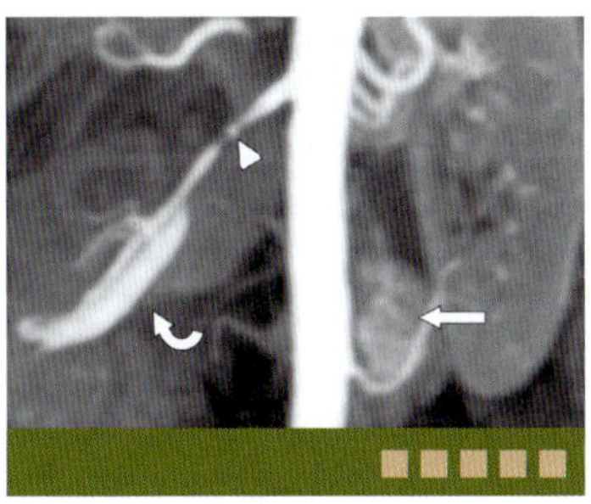

E. MRA shows left para-aortic hypervascular lesion (arrow). Right renal artery stenosis is seen (arrowhead) with renal arteriovenous fistula (curved arrow).

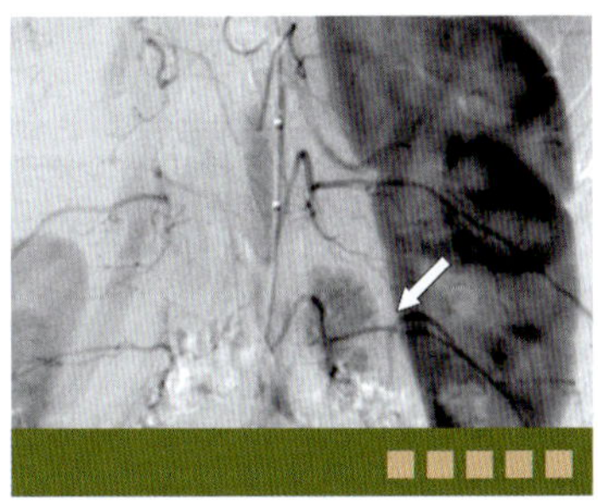

F. Angiogram shows the mass is hypervascular (arrow).

IMAGE KEY

Common

Rare

Typical

Unusual

DIFFERENTIAL DIAGNOSES IMAGES (G-H)

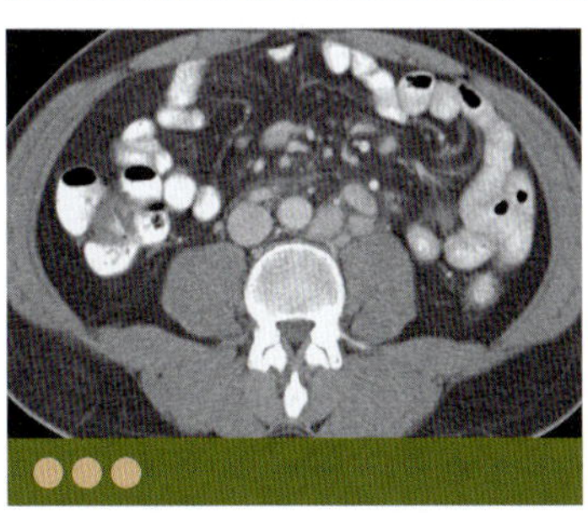

G. Lymphoma: Axial CECT shows multiple retroperitoneal lymph nodes in a para-aortic location in patient with a history of lymphoma. The patient did not have symptoms of hypertension.

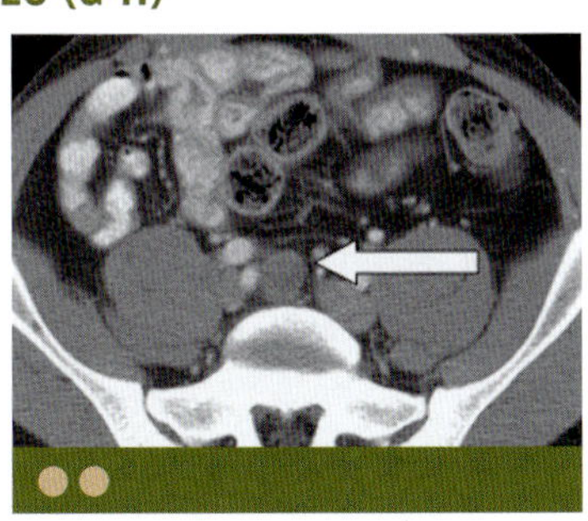

H. Testicular cancer metastasis: Axial CECT shows lymph node below the level of the aortic bifurcation in patient with seminoma.

Figures D, E, and F are of the same patient.

14–11 Adrenal Myelolipoma

Frank H. Miller

PRESENTATION

Incidental adrenal mass.

FINDINGS

CECT shows right adrenal mass predominately containing fat.

DIFFERENTIAL DIAGNOSES

- *Adenoma*: Does not show macroscopic fat.
- *Metastasis*: Does not show macroscopic fat.
- *Retroperitoneal liposarcoma*: Would not arise from adrenal gland.
- *Adrenal cortical carcinoma*: Does not show mass completely composed of macroscopic fat.
- *Exophytic renal angiomyolipoma*: Would arise from kidney.

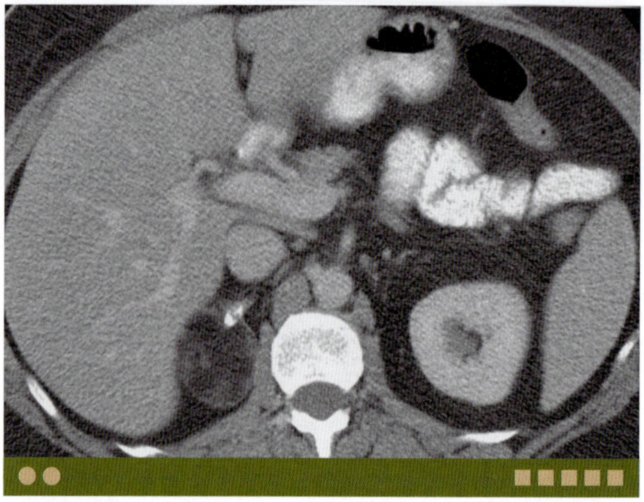

A. Axial CECT shows right adrenal mass that is predominately fat-containing and has associated calcification.

COMMENTS

Adrenal myelolipomas are uncommon benign neoplasms, which have mature fat and hematopoietic tissue in varying proportions. They are generally asymptomatic and detected incidentally on imaging studies and are hormonally inactive. They can rarely be associated with symptoms such as back or flank pain when large or associated with hemorrhage.

Detection of macroscopic fat within an adrenal mass on imaging establishes the diagnosis. On ultrasound, they may be of increased echogenicity from adipose tissue. The diagnosis is easily made, using CT scans and detecting negative HU caused by fat. The presence of fat is easily made visually when compared to subcutaneous or intra-abdominal fat. The diagnosis with MR is best made using frequency selective fat-suppressed sequences as seen in this example where the fat loses signal on fat-suppressed sequences. The use of in-phase and opposed-phase images may not be effective as there may not be fat and water in the same voxel. In addition, adrenal adenomas are more commonly the cause of lesions that drop in signal on opposed-phase imaging. Enhancement of the lesion may be seen as a result of the vascular nature of the hematopoietic component of the lesions. The diagnosis should be suspected in adrenal lesions with macroscopic fat. Because of the enhancement of the lesions, the diagnosis may be not made correctly on MR and the areas of fat may be less conspicuous to the radiologist. The lesions may also show calcifications. Myelolipomas generally do not require surgery unless patients are symptomatic. The lesions may grow slowly which is not an indication for surgery.

PEARLS

- **Adrenal lesions with macroscopic fat is highly suggestive of adrenal myelolipoma.**
- **Adrenal myelolipomas can be diagnosed on the basis of macroscopic fat.**
- **Adrenal myelolipoma are benign lesions that do not require further workup.**
- **Compare frequency selective fat-suppressed images with nonfat-suppressed images on MRI for fat.**
- **Macroscopic fat may not drop in signal on opposed-phase imaging.**

ADDITIONAL IMAGES (B-E)

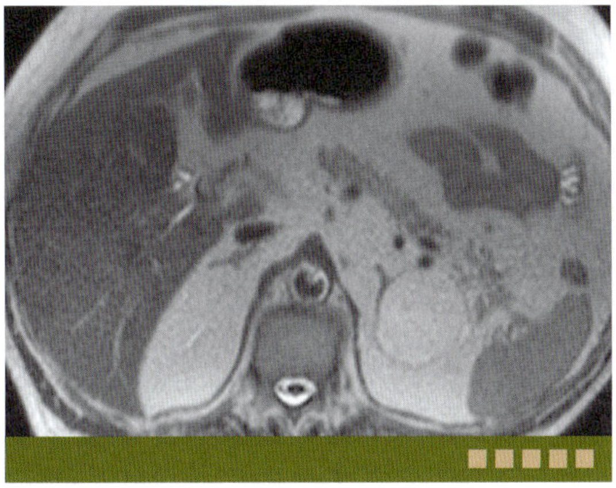

B. Axial T2-WI shows left adrenal lesion with high-signal intensity.

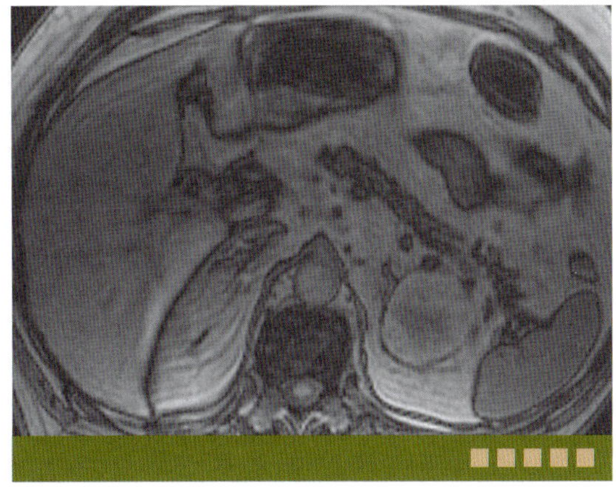

C. Axial opposed-phase T1-WI shows that the lesion does not drop in signal on the opposed-phase images as it contains macroscopic fat.

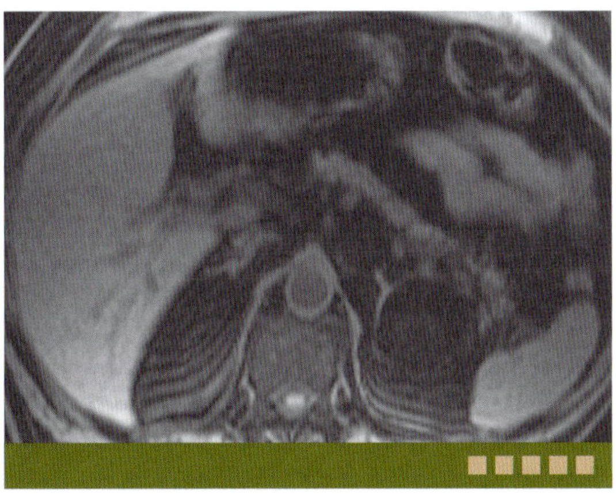

D. Axial frequency selective fat-suppressed T1-WI shows a drop in signal intensity because of the fat being suppressed in the myelolipoma.

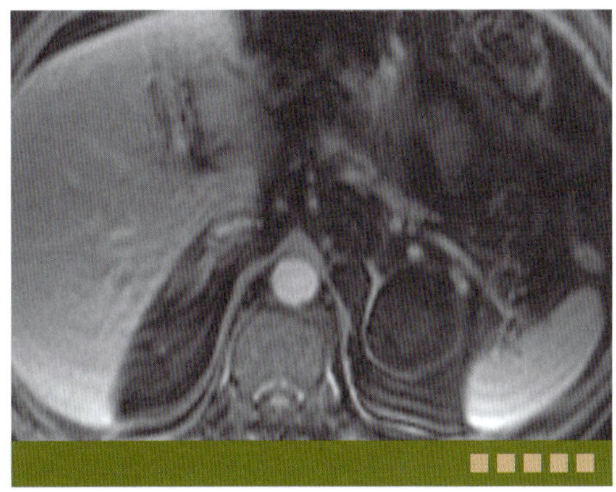

E. Axial contrast-enhanced T1-WI shows no enhancement of the adrenal myelolipoma.

DIFFERENTIAL DIAGNOSES IMAGES (F-G)

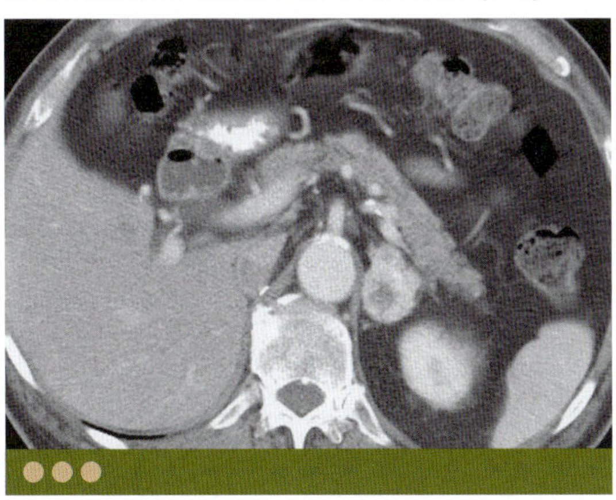

F. Adrenal metastasis: Axial CECT shows enhancing adrenal lesion proven to be metastasis from lung cancer. Note that the lesion does not contain fat.

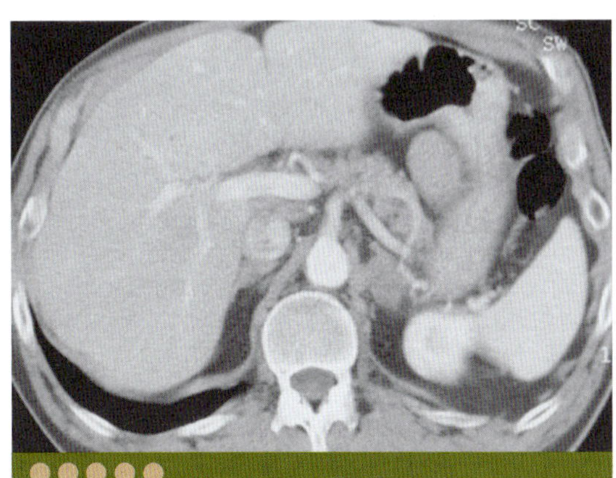

G. Bilateral adrenal adenomas: Axial CECT shows bilateral enhancing adrenal lesions that had microscopic fat on MR. The lesions do not contain macroscopic fat on CT to suggest myelolipoma.

IMAGE KEY

Common

Rare

Typical

Unusual

14–12 Adrenal Cortical Carcinoma

Frank H. Miller

PRESENTATION

Asymptomatic with large mass on imaging; most frequent clinical presentation is rapidly progressive Cushing syndrome with or without virilization.

FINDINGS

Nonspecific 4-cm, left adrenal mass and liver mass.

DIFFERENTIAL DIAGNOSES

- *Metastasis*: Can have similar appearance. Differentiate based on history or extra-adrenal malignancy but may require biopsy if not known malignancy.
- *Pheochromocytoma*: Associated with history of hypertension; classically vascular and hyperintense on T2 but can look like adrenal cortical carcinoma; distinguished on the basis of laboratory and clinical findings
- *Atypical (lipid-poor) adenoma*: Indistinguishable in this patient based on imaging appearance but tends to be small and not infiltrative or invade vessels and not associated with liver mass

COMMENTS

Adrenal cortical carcinomas are extremely rare with an incidence of 1 to 2 per million people. They are extremely aggressive with generally a poor prognosis. They usually grow rapidly and are large at diagnosis with the majority being larger than 6 cm. Approximately 10% are bilateral. Patients with adrenal cortical carcinoma usually present with pain and a palpable mass and more than 50% present with endocrinopathy including virilization or Cushing syndrome. Patients often present in the fourth or fifth decade of life.

On CT, the lesions have an attenuation value of greater than 10 HU on unenhanced CT. The lesions are generally heterogeneous and infiltrative with irregular margins. Necrosis and calcifications are common. Local invasion or tumor extension involving the inferior vena cava (IVC), heart, and metastases to the lung and liver may be seen. Vascular extension is suggestive of the diagnosis. There may be associated lymphadenopathy.

On MR, adrenal cortical carcinoma is often intermediate SI on T1-WI and shows mixed intermediate and high-signal intensity on T2-WI. These lesions are often large, with central necrosis. Some lesions may have small foci of lipid and lose signal on opposed-phase images, but generally, lipid would be only a small focus of the mass. Generally adrenal cortical carcinoma are larger lesions (>5 cm) than adenomas and more infiltrative and heterogeneous. Contrast-enhancement with gadolinium is helpful to detect adjacent structure invasion and vascular invasion.

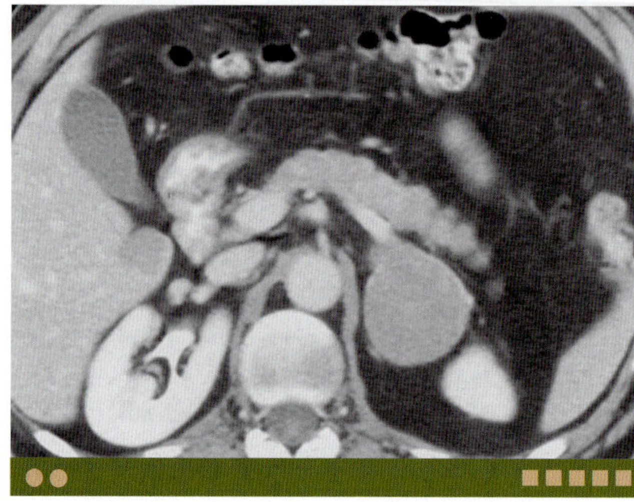

A. Axial CECT shows nonspecific left adrenal mass and hepatic mass.

Adrenal cortical carcinomas, similar to renal cell carcinoma or hepatocellular carcinoma, tend to invade veins including extending into the renal vein, IVC, or the right atrium. When staging these tumors, it is important to examine the chest with CT and liver with CT or MR to evaluate for metastases.

PEARLS

- **Adrenal cell carcinomas are rare but have a poor prognosis.**
- **Adrenal carcinomas tend to grow rapidly and present as large heterogeneous adrenal masses often with necrosis, hemorrhage, and calcifications.**
- **Lesions that do not lose signal on opposed-phase images are not lipid-rich adenomas.**
- **Lesions that do not lose signal on opposed-phase images may represent lipid-poor adenomas, pheochromocytoma, metastatic lesions, or adrenal cortical carcinoma.**
- **Adrenal masses that invade vessels should suggest adrenal cell carcinoma.**

ADDITIONAL IMAGES (B-F)

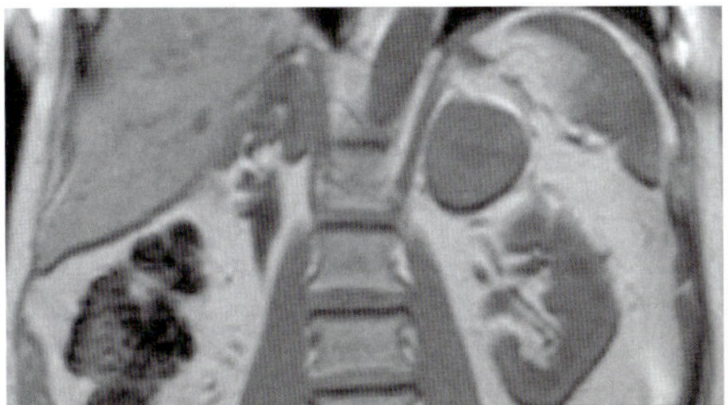

B. Coronal in-phase T1-WI shows left adrenal mass is similar in signal intensity to the spleen and liver.

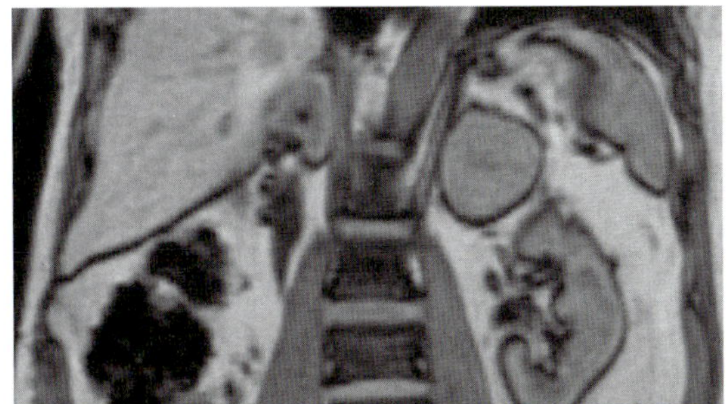

C. Coronal opposed-phase T1-WI shows left adrenal mass does not drop in signal. Unlike lipid-rich adenoma, this lesion does not drop in signal intensity. With the presence of a liver lesion, it is suspicious for adrenal cell carcinoma or metastasis to the adrenal. Biopsy confirmed adrenal cell carcinoma with liver metastasis.

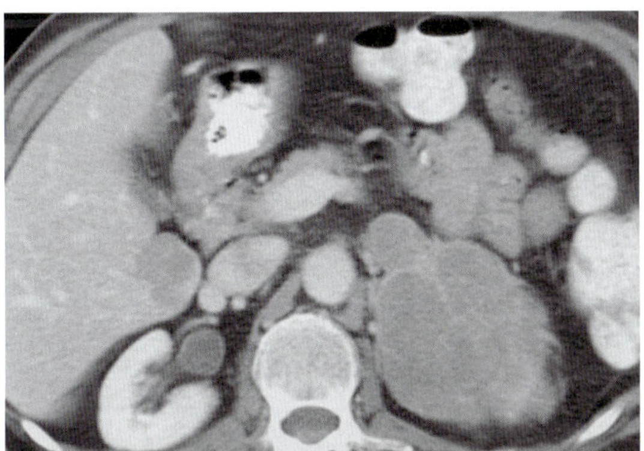

D. Follow-up axial CECT scan shows growth and the more typical appearance of adrenal cell carcinoma as a large heterogeneous infiltrative mass. This case is unusual as most adrenal cell carcinomas are larger than 6 cm and appear more infiltrative.

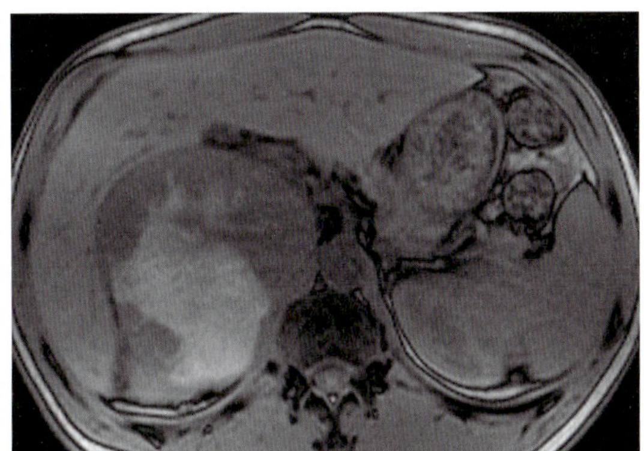

E. Adrenal cell carcinoma with hemorrhage. Axial T1-WI shows right adrenal mass with areas of increased signal intensity from hemorrhage.

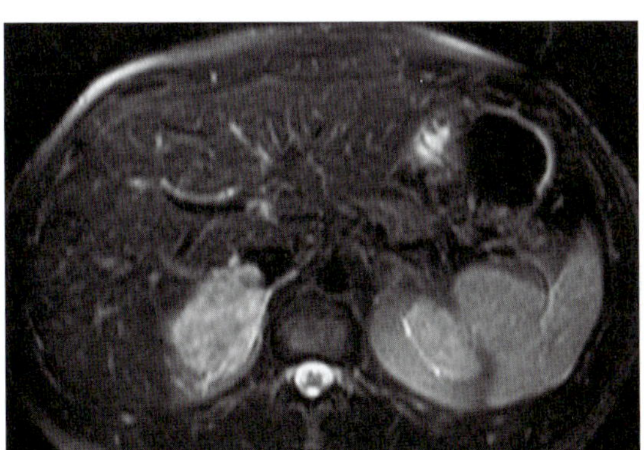

F. Adrenal cell carcinoma with invasion of IVC. Axial T2-WI shows increased signal adrenal lesion with invasion of the IVC. Adrenal cell carcinoma is one of few adrenal tumors to invade the IVC.

DIFFERENTIAL DIAGNOSES IMAGE

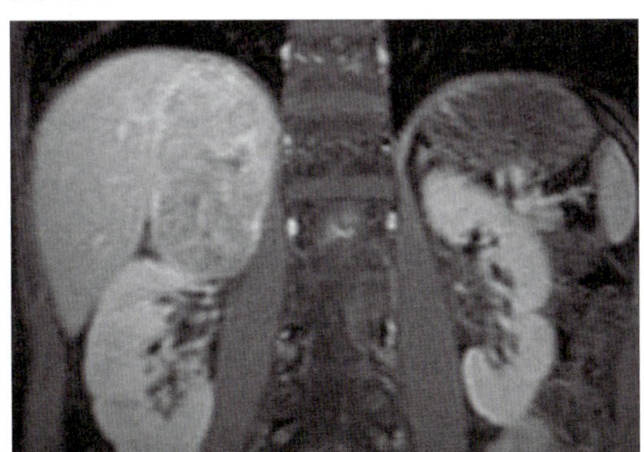

G. Pheochromocytoma: Coronal contrast-enhanced T1-WI shows solid enhancing right adrenal lesion. The imaging appearance of pheochromocytoma mimics other adrenal lesions. The distinction requires a clinical history of hypertension and biochemical evidence of pheochromocytoma.

IMAGE KEY

Common

Rare

Typical

Unusual

14–13 Adrenal Lymphoma

Frank H. Miller

PRESENTATION

History of non-Hodgkin lymphoma.

FINDINGS

Homogeneous bilateral adrenal masses.

DIFFERENTIAL DIAGNOSES

- *Adrenal hemorrhage*: Generally higher density attributed to hemorrhage; history of anticoagulation or bleeding diathesis helps differentiate.
- *Adrenal metastases:* Can look similar; differentiated on the basis of history.
- *Adrenal adenoma*: Generally low density from microscopic fat on unenhanced CT but can look similar following contrast.

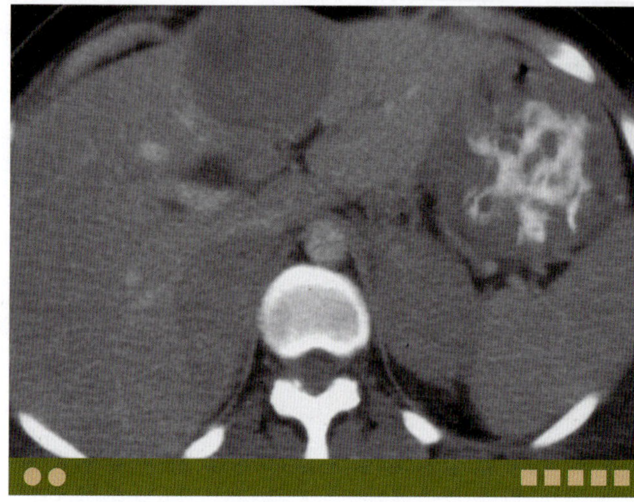

A. Axial CECT shows large bilateral homogeneously enhancing masses similar to muscle density with a solid liver mass in young patients with AIDS. Biopsy showed lymphoma.

COMMENTS

Adrenal lymphoma generally is attributed to secondary involvement of systemic lymphoma and not because of primary adrenal lymphoma. Most commonly, the adrenal gland is involved by non-Hodgkin lymphoma instead of Hodgkin disease. Adrenal lymphoma has been reported at autopsy in 25% of the patients with lymphoma but only 4% are prospectively seen on imaging studies. Primary adrenal lymphoma is very rare and has a poor outcome.

Adrenal lymphoma on CT or MR is seen most often as large, often homogenous adrenal masses with generally mild enhancement after contrast material. Bilateral involvement is seen in one-third to half of the patients. There is often associated lymphadenopathy, but this is not always seen. The shape of the adrenal gland can be preserved with diffuse enlargement or may present with solid adrenal masses or nodularity. On CT, the masses generally show hypoenhancement following contrast material. When small, they are often homogenous, but when larger, may be heterogeneous. Using MR, adrenal lymphoma is seen as low signal on T1-WI and heterogeneous high-signal intensity on T2-WI but is generally nonspecific. Unlike adenomas, signal drop-off is not seen on the opposed-phase images. When involving both adrenal glands, adrenal insufficiency may develop. Calcifications in adrenal lymphoma are rare unless treated similar to other sites of lymphoma. Changes more suggestive of lymphoma compared to other adrenal malignancies include very rapid change in size over short interval or response to medical therapy.

PEARLS

- **Adrenal lymphoma is most commonly seen in patients with history of non-Hodgkin lymphoma.**
- **The appearance on CT and MR may be nonspecific.**
- **Unlike adrenal adenomas, lesions from adrenal lymphoma are not very low density on unenhanced CT and do not drop in signal on opposed-phase images as they do not contain fat.**
- **Changes suggestive of lymphoma include very rapid change in size over short interval or response to medical therapy.**

ADDITIONAL IMAGES (B-C)

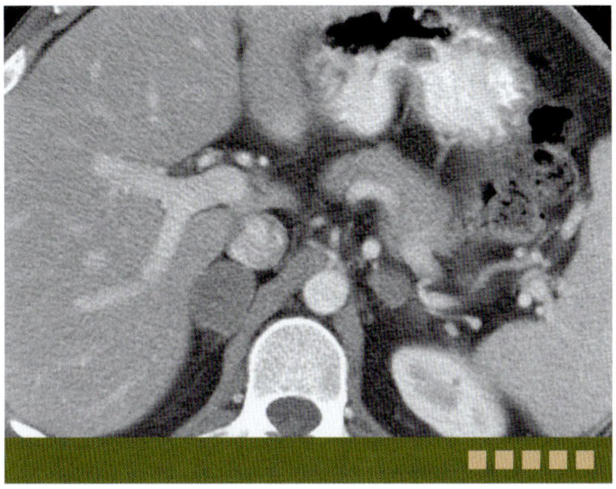

B. Axial CECT scan in a different patient shows bilateral adrenal masses which are homogenously hypoenhancing a patient with non-Hodgkin lymphoma.

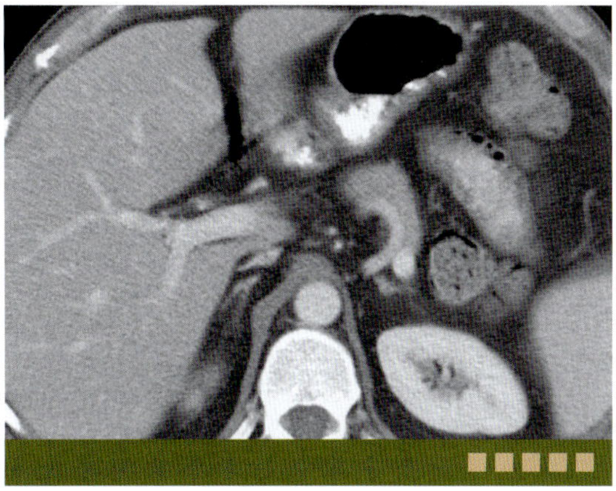

C. Follow-up axial CECT scan obtained 6 weeks later after starting chemotherapy shows resolution of the adrenal masses.

DIFFERENTIAL DIAGNOSES IMAGES (D-F)

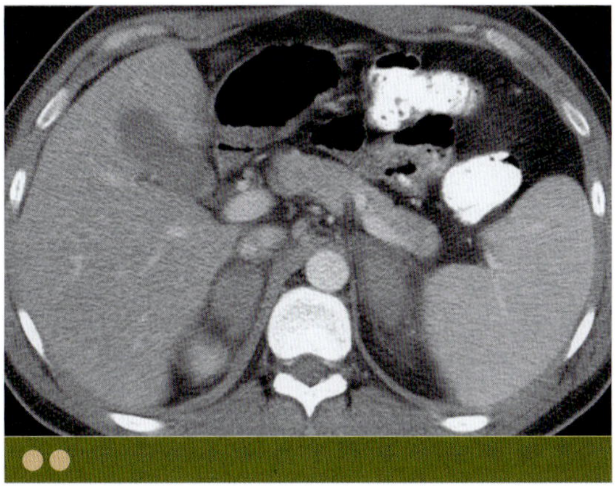

D. Adrenal hemorrhage: Axial CECT shows bilateral adrenal masses from hemorrhage into the adrenal glands. There is some adjacent inflammatory stranding. The history of anticoagulation in this patient helps differentiate from lymphoma or metastases.

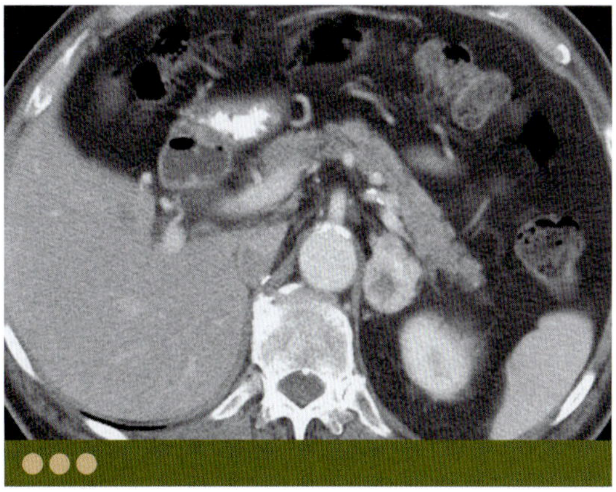

E. Adrenal metastasis: Axial CECT shows nonspecific enhancing lesion of the left adrenal gland from metastasis from lung cancer. The history of malignancy helps differentiate from lymphoma.

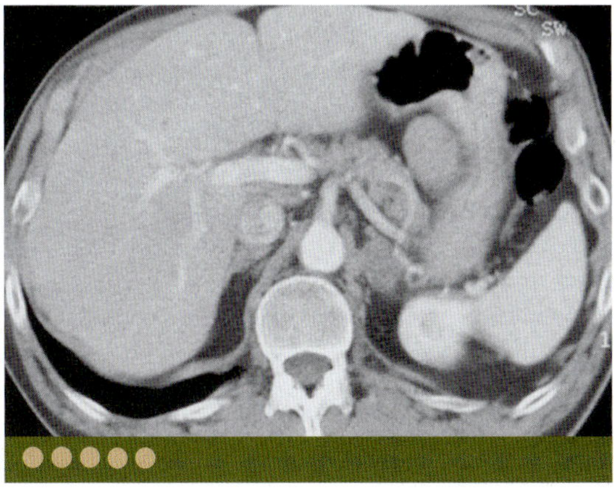

F. Adrenal adenomas: Axial CECT shows nonspecific enhancing adrenal masses from adenomas. Unenhanced CT or chemical shift MR is helpful to show the presence of fat from lipid-rich adenomas.

Figures B and C are of the same patient.

IMAGE KEY

Common

Rare

Typical

Unusual

14–14 Adrenal Neuroblastoma

Frank H. Miller

PRESENTATION

Often asymptomatic until invades or displaces adjacent organs or metastasizes; may present with pain or palpable mass; may cause paraneoplastic syndrome.

FINDINGS

Heterogeneous adrenal mass.

DIFFERENTIAL DIAGNOSES

- *Adrenal ganglioneuroma*: Tends to be more homogeneous.
- *Adrenal cell carcinoma*: Can look the same; often contains hemorrhage and necrosis; may invade vessels.
- *Pheochromocytoma*: Can look similar on imaging studies; history of hypertension and laboratory findings may help; distinction may require pathology.
- *Adrenal metastases*: Can appear heterogeneous similar to neuroblastomas; generally older age group and known malignancy.
- *Adrenal adenoma*: Presence of lipid; if present, helps distinguish; tends to be homogeneous.

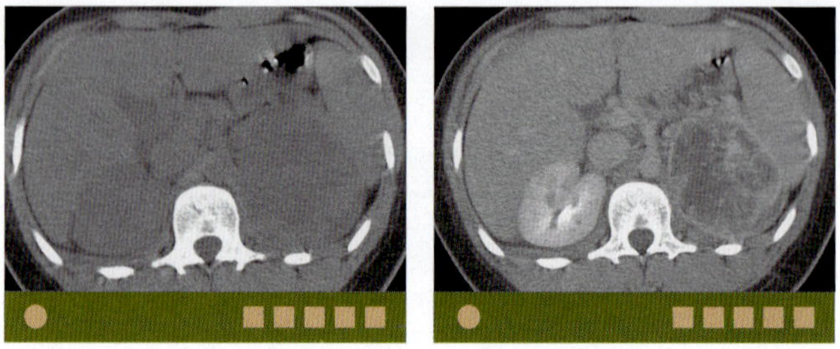

A. Axial NECT shows heterogeneous left adrenal mass in 18-year-old male.
B. Axial CECT shows heterogeneous enhancement of the mass.

COMMENTS

Adrenal ganglioneuromas, neuroblastoma, and ganglioneuroblastoma arise from the neural crest cells from the adrenal medulla and have a spectrum of malignant potential. Adrenal neuroblastomas are the most undifferentiated and aggressive. Ganglioneuromas are benign and ganglioneuroblastomas are intermediate in malignant potential. Two-thirds of neuroblastomas arise in the abdomen with two-thirds of these arising from the adrenal glands.

Adrenal neuroblastomas are the second most common pediatric abdominal mass after Wilms tumor. They may involve the neural crest of the medulla of the adrenal gland or extend along the sympathetic chain. They are rare in adults. Ganglioneuromas are more common in adolescents and young adults.

On imaging studies, neuroblastomas tend to be heterogeneous as a result of areas of necrosis or hemorrhage, whereas ganglioneuromas tend to be more homogeneous. On CT scans, they contain calcifications in about 85% of patients that tend to be coarse and amorphous. In contrast, the calcifications of ganglioneuromas tend to be discrete and punctuate. These calcifications are not easily diagnosed on MR. Neuroblastomas often displace the kidneys inferiorly. On MR, neuroblastomas often are heterogeneous signal intensity and seen as hypointense on T1-WI and hyperintense on T2-WI as a result of necrosis. Areas of hemorrhage are often seen as high-signal intensity on T1-WI as a result of methemoglobin. Imaging studies are also helpful to show tumor involvement of the liver, retroperitoneal lymph nodes, and bone. The appearance of neuroblastomas is nonspecific and biopsy or surgical resection is required for the diagnosis.

PEARLS

- **Adrenal ganglioneuromas, neuroblastoma, and ganglioneuroblastoma arise from the neural crest cells from the adrenal medulla.**
- **Neuroblastomas are the most undifferentiated and aggressive.**
- **Neuroblastomas are more common in children and rare in adults.**
- **Neuroblastomas tend to be heterogeneous from necrosis or hemorrhage.**
- **Biopsy or surgical resection is required for the diagnosis.**

ADDITIONAL IMAGES (C-D)

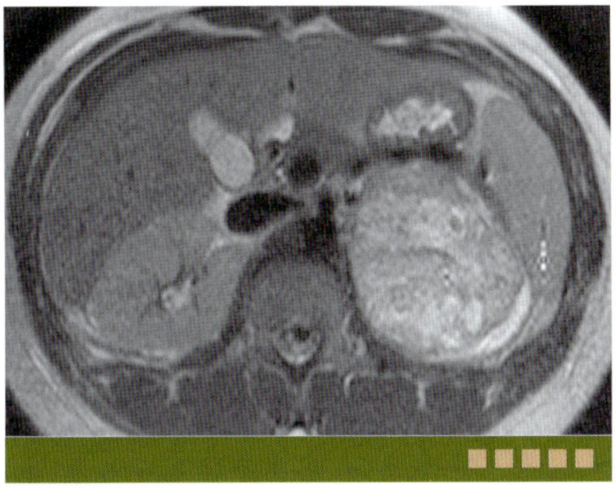

C. Axial T2-WI shows lesion is increased signal intensity with focal areas of high signal from necrosis. There is perilesional fluid.

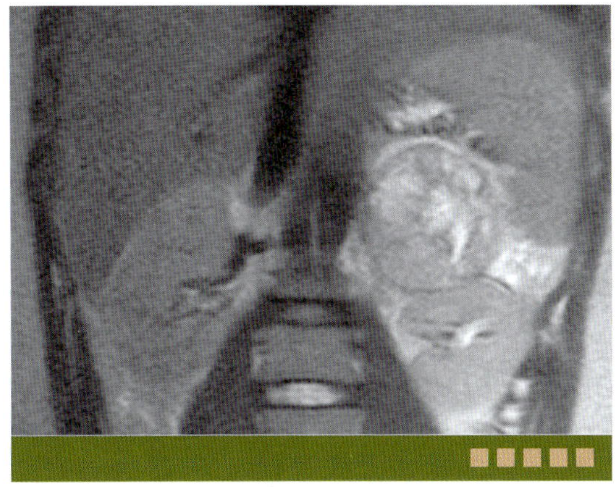

D. Coronal T2-WI shows left adrenal lesion is heterogeneous and displaces the left kidney inferiorly. The patient prior to surgery was suspected to have a pheochromocytoma as had elevated metanephrines and normatenephrines. Surgical histology showed neuroblastoma, which can produce catecholamines.

DIFFERENTIAL DIAGNOSES IMAGES (E-H)

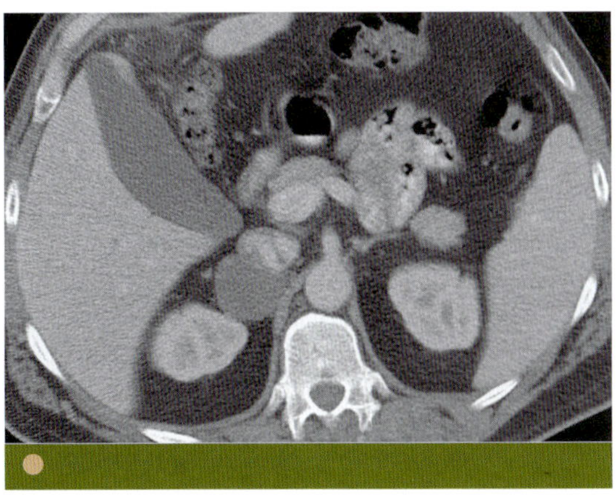

E. Adrenal ganglioneuroma: Axial CECT shows a right adrenal lesion from ganglioneuroma. Adrenal ganglioneuromas tend to be more homogeneous (as seen in this example) than neuroblastomas.

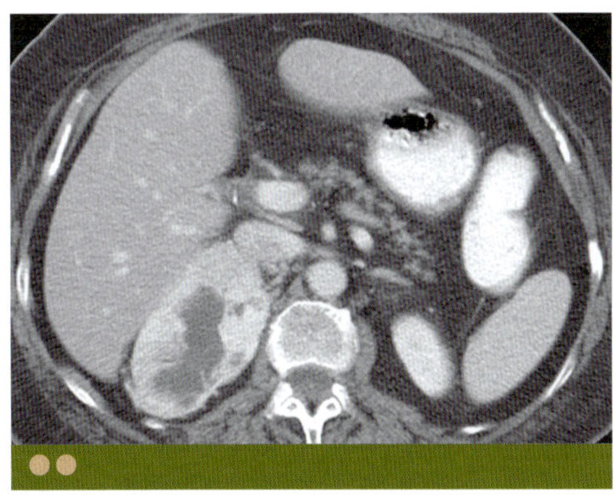

F. Adrenal pheochromocytoma: Axial CECT shows large heterogeneous mass that looks similar on imaging to the neuroblastomas. These lesions are more common in adults than neuroblastomas. Clinical findings help distinguish but surgical resection often required.

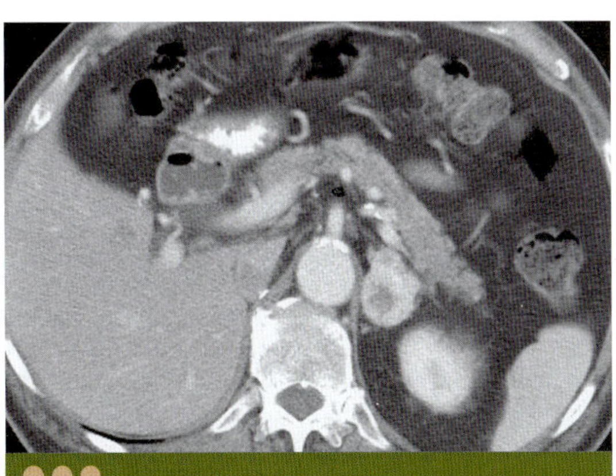

G. Adrenal metastasis from lung cancer: Axial CECT scan shows heterogeneous enhancing mass of the left adrenal gland with peripheral enhancement. The older age and associated lung cancer helps distinguish from neuroblastomas, although neuroblastomas can look similar on imaging studies.

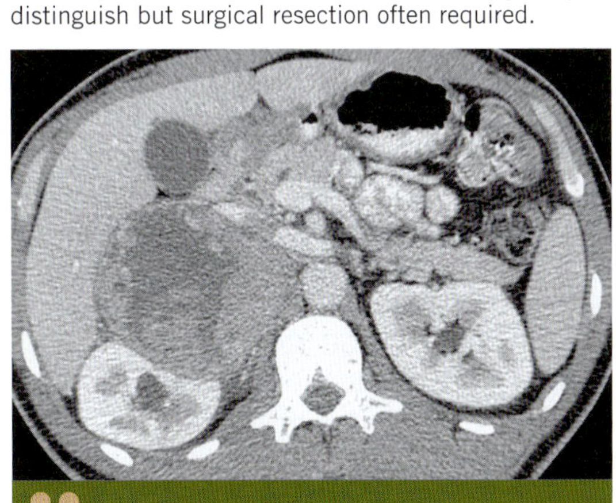

H. Adrenal cell carcinoma: Axial CECT shows large right heterogeneous mass that looks similar to neuroblastomas. It is generally seen in older age group and appears heterogeneous as may contain hemorrhage and necrosis.

IMAGE KEY

Common

Rare

Typical

Unusual

14–15 Adrenal Hemangioma

Frank H. Miller

PRESENTATION

Generally asymptomatic detected on imaging studies; may rarely present with abdominal pain attributed to mass effect or hemorrhage.

FINDINGS

Adrenal lesion that is of high signal on T2-WI.

DIFFERENTIAL DIAGNOSES

- *Pheochomocytoma*: Often high signal on T2-WI. Differentiate on the basis of clinical and laboratory findings.
- *Adrenal cyst*: May be of high signal on T2-WI but does not enhance.
- *Primary adrenal cortical carcinoma:* Often large with necrotic and hemorrhagic components; may invade veins.
- *Metastasis*: Often known malignancy; generally different appearance on imaging studies.

COMMENTS

Adrenal hemangiomas are very rare tumors. They are most commonly seen in patients between the ages of 50 and 70 years and have a female predominance. They may be solitary or multiple. They may be associated with Osler-Weber-Rendu disease, Sturge-Weber syndrome, and von Hippel-Lindau disease. They arise from the adrenal cortex. Pathologically, they most commonly are cavernous and rarely capillary. They contain dilated peripheral vascular spaces. When large, they may contain central necrosis, hemorrhage, calcifications, and/or fibrosis.

Adrenal hemangiomas generally do not cause symptoms. They may cause symptoms as a result of mass effect or bleeding, and patients present with abdominal pain. On plain radiographs, they may show punctuate and stippled calcifications when large. Imaging features seen on CT include the typical, calcified phlebolith-like calcifications and peripheral enhancement. Delayed filling-in of the lesion seen in hepatic hemangiomas may not be seen in adrenal hemangiomas because of the more commonly associated necrotic and fibrotic regions in the tumor. Sonographic findings include a well-circumscribed mass with heterogeneous echogenicity that may show cystic areas. There may be hyperechoic septa. On MR, the lesions usually are hypointense on T1-WI and hyperintense on T2-WI similar to hemangiomas in the liver. Some masses may have hemorrhagic components seen as high-signal intensity on T1-WI. Following contrast, the lesions may show peripheral nodular enhancement with centripetal filling-in of contrast on delayed imaging. This enhancement pattern is not typical of other tumors.

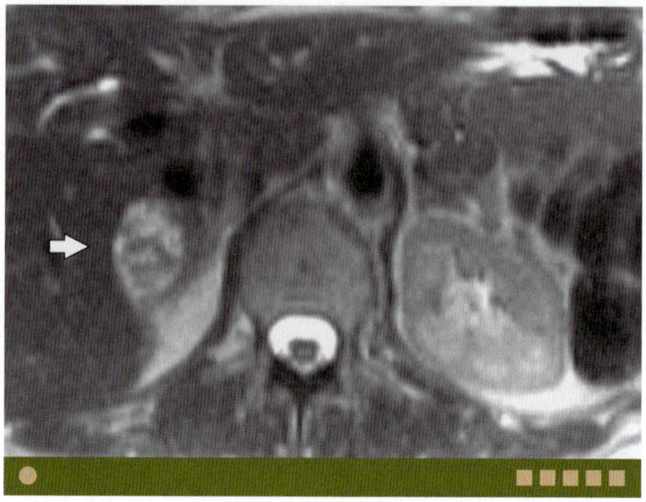

A. Collision tumor attributed to lateral hemangioma and medial adrenal adenoma. Axial T2-WI shows the lateral aspect of the lesion is of high-signal intensity (arrow) proven to be adrenal hemangioma. The medial aspect is not of high-signal intensity.

PEARLS

- **Adrenal hemangioma is a rare tumor of the adrenal cortex.**
- **Adrenal hemangioma tends to be detected incidentally on imaging studies.**
- **Adrenal hemangiomas may show phlebolith-like calcifications.**
- **Adrenal hemangiomas may show peripheral centripetal enhancement with progressive filling-in which is not generally seen in other tumors.**
- **On MR, hemangiomas are generally hypointense on T1-WI and hyperintense on T2-WI.**

ADDITIONAL IMAGES (B-E)

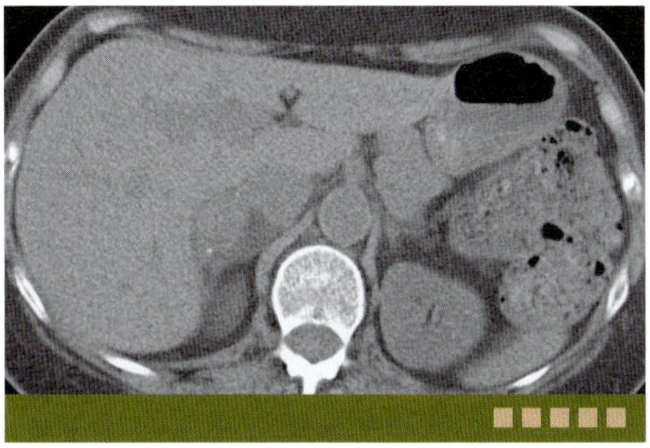

B. Axial NECT shows right adrenal mass with the lateral portion having an associated calcification.

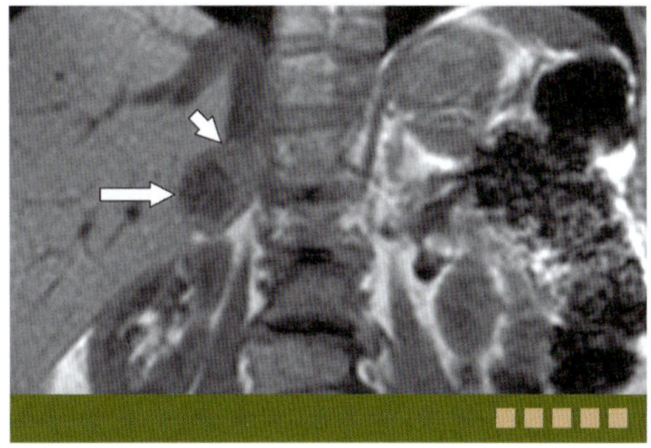

C. Coronal in-phase image shows lesion that is heterogeneous with the more lateral aspect (long arrow) hypointense and the medial aspect (small arrow) isointense to the liver.

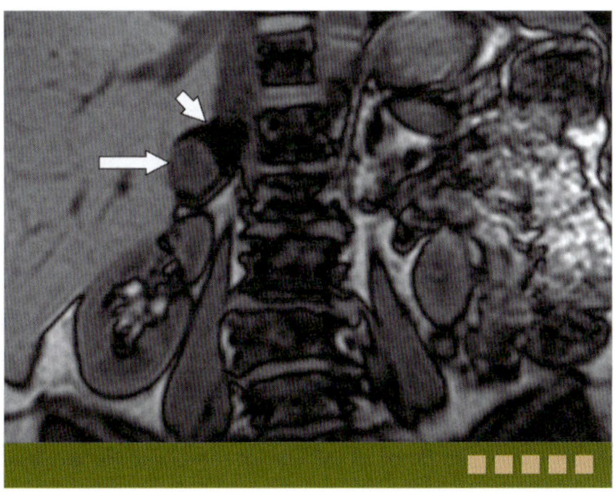

D. Coronal opposed-phase image shows the medial lesion drops in signal (small arrow) from an adrenal adenoma while the lateral part of the lesion (long arrow) does not drop in signal intensity.

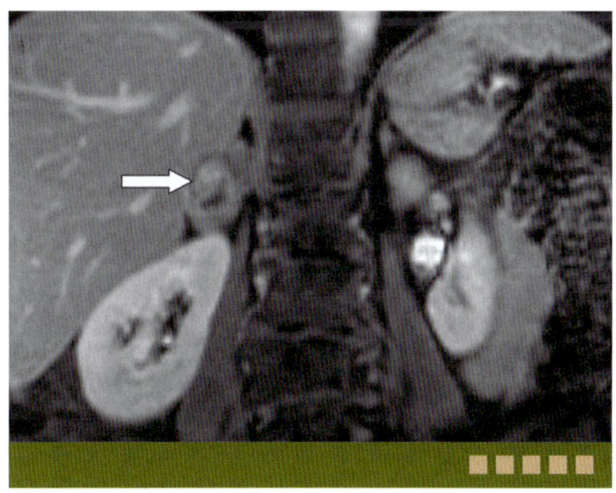

E. Coronal contrast-enhanced T1-WI shows progressive enhancement of the adrenal hemangioma. The lesion is a collision tumor with the medial lesion proven to be an adrenal adenoma.

IMAGE KEY

Common

Rare

Typical

Unusual

DIFFERENTIAL DIAGNOSES IMAGES (F-G)

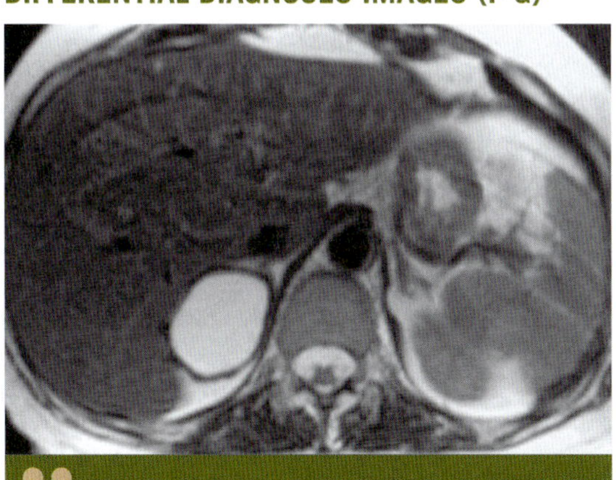

F. Adrenal cyst: Axial T2-WI shows lesion that is high signal on T2-WI. No enhancement was seen after contrast. Hemangiomas typically enhance.

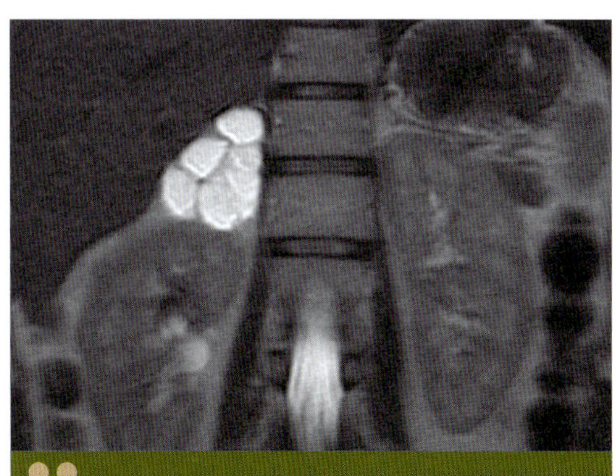

G. Cystic pheochromocytoma: On coronal T2-WI, the right adrenal mass is of high-signal intensity with septations. The patient had a history of hypertension.

14–16 Adrenal Cyst

Frank H. Miller

PRESENTATION

Incidental adrenal mass.

FINDINGS

Right adrenal mass that is of low signal on T1, high signal on T2, and does not enhance.

DIFFERENTIAL DIAGNOSES

- *Adrenal pheochromocytoma*: Distinguish on the basis of the history of hypertension and elevated abnormal labs, generally more complex and solid component.
- *Adrenal lymphangioma*: Can look the same.
- *Adrenal metastases*: More solid components.
- *Adrenal adenoma*: Not generally fluid-containing, although can be of low density on CT.

COMMENTS

Adrenal cysts are uncommon and generally incidental findings on imaging studies. They may be congenital but generally are from prior hemorrhage or trauma. They have been characterized as endothelial, epithelial, parasitic, and pseudocysts. Adrenal pseudocysts are the result of prior hemorrhage or infection.

Adrenal cysts are rare with an incidence of 0.06% to 0.18% in autopsy studies. Of adrenal cysts, approximately 45% are endothelial, 39% are pseudocysts, 9% are epithelial, and 7% are parasitic. Other studies have suggested that pseudocysts from prior hemorrhage are the main cause.

Simple endothelial cysts are generally thin-walled and fluid density on CT unless there has been prior hemorrhage. On MR, the fluid is seen as of low-signal intensity on T1-WI and of high-signal intensity on T2-WI. Pseudocysts may appear heterogeneous because of its complexity related to hemorrhage, septations, and calcifications. Hemorrhage may be seen as increased density on CT relative to simple fluid and may have variable signal intensities on T1- and T2-WI based on the stage of hemorrhage. Calcifications, especially of the wall, are easily seen on CT but may be difficult to detect on MR. The wall of adrenal cysts should be smooth and thin, measuring less than 3 mm. They may occasionally have septations. No enhancement should be seen on contrast-enhanced CT or MR of the internal portion of the adrenal cyst although the wall and septa may enhance.

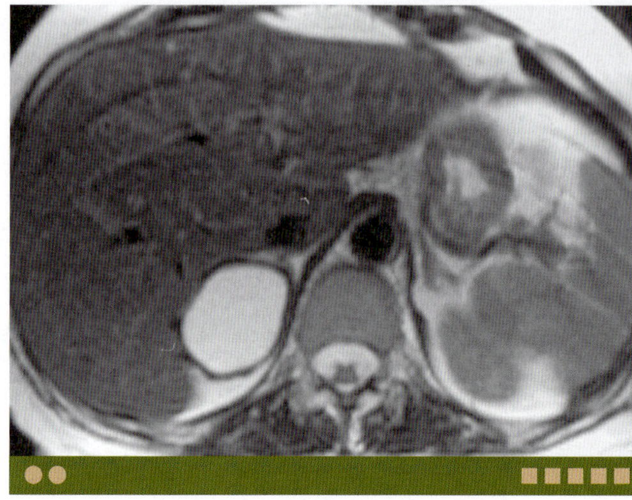

A. Axial T2-WI shows a high-signal intensity lesion measuring 4 cm from an adrenal cyst.

PEARLS

- **Adrenal cysts are uncommon and generally incidentally detected.**
- **Adrenal cysts may be congenital but generally are because of prior hemorrhage or trauma.**
- **Adrenal cysts are fluid density on CT and fluid signal intensity on MR.**
- **Pseudocysts may be more complex because of hemorrhage, septations, or calcifications.**

CHAPTER 14
Adrenal Gland

CASE
Adrenal Cyst

ADDITIONAL IMAGES (B-C)

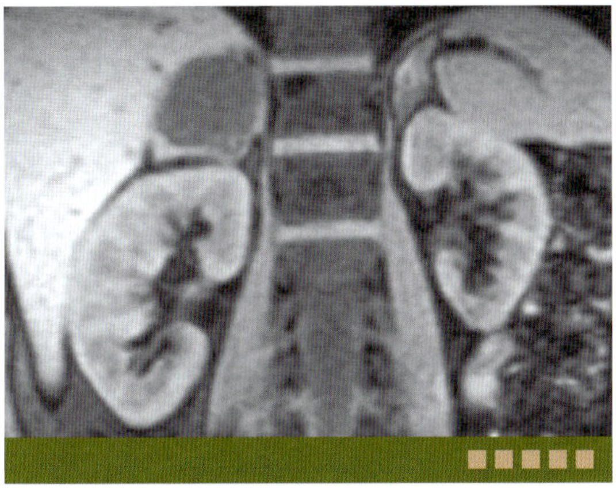

B. Coronal T1-WI shows low-signal intensity lesion of right adrenal gland from fluid in adrenal cyst. There is no high-signal material to suggest proteinaceous or hemorrhagic material.

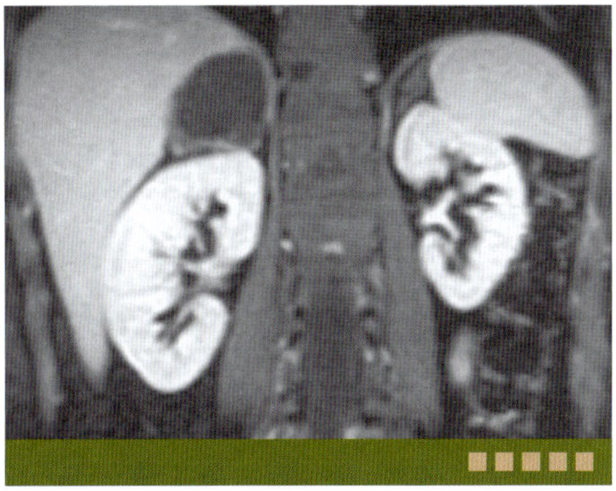

C. Coronal contrast-enhanced TI-WI shows no evidence of lesion enhancement. Coronal image nicely shows the suprarenal location of the adrenal mass.

DIFFERENTIAL DIAGNOSES IMAGES (D-E)

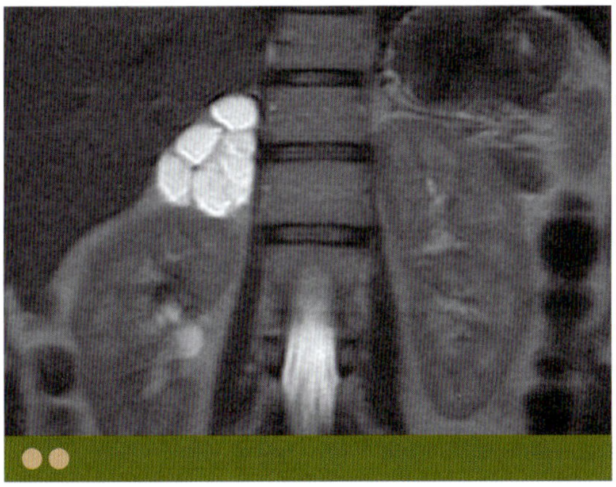

D. Pheochromocytoma: Coronal T2 shows multiple septations within lesion. The patient has a history of hypertension and lesion was proven to be pheochromocytoma. Lesion is more complex than simple adrenal cyst.

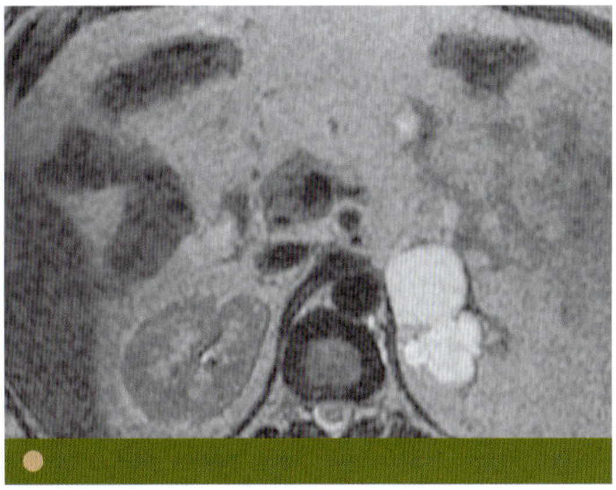

E. Lymphangioma: Axial T2-WI shows high-signal intensity left adrenal lesion proven to be lymphangioma.

IMAGE KEY

Common

Rare

Typical

Unusual

14–17 Adrenal Lymphangioma

Frank H. Miller

PRESENTATION

Incidental adrenal mass.

FINDINGS

CT shows hypodense left adrenal mass that measured fluid density and has peripheral calcifications.

DIFFERENTIAL DIAGNOSES

- *Adrenal cyst*: May be similar on imaging studies.
- *Adrenal pseudocysts*: May be similar on imaging studies.
- *Cystic pheochromocytoma*: Often can be distinguished on the basis of a history of hypertension or some complexity to the lesion.

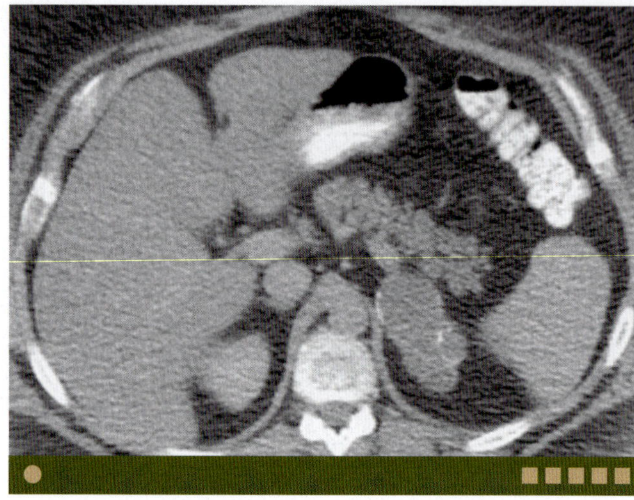

A. Axial NECT shows hypodense mass with peripheral calcifications in the left adrenal gland.

COMMENTS

Cystic lymphangiomas of the adrenal gland are rare and asymptomatic. They are generally "incidentalomas" seen more and more frequently as patients are scanned for various reasons with improvements in imaging techniques. They may also be incidentally detected at surgery.

Lymphangiomas can be seen at all ages with a peak incidence in the third to sixth decades of life. Lymphangiomas can be seen most commonly in the mesentery of the small intestine, omentum, or retroperitoneum. Involvement of the adrenal gland is less common.

On CT scans, lymphangiomas are seen as fluid density masses of the adrenal gland. On MR, because of their fluid content, the lesions are seen as low-signal intensity on T1-WI and high-signal intensity on T2-WI. They, typically, have a thin wall. Following contrast, there, generally, is not any significant internal enhancement. MR in the coronal and sagittal plane and MDCT reformatted images may be helpful to confirm the origin of the masses.

Other causes of adrenal cystic lesions include adrenal cysts and pseudocysts that can appear similarly on imaging studies. All these lesions are generally asymptomatic. When large, they may cause symptoms associated with mass effect, which may include pain or gastrointestinal symptoms. The lesions can usually be distinguished from cystic pheochromocytomas on the basis of lack of hypertension or laboratory findings to suggest pheochromocytoma.

Surgical removal may be indicated when large and complicated to confirm diagnosis or relieve symptoms.

PEARLS

- **Adrenal lymphangiomas are cystic lesions of the adrenal gland on imaging studies.**
- **Adrenal lymphangiomas are not able to be distinguished from other cystic adrenal lesions on imaging studies.**

ADDITIONAL IMAGES (B-C)

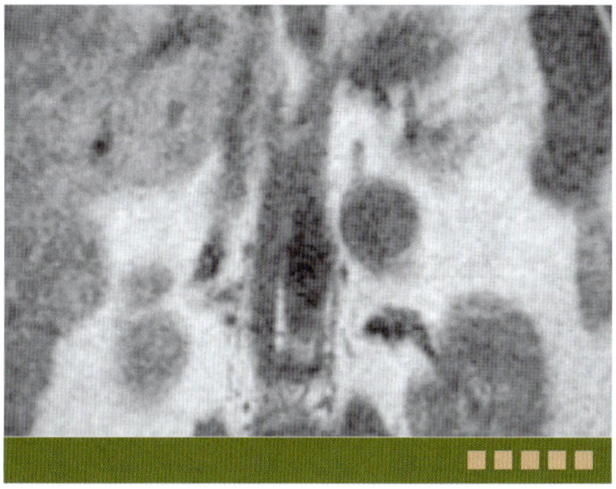

B. Coronal T1-WI shows hypointense lesion in the left adrenal gland.

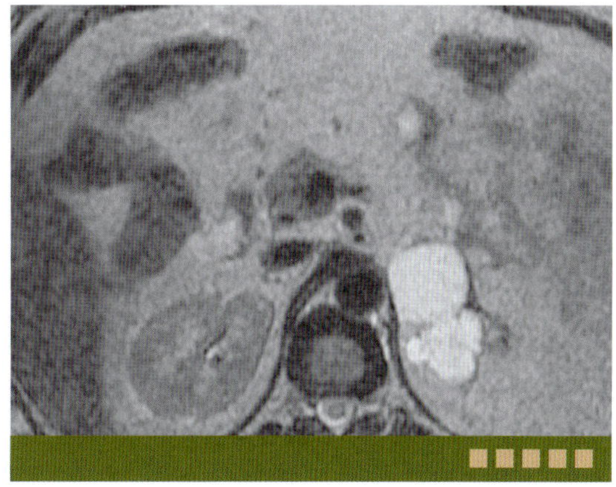

C. Axial T2-WI shows high-signal intensity lesion in the left adrenal gland. The patient had no history of trauma or hypertension. The lesion was resected and was a lymphangioma.

DIFFERENTIAL DIAGNOSES IMAGES (D-F)

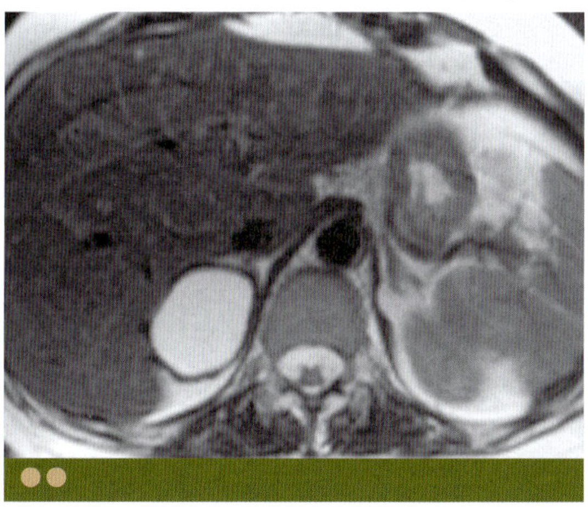

D. Adrenal cyst: Axial T2-WI shows fluid-containing lesion from right adrenal cyst.

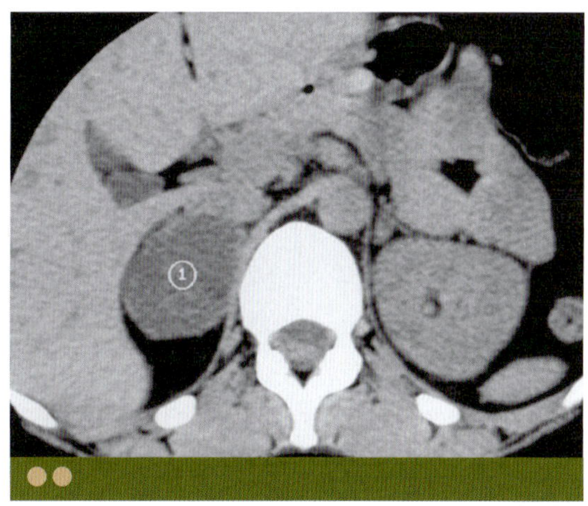

E. Cystic pheochromocytoma: Axial NECT shows right adrenal mass that measures fluid density.

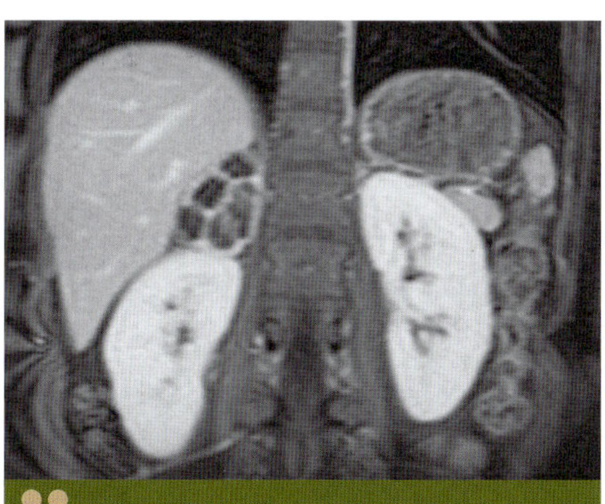

F. Cystic pheochromocytoma: Coronal contrast-enhanced T1-WI from the same patient as from Figure E. shows multiple septations within the mass. The patient had a history of hypertension.

IMAGE KEY

Common

Rare

Typical

Unusual

14–18 Adrenal Ganglioneuroma

Frank H. Miller

PRESENTATION

Right upper quadrant and epigastric pain with nonspecific mass seen on CT.

FINDINGS

Homogenous hypodense mass that is suprarenal in location and difficult to assess if arises from adrenal or adjacent to adrenal.

DIFFERENTIAL DIAGNOSES

- *Adrenal adenoma*: When contains lipid, drops in signal on opposed-phase MR images, low density on unenhanced CT.
- *Adrenal metastasis*: Differentiated based on history; can be nonspecific on imaging studies.
- *Adrenal pheochromocytoma*: Differentiated based on history; often hypervascular and high-signal intensity on T2-WI but can be of variable appearance.
- *Adrenal cell carcinoma*: Often large and heterogeneous.
- *Adrenal myelolipoma*: Characteristically has macroscopic fat.

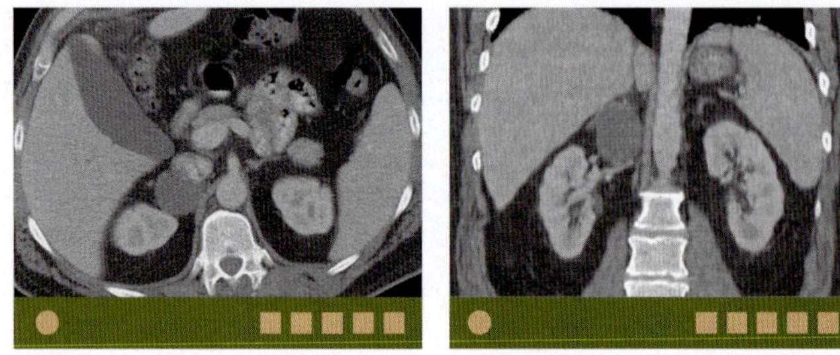

A. Axial CECT shows mass that is homogenously hypodense and is difficult to assess if arising from the adrenal gland or just adjacent to the adrenal gland.
B. Coronal reformatted CECT shows the relationship of the mass to the adrenal gland.

COMMENTS

Adrenal ganglioneuromas are uncommon benign lesions that occur more frequently in adults than in children. Adrenal ganglioneuromas, neuroblastoma, and ganglioneuroblastoma arise from the neural crest cells from the adrenal medulla and have a spectrum of malignant potential. Ganglioneuromas can arise in the posterior mediastinum as well as throughout the retroperitoneum, pelvis, gastrointestinal tract, and mesentery.

Ganglioneuromas are typically slow growing and incidentally discovered on imaging studies. They may produce symptoms depending on their size and location including as a mass or abdominal pain.

Neuroblastomas tend to arise in young children under the age of 5 years. These tumors tend to be aggressive and large at diagnosis. They often extend into the neural foramina. Ganglioneuroblastomas tend to be intermediate in malignant potential relative to neuroblastoma and ganglioneuroma and occur in patients of older age than neuroblastomas.

Ganglioneuromas on sonography tend to be homogenously hypoechoic. On CT, they are fairly homogenous and well defined. They show mild enhancement and may have punctate calcifications. They can have an infiltrative appearance and be difficult to distinguish from more malignant types. On MR imaging, they tend to be intermediate signal intensity on T1-WI and intermediate to high-signal intensity on T2-WI. Unlike adenomas, they do not contain intracellular lipid, and therefore, do not lose signal on opposed-phase images. Lack of growth over time or excision is required to show they are not malignant or confirm the diagnosis.

PEARLS

- **Adrenal ganglioneuromas are benign lesions.**
- **Adrenal ganglioneuromas occur more frequently in adults than in children.**
- **Ganglioneuromas are well-defined masses.**
- **Ganglioneuromas are of low-density, homogeneous on unenhanced CT, and show mild enhancement.**
- **On MR, they are homogeneous hypointense to intermediate intensity on T1-WI and intermediate- to high-signal intensity on T2-WI.**

ADDITIONAL IMAGES (C-E)

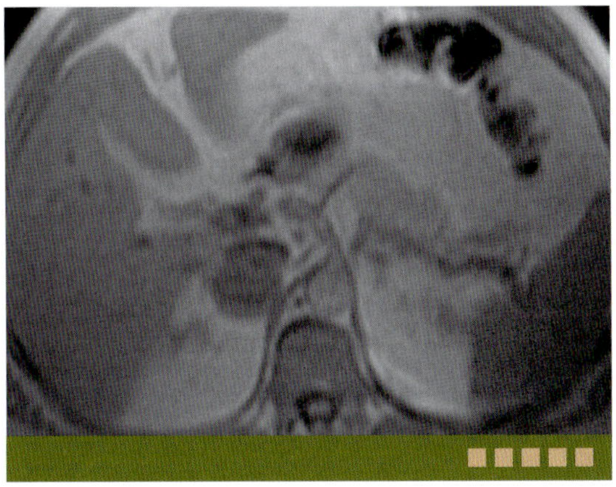

C. Axial in-phase T1-WI shows the adrenal lesion is homogeneous and isointense to the spleen.

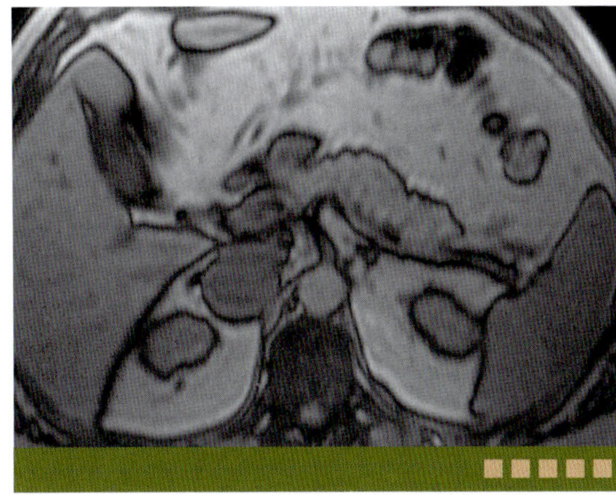

D. Axial opposed-phase T1-WI shows no drop in signal relative to the spleen to suggest that it represents an adenoma. The image can be identified as opposed-phase as the organs are etched in black.

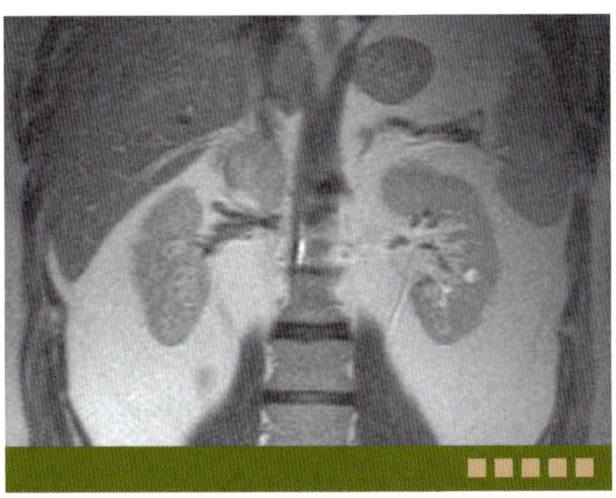

E. Coronal T2-WI shows the lesion is similar in signal intensity to the spleen. The lesion is relatively nonspecific in appearance. Surgical resection showed that it was a ganglioneuroma.

DIFFERENTIAL DIAGNOSES IMAGES (F-H)

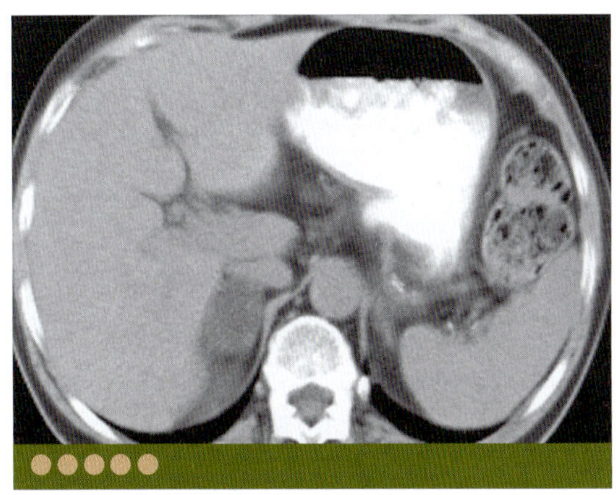

F. Adrenal adenoma: Axial NECT shows hypodense lesion that measures less than 10 HU.

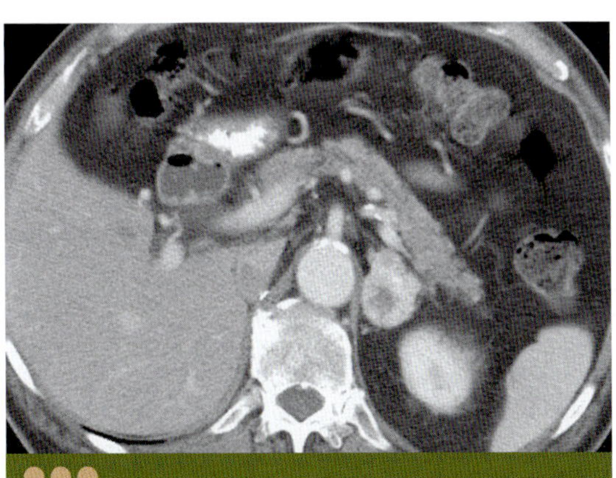

G. Adrenal metastasis from lung cancer: Axial CECT shows heterogeneously enhancing adrenal lesion in a patient with lung cancer from metastasis.

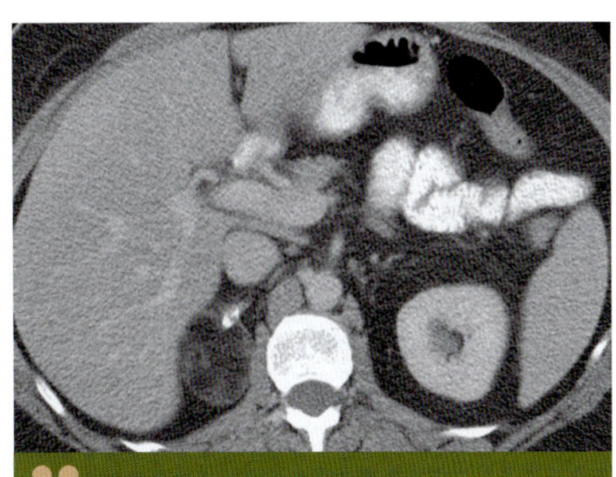

H. Adrenal myelolipoma: Axial CECT shows right adrenal lesion with calcification and fat. The presence of fat makes the diagnosis of myelolipoma.

IMAGE KEY

Common

Rare

Typical

Unusual

14–19 Adrenal Hemorrhage without Mass

Frank H. Miller

PRESENTATION

History of trauma.

FINDINGS

Right adrenal mass that is high density on unenhanced CT from hemorrhage. Contrast-enhanced image is nonspecific.

DIFFERENTIAL DIAGNOSES

- *Adrenal metastases*: Can be hemorrhagic; clinical history may help differentiate; enhancing mass may suggest malignancy; follow-up imaging may help as adrenal hemorrhage based on nonmalignant cause often resolves.
- *Adrenal pheochromocytoma with hemorrhage*: Clinical findings help distinguish.
- *Adrenal cortical carcinoma*: Large mass which may have central necrosis and hemorrhage; may invade veins.
- *Adrenal adenoma*: Generally low density from microscopic fat on unenhanced CT, although can look similar on CECT.

COMMENTS

Adrenal hemorrhage is usually attributed to trauma but can also be caused by adrenal masses that bleed, anticoagulants and coagulopathies, liver transplantation, sepsis, or hypotension. Traumatic adrenal hematomas occur on the right in up to 90% of the cases. The right adrenal may be involved more frequently because of compression of the adrenal between the liver and spine by blunt trauma. Patients with liver transplantation may develop hemorrhagic infarction and hematomas as a result of surgery involving the right adrenal vein.

An underlying mass as a cause for adrenal hemorrhage must be considered especially in patients without a discrete cause for hemorrhage. Adrenal hemorrhage may also be caused by underlying masses including metastases, adrenal cell carcinoma, pheochromocytoma, adenomas, and other adrenal masses.

Adrenal hemorrhagic masses are bilateral in up to 20% of the patients. When bilateral, signs of adrenal failure (Addison disease) should be evaluated for as the diagnosis may not be suspected clinically and can lead to significant morbidity and mortality. Causes for bilateral involvement include severe stress caused by sepsis, burns, surgery, and complicated pregnancy.

The imaging appearance of adrenal hematomas will vary depending on their chronicity. On ultrasound, adrenal hemorrhage may be hyperechoic especially when acute. Over time, the lesion becomes cystic. CT shows the

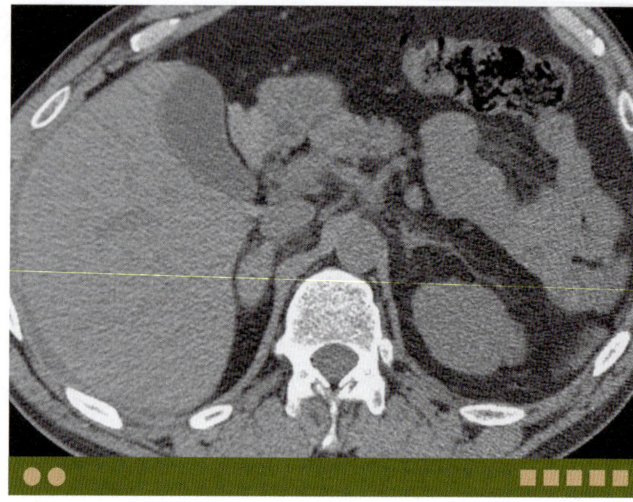

A. Axial NECT shows high-density right adrenal mass from adrenal hemorrhage.

adrenal masses are hyperdense on unenhanced images from hemorrhage when acute. Over time, the density of the adrenal gland may decrease and the lesion may become cystic or resolve. Calcifications may develop when several months old. Areas of enhancement within the lesion may suggest a hemorrhagic neoplasm. If there is enhancement or reason to suspect malignancy, biopsy or surgery may be required for distinction.

MR is the most accurate method to detect and characterize adrenal hemorrhage.

Because of the presence of methemoglobin, subacute hemorrhage is seen as high-signal intensity on T1-WI with a specific finding of a high-signal intensity rim sign as a result of methemoglobin. When more chronic, the hemorrhage is seen as hyperintense on T1- and T2-WI from free methemoglobin with a hypointense rim from hemosiderin.

PEARLS

- **Adrenal hemorrhage is most commonly related to trauma.**
- **A hyperdense lesion of adrenal gland on unenhanced CT suggests hemorrhage.**
- **Adrenal mass that is hyperintense on T1-weighted MR images suggests hemorrhage, especially if it does not suppress on fat-suppressed imaging.**
- **A hypointense rim on MR caused by hemorrhage may be seen as a result of hemosiderin.**

ADDITIONAL IMAGES (B-D)

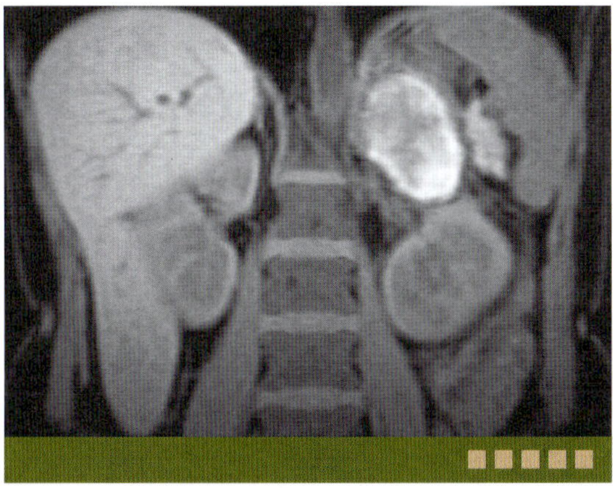

B. Coronal T1-WI shows high-signal intensity large left adrenal mass from hemorrhage.

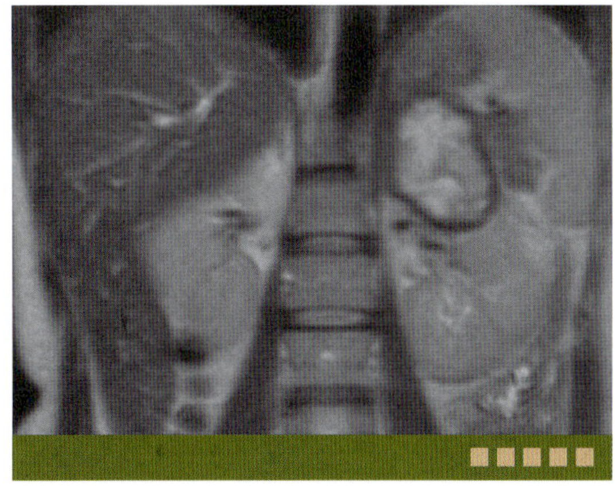

C. Coronal T2-WI shows that the mass has low-signal intensity peripheral rim from hemosiderin confirming adrenal hemorrhage.

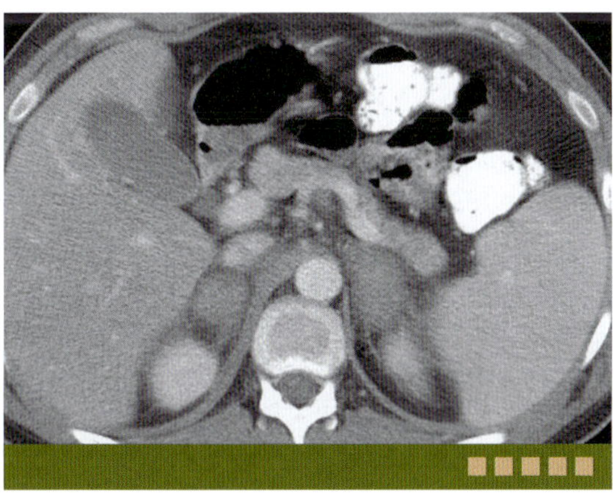

D. Axial CECT scan shows bilateral hemorrhagic adrenal masses related to anticoagulation. On CECT, the appearance is nonspecific. There is some adjacent inflammatory stranding. The history of anticoagulation in this patient helps differentiate from lymphoma or metastases.

DIFFERENTIAL DIAGNOSES IMAGES (E-G)

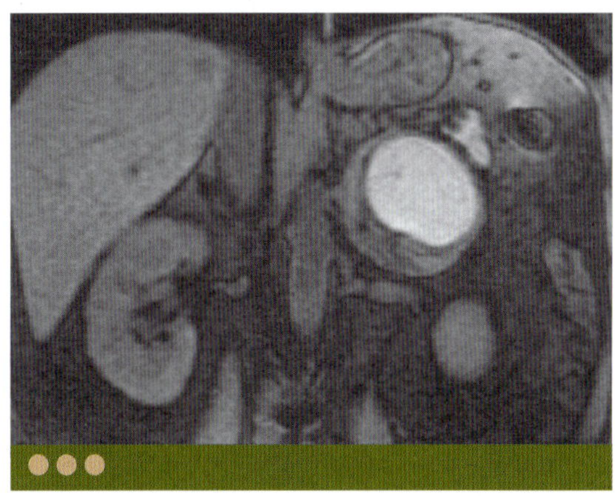

E. Pheochromocytoma: Coronal unenhanced T1-WI shows large high-signal intensity lesion from pheochromocytoma. The patient had a history of hypertension which was helpful in differential diagnoses and proven to be pheochromocytoma.

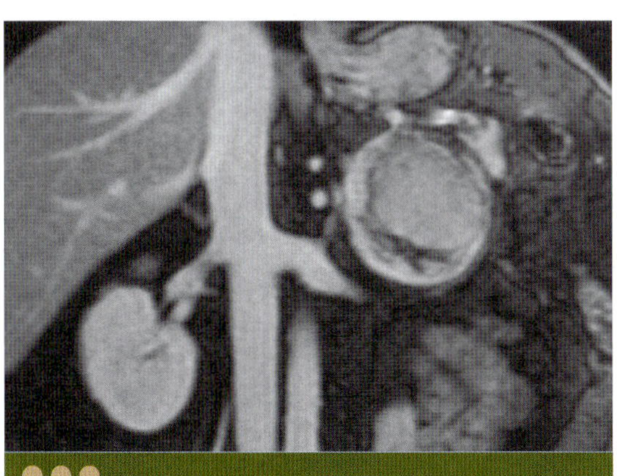

F. Pheochromocytoma: Coronal contrast-enhanced T1-WI in the same patient as in Figure E shows enhancement of the peripheral portion of the adrenal mass with the hemorrhagic component not enhancing.

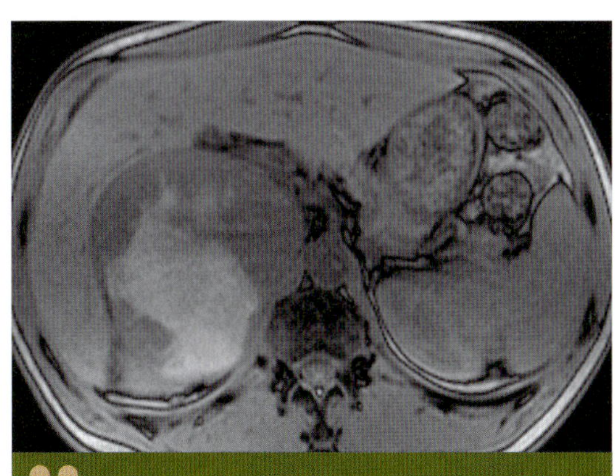

G. Adrenal cell carcinoma: Axial unenhanced T1-WI shows areas of high-signal intensity caused by hemorrhage.

Figures B and C are the same patient.
Figures E and F are the same patient.

IMAGE KEY

Common

Rare

Typical

Unusual

14-20 Adrenal Gland Trauma

Nancy A. Hammond

PRESENTATION

Trauma.

FINDINGS

Hematoma in the left suprarenal space with active extravasation of contrast material.

DIFFERENTIAL DIAGNOSIS

None

COMMENTS

Trauma to the adrenal gland is an uncommon injury. It is usually seen in the setting of blunt abdominal trauma and associated with significant trauma to other abdominal organs. As a result of the small size of the adrenal glands and their protected retroperitoneal location, the adrenal glands are usually spared in the setting of trauma. Two mechanisms of injury have been proposed: severe hyperextension and lateral compressive force, both resulting in compression of the gland against the spine.

Studies have reported the incidence of adrenal injury in the setting of trauma to be approximately 2%. The rate of adrenal injury seen at autopsy is reported to be 28% in patients with significant abdominal trauma. One study found the right adrenal gland to be more commonly injured than the left. Regardless of the side, ipsilateral rib fractures and injury to the ipsilateral visceral structure (liver and spleen) are commonly seen. Isolated adrenal hematoma is exceedingly rare and should prompt a search for additional injuries.

Contrast-enhanced CT is the modality of choice in the setting of trauma. Adrenal gland injuries appear as round or oval masses centered in the adrenal gland. As incidental adrenal adenomas are a common occurrence, the distinction between an adenoma and hematoma should be considered. Typically, a hematoma demonstrates higher attenuation than that of an adenoma with an average attenuation value reported as 52 HU. If the distinction between a hematoma and an adenoma cannot be made on routine contrast-enhanced imaging, 15 minutes delayed images can be obtained in clinically stable patients. Adenomas demonstrate significant washout while hematomas do not. Other reported findings on CT of adrenal trauma include irregular, diffuse suprarenal hemorrhage with obliteration of the adrenal gland and uniform enlargement of the adrenal gland with indistinct margins. Periadrenal findings include high-density stranding in the adjacent fat, adjacent focal hematomas, and hemorrhage in the posterior pararenal space. The presence of active extravasation of contrast material in the adrenal bed is consistent with active bleeding and is associated with higher morbidity and mortality.

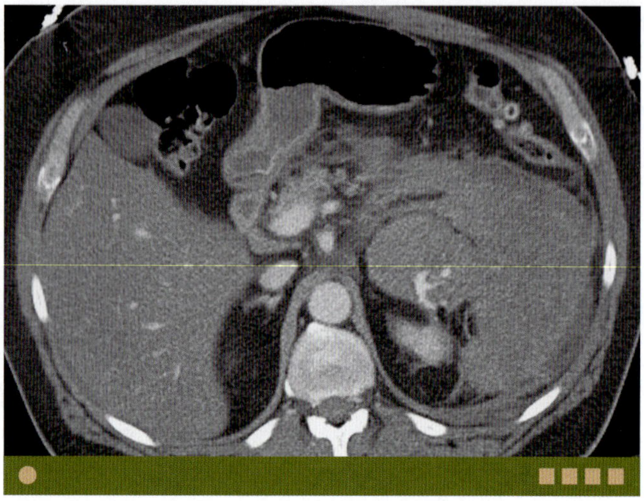

A. Axial CECT shows a mildly hyperdense collection in the left suprarenal region centered in the expected location of the left adrenal gland compatible with an adrenal gland hematoma. A focal area of high attenuation within this hematoma is compatible with active extravasation and acute hemorrhage. Note the normal appearing right adrenal gland. Atypically, no additional injuries were identified in this patient.

Treatment of adrenal gland injuries is based on the patient's stability, associated injuries, and viability of the gland during surgical exploration. Interventional angiography can be employed in patients with active extravasation. Conservative treatment with close follow-up is utilized in isolated trauma with limited hemorrhage.

PEARLS

- **Traumatic injury to the adrenal gland is uncommon and usually associated with significant intra-abdominal trauma.**
- **The right adrenal gland is more commonly injured than the left.**
- **The most common CT finding is a hyperattenuating round or oval mass centered in the adrenal gland.**

ADDITIONAL IMAGES (B-E)

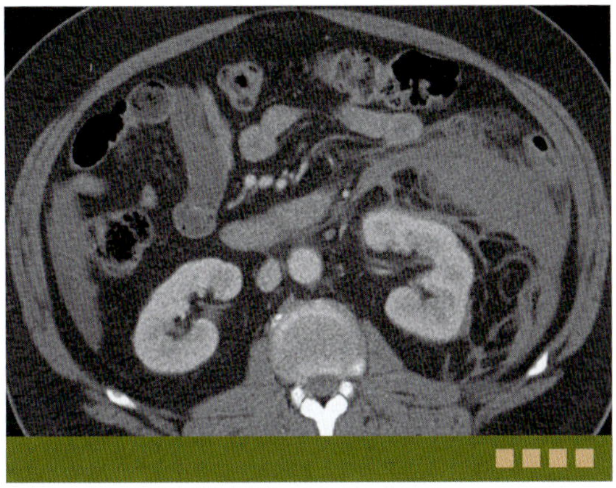

B. Axial CECT in the same patient obtained more inferiorly shows the extent of the hematoma extending into the anterior pararenal space and perinephric space and inferiorly along the lateroconal fascia.

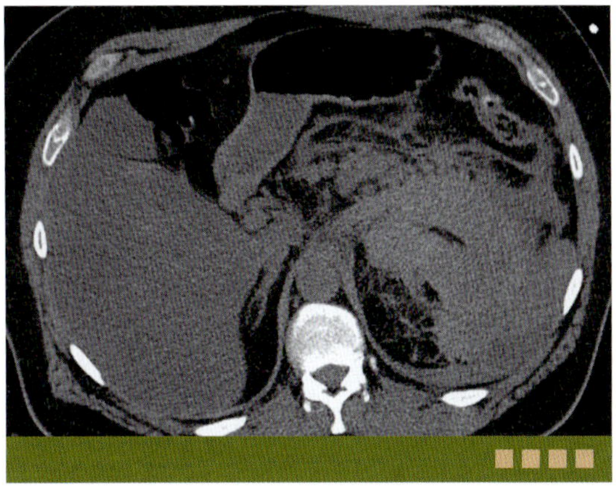

C. Axial NECT shows the characteristic high attenuation of an acute hematoma.

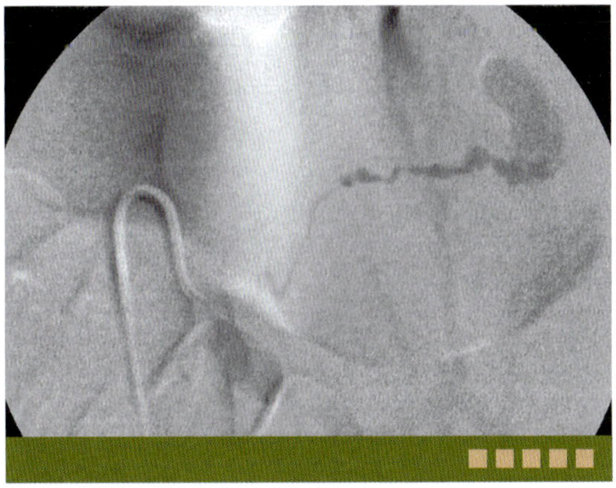

D. Selective angiogram shows active extravasation of contrast material from a left adrenal artery. From the tortuosity of this vessel and the super-selective nature of it, embolization was not achievable via percutaneous methods.

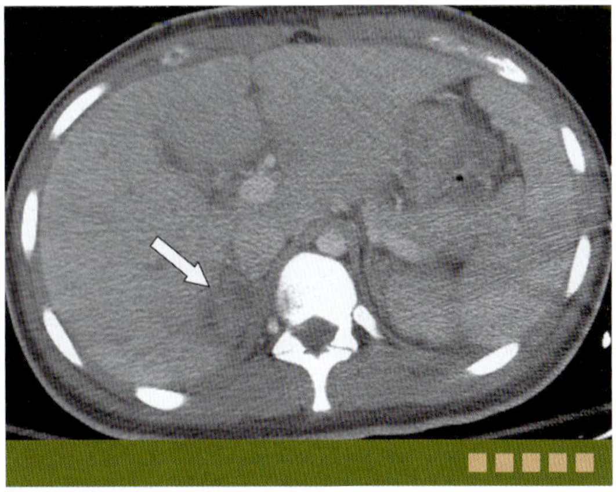

E. Axial CECT shows a more characteristic appearance of an adrenal gland hematoma in a trauma patient (arrow). The patient also had multiple hepatic lacerations.

IMAGE KEY

Common

Rare

Typical

Unusual

14–21 Adrenal Hyperplasia

Frank H. Miller

PRESENTATION

- Asymptomatic, detected on imaging studies.
- Cushing syndrome-hypercortisolism.
- Conn syndrome-hypertension, hypokalemia.

FINDINGS

Bilaterally enlarged adrenal glands that maintain the adrenal shape.

DIFFERENTIAL DIAGNOSES

Other causes of enlarged adrenal glands:

- *Metastases*: Differ as more focal masses and differ on the basis of history.
- *Lymphomas*: Differ on the basis of history but generally more focal masses.
- *Hemorrhages*: Differ based on history; do not maintain adrenal shape and differ in density and signal intensity.
- *Pheochromocytomas*: Bilateral in 10%; seen as masses and do not maintain adrenal shape, associated with hypertension.
- *Adenomas*: Focal lesions drop in signal intensity, can rarely mimic nodular adrenal hyperplasia.

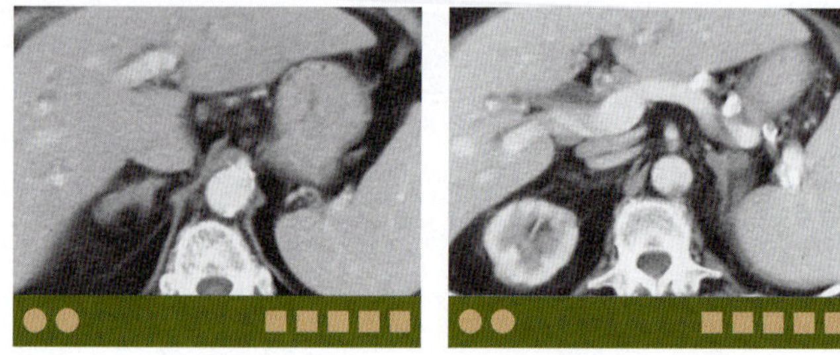

A. Axial CECT shows enlarged nodular right adrenal gland.
B. Axial CECT shows enlarged nodular left adrenal gland.

COMMENTS

Adrenal hyperplasia is bilaterally diffusely enlarged adrenal glands and can be attributed to primary or secondary causes. Secondary causes are associated with elevated levels of ACTH. Adrenal hyperplasia causes approximately 75% of the cases of Cushing syndrome and 20% of those of Conn syndrome. Cushing syndrome is associated with overproduction of ACTH generally by a pituitary adenoma that needs to be identified; an ACTH-producing tumor elsewhere in the body is a less likely cause. Conn syndrome is generally associated with hyperfunctioning adrenal adenoma and less commonly associated with adrenal hyperplasia.

Adrenal hyperplasia is seen as enlarged limbs of one or usually both adrenal gland, greater than 10 mm in width. Approximately 30% to 50% of those patients with biochemical evidence of adrenal hyperplasia have normal anatomic appearance on CT and MR. In over half the patients, the adrenal glands are enlarged diffusely with a normal shape to the adrenal gland. Less commonly adrenal hyperplasia can appear nodular or multinodular and mimic adenomas.

The differential diagnosis of bilaterally enlarged adrenal glands include causes of bilateral adrenal enlargement generally because of masses, including adenomas, metastases, hemorrhage, and pheochromocytomas. These masses, however, generally differ from hyperplasia as they appear as focal masses and not diffusely enlarged adrenal glands, and generally, do not maintain the shape of the adrenal glands. Infections such as tuberculosis or histoplasmosis can generally be distinguished based on clinical findings and are seen as low-density masses and often associated with calcifications and peripheral contrast enhancement.

Adrenal hyperplasia is generally treated medically unlike hyperfunctioning adrenal adenomas that are treated surgically. Massive macronodular hyperplasia is a rare form of hyperplasia with multiple nodules ranging from several millimeters to 5 cm. These are not associated with elevated levels of ACTH. The treatment is bilateral adrenalectomy.

PEARLS

- **Adrenal hyperplasia is associated with Cushing syndrome and Conn syndrome.**
- **Suspect adrenal hyperplasia when bilaterally enlarged adrenal glands that maintain shape and lack mass.**
- **Adrenal hyperplasia may have normal adrenal gland in 30% to 50%.**
- **Adrenal hyperplasia is generally treated medically unlike hyperfunctioning adrenal adenomas that are treated surgically.**

ADDITIONAL IMAGES (C-D)

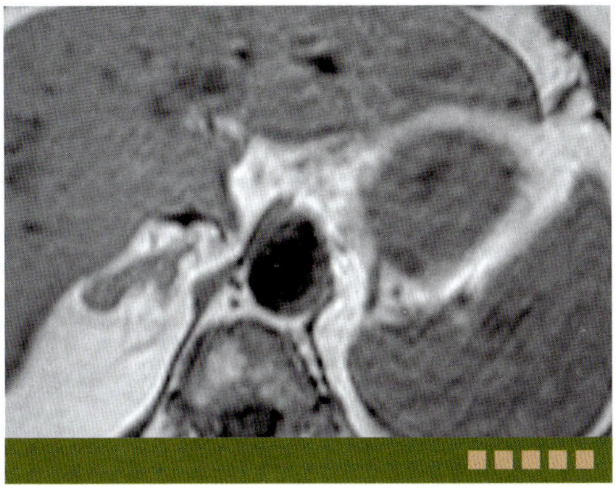

C. Adrenal hyperplasia. Axial in-phase MR image shows enlarged right adrenal gland that maintains its shape because of adrenal hyperplasia.

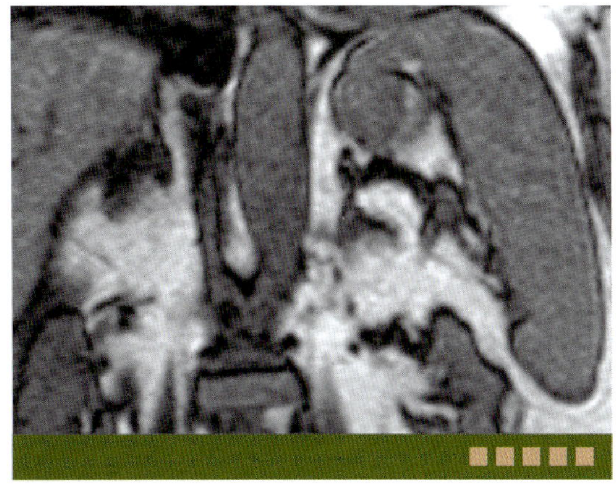

D. Adrenal hyperplasia. Coronal opposed-phase MR image shows enlarged right and left adrenal gland from hyperplasia.

DIFFERENTIAL DIAGNOSES IMAGES (E-H)

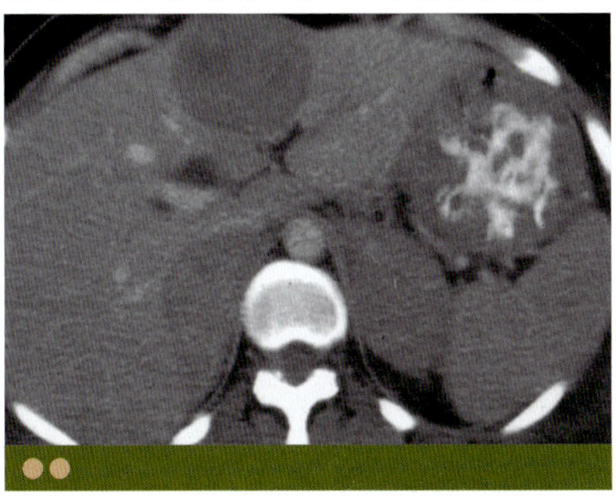

E. 45-year-old male with AIDS and non-Hodgkin lymphoma: Axial CECT shows large bilateral homogeneously enhancing renal masses and solid liver mass.

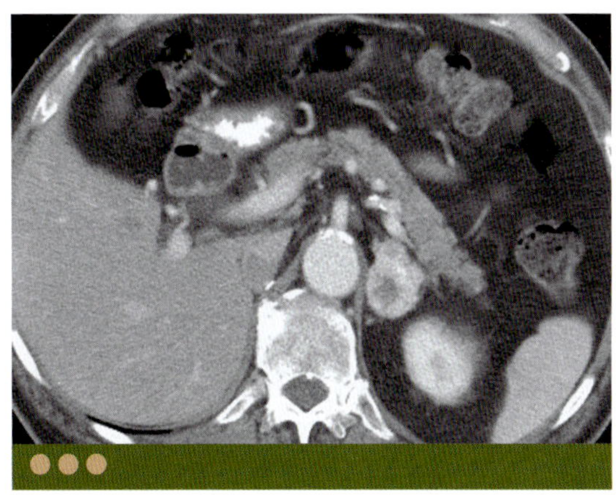

F. Adrenal metastasis: Axial CECT shows nonspecific enhancing lesion of the left adrenal gland from metastasis from lung cancer. The history of malignancy helps in the diagnosis.

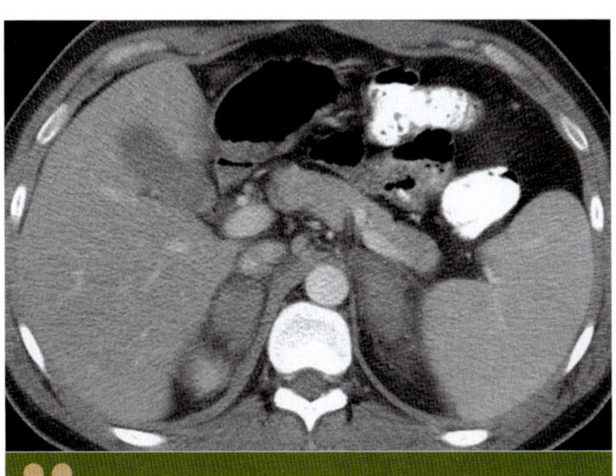

G. Adrenal hemorrhage: Axial CECT shows bilateral adrenal masses caused by hemorrhage into the adrenal glands. There is some adjacent inflammatory stranding. The history of anticoagulation in this patient helps in the diagnosis.

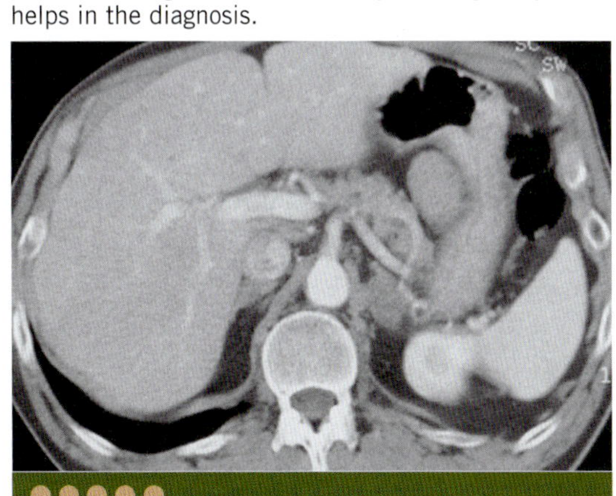

H. Bilateral adrenal adenomas: Axial CECT shows nonspecific enhancing adrenal masses from adenomas. Unenhanced CT or chemical shift MR is helpful to show the presence of fat seen in lipid-rich adenomas.

IMAGE KEY

Common

Rare

Typical

Unusual

14–22 Adrenal Insufficiency

Frank H. Miller

PRESENTATION

Adrenal insufficiency; symptoms include weakness, skin hyperpigmentation, weight loss, and abdominal pain.

FINDINGS

Atrophic adrenal glands.

DIFFERENTIAL DIAGNOSIS

- *Adrenal hyperplasia*: Seen as enlarged not atrophic glands.

COMMENTS

Adrenal insufficiency can be attributed to primary and secondary causes. Primary adrenal insufficiency or Addison disease is because of adrenal abnormality where there is a marked loss of adrenal tissue. Secondary abnormalities are because of abnormalities of the hypothalamus or pituitary gland where the adrenal gland does not receive stimulation from ACTH.

Primary adrenal insufficiency requires at least 90% of the gland to be destroyed. The most common cause of primary adrenal insufficiency is autoimmune disease. Tuberculosis used to be the most common cause in the United States. Adrenal insufficiency can also be because of metastases especially from lung cancer, hepatomas, and lymphoma; however, metastases are rarely associated with adrenal insufficiency as it requires a large amount of destruction of the adrenal cortex. Other causes include adrenal hemorrhage, infection such as histoplasmosis and blastomycosis, and sarcoidosis. ACTH stimulation testing shows in secondary adrenal insufficiency that serum cortisol levels do not rise after ACTH administration.

Imaging findings are variable depending on the cause. Plain abdominal radiographs and CT may show adrenal calcification as a result of tuberculosis or histoplasmosis. Involvement is often bilateral. In autoimmune adrenal insufficiency, CT scans may show significant atrophy. Adrenal hemorrhage can be diagnosed by the increased density on CT and increased T1 signal intensity on MR imaging.

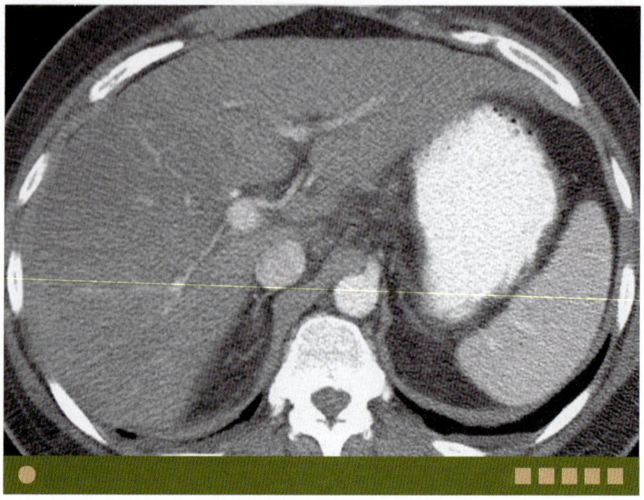

A. Axial CECT shows atrophic right adrenal gland.

PEARLS

- **Adrenal insufficiency may be primary or secondary.**
- **Causes of primary adrenal insufficiency include autoimmune disease, tuberculosis, histoplasmosis, tumors, and hemorrhage.**
- **CT and MR can show the presence of hemorrhage, masses, or calcifications depending on the etiology.**
- **In autoimmune disease, there may be significant cortical atrophy with very small adrenal glands.**

ADDITIONAL IMAGES (B-E)

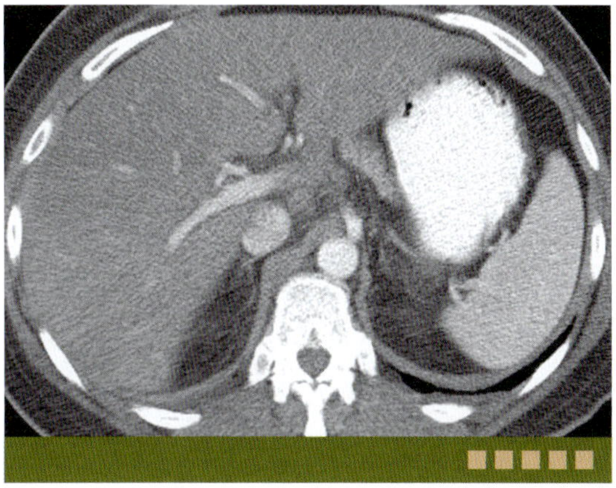

B. Axial CECT shows atrophy of both adrenal glands in the same patient as Figure A with adrenal insufficiency.

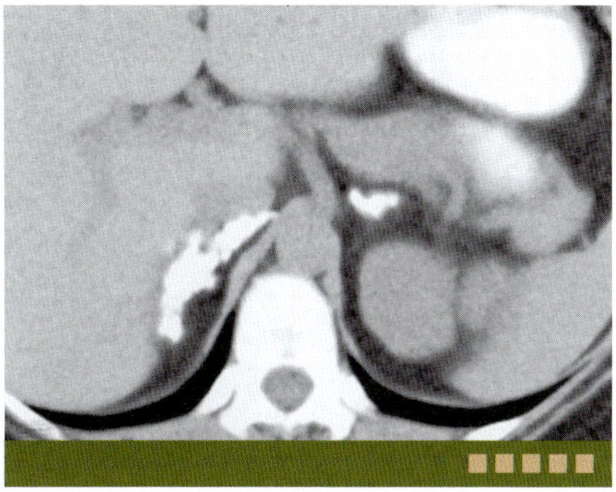

C. Axial NECT shows bilateral adrenal calcifications because of histoplasmosis.

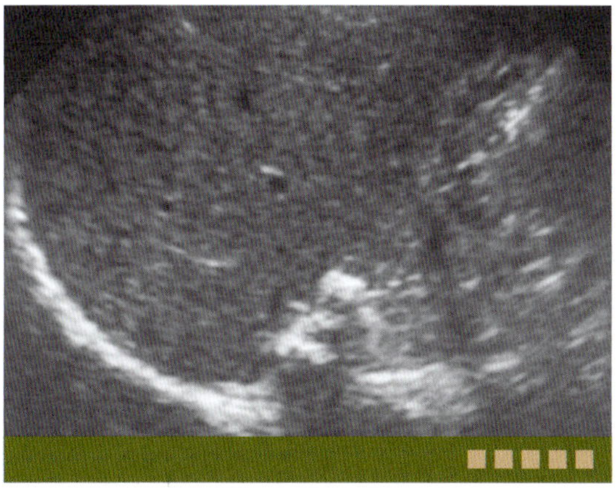

D. Longitudinal sonogram shows right adrenal gland with echogenic foci from calcifications.

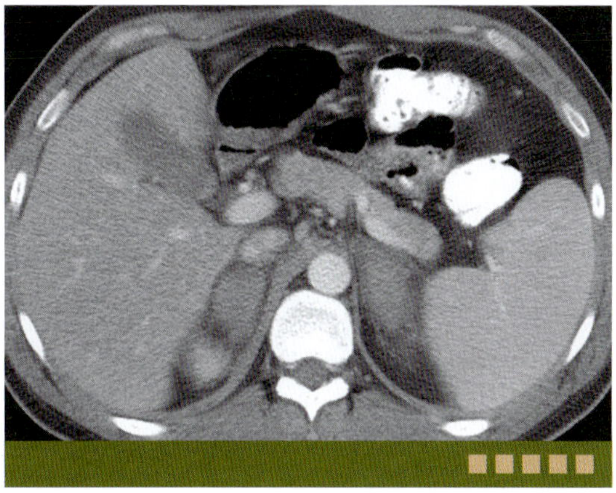

E. Adrenal hemorrhage. Bilateral increased density adrenal masses caused by adrenal hemorrhage, which can be a cause of adrenal insufficiency.

DIFFERENTIAL DIAGNOSIS IMAGE

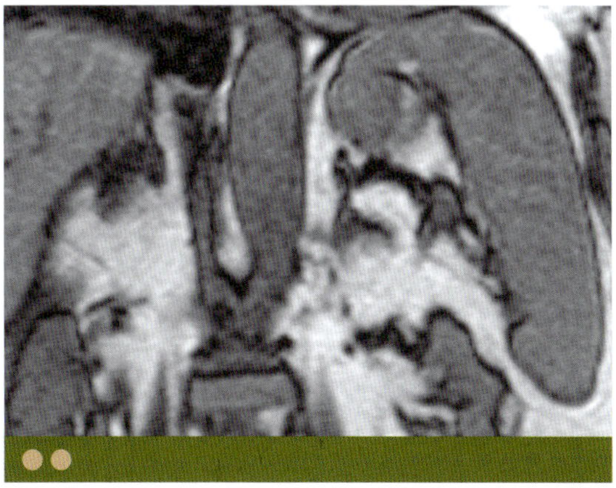

F. Adrenal hyperplasia: Coronal opposed-phase image shows bilateral enlarged adrenal glands with signal loss.

Figures C and D are the same patient and are different from A and B.

IMAGE KEY

Common

Rare

Typical

Unusual

CHAPTER 15

RETROPERITONEUM

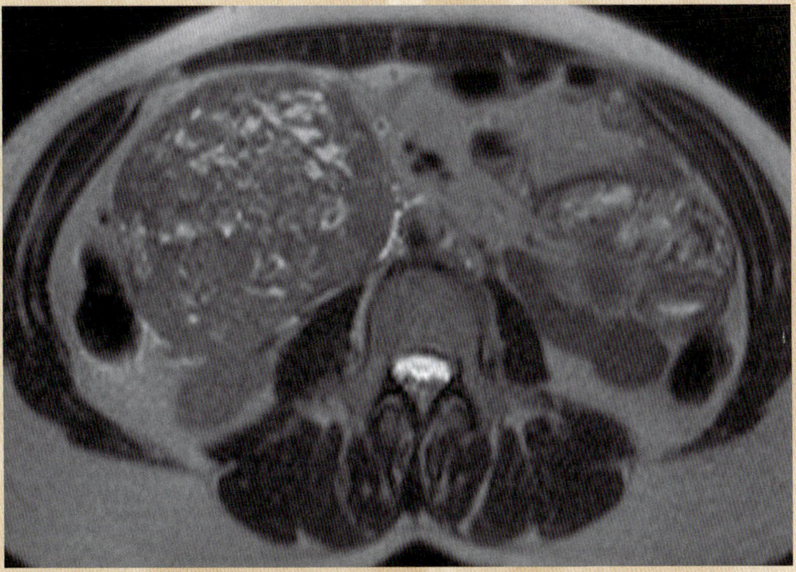

15–1 Retroperitoneal Leiomyosarcoma

Paul Nikolaidis

PRESENTATION

Abdominal mass/fullness, abdominal and back pain; lower extremity swelling.

FINDINGS

Large heterogeneous retroperitoneal mass with numerous small areas of cystic degeneration and necrosis.

DIFFERENTIAL DIAGNOSES

- *Malignant fibrous histiocytoma (MFH)*: Typically moderately hypervascular; may be more heterogeneous and contain calcifications.
- *Schwannoma*: Well demarcated round or oval masses that frequently demonstrate prominent hypodense (on CT) or hyperintense (on T2-WI) areas from cystic degeneration. Schwannomas may have calcifications on CT.
- *Metastases*: Differentiation may be very difficult. Metastatic lesions of the retroperitoneum may have overlapping features with primary malignancies.
- *Ganglioneuroma*: Generally more hypodense (on CT) with only mild-to-moderate postcontrast enhancement and occasional calcifications.
- *Lymphoma*: Usually a more homogeneous appearing mass, which may be more uniformly hypovascular; adenopathy may be present in other distant locations.

COMMENTS

Leiomyosarcomas are the second most common primary retroperitoneal neoplasms. They typically do not present until late, when patients become symptomatic because of compression of adjacent structures. Symptoms are nonspecific and can include abdominal and back pain, lower extremity swelling, weight loss, anorexia, nausea, and urinary obstruction/frequency.

Retroperitoneal leiomyosarcomas are often large (averaging 11 cm in diameter in one series) and heterogeneous. They often show areas of cystic degeneration and central necrosis, more commonly than other sarcomas. Fat and calcifications are not present.

On CT, they are typically large masses that are isodense to muscle, with areas of lower density representing necrosis.

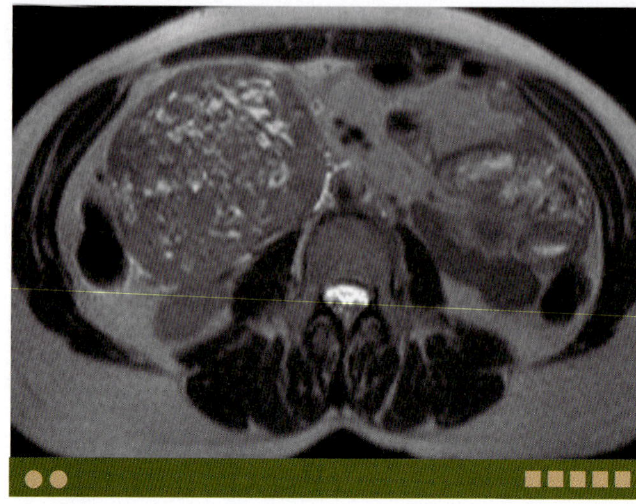

A. Axial T2-WI shows a large right-sided retroperitoneal mass with multiple T2-bright foci, corresponding to areas of cystic degeneration.

On MRI, they usually show heterogeneous low-to-intermediate signal on T1-WI and areas of intermediate-to-high signal on T2-WI, depending on the amount of cystic degeneration or necrosis present. Moderate contrast enhancement is seen at the periphery of the large lesions, whereas smaller lesions may show more uniform enhancement.

The treatment of choice is surgery, although complete excision is often impossible and debulking procedures may be required for recurrences. As a general rule, these neoplasms do not respond well to chemotherapy or radiation.

PEARLS

- **Second most common primary retroperitoneal neoplasm after liposarcoma.**
- **Heterogeneous, large masses with areas of necrosis.**
- **Do not have calcifications.**
- **Areas of lower attenuation on CT and higher signal on T2-weighted MR are often seen, corresponding to areas of necrosis.**

ADDITIONAL IMAGES (B-C)

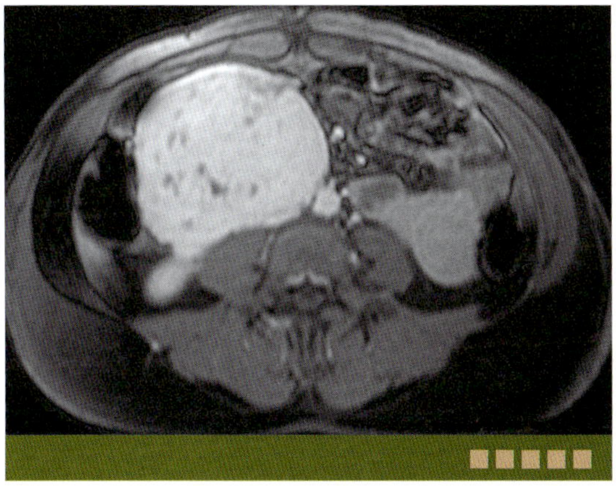

B. Corresponding axial postcontrast T1-WI shows that the mass enhances avidly, with the exception of the small areas of cystic degeneration.

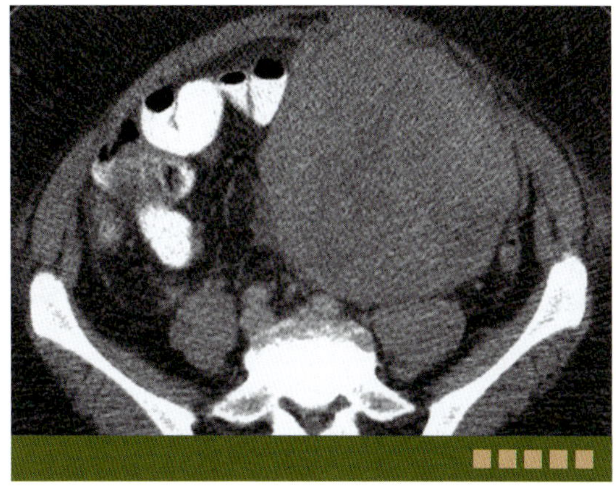

C. Axial CECT on a different patient shows a large, predominately solid, left-sided retroperitoneal mass extending into the pelvis. A few areas of relative hypodensity correspond to subtle areas of degeneration.

DIFFERENTIAL DIAGNOSES IMAGES (D-F)

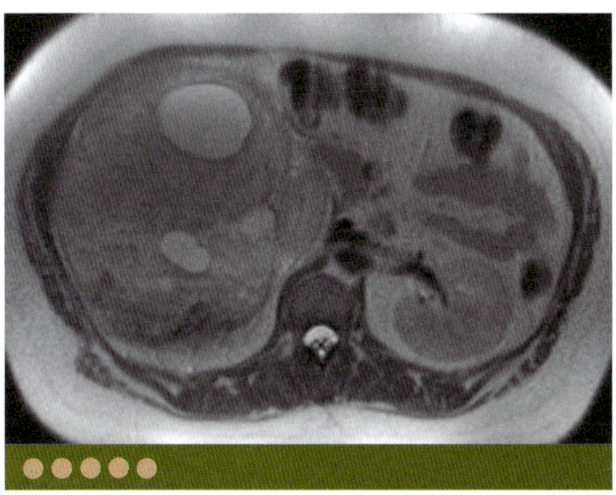

D. Malignant fibrous histiocytoma (MFH): Axial T2-WI shows a large right-sided retroperitoneal mass. The majority of the mass is isointense to soft tissue but slightly heterogeneous; there are rounded areas of high signal from necrosis.

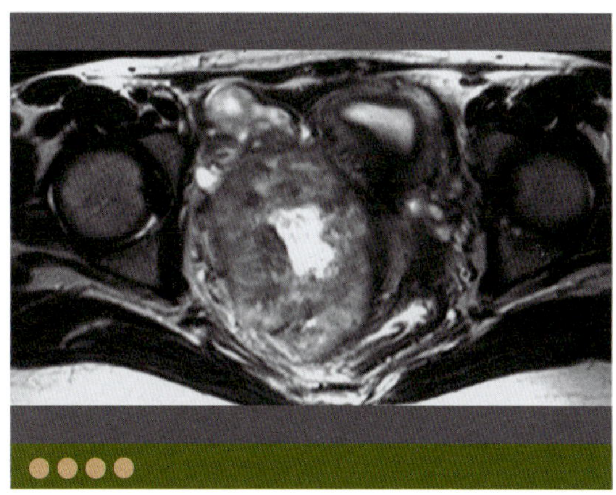

E. Schwannoma: Axial T2-WI shows a large heterogeneous, centrally hyperintense mass in the pelvis. It displaces the right ovary anteriorly and the uterus anterolaterally. This was shown on biopsy to represent a Schwannoma. (*Image courtesy of Dr Antonis Drevelengas, Interbalkan Hospital, Thessaloniki, Greece*).

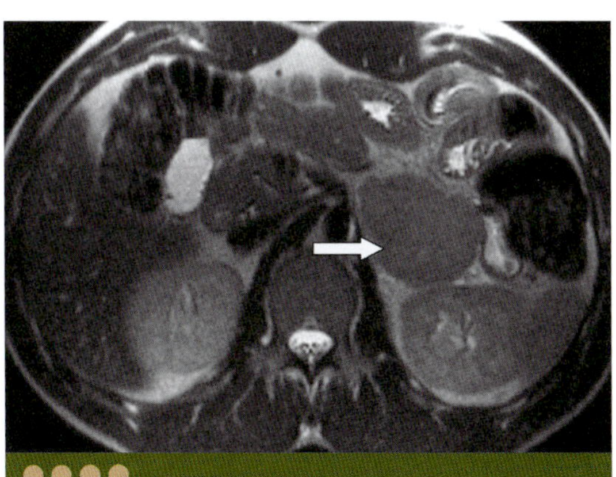

F. Metastasis: Axial T2-WI shows a left-sided retroperitoneal mass (arrow). The mass is uniformly hypointense without areas of degeneration or necrosis. On biopsy, it was shown to represent a metastasis from testicular carcinoma.

IMAGE KEY

Common

Rare

Typical

Unusual

15–2 Leiomyosarcoma of the Inferior Vena Cava

Nancy A. Hammond

PRESENTATION

Lower extremity swelling, abdominal pain, and palpable mass.

FINDINGS

Enhancing mass in the inferior vena cava (IVC).

DIFFERENTIAL DIAGNOSES

- *Bland IVC thrombus*: Nonenhancing clot in the IVC.
- *Tumor thrombus*: RCC is most common with extension of the tumor thrombus from involved kidney via the renal vein.

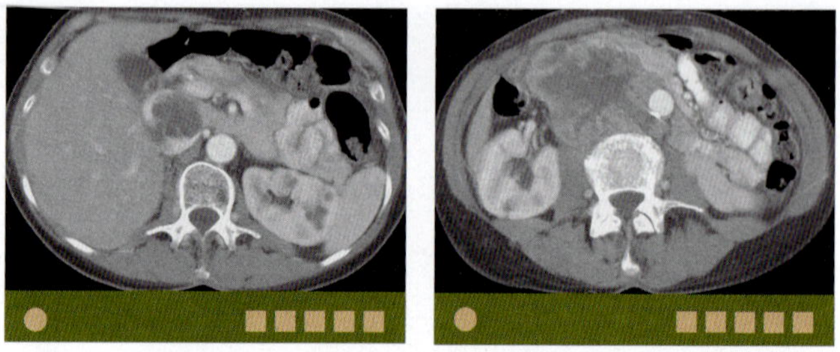

A. Axial CECT at the level of the left renal vein shows a low-density mass with some peripheral enhancement and expansion of the IVC. The renal vein is not involved.
B. Axial CECT in the same patient more inferiorly shows the extent of the mass arising from the IVC. Heterogenous enhancement with areas of low attenuation compatible with necrosis is present. A normal IVC is not appreciated at this level. Retroperitoneal extension may be present.

COMMENTS

Leiomyosarcoma of the IVC is an uncommon tumor seen more frequently in women than men with the average age of presentation in the sixth decade. Clinically, patients can present with abdominal pain, palpable abdominal mass, lower extremity edema, weight loss, and Budd-Chiari syndrome. Though the prognosis is generally poor, lesions located in the upper IVC segment have a particularly poor prognosis because of technical difficulties of achieving a radical resection of the tumor. Tumors involving the mid and lower segments of the IVC tend to have a better prognosis than those involving the upper segment of the IVC.

CT and MRI typically show an intraluminal IVC mass. Contrast-enhanced studies show heterogeneous enhancement of the mass with areas of necrosis often present. The presence of enhancement helps to distinguish this mass from bland thrombus. Extravascular extension into the retroperitoneum may or may not be present. In cases of tumors involving the mid portion of the IVC, renal vein involvement may also be present and should be evaluated for.

Leiomyosacroma of the IVC has an overall very poor prognosis and the optimal treatment regimen has not been established. Surgery in combination with chemotherapy and possibly radiation therapy is generally not curative but offers the best chance for prolonged survival.

PEARLS

- **Uncommon retroperitoneal tumor seen more commonly in women than men.**
- **Poor prognosis.**
- **Enhancing tumor within the IVC.**

ADDITIONAL IMAGES (C-E)

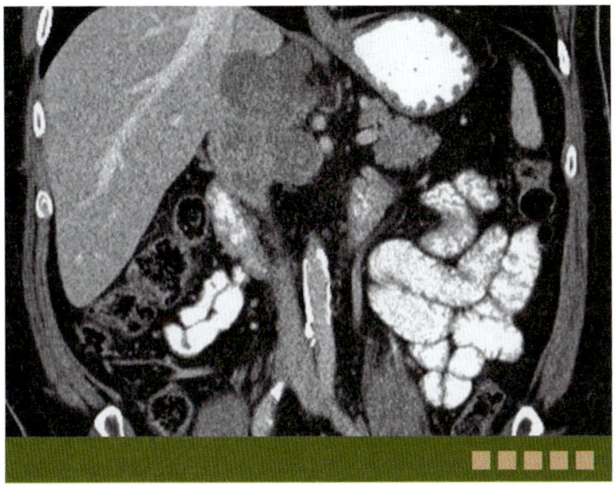

C. Coronal CECT in a different patient shows a heterogeneously enhancing retroperitoneal mass in the expected location of the IVC. A normal appearing IVC is seen more inferiorly.

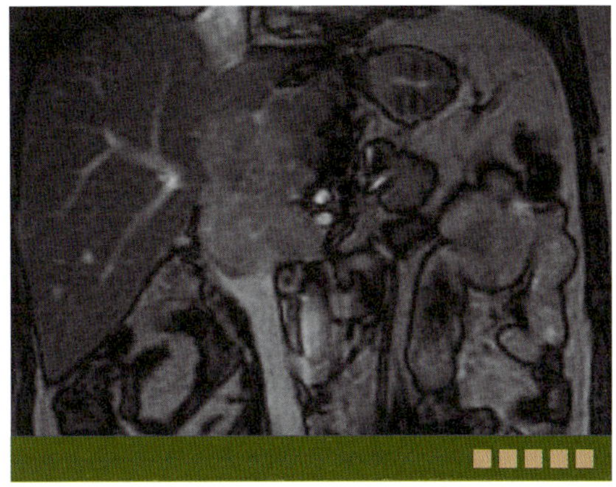

D. Coronal T2-WI in the same patient as Figure C shows a hyperintense mass expanding the IVC. Biopsy proved this to represent an IVC leimyosarcoma.

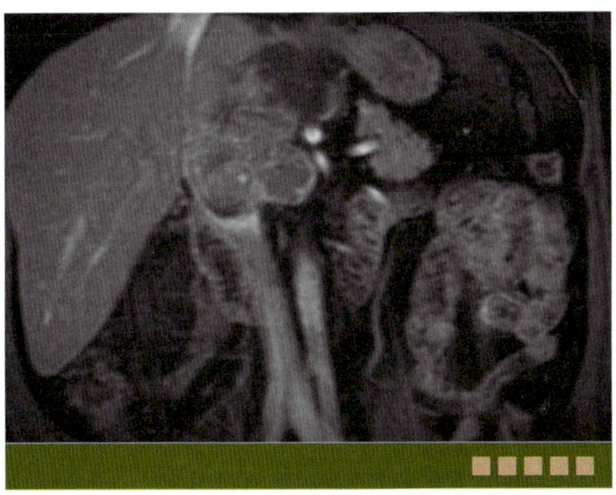

E. Coronal contrast-enhanced T1-WI shows the heterogeneous enhancement of this mass with areas of necrosis.

DIFFERENTIAL DIAGNOSES IMAGES (F-H)

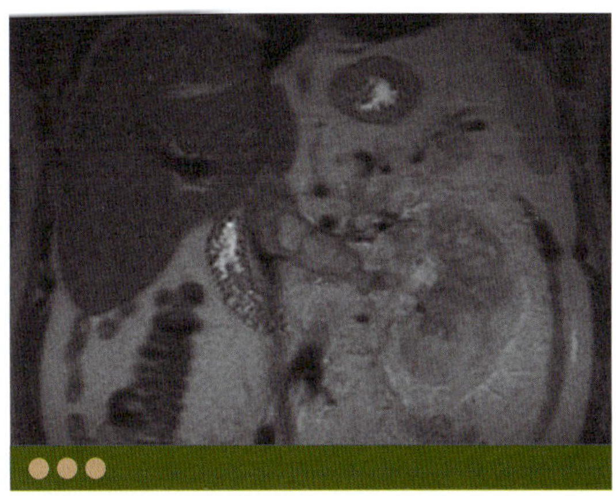

F. Tumor thrombus: Coronal T2-WI shows hyperintense tumor thrombus from a mass in the left kidney extending into the left renal vein and IVC compatible with venous extension of a renal cell carcinoma.

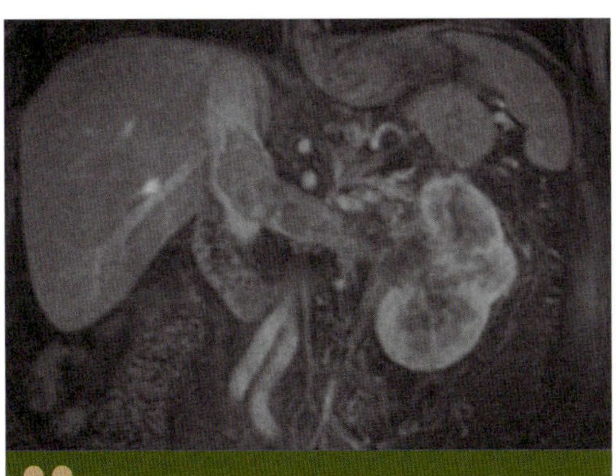

G. Tumor thrombus: Coronal contrast-enhanced T1-WI in the same patient as Figure F shows enhancement of the renal mass and tumor thrombus.

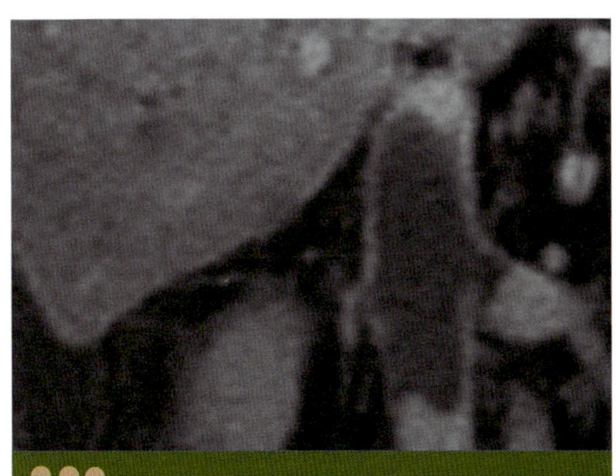

H. Bland thrombus: Coronal contrast-enhanced T1-WI shows nonenhancing thrombus in the IVC at the level of the renal veins. The patient is a liver transplant recipient with an IVC anastomotic stenosis.

IMAGE KEY

Common

Rare

Typical

Unusual

15–3 Intravenous Leiomyomatosis

David D. Casalino

PRESENTATION

Lower extremity edema and history of uterine fibroids.

FINDINGS

CT shows a mass in the IVC and involving the right common and internal iliac veins.

DIFFERENTIAL DIAGNOSES

- *Bland thrombus*: Patient may have known coagulopathy or risk factor for vascular thrombosis; no enhancement; may be hyperdense when acute; signal intensity on MR will depend on the age of the thrombus.
- *Renal, adrenal, hepatic and pancreatic tumors with venous invasion*: Primary tumor is usually apparent on imaging.
- *Retroperitoneal leiomyosarcoma*: Uncommon; primarily in women, fifth or sixth decade of life; rarely entirely intravascular; may not be able to distinguish from intravenous leiomyomatosis (IVL) if completely intraluminal and involving the entire IVC.
- *Leiomyosarcoma of the uterus and low-grade endometrial stromal sarcoma (LGESS) with gross venous invasion*: Rare occurrences with only a few case reports of each in the literature.

COMMENTS

IVL is a rare, benign smooth muscle tumor that spreads intravenously and originates from either smooth muscle of the venous wall or a uterine leiomyoma that has infiltrated a vein. IVL is usually limited to the uterus and, as a result, may be an incidental diagnosis after routine hysterectomy. IVL may extend through uterine and ovarian veins, through iliac veins, and into the IVC and heart. Extension into the renal veins, adrenal veins, and pulmonary arteries has also been reported. The majority of patients with IVL are white, premenopausal, and parous. Patients with IVL may present with symptoms related to uterine leiomyoma, venous occlusion, cardiac failure, or pulmonary involvement or sudden death related to tumor extension into the right atrium.

Imaging of IVL may include ultrasound and CT, but MR is particularly helpful because of multiplanar imaging capability, ease of MR arteriography and venography and ability to evaluate the extent of tumor. On CT, the tumor usually shows prominent homogeneous enhancement. The tumor may not be apparent or may be indistinguishable from bland thrombus if contrast is not administered. On T1-weighted MR imaging, the tumor may be heterogeneous or homogeneous and is usually hypointense compared to normal muscle tissue. On T2-weighted imaging, the tumor is usually heterogeneous and slightly hyperintense. On postcontrast imaging, the tumor shows prominent homogeneous enhancement.

Complete surgical excision is the treatment of choice and includes the affected veins, uterus, and ovaries owing to the estrogen dependence of the tumor. Antiestrogens may be given when tumor is unresectable or to control for incomplete resection or recurrence of the tumor. Because IVL may recur after resection, long-term follow-up of patients is recommended and generally includes imaging.

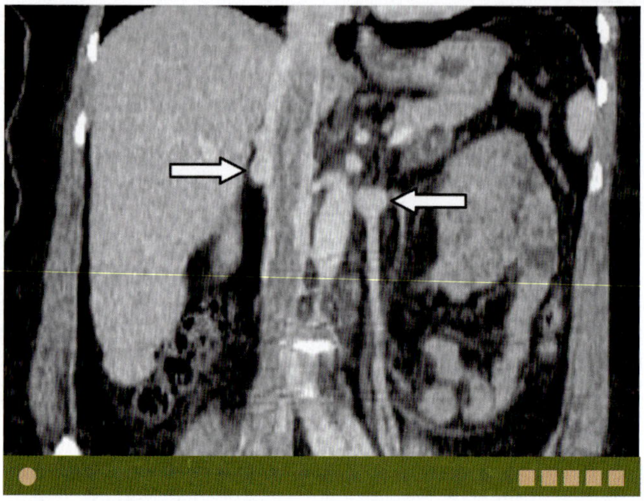

A. Coronal CECT shows a mass in the IVC and involving the right common and internal iliac veins. The renal veins (arrows) do not contain tumor.

PEARLS

- **IVL should be considered in a patient with uterine fibroids or history of uterine fibroids and intravenous tumor involving pelvic veins.**
- **Histopathologic diagnosis must be made because leiomyosarcomas of the retroperitoneum and uterus and LGESS may be associated with similar imaging findings.**
- **MR imaging offers advantages over ultrasonography and CT, particularly in surgical planning and posttreatment assessment.**
- **IVL will show prominent enhancement.**

ADDITIONAL IMAGES (B-D)

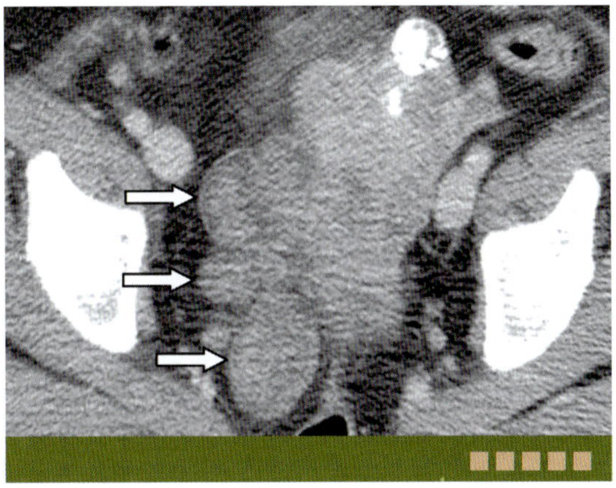

B. Axial CECT shows multinodular, enhancing tumor (arrows) in the right pelvis. This tumor is contiguous with the tumor in the right iliac veins and adjacent to the uterus, which has multiple leiomyomas.

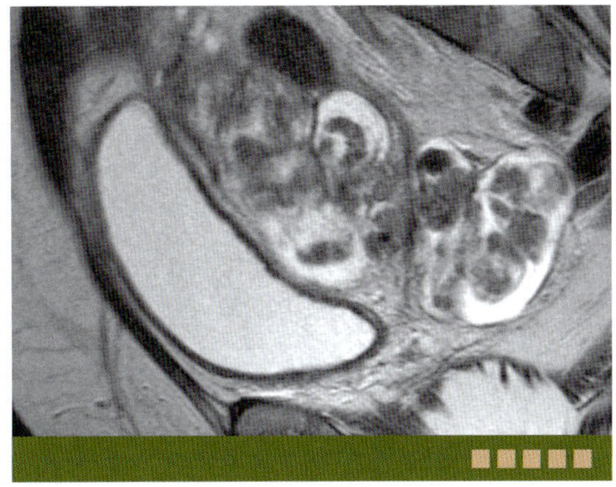

C. Sagittal T2-WI, 4 cm right of midline, shows a tangle of tubular structures, which represent dilated, tortuous pelvic veins, filled with heterogeneous tumor.

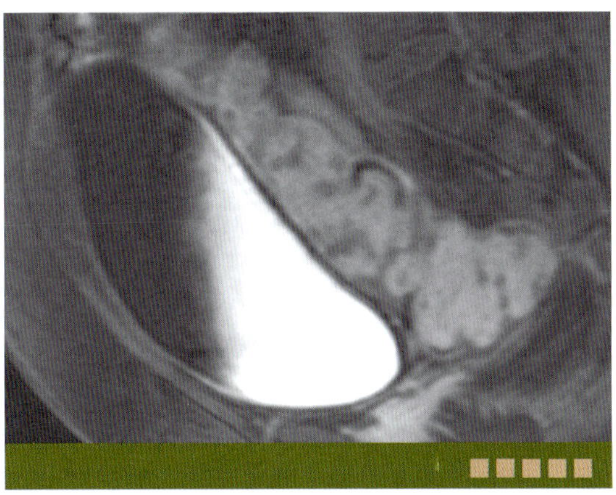

D. Sagittal contrast-enhanced T1-WI, at the same level, shows diffuse enhancement of the tumor.

DIFFERENTIAL DIAGNOSES IMAGES (E-G)

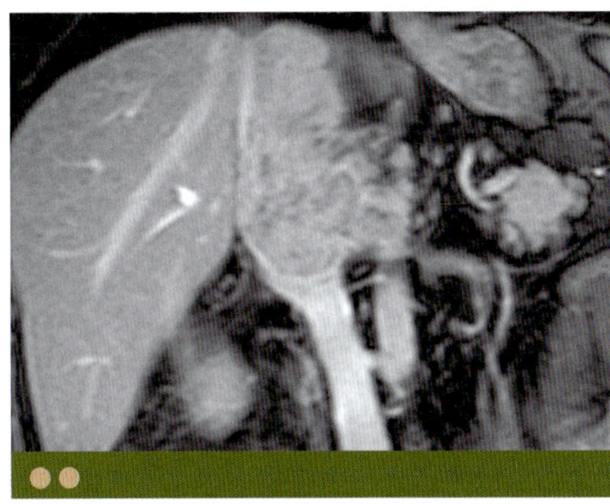

E. Retroperitoneal leiomyosarcoma: Coronal contrast-enhanced T1-WI shows a large, heterogeneously enhancing mass that is partial intraluminal and partial extraluminal and is not arising from a solid organ. These findings are virtually pathognomonic for a retroperitoneal leiomyosarcoma.

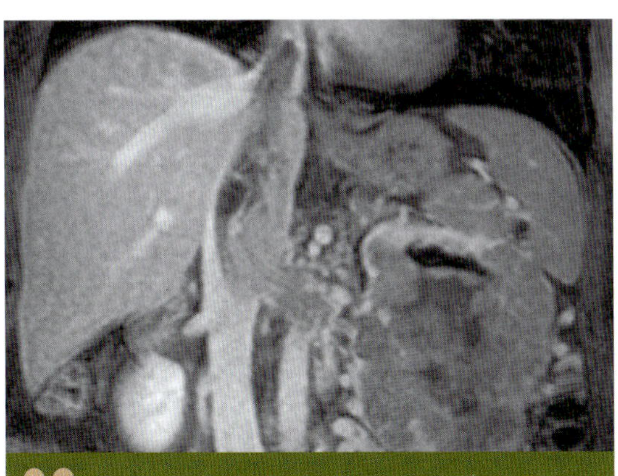

F. Tumor thrombus from RCC: Coronal contrast-enhanced T1-WI shows a large, heterogeneously enhancing left renal mass that extends into the renal vein, IVC, and right atrium.

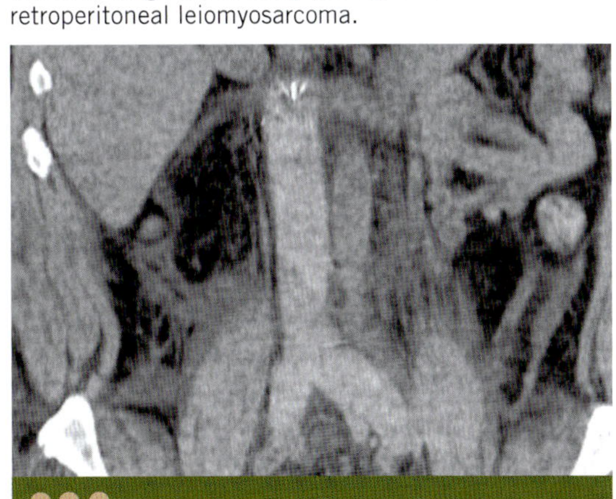

G. Bland thrombus: Coronal NECT shows hyperdense thrombus expanding the IVC and common iliac veins in a severely injured trauma patient, who has an IVC filter.

IMAGE KEY

Common
●●●●●
●●●●
●●●
●●
●
Rare

Typical
■■■■■
■■■■
■■■
■■
■
Unusual

15–4 Retroperitoneal Liposarcoma

Paul Nikolaidis

PRESENTATION

Abdominal mass/fullness, abdominal and back pain, lower extremity swelling.

FINDINGS

CT shows a large fatty retroperitoneal mass which causes significant displacement of surrounding organs.

DIFFERENTIAL DIAGNOSES

- *Renal angiomyolipoma*: An angiomyolipoma may enlarge significantly; usually the presence of a "claw sign" at its interface with the renal parenchyma should indicate its renal origin.
- *Fat necrosis or inflammation*: There may be history of surgery, and there should be no significant mass effect on adjacent organs.
- *Adrenal myelolipoma*: A myelolipoma may enlarge significantly, and in some instances, it may be difficult to determine that it originates from the adrenal gland.
- *Other retroperitoneal sarcomas*: In cases where there are no fatty elements in a liposarcoma (eg, pleomorphic subtype), it will be indistinguishable from several other neoplasms, necessitating biopsy for definitive diagnosis.

COMMENTS

Liposarcomas are the most common malignant primary retroperitoneal neoplasm. They are divided into several categories, including lipogenic, myxoid, pleomorphic, and round cell (ranging from well-differentiated to poorly differentiated). The classic distinguishing characteristic of liposarcomas is the presence of fat, although this is more reliably found in the lipogenic subtype and only variably present in the high-grade pleomorphic type. Liposarcomas tend to displace, rather than invade, surrounding structures. On CT, a lipogenic liposarcoma may be indistinguishable from a benign lipoma, although it typically contains solid or infiltrative enhancing components in addition to the low attenuation fat found in lipomas. The lipogenic form does not metastasize, but may very rarely dedifferentiate to a more aggressive type with metastatic potential. Myxoid liposarcomas may show areas of low (fluid) density on CT. They rarely occur in the retroperitoneum. The myxoid component is also isointense to fluid on MR. Pleomorphic liposarcomas have soft tissue density similar to muscle on CT. On T1-weighted MR images, pleomorphic liposarcomas have signal similar to muscle; however on T2-WI, they typically show higher intensity. Higher grade liposarcomas may not contain macroscopic fat, rendering them indistinguishable from other solid neoplasms such as leiomyosarcoma and MFH.

Complete surgical resection is necessary. Complete excision is often impossible and debulking procedures may be required for recurrence. They frequently recur and metastasize, and close follow-up imaging is needed.

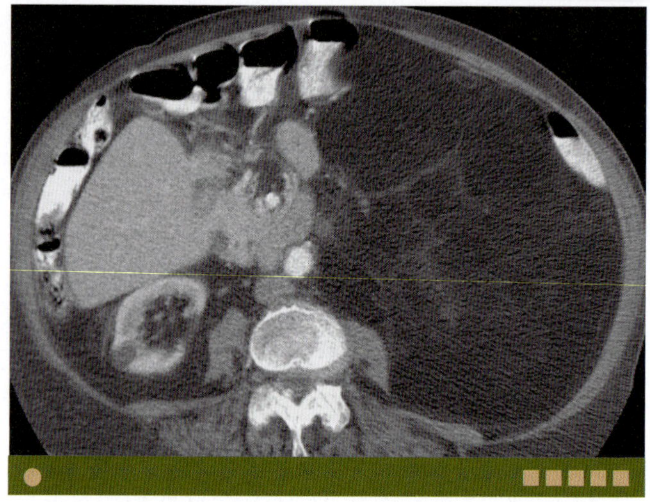

A. Axial CECT shows a large fatty retroperitoneal mass with very few linear and solid components. It causes significant displacement of surrounding structures.

PEARLS

- **Liposarcomas tend to displace, rather than invade, surrounding organs.**
- **Not all liposarcomas are pure fat in density.**
- **Some liposarcomas may not contain fat and may be indistinguishable from leiomyosarcoma and MFH.**
- **Treatment of choice is surgery, although complete excision is often impossible and debulking procedures may be required for recurrence.**

ADDITIONAL IMAGES (B-D)

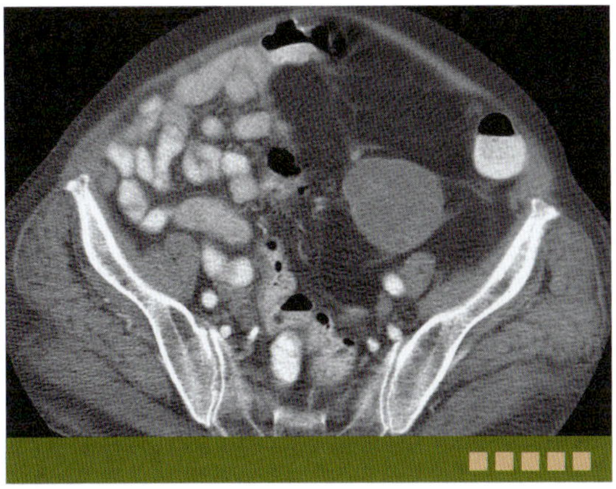

B. Axial CECT on the same patient shows that the large retroperitoneal mass extends into the pelvis, where an approximately 4-cm, nonfatty, soft-tissue nodule is seen anterior to the left common iliac vessels.

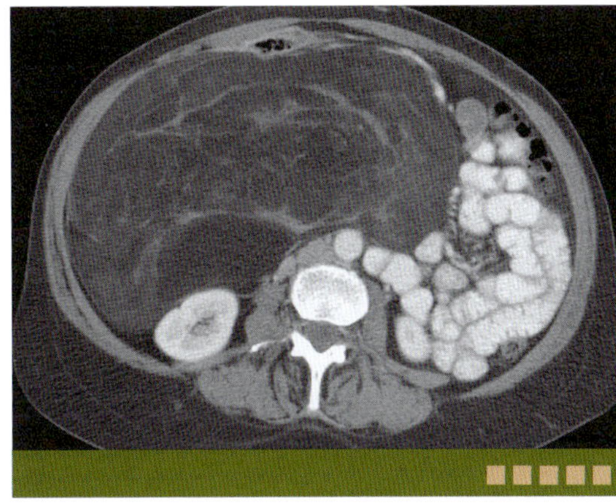

C. Axial CECT on a different patient shows a large fatty mass anterior to the right kidney extending to the left of midline. Note the areas of fat stranding and the numerous thin and slightly thickened linear hyperdense striations within the mass.

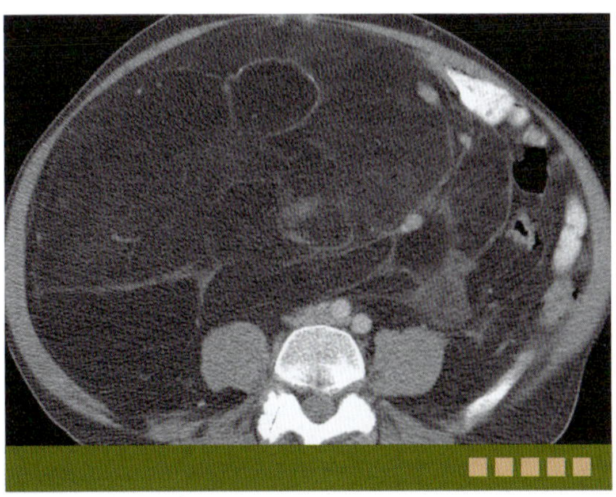

D. Axial CECT on a different patient shows a very large predominately fatty mass occupying almost the entire abdominal cavity. It significantly displaces the bowel toward the left.

DIFFERENTIAL DIAGNOSES IMAGES (E-G)

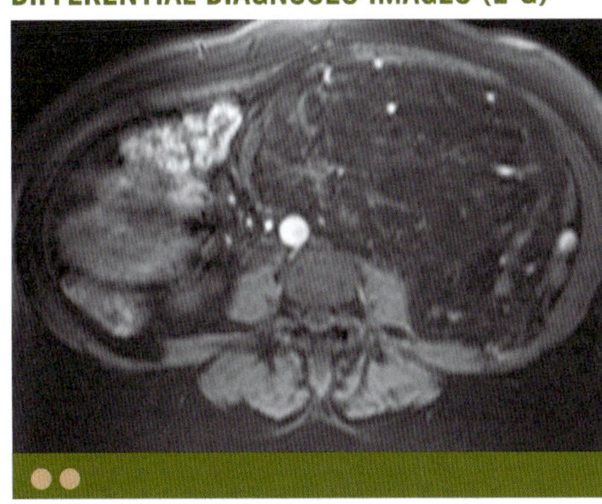

E. Large renal angiomyolipoma: Axial contrast-enhanced T1-WI shows a large, predominately fatty, left-sided retroperitoneal mass containing several vessels and striations, indistinguishable from a liposarcoma.

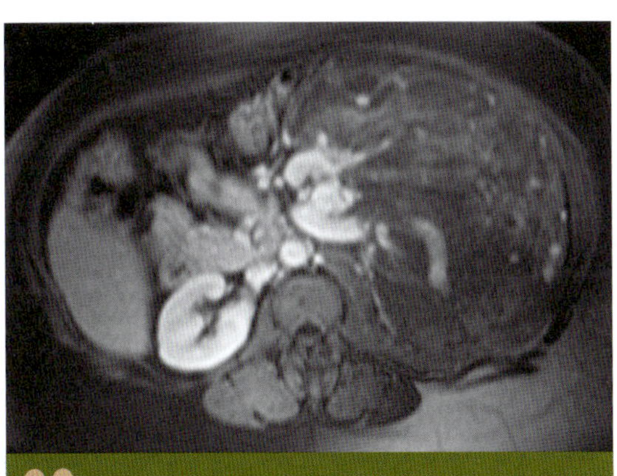

F. Large renal angiomyolipoma: Axial contrast-enhanced T1-WI on the same patient obtained further superiorly shows that the large fatty mass emanates from the left kidney. This mass was successfully resected surgically.

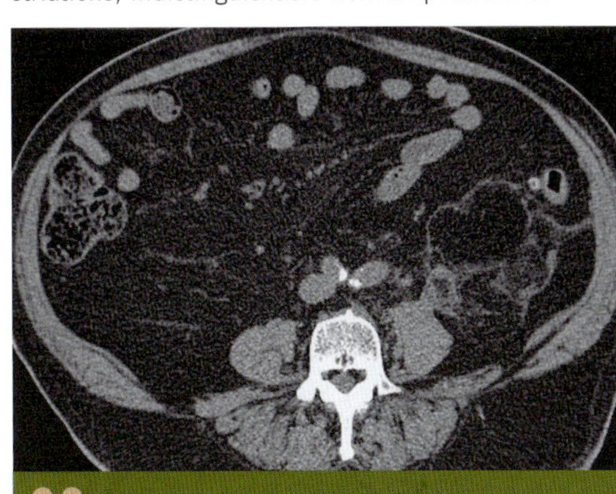

G. Retroperitoneal fat necrosis/scarring following nephrectomy: Axial NECT on a patient with history of left nephrectomy for renal cell carcinoma shows an apparent complex fatty lesion similar to a liposarcoma. This merely represented an area of postsurgical scarring and was stable on subsequent CT examinations.

IMAGE KEY

Common

Rare

Typical

Unusual

15–5 Retroperitoneal Malignant Fibrous Histiocytoma

Paul Nikolaidis

PRESENTATION

Abdominal mass/fullness; abdominal and back pain; lower extremity swelling.

FINDINGS

MR shows a large, heterogeneous retroperitoneal mass with moderate enhancement and a few areas of necrosis.

DIFFERENTIAL DIAGNOSES

- *Leiomyosarcoma*: May show cystic degeneration and central necrosis more commonly than other sarcomas; fat and calcifications are not typically present.
- *Lymphoma*: Usually a more homogeneous appearing mass; may be more uniformly hypovascular; adenopathy may be present in other distant locations.
- *Other primary or metastatic retroperitoneal neoplasms*: Differentiation is often difficult. Several primary and metastatic malignant lesions of the retroperitoneum may have overlapping features.

COMMENTS

Malignant fibrous histiocytoma (MFH) is the third most common retroperitoneal sarcoma. It is divided into four major subtypes: storiform-pleomorphic, myxoid, giant cell, and inflammatory. Many rare mesenchymal tumors that were classified under different names in the past now fall under the umbrella of MFH. They typically do not present until late, when patients become symptomatic from compression of adjacent structures. Symptoms are nonspecific and can include abdominal and back pain, lower extremity swelling, weight loss, anorexia, nausea, and urinary obstruction/frequency.

On CT, MFHs are typically heterogeneous masses which show at least moderate enhancement. They do not contain fat, but may contain calcifications, which are very rare in liposarcomas and leiomyosarcomas, and therefore, can be a useful distinguishing characteristic. However, calcification is only found in approximately 25% of the cases of MFH, limiting its usefulness.

On MR, they are usually large, heterogeneous masses which may show low-to-intermediate signal on T1-WI and areas of high signal on T2-WI. MFHs are moderately hypervascular following gadolinium administration.

Treatment of choice is surgery, although complete excision is typically not feasible and subsequent debulking procedures may be required. They usually do not respond well to chemotherapy or radiation and 5-year survival is poor.

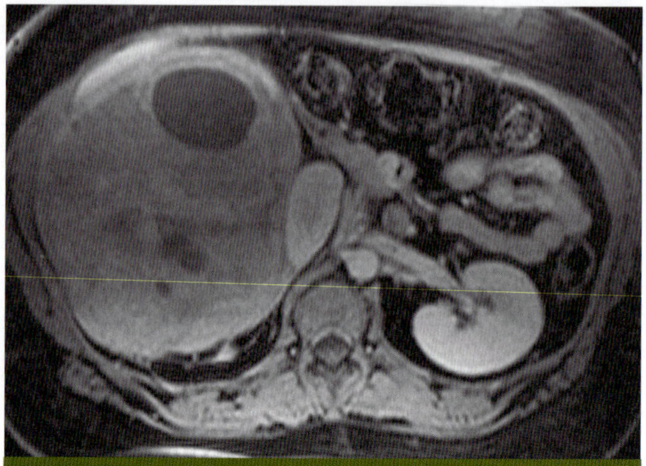

A. Axial contrast-enhanced T1-WI shows a large right-sided retroperitoneal mass. The majority of the mass enhances but there are areas of nonenhancement from necrosis.

PEARLS

- **Third most common primary retroperitoneal neoplasm after liposarcoma and leiomyosarcoma.**
- **Heterogeneous masses that may contain calcification on CT (in approximately 25% of the cases).**
- **They enhance on CT and MR.**
- **Treatment of choice is surgery, although complete excision is often impossible.**
- **Generally do not respond well to treatment with a poor 5-year survival rate.**

ADDITIONAL IMAGES (B-C)

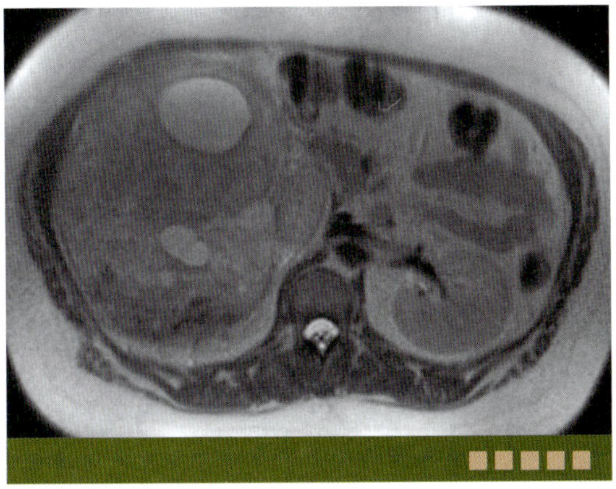

B. Corresponding T2-WI shows the large retroperitoneal mass with rounded hyperintense foci corresponding to areas of necrosis and cystic degeneration.

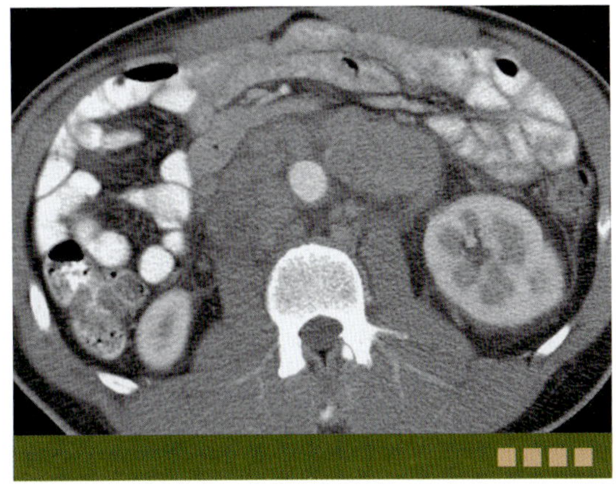

C. Contrast-enhanced CT scan on a different patient shows a dominant left para-aortic mass with extensive surrounding lymphadenopathy. This mass was shown to represent a retroperitoneal MFH. This appearance is indistinguishable from lymphoma or other metastatic neoplasms.

DIFFERENTIAL DIAGNOSES IMAGES (D-F)

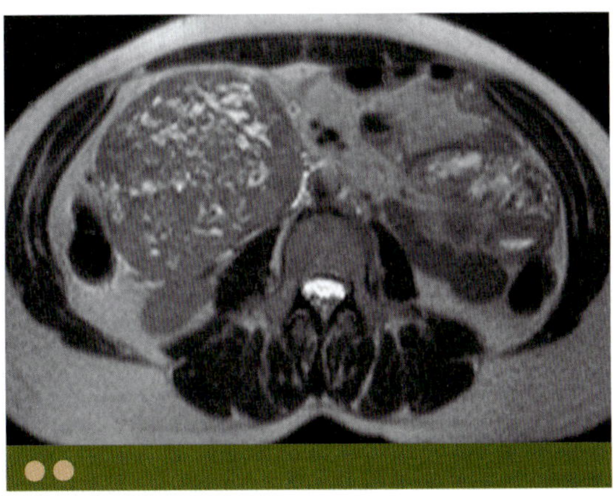

D. Leiomyosarcoma: Axial T2-WI shows a large right-sided retroperitoneal mass with multiple T2-bright foci, corresponding to areas of cystic degeneration.

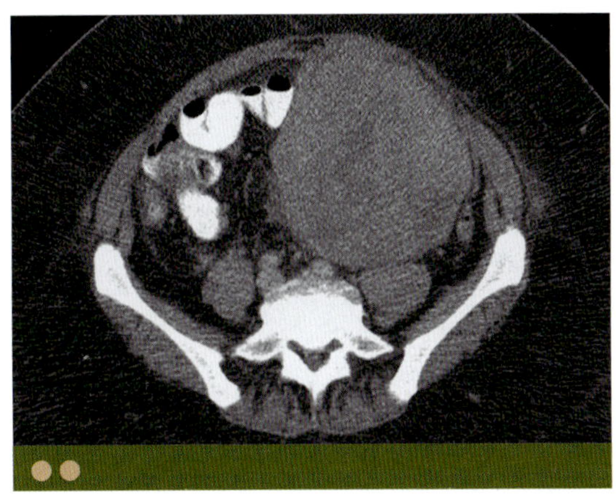

E. Leiomyosarcoma: Axial CECT on a different patient shows a large, predominately solid, left-sided retroperitoneal mass extending into the pelvis. A few areas of relative hypodensity correspond to subtle areas of cystic degeneration.

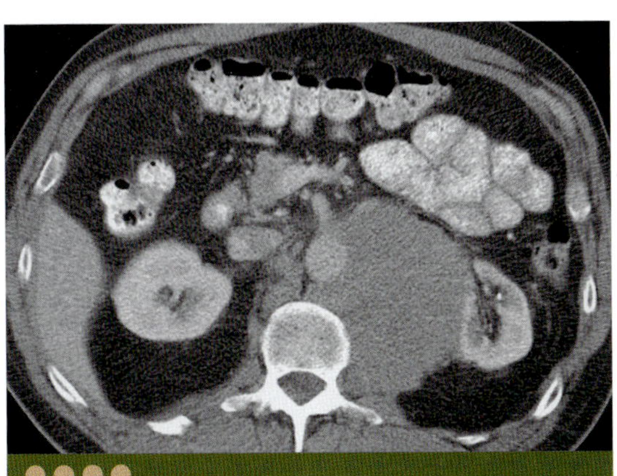

F. Lymphoma: Axial CECT shows a large left-sided retroperitoneal mass, which is inseparable from the aorta. It also displaces the left kidney laterally. This was shown on biopsy to represent lymphoma.

IMAGE KEY

Common

Rare

Typical

Unusual

15–6 Retroperitoneal Lymphoma

Paul Nikolaidis

PRESENTATION

Fever, weight loss, and anorexia.

FINDINGS

CT shows a large midline mildly enhancing retroperitoneal soft tissue mass completely surrounding the aorta.

DIFFERENTIAL DIAGNOSES

- *Retroperitoneal fibrosis*: Confluent soft tissue is seen surrounding the aorta; may be indistinguishable on imaging rendering biopsy necessary.
- *Metastatic lymphadenopathy*: Often difficult to distinguish, unless biopsied. Patients may have a known primary malignancy (ie, cervical, endometrial or prostate cancer).
- *Castleman disease*: Markedly hyperenhancing nodes primarily in the mediastinum; biopsy usually necessary.
- *Retroperitoneal hemorrhage*: Areas of hemorrhage may be more ill-defined in contrast to more discrete retroperitoneal soft tissue masses.
- *Primary soft tissue sarcomas*: May present as a large solid retroperitoneal mass; in some cases there may be areas of cystic degeneration (leiomyosarcoma), heterogeneity and possible calcifications (MFH).

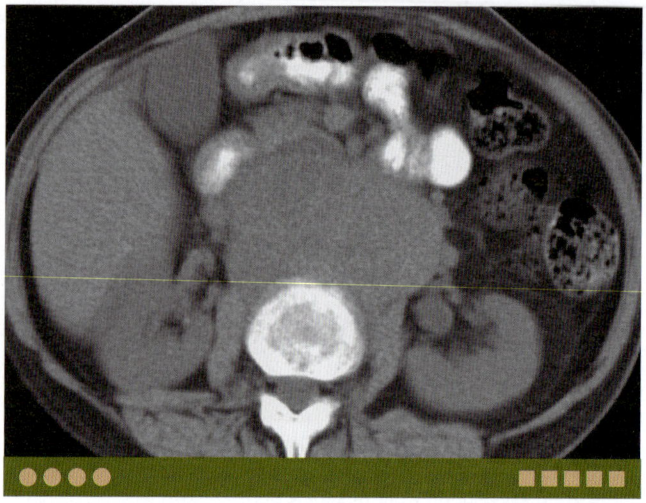

A. Axial noncontrast CT of the abdomen shows a large midline retroperitoneal mass surrounding the aorta. The mass is approximately isodense to the kidneys on this noncontrast examination.

COMMENTS

Lymphomas are a malignancy of lymphoid cell origin. Their presentation, manifestations and prognosis largely depend on histologic subtype and stage. Non-Hodgkin lymphoma may often manifest as adenopathy and/or extranodal disease, unlike Hodgkin lymphoma, which primarily affects nodal chains, with extranodal disease being a late manifestation of widespread disease. Staging of lymphoma is largely dependent on the extent of nodal involvement. The Ann Arbor system for staging Hodgkin lymphoma, increases the stage of the disease as more nodes and more locations become involved. Advancing stage alters the treatment options and prognosis. Retroperitoneal lymphadenopathy is frequent in lymphoma.

CT is excellent for diagnosing and staging lymphoma involving the retroperitoneum and elsewhere. Mild contrast enhancement is typically seen, and lymph node enlargement is usually assessed by measuring the short axis diameter. Fluorine-18-deoxyglucose positron emission tomography (FDG-PET) can be overlaid with traditional CT images for added accuracy in staging when compared to the same images viewed side-by-side. FDG-PET shows increased uptake in Hodgkin lymphoma and several types of non-Hodgkin lymphoma. MR also allows for easy identification of enlarged lymph nodes, particularly on spin echo T1-WI and heavily T2-weighted sequences.

PEARLS

- **The retroperitoneum is commonly involved in patients with lymphoma.**
- **Staging of lymphoma and treatment planning is largely dependent on the extent of nodal involvement.**
- **CT is excellent for diagnosing and staging lymphoma; enlarged nodes usually show mild enhancement but may also be necrotic.**
- **CT combined with FDG-PET further increases diagnostic accuracy.**

ADDITIONAL IMAGES (B-C)

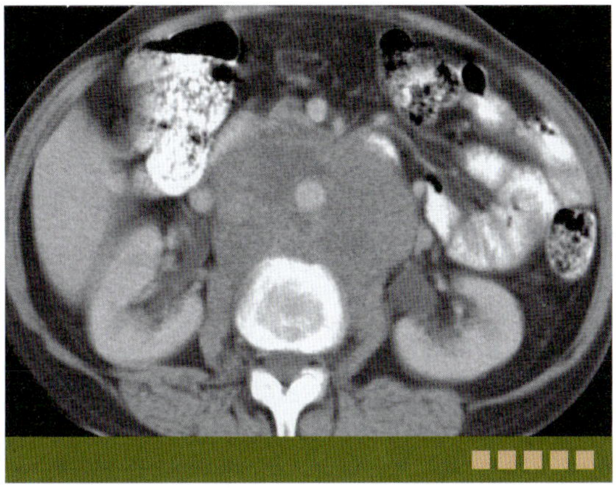

B. Corresponding axial CECT on the same patient shows a large soft tissue mass which enhances less than the liver and kidneys. There are some areas of further decreased enhancement immediately to the right of the aorta, likely from necrosis. The mass surrounds the aorta entirely, which it also displaces anteriorly.

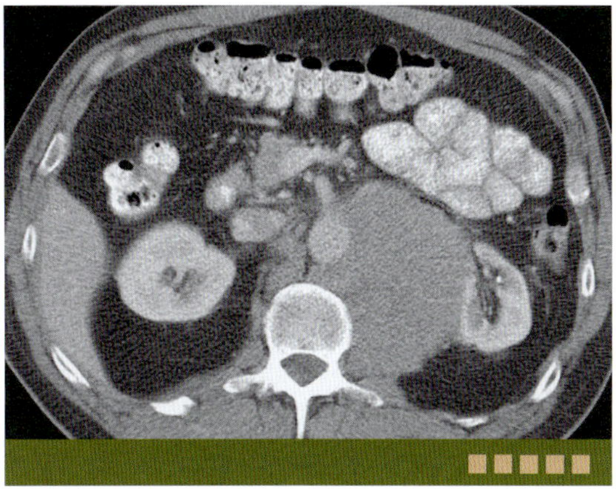

C. Axial CECT on another patient shows a large left-sided retroperitoneal mass which surrounds a significant portion of the aorta and portion of the superior mesenteric artery. It also displaces the left kidney laterally. It enhances to a lesser degree than the kidneys and liver.

DIFFERENTIAL DIAGNOSES IMAGES (D-E)

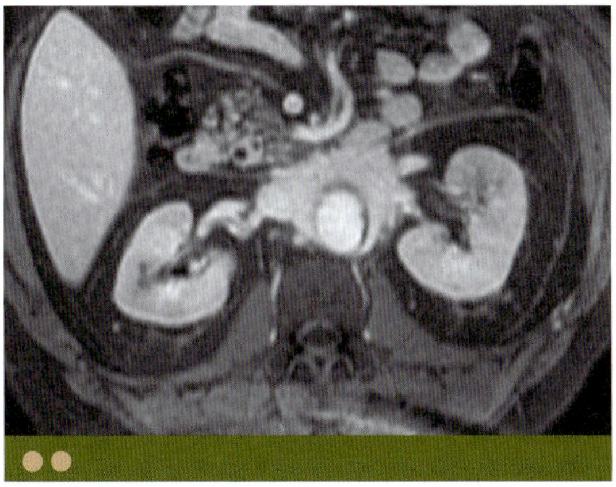

D. Retroperitoneal fibrosis: Axial contrast-enhanced T1-WI shows an enhancing soft tissue mass surrounding a significant portion of the aorta. This was biopsy proven to represent RPF.

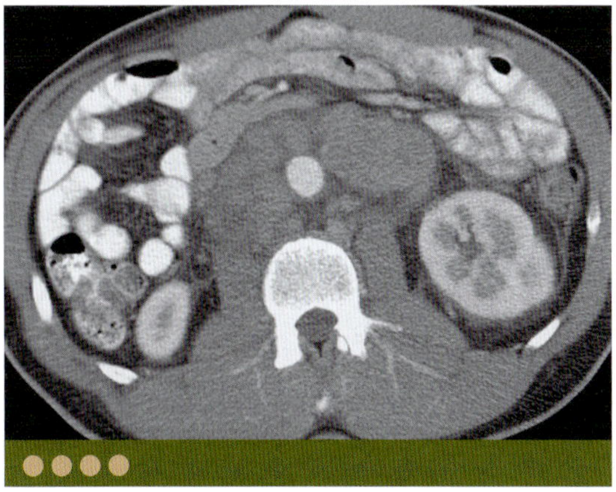

E. Retroperitoneal metastases: Axial CECT on a patient with a history of a primary sarcoma of the right thigh shows significant retroperitoneal lymphadenopathy surrounding and slightly lifting the aorta anteriorly. This appearance is indistinguishable from lymphoma on imaging.

IMAGE KEY

Common
●●●●●
●●●●
●●●
●●
●
Rare

Typical
■■■■■
■■■■
■■■
■■
■
Unusual

15–7 Retroperitoneal Metastases

Paul Nikolaidis

PRESENTATION

Asymptomatic, weight loss, ureteral obstruction.

FINDINGS

Enlarged, enhancing retroperitoneal lymph nodes in a patient with history of a right thigh sarcoma.

DIFFERENTIAL DIAGNOSES

- *Castleman disease*: Rare entity, with avidly enhancing nodes or soft tissue masses involving primarily the mediastinum but also seen in the retroperitoneum; biopsy is usually necessary.
- *Mycobacterial infection*: Typically hypodense, necrotic nodes in immune deficient patients, because of TB or MAI infection.
- *Reactive adenopathy*: May enhance to the same degree as malignant adenopathy; nodes are generally not significantly enlarged, but may be impossible to distinguish on imaging.
- *Retroperitoneal fibrosis*: Confluent soft tissue surrounding the aorta; in many instances biopsy is necessary. Benign and (less frequently) malignant causes of RPF have been described.
- *Primary retroperitoneal neoplasms*: May present as a large solitary retroperitoneal mass in patients without a history of any other primary malignancy.

COMMENTS

Metastatic lymphadenopathy in the retroperitoneum is most commonly associated with testicular cancer which characteristically spreads to the para-aortic nodes, but can also occur in renal, bladder, prostate, cervical, and ovarian cancer. Retroperitoneal lymphatic spread may also occur with cancers of the pancreas, breast and colon. Metastases must be differentiated from primary tumors that also arise in the retroperitoneal space (sarcomas, germ cell tumors, lymphomas). Malignant retroperitoneal masses may also occur from direct invasion from adjacent primary intra-abdominal neoplasms, including the pancreas, stomach, and duodenum.

Less commonly, patients may present with malignant RPF (approximately 8% of the patients with RPF). In addition to lymphomas, this occurs with sarcomas, and many carcinomas, including breast, lung, stomach, colon, bladder, prostate, and cervical cancer. This is because of a marked desmoplastic response to metastatic tumor cells. Malignant RPF may be distinguished from retroperitoneal lymph node metastases as the ureter is typically displaced medially.

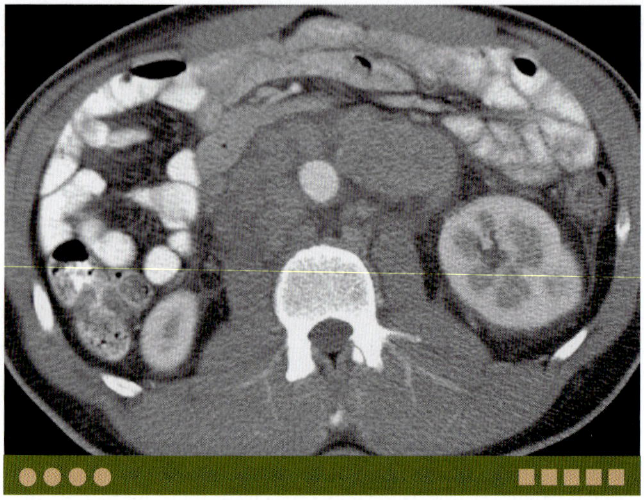

A. Axial CECT shows extensive metastatic retroperitoneal adenopathy. The patient had a known primary sarcoma of the right thigh.

Cross-sectional imaging (CT and MR) are the preferred modalities for the evaluation of retroperitoneal metastases. Metastases can infiltrate the lymph nodes without enlarging them, thus making diagnosis by CT size criteria alone difficult. CT, combined with FDG-PET, further increases diagnostic accuracy in PET-avid metastases; MR lymphangiography with USPIO may also aid in the diagnosis. In many instances, staging lymphadenectomy is required for accurate diagnosis.

PEARLS

- **Usually from pelvic malignancies, most commonly testicular cancer.**
- **Malignant RPF may occur because of a desmoplastic response to metastatic tumor cells.**
- **CT and MR are excellent modalities; however involved nodes may not be enlarged by size criteria.**
- **CT with FDG-PET increases diagnostic accuracy in PET-avid malignancies.**

ADDITIONAL IMAGES (B-C)

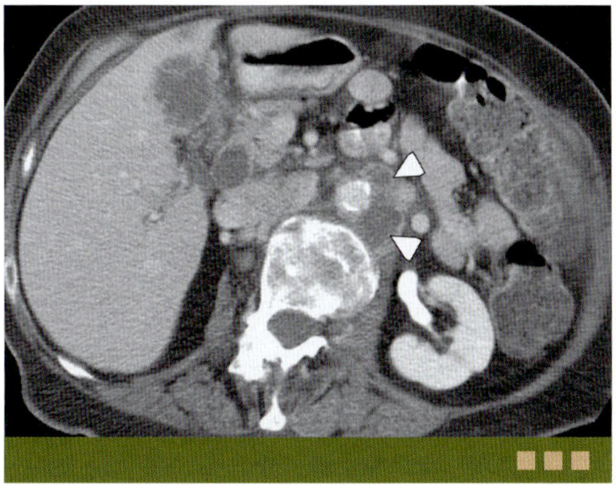

B. Axial CECT on a different patient with a history of colon cancer shows necrotic retroperitoneal adenopathy (arrowheads).

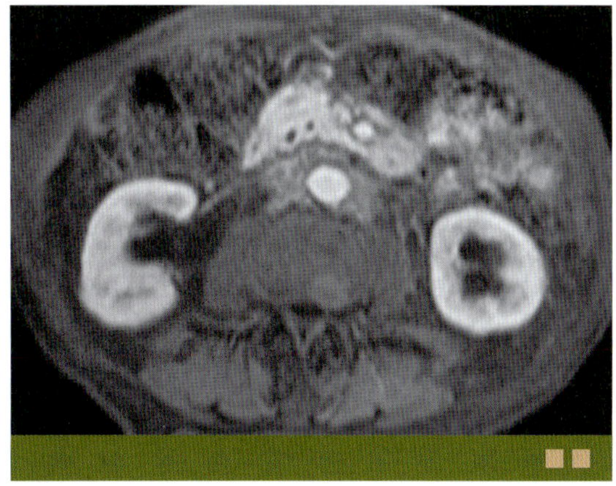

C. Axial contrast-enhanced T1-WI, shows a confluent soft tissue mass surrounding the aorta, indistinguishable from RPF. CT-guided biopsy confirmed metastatic bladder cancer.

DIFFERENTIAL DIAGNOSES IMAGES (D-G)

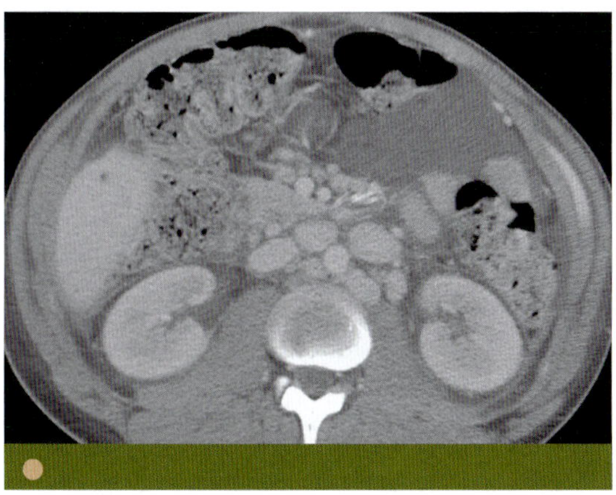

D. Castleman disease: Axial CECT on a 40- year-old male patient shows multiple enhancing retroperitoneal lymph nodes. These were biopsy proven to be attributable to Castleman disease.

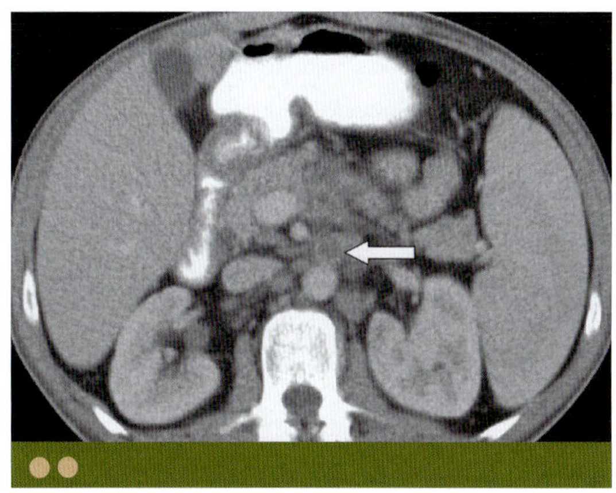

E. Mycobacterial infection: Axial CECT shows retroperitoneal adenopathy, and several lymph nodes are centrally hypodense (arrow). The patient had no known primary malignancy, but was immune compromised. This was biopsy proven to be secondary to MAI.

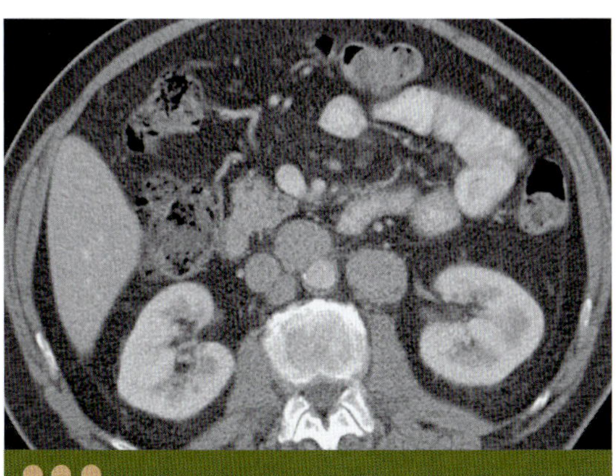

F. Reactive lymph nodes: Axial CECT on a different patient shows retroperitoneal adenopathy. Lymphoma was suspected and a percutaneous biopsy was performed. These lymph nodes were shown to be reactive.

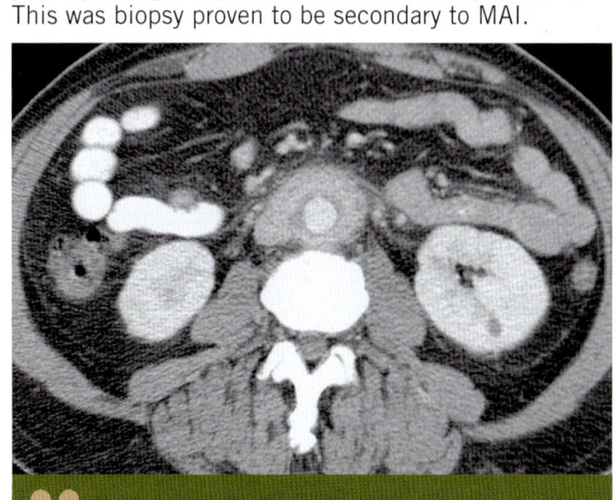

G. Retroperitoneal fibrosis: Axial CECT shows an enhancing retroperitoneal mass, which encircles the abdominal aorta. This was biopsy proven to represent RPF.

IMAGE KEY

Common

Rare

Typical

Unusual

15–8 Retroperitoneal Schwannoma

Paul Nikolaidis

PRESENTATION

Typically asymptomatic; incidentally discovered on imaging.

FINDINGS

CT shows a well-demarcated round peripherally enhancing mass with an area of central hypodensity from cystic degeneration.

DIFFERENTIAL DIAGNOSES

- *Leiomyosarcoma*: Typically a large solid mass with areas of cystic degeneration and central necrosis; may be difficult to distinguish.
- *Lymphoma*: Adenopathy may be present in other locations.
- *Retroperitoneal metastases*: Metastatic lesions of the retroperitoneum may have overlapping features.
- *MFH*: Generally a moderately hypervascular mass, more heterogeneous, and may contain calcifications.
- *Ganglioneuroma*: Typically an oval, crescentic, or lobulated hypodense mass with only mild-to-moderate postcontrast enhancement. There are occasional calcifications; they classically surround vessels without compressing their lumina.

COMMENTS

Schwannomas are benign nerve sheath tumors. They are typically seen in patients aged 20 to 50 and are more common in females. Schwannomas are almost always slow-growing and nonaggressive. They are often located in the head and neck as well as the flexor surfaces of the extremities, but may also be found in the pelvis and retroperitoneum. Schwannomas comprise 6% of the primary retroperitoneal tumors, and are usually located in the paravertebral regions, adjacent to the kidney, or in the presacral pelvic retroperitoneum. Though most Schwannomas are generally under 5 cm in diameter, those occuring in the retroperitoneum may become quite large over time.

On CT, retroperitoneal schwannomas are well-demarcated round or oval masses that frequently demonstrate prominent hypodense areas relating to cystic degeneration. They may have calcifications. They have smooth, well-defined borders. Following contrast administration, they demonstrate variable homogeneous or heterogeneous enhancement, depending on the extent of cellularity, degeneration, and hemorrhage.

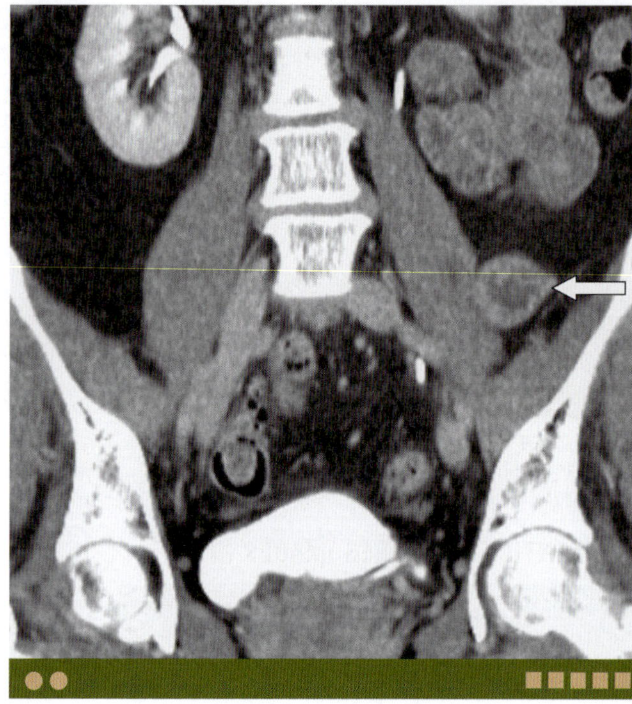

A. Coronal CECT reformation shows a centrally necrotic, peripherally enhancing mass adjacent to the left psoas (arrow). A faint fat plane between the mass and the psoas is present.

The MR appearance of retroperitoneal schwannomas is also variable, depending on the amount of solid and cystic components. Solid components are usually isointense to skeletal muscle on T1-WI. On T2-WI schwannomas are usually hyperintense, but may also be isointense to skeletal muscle.

Complete surgical resection is usually curative.

PEARLS

- **Typically have smooth, well-defined borders and an ovoid or spherical shape.**
- **Solid schwannomas are generally homogeneous masses without fat, sometimes with cystic degeneration.**
- **Usually enhance avidly following contrast administration (except for cystic spaces).**
- **Cystic schwannomas show areas of lower attenuation on CT and higher signal on T2-weighted MR.**

ADDITIONAL IMAGES (B-D)

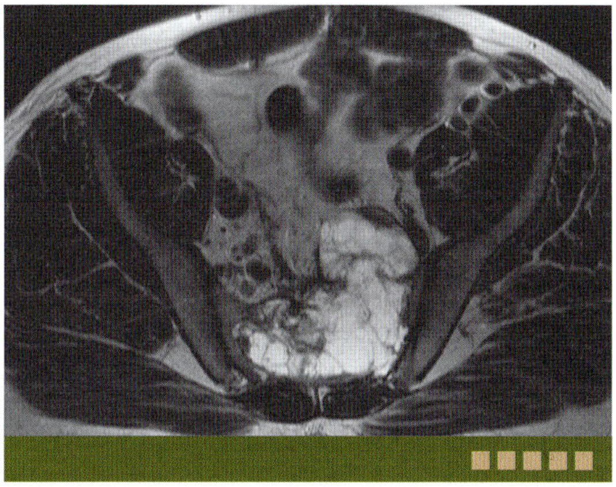

B. Axial T2-WI shows a large predominately hyperintense mass which appears cystic emanating from the left sacrum.

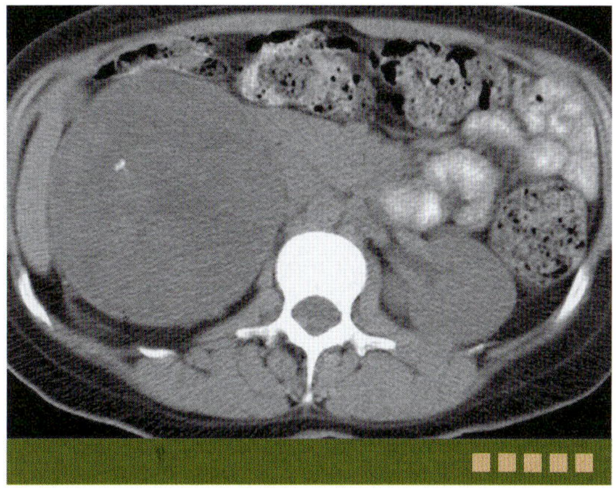

C. Axial NECT on a different patient shows a large, right-sided retroperitoneal mass containing at least one calcification.

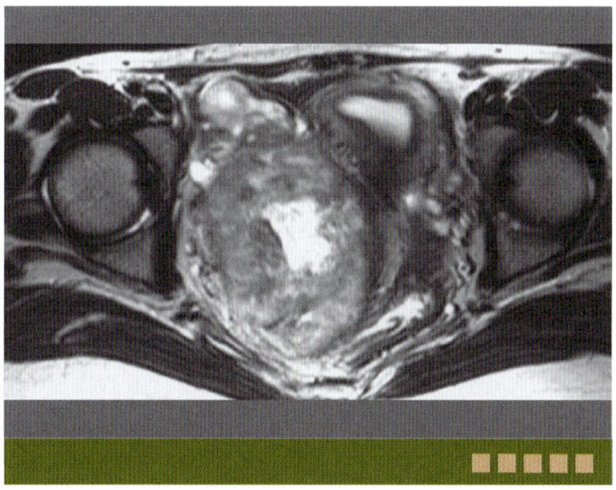

D. Axial T2-WI on another patient shows a large heterogeneous, centrally hyperintense mass in the pelvis. It displaces the right ovary anteriorly and the uterus anterolaterally. (*Image courtesy of Dr Antonis Drevelengas, Interbalkan Hospital, Thessaloniki, Greece*).

DIFFERENTIAL DIAGNOSES IMAGES (E-G)

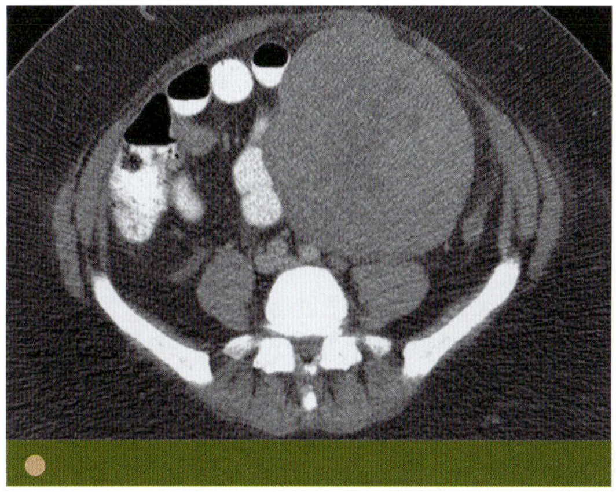

E. Leiomyosarcoma: Axial CECT on a different patient shows a large left-sided mass, which is predominantly solid. A few subtle areas of hypodensity correspond to areas of cystic degeneration.

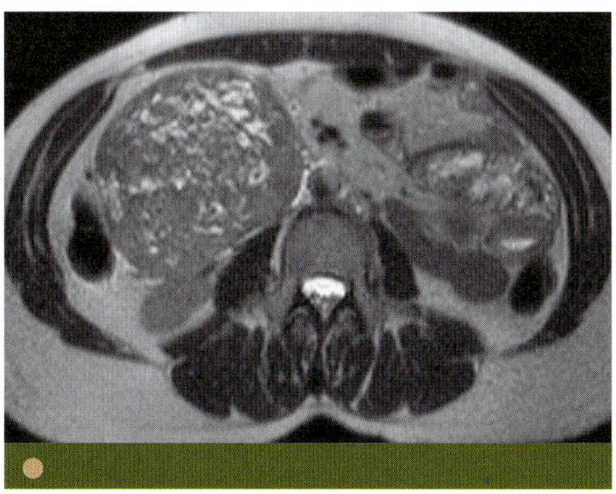

F. Leiomyosarcoma: Axial T2-WI shows a large right-sided retroperitoneal mass with multiple T2-bright foci, corresponding to areas of cystic degeneration.

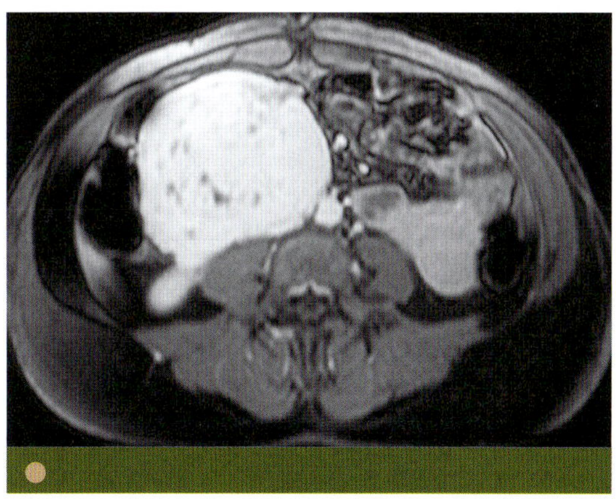

G. Leiomyosarcoma: Corresponding contrast-enhanced T1-WI shows avid enhancement of the majority of the mass. The small foci of degeneration do not enhance.

IMAGE KEY

Common

●●●●●
●●●●
●●●
●●
●

Rare

Typical

■■■■■
■■■■
■■■
■■
■

Unusual

15–9 Retroperitoneal Ganglioneuroma

Paul Nikolaidis

PRESENTATION

Abdominal pain, palpable mass, some patients present with diarrhea.

FINDINGS

CT shows a lobulated relatively hypodense (and hypointense on T1-WI) mass showing only mild enhancement. The mass completely encircles several blood vessels.

DIFFERENTIAL DIAGNOSES

- *Schwannomas*: Typically more heterogeneous in appearance, with both solid and cystic components. They both may occasionally contain calcifications.
- *Lymphoma*: Lymphoma is usually not as hypodense and hypovascular (unless there is necrosis); adenopathy is often present in other locations.
- *Retroperitoneal metastases*: Metastatic lesions of the retroperitoneum may have overlapping features, particularly if relatively hypodense with only mild enhancement.
- *MFH*: Generally a moderately hypervascular mass, more heterogeneous, and may contain calcifications.
- *Leiomyosarcoma*: Typically a large solid mass with areas of cystic degeneration and central necrosis.

COMMENTS

Ganglioneuromas are benign, slow-growing tumors arising from the sympathetic nervous system. They are composed of mature Schwann cells, ganglion cells, and nerve fibers. They are most commonly found in the retroperitoneum or posterior mediastinum, arising from the paravertebral sympathetic chain. They tend to be larger, more rounded, and may contain calcifications more frequently than nerve sheath tumors. Although retroperitoneal ganglioneuromas are usually asymptomatic, they may occasionally present with abdominal pain, a palpable mass, or diarrhea resulting from vasoactive intestinal peptide secretion.

CT precisely delineates these lesions and their relationship to the blood vessels. CT features of ganglioneuroma include an oval, crescentic, or lobulated hypodense mass with only mild-to-moderate postcontrast enhancement. On precontrast images, their attenuation is lower than skeletal muscle. There are occasional calcifications. They classically grow by extending into spaces between preexisting structures and surround vessels without compressing their lumina. Even though ganglioneuromas may encircle the vasculature, they are encapsulated tumors which rarely invade the vessel wall.

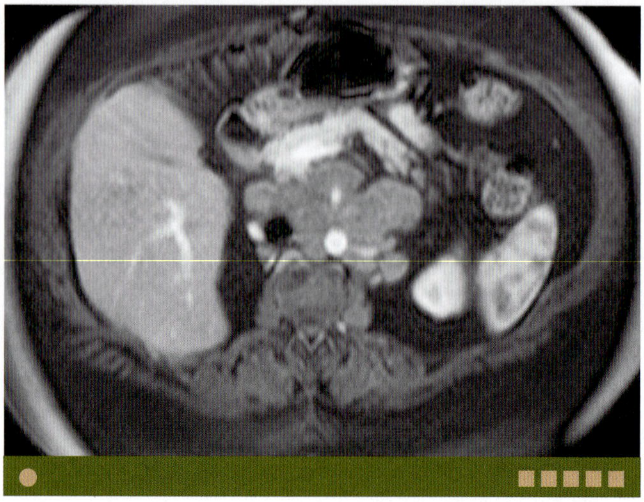

A. Contrast-enhanced T1-WI shows a relatively hypovascular lobulated retroperitoneal mass, which surrounds the aorta and surrounding vessels.

On MR, ganglioneuromas are hypointense on T1-WI, and markedly hyperintense on T2-WI. A whorled appearance of the tumor may be seen, which histologically corresponds to interlacing Schwann cells and collagen fibers. Following gadolinium administration, they are relatively hypovascular and only gradually accumulate contrast over time owing to their high myxoid composition.

As these tumors do not invade the surrounding vasculature, complete surgical resection is often curative.

PEARLS

- **Ganglioneuromas are benign, slow-growing tumors arising from the sympathetic nervous system.**
- **Occasionally present with diarrhea resulting from vasoactive intestinal peptide secretion.**
- **On CT, they are relatively hypodense lesions with occasional calcifications which show only mild enhancement.**
- **On MR, they are hypointense on T1-WI, and hyperintense on T2-WI.**

ADDITIONAL IMAGES (B-D)

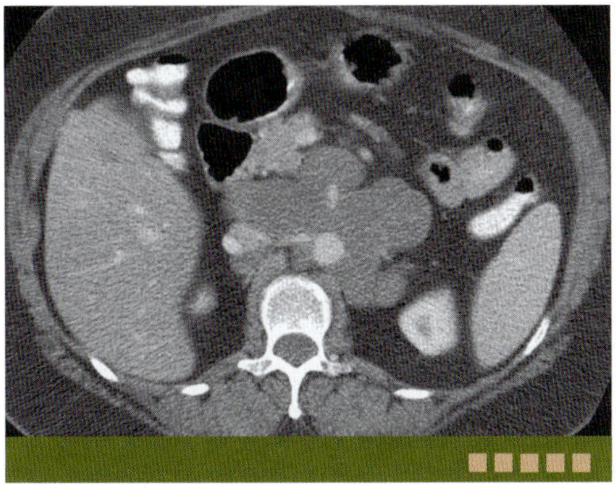

B. Axial CECT on the same patient shows the lobulated, relatively hypodense and hypo-enhancing mass, which was a biopsy proven retroperitoneal ganglioneuroma.

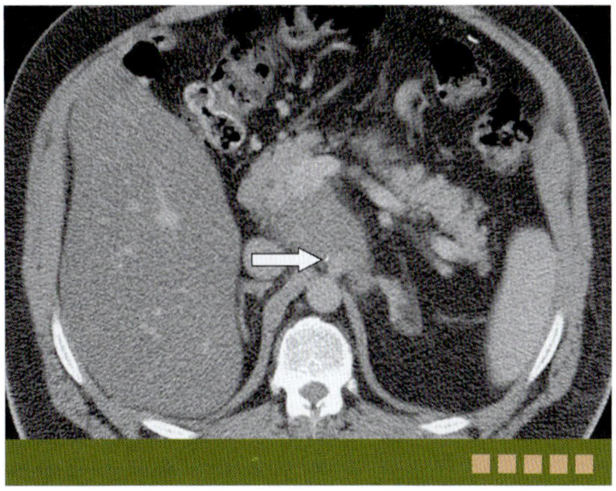

C. Axial CECT on another patient with a biopsy-proven ganglioneuroma shows a relatively hypodense and hypo-enhancing mass with a single calcification adjacent to the superior mesenteric artery (arrow).

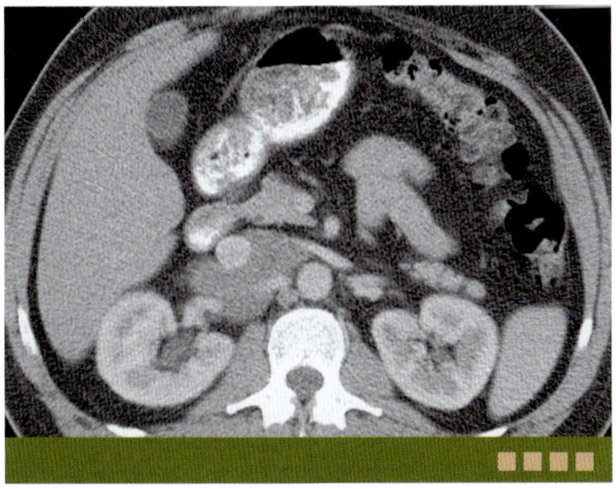

D. Axial CECT on another patient shows a similar appearing retroperitoneal lesion. Note how this lesion also surrounds but does not narrow or invade the regional blood vessels.

DIFFERENTIAL DIAGNOSES IMAGES (E-G)

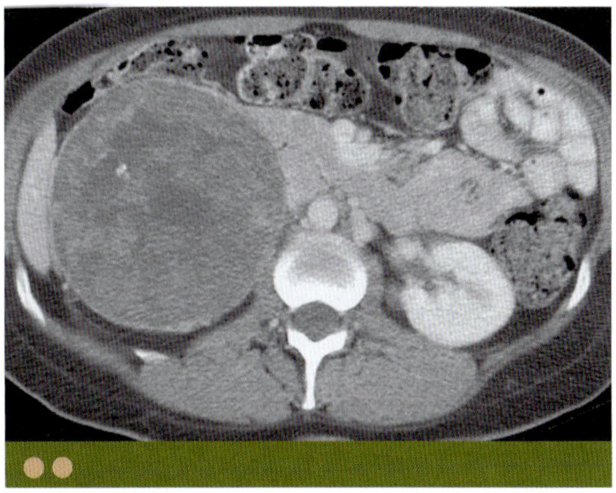

E. Schwannoma: Axial CECT shows a large round, relatively hypodense and hypo-enhancing retroperitoneal schwannoma. It contains a few areas of lower attenuation corresponding to areas of cystic degeneration and a few calcifications.

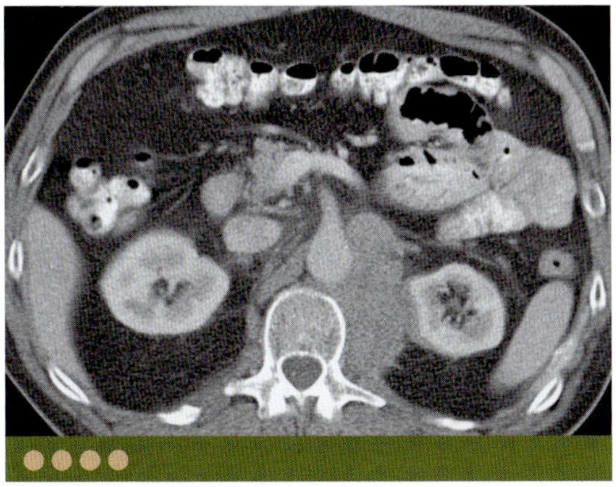

F. Lymphoma: Axial CECT shows a less well-defined left retroperitoneal mass which is slightly higher in attenuation and shows mild enhancement. This lesion also abuts a portion of the aorta and the left kidney.

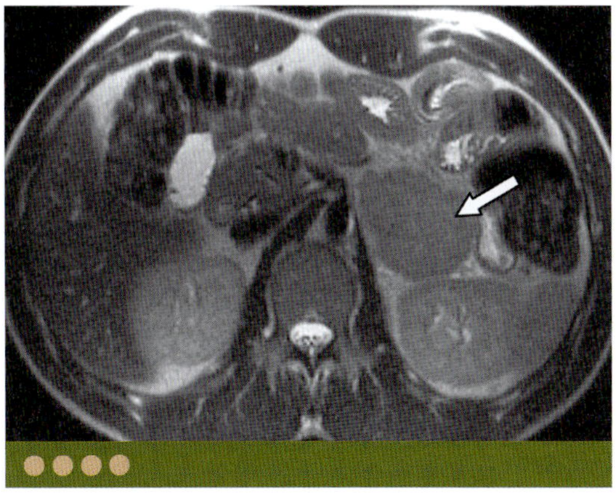

G. Metastasis: Axial T2-WI shows an oval retroperitoneal mass anterior to the left kidney (arrow). This represented a metastatic lesion from testicular carcinoma.

IMAGE KEY

Common

Rare

Typical

Unusual

15–10 Retroperitoneal Lymphangioma

Paul Nikolaidis

PRESENTATION

Incidental finding on imaging, rarely presents with pain or obstruction.

FINDINGS

CT shows a fluid density retroperitoneal lesion, with very faint septations and no enhancing components.

DIFFERENTIAL DIAGNOSES

- *Retroperitoneal cyst*: Cysts of enteric or bronchogenic origin may be entirely indistinguishable on imaging; diagnosis may only be made on histologic analysis on the basis of the composition of the cyst wall.
- *Pancreatic pseudocysts*: Patients usually have a history of prior pancreatitis. They are usually multiple, more irregularly shaped, and may have thick walls.
- *Pancreatic cystic lesions*: Exophytic cysts of pancreatic origin may be difficult to diagnose unless their relationship to the pancreas is apparent on imaging.
- *Lymphocele*: Patients usually have a history of surgery near the area where the lesion is located; they often occur in the pelvis.

COMMENTS

Retroperitoneal lymphangiomas are uncommon benign mesenchymal neoplasms that are histologically characterized by intercommunicating endothelium-lined spaces. They are usually found incidentally on imaging, surgery, or autopsy. Lymphangiomas are classified into three groups depending on the size of the lymphatic spaces: capillary (or simple), cavernous and cystic. Their contents may be serous or chylous fluid, and they may contain protein or lipoid material.

Lymphangiomas are seen more commonly in men and can occur at any age. Although most occur in the neck (75% of the cases) and axillary regions (20%), they can also be found in the retroperitoneum. Retroperitoneal lymphangiomas are often asymptomatic and incidentally discovered during imaging or at surgery performed for unrelated conditions.

CT provides valuable information regarding size, composition, and their anatomical relationship to surrounding structures. They are typically well-circumscribed, elongated, unicameral, or septated fluid density lesions which do not enhance following contrast administration. Fat

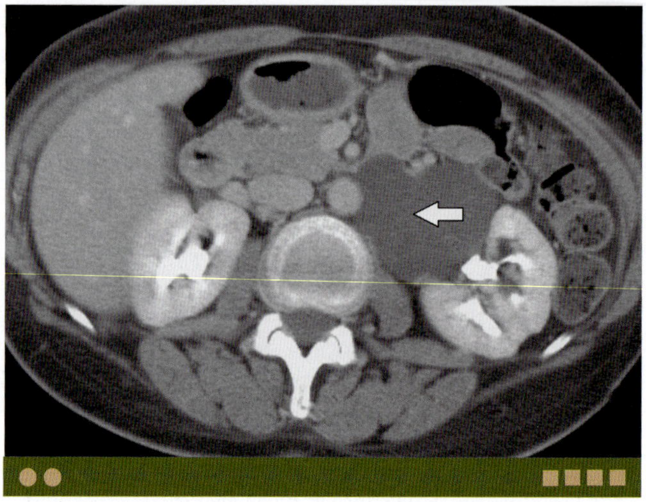

A. Axial CECT shows a fluid density retroperitoneal lesion near the left renal hilum, with a few faint internal septations (arrow) and no enhancing components. It exerts mild mass effect on the left renal collecting system and displaces the kidney laterally.

content may be identified on CT if there is enough present to sufficiently decrease attenuation to negative Hounsfield levels; in most instances fat mixed with fluid is difficult to identify on CT. Lymphangiomas may have a thin enhancing wall, and in a few instances, they may contain septations, mural nodules, or calcifications. Lymphangiomas do not typically displace or compress adjacent structures.

MR also allows for easy identification of lymphangiomas, particularly on T2-WI. Because of their fluid content, they are typically high signal on T2-WI and low on T1-WI, unless complicated by hemorrhage. The presence of fat content may be shown on chemically selective fat-saturated and chemical shift MR sequences.

PEARLS

- **Lymphangiomas typically occur in the neck and axillary regions, but few occur in the retroperitoneum.**
- **Thought to represent either congenital or acquired lesions.**
- **On CT and MR, they appear as well-circumscribed, nonenhancing simple or complex cystic lesions.**
- **On MR, they are typically T2-hyperintense and T1-hypointense, and fat content may be demonstrated on fat-saturated and chemical shift sequences.**

ADDITIONAL IMAGES (B-D)

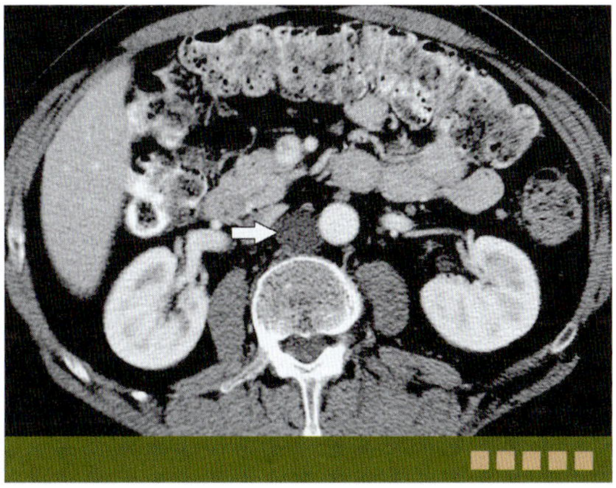

B. Axial CECT on another patient shows a low-density lesion in the right para-aortic region (arrow). Region of interest attenuation measurements ranged from –4 to +3 Hounsfield units.

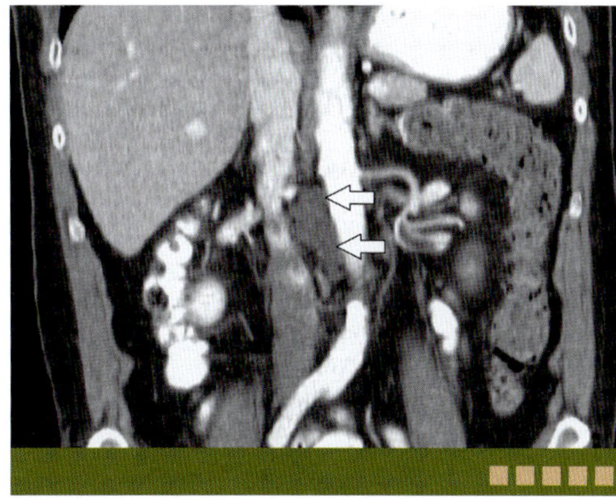

C. Corresponding coronal CECT reformation on the same patient better delineates the elongated retroperitoneal cystic mass (arrows) that contains few very faint internal septations.

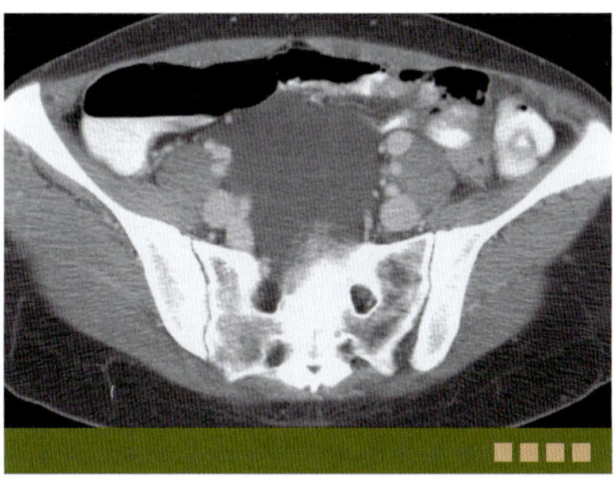

D. Axial CECT on another patient shows a large low-density retroperitoneal lesion which extends into the pelvis, adjacent to the iliac vasculature. The patient had no history of prior surgery. Chylous fluid was demonstrated on aspiration.

DIFFERENTIAL DIAGNOSES IMAGES (E-G)

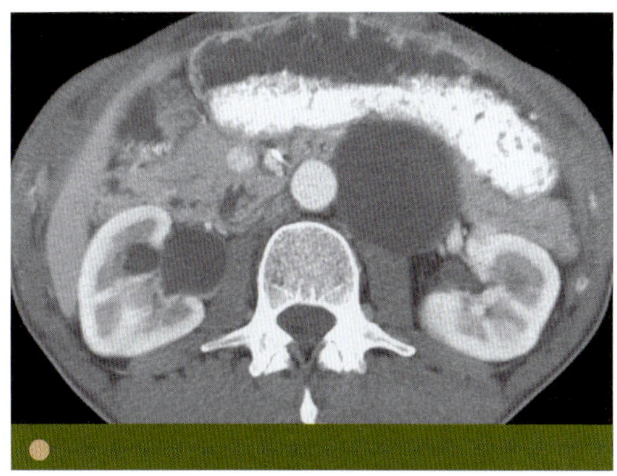

E. Retroperitoneal cyst (enteric duplication cyst): Axial CECT shows a large left-sided, cystic retroperitoneal lesion. On histologic analysis, the cyst wall showed the stratified mucosal pattern of the gastrointestinal tract.

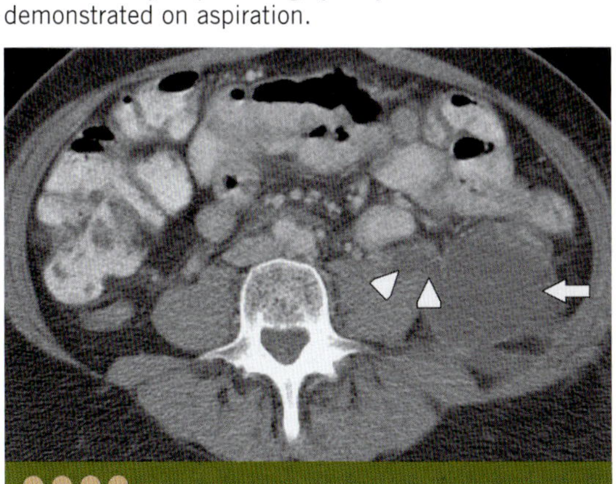

F. Pancreatic pseudocyst/fluid collection: Axial CECT in a patient with pancreatitis shows an irregularly outlined cystic retroperitoneal lesion (arrow) with a mildly thickened, enhancing wall. This lesion also extends into the psoas muscle (arrowheads).

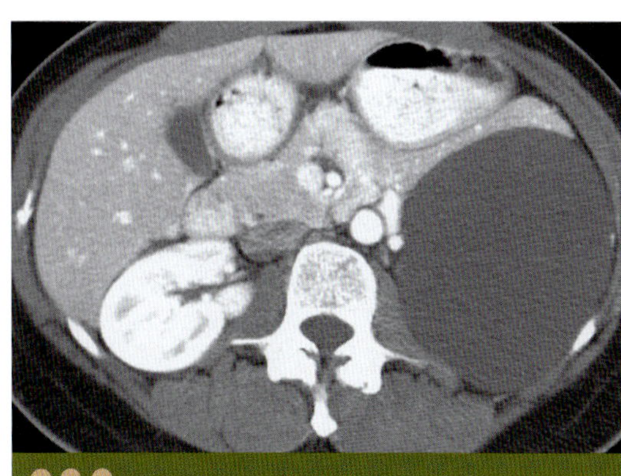

G. Pancreatic cystadenoma: Axial CECT shows a large hypodense cyst that appears to arise from the tail of the pancreas. This was aspirated on endoscopic ultrasound and fluid analysis was compatible with a mucinous cystadenoma.

IMAGE KEY

Common

Rare

Typical

Unusual

15–11 Retroperitoneal Fibrosis

Paul Nikolaidis

PRESENTATION

Pain, weight loss, and anorexia.

FINDINGS

CT shows a midline enhancing retroperitoneal soft tissue mass surrounding the aorta.

DIFFERENTIAL DIAGNOSES

- *Retroperitoneal lymphoma*: More discrete lymph nodes and nodal masses may be seen surrounding the aorta; there may be lymphadenopathy elsewhere. Ureters may be displaced laterally. However, in many instances indistinguishable from fibrosis, necessitating biopsy.
- *Metastatic lymphadenopathy*: Usually more discrete lymph nodes and nodal masses are seen surrounding the aorta; there may be lymphadenopathy elsewhere. Patients may have a known primary malignancy. In several cases, there are overlapping imaging features and the nodal mass is confluent.
- *Inflammatory aortic aneurysm*: Inflammatory or fibrotic changes in the periaortic region are seen in conjunction with an abdominal aneurysm.

COMMENTS

Retroperitoneal fibrosis (RPF) is a chronic inflammatory disease of unknown etiology. About two-thirds of cases are idiopathic, but the remaining cases are secondary to medications, neoplasms, infections, and other causes. Patients may present with vague, nonspecific complaints such as poorly localized pain, anorexia, nausea, and weight loss.

CT is generally the imaging modality of choice; it may also successfully guide percutaneous biopsy. RPF appears as a homogeneous mass or plaque encasing the aorta, iliac arteries and IVC, which may spread laterally to involve the ureters. Organs are generally not displaced unless the mass is malignant in origin, when enlarged lymph nodes may be present. Attenuation is isodense with muscle. Areas of RPF may show enhancement early in disease, when inflammation is more prevalent. MR appearance is similar to that of CT. RPF is generally hypointense on T1-WI. On T2-WI, it is usually hyperintense early, secondary to inflammation and edema. The affected areas may become hypointense later in the disease course, from underlying progressive fibrosis. Malignant etiologies may cause T2-WI to demonstrate less homogeneous signal.

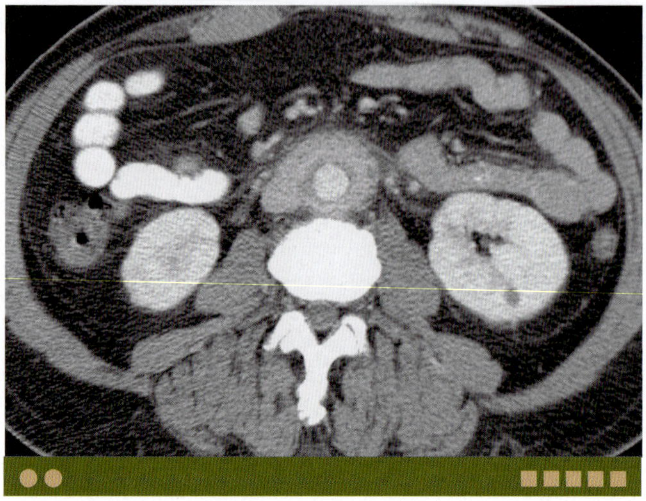

A. Axial CECT of the abdomen shows an enhancing circumferential soft tissue mass surrounding the aorta.

If the patient has hydronephrosis, it should be treated either by ureteral stent placement or surgical ureterolysis. In ureterolysis, the ureters are released from the area of fibrosis and are moved into the peritoneal cavity; to separate the ureters from the fibrosis, a peritoneal flap or omental fat or artificial material may be utilized. Immunosuppressive drugs, such as azathioprine and cyclophosphamide, have also been used in the treatment. The use of steroids in the treatment of RPF remains controversial.

PEARLS

- **RPF is a chronic inflammatory disease of unknown etiology.**
- **Patients may have vague, nonspecific symptoms including anorexia, nausea, and weight loss.**
- **CT and MR are excellent for diagnosing RPF; however, in many instances biopsy is necessary.**
- **On T2-WI, the affected areas may show high signal early in the course of disease and low signal later.**

ADDITIONAL IMAGES (B-C)

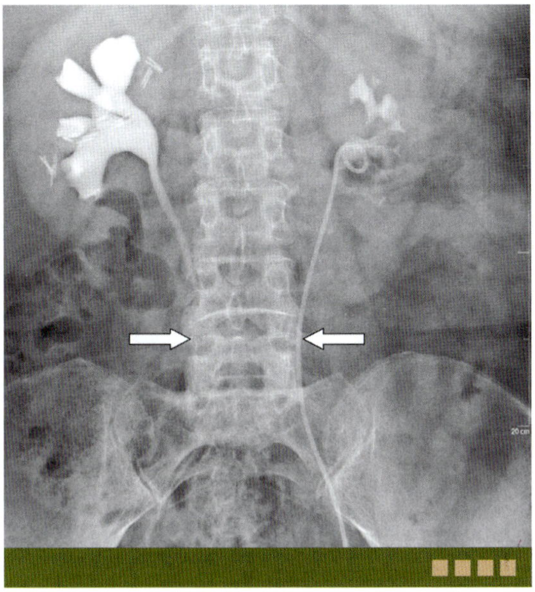

B. IVU shows medial displacement of both ureters owing to RPF (arrows). Note that this process has caused right-sided hydronephrosis. A stent was placed in the left ureter to relieve the hydronephrosis.

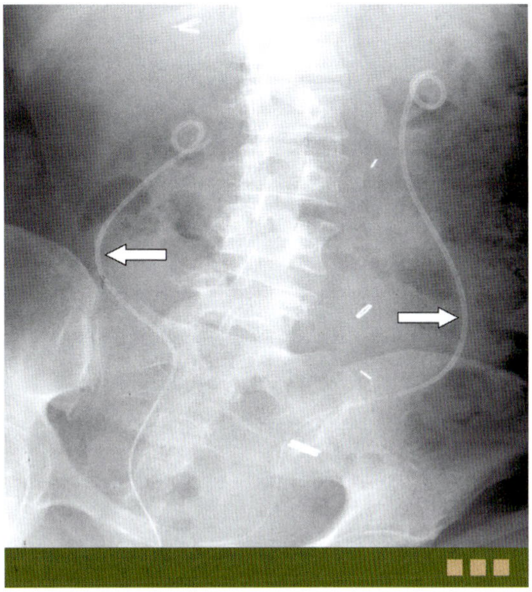

C. Abdominal plain radiograph shows bilateral ureteral stents with lateral deviation of the midportion of both ureters (arrows), a typical appearance after ureterolysis and lateral transposition of the ureters for the treatment of RPF.

IMAGE KEY

Common

Rare

Typical

Unusual

DIFFERENTIAL DIAGNOSES IMAGES (D-E)

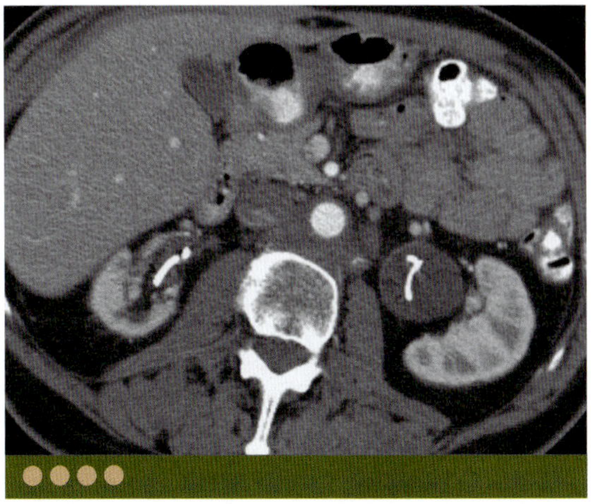

D. Lymphoma: Axial CECT on another patient shows a confluent soft tissue mass surrounding the abdominal aorta. There is bilateral hydronephrosis, necessitating placement of ureteral stents. Imaging features are similar to what would be encountered in RPF. This was shown on biopsy to represent lymphoma. RPF occurs in the setting of neoplasms.

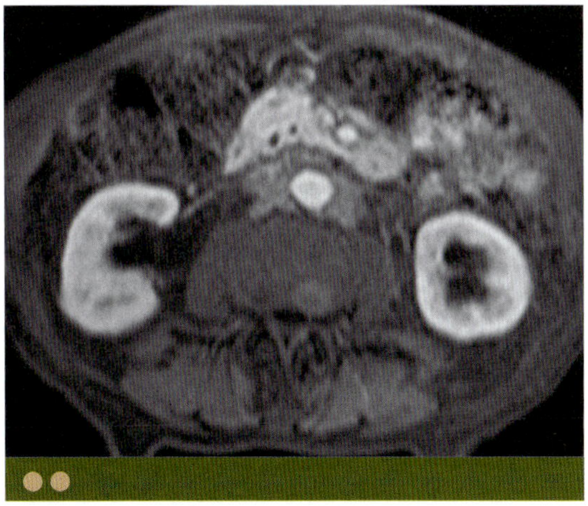

E. Metastases from bladder carcinoma: Axial contrast-enhanced T1-WI shows a confluent soft tissue mass surrounding the aorta. By imaging, its appearance is indistinguishable from RPF. The patient had a history of bladder carcinoma and percutaneous CT-guided biopsy revealed metastatic disease to the retroperitoneum.

15–12 Extramedullary Hematopoiesis

Frank H. Miller

PRESENTATION

Generally painless and asymptomatic; reported cases of nephrotic syndrome and renal failure when obstructive.

FINDINGS

CT shows bilateral homogeneous perirenal and parapelvic masses and splenomegaly.

DIFFERENTIAL DIAGNOSES

- *Perirenal lymphoma*: Different history; typically history of lymphoma and not other findings of extramedullary hematopoiesis.
- *Perinephric infection*: Distinguished on the basis of history, fevers, chills, elevated white blood count, pyuria.
- *Perinephric metastases*: Typically history of metastases.
- *Perinephric hematoma*: Generally history of trauma or underlying mass that bled.

COMMENTS

Extramedullary hematopoiesis is a result of the body attempting to create red blood cells because of bone marrow hematopoietic insufficiency. It is often associated with myelofibrosis, hemoglobinopathies, and bone marrow tumors. Common sites of extramedullary hematopoiesis include paraspinal tissues, liver, and spleen. It has also been reported in the adrenal gland, bowel, and breast and rarely involves the kidney.

Extramedullary hematopoiesis can lead to renal failure with ureteral obstruction and hydronephrosis and renal parenchymal involvement. The diagnosis is important as it may respond to radiation therapy. Parapelvic or perirenal involvement may be seen. Extramedullary hematopoiesis may surround the kidney but does not generally distort it.

The imaging features are often not specific and biopsy may be required for the diagnosis. The diagnosis should be suspected based on the appropriate clinical scenario. When involving the kidney, there are three main types: parenchymal, intrapelvic and perirenal. When parenchymal, the kidney may be diffusely enlarged or have solitary or multiple renal masses. Pelvic involvement may be isolated or associated with extension from the parenchymal masses. Perirenal type includes hypodense mass or nodules surrounding or encasing the kidneys which are hypovascular. Biopsy may be needed to distinguish extramedullary hematopoiesis from lymphoma or uroepithelial tumors. Features that should increase suspicion include patients with underlying hematologic disorders especially when associated with paraspinal masses because of extramedullary hematopoiesis.

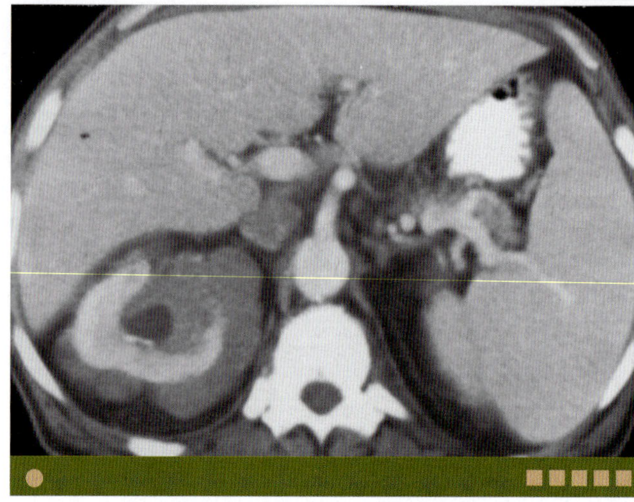

A. CECT shows hypodense mass that surrounds the kidney and renal pelvis but does not invade it. The spleen was enlarged.

PEARLS

- **Extramedullary hematopoiesis should be considered in patients with myeloproliferative disorder or chronic severe anemia like thalassemia and renal or perirenal masses.**
- **Extramedullary hematopoiesis should be considered in patients with associated paraspinal masses.**
- **Biopsy may be required to distinguish extramedullary hematopoiesis from lymphoma or other malignancies.**

ADDITIONAL IMAGE

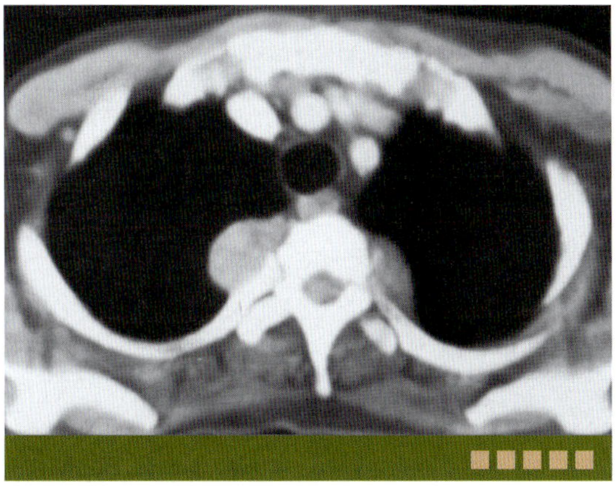

B. CECT shows bilateral paraspinal tissue because of extramedullary hematopoiesis.

DIFFERENTIAL DIAGNOSES IMAGES (C-E)

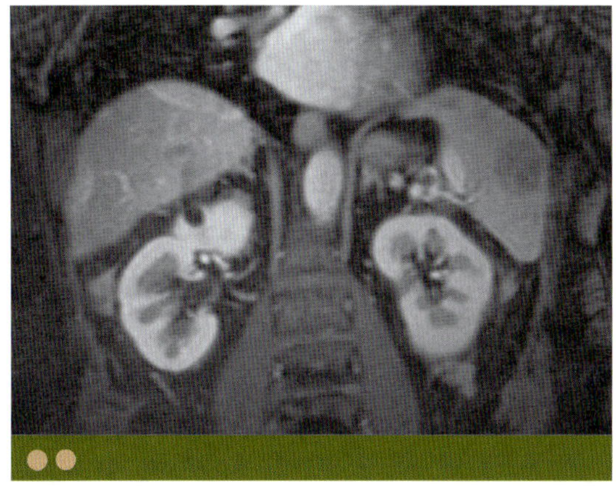

C. Non-Hodgkin lymphoma: Coronal contrast-enhanced T1-WI, shows normal kidneys with enhancing perinephric soft tissue because of non-Hodgkin lymphoma. Perinephric enhancing masses is one of the presentations of lymphoma.

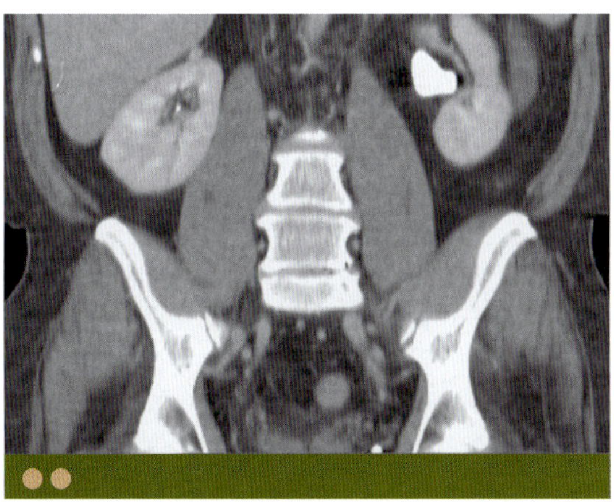

D. Perirenal non-Hodgkin lymphoma: Coronal CECT shows focal mass because of perirenal lymphoma at surgical resection. Appearance is nonspecific.

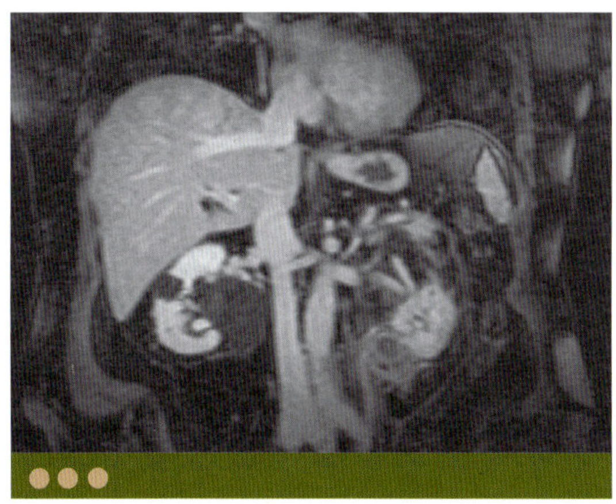

E. Acute pyelonephritis: Coronal contrast-enhanced T1-WI, shows perinephric inflammation from acute pyelonephritis. The clinical history of fevers and chills helps distinguish it from other entities.

IMAGE KEY

Common

Rare

Typical

Unusual

15–13 Inflammatory Aneurysm of the Abdominal Aorta

Paul Nikolaidis

PRESENTATION

Fatigue, abdominal, or back pain.

FINDINGS

CT shows an enhancing soft tissue mass surrounding the abdominal aorta.

DIFFERENTIAL DIAGNOSES

- *Atherosclerotic abdominal aortic aneurysm*: Simple atherosclerotic aneurysms have a smooth wall with peripheral calcification. The lack of a surrounding inflammatory soft tissue component should differentiate them from IAA.
- *Aortic rupture*: Ruptured AAA will appear as a retroperitoneal hematoma seen along with an abdominal aortic aneurysm. Periaortic hemorrhage may extend into the perirenal space, the pararenal space, or both. Extension into the peritoneum may also occur.
- *Retroperitoneal fibrosis*: Confluent soft tissue is seen surrounding the aorta in the absence of an aortic aneurysm.

COMMENTS

Inflammatory aortic aneurysm (IAA) is a distinct type of aneurysm usually involving the infrarenal abdominal aorta. They constitute approximately 5% of all infrarenal abdominal aortic aneurysms. Rarely, they may involve the descending thoracic aorta. A thickened aneurysm wall, peri-aneurysmal fibrosis, and dense adhesions to adjacent abdominal organs such as the duodenum, IVC, and ureter are characteristic of IAA. Patients may present with fatigue, malaise, abdominal or back pain. An elevated sedimentation rate (ESR) is typically seen. The mean age of patients with IAA is 65, which is approximately 5 to 10 years younger than patients with noninflammatory aneurysms.

CT will often show a thickened, calcified aortic wall surrounded by a low-attenuation soft tissue mass. The surrounding circumferential periaortic mass represents the outer fibrotic plaque. It demonstrates soft tissue attenuation and may extend inferolaterally toward the psoas or iliac arteries. Typically, the surrounding area of fibrosis is thicker anteriorly and laterally, with relative sparing of the posterior wall. The inflammatory mass enhances on CECT, but to a lesser extent than the intravascular contrast. When intraluminal thrombus is present, a classic four-layered appearance is seen: the enhanced lumen; the nonenhanced thrombus; the focally calcified, nonenhanced aortic wall; and the enhanced periaortic fibrotic plaque.

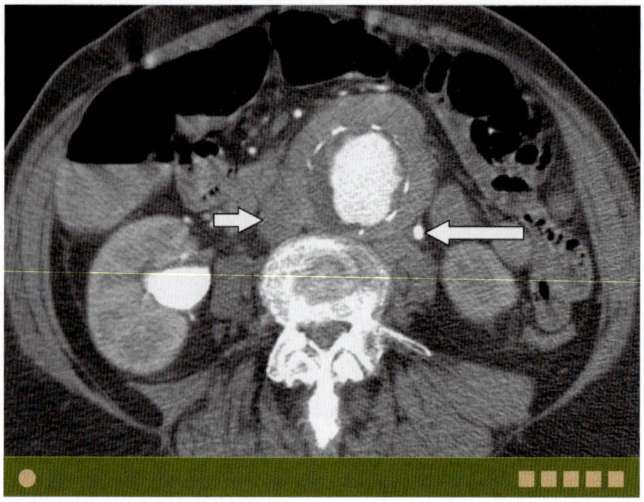

A. Axial CECT shows the classic four-layered appearance of an inflammatory aneurysm: the central contrast-enhanced lumen; the nonenhancing thrombus; the focally calcified aortic wall; and the outer layer of enhancing periaortic fibrosis. Note the thick layer of perianeurysmal fibrosis inseparable from the IVC (short arrow) and close to the left ureter (long arrow).

MR also characterizes IAA, perhaps with greater sensitivity than CT. Following gadolinium administration, the fibrotic plaque enhances and can be separated from the mural thrombus. On fat-saturated and conventional T2-WI, alternating layers of high and low signal within the fibrotic plaque may be seen, thought to represent alternating layers of fibrosis and inflammation.

It is important to correctly diagnose inflammatory abdominal aortic aneurysms as their surgical repair is associated with higher morbidity and mortality. This is, in part, because of their adherence to neighboring structures, rendering it more difficult to mobilize the aneurysm at surgery. Endovascular approaches are now favored.

PEARLS

- **A distinct type of aneurysm usually involving the infrarenal abdominal aorta.**
- **Characterized by peri-aneurysmal fibrosis and dense adhesions to adjacent organs.**
- **CT and MR are both excellent for diagnosing IAA.**
- **On T2-WI alternating layers of high and low signal are typically seen within the fibrotic plaque.**

ADDITIONAL IMAGES (B-D)

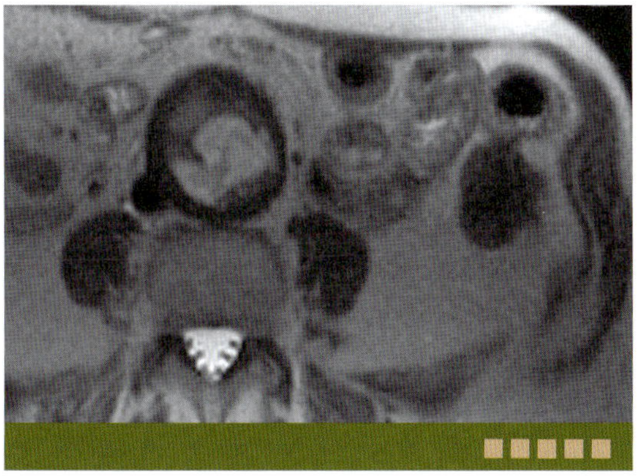

B. Axial T2-WI on a different patient with an inflammatory aortic aneurysm shows the classic pattern of alternating layers of high and low signal within the fibrotic plaque, representing alternating layers of fibrosis and inflammation. The outer layer of periaortic fibrosis is uniformly low in signal intensity.

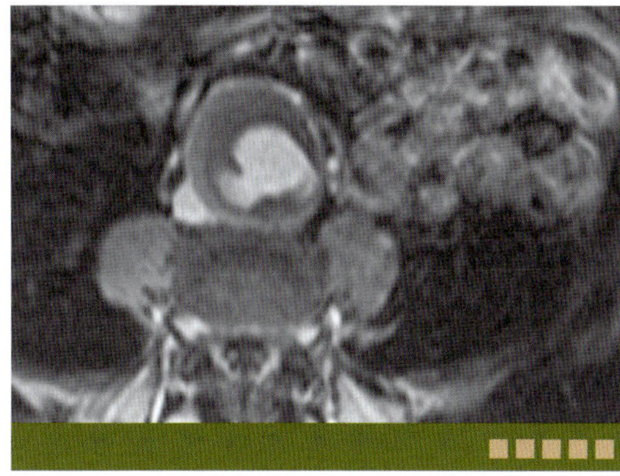

C. Corresponding axial contrast-enhanced T1-WI on the same patient shows a thin circumferential layer of enhancement representing the perianeurysmal fibrotic plaque.

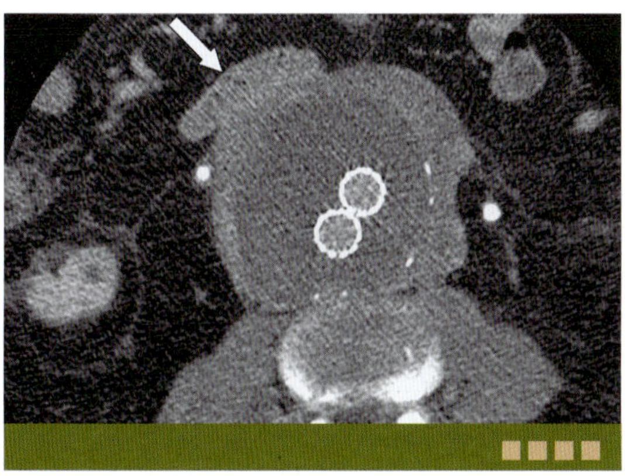

D. Axial CECT on another patient with history of a treated inflammatory aortic aneurysm shows an endograft within the aneurysm. The stent was placed approximately five months prior to the CT. There is continued mild enhancement of the layer of perianeurysmal fibrosis which remains inseparable from the duodenum (arrow).

DIFFERENTIAL DIAGNOSES IMAGES (E-G)

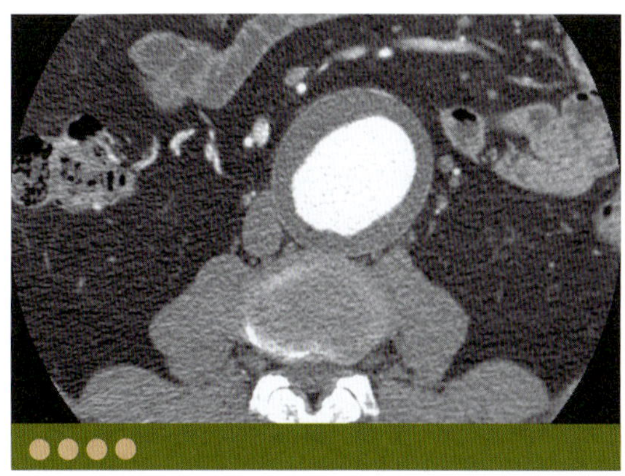

E. Simple atherosclerotic abdominal aortic aneurysm: Axial CECT on another patient shows an aneurysm with a smooth, thin wall and peripheral atherosclerotic calcification. Mural thrombus is seen within the lumen of the aorta. The lack of surrounding inflammatory soft tissue differentiates this from an inflammatory aortic aneurysm.

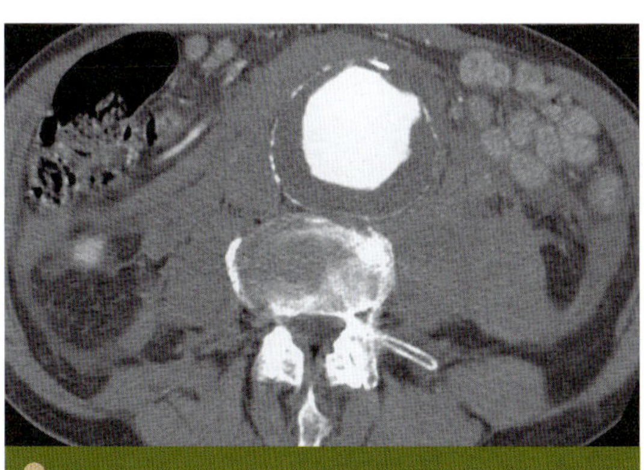

F. Ruptured abdominal aortic aneurysm: Axial CECT of the abdomen shows a ruptured abdominal aortic aneurysm with a large retroperitoneal hematoma.

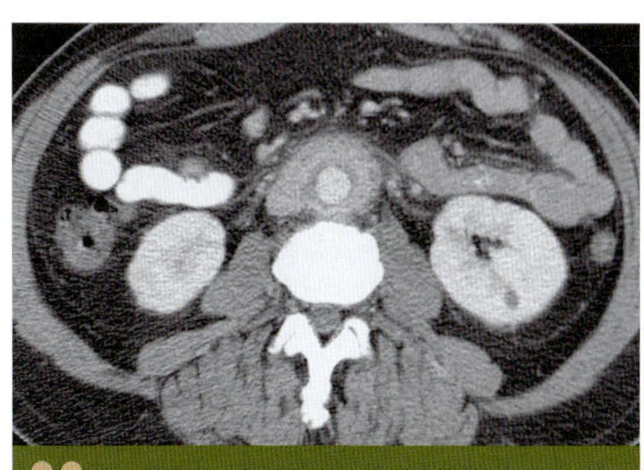

G. Retroperitoneal fibrosis: Axial CECT shows an enhancing soft tissue mass surrounding a significant portion of the (normal caliber) abdominal aorta.

IMAGE KEY

Common

Rare

Typical

Unusual

15–14 Ruptured Abdominal Aortic Aneurysm

Paul Nikolaidis

PRESENTATION

Hypogastric pain, pain in the lower back, and hypotension.

FINDINGS

CT shows a large abdominal aortic aneurysm along with extensive retroperitoneal hemorrhage.

DIFFERENTIAL DIAGNOSES

- *Inflammatory aortic aneurysm*: Peri-aneurysmal fibrosis in inflammatory aortic aneurysms is manifested by smoother, circumferential soft tissue encircling the aorta, without associated retroperitoneal hemorrhage.
- *Retroperitoneal fibrosis*: Confluent enhancing soft tissue is seen surrounding the aorta. There is no retroperitoneal hemorrhage.

COMMENTS

The risk of aortic aneurysm rupture increases with aneurysm size. For aneurysms that are 4 to 5 cm in size the incidence of rupture is 1% to 3% per year. For aneurysms measuring 5 to 7 cm, the risk increases to 6% to 11%. For those exceeding 7 cm, the risk of rupture is greater than 20%. Prompt diagnosis of rupture and impending rupture is imperative. The most common site of rupture is from the posterolateral aspect of the aorta, which results in hemorrhage into the retroperitoneal space. The most common presenting symptoms are hypogastric and lower back pain and hypotension.

The sensitivity of ultrasound in detecting rupture of an AAA is low. Sonography may be useful, however, in the setting of an unstable hypotensive patient to rapidly evaluate for the presence of an abdominal aortic aneurysm.

CECT is the procedure of choice for suspected rupture for the hemodynamically stable patient. Most ruptures appear as a retroperitoneal hematoma seen along with an abdominal aortic aneurysm. On CECT, active extravasation of contrast may be seen, but that is unlikely as the patient would probably extravasate to death.

In most instances, the exact site rupture is not visible on imaging. Discontinuity of the aortic wall or a focal gap in otherwise continuous circumferential wall calcifications may show the location of a rupture. There is typically a delay of several hours between the initial intramural hemorrhage and frank extravasation into the periaortic soft tissues.

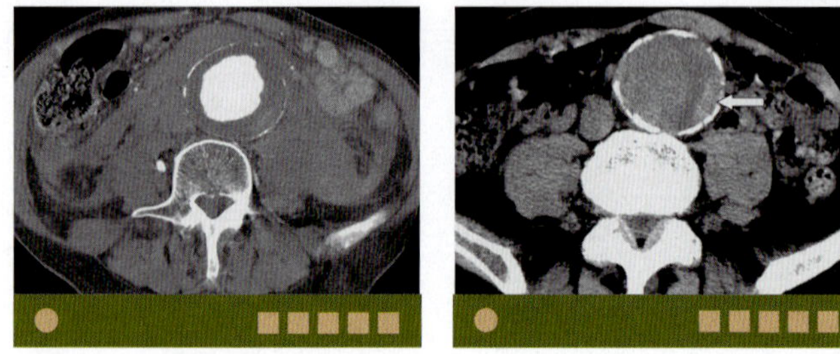

A. Axial CECT of the abdomen shows a ruptured abdominal aortic aneurysm with a large retroperitoneal hematoma.
B. Axial NECT on the same patient that was obtained two weeks previously shows a peripheral hyperdense crescent within mural thrombus (arrow). The hyperattenuating crescent is an important sign of impending rupture.

Contained or impending ruptures are more difficult to identify. Imaging features suggestive of instability or impending rupture include a sudden increase in aneurysm size, a low thrombus-to-lumen ratio, and the presence of hemorrhage into a mural thrombus. Acute intramural hemorrhage should be recognized immediately and appears as a peripheral crescent-shaped hyperdense focus within the aortic wall or mural thrombus. It is best seen on noncontrast CT or MR. "Draping" of the posterior aspect of an aneurysmal aorta over the vertebrae (when the posterior aortic wall is not distinctly identified or closely follows the contour of adjacent vertebral bodies) is a sign of a contained rupture.

The overall mortality rate for ruptured abdominal aortic aneurysms is 80%. Emergent open surgery is often warranted. Endovascular repair techniques are now increasingly utilized, particularly for elective cases when patients are stable or at high risk for open surgery.

PEARLS

- **The incidence of rupture increases with aneurysm size.**
- **The mortality rate is 80%, and immediate diagnosis is imperative.**
- **CT and MR are both excellent for diagnosing ruptured aneurysms.**
- **Contained or impending ruptures are more difficult to identify.**

ADDITIONAL IMAGES (C-E)

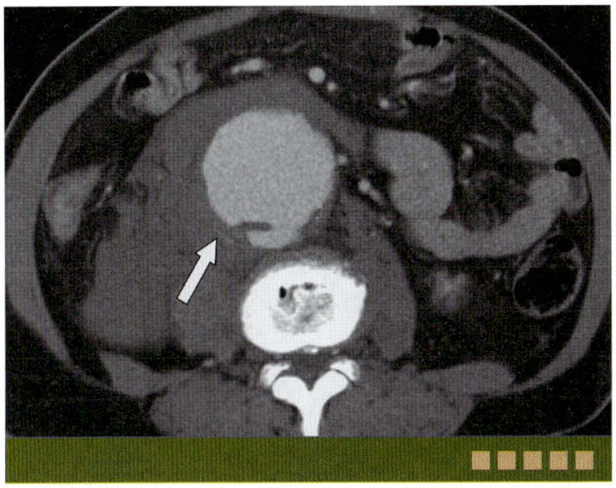

C. Axial CECT on a different patient with a ruptured aortic aneurysm shows the site of the aortic rupture. Faint arterial extravasation is seen (arrow). A right-sided retroperitoneal hematoma is present.

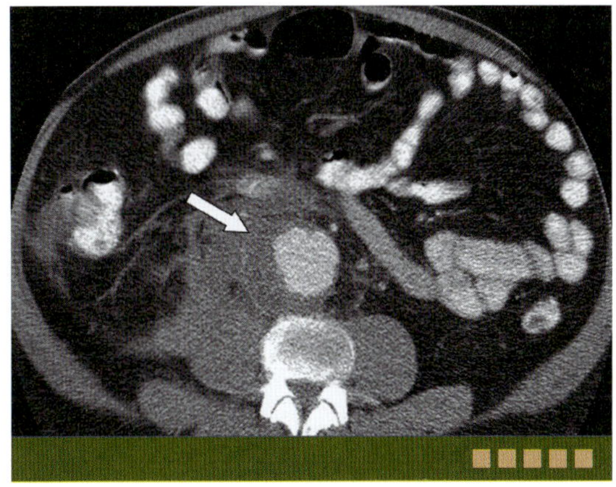

D. Axial CECT on another patient with a ruptured aortic aneurysm shows a right-sided retroperitoneal hematoma. The site of aortic rupture is likely the small area of discontinuity of the aortic wall (arrow).

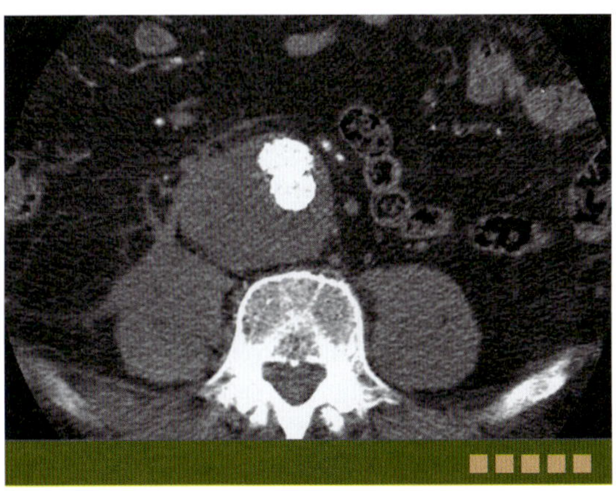

E. Axial CECT on the same patient 1 year after the aortic rupture. An Endograft is now seen within the aneurysm.

DIFFERENTIAL DIAGNOSES IMAGES (F-H)

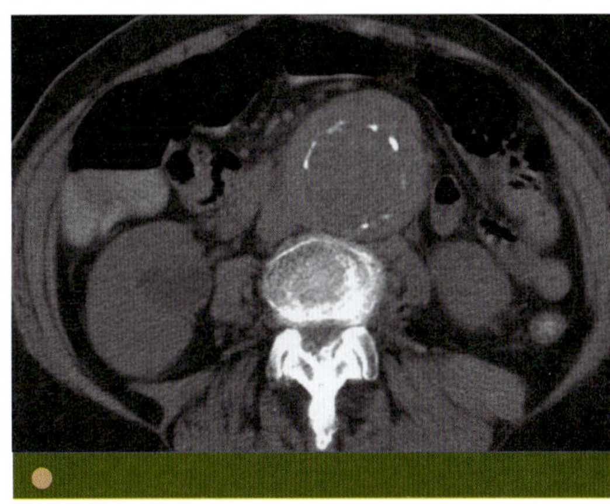

F. Inflammatory aneurysm of the abdominal aorta: Axial NECT of the abdomen shows circumferential soft tissue surrounding the aortic aneurysm.

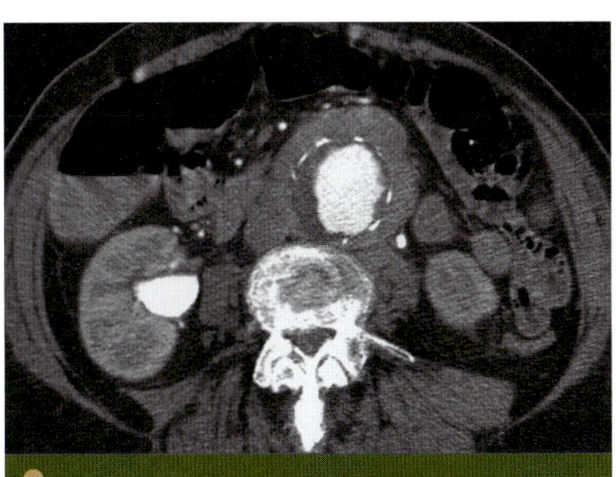

G. Inflammatory aneurysm of the abdominal aorta: Corresponding axial CECT shows the classic four-layered appearance of an inflammatory aneurysm.

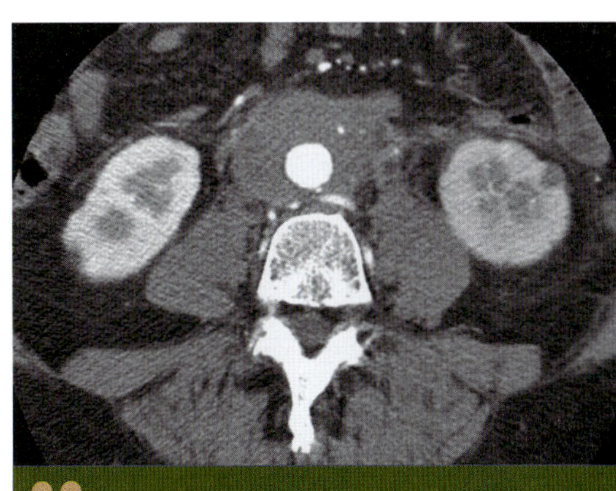

H. Retroperitoneal fibrosis: Axial CECT shows confluent enhancing soft tissue surrounding the abdominal aorta that is normal in caliber.

IMAGE KEY

Common

Rare

Typical

Unusual

15–15 Retroperitoneal Hemorrhage

Paul Nikolaidis

PRESENTATION

Asymptomatic, sudden onset abdominal pain, and falling hematocrit.

FINDINGS

CT shows an ill-defined nonenhancing retroperitoneal mass which is hyperdense on precontrast images.

DIFFERENTIAL DIAGNOSES

- *Retroperitoneal fluid collections (pancreatitis, abscesses)*: Usually more hypodense (especially compared to acute hemorrhage). May have an enhancing peripheral rim. Follow-up imaging is often appropriate to show resolution or guide management.
- *Retroperitoneal tumors or adenopathy*: Neoplastic lesions are usually more discrete (with the exception of lymphoma) and may show mild or moderate enhancement; PET or biopsy scan may confirm a neoplasm.

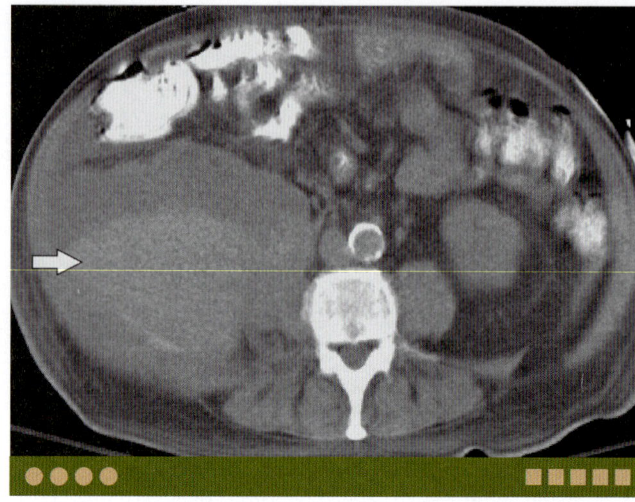

A. Axial NECT shows a large retroperitoneal lesion with mixed density elements. There is a large hyperdense component (arrow). The presence of high density on a nonenhanced study suggests hemorrhage.

COMMENTS

Retroperitoneal hemorrhage most often occurs in patients on anticoagulation therapy. It usually results from a venous bleed. Additional etiologies include trauma, ruptured aortic or renal artery aneurysm, and renal, adrenal, or other retroperitoneal neoplasms. Though typically asymptomatic, patients may present with sudden onset abdominal or flank pain, or with a palpable mass and falling hematocrit. Additional more vague signs and symptoms may include thigh pain, low grade fever, or hypoactive bowel sounds. In such instances, evaluation with cross-sectional imaging becomes important.

CT is the most widely utilized modality for diagnosing and localizing retroperitoneal hemorrhage. Normally, there is sharp delineation of the retroperitoneal structures by surrounding extraperitoneal fat. Retroperitoneal hemorrhage can be detected on CT as an abnormal soft tissue density which may obscure, displace, enlarge or compress surrounding normal retroperitoneal structures. Areas of hemorrhage may be more ill-defined, in contrast to more discrete retroperitoneal neoplasms. Acute hemorrhage typically has a homogeneous attenuation of 50 to 80 HU. Without IV contrast, the area of hemorrhage can be distinguished from the normal retroperitoneal structures by its high attenuation. On CECT, most hematomas are readily identified; in rare instances, it may be more difficult to recognize subtle retroperitoneal hemorrhage.

Unless (in rare instances) there is active bleeding or extravasation of contrast, the hematoma will not enhance. In subacute hematomas, approximately 5 to 15 days after hemorrhage, foci of high attenuation are usually surrounded by areas of lower (fluid) density. Chronic hematomas may appear as a low-density mass with a thick, dense rim; some may develop peripheral calcifications.

PEARLS

- **Etiologies include anticoagulation therapy, trauma, ruptured aneurysms, and retroperitoneal neoplasms.**
- **Acute hemorrhage is hyperdense on precontrast CT.**
- **Subacute hemorrhage may show areas of lower density or liquefaction.**
- **Chronic hematomas may appear as a low-density mass with a thick, dense rim or peripheral calcification.**

ADDITIONAL IMAGES (B-D)

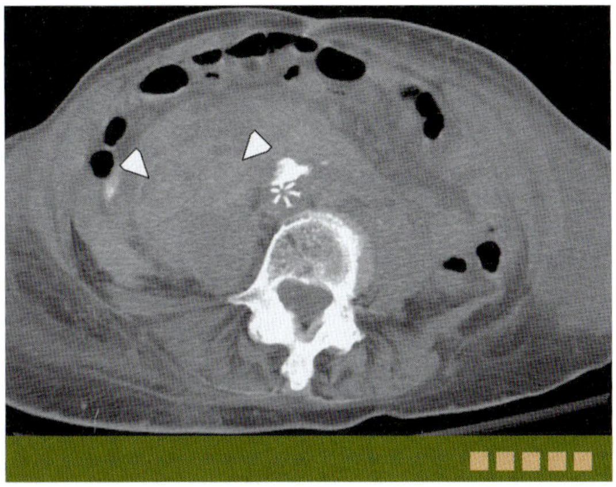

B. Axial NECT on another patient shows a large retroperitoneal hematoma which crosses the midline. It contains several hyperdense components (arrowheads).

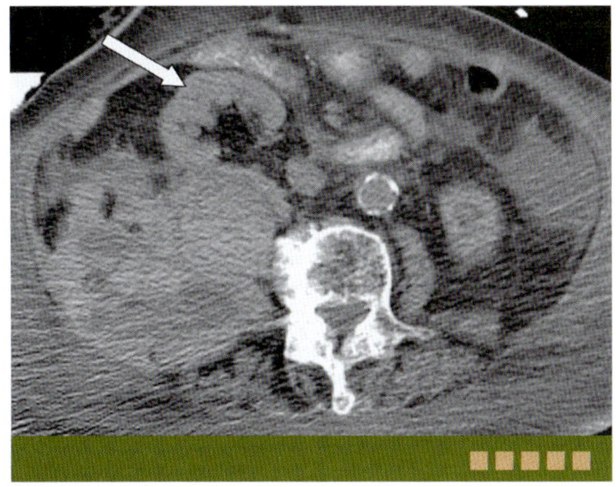

C. Axial NECT on a different patient shows a mixed density, right-sided retroperitoneal hematoma. It displaces the right kidney anteriorly (arrow).

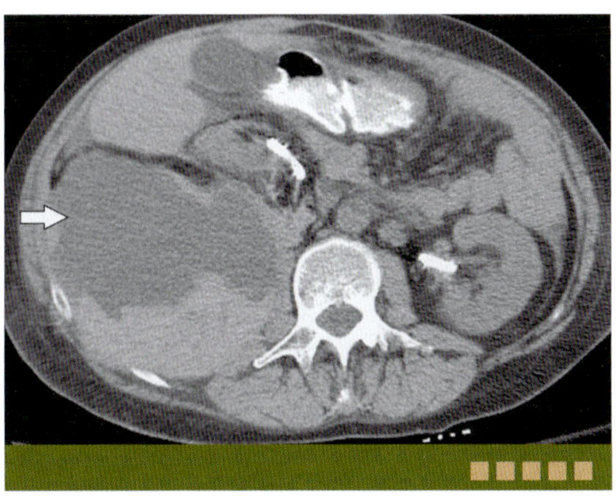

D. Axial NECT on a different patient shows a subacute retroperitoneal hematoma. Note the large amount of hypodense serum (arrow).

DIFFERENTIAL DIAGNOSES IMAGES (E-G)

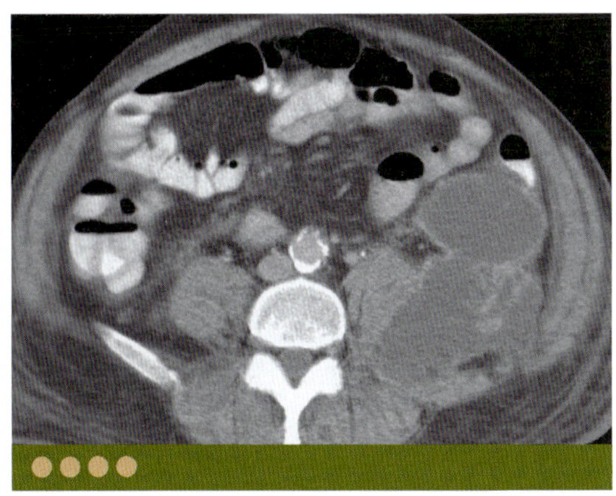

E. Pancreatitis with retroperitoneal fluid collections: Axial CECT shows a retroperitoneal fluid collection from fluid that originated from the inflamed pancreas.

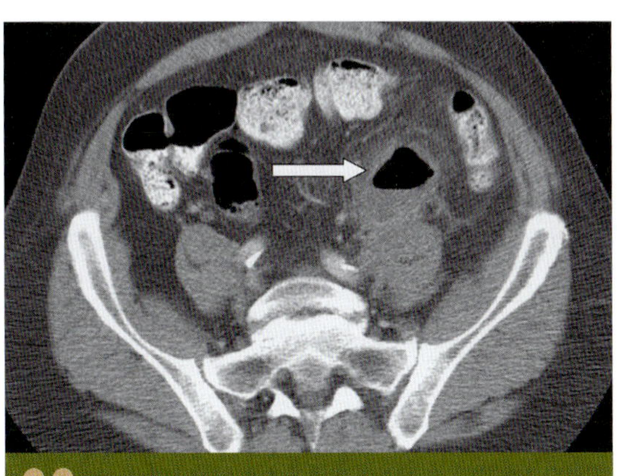

F. Retroperitoneal abscess: Axial CECT on a patient with diverticulitis shows a thick-walled fluid collection anterior to the left psoas muscle containing air (arrow).

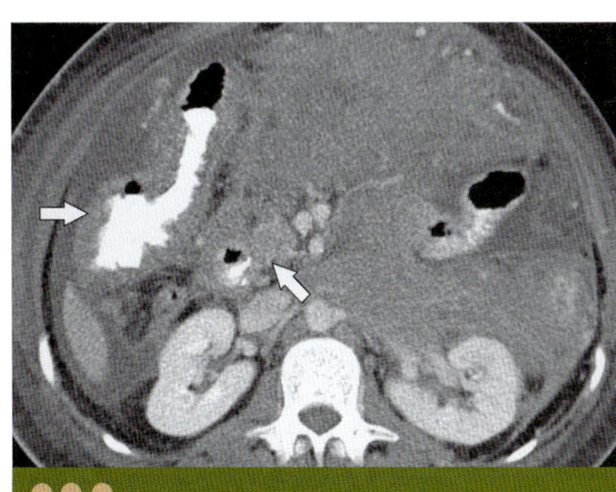

G. Lymphoma: Axial CECT shows a large enhancing mass occupying large portion of the retroperitoneum and mesentery. Note the gastric and duodenal wall thickening (arrows).

IMAGE KEY

Common

Rare

Typical

Unusual

15–16 Retroperitoneal Abscess

Paul Nikolaidis

PRESENTATION

Malaise, fever, and weight loss.

FINDINGS

CT shows a thick-walled fluid collection anterior to the left psoas muscle containing air.

DIFFERENTIAL DIAGNOSES

- *Retroperitoneal fluid collections from pancreatitis*: Sterile fluid collections from pancreatitis may be difficult to distinguish from abscesses. The presence of gas is suggestive of infection.
- *Retroperitoneal hemorrhage*: Usually will have hyperdense components, especially if acute or subacute. Abscesses are more likely to have an enhancing peripheral rim; the presence of gas is pathognomonic.
- *Necrotic retroperitoneal tumors or adenopathy*: Patients often have a history of malignancy. There may be a larger solid component.

COMMENTS

Although retroperitoneal abscesses are uncommon, they may be associated with significant morbidity and mortality. Given their confined location in the retroperitoneum, they may present with mild symptoms and subtle clinical signs, resulting in a delay in diagnosis. The clinical presentation is often an insidious and nonspecific onset of malaise, fever, nausea, and weight loss. Psoas abscesses appear to be more commonly associated with pain.

Patients may have coexisting disorders, particularly diabetes, renal failure, and hepatic disease. Retroperitoneal abscesses originating from the kidney often occur in the perirenal space. Other causes include trauma, perforated cancers, diverticulitis, and pancreatitis. Intramuscular abscesses, particularly involving the psoas may also occur, frequently encountered in patients with Crohn disease or perforated malignancies of the GI tract. Extension into the retroperitoneum may occur with infection from TB; there may be superimposed spinal involvement.

Retroperitoneal abscesses may be seen on CT and MR and less reliably on ultrasound. CT is generally the preferred modality, as gas is more readily identified. CT is more sensitive and specific and is diagnostic in more than 95%.

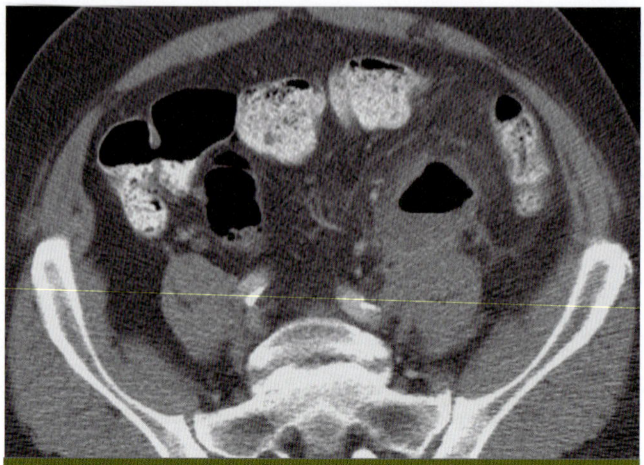

A. Axial CECT shows a thick-walled fluid collection anterior to the left psoas muscle containing air. There is surrounding fat stranding. This represents a retroperitoneal abscess in a patient with perforated acute diverticulitis.

Prompt diagnosis and treatment are necessary as the mortality rate has been reported to be as high as 17% with deaths ensuing from sepsis. CT-guided drainage is usually the treatment of choice, although ultrasound guidance may be successfully used in many instances. Antibiotics alone usually will not suffice. Pathogens are usually polymicrobial with gram negative organisms, particularly *Proteus* and *Escherichia.* However, the incidence of abscesses owing to gram-positive cocci, *Candida* and tuberculosis has increased in recent years, particularly in immunosuppressed patients.

PEARLS

- **Retroperitoneal abscesses are uncommon but associated with significant morbidity and mortality.**
- **Patients present later than those with intra-abdominal abscesses.**
- **CT is the most sensitive and specific technique for their detection.**
- **Image-guided drainage is usually the treatment of choice.**

ADDITIONAL IMAGES (B-D)

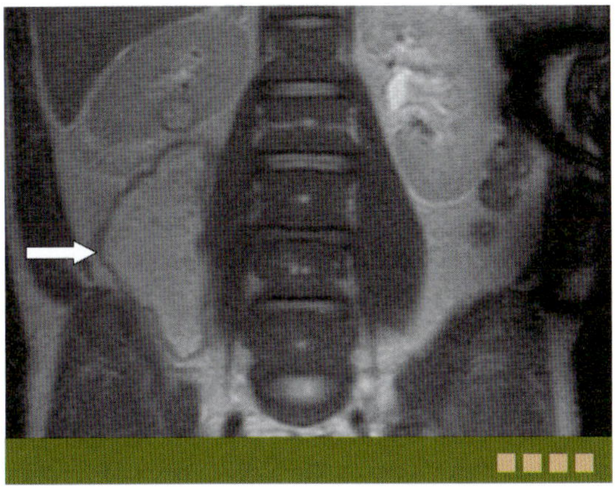

B. Coronal T2-WI in a patient with HIV shows a large abscess below the right kidney (arrow). It has a slightly thickened hypointense wall. This was successfully treated with CT-guided drainage.

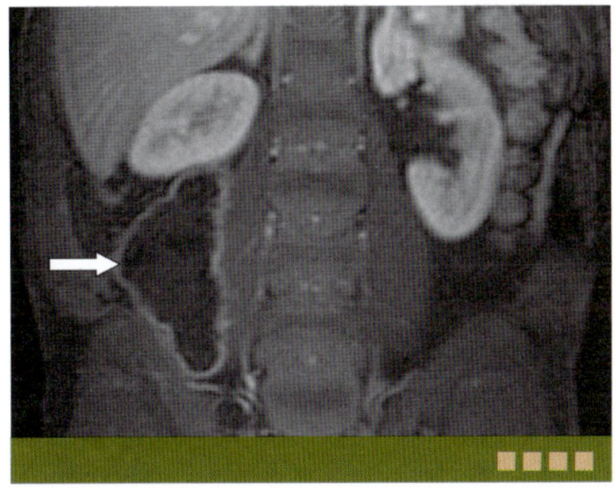

C. Coronal contrast-enhanced T1-WI on the same patient shows the enhancement of the wall of the abscess. Its contents are nonenhancing.

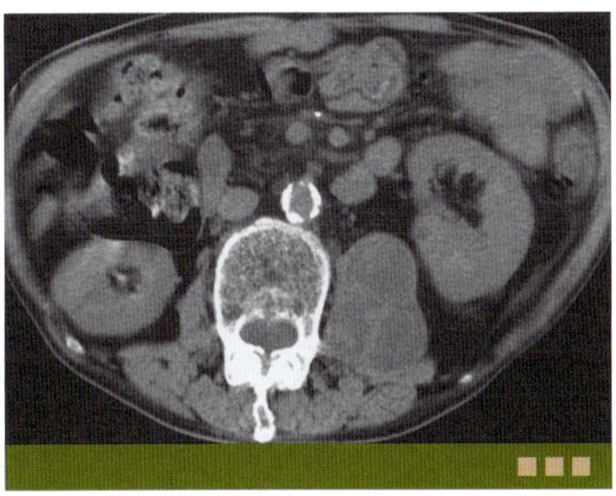

D. Axial CECT on a different patient shows a complex multicompartment fluid collection involving the left psoas muscle. Image-guided aspiration and drainage confirmed tuberculous infection. (*Image courtesy of Dr Antonis Drevelengas, Interbalkan Hospital, Thessaloniki, Greece.*)

DIFFERENTIAL DIAGNOSES IMAGES (E-G)

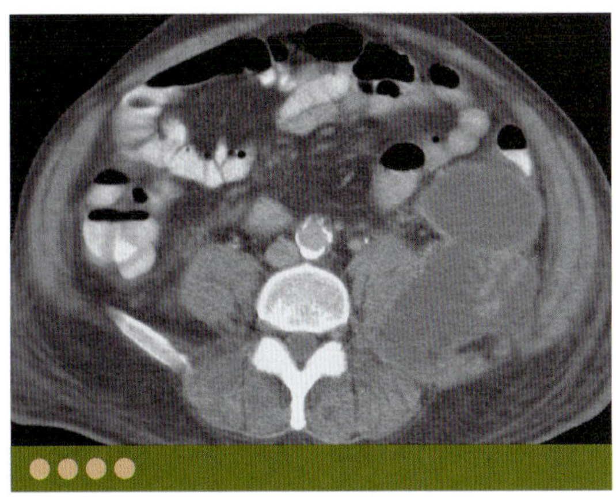

E. Retroperitoneal fluid collection from acute pancreatitis: Axial CECT shows a complex, peripherally enhancing cystic lesion that also involves the left psoas muscle. The patient had a recent history of acute pancreatitis.

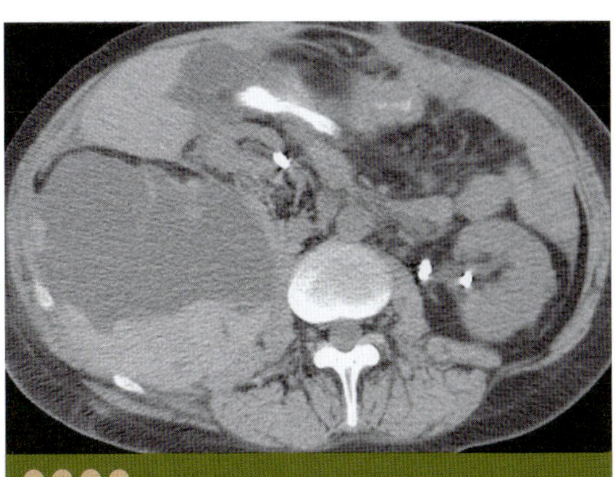

F. Retroperitoneal hematoma: Axial nonenhanced CT shows a large right retroperitoneal hematoma with mixed density elements, including layering high-density contents.

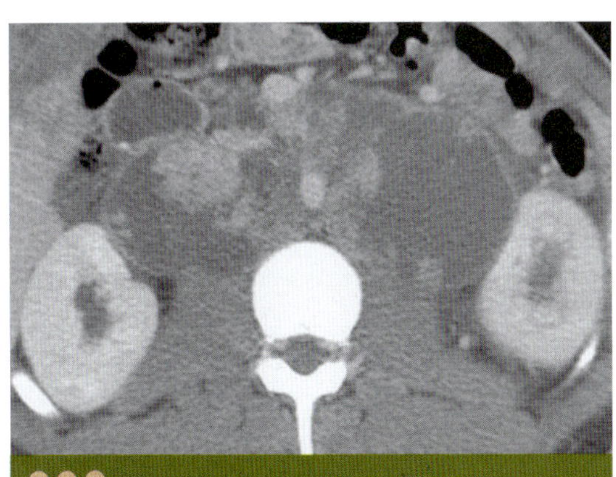

G. Retroperitoneal metastases: Axial CECT on a patient with history of testicular germ cell tumor shows extensive necrotic retroperitoneal adenopathy surrounding the aorta.

IMAGE KEY

Common

Rare

Typical

Unusual

CHAPTER 16

FEMALE PELVIS

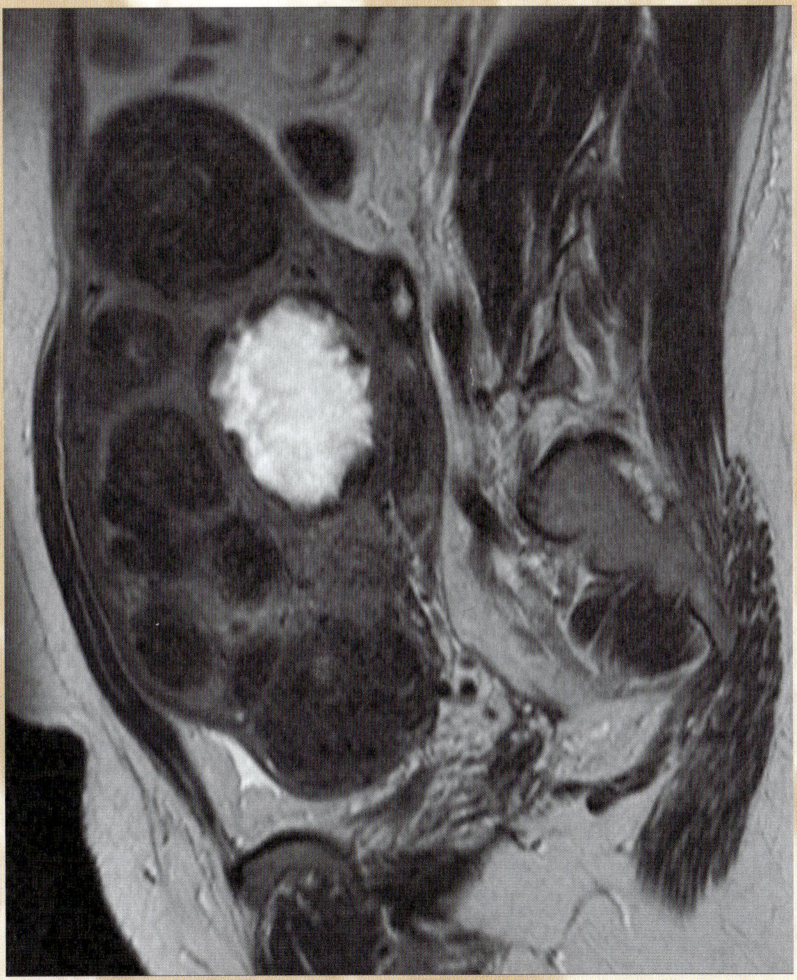

Part 1

Uterus

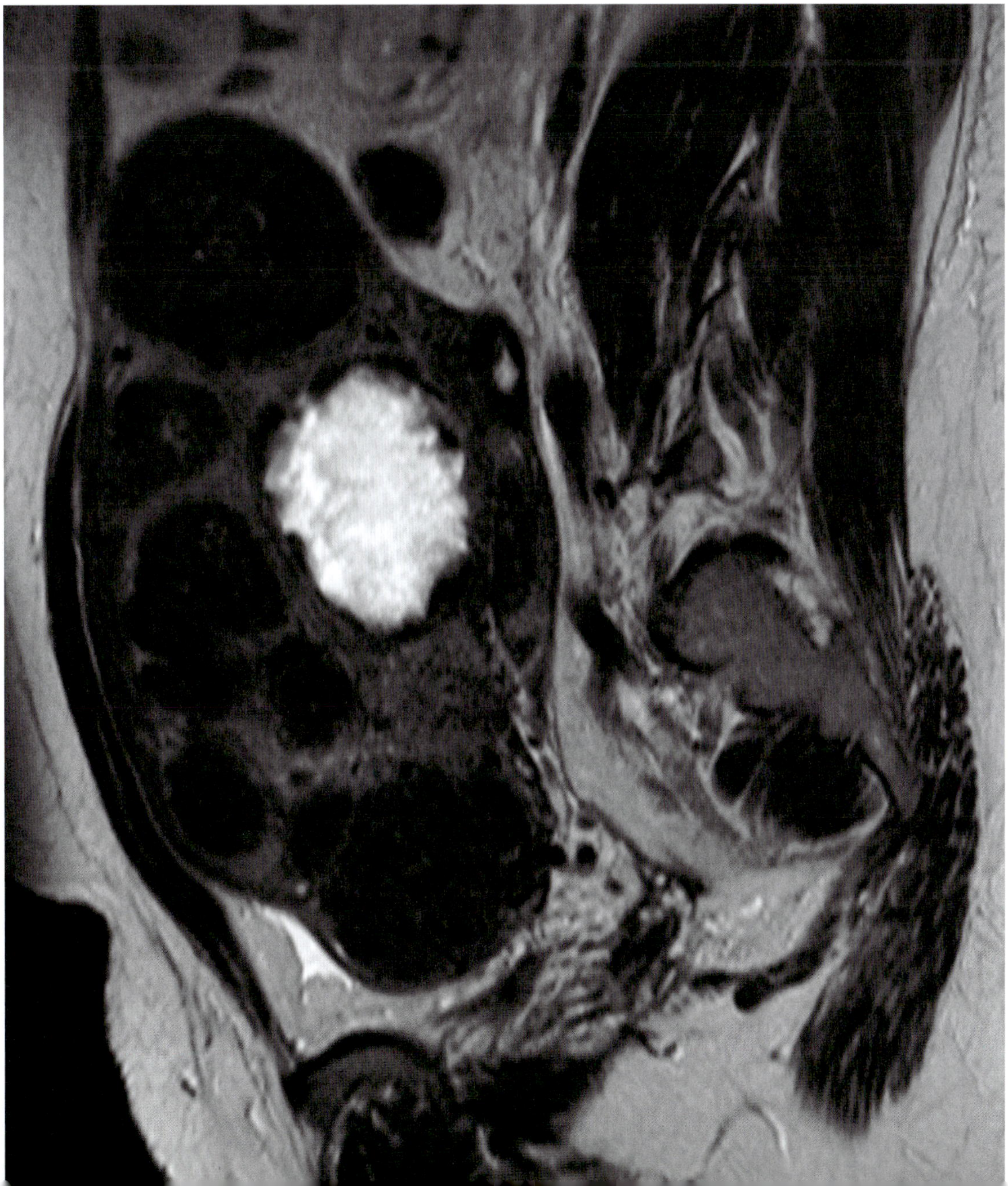

16–1 Uterine Fibroids—General

Paul Nikolaidis

PRESENTATION

Menorrhagia, pelvic pain, pressure.

FINDINGS

The uterus is enlarged and contains numerous well-circumscribed lesions that demonstrate homogenously low-signal intensity on T2-WI.

DIFFERENTIAL DIAGNOSES

- *Focal adenomyosis/adenomyomas*: Lesions are less well defined than fibroids, usually with a poorly defined border, minimal mass effect, and an elliptical rather than round configuration. Characteristic punctate T2-bright foci are typically present.
- *Uterine leiomyosarcoma*: While often indistinguishable from uterine fibroids, these rare lesions may show rapid enlargement and large areas of increased heterogeneity and necrosis.

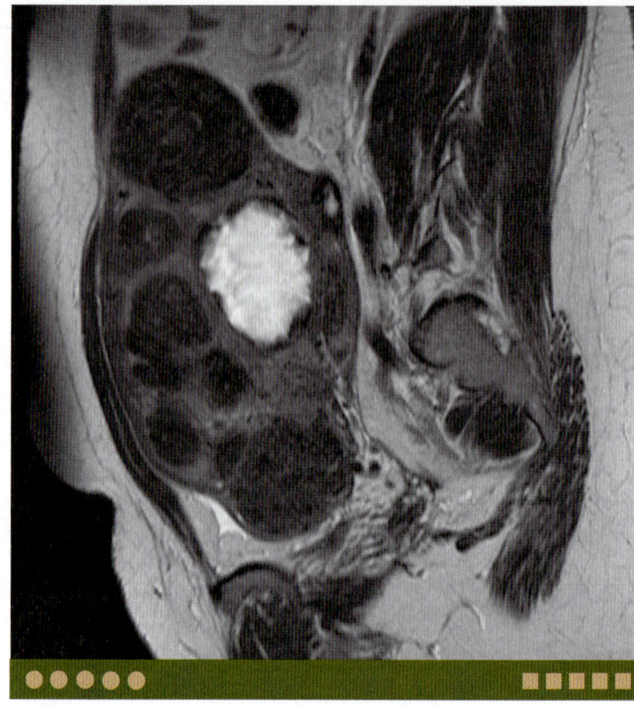

A. Sagittal T2-WI shows an enlarged uterus containing several T2 hypointense fibroids in addition to one that is hyperintense, presumably secondary to degeneration. Classically, fibroids are hypointense on T2-WI.

COMMENTS

Fibroids are the most common tumors in the uterus and occur in young and middle-aged females, with an incidence of approximately 20% to 30%. They are composed of whorled bundles of smooth muscle fibers separated by variable amounts of interspersed connective tissue and collagen. Their growth is promoted by estrogen. While most women with fibroids are asymptomatic, they may present with bleeding, pain, infertility, or a palpable mass.

Fibroids are classified as submucosal, intramural and subserosal. Submucosal fibroids protrude into the uterine cavity, distorting the endometrial cavity. Intramural fibroids are contained within the myometrium. Subserosal fibroids extend to and deform the peritoneal covering of the uterus.

On sonography, fibroids are typically well-defined, slightly heterogeneous and hypoechoic. They attenuate the ultrasound beam causing variable degrees of acoustic shadowing. They often show edge shadows and may have linear or chunky calcifications. If degenerated they may contain cystic, anechoic foci.

On CT, uterine fibroids appear either homogeneous or heterogeneous. Calcification or cystic changes may be seen in 3% to 10% of all fibroids, especially larger lesions. Smaller lesions may be inconspicuous.

MR is highly accurate, sensitive, and specific. Non-degenerated uterine fibroids appear as well-circumscribed masses of homogenously decreased signal intensity on T2-WI. On T1-weighted imaging, they are generally isointense to myometrium, unless they have undergone hemorrhagic degeneration in which case they are hyperintense. Unless degenerated or previously embolized, they enhance following gadolinium administration. More cellular fibroids may demonstrate higher signal intensity on T2-weighted sequences.

PEARLS

- **Fibroids are very common benign tumors.**
- **Growth is promoted by estrogen.**
- **On sonography they are slightly heterogeneous, hypoechoic and attenuate the ultrasound beam.**
- **T2-weighted MR will show low intensity and sharp borders, unless hypercellular, degenerated, or hemorrhagic.**

ADDITIONAL IMAGES (B-D)

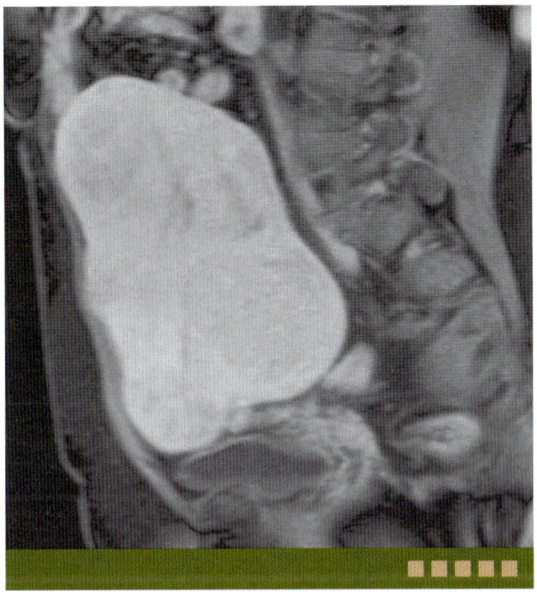

B. Sagittal contrast-enhanced T1-WI on a different patient shows a lobulated, enlarged uterus containing numerous enhancing round lesions compatible with fibroids.

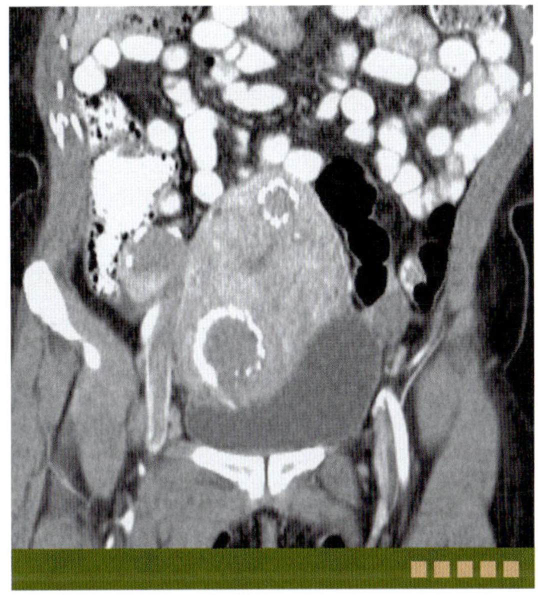

C. Coronal CECT reformation shows an enlarged uterus with two degenerated peripherally calcified fibroids. Note that there is no central enhancement of these fibroids.

DIFFERENTIAL DIAGNOSES IMAGES (D-E)

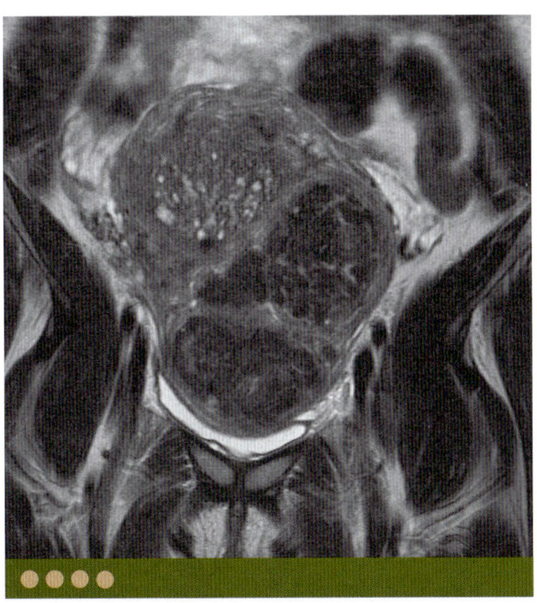

D. Fibroids and coexistant adenomyoma: Coronal T2-WI shows several T2 hypointense uterine fibroids in the mid and lower portion of an enlarged uterus. Superiorally, there is a focal adenomyoma, which is less well circumscribed, not as hypointense, and shows numerous T2-bright foci.

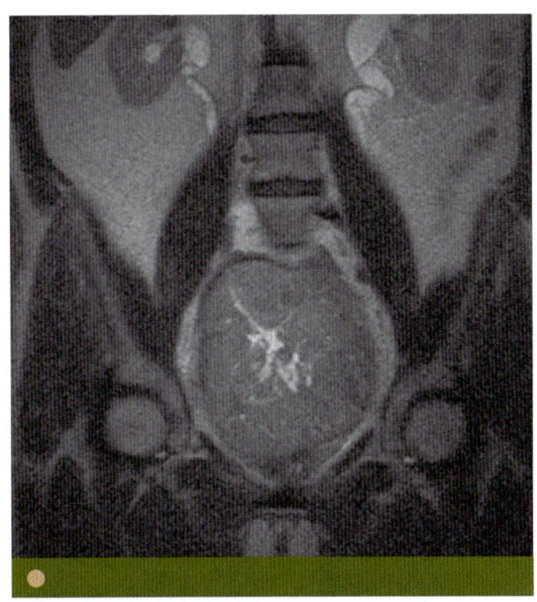

E. Leiomyosarcoma: Coronal T2-WI shows that the uterus is almost entirely replaced by a relatively hypointense mass with central linear foci of high-signal intensity. This mass was rapidly growing and on hysterectomy was shown to represent a large uterine leiomyosarcoma. Note that there is bilateral hydronephrosis and hydroureter.

IMAGE KEY

Common

Rare

Typical

Unusual

16–2 Submucosal Uterine Fibroids

Paul Nikolaidis

PRESENTATION

Menorrhagia, infertility, may be asymptomatic.

FINDINGS

A well-circumscribed lesion is seen projecting into the endometrial cavity, demonstrating homogeneously low-signal intensity on T2-WI.

DIFFERENTIAL DIAGNOSES

- *Endometrial carcinoma*: On MR, endometrial carcinoma is mildly hyperintense, heterogenous, and generally will enhance less than fibroids (unless degenerated). There may be disruption of the junctional zone and myometrial invasion.
- *Endometrial polyp*: On T2-WI, polyps are usually mildly hyperintense, sometimes with a central low-signal focus.

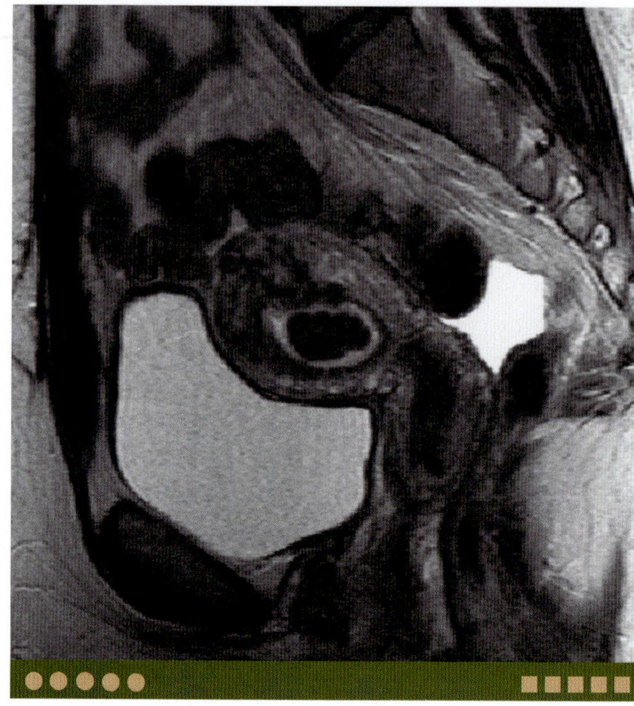

A. Sagittal T2-WI shows a large hypointense mass within the endometrial cavity surrounded by a thin layer of endometrium.

COMMENTS

Leiomyomas are classified as submucosal, intramural, and subserosal. Submucosal leiomyomas protrude into the uterine cavity, distorting the endometrium. They occur less frequently than other types of fibroids, but are more likely to be symptomatic as they may cause bleeding and infertility.

On sonography, submucosal fibroids are typically well defined, slightly heterogeneous hypoechoic lesions that indent and distort the myometrium. If larger, they may attenuate the ultrasound beam and cause variable degrees of acoustic shadowing. They often show edge shadows. Hysterosonography is more sensitive for the detection and characterization of submucosal fibroids than conventional gray-scale transvaginal sonography. Ultrasonography is less sensitive in the setting of an enlarged, myomatous uterus containing multiple fibroids. Furthermore, in some patients the endometrium may be very distorted or difficult to visualize.

MR imaging is highly accurate, sensitive, and specific for the evaluation of the exact location of uterine fibroids. It allows the precise demonstration of the endometrium and uterine zonal anatomy to assist in defining each fibroid as submucosal, intramural, or subserosal. Determining the exact location of fibroids is important for treatment and follow-up purposes. MR allows for more precise delineation of the size and location of fibroids than sonography, especially in larger patients or when the uterus is significantly enlarged. Nondegenerated uterine fibroids appear as well-circumscribed masses of homogenously decreased signal intensity when compared with normal myometrium on T2-WI. More cellular fibroids, composed primarily of compact smooth muscle cells with little or no collagen, demonstrate relatively higher signal intensity on T2-WI with avid enhancement on postcontrast images.

Purely submucosal uterine fibroids, particularly when they have a small stalk, are typically amenable to hysteroscopic resection.

PEARLS

- **Submucosal leiomyomas protrude into and distort the endometrial cavity.**
- **They may be symptomatic causing bleeding and infertility.**
- **Generally, MR allows for more precise delineation of submucosal fibroids than sonography.**

ADDITIONAL IMAGES (B-C)

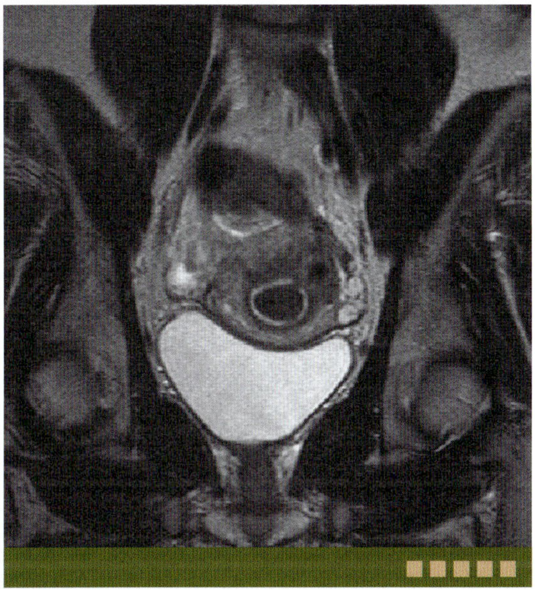

B. Corresponding coronal T2-WI shows the majority of the submucosal fibroid to be surrounded by a thin portion of endometrium except for the location of the small stalk.

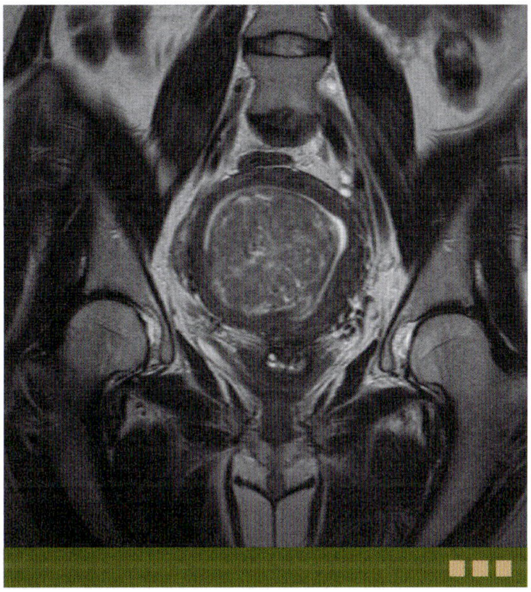

C. Coronal T2-WI on a different patient shows a large submucosal fibroid. It does not have the characteristic low-signal intensity on T2-WI, as a result of areas of degeneration.

DIFFERENTIAL DIAGNOSES IMAGES (D-E)

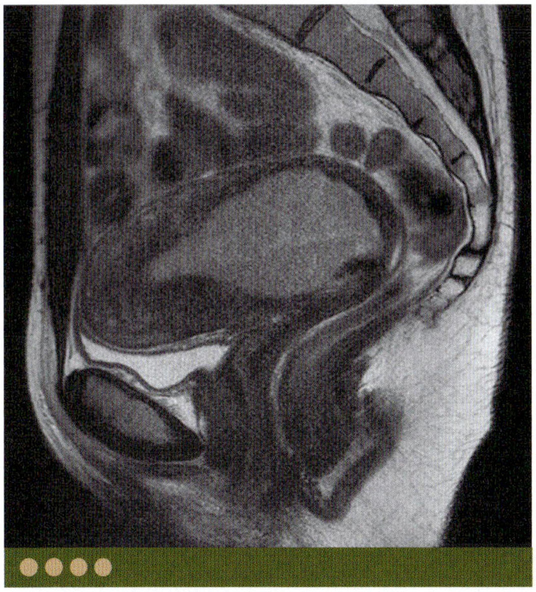

D. Endometrial carcinoma: Sagittal T2-WI on a patient with vaginal bleeding shows a mildly hyperintense lesion. It expands the lower part of the endometrial cavity. It is also extends into the cervical cavity. This represented a large endometrial carcinoma.

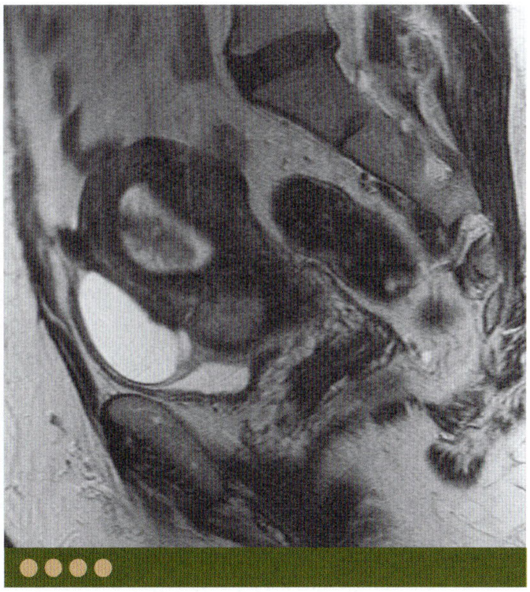

E. Endometrial polyp: Sagittal T2-WI on a patient with vaginal bleeding shows a mildly hyperintense endometrial mass with a central area of lower signal. This was shown on subsequent hysteroscopy and biopsy to represent an endometrial polyp.

IMAGE KEY

Common

Rare

Typical

Unusual

16–3 Subserosal Uterine Fibroids

Paul Nikolaidis

PRESENTATION

Palpable mass, pelvic fullness, urinary symptoms.

FINDINGS

A well-circumscribed pelvic mass located immediately adjacent to the uterus, with uniformly low-signal intensity on T2-WI.

DIFFERENTIAL DIAGNOSIS

- *Ovarian fibroma*: Has same signal characteristics as a uterine fibroid (hypointense on T2-WI); it should be shown to be connected to the ovary and separate from the uterus.

COMMENTS

Subserosal leiomyomas extend to and deform the peritoneal covering of the uterus. They may present as a palpable mass or with symptoms of pain or pressure on adjacent organs. If pressing on the bladder, patients may present with urinary symptoms. If pedunculated, patients may present with acute pain secondary to torsion.

On sonography, subserosal fibroids typically are well defined, slightly heterogeneous hypoechoic lesions that are inseparable from the uterus. Their attachment to the uterus is usually evident, but in some cases where there is a very thin stalk, it may not be visualized sonographically. They attenuate the ultrasound beam causing variable degrees of acoustic shadowing. They often show edge shadows, may have linear or chunky calcifications, and may contain anechoic, cystic foci, if degenerated.

MR imaging is highly accurate, sensitive, and specific in the evaluation of subserosal uterine fibroids, as it allows their exact localization. MR also nicely demonstrates the size of the stalk or attachment to the uterus, and the exact relationship of the fibroid to the adjacent pelvic viscera. Nondegenerated subserosal fibroids appear as well-circumscribed masses of homogeneous low-signal intensity when compared to normal myometrium on T2-WI. More cellular fibroids demonstrate higher signal intensity on T2-WI, with avid enhancement on postcontrast images. Degenerated subserosal fibroids appear as well-circumscribed masses of variable, often high, signal on T2-WI and may not enhance on postcontrast images.

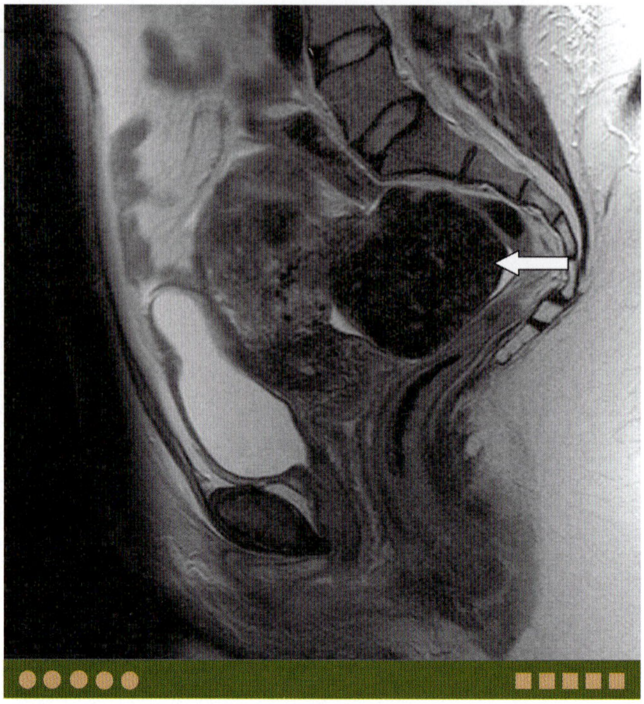

A. Sagittal T2-WI shows a large hypointense mass immediately posterior to the uterus (arrow). It has a broad-based attachment to the uterus. Additional smaller intramural fibroids are also present.

PEARLS

- **Extend to and deform the peritoneal covering of the uterus.**
- **Often asymptomatic unless they become quite enlarged or undergo torsion.**
- **The differentiation between a subserosal fibroid and an adnexal mass (especially in the setting of torsion) is very important.**
- **MR is the best modality for the identification and most precise delineation of subserosal fibroids.**

ADDITIONAL IMAGES (B-D)

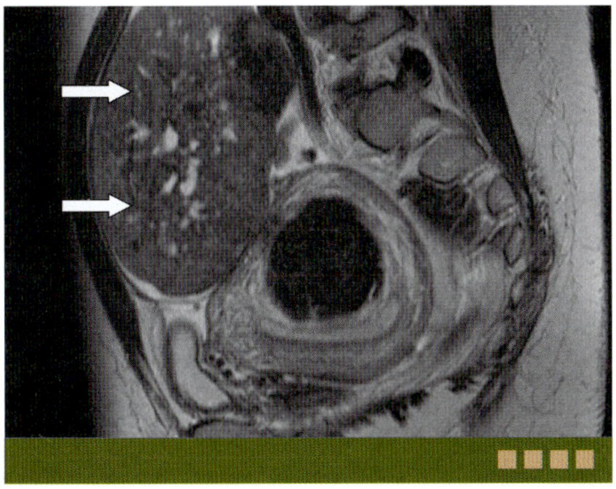

B. Sagittal T2-WI on a different patient shows a pedunculated subserosal uterine fibroid (arrows). Note the presence of multiple T2-hyperintense foci within the mass, representing foci of degeneration.

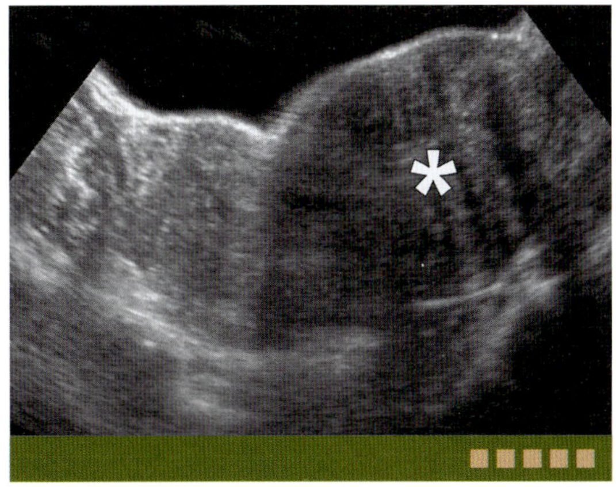

C. Transverse transabdominal sonogram shows a 7 cm heterogeneous solid pelvic mass (asterisk) immediately adjacent to the uterus. It attenuates the sound beam.

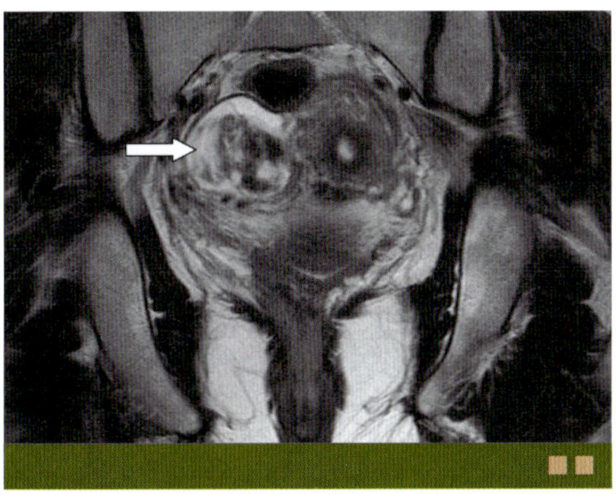

D. Coronal T2-WI on another patient with acute onset of right pelvic pain shows a round heterogeneous mass (arrow) with predominantly high T2-signal. It is connected to the uterus. This represents a torsed/degenerated subserosal uterine fibroid.

DIFFERENTIAL DIAGNOSIS IMAGES (E-G)

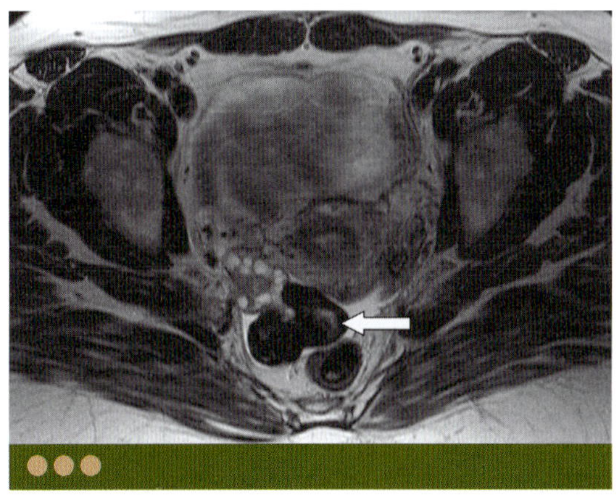

E. Ovarian fibroma: Axial T2-WI shows a hypointense mass immediately posterior to the right ovary (arrow). Note that this hypointense mass is connected to the right ovary and not the uterus.

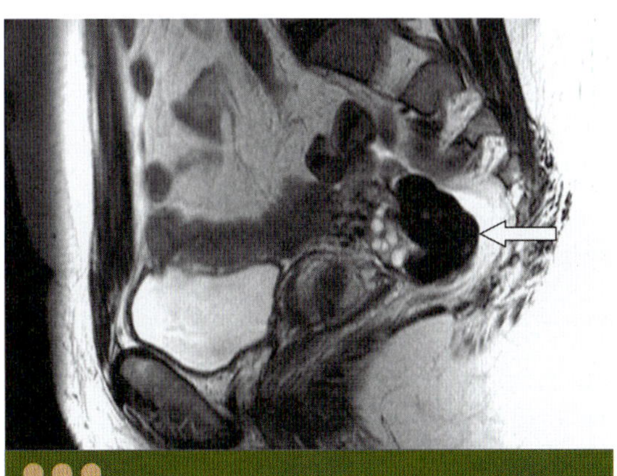

F. Ovarian fibroma: Corresponding sagittal T2-WI again shows the hypointense mass immediately posterior to the right ovary (arrow).

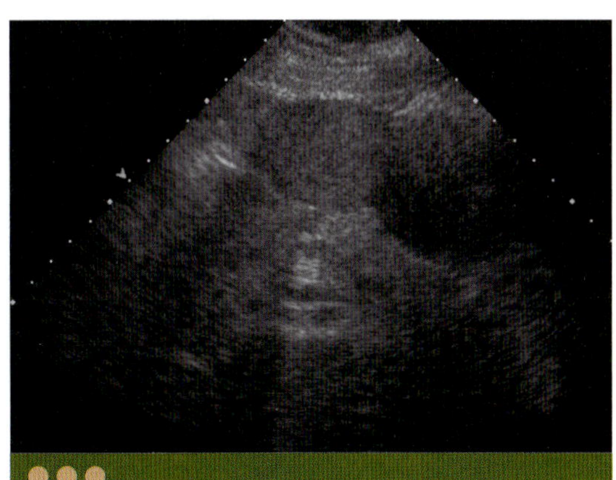

G. Ovarian fibroma: Transvaginal sonogram shows a homogeneous solid lesion corresponding to an ovarian fibroma.

IMAGE KEY

Common

Rare

Typical

Unusual

16–4 Uterine Artery Embolization

Paul Nikolaidis

PRESENTATION

Treatment option for patients with bulk symptoms; menorrhagia.

FINDINGS

Post uterine artery embolization (UAE) MR images compared to the pre-UAE MR show a decrease in fibroid and uterine size. Treated fibroids no longer enhance.

DIFFERENTIAL DIAGNOSIS

None

COMMENTS

Fibroids are the most common tumors in the uterus with an incidence of more than 20% to 30%. While most women are asymptomatic, they may present with significant bleeding, pain, or pressure on adjacent organs. Until recently, the main treatment options were surgical (myomectomy or hysterectomy) or hormonal treatment. The application of UAE to the treatment of uterine fibroids was first described in 1995. It has since grown exponentially, and an estimated 25,000 patients were treated in 2008.

UAE results in the infarction of fibroids by injecting a particulate embolization agent into the main uterine arteries. The hypervascular nature of fibroids causes the embolization agents to preferentially target the fibroids, with relative sparing of the normal myometrium, ultimately resulting in infarction, coagulation necrosis, retraction, and shrinkage of the fibroids.

Clinical studies have reported a success rate of about 81% to 94% in curing menorrhagia symptoms, and an average reduction in fibroid volume ranging between 35% and 70%. UAE is best suited for premenopausal women with symptomatic fibroids and no plans for childbearing. It is also appropriate for postmenopausal women, but only for bulk symptoms, not menorrhagia, which may have a different cause.

Prior to the procedure, a baseline MR examination should be performed to evaluate the size, location, and enhancement characteristics of fibroids. The preprocedure MR is also important in the detection of any other uterine or extrauterine pathology (such as adenomyosis, endometriosis, endometrial, other pelvic lesions). Follow-up of patients after UAE consists of both clinical and imaging follow-up. A routine follow-up MR is usually done at 3 months after the procedure. Treated fibroids should show a decrease in size and should no longer enhance. MR should also be obtained if a complication is suspected, or if the patient presents with symptoms, including significant pain or signs of infection.

UAE is generally a very safe procedure that is well tolerated. Severe complications, requiring major treatment or readmission occur in approximately 1.3%. One potentially severe complication is fibroid expulsion with associated infection. Expulsion is usually self-limited and occurs at 2 weeks to 6 months following UAE. If there is associated infection, patients may present with pain, fever, vaginal bleeding or discharge, and tissue passage. Management usually consists of antibiotics, pain medications, and observation. If the patient becomes septic, or if the fibroid has not passed within 2 to 4 days, hysteroscopic-assisted removal should be considered; in more severe cases, emergent hysterectomy may be required.

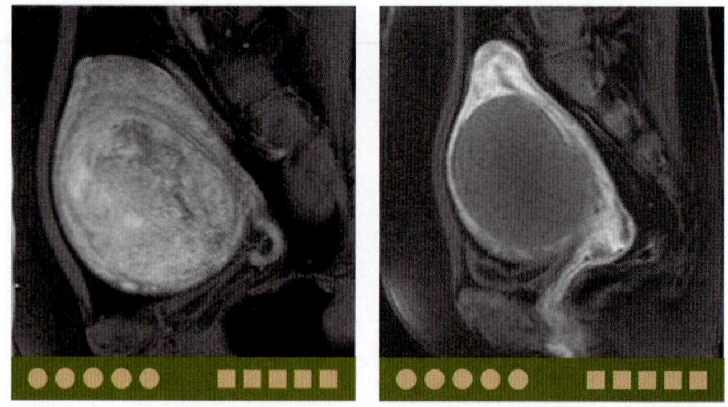

A. Sagittal contrast-enhanced T1-WI shows an enlarged uterus with a dominant 9-cm enhancing fibroid.
B. Sagittal contrast-enhanced T1-WI 4 months following UAE. The uterus is smaller and the fibroid no longer enhances.

PEARLS

- **UAE is a safe and effective treatment alternative to surgery for symptomatic fibroids.**
- **Preprocedure MR should be routinely obtained.**
- **MR is also useful in routine follow-up and evaluation of potential complications.**

ADDITIONAL IMAGES (C-F)

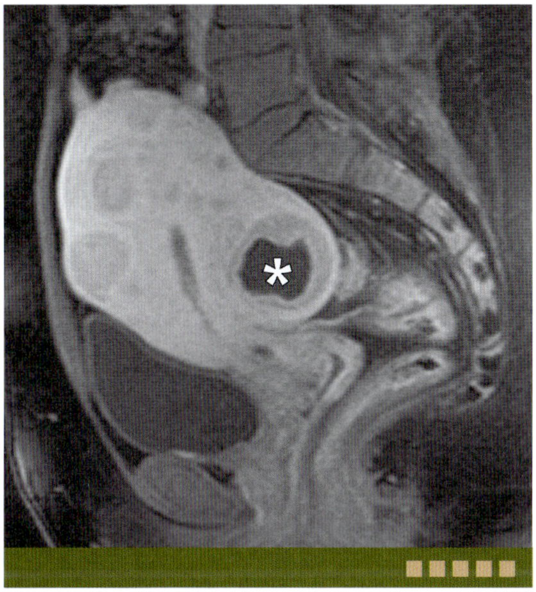

C. Sagittal contrast-enhanced T1-WI on another patient shows numerous fibroids within an enlarged uterus. All but one (asterisk) enhance.

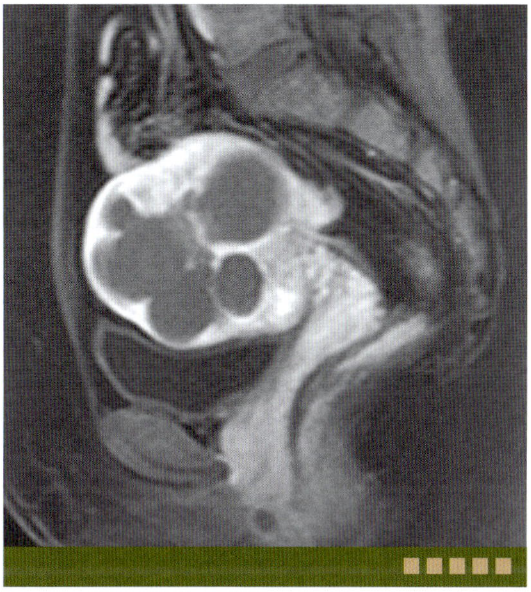

D. Sagittal contrast-enhanced T1-WI on the same patient obtained 6 months following UAE. The uterus has decreased in size. All fibroids no longer enhance.

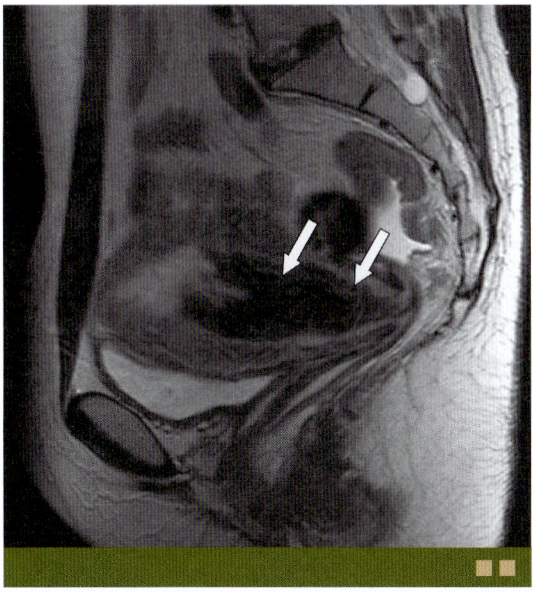

E. Sagittal T2-WI on a patient who underwent UAE 4 months prior shows an oblong uterine fibroid that fills the lower portion of the uterine cavity and extends into the cervix (arrows). The fibroid is about to be expelled from the endometrial cavity, one of the most important complications of UAE.

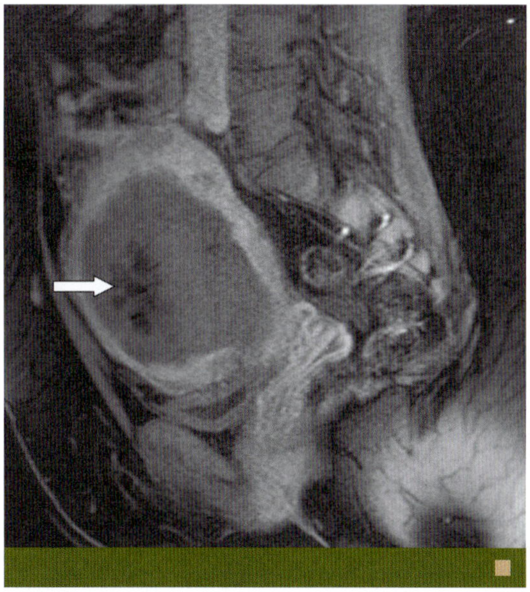

F. Sagittal contrast-enhanced T1-WI in another patient who underwent UAE 2 months prior shows a large nonenhancing uterine fibroid. Foci of low-signal intensity correspond to air (arrow). The patient, who was septic, underwent hysterectomy, and an infected fibroid was confirmed on pathology.

IMAGE KEY

Common

Rare

Typical

Unusual

16–5 Uterine Lipoleiomyoma

Paul Nikolaidis

PRESENTATION

Usually asymptomatic.

FINDINGS

Transabdominal and transvaginal sonography shows a hyperechoic shadowing mass within the uterus.

DIFFERENTIAL DIAGNOSES

- *Ovarian dermoid*: Sonographic features are identical; however, lesions are of ovarian origin and not intrauterine in location.
- *Uterine fibroid (leiomyoma)*: Lipoleiomyomas are distinguished from uterine fibroids on sonography by their uniformly hyperechoic appearance. On CT and MR, the identification of fat within the lipoleiomyoma is diagnostic.

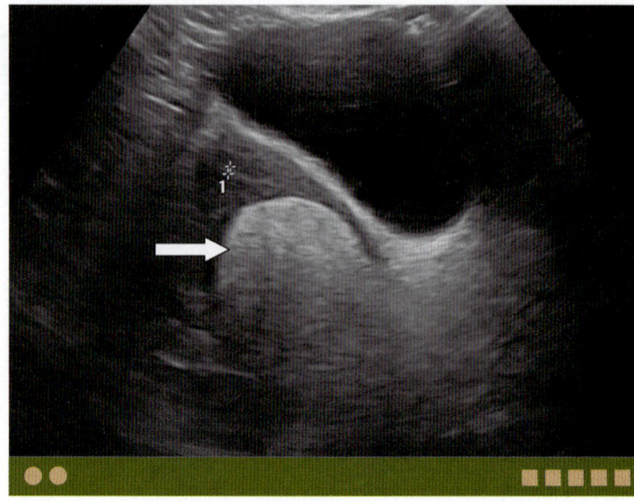

A. Sagittal transabdominal sonogram shows a large hyperechoic uterine lesion (arrow) with extensive shadowing. Note the adjacent thin endometrial stripe (calipers).

COMMENTS

Lipoleiomyomas are rare benign uterine tumors that occur in older females, with a reported incidence of 0.03% to 0.2%. Most patients are asymptomatic. They are composed of fatty elements, bundles of smooth muscle fibers and fibrous tissue. Proposed etiologic theories include metaplasia from smooth muscle or connective tissue and proliferation of lipid tissue within embryonic rests. Patients may have coexisting fibroids.

Lipoleiomyomas usually have pathognomonic features on sonography. The characteristic appearance is a markedly hyperechoic myometrial mass with significant associated shadowing. The equivalent of the "tip of the iceberg" sign seen with ovarian dermoids is often present.

On CT, they appear as well circumscribed predominantly fatty masses, often with some areas of nonfatty tissue. On CECT, they may show areas of mildly heterogeneous enhancement and a well-defined border. Unlike fibroids, they do not have areas of calcification or cystic change.

On MR, lipoleiomyomas appear as well-circumscribed masses that are hyperintense on T1-WI. A few hypointense thin bands of smooth muscle and fibrous tissue are usually seen traversing the predominantly fatty lesion. Signal dropout should be present on fat-suppressed sequences. Following gadolinium administration, enhancing amorphous bands of tissue are seen within the fatty mass. In some cases, the lesion will have an enhancing capsule.

PEARLS

- **Rare benign predominantly fatty tumors of the uterus.**
- **Occur in older patients, usually asymptomatic.**
- **On sonography, markedly hyperechoic shadowing myometrial lesions.**
- **On CT and MR, predominantly fatty masses with enhancing bands of smooth muscle and fibrous tissue.**

ADDITIONAL IMAGES (B-D)

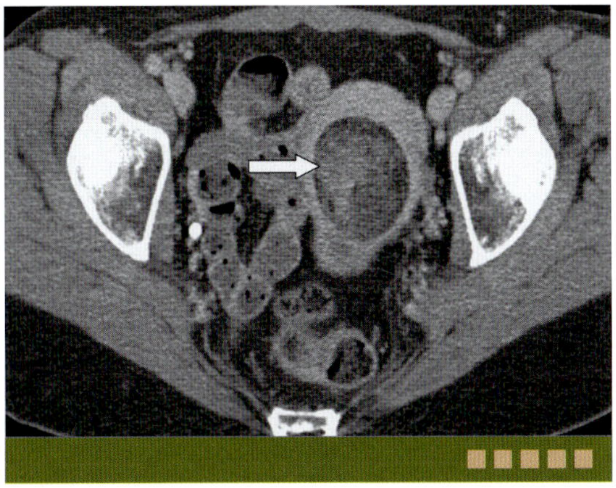

B. Axial CECT on the same patient shows a predominantly fatty myometrial mass with internal enhancing soft tissue components (arrow). Note that there is slight capsular enhancement.

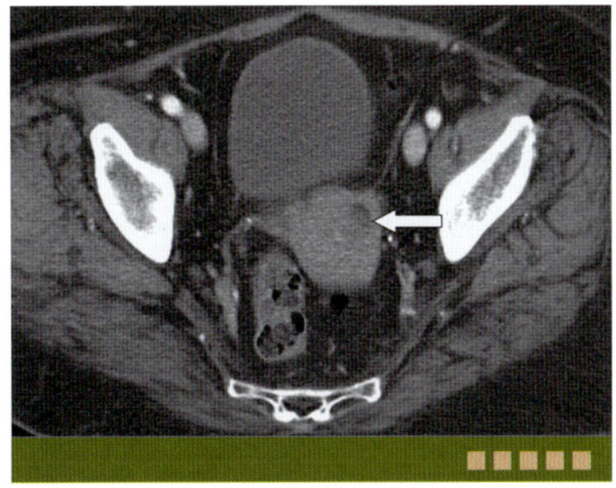

C. Axial CECT on another patient shows a small myometrial mass (arrow) with fatty elements (confirmed by negative Hounsfield attenuation units).

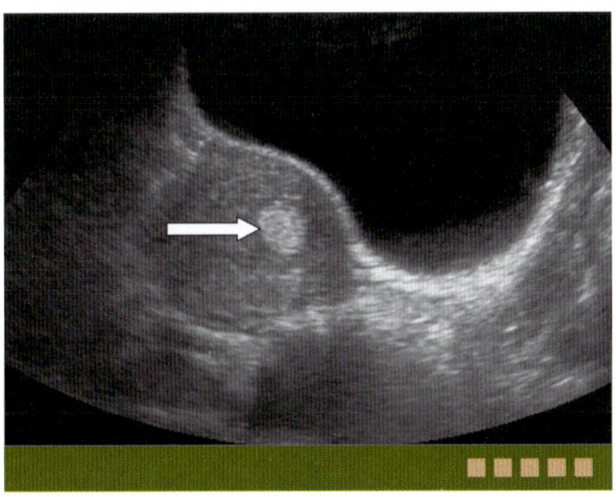

D. Corresponding sagittal transabdominal pelvic sonogram shows the markedly hyperechoic small uterine lipoleiomyoma (arrow).

DIFFERENTIAL DIAGNOSES IMAGES (E-G)

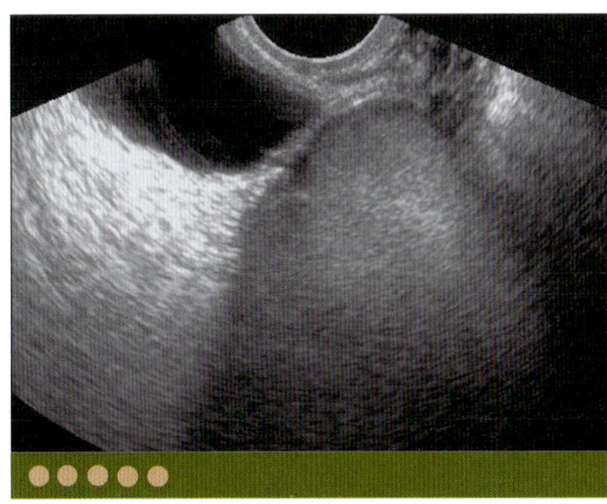

E. Ovarian dermoid: Transvaginal sonogram shows a large hyperechoic lesion with extensive shadowing. Sonographic features are similar to a lipoleiomyoma, but this lesion is located in the left adnexa, adjacent to the uterus.

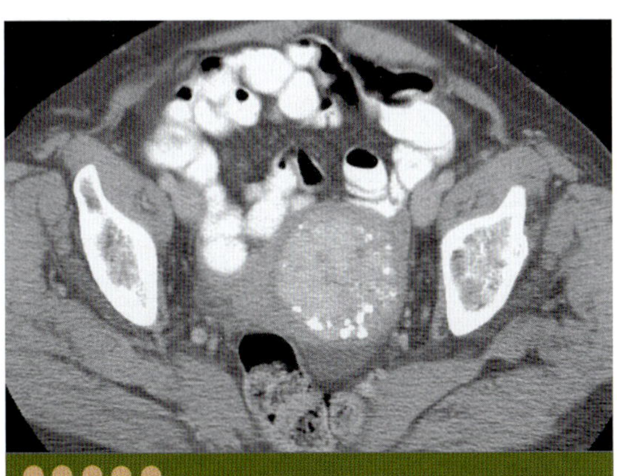

F. Uterine fibroid (leiomyoma): Axial CECT shows a peripherally calcified, enhancing intramural fibroid. Note that there are a few small internal areas of low attenuation, corresponding to areas of cystic degeneration (not fatty tissue by Hounsfield units [HU]). Lipoleiomyomas are not known to calcify.

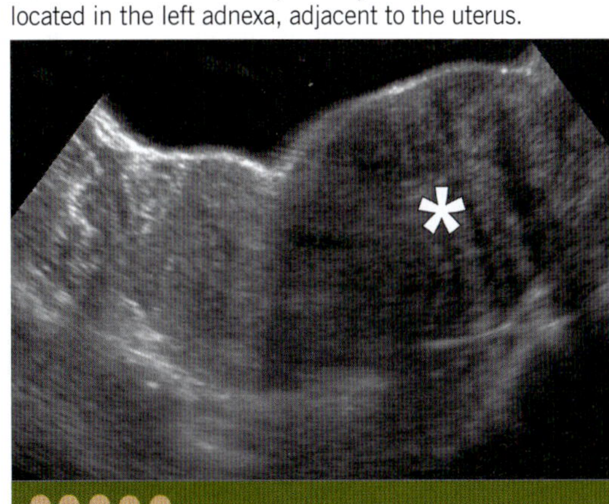

G. Uterine fibroid (leiomyoma): Transverse transabdominal sonogram shows a 7 cm heterogeneous solid uterine mass (arrowhead). It is isoechoic to slightly hypoechoic. It also attenuates the sound beam. This was shown on MR to represent a large uterine fibroid. A lipoleiomyoma would be markedly hyperechoic with significant shadowing.

IMAGE KEY

Common

Rare

Typical

Unusual

16–6 Uterine Leiomyosarcoma

Paul Nikolaidis

PRESENTATION

Pelvic mass/fullness, abdominal and back pain.

FINDINGS

MR demonstrates a large heterogeneous, necrotic uterine mass.

DIFFERENTIAL DIAGNOSES

- *Uterine fibroids*: Uterine leiomyosarcoma should be considered if there has been rapid growth, if more than 50% of a fibroid demonstrates high-signal intensity on T2-WI, if T1-hyperintense foci are present, or if large necrotic areas are seen on postcontrast imaging.
- *Advanced endometrial carcinoma or sarcoma*: May be impossible to distinguish from a leiomyosarcoma.

COMMENTS

Uterine leiomyosarcoma (LMS) represents the most frequent type of pure uterine sarcomas, accounting for 42% to 60% of uterine sarcomas and 1% to 8% of all uterine malignancies. Uterine LMS is more prone to metastasize to distant organs (lungs, liver, kidney) than endometrial cancer. They usually occur in postmenopausal women. Several cases have been reported in women of reproductive age.

Differentiating uterine LMS from uterine fibroids may be difficult. The prevalence of sarcomatous degeneration in patients with fibroids is less than 1%. There are no reliable imaging criteria to help distinguish sarcomatous degeneration from other types of degeneration. One recent study suggested that LMS should be considered if more than 50% of a fibroid demonstrates high-signal intensity on T2-WI, if there are high-signal intensity areas of any size on T1-WI, or if there are any avascular, pocket-like areas on contrast-enhanced imaging.

In the clinical setting, leiomyosarcoma should be considered when there is rapid fibroid growth in a postmenopausal woman. Unfortunately, in some cases leiomyosarcomas will be presumed to represent fibroids and may be inadvertently followed clinically or embolized.

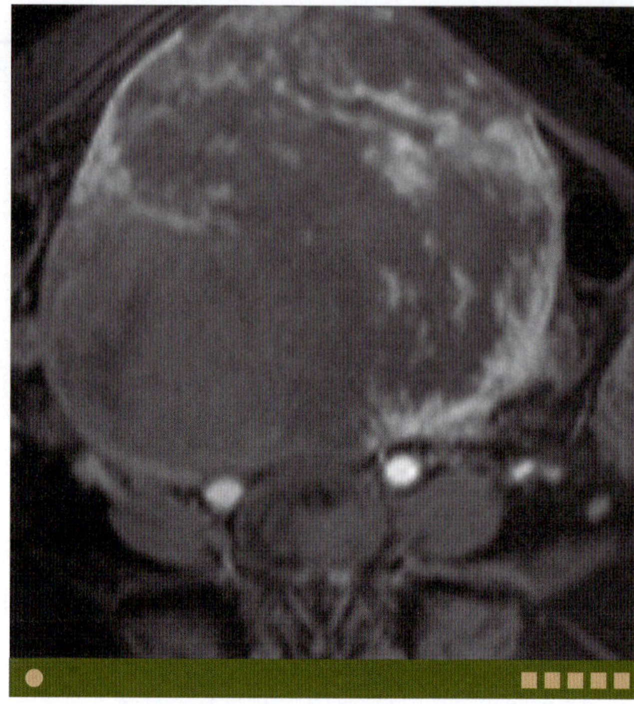

A. Axial contrast-enhanced T1-WI shows a large necrotic uterine mass with only a few intervening strands of enhancing tissue.

The most important prognostic factor is the stage of the disease. While an almost 80% 5-year survival rate has been reported in patients with stage I LMS, prognosis for patients with more advanced disease is very poor. Most patients will present with later stage disease.

PEARLS

- **Most frequent type of pure uterine sarcoma.**
- **Usually occur in postmenopausal women.**
- **Leiomyosarcoma should be considered when there is rapid growth of a fibroid, particularly in a postmenopausal woman.**
- **There are no consistent, reliable imaging criteria to distinguish sarcomatous degeneration from other types of degeneration.**

ADDITIONAL IMAGES (B-C)

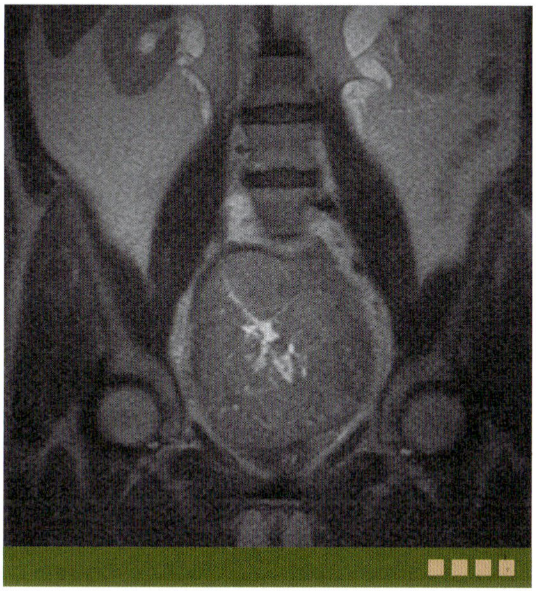

B. Coronal T2-WI on a different patient shows a large uterine mass with central areas of increased signal. Note how this mass causes bilateral hydronephrosis.

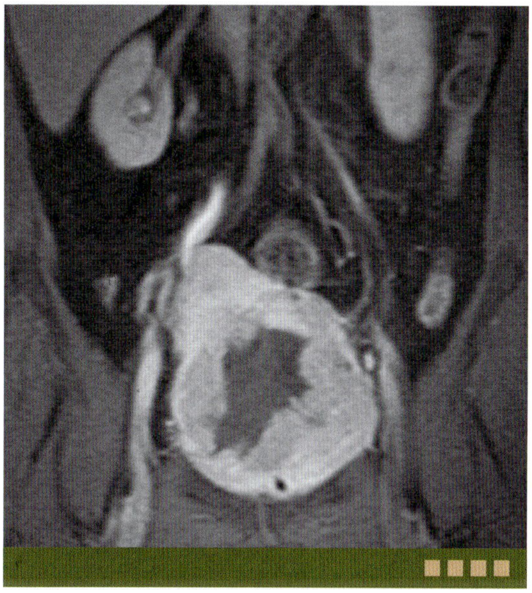

C. Corresponding coronal contrast-enhanced T1-WI on the same patient shows central areas of necrosis. This would be difficult to distinguish from a degenerated or incompletely embolized uterine fibroid.

DIFFERENTIAL DIAGNOSES IMAGES (D-E)

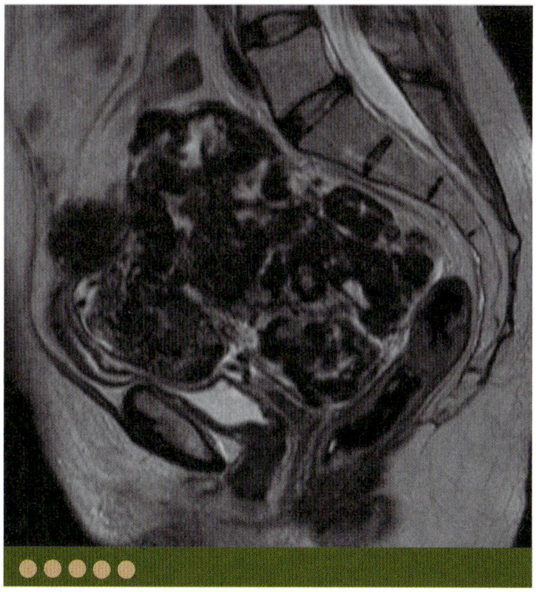

D. Uterine fibroids: Sagittal T2-WI shows multiple irregularly outlined uterine fibroids, enlarging, and distorting the shape of the uterus. A few foci of high-signal intensity relating to degeneration are seen.

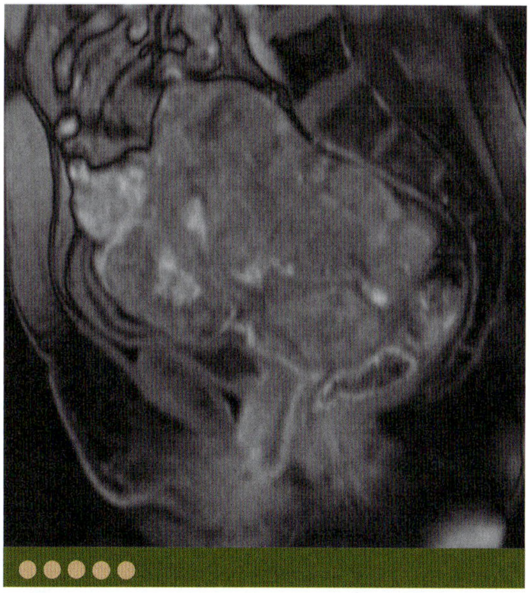

E. Uterine fibroids: Corresponding sagittal contrast-enhanced T1-WI shows a heterogeneous pattern of enhancement of the uterine fibroids. They are mostly relatively hypovascular.

IMAGE KEY

Common

Rare

Typical

Unusual

16–7 Diffuse Adenomyosis

Paul Nikolaidis

PRESENTATION

Heavy menstrual bleeding, bulk symptoms, enlarged uterus.

FINDINGS

A markedly thickened hypointense junctional zone is seen containing multiple punctate T2-bright foci.

DIFFERENTIAL DIAGNOSIS

None

COMMENTS

Adenomyosis is a process in which ectopic endometrial glands and stroma extend deep into the myometrium, with associated smooth muscle hypertrophy. The estimated incidence of adenomyosis varies widely, reported to be between 5% and 70% in different surgical series. Symptoms are present in about a third of patients. They are usually nonspecific, including dysmenorrhea, menorrhagia, bulk symptoms and pelvic pain. Similar symptoms are also encountered with fibroids, dysfunctional bleeding, or even endometriosis. Up to 80% of women with adenomyosis have other coexisting pelvic disease, making diagnosis a challenge.

Ultrasound usually shows enlargement of the uterus, heterogeneity and characteristic foci of decreased echogenicity within the myometrium (representing the ectopic endometrial glands). Echogenic linear striations may also be seen within the myometrium.

MR is very sensitive in the detection of adenomyosis. Diffuse adenomyosis appears as thickening of the entire junctional zone (measuring more than 12 mm) on T2-WI. In many instances, there are embedded T2-bright foci, corresponding to islands of ectopic endometrial tissue and cystic dilatation of glands. When menstrual hemorrhage occurs within these ectopic endometrial tissues, they may show high-signal intensity on T1-WI.

Reduction of heavy menstrual bleeding can be achieved with GnRH agonists such as Lupron. UAE remains controversial in the treatment of isolated adenomyosis, without coexisting fibroids. Hysterectomy is still considered by many to be the only permanent treatment for symptomatic adenomyosis.

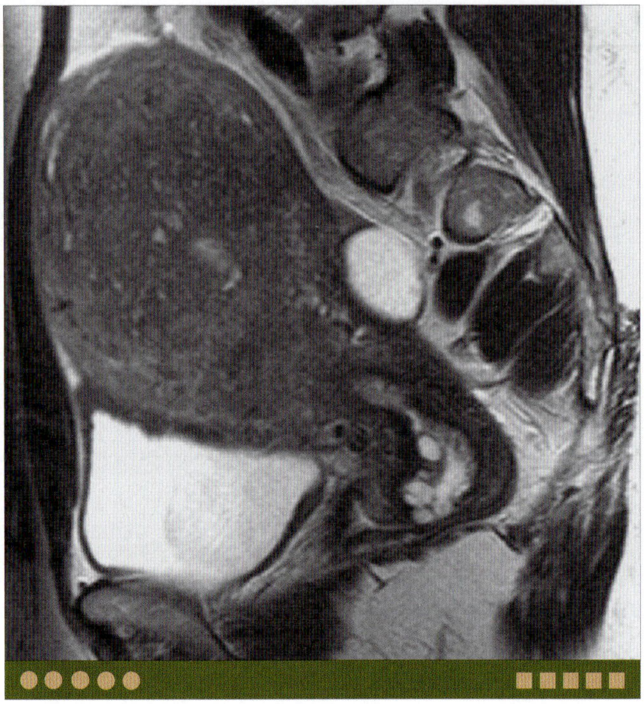

A. Sagittal T2-WI shows an enlarged uterus with a markedly thickened junctional zone, containing numerous characteristic small hyperintense foci.

PEARLS

- **Endometrial glands and stroma extend deep within the myometrium diffusely throughout the uterus.**
- **Symptoms are usually nonspecific and include dysmenorrhea, menorrhagia, and bulk symptoms or pain.**
- **On sonography, the uterus is typically enlarged and heterogeneous with small anechoic or hypoechoic foci.**
- **MR classically shows thickening of the junctional zone, often with characteristic small foci of high signal on T2-WI.**

ADDITIONAL IMAGES (B-E)

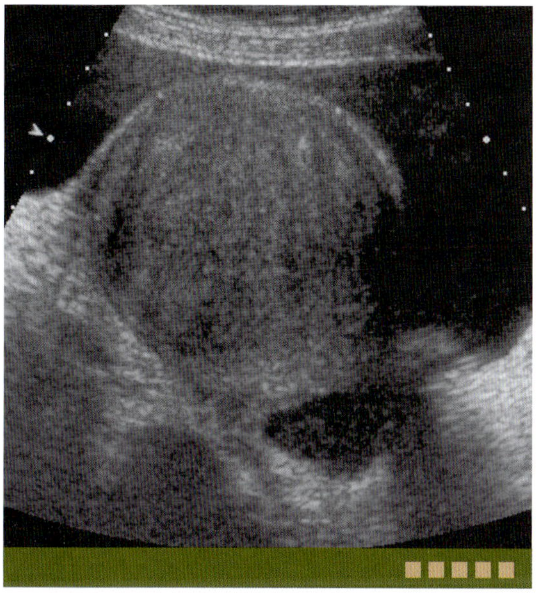

B. Transverse transabdominal pelvic sonogram again shows an enlarged, globular uterus with numerous punctate anechoic and hypoechoic foci.

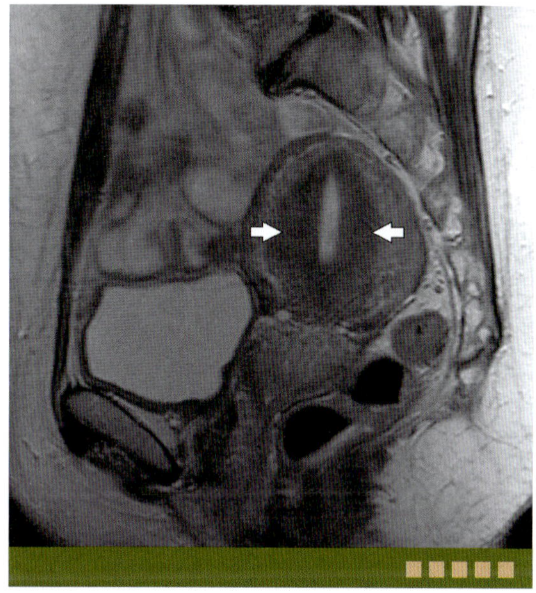

C. Sagittal T2-WI on a different patient with diffuse adenomyosis shows widening of the hypointense junctional zone (arrows), which measures up to 19 mm.

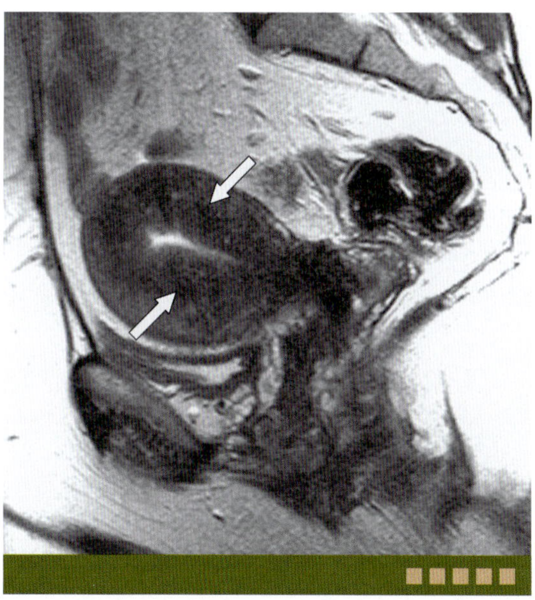

D. Sagittal T2-WI on a different patient with diffuse adenomyosis shows the junctional zone is relatively indistinct and widened measuring up to 17 mm (arrows). A few small hyperintense foci are also seen.

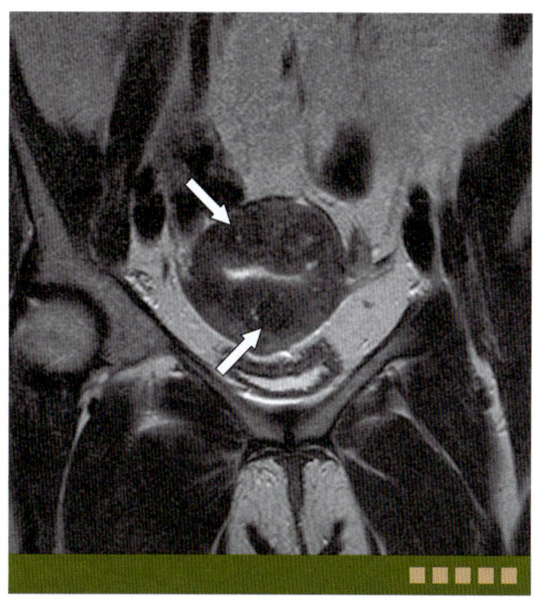

E. Coronal T2-WI on the same patient again shows an indistinct and widened junctional zone that extends well into the outer myometrium (arrows).

IMAGE KEY

Common

Rare

Typical

Unusual

16–8 Focal Adenomyosis and Adenomyoma

Paul Nikolaidis

PRESENTATION

Heavy menstrual bleeding, bulk symptoms, enlarged uterus on pelvic examination.

FINDINGS

T2-WI shows a hypointense myometrial mass with small internal T2-bright foci.

DIFFERENTIAL DIAGNOSIS

- *Uterine fibroid*: May be difficult to distinguish from an adenomyoma. Fibroids are usually better defined, rounder, and with sharper borders. Adenomyomas should be inseparable from the junctional zone. Adenomyomas may also show the characteristic small T2-hyperintense foci.

COMMENTS

Adenomyosis is most commonly diffuse but may also occur as a focal mass. Two forms of focal adenomyosis have been described: (1) focal adenomyosis, which is typically restricted to only one side of the uterus and (2) adenomyoma, which is a more localized, circumscribed form of adenomyosis. Some authors prefer not to use the term "adenomyoma" but simply use the term focal adenomyosis as there are other distinct pathologic entities described as adenomyomas.

The best modality for detection and characterization of these more localized forms of adenomyosis is MR. Areas of focal adenomyosis are typically restricted to only one side of the uterus. They are low-signal intensity on T2-WI. The junctional zone is either indistinct or abnormally widened. Characteristic T2-bright foci are typically present, corresponding to islands of ectopic endometrial glands with cystic dilatation.

More circumscribed areas of adenomyosis (adenomyomas) may pose a greater diagnostic challenge.

On MR, adenomyomas are usually less well-defined lesions without sharp borders, and an irregular interface with the myometrium. They generally exert minimal mass effect. Adenomyomas are of low-signal intensity on T2-WI. The characteristic punctate T2-bright foci, representing ectopic endometrial tissue and cystic dilatation of endometrial glands may be present, but not always, rendering diagnosis more difficult. In general, adenomyomas enhance less avidly than fibroids following gadolinium administration.

In patients that are asymptomatic, no treatment is necessary. Temporary relief of heavy menstrual bleeding can be achieved with GnRH agonists such as Lupron. Uterine artery embolization remains controversial in the treatment of isolated adenomyosis. Hysterectomy is currently considered by many to be the only permanent treatment for symptomatic adenomyosis.

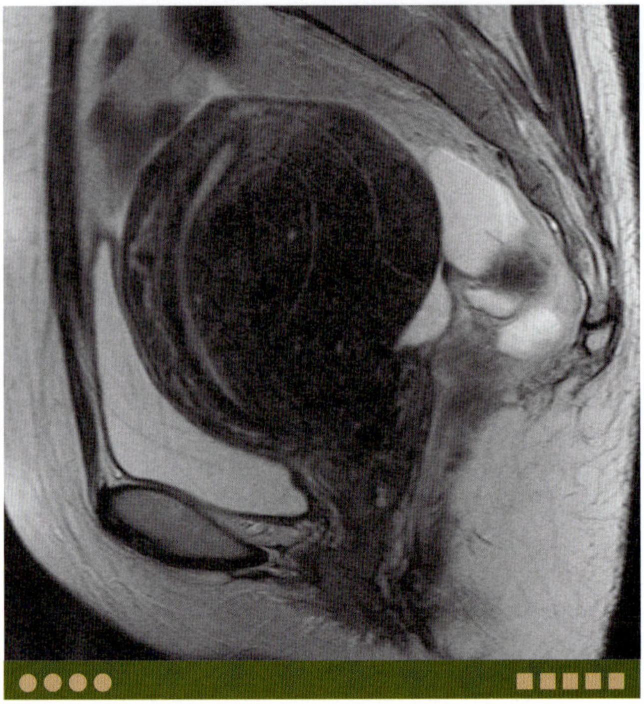

A. Sagittal T2-WI shows a large hypointense oval area of low-signal intensity in the posterior aspect of the uterus, with a few small hyperintense foci. Note how this area of focal adenomyosis is not very well circumscribed, and is somewhat ovoid in shape.

PEARLS

- **Two forms of focal adenomyosis have been described: adenomyoma (a localized, circumscribed form of adenomyosis) and focal adenomyosis (affecting only one side of the uterus).**
- **Symptoms are usually nonspecific and include dysmenorrhea, menorrhagia, and pelvic pain.**
- **On sonography, may be difficult to distinguish from fibroids.**
- **MR is usually diagnostic as it allows for a more detailed depiction of the uterus and excellent delineation of zonal anatomy.**

ADDITIONAL IMAGES (B-C)

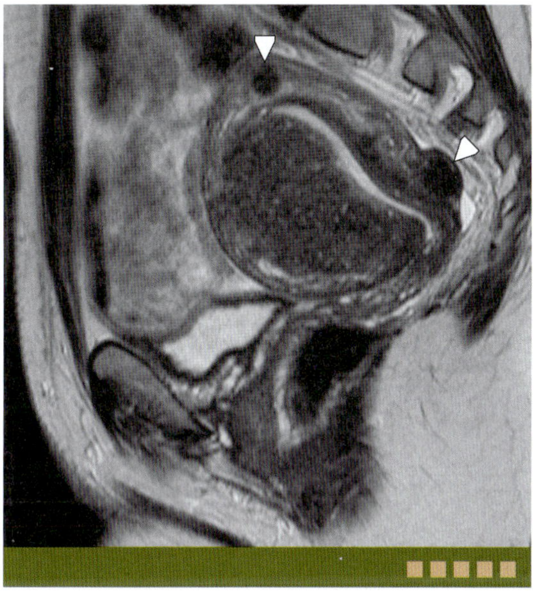

B. Sagittal T2-WI on a different patient shows an area of focal adenomyosis in the anterior aspect of the uterus. Again, characteristic T2-bright foci are seen. Note the presence of two small fibroids (arrowheads).

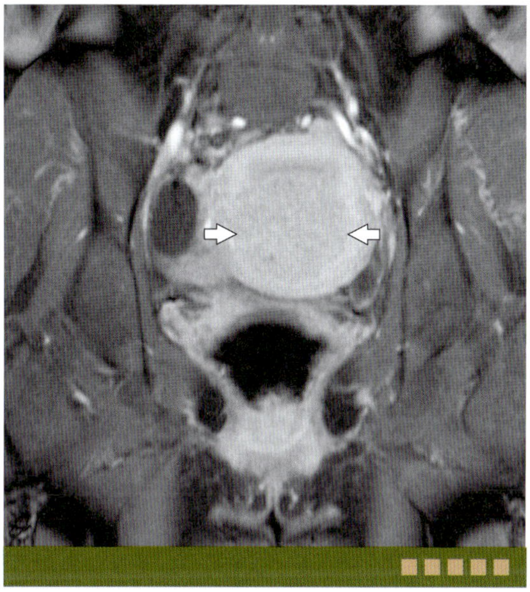

C. Coronal contrast-enhanced T1-WI on the same patient again shows an area of focal adenomyosis inferior to the endometrial cavity (arrows). Note the faint subtle foci of nonenhancement, corresponding to areas of cystic dilatation of endometrial glands.

DIFFERENTIAL DIAGNOSIS IMAGES (D-E)

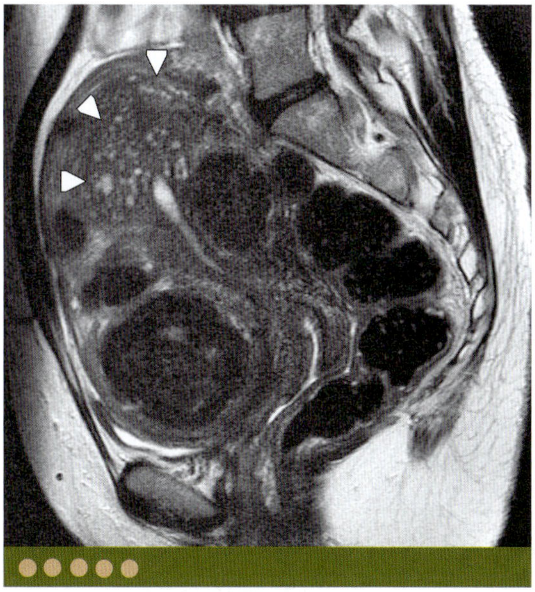

D. Uterine Fibroids (with coexistent adenomyoma): Sagittal T2-WI shows numerous well-defined hypointense fibroids. The coexistent adenomyoma in the superior aspect of the uterus (arrowheads) shows the classic T2-hyperintense foci. Also note how the adenomyoma is indistinguishable from the junctional zone.

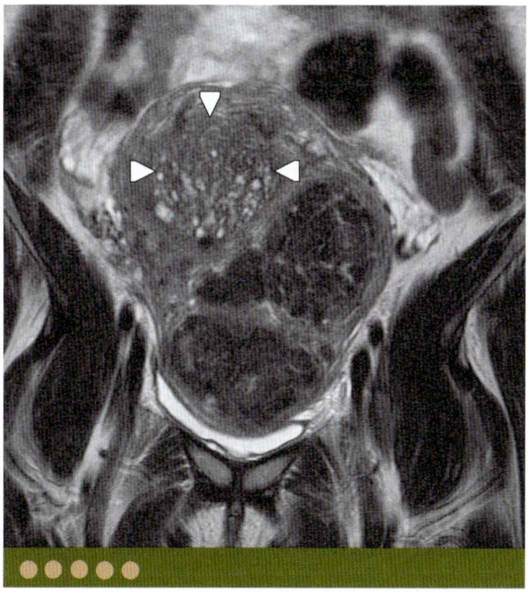

E. Uterine Fibroids (with coexistent adenomyoma): Coronal T2-WI on the same patient again shows fibroids in the mid- and lower portion of the uterus and an adenomyoma superiorly (arrowheads). Again, note the characteristic small T2-hyperintense foci, a classic finding in adenomyosis.

IMAGE KEY

Common

Rare

Typical

Unusual

16-9 Endometrial Hyperplasia

Paul Nikolaidis

PRESENTATION

Prolonged/irregular menstrual cycles, postmenopausal bleeding, or anovulatory cycles in younger women.

FINDINGS

A hyperintense mass similar to the endometrium is seen on T2-WI containing a few small cystic foci. Peak enhancement was at 2 minutes following contrast administration.

DIFFERENTIAL DIAGNOSES

- *Endometrial carcinoma*: On MR, carcinoma is heterogeneous and mildly hyperintense on T2-WI; relatively hypoenhancing following gadolinium, particularly in later phases. Myometrial thinning, invasion, or necrosis suggests cancer.
- *Endometrial polyp*: On T2-WI, they may be mildly hyperintense, often with a central hypointense focus, representing the central fibrous core of the polyp.
- *Submucosal fibroids*: On MR, fibroids are classically low-signal intensity on T2-WI, although may be hyperintense if degenerated.

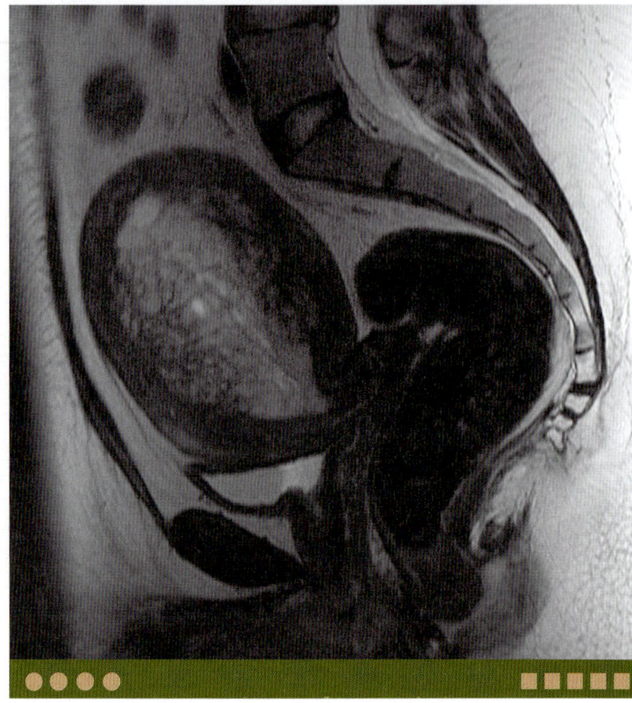

A. Sagittal T2-WI on a patient with vaginal bleeding shows a large, slightly heterogenous, mildly hyperintense mass expanding the endometrial cavity.

COMMENTS

Endometrial hyperplasia refers to an abnormal proliferation of endometrial stroma and glands secondary to stimulation by estrogen. It represents a spectrum of endometrial changes ranging from hyperplasia without cytological atypia to hyperplasia with cytological atypia (atypical hyperplasia). Young women with anovulatory cycles may have a mild and reversible form of cystic endometrial hyperplasia. Older women, in contrast, tend to have adenomatous hyperplasia. Endometrial hyperplasia should be suspected in the setting of prolonged or irregular menstrual cycles and in cases of postmenopausal bleeding.

On ultrasound, all types of endometrial hyperplasia can cause diffusely smooth hyperechoic endometrial thickening. In postmenopausal patients, it can only reliably be excluded if the endometrium measures less than 5 mm. Endometrial hyperplasia may cause focal or asymmetric thickening and irregularity of the endometrial surface, and be indistinguishable from endometrial carcinoma.

On MR, hyperplasia demonstrates high-signal intensity on T2-WI, similar to endometrium. Small cystic components may be better seen on contrast-enhanced images. On dynamic contrast-enhanced MR, endometrial hyperplasia characteristically reaches peak enhancement 2 to 3 minutes following contrast administration with intense and persistent enhancement. In contrast, endometrial carcinoma demonstrates early mild enhancement (<1 minute) and late gradual washout.

A definitive diagnosis can only be made with biopsy, as imaging alone often cannot accurately differentiate between hyperplasia and carcinoma.

PEARLS

- **Encompasses a spectrum of endometrial changes ranging from hyperplasia without cytological atypia to hyperplasia with cytological atypia.**
- **Definitive diagnosis is usually made with biopsy.**
- **On sonography, there is diffuse smooth (and less commonly more focal) hyperechoic thickening of the endometrium.**
- **On dynamic MR studies, characteristically reaches peak enhancement at 2 to 3 mininutes with intense and persistent enhancement.**

ADDITIONAL IMAGES (B-C)

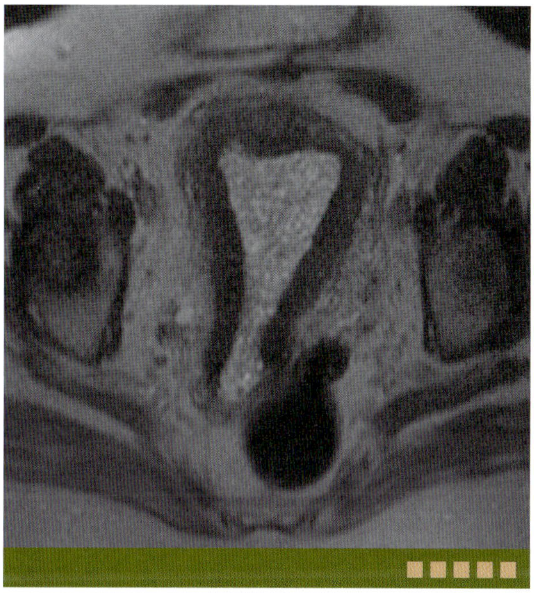

B. Axial T2-WI on a different patient shows an expanded mildly hyperintense endometrium. There is the appearance of numerous small cystic foci, as well. The patient had a 3-month history of vaginal bleeding and endometrial biopsy showed hyperplasia.

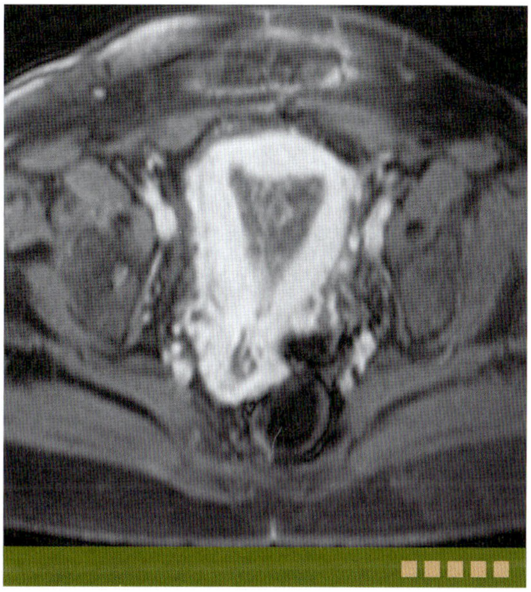

C. Corresponding contrast-enhanced axial T1-WI on the same patient shows only mild early enhancement of the endometrium. The small nonenhancing foci represent areas of cystic change, a common finding in endometrial hyperplasia.

DIFFERENTIAL DIAGNOSES IMAGES (D-E)

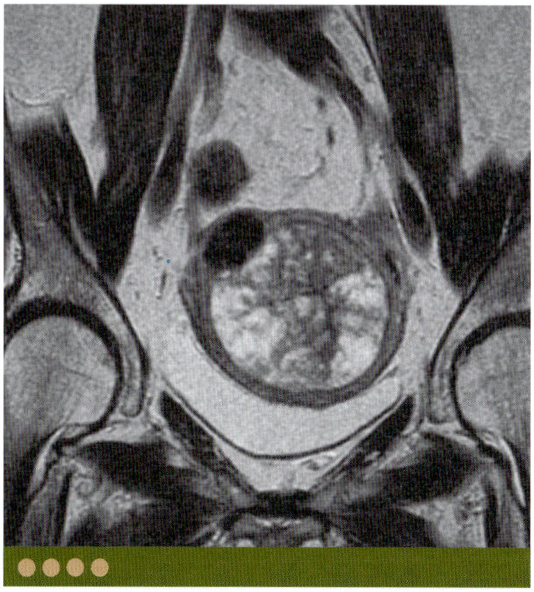

D. Endometrial carcinoma: Coronal T2-WI shows a large predominately hyperintense but heterogeneous mass expanding the endometrial cavity. Because of the excessive heterogeneity, biopsy was recommended which showed endometrial carcinoma. There is no evidence of myometrial invasion.

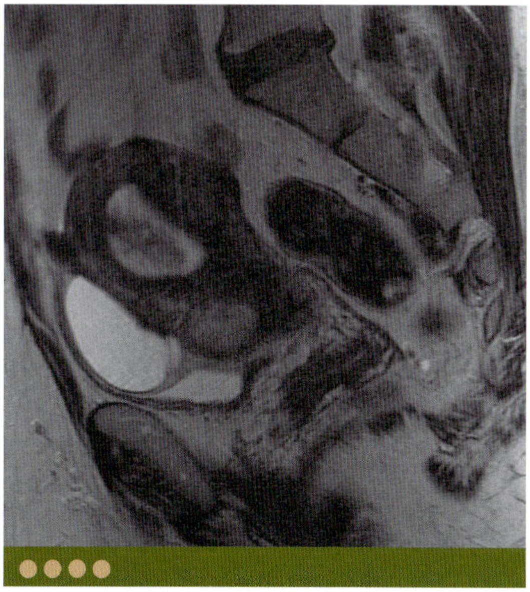

E. Endometrial polyp: Sagittal T2-WI shows a hyperintense mass within the endometrial cavity with a central area of low-signal intensity. The area of hypointensity likely corresponds to the central fibrous core of the endometrial polyp.

IMAGE KEY

Common

Rare

Typical

Unusual

16–10 Endometrial Changes from Tamoxifen

Paul Nikolaidis

PRESENTATION

Postmenopausal bleeding, history of breast cancer.

FINDINGS

Transvaginal sonography shows a homogeneously thickened endometrium with cystic changes.

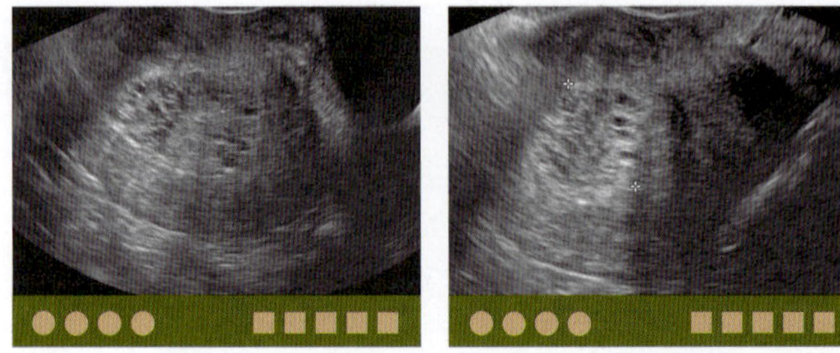

A. and **B.** Transverse (A) and sagittal (B) transvaginal sonograms of the uterus show a thickened hyperechoic endometrium with numerous small cystic foci.

DIFFERENTIAL DIAGNOSES

- *Endometrial hyperplasia*: Usually smooth, diffuse endometrial thickening. Cystic changes may be also present.
- *Endometrial carcinoma*: Typically a more ill-defined, heterogeneous lesion that cannot be clearly separated from the underlying endometrium. Biopsy is generally indicated since they often have overlapping imaging features, and because carcinomas may coexist with changes from tamoxifen.
- *Endometrial polyps*: The most frequently encountered sonographic abnormality leading to biopsy; often impossible to distinguish. Biopsy is generally indicated.

COMMENTS

Tamoxifen is an anti-estrogen agent that binds to estrogen receptors. It is widely used as an adjunct chemotherapy agent in women with breast cancer. However, in addition to its anti-estrogen effects on breast tissue, tamoxifen is a weak estrogen agonist on endometrial tissue in postmenopausal women. Long-term use is associated with an increased number of endometrial lesions, including proliferative endometrium, endometrial hyperplasia, polyps, and carcinoma. An increased incidence of fibroids and adenomyosis has also been described. Approximately 50% of the women who use tamoxifen develop uterine abnormalities after 6 to 36 months of treatment.

Transvaginal ultrasound (TVUS) and hysterosonography are the main imaging modalities for the diagnosis of endometrial abnormalities. The normal appearance of the atrophic postmenopausal endometrium on sonography is thin, homogeneous, and echogenic. Asymptomatic postmenopausal women on tamoxifen have a thicker endometrium. Classic changes in patients on tamoxifen include a thickened (homogeneous or heterogeneous) endometrium with cystic changes. However, a homogeneously or heterogeneously thickened endometrium without cystic changes may be encountered. The most appropriate "cut off" value for detecting endometrial abnormalities in asymptomatic women, while avoiding a high false positive rate, lies somewhere between 8 and 10 mm. Polyps are the most frequent abnormality on sonography leading to biopsy (80% in one recent large series).

MR should show a mildly hyperintense endometrium on T2-WI, often with more focal bright, cystic foci. The thickened endometrium should enhance on postcontrast T1-WI, while the cystic foci should not.

Regardless of exact imaging features, biopsy is generally indicated, as there may be overlap in imaging features with malignancy, but also because carcinomas and changes from tamoxifen may coexist.

PEARLS

- **Tamoxifen is a weak estrogen agonist on endometrial tissue in postmenopausal women.**
- **Long-term use of tamoxifen can cause several uterine abnormalities.**
- **On sonography or MR, cystic changes are classic, but a homogeneously or heterogeneously thickened endometrium without cystic changes may be encountered.**
- **Biopsy is often indicated, as there is an overlap in imaging features with endometrial carcinoma.**

ADDITIONAL IMAGES (C-E)

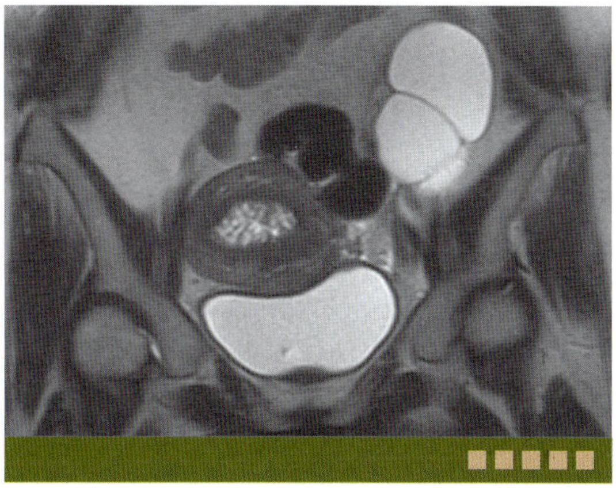

C. Sagittal T2-WI on the same patient shows a thickened endometrium with numerous cystic foci. Note the coexisting left adnexal cystic mass.

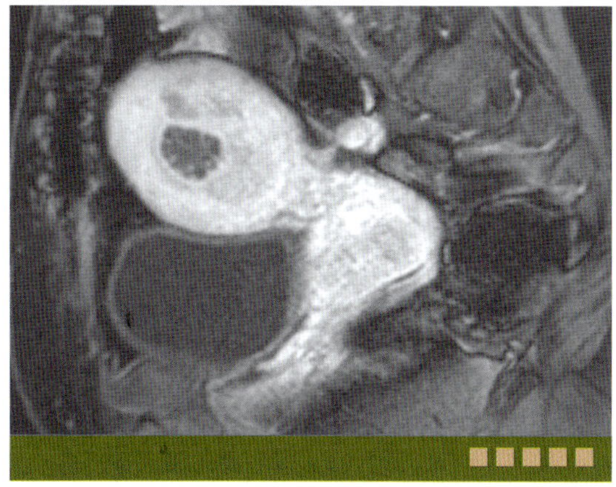

D. Corresponding contrast-enhanced sagittal T1-WI shows that the areas of cystic change do not enhance.

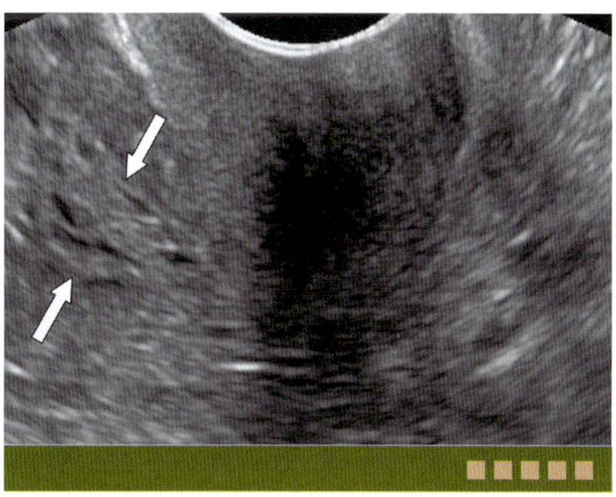

E. Sagittal transvaginal sonogram of the uterus on a different patient with history of breast cancer (on tamoxifen for 3 years) shows a thickened hyperechoic endometrium with numerous small cystic foci (arrow).

DIFFERENTIAL DIAGNOSES IMAGES (F-H)

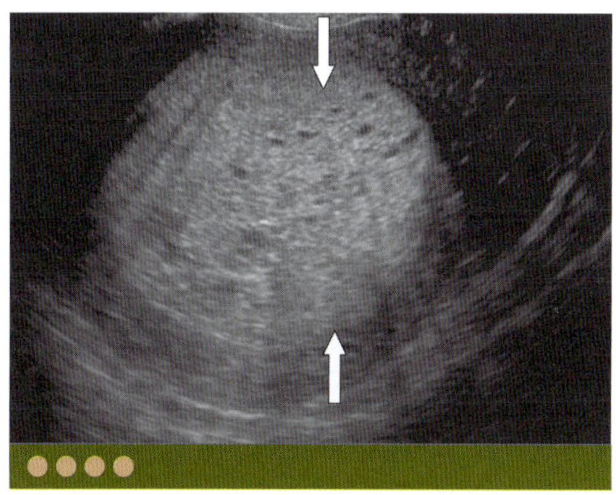

F. Endometrial hyperplasia: Longitudinal transabdominal sonogram shows a markedly thickened echogenic endometrium with few small anechoic foci (arrows). Repeated biopsies showed only hyperplasia.

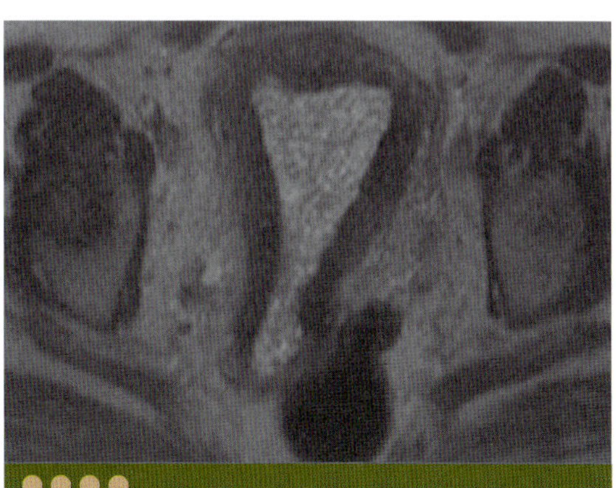

G. Endometrial hyperplasia: Axial T2-WI on another patient shows an abnormally widened hyperintense endometrium. Biopsy showed endometrial hyperplasia.

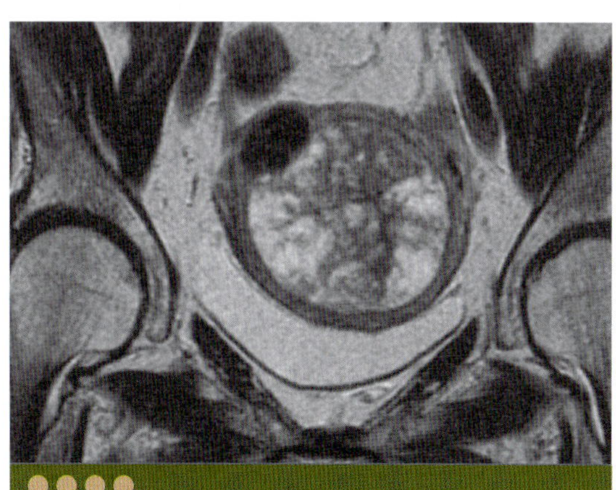

H. Endometrial cancer: Coronal T2-WI shows a large predominately hyperintense heterogeneous mass expanding the endometrial cavity.

IMAGE KEY

Common

Rare

Typical

Unusual

16–11 Endometrial Cancer

Paul Nikolaidis

PRESENTATION

Postmenopausal vaginal bleeding, obesity, and history of unopposed estrogen replacement therapy.

FINDINGS

MR shows a hyperintense, heterogeneous lesion on T2-WI expanding the endometrial cavity.

DIFFERENTIAL DIAGNOSES

- *Submucosal fibroid*: Fibroids are classically dark on T2-WI, unless degenerated when they may be heterogeneously hyperintense; they should be shown to be separate from the endometrium and junctional zone.
- *Endometrial polyp*: Several overlapping features; no myometrial invasion or necrosis; polyps may be less heterogeneous. Biopsy is usually required.
- *Endometrial hyperplasia*: On dynamic MR, hyperplasia reaches peak enhancement 2 to 3 minutes following contrast and shows intense and persistent enhancement.

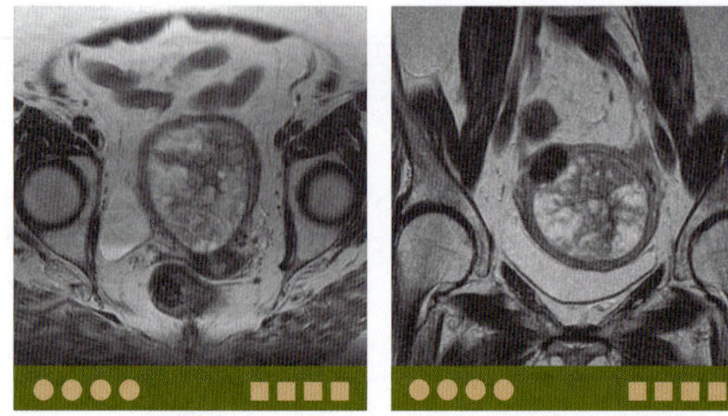

A. and **B.** Axial (A) and coronal (B) T2-WI show a large hyperintense lesion expanding the endometrial cavity. The hypointense thinned junctional zone is well seen.

COMMENTS

Endometrial carcinoma is the most common female genital tract malignancy with a peak incidence between 50 and 70 years of age. Known risk factors include obesity, nulliparity, polycystic ovary disease, unopposed estrogen replacement therapy, and endometrial hyperplasia. Up to 90% of patients present with vaginal bleeding.

On sonography, endometrial carcinoma is typically an ill-defined, heterogeneous echogenic lesion that cannot be separated from the underlying endometrium. Arterial waveforms are usually detected on Doppler interrogation. Blood is often seen in the endometrial cavity.

On MR, lesions are mildly hyperintense on T2-WI, but less than normal endometrium. Segmental thinning or disruption of the junctional zone may be seen and interruption of the T2-dark junctional zone is highly suggestive of myometrial invasion. The junctional zone may be very difficult to visualize in postmenopausal women, however. Following IV gadolinium administration lesions show poor enhancement compared to the myometrium, a finding which can help outline the depth of invasion.

The depth of myometrial invasion is critical in patients with endometrial carcinoma, affecting survival rates and dictating clinical management.

PEARLS

- **Most common female genital tract malignancy with peak incidence between 50 and 70 years of age.**
- **On sonography, they are typically ill-defined, heterogeneous echogenic lesions inseparable from the underlying endometrium.**
- **On MR, lesions are mildly hyperintense but less than normal endometrium on T2-WI.**
- **Following IV gadolinium administration lesions enhance less than the surrounding normal myometrium.**

ADDITIONAL IMAGES (C-D)

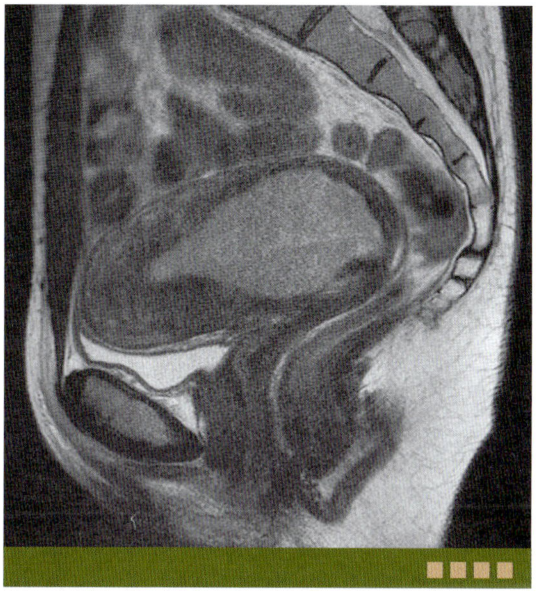

C. Sagittal T2-WI shows a large hyperintense lesion centered in the lower portion of the endometrial cavity and extending into the cervix.

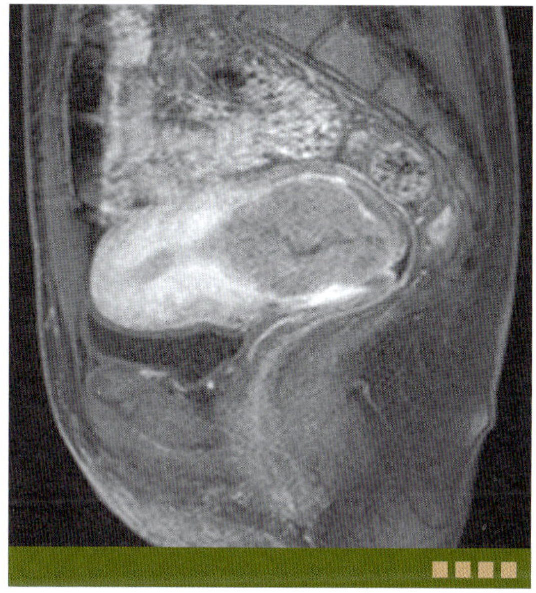

D. Corresponding sagittal contrast-enhanced T1-WI shows that the large endometrial mass enhances less than the surrounding myometrium.

DIFFERENTIAL DIAGNOSES IMAGES (E-F)

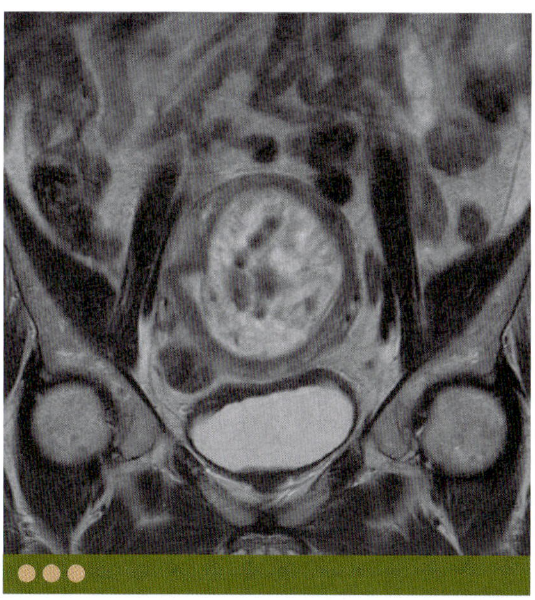

E. Degenerated submucosal leiomyoma: Coronal T2-WI shows a large heterogeneously hyperintense mass that occupies the endometrial cavity but is separate from the endometrium.

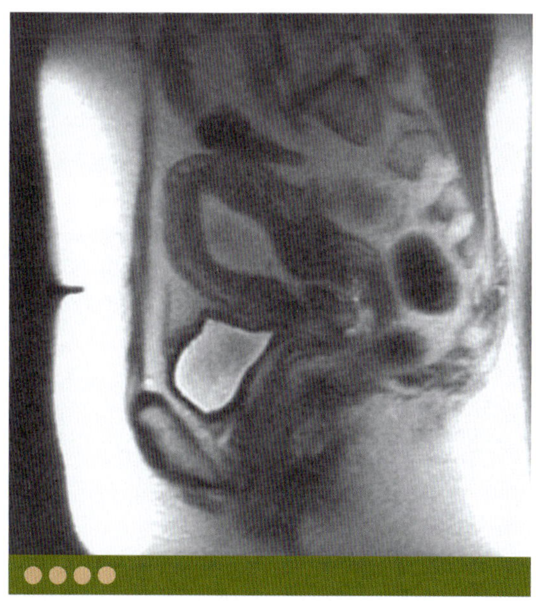

F. Endometrial polyp: Sagittal T2-WI shows a small, mildly hyperintense, endometrial mass. It contains a subtle central area of lower signal representing its fibrous core.

IMAGE KEY

Common

Rare

Typical

Unusual

16–12 Malignant Mixed Müllerian Tumors (Uterine Carcinosarcoma)

Paul Nikolaidis

PRESENTATION

Vaginal bleeding, discharge, and pelvic mass.

FINDINGS

MR shows a large heterogeneous lesion with large areas of necrosis extending from the endometrial cavity through the myometrium, also with extension to the cervix and vagina.

DIFFERENTIAL DIAGNOSES

- *Other uterine sarcomas*: It is virtually impossible to distinguish between a malignant mixed Müllerian tumor (MMMT) and other uterine sarcomas including leiomyosarcomas and endometrial stromal sarcomas.
- *Endometrial carcinoma*: Late-stage advanced endometrial adenocarcinoma may also be impossible to distinguish from an MMMT on imaging. Patients also have similar risk factors and clinical presentations.
- *Uterine fibroids*: May be difficult to distinguish an MMMT from large, heterogeneous degenerated fibroids. Findings that may suggest MMMT include rapid growth, areas of more heterogeneous high signal on T2-WI, and T1-hyperintense foci.

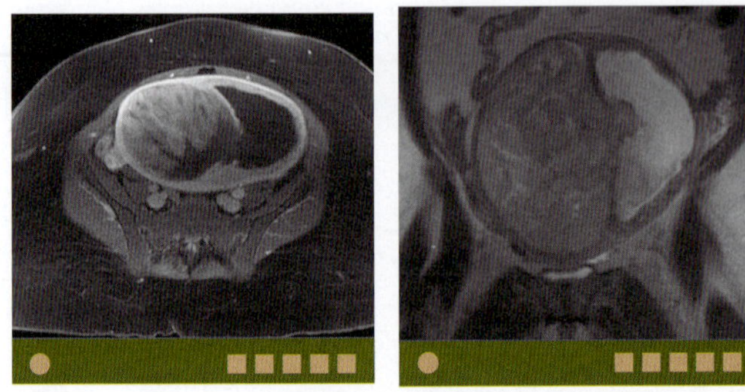

A. Axial contrast-enhanced T1-WI shows a large heterogeneously enhancing lesion extending from the right side of the endometrial cavity and invading through the myometrium. The endometrial cavity is obstructed and distended.
B. Corresponding coronal T2-WI shows that the large mass is mildly hyperintense.

COMMENTS

Uterine sarcomas are rare, comprising approximately 5% of uterine malignancies. Uterine sarcomas include primary malignant mixed müllerian (mesodermal) tumors, also known as carcinosarcomas, along with leiomyosarcomas and endometrial stromal sarcomas. Although MMMTs can originate anywhere along the lower female genital tract, they most commonly arise in the uterus. They typically occur in postmenopausal women. They differ histologically from other uterine sarcomas in that they contain both epithelial and stromal elements, whereas the other uterine sarcomas do not contain epithelial elements. The epithelial component predominates in metastatic lesions.

Compared to endometrial adenocarcinomas, these sarcomas behave even more aggressively and are associated with a poorer prognosis. Risk factors overlap with those for endometrial carcinoma and include excess estrogen exposure, chronic tamoxifen use, nulliparity, and prior pelvic irradiation.

On CT, dilatation of the endometrial cavity is present in almost all cases. An ill-defined mass is usually seen within the endometrial cavity, often with significant myometrial invasion and even extrauterine extension.

The typical MR features of MMMT include scattered areas of high-signal intensity on T1-WI and a heterogeneous appearance on T2-WI with areas of intermediate or high signal. Masses show heterogeneous but avid enhancement on gadolinium-enhanced images. Deep myometrial invasion will often be evident. However, imaging findings are not very specific.

Comparing to endometrial adenocarcinomas, these sarcomas behave more aggressively. The prognosis is poor, with 5-year survival rates of less than 20%. No adjuvant therapy has been shown to be effective, and treatment of persistent or recurrent tumor by chemotherapy or radiation almost always will not result in cure. Prognosis is better when there is limited myometrial and cervical involvement and absence of vascular invasion within the endometrium. Five-year survival of around 50% has been reported in women with stage I disease.

PEARLS

- **MMMTs are rare sarcomas that most commonly arise in the uterus.**
- **These aggressive neoplasms typically occur in postmenopausal women.**
- **Imaging may not reliably distinguish between MMMT, other uterine sarcomas, endometrial cancer, and even degenerated fibroids.**
- **Areas of hyperintensity are seen on T1-WI and heterogeneous areas of iso- or hyperintensity on T2-WI.**

ADDITIONAL IMAGES (C-E)

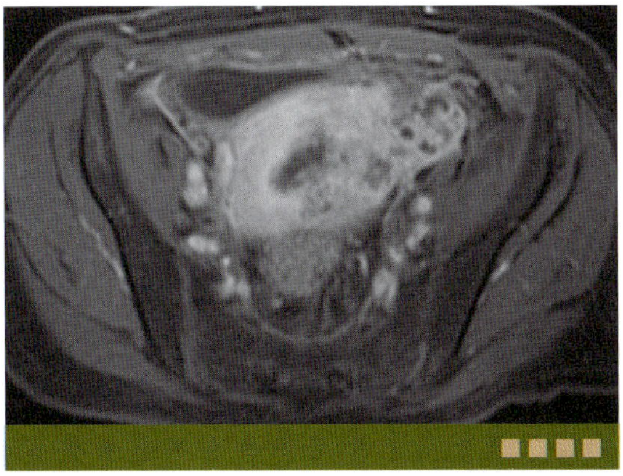

C. Axial contrast-enhanced T1-WI on another patient shows a large heterogeneous lesion with large areas of necrosis invading through the myometrium.

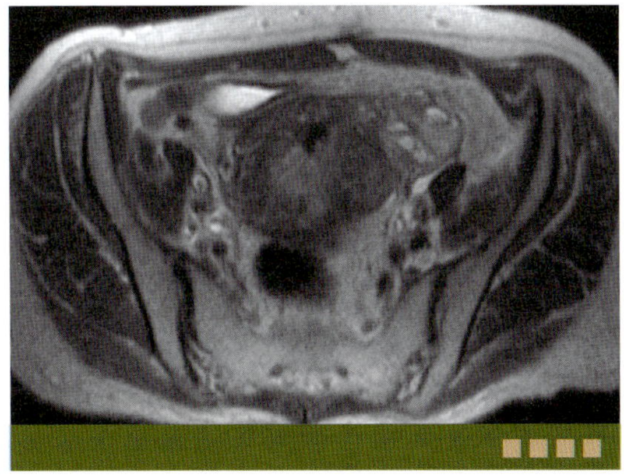

D. Corresponding axial T2-WI shows the mass is ill-defined and hyperintense.

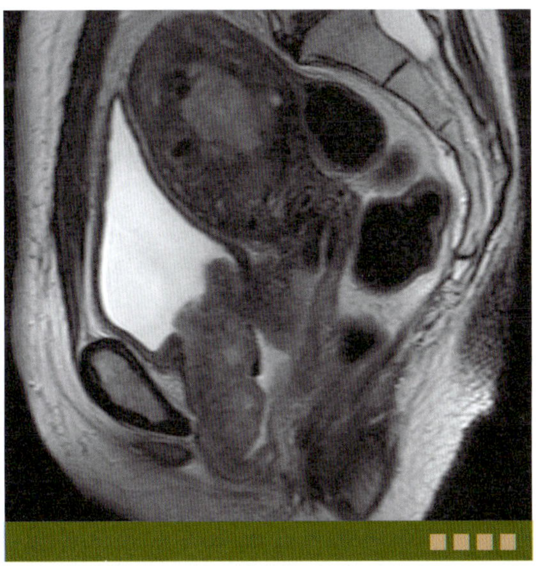

E. Sagittal contrast-enhanced T2-WI on the same patient shows the extent of neoplastic involvement. Tumor has extended through the cervix and vagina.

DIFFERENTIAL DIAGNOSES IMAGES (F-H)

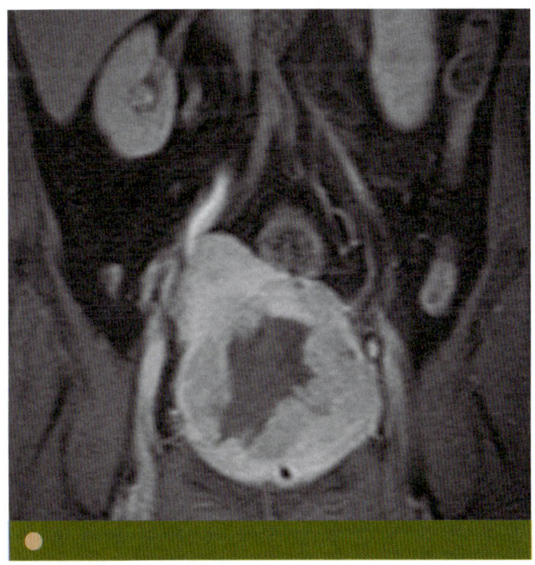

F. Uterine leiomyosarcoma: Coronal contrast-enhanced T1-WI shows a large uterine mass with central necrosis. It is difficult to distinguish from MMMT.

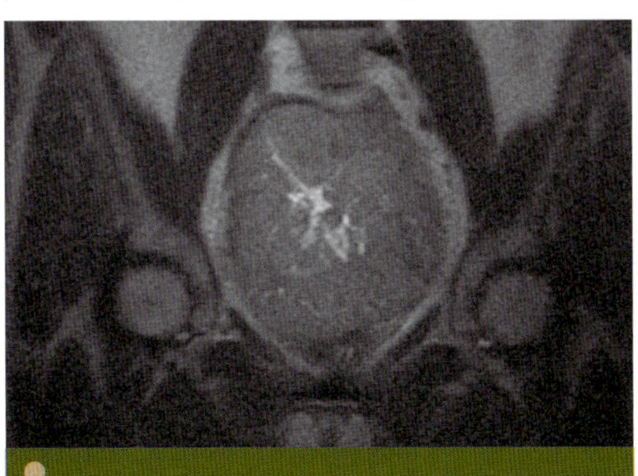

G. Uterine leiomyosarcoma: Coronal T2-WI on the same patient shows few central areas of increased signal within the mass.

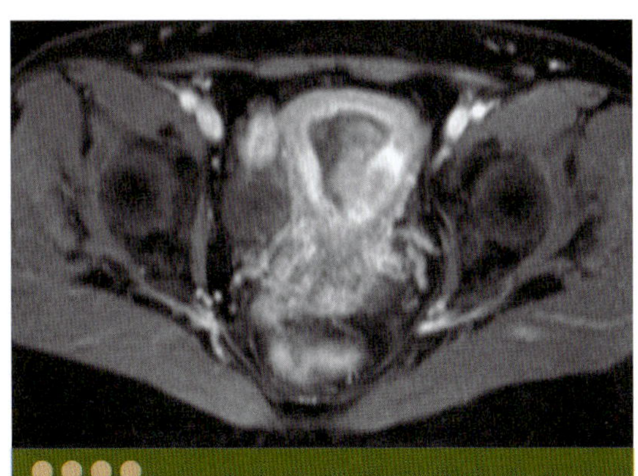

H. Endometrial cancer (adenocarcinoma): Axial contrast-enhanced T1-WI shows an enhancing endometrial mass that invades the myometrium.

IMAGE KEY

Common

●●●●●
●●●●
●●●
●●
●

Rare

Typical

■■■■■
■■■■
■■■
■■
■

Unusual

16–13 Müllerian Agenesis/Hypoplasia and the Mayer-Rokitansky-Kuster Hauser (MRKH) Syndrome

Paul Nikolaidis

PRESENTATION

Primary amenorrhea, dyspareunia.

FINDINGS

MR shows complete absence of the uterus and vagina.

DIFFERENTIAL DIAGNOSIS

None

COMMENTS

Type I müllerian anomalies under the American Fertility Society classification (Müllerian agenesis and hypoplasia) encompass variable degrees of early failure to form the Müllerian ducts. Complete vaginal agenesis is the common presentation. This is known as the Mayer-Rokitansky-Kuster-Hauser syndrome (MRKH). Approximately 90% of patients have associated uterine agenesis, whereas 10% have a small rudimentary uterus, with or without an associated obstructed endometrial segment. In nearly 95% of MRKH patients, the vagina is completely absent from the introitus. In the remaining 5%, a blind upper portion of the vagina is present.

Women with MRKH have a 46 XX karyotype, female secondary sexual characteristics and normal ovarian function, including cyclic ovulation, but have absence or hypoplasia of the vagina. One in three women with MRKH will have associated abnormalities of the genitourinary (GU) tract including unilateral renal agenesis, ectopia of one or both kidneys, and horseshoe kidney. One in ten patients have skeletal anomalies, including cervico-thoracic anomalies, asymmetric, fused or wedged vertebrae, scoliosis, and Klippel-Feil anomaly.

Ovarian function is typically preserved because ovaries are derived from the primitive ectoderm. Patients will often present with primary amenorrhea, inability to have intercourse secondary to dyspareunia, or voiding difficulties.

On MR, uterine agenesis and hypoplasia are best delineated on sagittal T2-WI, whereas vaginal agenesis is best demonstrated on axial images. Complete agenesis results in no identifiable uterus. Uterine hypoplasia demonstrates a small uterus often with abnormal low-signal intensity myometrium on T2-WI and poorly delineated zonal anatomy. The endometrial cavity and the myometrium are diminutive.

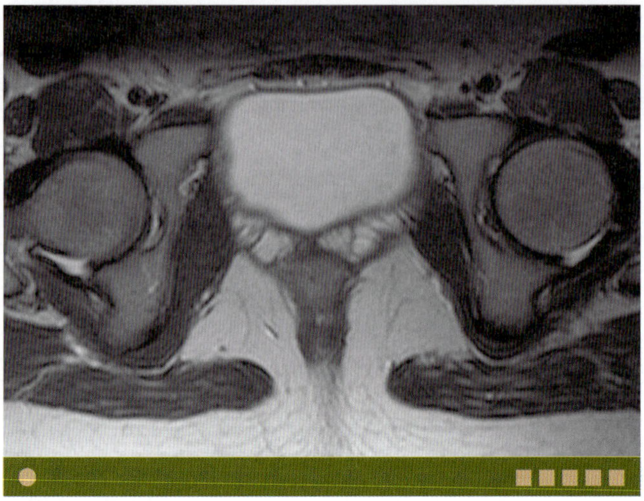

A. Axial T2-WI through the lower pelvis shows complete absence of any tissue (representing a vagina) between the rectum and bladder.

Treatment is usually delayed until the patient is about to start sexual activity. Vaginal dilatation and reconstruction is usually performed, especially in patients with an obstructed uterus; however, reproductive potential is virtually absent. In addition, it is important to manage psychological symptoms as these syndromes are associated with anxiety about femininity and physical image.

PEARLS

- **Attributed to early failure in the formation of the Müllerian ducts.**
- **Associated upper tract GU anomalies include unilateral renal agenesis, renal ectopia, or fusion anomalies.**
- **Uterine agenesis and hypoplasia is best seen on sagittal T2-WI.**
- **Vaginal agenesis or the hypoplastic remnant vagina is best demonstrated on axial T2-WI.**

ADDITIONAL IMAGES (B-G)

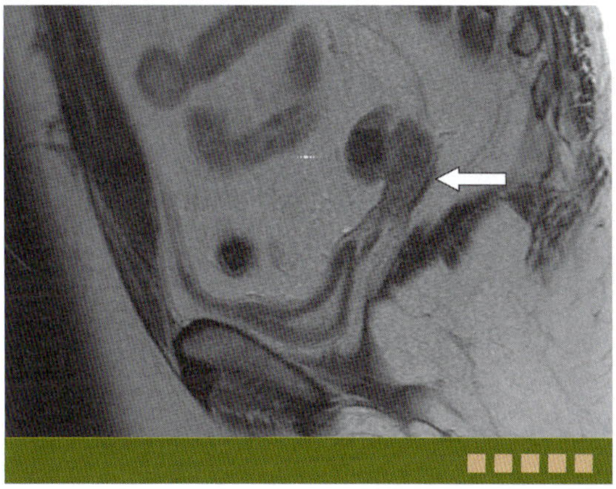

B. Sagittal T2-WI on another young female with amenorrhea shows an abnormal markedly hypoplastic uterus (arrow). Note absence of the majority of the vagina between the rectum and bladder. A small portion of remnant vagina is present just below the level of the cervix.

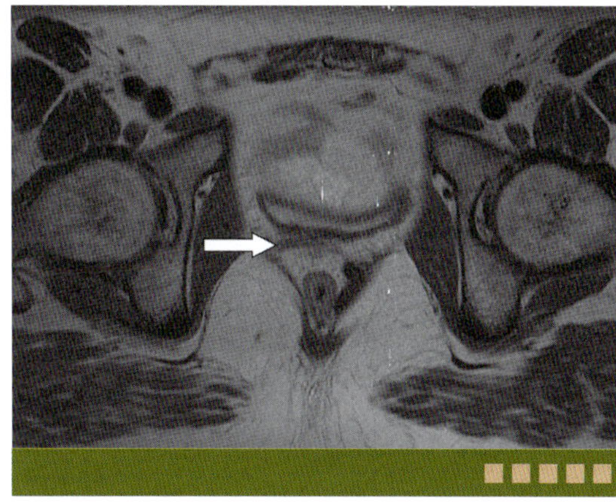

C. Corresponding axial T2-WI better shows the small blind upper portion of the vagina (arrow). Approximately 5% of patients with MRKH will have a blind upper one-third of the vagina, better seen on axial (not sagittal) T2-WI.

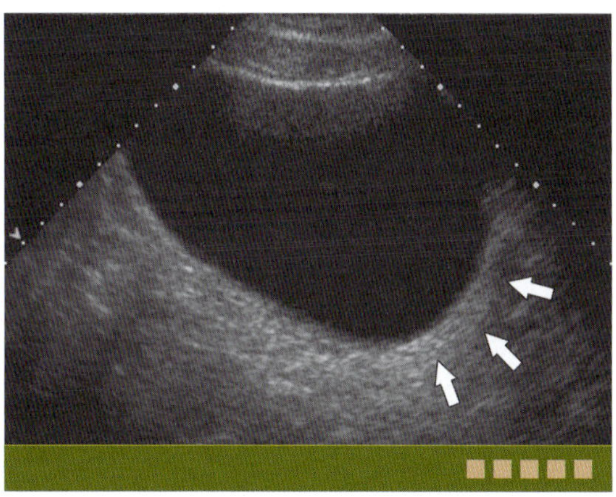

D. Sagittal transabdominal ultrasound on another patient with MRKH shows complete absence of any tissue in the expected location of the cervix and uterus.

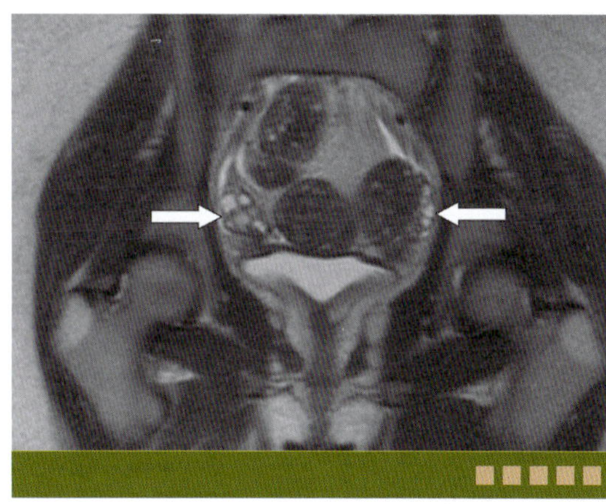

E. Coronal T2-WI on the same patient shows bilateral normal ovaries (arrows). Most women with MRKH have normal ovaries and develop secondary sexual characteristics.

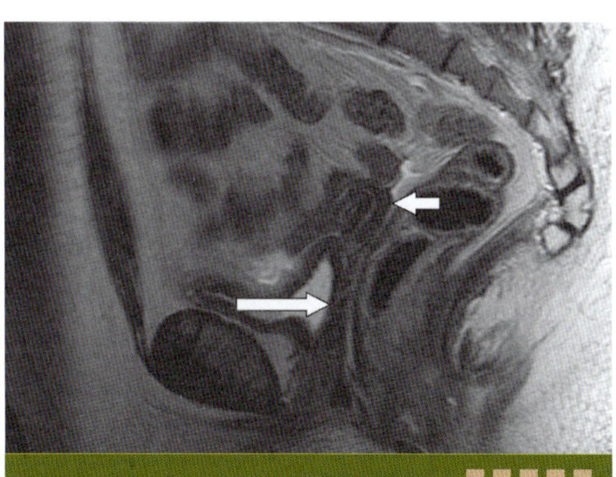

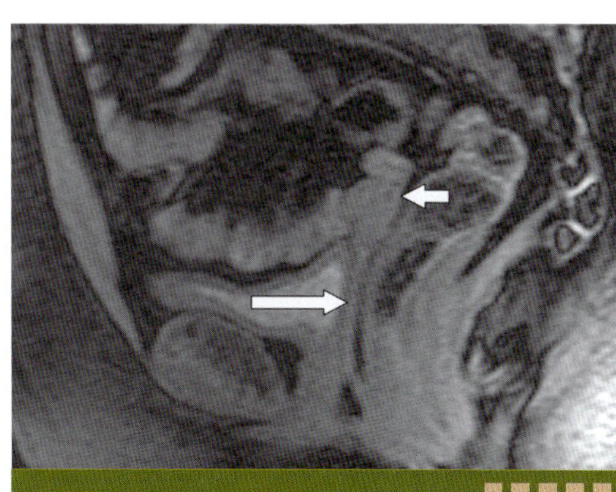

F. and **G.** Sagittal T2-WI (E) and contrast-enhanced T1-WI (F) on another patient shows a hypoplastic uterus (short arrow). Note the presence of a small portion of remnant vagina between the bladder and rectum (long arrow).

IMAGE KEY

Common

Rare

Typical

Unusual

16–14 Endometrioma

Paul Nikolaidis

PRESENTATION

Cyclical pelvic pain.

FINDINGS

MR shows a rounded adnexal lesion that shows uniform low-signal intensity on T2-WI and is markedly hyperintense on fat suppressed noncontrast T1-WI.

DIFFERENTIAL DIAGNOSES

- *Hemorrhagic ovarian cyst*: On sonography, they have a classic appearance including a reticulated pattern with linear fibrin strands or a retracting clot. May be more difficult to distinguish on MR.
- *Ovarian dermoid*: Dermoids are also hyperintense on T1-WI, but contrary to endometriomas, they become hypointense on fat-suppressed T1 sequences. On T2-WI, dermoids are generally isointense to fat seen elsewhere in the pelvis.

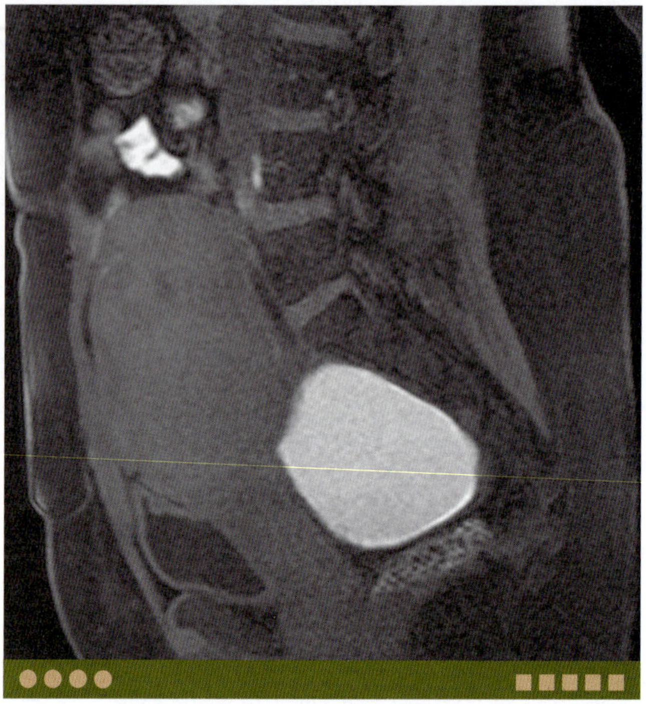

A. Sagittal fat-suppressed noncontrast T1-WI shows a large hyperintense oval mass posterior to the uterus and cervix.

COMMENTS

Endometriosis is defined by the presence of ectopic endometrial glands and stroma outside the uterus. Symptoms are often debilitating and include pelvic pain, dysmenorrhea, dyspareunia, dyschezia, and urinary symptoms. Pelvic endometriosis commonly involves the peritoneum, ovaries, and uterine ligaments. An endometrioma is a cyst that contains hemorrhagic products, which usually arises at the ovary. It may be bilateral.

Ultrasound is highly sensitive for the detection of ovarian endometriotic cysts (endometriomas). The classic sonographic appearance is a cystic structure with homogeneous low-level echoes, sometimes referred to as a "ground glass" appearance. Endometriomas tend to have more homogeneous internal echoes as opposed to the more heterogeneous and reticular pattern in hemorrhagic cysts. Less frequently, endometriomas may be multilocular, with areas of anechoic fluid and other areas of complex fluid, separated by septations. Fluid–fluid levels may be seen in a few instances.

MR is highly accurate in the diagnosis of endometriomas. An advantage over ultrasound is its ability to detect additional areas of endometriosis, including very small implants or involvement of the deep pelvis, cul de sac, bladder, and rectosigmoid. Endometriomas are hyperintense on spin-echo T1-WI, and in particular, on fat-suppressed T1-WI. On T2-WI, they may be hyperintense, but often demonstrate a relative decrease in signal intensity referred to as "T2 shading."

PEARLS

- **An endometrioma is a cyst that contains hemorrhagic products.**
- **On sonography, they classically contain homogeneous internal low-level echoes.**
- **Lower signal intensity referred to as "shading" may be seen on T2-weighted images.**
- **They are markedly hyperintense on fat-saturated T1-weighted images.**

ADDITIONAL IMAGES (B-D)

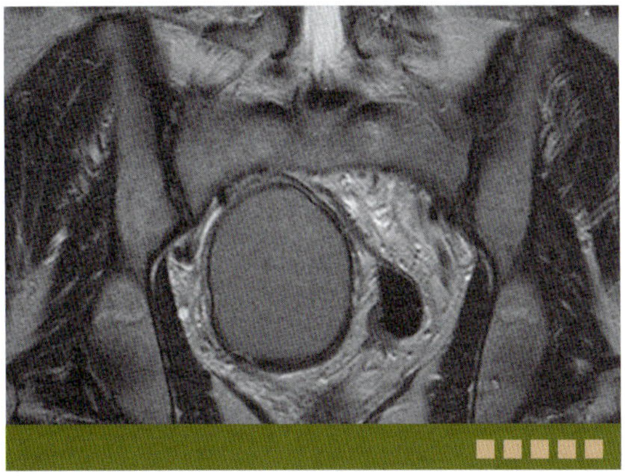

B. Coronal T2-WI on the same patient as A shows uniform low-signal intensity of the endometrioma on this sequence. This is referred to as T2 shading.

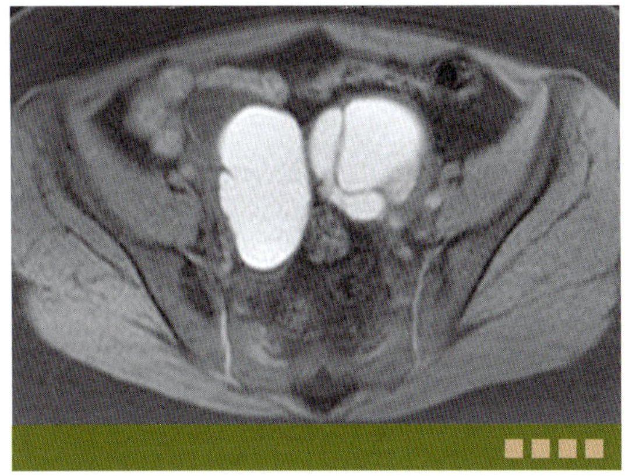

C. Axial fat-suppressed noncontrast T1-WI shows bilateral endometriomas. There was also endometriosis of the left fallopian tube.

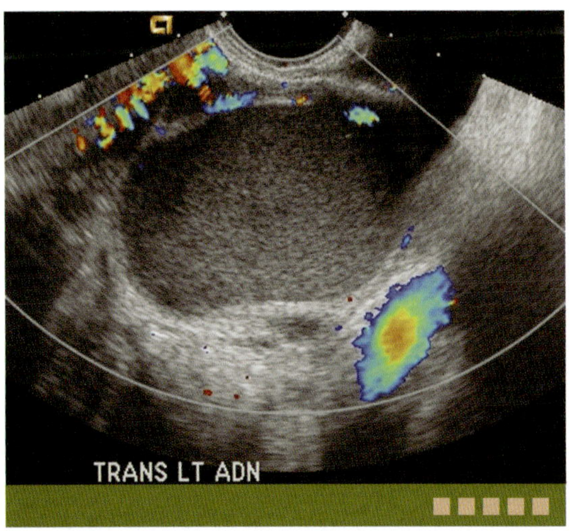

D. Transvaginal color Doppler sonogram in a different patient shows a left ovarian lesion with uniform low-level echoes. It is completely avascular. This persisted on a follow-up study 9 weeks later and was shown to represent an endometrioma on laparoscopy.

DIFFERENTIAL DIAGNOSES IMAGES (E-G)

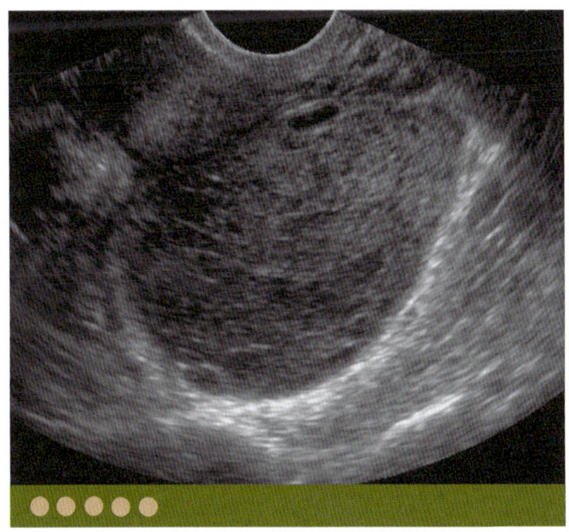

E. Hemorrhagic ovarian cyst: Transvaginal sonogram shows a left ovarian lesion with some heterogeneity and fine septations arranged in a reticular pattern. This was presumed to represent a hemorrhagic ovarian cyst and resolved on a subsequent follow-up study obtained 2 months later.

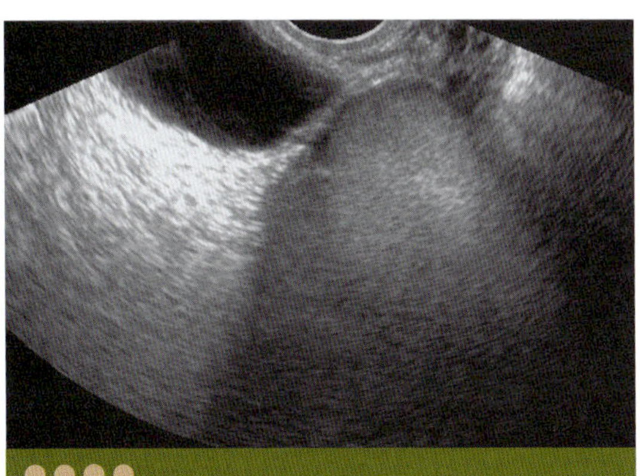

F. Ovarian dermoid: Transvaginal sonogram shows a large hyperechoic left ovarian lesion with poor distal transmission of the sound wave and shadowing.

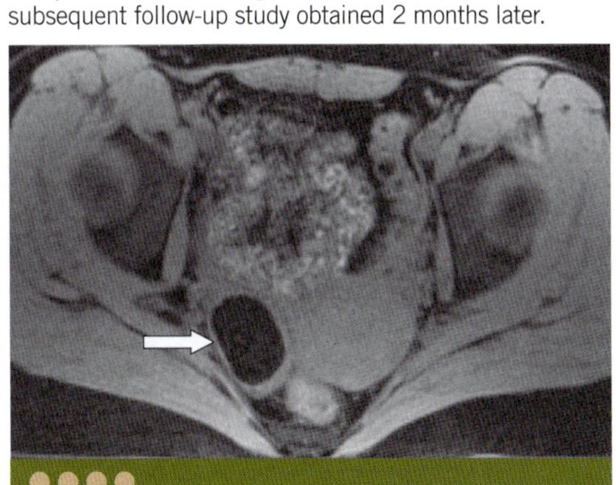

G. Ovarian dermoid: Axial fat-suppressed noncontrast T1-WI shows a right ovarian lesion that shows signal drop because of fat suppression. If this was an endometrioma, it would be bright on this sequence.

IMAGE KEY

Common

Rare

Typical

Unusual

16–15 Deep Pelvic Endometriosis

Paul Nikolaidis

PRESENTATION

Chronic pelvic pain, dysmenorrhea, and dyspareunia.

FINDINGS

MR of the pelvis shows small hyperintense foci in the deep pelvis on noncontrast fat-suppressed T1-WI sequences.

DIFFERENTIAL DIAGNOSIS

None

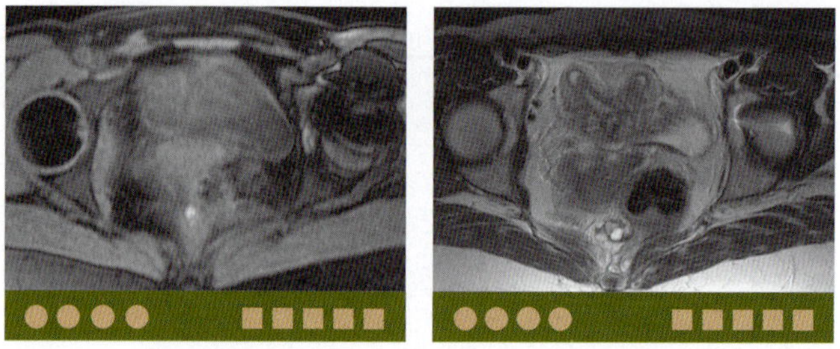

A. and **B.** Axial fat-saturated nonenhanced T1-WI (A) and T2-WI (B) show foci of high-signal intensity representing endometriotic lesions in the posterior deep pelvis, adjacent to the rectum.

COMMENTS

Endometriosis is defined by the presence of ectopic endometrial glands and stroma outside the uterus. Symptoms are often debilitating and include pelvic pain, dysmenorrhea, dyspareunia, dyschezia, and urinary symptoms. Deep pelvic endometriosis involves the uterosacral ligaments, pouch of Douglas (which may be obliterated), torus uterinus, vagina and recto-sigmoid colon. It is often associated with peritoneal and ovarian lesions. In cases of long-standing or severe disease, there is usually significant associated proliferation of smooth muscle cells and fibrosis.

The gold standard in the diagnosis of endometriosis is laparoscopy. While ultrasound is highly sensitive for the detection of ovarian endometriotic cysts (endometriomas) and larger anterior pelvic lesions or bladder lesions, its sensitivity and specificity in the detection of implants in deep pelvic endometriosis is significantly lower.

MR is the best imaging modality for the detection of endometriosis and the assessment of the extent of pelvic involvement. It is highly accurate for both anterior and posterior pelvic endometriosis and enables accurate pre-operative planning. Foci of deep pelvic endometriosis are hyperintense on spin-echo T1-WI and are most readily conspicuous on fat-suppressed gradient echo T1 sequences. In addition, T2 hyperintense or hypointense nodules may be present. Associated fibrotic changes may be present. They are typically hypointense on both T1-WI and T2-WI.

Laparoscopic surgery with lysis of adhesions is often the treatment of choice. Pre-operative MR assists the gynecologic surgeon in the planning of surgery.

PEARLS

- **Usually involves the uterosacral ligaments, pouch of Douglas, vagina, and rectosigmoid colon.**
- **Deep pelvic endometriotic lesions may be missed on sonography.**
- **MR is excellent in identifying the presence and extent of deep pelvic endometriosis.**
- **Noncontrast fat-saturated T1-WI is the best MR sequence; foci of deep pelvic endometriosis are most conspicuous.**

ADDITIONAL IMAGES (C-H)

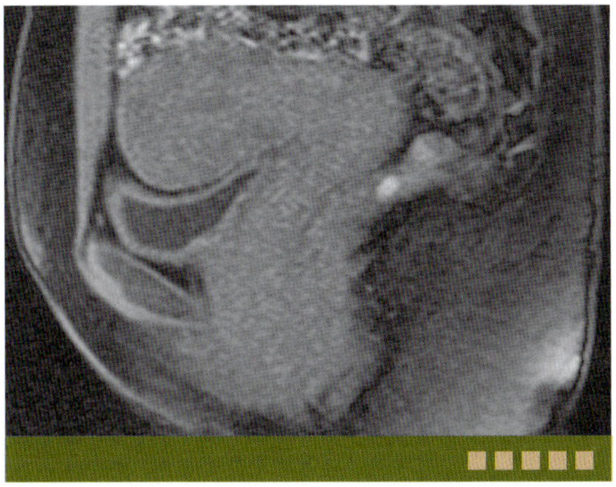

C. Sagittal fat-saturated, nonenhanced T1-WI on the same patient nicely shows the focus of endometriosis in the deep pelvis.

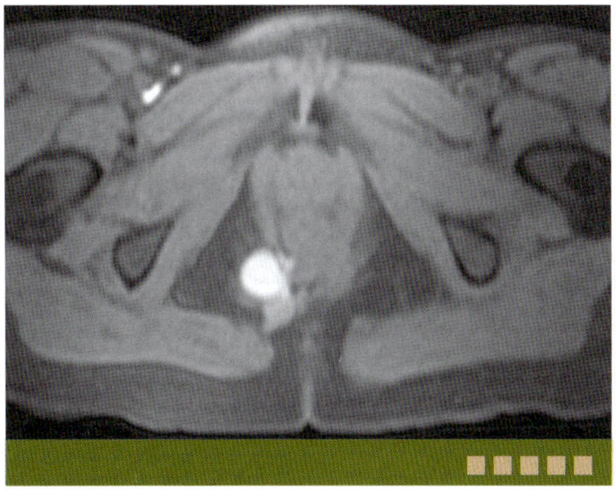

D. Axial fat-saturated, nonenhanced T1-WI shows high-signal lesions in the ischiorectal fossa in another patient with history of endometriosis.

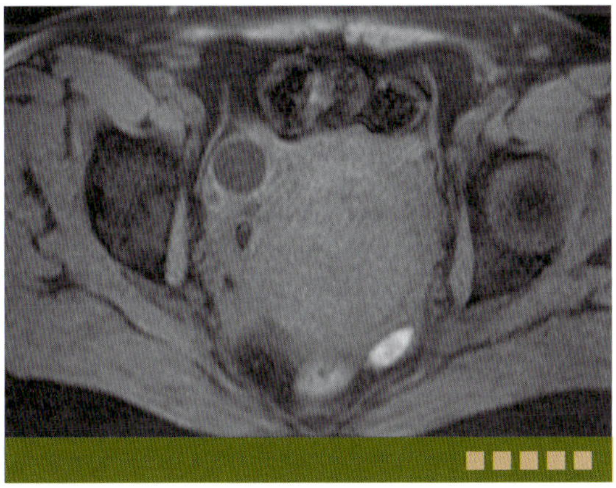

E. Axial fat-saturated nonenhanced T1-WI in another patient with endometriosis shows a high-signal lesion in the cul de sac.

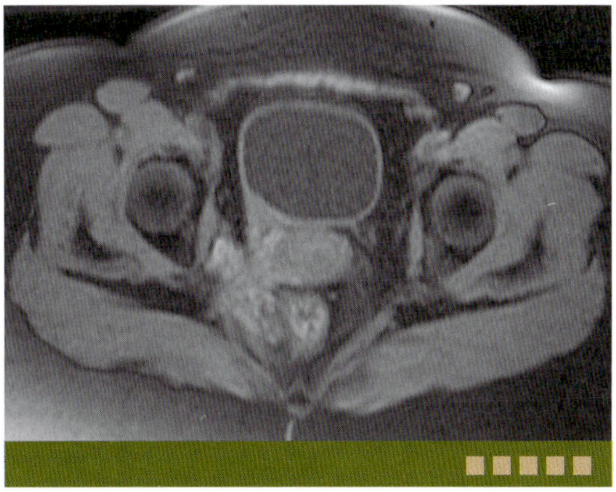

F. Axial fat-saturated nonenhanced T1-WI in a patient with a long-standing history of endometriosis shows a stellate soft tissue lesion in the posterior right pelvis with a few scattered foci of high signal.

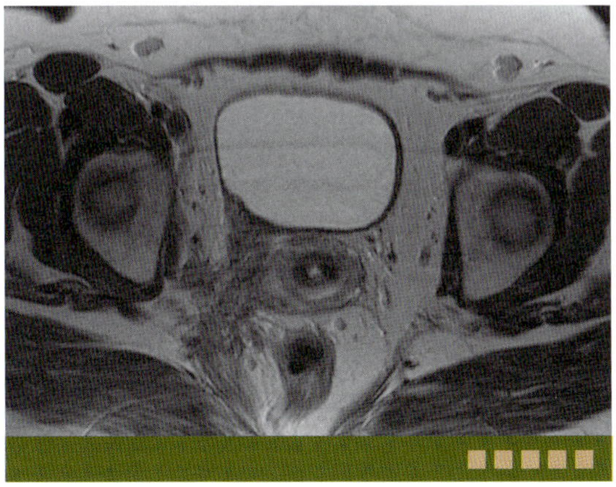

G. Axial T2-WI on the same patient shows the stellate soft tissue lesion in the posterior pelvis to be predominantly hypointense. This is a result of extensive fibrosis.

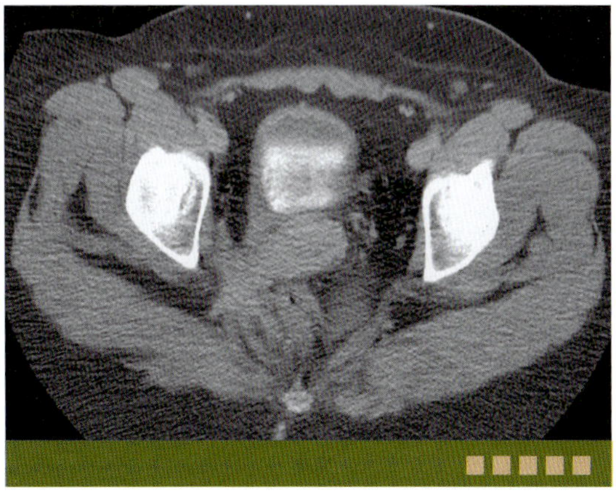

H. Axial CECT on the same patient shows the stellate soft tissue lesion in the posterior pelvis, representing extensive fibrosis as a result of chronic deep pelvic endometriosis with severe inflammation and scarring.

IMAGE KEY

Common

Rare

Typical

Unusual

16–16 Pelvic Congestion Syndrome

Nancy A. Hammond

PRESENTATION

Chronic pelvic pain.

FINDINGS

Prominent pelvic venous structures.

DIFFERENTIAL DIAGNOSIS

- *Pelvic varicosities secondary to upstream obstruction*: Thrombosis or occlusion of the IVC or portal hypertension.

COMMENTS

Pelvic congestion syndrome is a cause of chronic pelvic pain (pain >6 months duration) associated with dilatation of the pelvic veins. Pelvic varicosities develop secondary to incompetence or lack of valves in the ovarian veins and other draining veins of the pelvis. This entity typically occurs in multiparous, premenopausal women. During pregnancy, there is significantly increased blood flow to the ovaries which can result in valve damage. This damage results in backflow of blood and the development of varices that cause pain. Symptoms include chronic pelvic pain that is worse with prolonged standing, after intercourse, and during menstruation. Before the diagnosis of pelvic congestion syndrome is made, other cause of chronic pelvic pain should be evaluated for and eliminated.

CT or MR demonstrates varicose veins around the uterus and ovaries. There may be retrograde filling of the ovarian veins. An ovarian vein diameter of greater than 5 mm has been suggested to be pathognomonic for pelvic congestion syndrome but this criterion has not been universally accepted. The uterus is enlarged with prominent vasculature in the myometrium. Pelvic ultrasound can also be used to diagnose pelvic congestion syndrome. Sonographic findings include prominent, dilated pelvic venous plexuses, dilatation of the ovarian veins with reversal of flow, and dilated arcuate veins crossing the uterine myometrium. Polycystic changes to the ovaries have also been reported. Traditionally, venography is considered the gold standard for diagnosing pelvic congestion syndrome but MR angiography is playing an increasing role.

Treatment is typically catheter directed venous embolization.

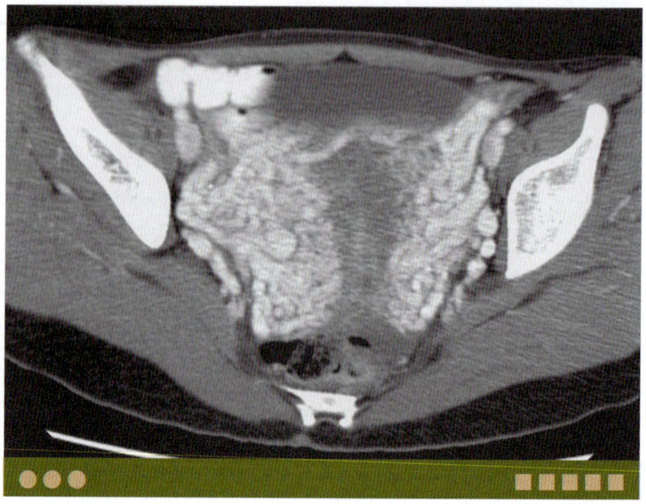

A. Axial CECT shows a markedly increased number of dilated parametrial vessels in this patient with chronic pelvic pain.

PEARLS

- **Usually seen in multiparous, premenopausal women.**
- **Imaging demonstrates prominent pelvic veins and ovarian veins and enlarged uterus.**
- **Treatment is venous embolization.**

ADDITIONAL IMAGES (B-E)

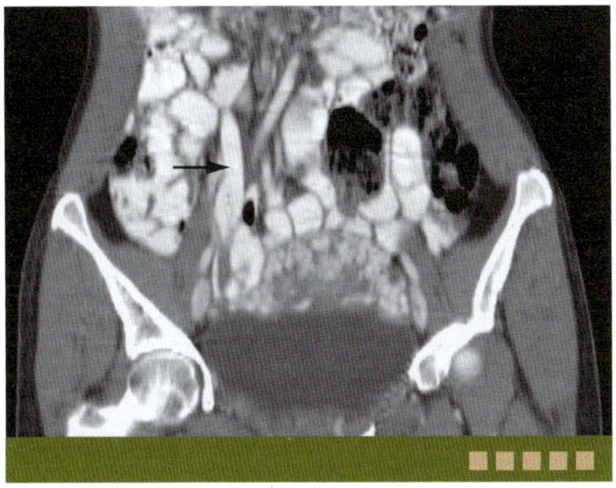

B. Coronal CECT in the same patient as Figure A further shows the prominent parametrial vessels and the dilated right ovarian vein (arrow).

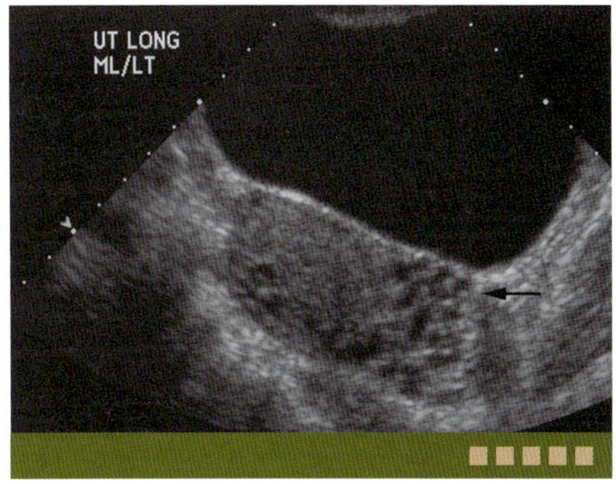

C. Longitudinal sonogram through the uterus shows multiple tubular anechoic structures surrounding the uterus (arrow).

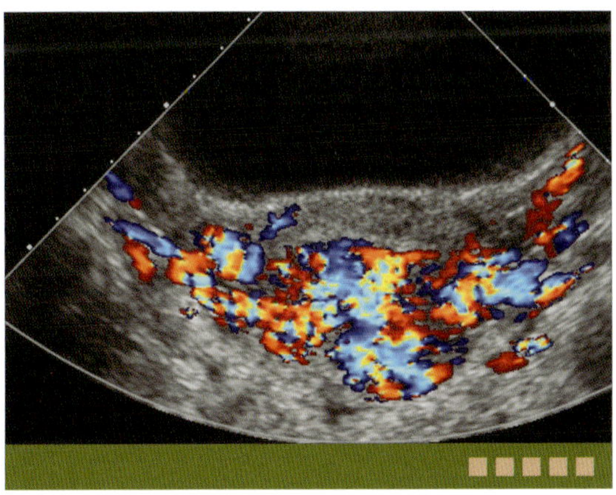

D. Transverse sonogram in the same patient as Figure C shows flow within the above-noted tubular structures compatible with multiple parametrial varicosities.

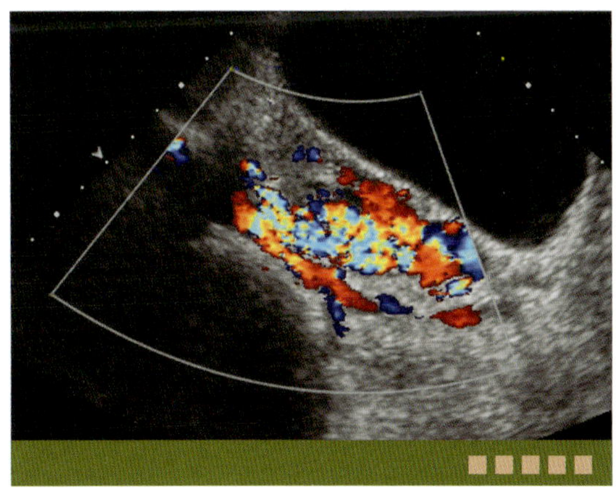

E. Longitudinal sonogram of the left ovary in the same patient shows prominent ovarian vessels. A similar finding was seen on the right.

IMAGE KEY

Common

Rare

Typical

Unusual

DIFFERENTIAL DIAGNOSIS IMAGES (F-G)

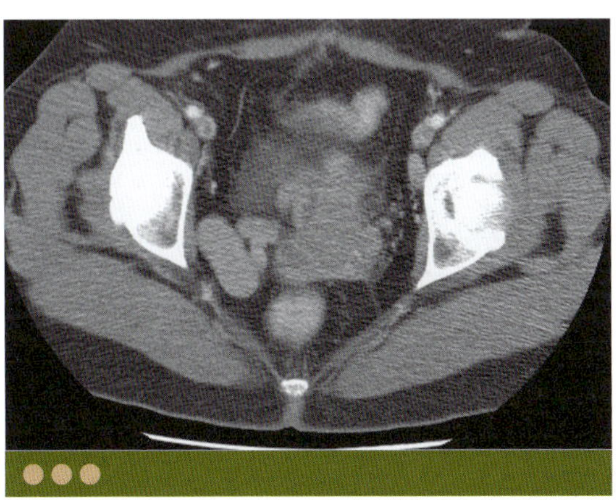

F. Pelvic collaterals IVC occlusion: Axial CECT shows dilated pelvic veins in the right hemipelvis.

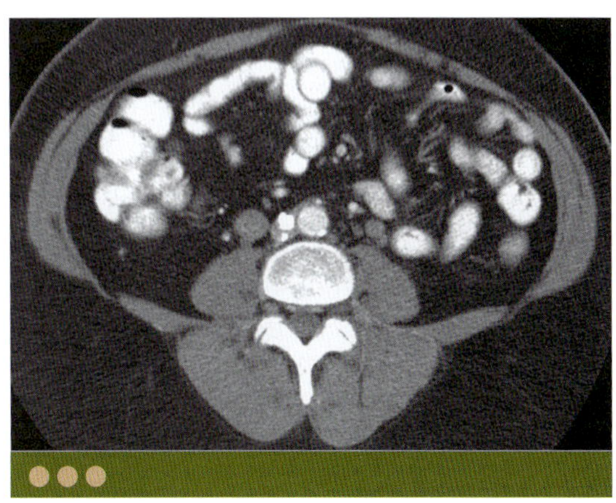

G. Axial CECT in the same patient as in Figure F obtained at a more superior level shows near complete to complete occlusion of the IVC by densely calcified thrombus.

16–17 Septate Uterus

Paul Nikolaidis

PRESENTATION

Infertility, history of spontaneous abortions.

FINDINGS

The uterus shows a mildly convex external contour and divergent uterine horns.

DIFFERENTIAL DIAGNOSIS

- *Bicornuate uterus*: Horns of a septate uterus have a more acute angle (<105°). On MR, a septate uterus should have no fundal indentation or a fundal indentation of less than 1.0 cm.

COMMENTS

A septate uterus occurs when there is partial or complete failure of resorption of the uterovaginal septum following fusion of the Müllerian ducts. This is the most common congenital uterine anomaly, representing approximately 55% of such anomalies. The septum may be composed of myometrial or fibrous tissue and can be either partial or complete (extending to the external cervical os). In 5% of cases, the septum may extend into the superior vagina. Differentiation between septate and bicornuate uteri is very important, as they are treated differently. An uncorrected septate uterus may result in spontaneous abortion in as many as 90% of pregnancies.

Hysterosalpingography (HSG) can help differentiate between septate and bicornuate uteri. If the two uterine cavities are not widely spaced with an angle between them of less than 105°, the uterus is more likely to be septate. With ultrasonography, a thin echogenic septum may be demonstrated.

MR is usually the only imaging modality that can almost always effectively differentiate between a bicornuate and septate uterus. Using features of both internal and external uterine anatomy, MR has been reported to be 100% sensitive and specific in the diagnosis of septate uterus. The external uterine contour of a septate uterus can be convex, flat, or mildly concave. A septate uterus may only have a fundal indentation of less than 1.0 cm, if any at all. The fundal segment of the septum is isointense to myometrium in all septa. In complete septa, the inferior segment of the septum is usually seen as a thin hypointense structure on T2-WI, because septa are more fibrous in composition inferiorly whereas mostly or entirely myometrial superiorly. Most partial septa are composed primarily of myometrium.

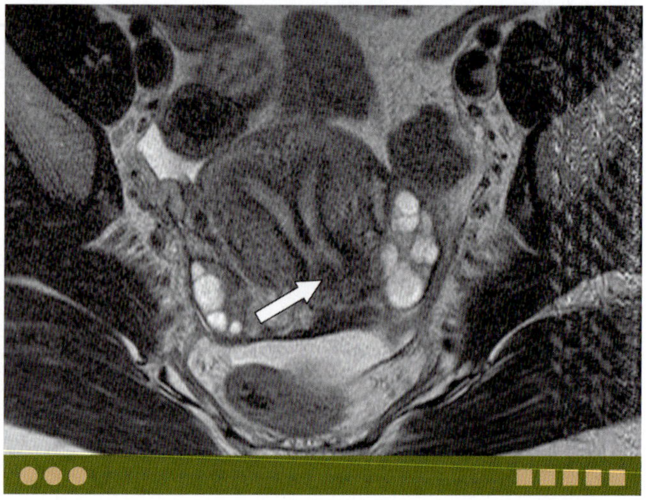

A. Axial T2-WI shows a septate uterus with a mildly convex external fundal contour and no fundal indentation. Portion of the hypointense dividing septum is also visualized inferiorly near the internal cervical os (arrow).

A septate uterus may be easily corrected hysteroscopically, by resecting the septum, resulting in an increase in live births of up to 86%. The length of the septum does not affect reproductive outcomes; both partial and complete septa have similar complication rates.

PEARLS

- **From failure of resorption of the uterovaginal septum.**
- **On HSG, the two uterine cavities should have an acute angle separating them (<105°).**
- **On MR, a septate uterus should have no external fundal indentation or a very small one (<1.0 cm).**
- **Easily corrected hysteroscopically.**

ADDITIONAL IMAGES (B-D)

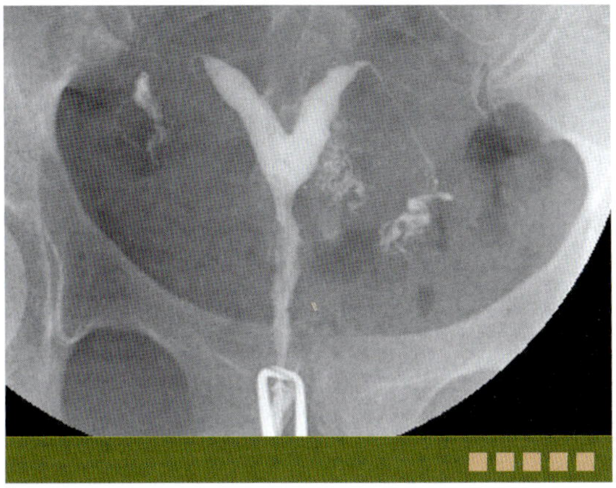

B. HSG on a patient with a septate uterus shows an acute angle between the uterine horns (67°).

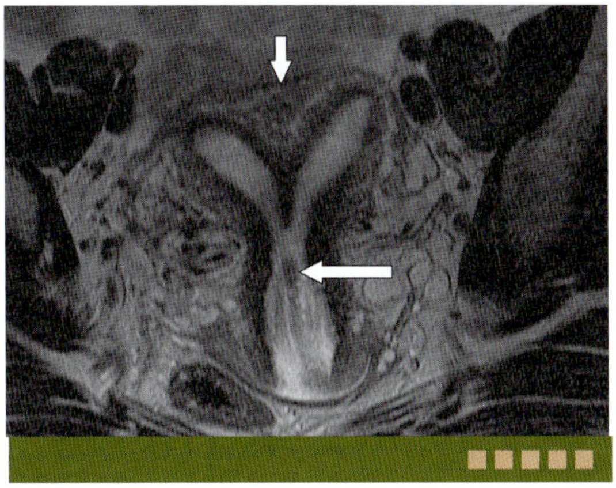

C. Axial T2-WI in another patient shows a septate uterus with a flat to minimally concave external fundal contour (short arrow). Portion of the dividing septum is also visualized inferiorly (long arrow).

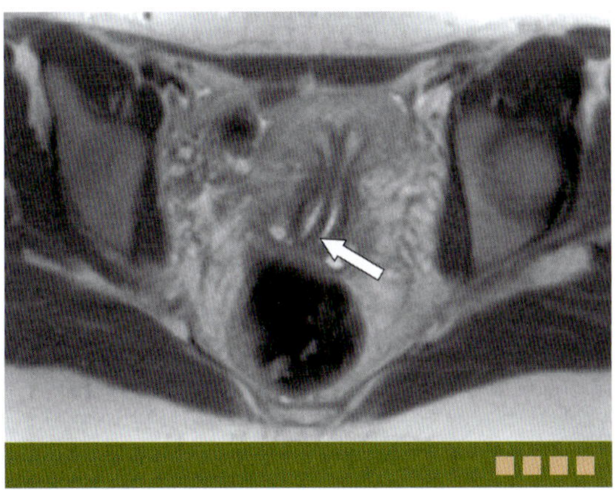

D. Axial T2-WI in another patient shows a septate uterus with a flat external fundal contour and no fundal indentation. The dividing septum is complete extending to the external cervical os (arrow).

DIFFERENTIAL DIAGNOSIS IMAGES (E-G)

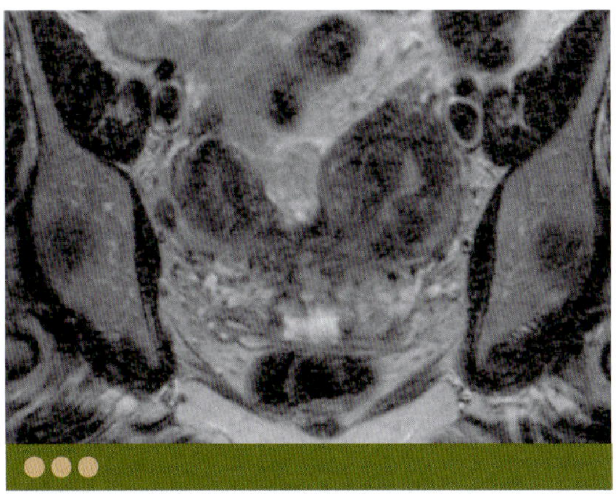

E. Bicornuate Uterus: Axial T2-WI shows a bicornuate uterus with widely divergent uterine horns. The proximal uterus is fused and a single cervix was present. There is a deep fundal indentation.

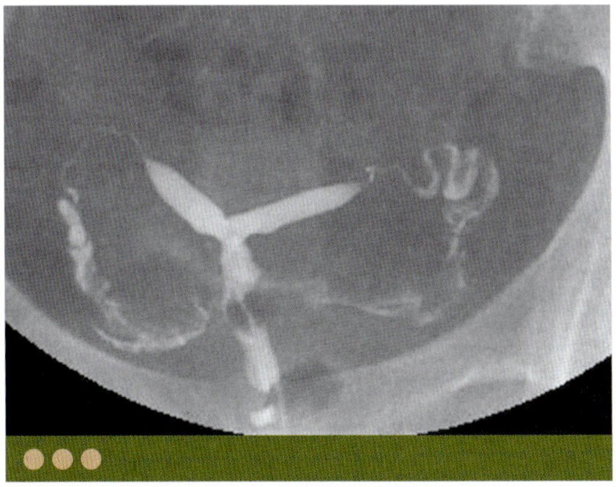

F. Bicornuate Uterus: HSG on the same patient shows two widely divergent uterine horns with an angle well over 105°. A single cervix was cannulated, distinguishing it from a uterus didelphys.

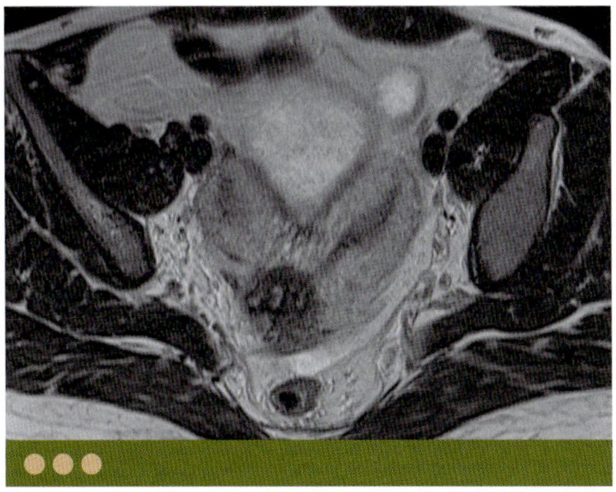

G. Bicornuate Uterus: Axial T2-WI on another patient with a bicornuate uterus shows the classic appearance of two widely divergent uterine horns that are fused proximally.

IMAGE KEY

Common

Rare

Typical

Unusual

16–18 Bicornuate Uterus

Paul Nikolaidis

PRESENTATION

Infertility, history of recurrent pregnancy losses.

FINDINGS

MR shows two divergent uterine horns and a significant external fundal cleft.

DIFFERENTIAL DIAGNOSES

- *Septate uterus*: On HSG, the two opacified uterine horns are not as widely divergent, with an angle of less than 105° separating them. On MR, the external uterine contour of a septate uterus can be convex, flat, or mildly concave and may only have a fundal indentation of less than 1.0 cm (if any at all).
- *Uterus didelphys*: The two horns and cervices are completely separate.

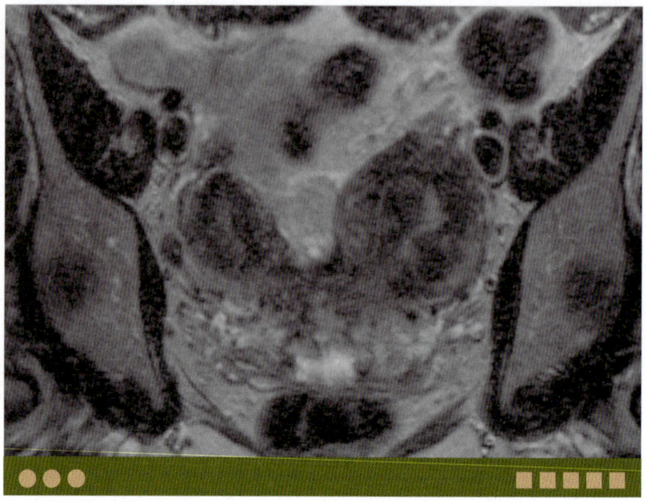

A. Axial T2-WI shows a bicornuate uterus with widely divergent uterine horns. The two horns are fused proximally. There is a deep fundal indentation.

COMMENTS

A bicornuate uterus has a single cervix but two uterine horns. It results from partial nonfusion of the Müllerian ducts, and specifically the uterovaginal horns at the level of the fundus. The central bridging myometrium may extend to the internal cervical os (uterus bicornuate unicollis) or all the way to the external cervical os (uterus bicornuate bicollis). A bicornuate bicollis uterus is associated with a duplicated cervix, although the two cervices are connected. A bicornuate bicollis uterus should be readily distinguished from a uterus didelphys as it demonstrates some degree of fusion between the two horns, whereas in a uterus didelphys the two horns and cervices are completely separate. Differentiation between bicornuate and septate uteri is sometimes more difficult and is very important, as management options are very different.

On HSG, if the two uterine cavities are widely spaced with an angle greater than 105°, the uterus is more likely to be bicornuate or didelphys than septate. HSG alone may not always be diagnostic since the external fundal contour is typically not visualized.

Sonography may demonstrate a double thickness myometrium, two hyperechoic endometrial complexes and most importantly a fundal cleft and divergent uterine horns.

MR is the only imaging modality that can almost always differentiate between a bicornuate and septate uterus. MR has been shown to be 100% accurate in the diagnosis of bicornuate uterus in a recent study. A bicornuate uterus has an external fundal indentation deeper than 1.0 cm, whereas a septate uterus has an indentation of either less than 1.0 cm or no indentation at all. Normal uterine zonal anatomy should be seen in both horns.

A bicornuate uterus has a lower rate of complications than the other Müllerian anomalies, but may require laparotomy for surgical correction. Surgical intervention may not be necessary in many cases, and the length of subsequent gestations may increase with increasing parity. Strassman metroplasty has been advocated in women with recurrent pregnancy losses who have no other potential reasons for infertility.

PEARLS

- **Because of partial nonfusion of the Müllerian ducts.**
- **A bicornuate uterus has a lower rate of complications but may require laparotomy for surgical correction.**
- **On HSG, the two uterine cavities are widely spaced with an angle of greater than 105°.**
- **On MR, a bicornuate uterus should have a fundal indentation greater than 1.0 cm.**

ADDITIONAL IMAGES (B-D)

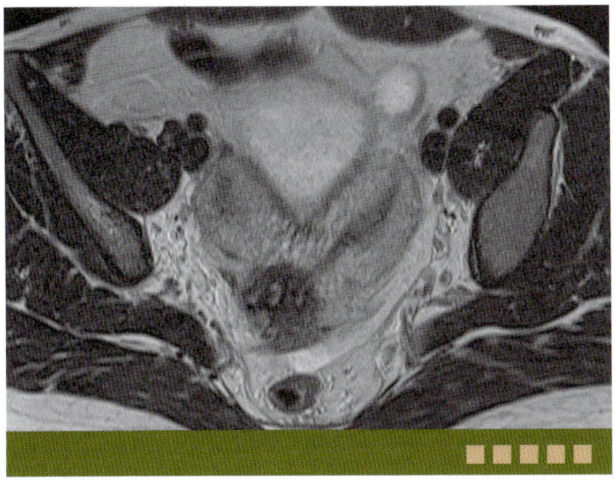

B. Axial T2-WI on another patient with a bicornuate uterus shows the classic appearance of two widely divergent uterine horns that are fused proximally.

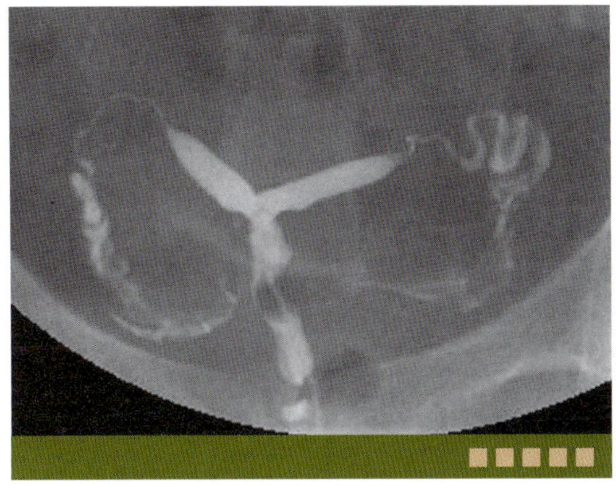

C. HSG on another patient shows the classic appearance of widely divergent uterine horns with opacification of both fallopian tubes.

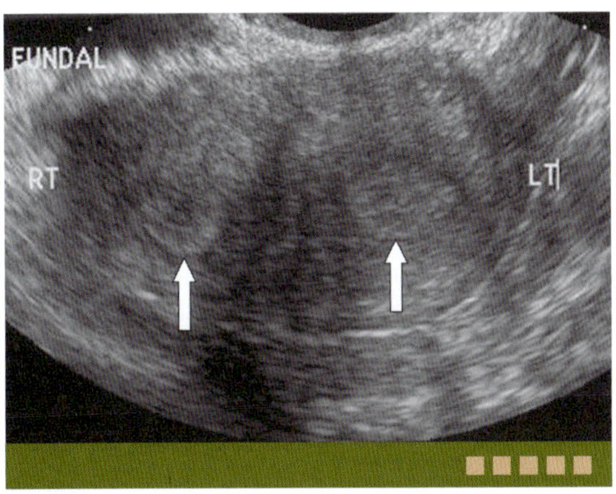

D. Transverse sonogram shows a double thickness myometrium and two hyperechoic endometrial complexes (arrows).

DIFFERENTIAL DIAGNOSES IMAGES (E-G)

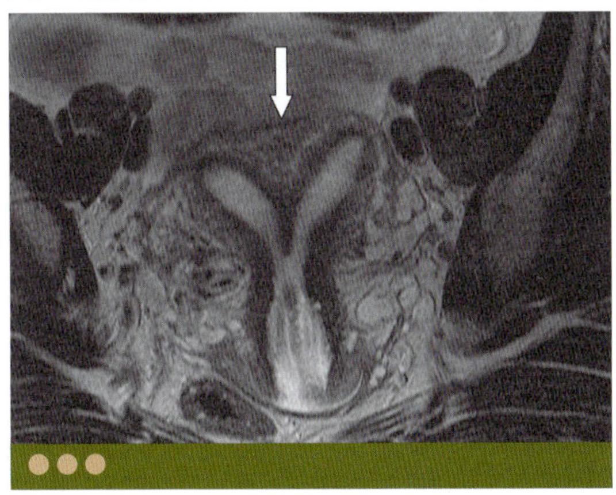

E. Septate Uterus: Axial T2-WI on another patient shows a septate uterus with a flat external fundal contour and no fundal indentation (arrow).

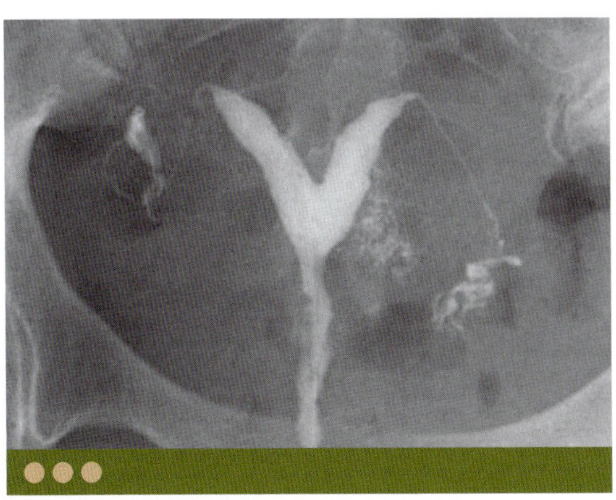

F. Septate Uterus: HSG on the same patient shows an acute angle between the uterine horns (67°). In a bicornuate uterus, the two horns would be more divergent with an angle exceeding 105°.

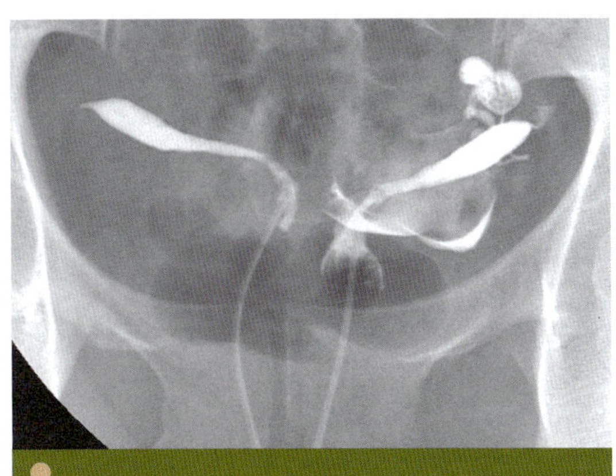

G. Uterus Didelphys: HSG shows simultaneous catheterization of two separate cervices and opacification of two widely divergent noncommunicating endometrial cavities.

IMAGE KEY

Common

Rare

Typical

Unusual

16–19 Unicornuate Uterus

Paul Nikolaidis

PRESENTATION

Infertility, history of spontaneous abortions.

FINDINGS

HSG shows a single uterine horn and fallopian tube. MR similarly demonstrates a single uterine horn. A second rudimentary horn was not seen in this case.

DIFFERENTIAL DIAGNOSIS

None

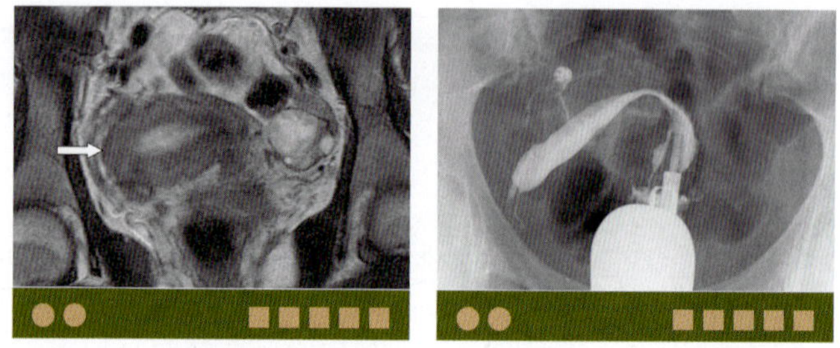

A. Sagittal T2-WI shows a unicornuate uterus with the classic "banana" shape and contour (arrow). There was no associated rudimentary horn.
B. Corresponding HSG shows the classic appearance of the deviated endometrial cavity with opacification of only one fallopian tube.

COMMENTS

A unicornuate uterus (American Fertility Society type II malformation), consists of a single uterine horn and fallopian tube. It is the result of complete, or almost complete, arrest of development of one of the paired Müllerian ducts. When not corrected, this anomaly is associated with a low rate of reproductive success, with a live birth rate of less than 50%. There is a high incidence of spontaneous abortion, premature birth, intrauterine growth retardation, and abnormal fetal lie. Other complications include dysmenorrhea, hematometra, and an increased incidence of endometriosis and ectopic pregnancies. Approximately 40% of the patients have associated renal anomalies (ipsilateral agenesis in approximately two-thirds, but also horseshoe or ectopic kidneys, duplications and cystic renal dysplasias may occur).

In two-thirds of the patients, the arrest in the development of one of the Müllerian ducts is not complete, and a rudimentary horn with or without functioning endometrium will be present. The prognosis and optimal management is dictated by whether or not there is a communicating rudimentary horn, and also whether it contains an endometrial lining. If the rudimentary horn becomes obstructed, the patient may present with an enlarging pelvic mass. These patients are prone to various gynecologic and obstetric complications (including miscarriage, ectopic pregnancy, abnormal fetal presentation, intrauterine growth retardation and premature labor) that may be avoided by surgical resection of the rudimentary horn and its tube. If there is a communicating rudimentary horn, surgery is also indicated because a pregnancy within such a horn is unlikely to be viable. If a noncommunicating rudimentary horn is present but without an endometrial lining, complications are unlikely, and surgery is generally not necessary.

A unicornuate uterus is well visualized on HSG as a single uterine horn and fallopian tube. MR is far superior for the identification and assessment of the degree of dilatation of a noncommunicating rudimentary horn. The uterus is elongated and slightly curved with a characteristic "banana" shape. Normal zonal anatomy is maintained, although uterine volume is decreased. The appearance of the rudimentary horn depends on whether endometrial tissue is present. In non-cavitary rudimentary horns, asymmetric soft tissue is seen at the base of the dominant horn. In cavitary rudimentary horns, variable amounts of hyperintense endometrial tissue are seen on T2-WI. All MR examinations performed for the evaluation of uterine anomalies should include a larger field of view T2-weighted sequence to include the kidneys. Frequent associated renal anomalies may then be identified. An undescended or ectopic ovary that attaches at an area above the common iliac vessels may also be seen in almost half of the patients with a unicornuate uterus.

PEARLS

- **Attributed to arrest in the development of one of the two müllerian ducts.**
- **If arrested development of the mullerian duct is incomplete, a rudimentary horn with or without functioning endometrium will be present.**
- **On HSG, a single uterine horn and fallopian tube is identified.**
- **MR allows for better identification of any associated rudimentary horn.**

ADDITIONAL IMAGES (C-H)

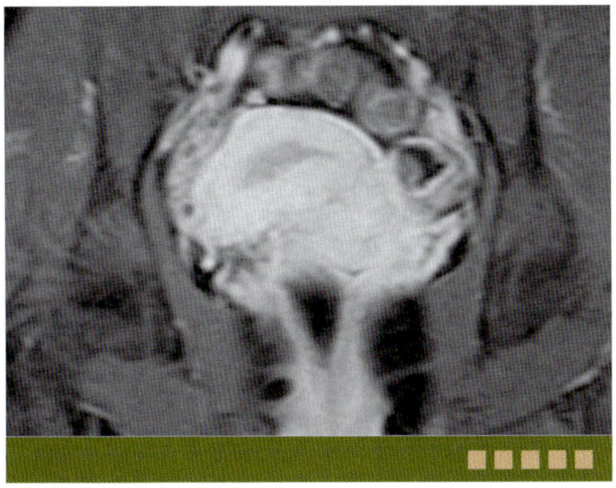

C. Corresponding sagittal contrast-enhanced T1-WI shows the classic shape and contour of a unicornuate uterus. Normal myometrial enhancement is seen.

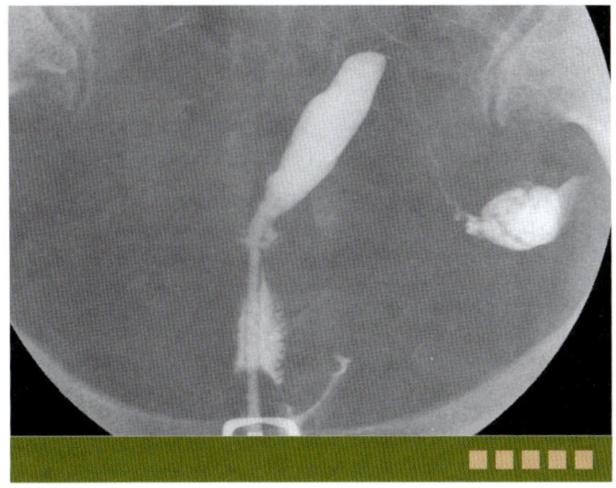

D. HSG on another patient shows the classic appearance of a deviated endometrial cavity with opacification of one fallopian tube. In this case, the uterine cavity is tilted toward the left.

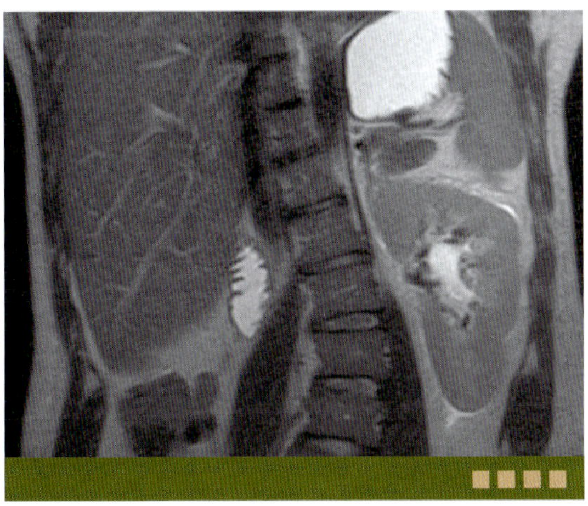

E. Coronal T2-WI in a patient with a unicornuate uterus shows associated congenital absence of the right kidney. Given the prevalence of associated renal anomalies, MR examinations should include a larger field of view T2-weighted sequence including the kidneys.

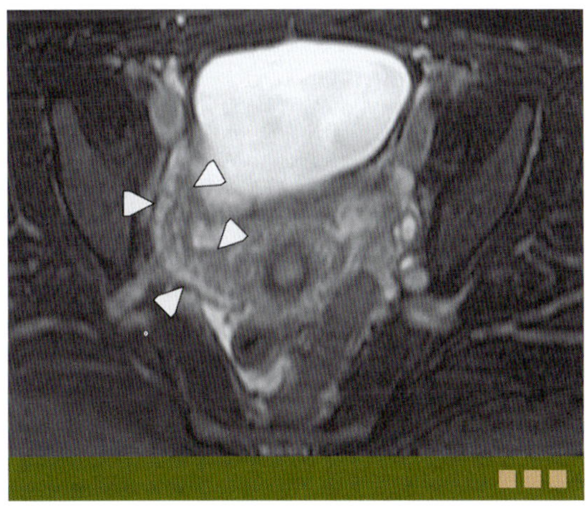

F. Axial T2-WI in another patient shows a unicornuate uterus with a small adjacent non-cavitary rudimentary horn on the right (arrowheads).

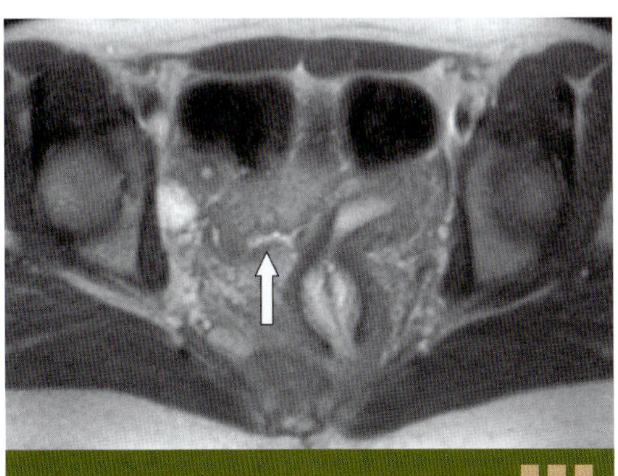

G. Axial T2-WI in another patient shows a unicornuate uterus with an adjacent cavitary rudimentary horn. A small amount of endometrial tissue is seen within the rudimentary horn, which did not clearly communicate (arrow).

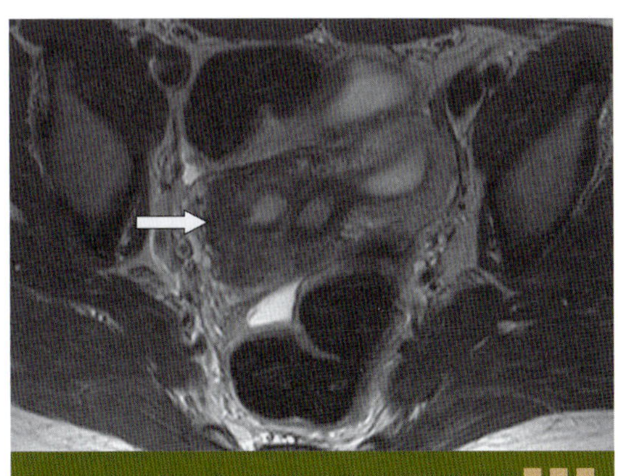

H. Axial T2-WI in another patient shows a unicornuate uterus with an adjacent communicating cavitary rudimentary horn (arrow).

IMAGE KEY

Common

Rare

Typical

Unusual

16–20 Uterus Didelphys

Paul Nikolaidis

PRESENTATION

Infertility, history of spontaneous abortions.

FINDINGS

HSG performed after cannulation of two cervices shows two separate divergent uterine cavities.

DIFFERENTIAL DIAGNOSES

- *Bicornuate uterus*: On HSG, the two cervices of a uterus didelphys must be cannulated and two divergent uterine cavities will be opacified. On MR, the two horns and cervices are completely separate.
- *Unicornuate uterus*: On HSG, if only one of the two cervices of a uterus didelphys is cannulated, then it may be mistaken for a unicornuate uterus.

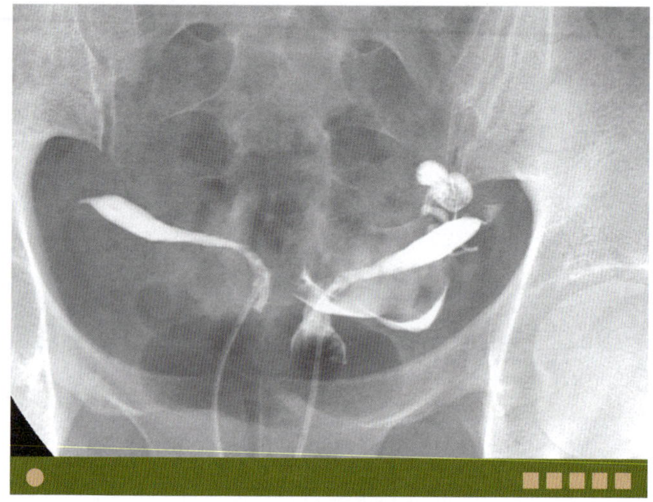

A. HSG shows simultaneous catheterization of two separate cervices and opacification of two widely divergent endometrial cavities that do not communicate. Findings are diagnostic of a uterus didelphys.

COMMENTS

Uterus didelphys (American Fertility Society type III malformation) is one of the least common congenital uterine anomalies. It consists of two entirely separate uterine horns and cervices. This anomaly results from complete nonfusion of both müllerian ducts during embryologic development. Both individual horns are fully developed and almost normal in size. By definition, two cervices must be present in all cases. A very minor degree of fusion may exist at the interface of the subjacent cervices.

Almost 75% of patients with a uterus didelphys may also have an associated vertical (transverse) dividing vaginal septum which may be further complicated by the presence of additional secondary fusion defects, such as a horizontal septum. Uterus didelphys has the highest association with transverse vaginal septa but similar septa may also be observed with other anomalies. While usually asymptomatic, few patients with such septa may develop obstruction of one of the horns and present with hematocolpos or dysmenorrhea.

HSG is diagnostic only if both cervices are identified and cannulated. Longitudinal or transverse vaginal septa may be present. MR is superior in the evaluation of these types of uterine duplications. Coronal T2-WI are excellent in showing the uterine and cervical duplications, while axial T2-WI may demonstrate the dividing vaginal septa seen in many patients.

Uterus didelphys is associated with one of the lowest live birth rates (40%-50%) of all major müllerian anomalies. In addition to an anatomic basis, these poor reproductive outcomes are also thought in part to be because of decreased vascularity of the uterine horns. Metroplasty is often considered for surgical repair in patients with recurrent pregnancy losses; however, since each horn is an almost fully developed uterus, it may carry a pregnancy to full term.

PEARLS

- **Attributed to complete nonfusion of the müllerian ducts.**
- **A uterus didelphys has a high rate of reproductive complications.**
- **On HSG, both cervices should be identified and cannulated in order to reach the correct diagnosis.**
- **On MR, two separate cervices and uterine horns should be seen and a vaginal septum may also be demonstrated.**

ADDITIONAL IMAGES (B-D)

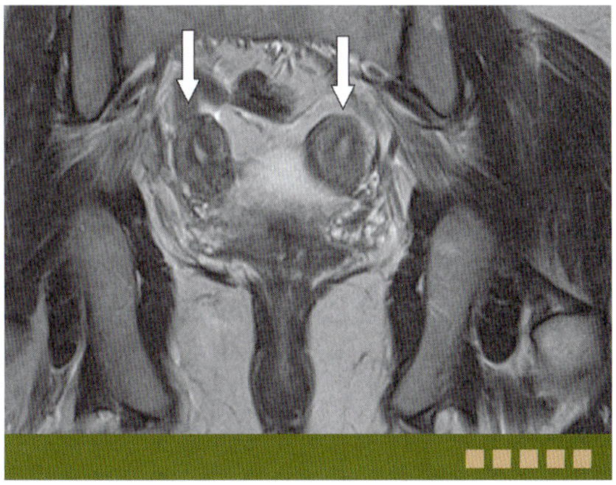

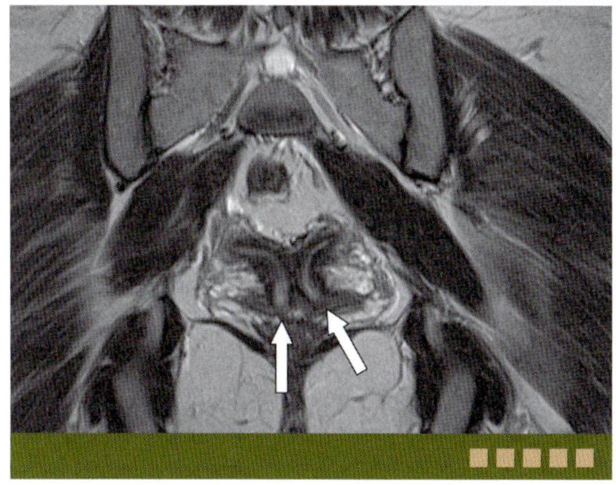

B. and **C.** Sequential coronal T2-WI on a patient with a uterus didelphys show two widely divergent uterine horns (top arrows) and completely separate cervices (bottom arrows).

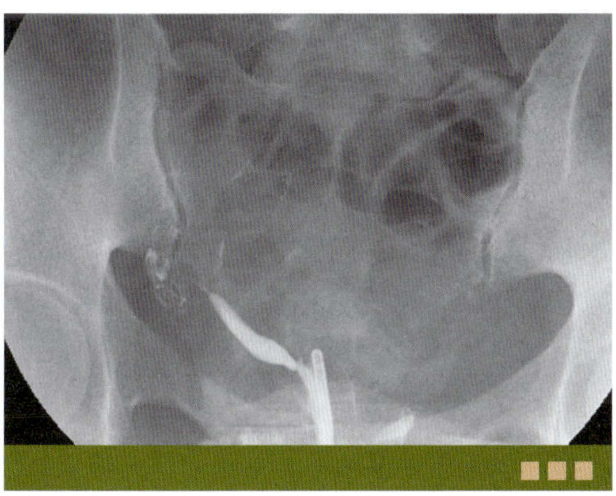

D. HSG of a uterus didelphys with cannulation of only one of the two cervices shows a deviated endometrial cavity and filling of one fallopian tube. If only one of the cervices of a uterus didelphys is cannulated, it may be mistaken for a unicornuate uterus.

DIFFERENTIAL DIAGNOSES IMAGES (E-G)

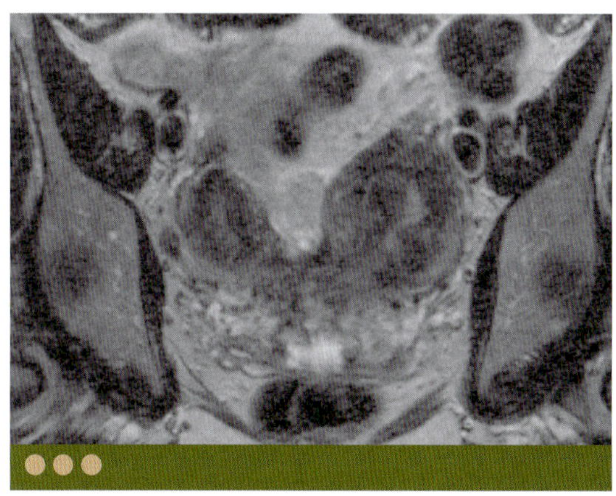

E. Bicornuate Uterus: Axial T2-WI shows a bicornuate uterus with widely divergent uterine horns. The proximal uterus is fused, and a single cervix was present.

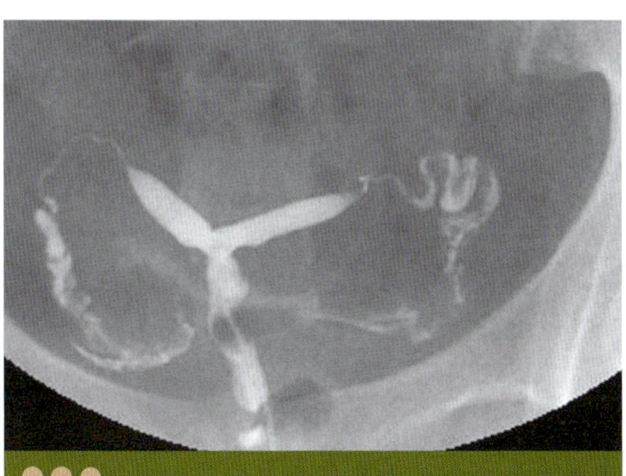

F. Bicornuate Uterus: HSG on the same patient shows two widely divergent uterine horns with an angle exceeding 105°. A single cervix was present, distinguishing it from a uterus didelphys.

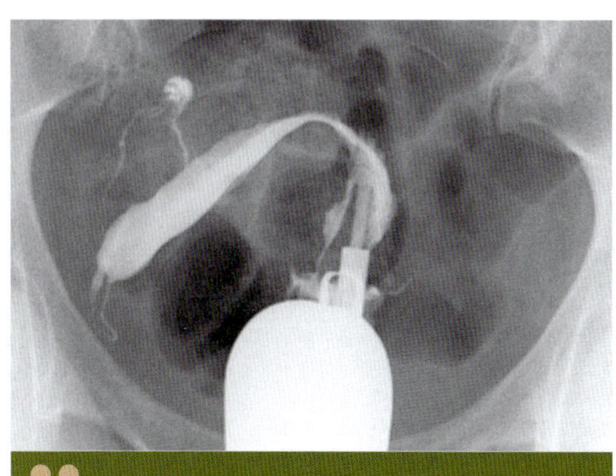

G. Unicornuate uterus: HSG shows a unicornuate uterus with a rightward deviated endometrial cavity and opacification of only one fallopian tube. If only one cervix of a uterus didelphys is cannulated, it may have a similar appearance and be mistaken for a unicornuate uterus.

IMAGE KEY

Common

Rare

Typical

Unusual

Part 2

Cervix

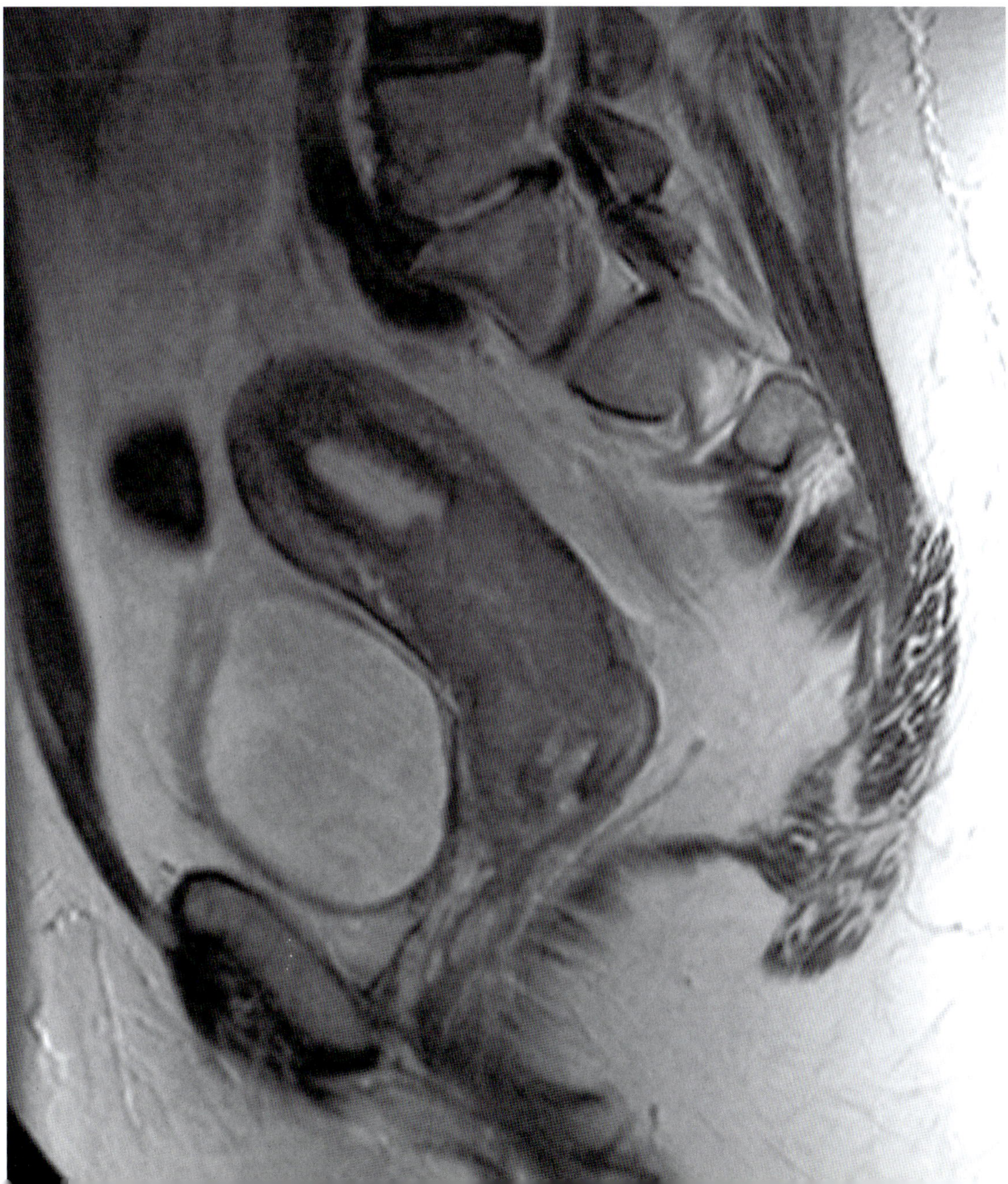

16–21 Cervical Cancer I and II

Nancy A. Hammond

PRESENTATION

Asymptomatic, vaginal bleeding, or vaginal discharge.

FINDINGS

T2-WI hyperintense cervical mass with enhancement on postcontrast sequences.

DIFFERENTIAL DIAGNOSIS

- *Cervical fibroid*: Well-defined T2-WI hypointense mass with variable enhancement.

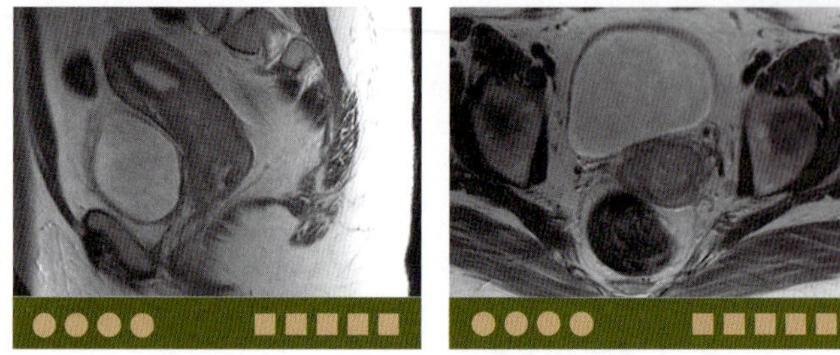

A. Sagittal T2-WI shows a hyperintense mass centered in the cervix and extending into the lower uterus. The outer wall of the cervix is maintained.
B. Axial T2-WI further shows the cervical mass with preservation of the outer cervical stroma.

COMMENTS

Cervical cancer is the third most common gynecologic malignancy in women in the United States. The mean age of women with cervical cancer is 50 years. It is associated with human papillomavirus infection. Most cancers are squamous cell origin (85%) with the remainder being adenocarcinomas. Asymptomatic patients are detected by routine Papanicolaou (PAP) smears, whereas symptomatic patients present with bleeding or vaginal discharge. Screening with PAP smears has decreased cervical cancer mortality by 70% in the past 50 years. Fortunately, the majority of cancers are confined to the cervical canal when discovered representing stage I disease. Risk factors for the development of cervical cancer include HPV infection, cigarette smoking, low socioeconomic status, and multiple sexual partners.

Cervical cancer is staged according to the International Federation of Gynecology and Obstetrics (FIGO) clinical classification. Accurate staging is essential as it influences patient management. Women with greater than Stage IIB disease are not surgical candidates and are treated with radiation. Stage IIB disease is defined as any tumor with parametrial invasion. Stage I tumors are confined to the cervix. Stage II tumors extend beyond the cervix. Stage III tumors invade the pelvic sidewall, obstruct the ureter, or invade the distal vagina. Stage IV tumors are characterized by extension beyond the true pelvis, invasion of the bladder or rectal mucosa, or distant metastases.

MR is an excellent modality in evaluating patients with known cervical cancer for primary staging. It can accurately stage the disease and is more accurate than CT. CT lacks the spatial resolution necessary for primary staging but is utilized in patients with advanced disease. On MRI, multiplanar T2-weighted sequences have been found to be the most useful for local staging. Cervical cancer appears as a T2-hyperintense lesion relative to the dark cervical stroma. Preservation of the black ring of cervical stroma virtually excludes parametrial invasion. It is important to note that disruption of the low-signal ring does not necessarily indicate parametrial extension as the outer cervical stroma may be preserved. However, when there is disruption of the stromal ring, patients have an 85% chance of parametrial invasion. Most studies have found that gadolinium enhanced sequences do not provide significant improvement in the primary staging of cervical cancer, however, are useful in evaluating lymphadenopathy and distal metastases.

Although not utilized as a diagnostic modality, cervical cancer appears as an inhomogeneous enlarged cervix on ultrasound. CT may also show an enlarged heterogeneous cervix. The primary mass typically is a low-density mass enlarging the cervix.

PEARLS

- **Cervical cancer is the third most common gynecological malignancy in women in the United States and has a known association with human papilloma virus (HPV).**
- **MR is a valuable tool in primary staging of women with cervical cancer.**
- **Stage IIB disease consists of parametrial extension and excludes the patient from surgical management.**

ADDITIONAL IMAGES (C-D)

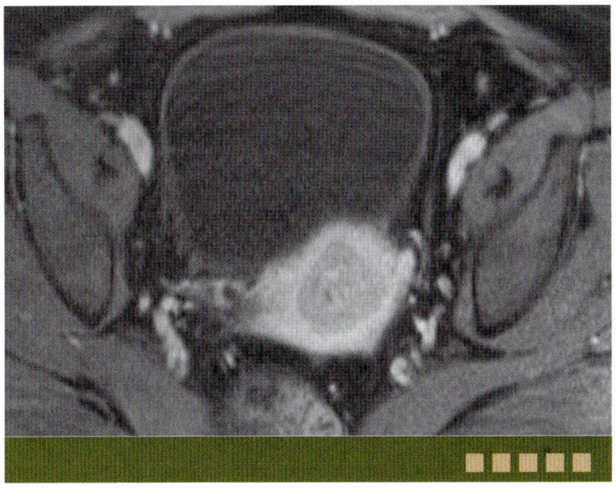

C. Axial contrast-enhanced T1-WI in the same patient shows the lesion in the cervix which enhances to a lesser degree than the adjacent normal cervical parenchyma. There is no evidence of parametrial extension.

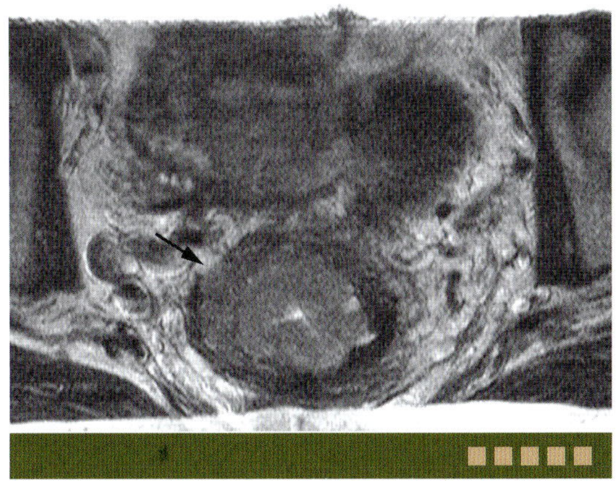

D. Axial T2-WI in a different patient also shows a hyperintense mass centered in the cervix with loss of the normal low-signal stroma (arrow) suggestive of parametrial invasion and stage IIB disease.

IMAGE KEY

Common

Rare

Typical

Unusual

DIFFERENTIAL DIAGNOSIS IMAGES (E-F)

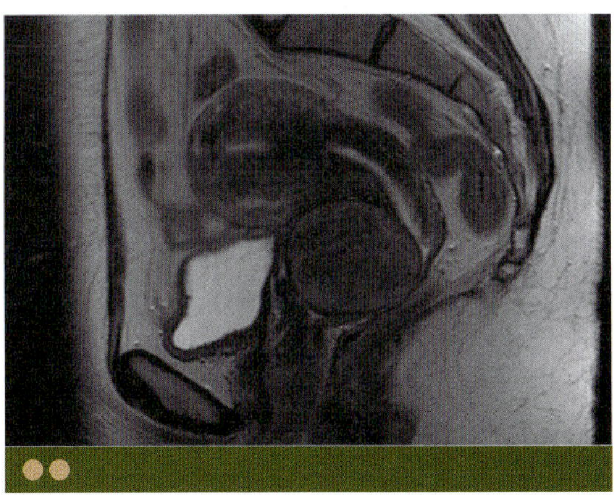

E. Cervical fibroid: Sagittal T2-WI shows a well-defined hypointense cervical mass consistent with a cervical fibroid.

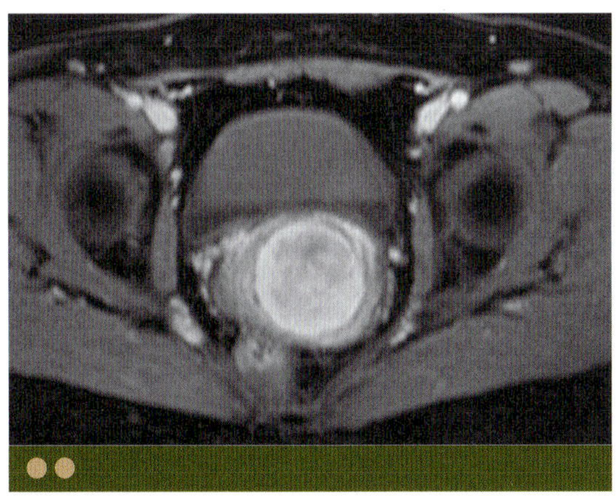

F. Cervical fibroid: Axial contrast-enhanced T1-WI in the same patient as Figure E shows the characteristic intense enhancement of a fibroid.

16–22 Cervical Cancer Stage III/IV

Nancy A. Hammond

PRESENTATION

Cervical mass on physical examination.

FINDINGS

Enlarged heterogeneous cervix on CT with pelvic lymphadenopathy.

DIFFERENTIAL DIAGNOSIS

- *Endometrial cancer*: Mass centered in the region of the uterus rather than the cervix. The two may be difficult to distinguish when large and involving both uterus and cervix.

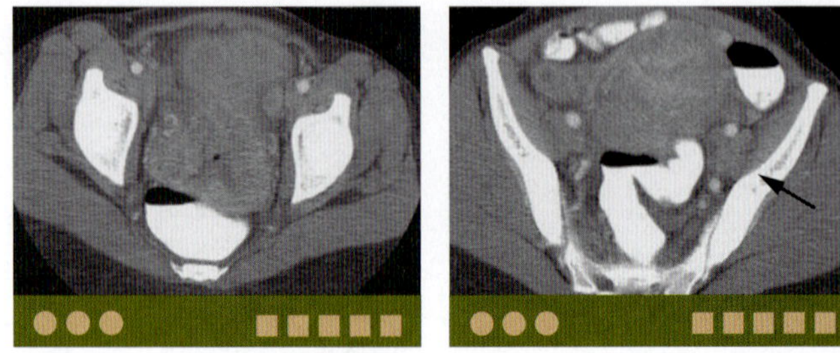

A. Axial CECT shows an enlarged heterogeneous cervix suggesting an underlying mass lesion.
B. Axial CECT in the same patient just superior to figure A shows lymphadenopathy along the left iliac chain compatible with metastases and advanced stage disease (arrow).

COMMENTS

Cervical cancer is the third most common gynecologic malignancy in women in the United States. As a result of screening of patients with the PAP smears, mortality from cervical cancer has decreased by 70% in the past 50 years. The majority of cancers are confined to the cervical canal when discovered representing stage I disease.

Cervical cancer is staged according to the International Federation of Gynecology and Obstetrics (FIGO) clinical classification. Stage I tumors are confined to the cervix. Stage II tumors extend beyond the cervix. Stage III tumors invade the pelvic sidewall, obstruct the ureter, or invade the distal vagina. Stage IV tumors are characterized by extension beyond the true pelvis, invasion of the bladder or rectal mucosa, or distant metastases. Stage IV disease is treated with chemotherapy and radiation therapy. MR can establish parametrial extension with an accuracy ranging from 75% to 95%. In women with non-surgical disease, localization of tumor and the presence or absence of ureteral obstruction aids in determining the extent of radiation therapy and the need for ureteral stenting.

In evaluating advanced disease, the presence of masses extending into the bladder lumen or sessile nodularity along the posterior bladder wall contiguous with the cervical mass suggests bladder extension. On MR, abnormally high signal within the normally low-signal posterior bladder wall and abnormal soft tissue in the uterovesical space suggests stage IVA disease. Importantly, contrast enhancement or abnormal signal in the uterovesical space may alternatively represent an inflammatory response to the cervical tumor rather than tumor extension.

While MRI more accurately stages local extension of cervical cancer, CT can be helpful in advanced stage disease demonstrating prominent parametrial or pelvic sidewall involvement, lymphadenopathy, hyrdronephrosis caused by ureteral involvement, and distant metastases. CT is frequently used in patients with suspected tumor recurrence. Recurrent disease can be difficult to distinguish from post-therapy fibrosis and may require biopsy.

PEARLS

- **Cervical cancer most commonly presents with Stage I disease because of screening with PAP smears.**
- **Disease Stage IIB and above are excluded from surgical treatment.**
- **MRI can accurately stage local extension of cervical cancer.**
- **CT is valuable in evaluating for distant metastases.**

ADDITIONAL IMAGES (C-G)

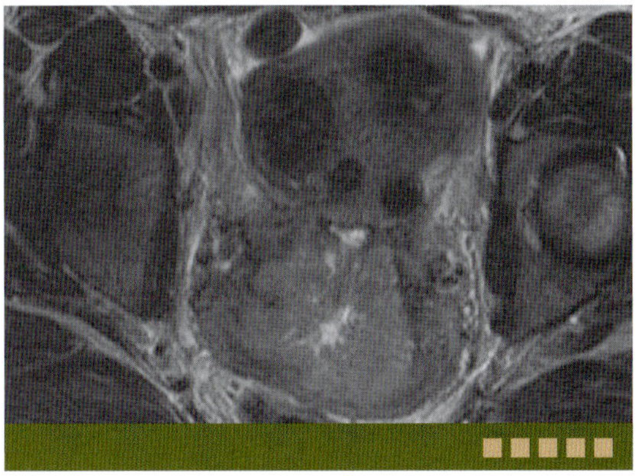

C. Axial T2-WI in the same patient shows a hyperintense mass centered in the cervix with loss of the normal hypointense cervical stroma anteriorly. Hypointense masses in the uterus are compatible with uterine fibroids.

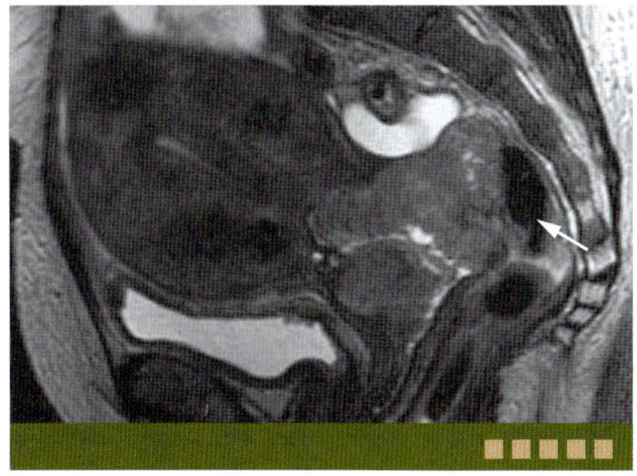

D. Sagittal T2-WI in the patient better shows the extent of the cervical mass clearly extending beyond the cervix posteriorly (arrow).

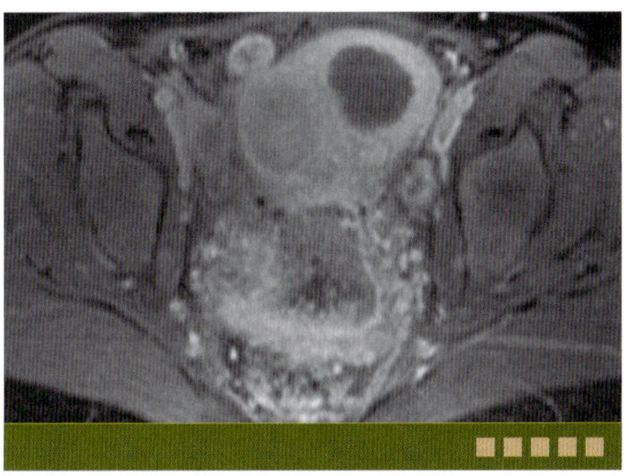

E. Axial contrast-enhanced T1-WI delineates the heterogeneously enhancing cervical mass. The enlarged left external iliac lymph node is also shown.

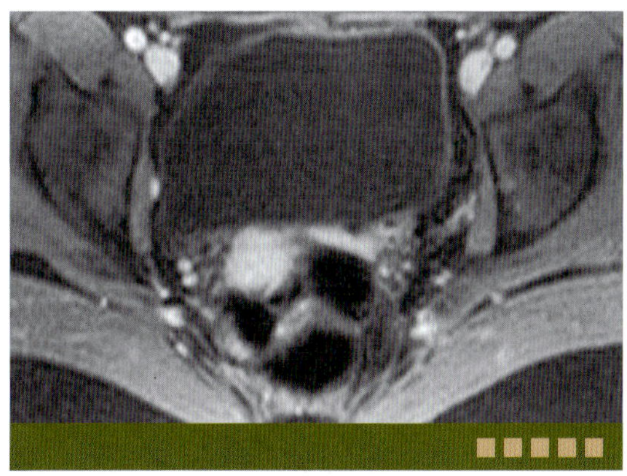

F. Axial contrast-enhanced T1-WI in a patient with a history of cervical cancer status post total hysterectomy shows an enhancing soft-tissue mass along the right vaginal cuff consistent with recurrent disease.

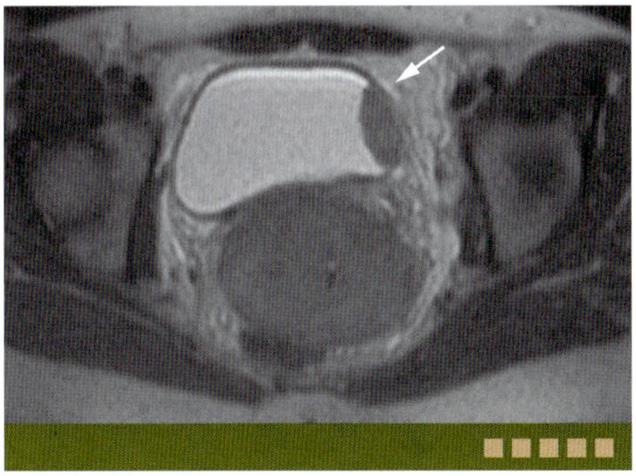

G. Axial T2-WI in a different patient shows a large hyperintense mass centered in the cervix. Additionally, a nodular mass is present along the left lateral aspect of the urinary bladder (arrow) with signal characteristics similar to that of the cervical mass consistent with metastatic disease.

DIFFERENTIAL DIAGNOSIS IMAGE

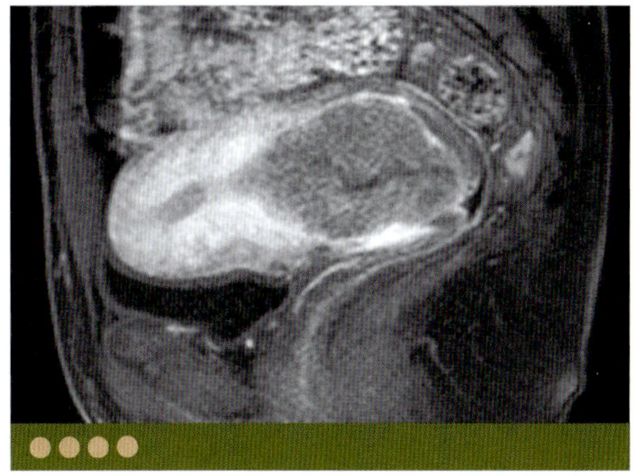

H. Endometrial cancer: Sagittal contrast enhanced T1-WI shows an enhancing mass centered in the lower uterine segment.

IMAGE KEY

Common

●●●●●
●●●●
●●●
●●
●

Rare

Typical

■■■■■
■■■■
■■■
■■
■

Unusual

16–23 Adenoma Malignum

Paul Nikolaidis

PRESENTATION

Watery vaginal discharge.

FINDINGS

MR shows a cervical lesion containing multiple, ill-defined small cysts with a few intervening solid components.

DIFFERENTIAL DIAGNOSES

- *Deep nabothian cysts*: Adenoma malignum usually contains numerous small cysts without a clear margin and may even exhibit solid parts. A solid enhancing portion may be seen.
- *Adenomatous hyperplasia of the endocervical glands*: Adenomatous hyperplasia does not deeply invade the cervical stroma.
- *Cervical cancer*: Multiple discrete cystic foci are generally not present, unless there are nabothian cysts near/in an area of cervical carcinoma.

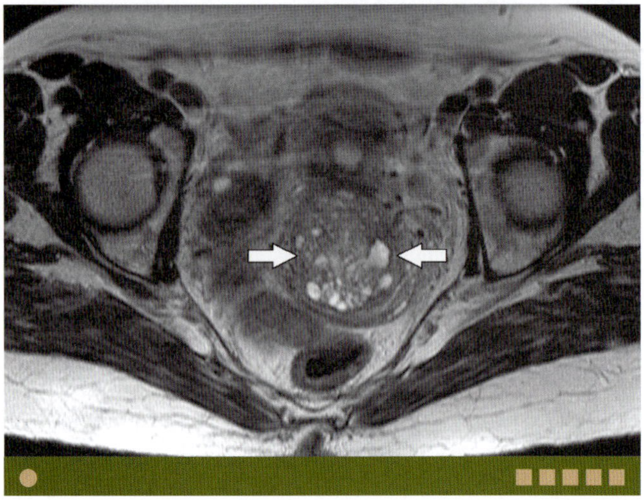

A. Axial T2-WI shows a cervical mass containing numerous small cystic structures (arrows).

COMMENTS

Adenoma malignum is a rare variant of cervical adenocarcinoma. Adenocarcinoma of the cervix accounts for only about 5% to 15% of all carcinomas of the cervix. The vast majority of cervical carcinomas are squamous cell carcinomas. Adenoma malignum is thought to represent only 3% of all cervical adenocarcinoma cases. This neoplasm usually arises from the columnar epithelial lining of the endocervical canal and tends to grow within the cervix, therefore, often making it difficult to detect via clinical vaginal examination. The most common initial symptom is a watery discharge. It is sometimes seen in association with other disease entities or syndromes, such as Peutz-Jeghers syndrome and mucinous tumor of the ovary.

Sonographically, adenoma malignum may appear as a hyperechoic mass mixed with multiple cysts. On CT, a low attenuation endocervical mass may be seen.

MR is the best imaging modality for the detection and characterization of adenoma malignum. Multiple cystic lesions are seen within the cervical stroma, if the cysts are large enough to be visualized. On T1-WI, the fluid within the cysts tends to be isointense or slightly hyperintense to the cervical stroma. On T2-WI, the cyst fluid is usually markedly hyperintense. On T2-WI, the cervical stroma surrounding the cystic mass may be hyperintense compared to the uterus. This is either because of the presence of tiny cysts not fully depicted on MR, or because of edema within the cervical stroma. Following gadolinium administration, a solid enhancing portion may be seen.

Adenoma malignum is associated with early dissemination, poor response to therapy and an unfavorable prognosis.

PEARLS

- **A rare variant of cervical adenocarcinoma (approximately 3% of adenocarcinomas).**
- **The most common initial symptom is a watery discharge.**
- **On MR, sometimes difficult to differentiate from deep nabothian cysts.**
- **Following IV gadolinium administration, a solid enhancing component may be seen.**

ADDITIONAL IMAGES (B-C)

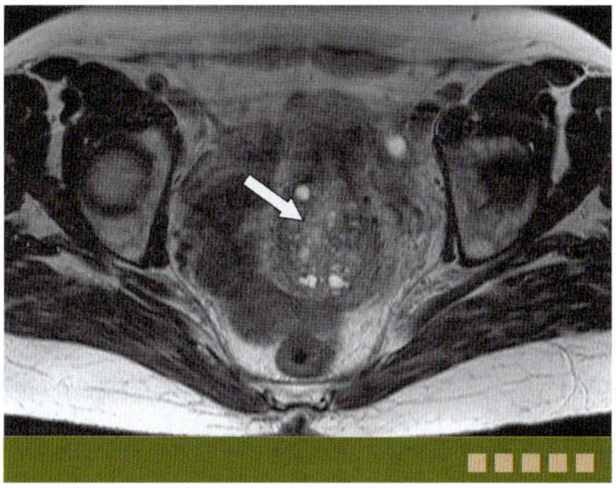

B. Additional axial T2-WI shows an area of more solid tissue centrally within the cervical mass, which is mildly hyperintense (arrow).

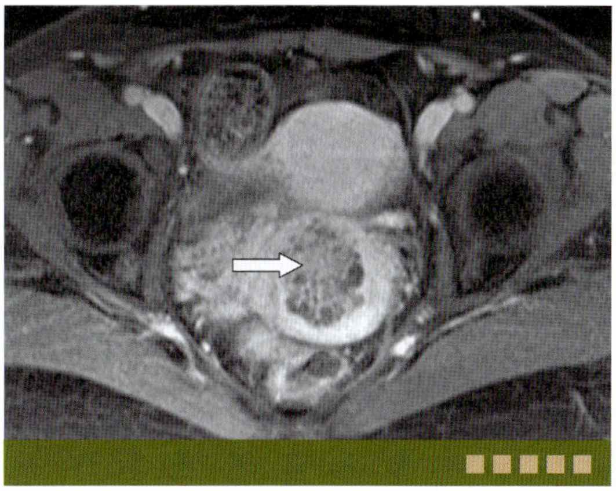

C. Corresponding axial contrast-enhanced T1-WI shows several areas of nonenhancement representing the small cystic foci, along with a central enhancing component (arrow).

DIFFERENTIAL DIAGNOSES IMAGES (D-G)

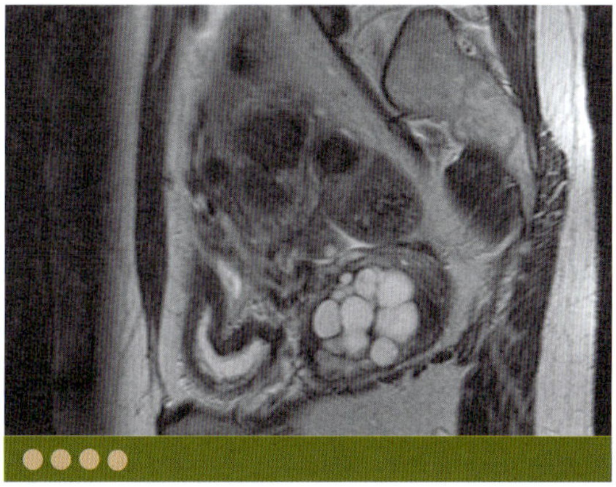

D. Multiple nabothian cysts: Sagittal T2-WI shows multiple well defined, relatively large cysts within the cervix, corresponding to deep nabothian cysts.

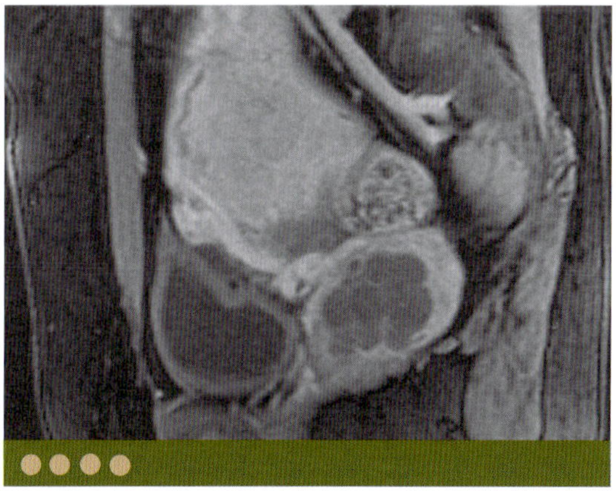

E. Multiple nabothian cysts: Corresponding sagittal contrast-enhanced T1-WI shows that the nabothian cysts do not enhance. Furthermore, there are no associated enhancing or solid components.

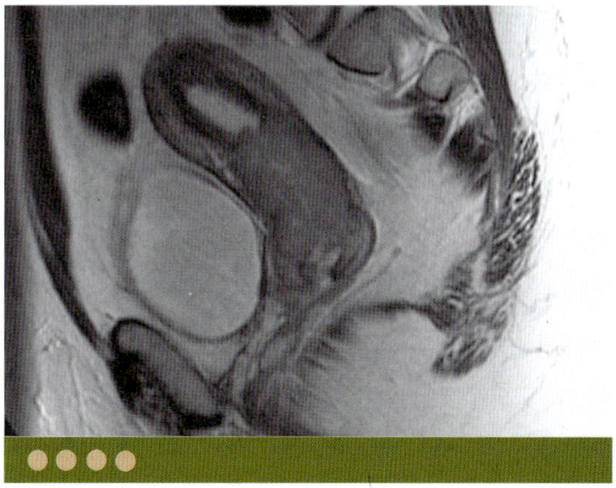

F. Cervical cancer: Sagittal T2-WI shows a large solid mass involving the cervix and lower uterus. There are no associated cystic components.

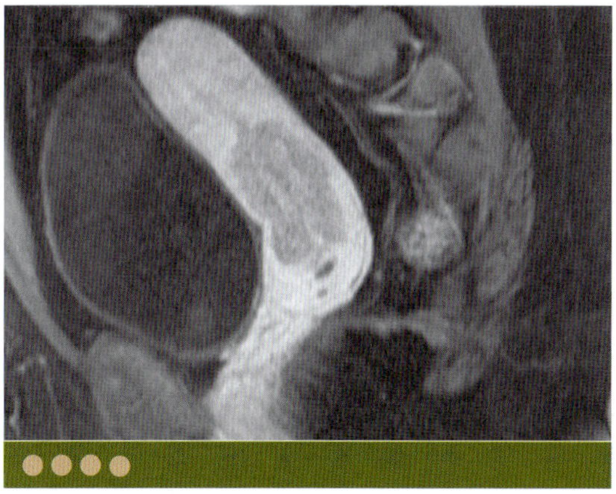

G. Cervical cancer: Corresponding sagittal T1-WI shows that the mass enhances to a lesser degree than the surrounding normal uterine and cervical tissue. There are no associated nonenhancing cystic components.

IMAGE KEY

Common

Rare

Typical

Unusual

16–24 Cervical Leiomyoma (Fibroid)

Paul Nikolaidis

PRESENTATION

Menorrhagia, dystocia, may be asymptomatic.

FINDINGS

A well-circumscribed T2-hypointense lesion is seen arising from the anterior aspect of the cervix.

DIFFERENTIAL DIAGNOSES

- *Cervical carcinoma*: Cervical cancer is more ill-defined, T2-hyperintense and will enhance less than adjacent normal cervix and uterus. There may be some overlap in imaging features with degenerated leiomyomas.
- *Uterine body leiomyoma*: In some cases, the exact origin of the leiomyoma is difficult to discern.

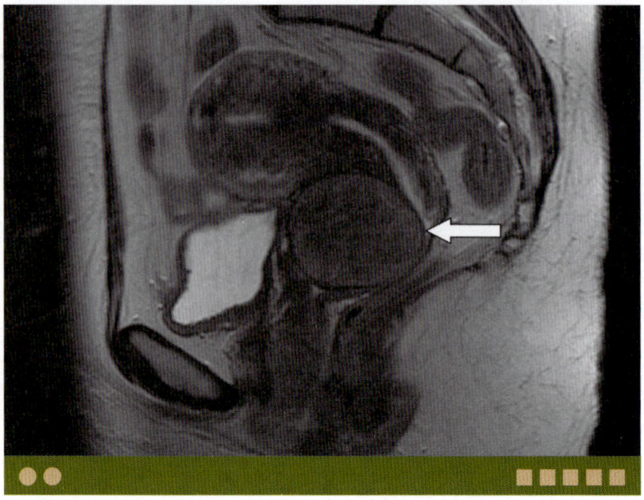

A. Sagittal T2-WI shows a large well-circumscribed hypointense mass arising from the anterior aspect of the cervix (arrow).

COMMENTS

The wide majority of uterine leiomyomas occur in the uterine body. The incidence of cervical leiomyomas is very low. They may be incidentally discovered on imaging. When symptomatic, cervical leiomyomas may present with hypermenorrhea, dysmenorrhea, or a pelvic mass. When submucosal, they may occasionally form polypoid tumors and protrude into the cervical canal or even the vagina. As they are located along the birth canal, they may cause maternal dystocia. They may occur along with other leiomyomas of the uterine body or in isolation.

Imaging findings are similar to uterine body leiomyomas. On sonography, they are typically well-defined, slightly heterogeneous hypoechoic lesions that will not be discovered unless the cervix is carefully scanned.

MR is highly accurate in determining the exact location of a cervical leiomyoma. Nondegenerated leiomyomas are well circumscribed masses of low-signal intensity. They enhance homogeneously. Hyaline degeneration is hypointense on T2-WI and is associated with lack of enhancement. Leiomyomas with cystic degeneration will be markedly hyperintense on T2-WI. The presence of high signal on T1-WI or T2-WI suggests degeneration, often hemorrhagic. This may occur in pregnancy.

Differentiation from cervical cancer is essential to avoid unnecessary surgery. If a cervical leiomyoma is symptomatic or complicates a pregnancy, resection is indicated.

PEARLS

- **Cervical leiomyomas occur infrequently comparing to leiomyomas of the uterine body.**
- **They may be symptomatic in pregnancy, causing dystocia.**
- **They must be differentiated from cervical malignancies.**
- **MR is ideal for precise delineation of cervical leiomyomas.**

ADDITIONAL IMAGES (B-D)

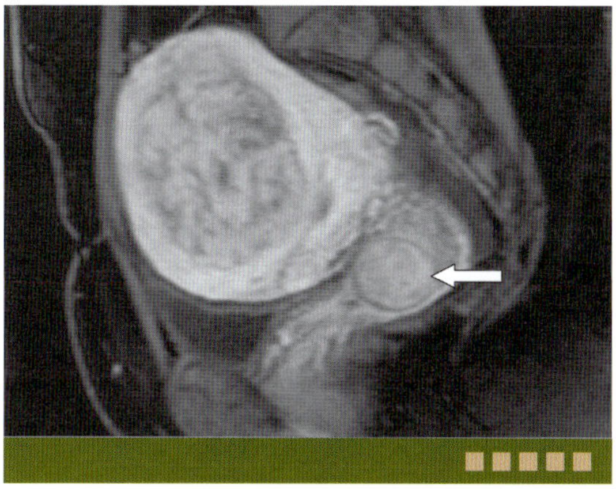

B. Axial contrast-enhanced T1-WI on another patient shows two leiomyomas, one in the uterine body and the other in the cervix (arrow). Note how well-circumscribed the cervical leiomyoma is. Both lesions enhance, but not very avidly.

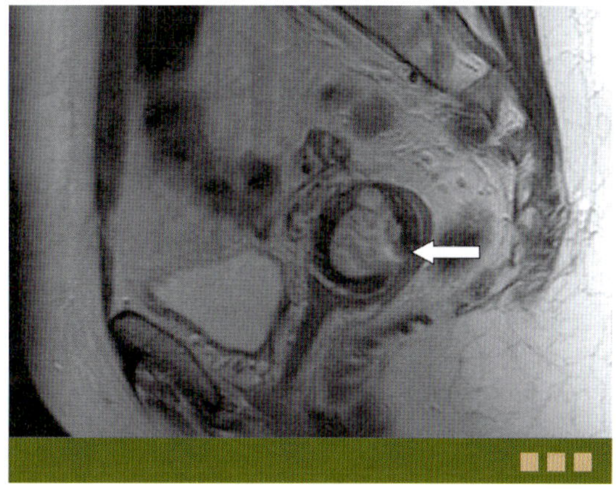

C. Sagittal T2-WI on another patient shows a rounded cervical lesion with a heterogeneous appearance on T2-WI, with large portion showing increased signal (arrow). Biopsy revealed a degenerating leiomyoma.

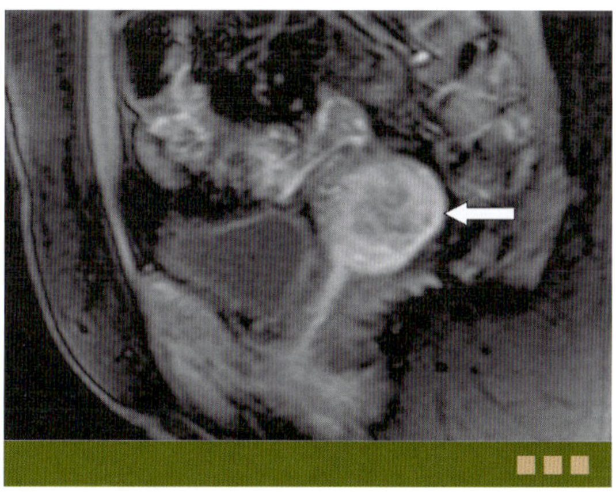

D. Corresponding sagittal contrast-enhanced T1-WI shows heterogeneous enhancement of the cervical leiomyoma.

DIFFERENTIAL DIAGNOSES IMAGES (E-G)

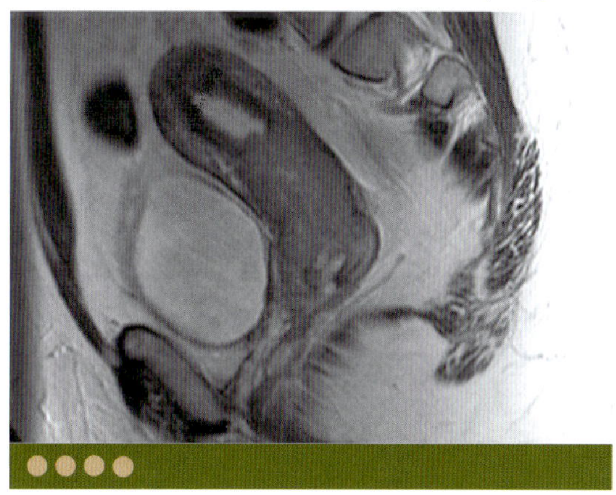

E. Cervical cancer: Sagittal T2-WI shows a mild hyperintense mass involving the cervix and lower uterus. There are some areas of mild heterogeneous signal. The mass is not as discrete as a typical cervical leiomyoma.

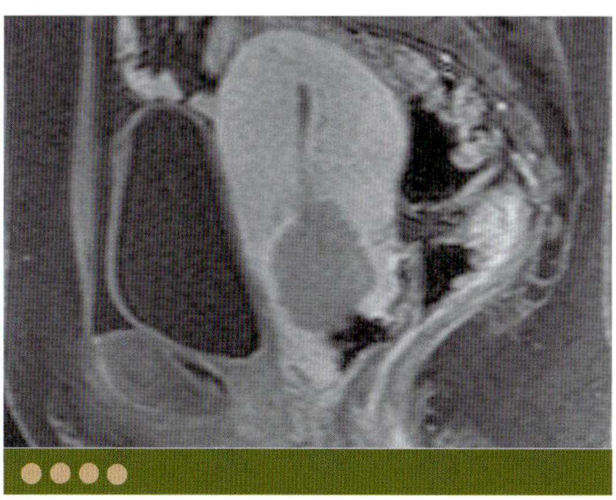

F. Cervical cancer: Sagittal contrast-enhanced T1-WI on another patient shows a mass enhancing to a lesser degree than the surrounding normal uterine and cervical tissue.

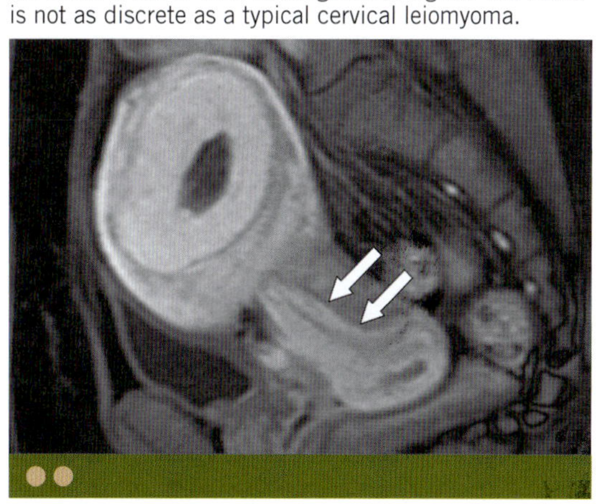

G. Atypical prolapsing uterine body leiomyoma: Sagittal contrast-enhanced T1-WI on another patient shows an enhancing lesion extending through the cervix into the vagina (arrows). This was shown on subsequent hysteroscopy and biopsy to represent an atypical leiomyoma arising from the uterine body and prolapsing through the cervix.

IMAGE KEY

Common

Rare

Typical

Unusual

Part 3

Vagina

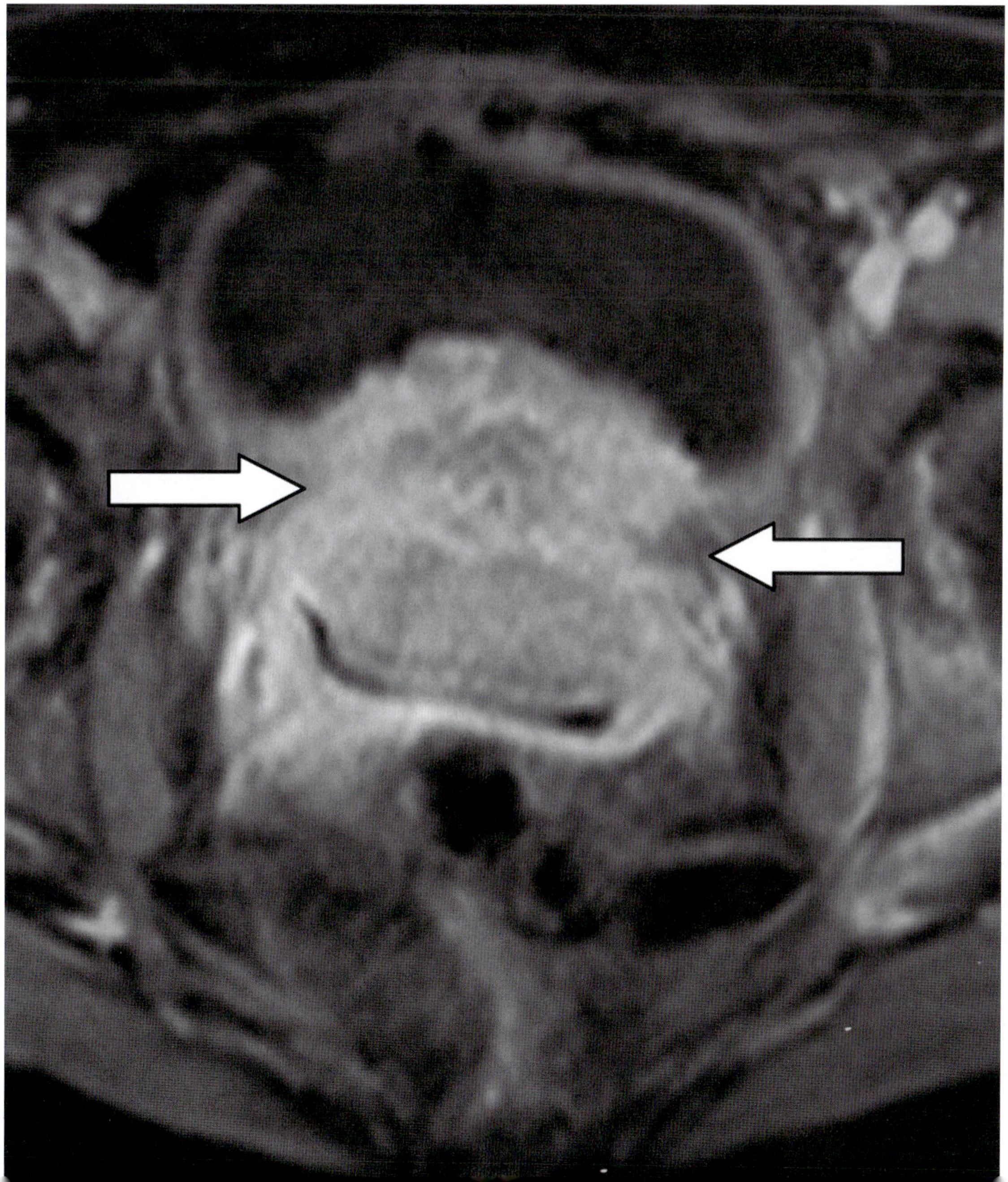

16–25 Primary Vaginal Cancer

Paul Nikolaidis

PRESENTATION

Vaginal bleeding, vaginal discharge.

FINDINGS

MR shows a large enhancing anterior vaginal mass extending into the bladder.

DIFFERENTIAL DIAGNOSES

- *Secondary neoplastic involvement*: Neoplastic involvement of the vagina is most frequently secondary to direct extension from adjacent structures, particularly the cervix, vulva, or rectum. Identification of the epicenter of the mass is, therefore, critical.
- *Vaginal leiomyoma*: Usually in the midline anterior vaginal wall; also typically smaller and better delineated. Classic MR features are homogeneous low signal on T1- and T2-WI (similar to myometrium).
- *Vaginal hemangioma*: Exceedingly rare, arise at infancy and grow slowly. Intermediate signal on T1-WI; on T2-WI may appear as high-signal intensity lobules, show flow voids and may even have fluid–fluid levels.

COMMENTS

Carcinoma of the vagina is one of the less common female genital tract malignancies with an incidence of 1% to 2%. Approximately two-thirds of the patients present with vaginal bleeding. The most common primary vaginal malignancy is squamous cell carcinoma (approximately 90% of cases) that typically occurs in elderly patients. There is an increased incidence with HPV infection. Approximately 5% of primary vaginal malignancies are adenocarcinomas. A rare variant known as clear cell adenocarcinoma occurs in women with diethylstilbestrol (DES) exposure.

The role of CT is limited to the evaluation of nodal and distant metastases. Lymphatic drainage of carcinomas involving the upper two-thirds of the vagina is via the pelvic lymph nodes, whereas tumors affecting the lower third drain via the inguinal nodal chains.

MR is more helpful in assessing the primary tumor and its relationship to adjacent structures, but is also useful in the evaluation of nodal involvement and distant metastases. Both primary and metastatic vaginal neoplasms demonstrate similar imaging characteristics. They are hypo- to isointense on T1-WI and intermediate- to high-signal intensity on T2-WI. Adenocarcinomas may demonstrate even higher signal on T2-WI than squamous cell carcinomas, because of mucin production.

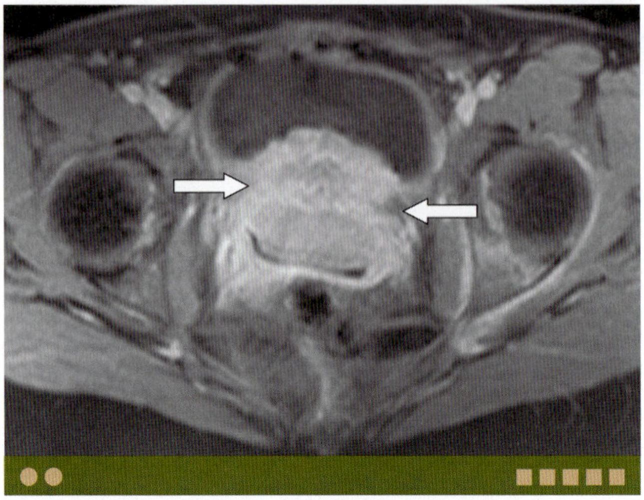

A. Axial contrast-enhanced T1-WI shows a large mass arising from the anterior wall of the vagina (arrows). It extends anteriorly into the bladder.

Staging is critical, affecting survival rates and dictating clinical management. Treatment for earlier stage disease that does not involve the pelvic sidewall (Stages I and II) consists of surgical excision and post-op radiation therapy. Advanced stage disease is usually treated with combination external beam with interstitial brachytherapy and/or chemotherapy.

PEARLS

- **Unusual female genital tract malignancies; 90% are squamous cell carcinoma.**
- **Clear cell adenocarcinoma of the vagina is associated with DES exposure.**
- **Role of CT generally limited to the evaluation of nodal or distant metastases.**
- **MR better delineates the vaginal tumor and can also assess metastatic disease.**

ADDITIONAL IMAGES (B-D)

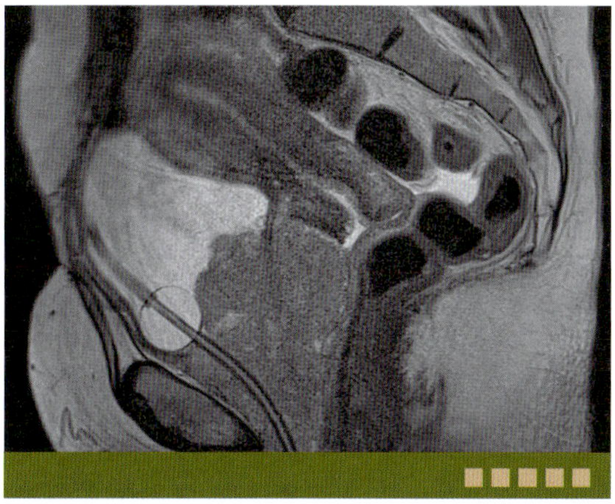

B. Corresponding sagittal T2-WI on the same patient shows a large vaginal mass, which has invaded the bladder and urethra.

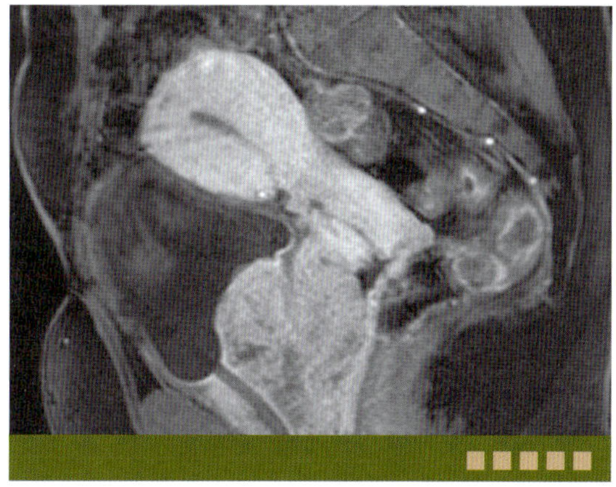

C. Corresponding sagittal contrast-enhanced T1-WI on the same patient shows the heterogeneously enhancing large vaginal mass.

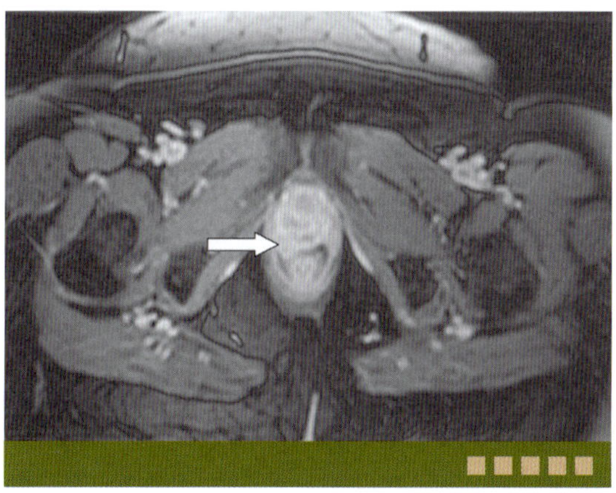

D. Axial contrast-enhanced T1-WI on a different patient shows an enhancing vaginal mass. Note that it extends posteriorly and invades the rectal serosa (arrow).

DIFFERENTIAL DIAGNOSES IMAGES (E-G)

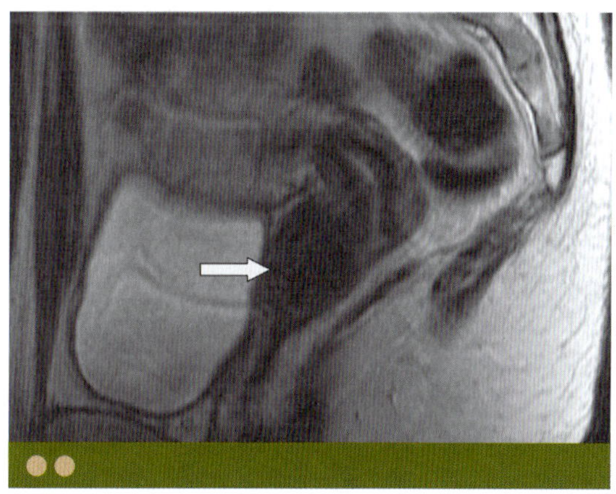

E. Vaginal leiomyoma: Sagittal T2-WI shows a well-circumscribed vaginal mass, which has uniform low-signal on T2 (arrow). Its signal intensity parallels that of a uterine leiomyoma.

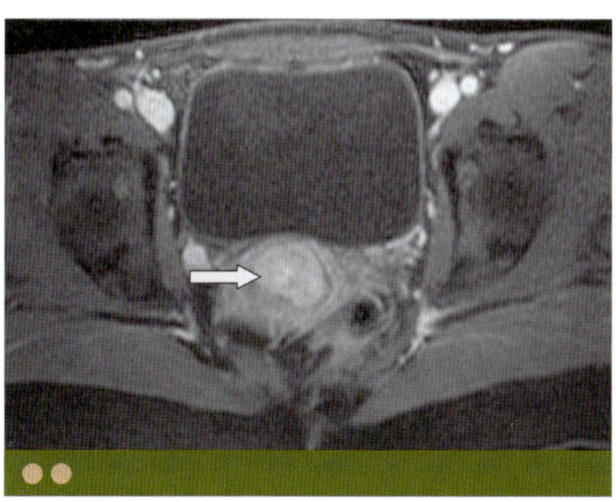

F. Vaginal leiomyoma: Corresponding axial contrast-enhanced T1-WI shows that the mass enhances avidly (arrow). It has well-defined borders.

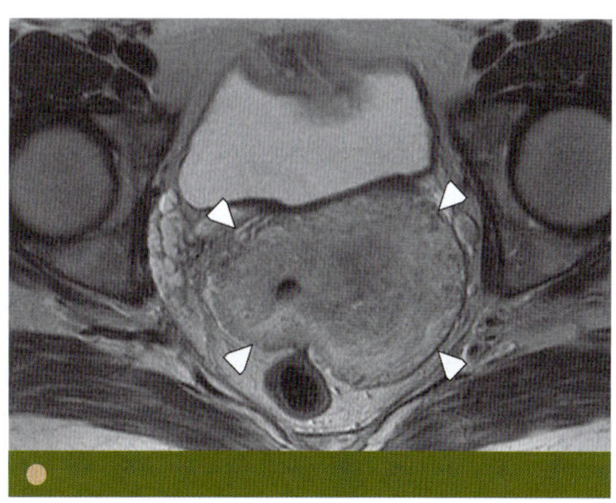

G. Vaginal hemangioma: Axial T2-WI shows a large vaginal mass in a patient who presented with a palpable mass on physical examination (arrowheads). On biopsy, this was shown to represent a large hemangioma—a rare lesion.

IMAGE KEY

Common
●●●●●
●●●●
●●●
●●
●
Rare

Typical
■■■■■
■■■■
■■■
■■
■
Unusual

16–26 Vaginal Hemangioma

Paul Nikolaidis

PRESENTATION

Vaginal mass.

FINDINGS

MR shows a large infiltrative vaginal mass.

DIFFERENTIAL DIAGNOSES

- *Vaginal cancer*: Neoplastic involvement of the vagina is most frequently secondary to adjacent malignancies. Vaginal cancer is typically hypo- to isointense on T1-WI and iso- to hyperintense on T2-WI; large areas of necrosis may be present.
- *Vaginal leiomyoma*: Typically round, well-delineated lesions. Classic MR features are homogeneously low signal on T1- and T2-WI (similar to the myometrium).

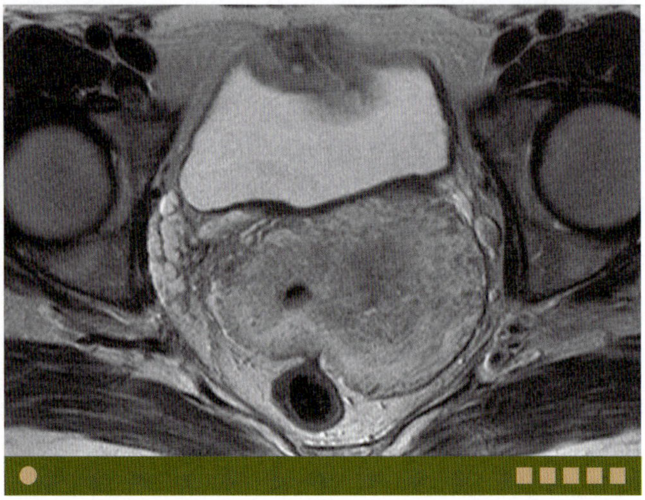

A. Axial T2-WI shows a large circumferential vaginal mass, which has also extended into the lower part of the cervix. The mass is predominantly hyperintense. Note small rounded internal areas of T2 hypointensity representing flow voids.

COMMENTS

Cavernous hemangiomas are common encapsulated lesions composed of cavernous vascular channels separated by connective tissue. These tumors are more often found in the liver, but may also occur in other parts of the body. In the pelvis, in addition to the vulva and vagina, they may occur with greater frequency in the uterine corpus, cervix, and/or in the fetus. They are usually asymptomatic and may be incidental findings discovered on imaging. Hemangiomas of the vagina are exceedingly rare lesions.

They microscopically and macroscopically resemble hemangiomas of the skin. Histologically, a cavernous hemangioma is encapsulated and composed of cavernous vascular channels separated by connective tissue. Hemangiomas can be present at birth or grow later in life.

Ultrasound findings are nonspecific. No significant increased vascularity is seen on color Doppler imaging despite the vascular nature of the lesion.

CT may delineate the areas of involvement, but not as well as MR. Vascular calcifications may be seen on CT. MR is generally preferable as it shows greater anatomic detail in the pelvis. The extent of the lesion is typically better defined, therefore, assisting in surgical planning. A vaginal hemangioma may show intermediate signal on T1-WI. On T2-WI, it will typically appear hyperintense. Discrete high-signal intensity lobules may be seen. On T2-WI, flow voids may be seen in the lesion. Larger lesions may even show fluid–fluid levels.

Typically, vaginal hemangiomas are small and cause few, if any symptoms. In such cases, they are generally followed clinically. If larger, or symptomatic, surgical excision may be considered. There are several reports of hemangiomas becoming apparent or symptomatic during gestation. This is thought to result from increased pelvic blood flow and increased estrogen levels during pregnancy.

PEARLS

- **Unusual female genital tract lesions that will more frequently occur in the uterine body and cervix.**
- **On histopathology, they resemble hemangiomas of the skin.**
- **On T2-WI, they are hyperintense, may contain flow voids and show fluid-fluid levels.**
- **May show delayed enhancement following gadolinium.**

ADDITIONAL IMAGES (B-C)

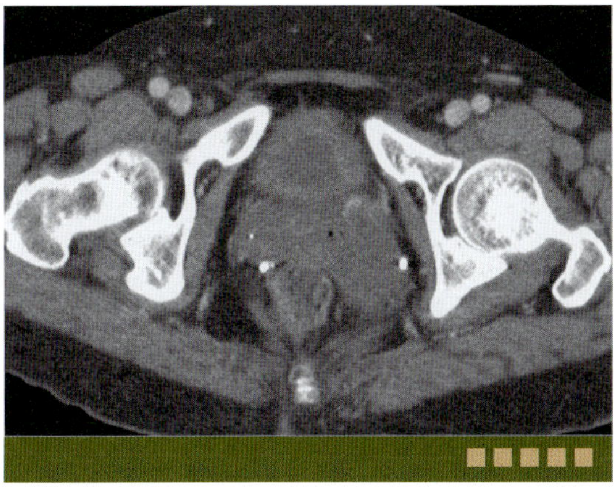

B. Corresponding axial CECT on the same patient shows the faintly enhancing circumferential vaginal mass. Few phleboliths are seen in its periphery.

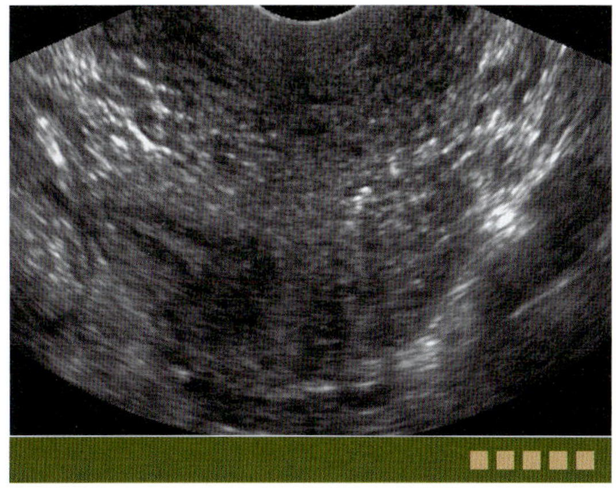

C. Transverse pelvic ultrasound on the same patient shows nonspecific heterogeneous tissue. There was no appreciable increased vascularity on color Doppler.

DIFFERENTIAL DIAGNOSES IMAGES (D-F)

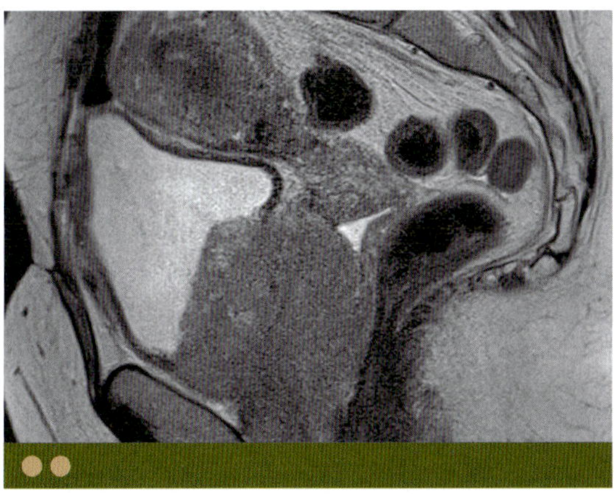

D. Vaginal cancer: Sagittal T2-WI shows a large predominantly isointense mass arising from the anterior wall of the vagina. It invades the bladder.

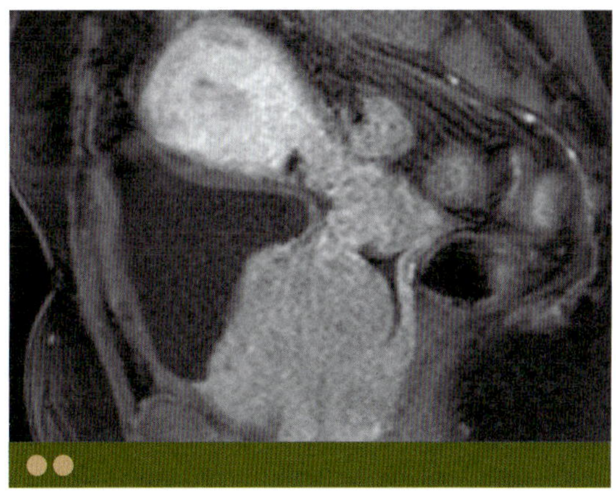

E. Vaginal cancer: Corresponding sagittal contrast-enhanced T1-WI obtained 60 seconds after gadolinium administration shows the large heterogeneously enhancing vaginal mass. It enhances less than the myometrium.

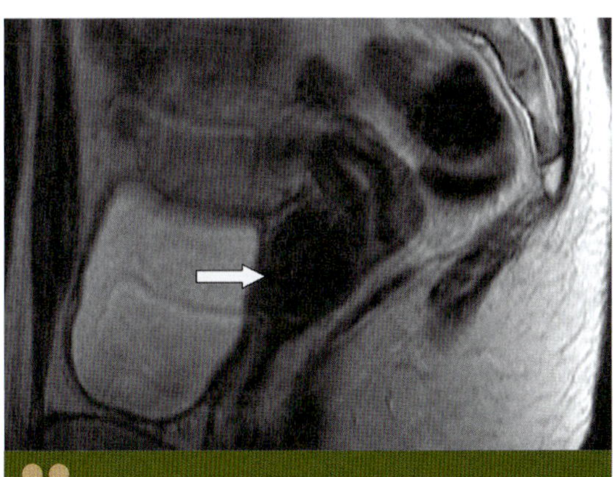

F. Vaginal leiomyoma: Sagittal T2-WI shows a well-circumscribed hypointense anterior vaginal mass (arrow). Its uniformly low-signal intensity parallels that of a classic uterine leiomyoma (fibroid).

IMAGE KEY

Common

Rare

Typical

Unusual

16–27 Vulvar Carcinoma

Paul Nikolaidis

PRESENTATION

Palpable or visible vulvar mass.

FINDINGS

MR shows a vulvar soft tissue mass without distal adenopathy.

DIFFERENTIAL DIAGNOSES

- *Vaginal or rectal cancer with spread to perineum*: Usually centered in the vagina or rectum; signal intensity and enhancement patterns may be similar.
- *Vulvar inflammation/abscess*: Inflammation and abscess formation may occur in patients that are immune compromised, have Crohn disease, or following radiation. Clinical history and examination are important. These should also be differentiated from Bartholin duct cysts and gland abscesses, Hidradenoma papilliferum, and epidermal inclusion cysts of the labia majora.
- *Postradiation changes*: High T2 signal and enhancement may be seen in the first 6 months after therapy, as a result of mucosal and intramuscular edema. Subsequently, fibrotic changes occur, with decreased T2 signal.
- *Vulvar angiomyxoma*: May be impossible to distinguish; usually higher T2 signal and a whorled pattern because of the high myxomatous content.

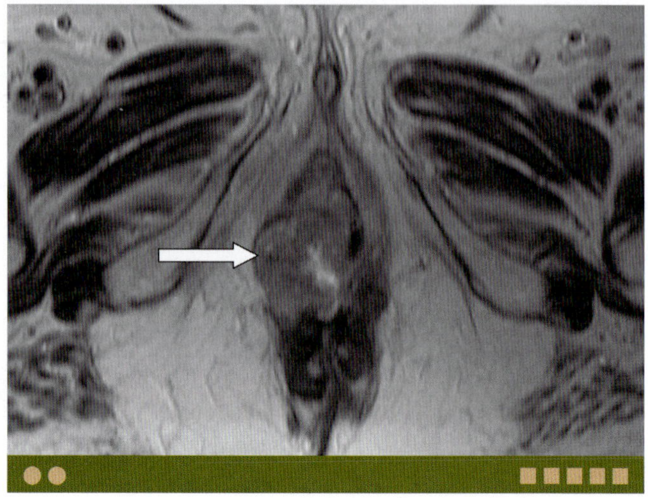

A. Axial T2-WI shows a lobulated soft-tissue mass in the vulva with low- to intermediate-signal intensity (arrow).

COMMENTS

The vulva is comprised of the mons pubis, the labia majora and minora, the clitoris, the vestibular bulb, vestibular glands and the vestibule of the vagina. Carcinoma of the vulva is a rare gynecologic cancer, with an incidence of less than 1/8 that of cervical cancer. Two-thirds of cases occur in elderly patients over 70. The most common subtype is squamous cell carcinoma (85%). One variant of squamous carcinoma is verrucous carcinoma which is well-differentiated, slow growing and does not metastasize. Other histological types include Bartholin gland cancer, sarcoma, basal cell carcinoma, and adenocarcinoma. Human papilloma virus (HPV)-positive tumors may occur in younger patients and may be multifocal.

Vulval cancer most commonly involves the labia, and may extend to the vagina, urethra, and rectum. It rarely extends beyond the pelvis. Metastatic spread initially occurs along the lymphatics, involving the inguinal, pelvic, iliac, and periaortic lymph nodes. Because carcinoma of the vulva is an external, clinically visible lesion, the main focus of imaging is to provide information regarding disease spread and particularly nodal involvement. The neoplasm may then be accurately staged for prognostic and treatment purposes. The most important prognostic factors are size of the primary tumor, depth of invasion and involvement of regional lymph nodes. Patients with negative groin nodes have a 90% survival rate compared to 50% when there are positive nodes.

CT may be limited in determining early nodal involvement in the pelvis and groin, as involved nodes may not meet the size criteria for pathologic enlargement. MR also allows for identification of lymphadenopathy, but conventional MR also relies on size criteria to detect nodal involvement. MR lymphangiography has shown promise in detecting nodal metastases and ultrasmall supraparamagnetic iron oxide (USPIO) has been successfully utilized. After infusion, macrophages in normal nodes will uptake the USPIO, reducing the signal intensity of normal nodes on T2* sequences because of the effects of iron oxide. Metastatic nodes will not take up USPIO and will continue to enhance, because malignant cells will replace the macrophages.

PEARLS

- **A rare gynecologic malignancy that usually presents as a visible or palpable mass.**
- **Most common histologic subtype is squamous cell carcinoma.**
- **Main role of imaging is to provide information regarding nodal involvement.**
- **MR lymphangiography utilizing USPIO may be useful in the earlier detection of nodal involvement.**

ADDITIONAL IMAGES (B-D)

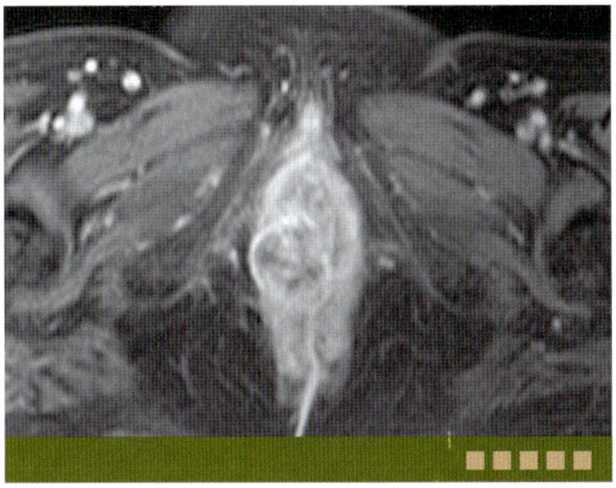

B. Corresponding axial contrast-enhanced T1-WI shows a heterogeneously enhancing mass with a central area of decreased enhancement and necrosis.

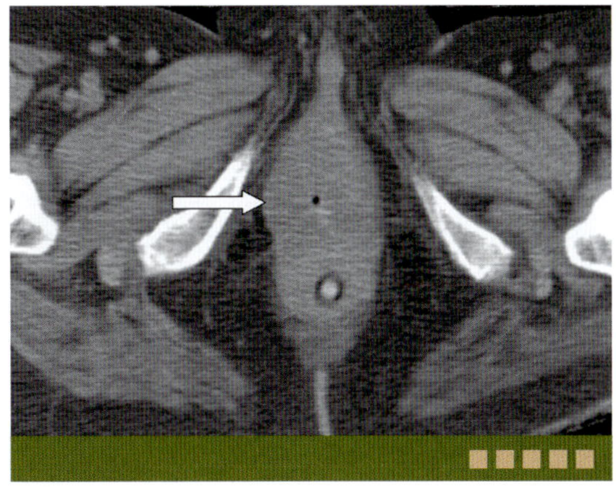

C. Corresponding axial CECT shows how the vulvar mass is more difficult to exactly delineate on CT than on MR (arrow).

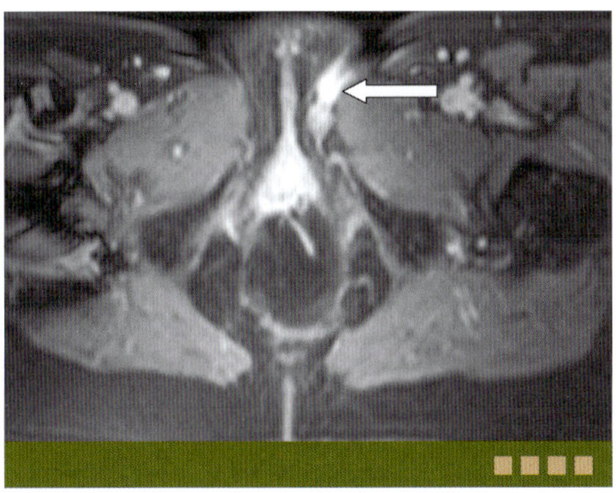

D. Axial contrast-enhanced T1-WI on another patient with vulvar carcinoma shows abnormal enhancing nodular tissue extending to the left groin (arrow).

DIFFERENTIAL DIAGNOSES IMAGES (E-G)

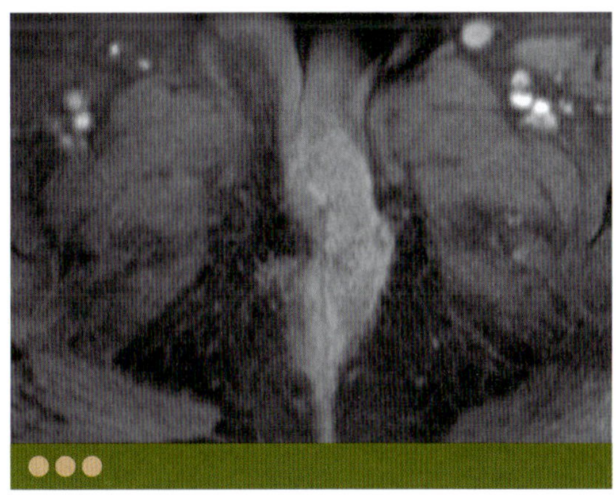

E. Rectal cancer with vulvar invasion: Axial contrast-enhanced T1-WI in a patient with rectal cancer shows a large soft tissue mass in the region of the vulva.

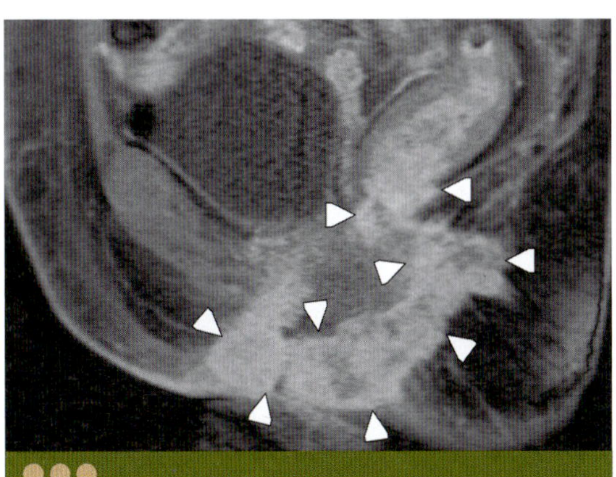

F. Rectal cancer with vulvar invasion: Corresponding sagittal contrast-enhanced T1-WI shows contiguous abnormal enhancing soft tissue extending from the rectum to the vulva and perineum (arrowheads).

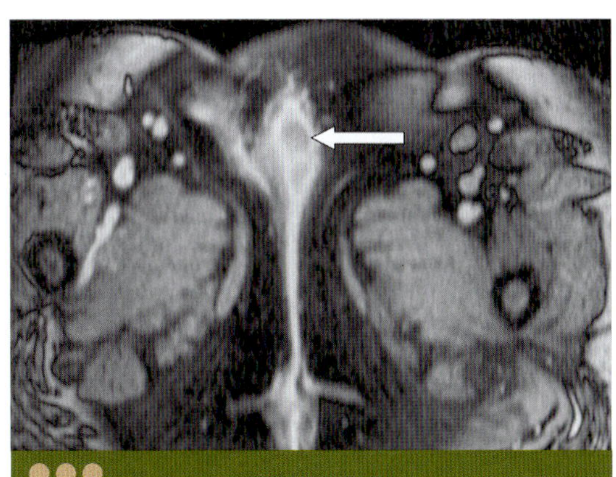

G. Vulvar inflammation and abscesses: Axial contrast-enhanced T1-WI in a patient with Crohn disease shows increased enhancement and small abscesses in the region of the vulva (arrow). In addition to abscesses, draining sinuses and vulvar or perineal ulcerations may occur in patients with Crohn disease.

IMAGE KEY

Common

Rare

Typical

Unusual

16–28 Gartner Duct Cyst

Nancy A. Hammond

PRESENTATION

Incidental finding on imaging.

FINDINGS

Cystic mass at the anterolateral aspect of the proximal vagina.

DIFFERENTIAL DIAGNOSES

- *Bartholin cyst*: Located in the posterolateral aspect of the distal vagina.
- *Urethral diverticulum*: Communicates with the urethra.

COMMENTS

Gartner duct cysts arise from the remnants of the embryologic mesonephric ducts. While cysts may form anywhere along the course of the mesonephric duct in the broad ligament and along the lateral wall of the uterus and vagina, they most characteristically are located in the anterolateral aspect of the proximal vagina. They may be single or multiple and can be associated with other anomalies of the genitourinary system.

Gartner duct cysts are typically small and asymptomatic but can become large and cause vaginal or urethral obstruction. Children with Gartner duct cysts can be symptomatic secondary to communication with an ectopic ureter of the cervix.

Sonographically, this entity appears as a well-circumscribed, thin-walled cystic mass in the anterolateral wall of the vagina. CT demonstrates a nonenhancing hypodense mass in the characteristic location. On MR, T1 signal depends on the presence of any intracystic protein or hemorrhage. A simple Gartner duct cyst is hypointense on T1-weighted sequences. If protein or hemorrhage is present, the cyst will be T1 hyperintense. T2-weighted sequences demonstrate a hyperintense mass. Unless complicated by infection, no enhancement is typically present. If infected, peripheral enhancement is present.

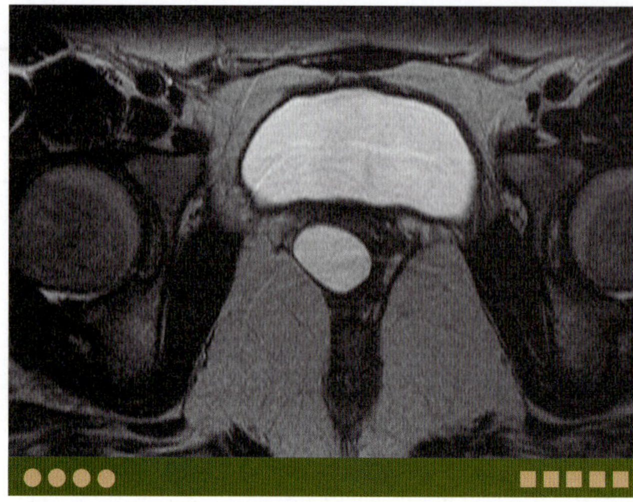

A. Axial T2-WI shows a hyperintense cystic mass in the anterolateral aspect of the proximal vagina in a typical location for a Gartner duct cyst.

PEARLS

- **Usually asymptomatic, incidental finding.**
- **Can be associated with other genitourinary anomalies.**
- **Occurs characteristically in the anterolateral wall of the proximal vagina.**
- **MR appearance depends on internal complexity.**

ADDITIONAL IMAGES (B-C)

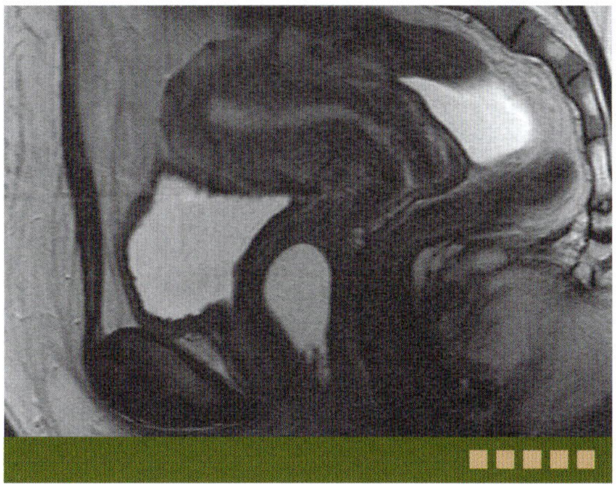

B. Sagittal T2-WI further shows the cystic vaginal mass.

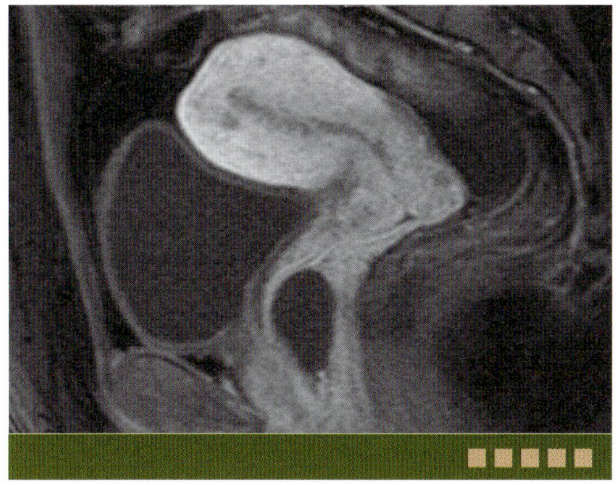

C. Sagittal contrast-enhanced T1-WI shows nonenhancement of the cystic lesion. No peripheral enhancement is present to suggest infection.

DIFFERENTIAL DIAGNOSES IMAGES (D-F)

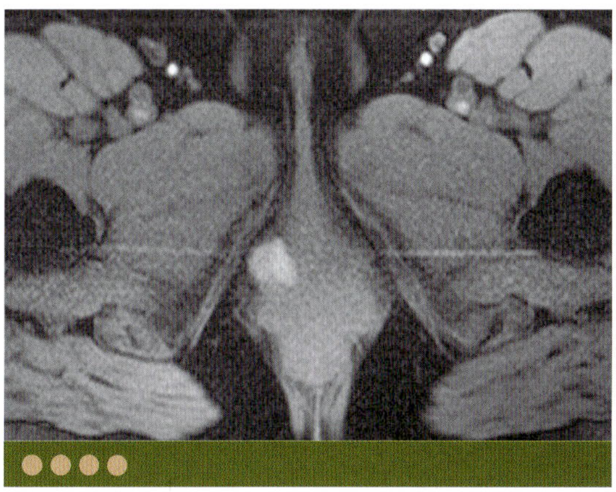

D. Bartholin cyst: Axial nonenhanced T1-WI in a different patient shows a hyperintense mass in the posterolateral aspect of the distal vagina. The lesion was hyperintense on T2-WI. The T1 hyperintensity was because of proteinaceous or hemorrhagic contents.

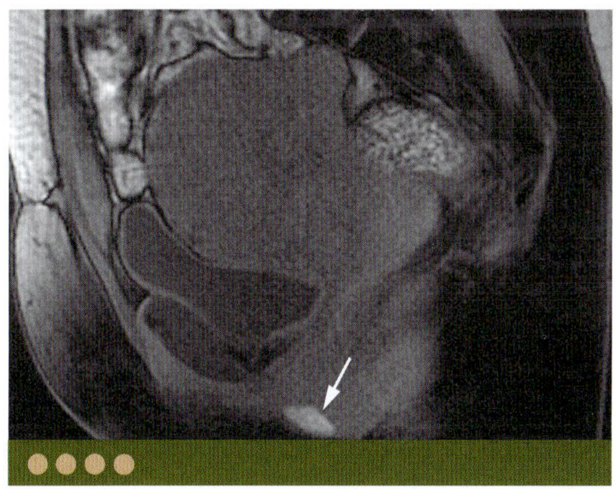

E. Bartholin cyst: Sagittal nonenhanced T1-WI in the same patient as that in Figure D shows the more inferior location of a Bartholin cyst compared to Gartner duct cyst (arrow).

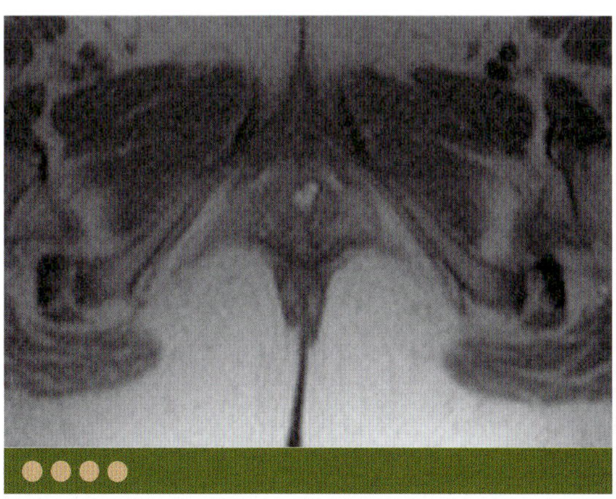

F. Urethral diverticulum: Axial T2-WI shows a small, midline hyperintense structure just anterior to the expected location of the urethra.

IMAGE KEY

Common

Rare

Typical

Unusual

16–29 Bartholin Cyst

Nancy A. Hammond

PRESENTATION

Incidental finding on imaging.

FINDINGS

Cystic mass in the posterolateral aspect of the distal vagina.

DIFFERENTIAL DIAGNOSES

- *Gartner duct cyst*: Located in the anterolateral aspect of the proximal vagina.
- *Malignant tumors of Bartholin gland*: The presence of solid enhancing component should raise possibility of malignant tumor.
- *Urethral diverticulum*: More centrally located, may see communication with urethra.

COMMENTS

Bartholin glands or the greater vestibular glands are located in the superficial fascia of the urogenital diaphragm on either side of the opening of the vagina. Each gland drains into the vestibule through a duct secreting lubricating mucus. When these ducts become obstructed, a painless swelling forms and results in a Bartholin cyst. Bartholin cysts can become large, measuring up to 5 to 6 cm, and result in the obstruction of the rectum. Bartholin cysts can usually be visualized and palpated on physical examination. Clinically, they are typically asymptomatic but can become infected.

Ultrasound demonstrates a well-defined cystic mass at the posterolateral aspect of the distal vagina. When uncomplicated, CT demonstrates a hypodense mass in a characteristic location. If infected, peripheral enhancement may be present. On MR, the T1 appearance depends on the presence of intracystic protein or hemorrhage which will appear as hyperintense. Simple cysts demonstrate T1 hypointensity. Like CT, peripheral enhancement is seen with infection. However, a solid enhancing component should not be present and should raise suspicion for a malignant tumor of Bartholin glands such as squamous cell tumor or adenoid cystic carcinoma. T2-weighted sequences demonstrate a well-circumscribed hyperintense lesion.

Treatment of Bartholin cyst depends on the size of the cyst, how painful it is, and whether it is infected. When large and symptomatic, surgical drainage may be necessary.

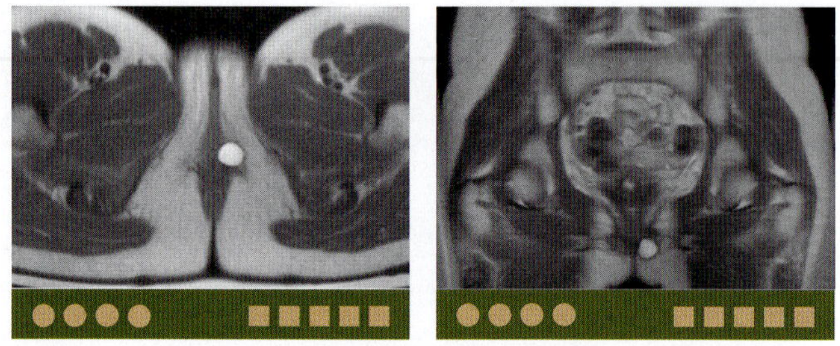

A. Axial T2-WI shows a hyperintense mass at the posterolateral aspect of the distal vagina compatible with a Bartholin cyst. **B.** Coronal T2-WI in the same patient shows the distal vaginal location of this lesion characteristic of a Bartholin cyst.

PEARLS

- **Bartholin cysts result from obstuction of the duct draining the gland to the vaginal vestibule.**
- **Typically asymptomatic but can become infected or obstructive.**
- **Located at the posterolateral aspect of the distal vagina.**

ADDITIONAL IMAGES (C-E)

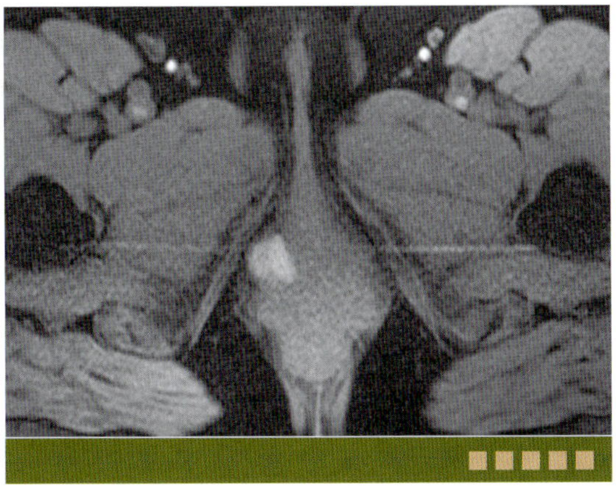

C. Axial T1-WI in a different patient shows a hyperintense lesion in the typical location for a Bartholin cyst. The lesion was hyperintense on T2-WI sequences. The T1 hyperintensity is consistent with either hemorrhagic or proteinaceous fluid.

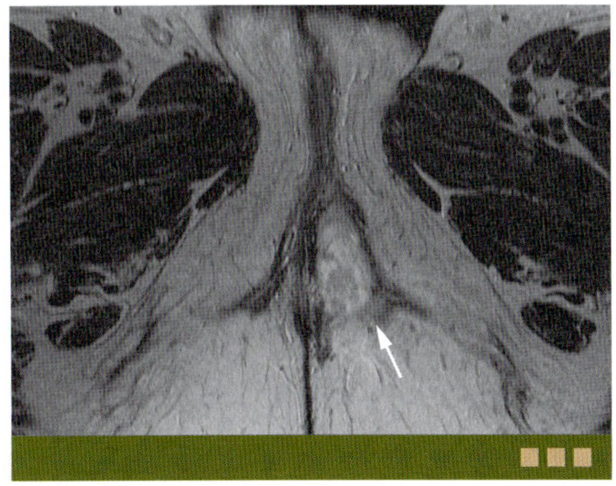

D. Axial T2-WI in a different patient shows a hyperintense lesion compatible with a Bartholin cyst. The ill-defined posterior margin and irregularity in the adjacent fat is suggestive of rupture of the cyst (arrow).

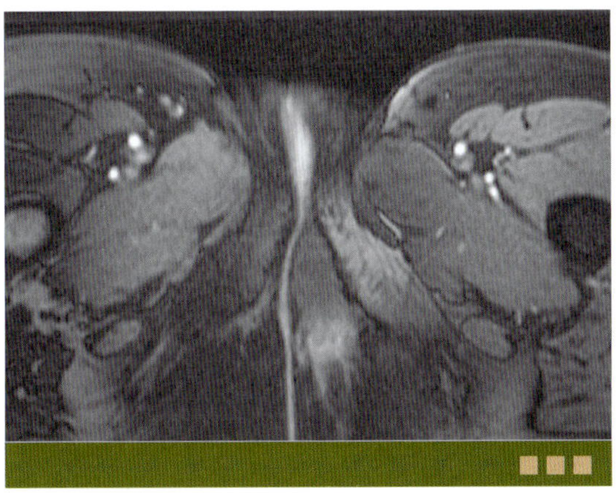

E. Axial contrast-enhanced T1-WI in the same patient as Figure D confirms the presence of rupture of the Bartholin cyst. The region of hyperintensity was present on nonenhanced images and consistent with areas of hemorrhage or proteinaceous fluid.

DIFFERENTIAL DIAGNOSES IMAGES (F-G)

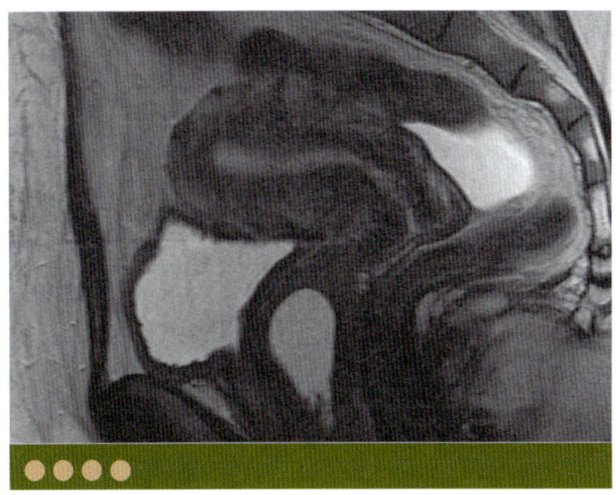

F. Gartner duct cyst: Sagittal T2-WI shows a cystic mass at the anterior aspect of the proximal vagina. Axial images confirmed its lateral location.

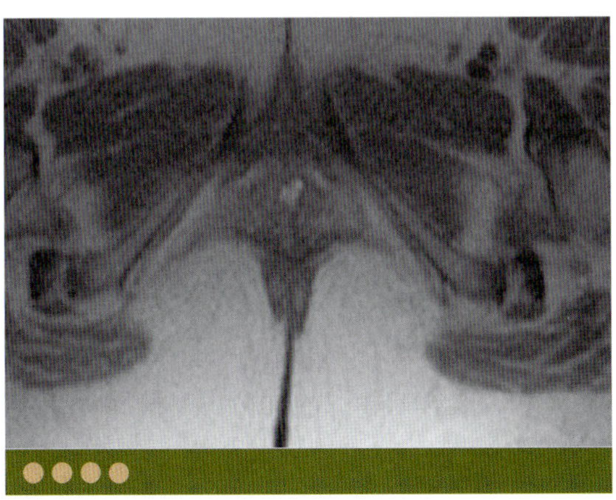

G. Urethral diverticulum: Axial T2-WI shows a centrally located hyperintense lesion just anterior to the expected location of the urethra compatible with a urethral diverticulum.

IMAGE KEY

Common

Rare

Typical

Unusual

Part 4

Ovary

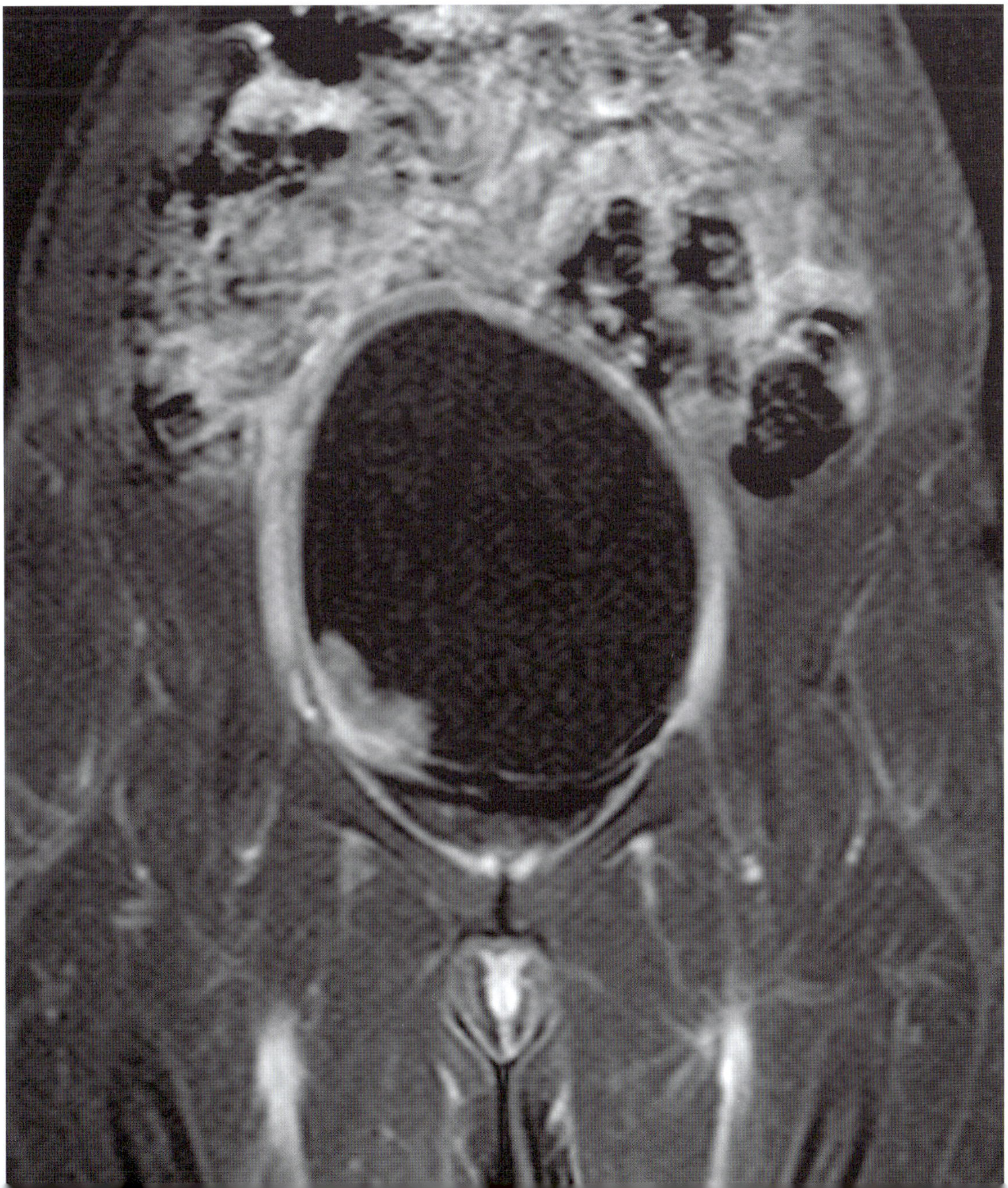

16–30 Ovarian Cancer

Nancy A. Hammond

PRESENTATION

Abdominal mass; bloating.

FINDINGS

Complex ovarian mass.

DIFFERENTIAL DIAGNOSIS

- *Benign ovarian cystic lesion*: Absence of internal solid components can aid in differentiating benign from malignant lesions. However, the distinction between the two can be difficult to make based on imaging.

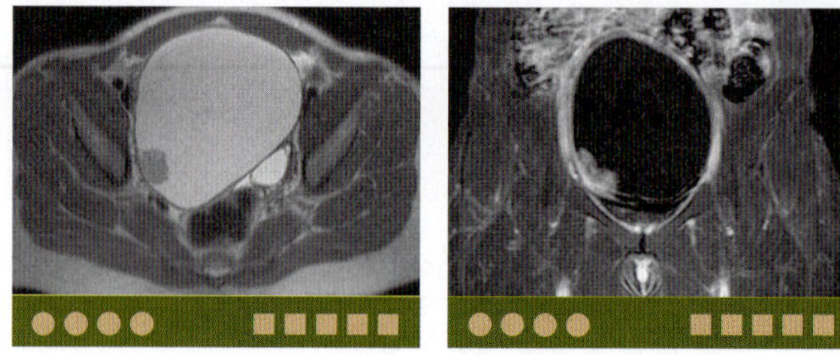

A. Axial T2-WI shows a unilocular cystic pelvic mass arising from the left adnexa with a solid mural nodule raising suspicion for malignant etiologies. This was pathologically proven to represent a serous cystadenocarcinoma.
B. Coronal contrast-enhanced T1-WI subtraction in the same patient confirms enhancement of the solid nodular component.

COMMENTS

Ovarian cancer is the second most common gynecologic malignancy in women in the United States and the most common cause of death of all gynecologic malignancies. Most patients present with stage III or greater disease.

Approximately 85% of all the ovarian cancers arise from the epithelial lining cells of the ovary. Among the malignant subtypes of epithelial neoplasms are serous cystadenocarcinoma (50%), mucinous cystadenocarcinoma (20%), endometrioid carcinoma (20%), and clear cell carcinoma (10%). Unlike the serous and mucinous subtypes which have benign counterparts, the endometrioid and clear cell variants are almost always malignant. The endometrioid type is bilateral 25% of the time. Most are mixed solid and cystic, but they can also be entirely solid. The endometrioid subtype is associated with endometriosis and endometrial hyperplasia. Clear cell lesions are typically unilocular cysts with mural nodules.

Ovarian cancer is more common in older (postmenopausal) women. Risk factors include nulliparity, infertility, late menopause, and family history. Screening for ovarian cancer with either transvaginal sonography or tumor markers has not been shown to decrease morbidity or mortality. The tumor marker CA-125 has been shown to be elevated in only 50% of women with stage I disease but can also be elevated in benign conditions including uterine leiomyoma, endometriosis, and pelvic inflammatory disease.

Sonography is the initial imaging modality in evaluating a suspected ovarian mass. Sonographic findings that raise suspicion for a malignant ovarian lesion include large size of lesion (>5cm), presence of solid components, mural nodules, internal papillary projections and/or thickened septations. CT findings of adnexal masses suggesting malignancy include size more than 5 cm, solid tumor components, thick enhancing septations, peritoneal implants, and ascites. Despite CT's low sensitivity for detection of small peritoneal implants, it is a good predictor of resectability, valuable in assessing residual or recurrent disease, and remains the imaging modality of choice in assessing for peritoneal spread. Omental caking, nodular peritoneal implants, scalloping of the liver surface and ascites are common findings.

MR can be helpful in evaluating adnexal masses found to be indeterminate by sonography. The MR characteristics of a malignant adenxal mass include large size of lesion (>5 cm) and the presence of solid components. MR is also valuable in evaluating for advanced disease.

Treatment of ovarian cancer includes total abdominal hysterectomy, bilateral oophorectomy, omentectomy, pelvic and para-aortic lymphadenectomy, peritoneal biopsy and removal of any implants, and chemotherapy. Some patients with advanced disease receive pre-operative chemotherapy when pre-operative imaging or direct inspection suggests that tumor debulking surgery would not be successful.

PEARLS

- **Ovarian cancer is the second most common gynecologic malignancy in women in the United States.**
- **The majority of cases arise from the epithelial lining with serous cystadenocarcinoma, the most common subtype.**
- **Sonography is considered the first line modality in evaluating the internal characteristics of an ovarian cyst with MR helpful for indeterminate lesions.**
- **Ovarian cancer is staged surgically but cross-sectional imaging can aid in determining resectability and in evaluating tumor recurrence.**

ADDITIONAL IMAGES (C-H)

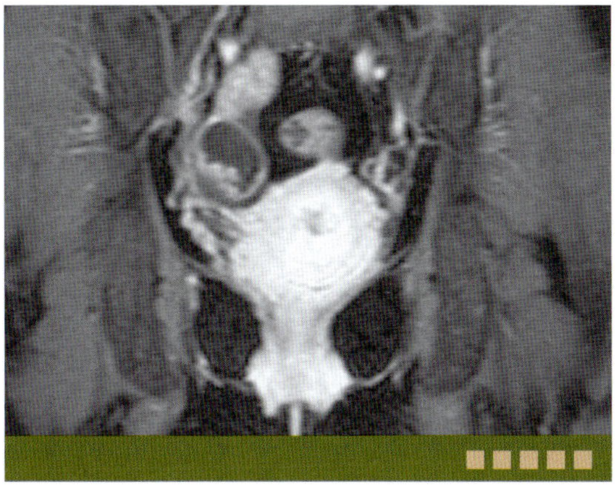

C. Coronal contrast-enhanced T1-WI shows an enhancing solid component to aright adenxal cystic mass. This lesion was found to represent a serous cystadenocarcinoma on surgical pathology.

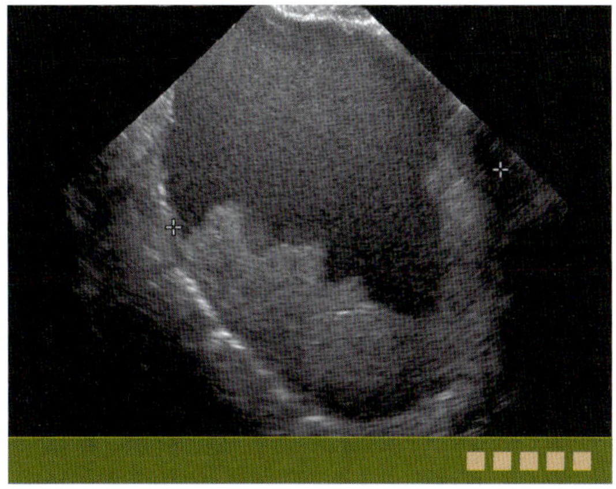

D. Transverse sonogram of the right ovary shows a complex cystic mass with internal echoes and a solid mural component. This was pathologically proven to represent a mucinous cystadenocarcinoma.

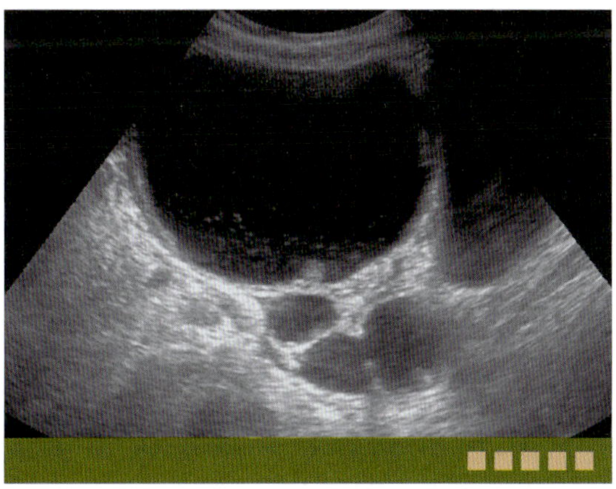

E. Longitudinal sonogram in a different patient shows a complex cystic mass arising from the left ovary with mural nodularity. This lesion was pathologically proven to represent a clear cell type of ovarian cancer.

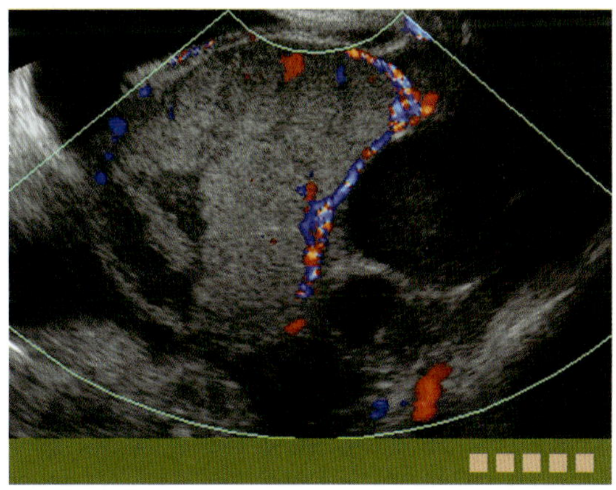

F. Transverse sonogram in a different patient shows a large solid and cystic mass arising from the right ovary. Doppler interrogation confirms blood flow in the solid component. Note the internal echoes within the cystic component. This lesion was pathologically proven to represent the endometrioid type of ovarian cancer.

IMAGE KEY

Common

Rare

Typical

Unusual

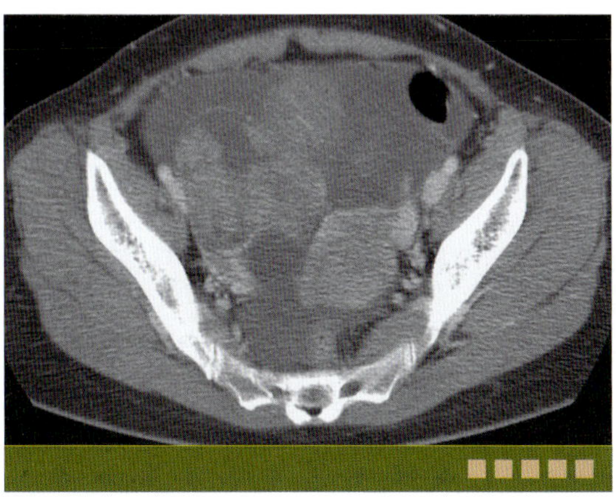

G. Axial CECT in the same patient as Figure F shows the CT appearance of the complex right ovarian mass with both solid and cystic components. A large amount of ascites is present in the pelvis as well.

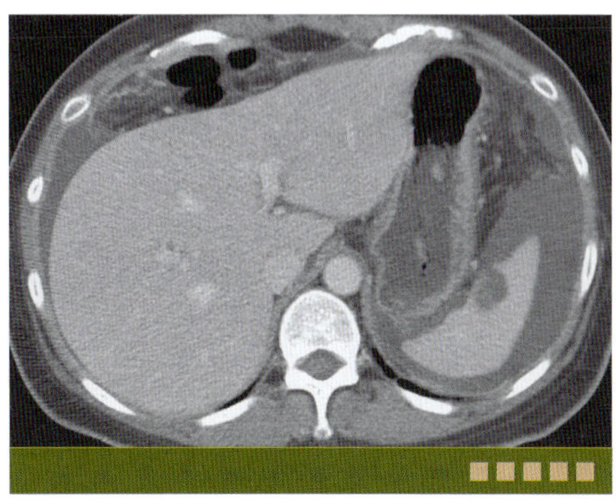

H. Axial CECT in the same patient as Figure G shows malignant ascites in the upper abdomen with thickening and nodularity to the peritoneal surface. Lesion is seen scalloping the splenic surface typical of ovarian metastases.

16–31 Ovarian Cystadenoma

Nancy A. Hammond

PRESENTATION

Abdominal mass.

FINDINGS

Cystic ovarian mass.

DIFFERENTIAL DIAGNOSES

- *Ovarian cystadenocarcinoma*: Presence of solid component, thick wall, mural nodules or papillary projections should raise suspicion for malignancy. Lesions less than 4 cm have a higher likelihood of malignancy
- *Functional ovarian cyst*: Simple appearing cyst with thin wall, can be large, may be difficult to distinguish from cystic ovarian neoplasm warranting follow-up study when suspected.
- *Paraovarian cyst*: Separate from ovary, can be large, thin-walled, and unilocular.
- *Peritoneal inclusion cyst*: History of prior surgical procedures, multiloculated cyst associated with the ovary, insinuates among peritoneal structures.
- *Tuboovarian abscess*: Complex cystic mass in a patient with pelvic infection.

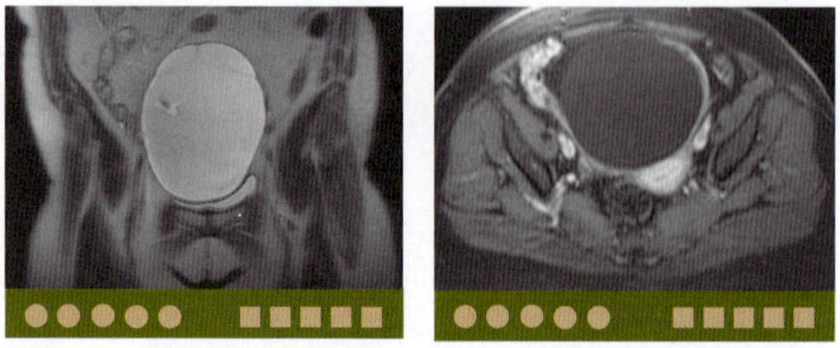

A. Coronal T2-WI shows a large unilocular, cystic mass in the pelvis. No septations or solid components are visualized on this image. **B.** Axial contrast-enhanced T1-WI further shows a simple appearing unilocular mass in the pelvis with a thin wall and without areas of internal enhancement or evidence of solid components.

COMMENTS

Ovarian cystadenomas are the most common benign ovarian neoplasms. These most commonly arise from the epithelial lining and are classified as either serous or mucinous tumors. Serous ovarian tumors account for approximately 25% of all benign ovarian neoplasms. Mucinous ovarian tumors represent approximately 20% of all benign ovarian neoplasms.

Serous cystadenomas are seen in a younger population (20-30 years old) than their malignant counterpart. They typically present as abdominal mass or increasing abdominal girth. Bilateral lesions are identified approximately 15% of the time. Mucinous cystadenomas occur most commonly in the third-to-fifth decade and are bilateral only about 2% to 10% of the time.

On imaging, serous cystadenomas are large cystic lesions with the average size reported to be 5 to 10 cm. They tend to be unilocular but may be multilocular. Serous cystadenomas can be indistinguishable from simple cyst but may also have thin septations and occasionally papillary projections. It is important to note that the presence of papillary projections is suggestive but not 100% specific for malignancy and can be seen in benign lesions. On MR, serous cystadenomas follows fluid signal on all sequences.

Mucinous lesions tend to be larger than their serous counterparts, are multiloculated, usually unilateral and do not have papillary projections. The size of a mucinous tumor does not correlate with malignancy. Sonographically, mucinous cystadenomas have thick and numerous septations. Internal echoes may be present as a result of debris. On MR, the appearance of the contents of the cysts depends on the degree of hydration of the intracellular and extracellular mucin. Hydrated mucin follows the signal of simple fluid on all sequences while viscus mucin has variable T2 signal and increased T1 signal. In the absence of metastatic disease, differentiating between benign, malignant, and borderline mucinous tumors on the basis of imaging can be difficult and is usually determined surgically.

PEARLS

- **Ovarian cystadenomas are the most common benign ovarian neoplasm.**
- **Serous cystadenomas are slightly more common than mucinous and are more likely to be bilateral.**
- **Serous cystadenomas tend to be unilocular, whereas mucinous cystadenomas tend to be multilocular.**
- **Large size, presence of thick, irregular wall, solid component, mural nodule, or papillary projections should raise suspicion for malignancy.**

ADDITIONAL IMAGES (C-E)

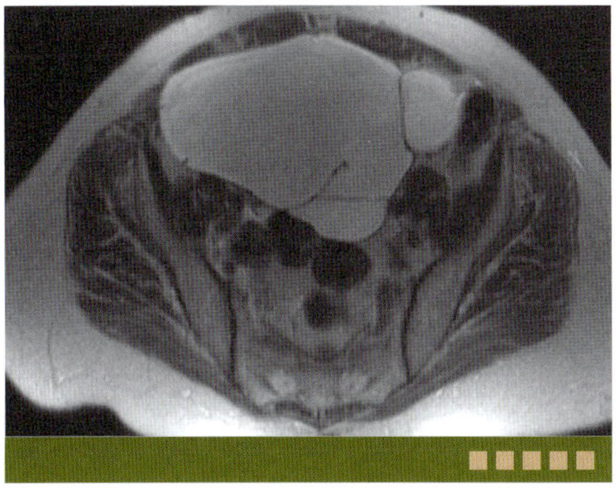

C. Axial T2-WI in the same patient shows a few thin septations within the lesion.

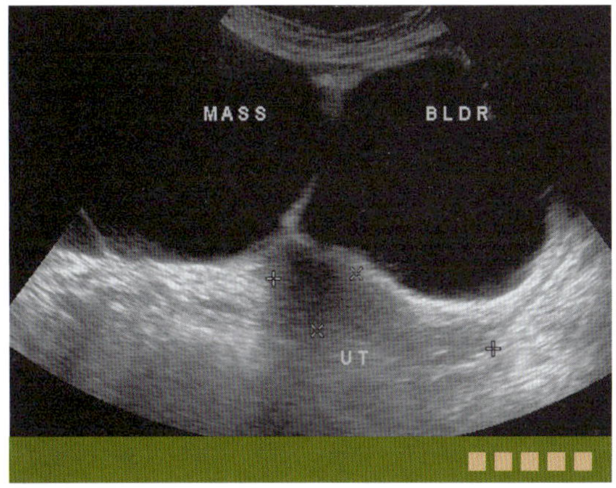

D. Longitudinal sonogram obtained transabdominally in the same patient shows a distended urinary bladder and a unilocular cystic mass just superior to the bladder.

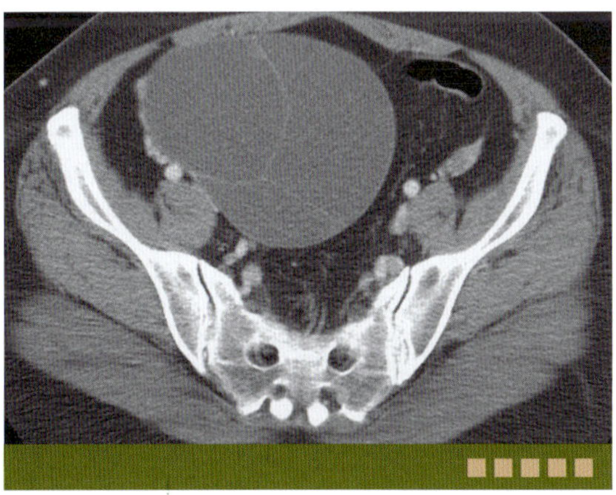

E. Axial CECT shows a multilocular cystic pelvic mass containing multiple internal septations consistent with a mucinous cystic ovarian neoplasm. This was pathologically confirmed to represent a mucinous cystadenoma.

DIFFERENTIAL DIAGNOSES IMAGES (F-H)

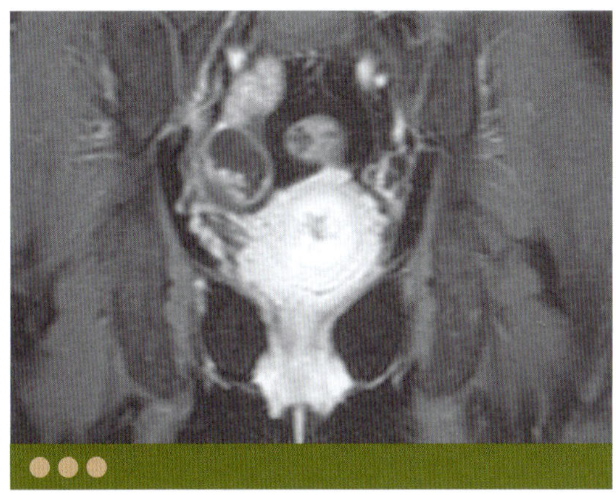

F. Serous cystadenocarcinoma: Coronal contrast-enhanced T1-WI shows a cystic mass arising from the right adnexa. Although this lesion is small, the presence of the solid, enhancing component at its inferior aspect is suggestive of malignancy.

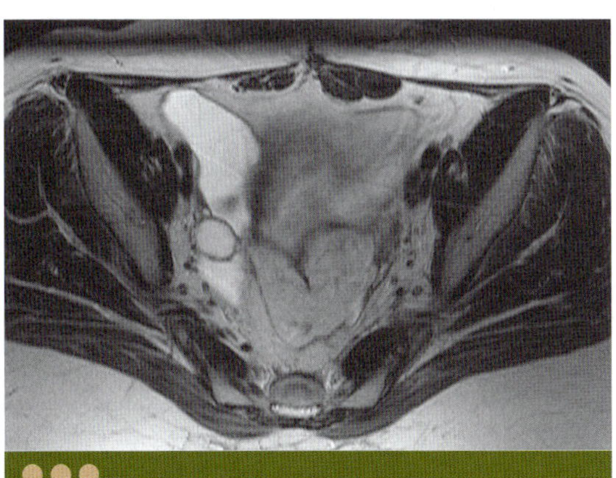

G. Peritoneal inclusion cyst: Axial T2-WI in a patient with a history of multiple abdominal surgeries shows a cystic mass associated with the right ovary. The mass conforms to the peritoneal spaces. No solid components are identified.

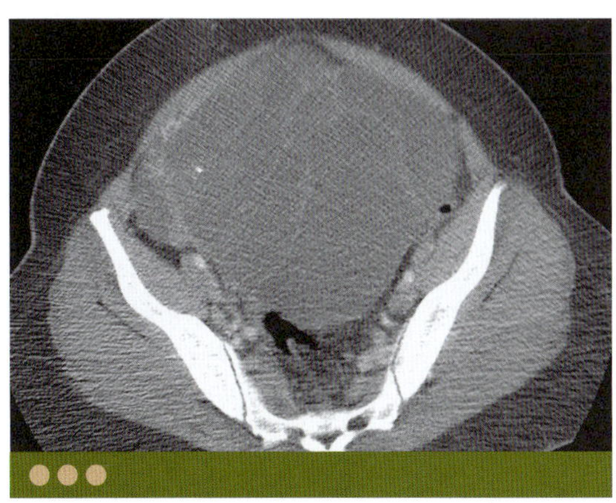

H. Mucinous cystadenocarcinoma: Axial CECT shows a complex cystic mass in the pelvis with multiple septations. Some of these appear thickened as noted along the right lateral aspect of the mass. A small amount of internal calcification is also present.

IMAGE KEY

Common

Rare

Typical

Unusual

16–32 Dermoid Cyst (Mature Cystic Teratoma)

Paul Nikolaidis

PRESENTATION

Typically asymptomatic, often incidental finding on imaging, rarely may cause pain resulting from rupture or torsion.

FINDINGS

CT shows a large complex adnexal mass containing fatty tissue (–80 HU), and several large calcifications, including teeth.

DIFFERENTIAL DIAGNOSES

- *Endometriomas*: Easy to distinguish on CT or ultrasound. On MR they are also hyperintense on T1-WI, but contrary to dermoids, they remain hyperintense on fat-suppressed T1 sequences.
- *Lipomas/liposarcomas*: Benign and malignant lipomatous lesions may also occur in the pelvis; typically will not be intimately associated with the ovary.

COMMENTS

Mature cystic teratomas, also known as dermoid cysts, are the most common benign ovarian tumor. They are typically asymptomatic and are usually found in women in their 20s and 30s. They are occasionally bilateral. They have the rare potential to become malignant. Because they are derived from totipotential germ cells, they can give rise to all types of cells necessary to form mature tissues, including hair, teeth, bone, sebaceous material, and neural tissue.

Mature cystic teratomas usually have pathognomonic features on sonography. The characteristic appearance is a complex, partially cystic lesion with one or more shadowing echogenic regions. In some cases, a fluid–fluid level may be seen. The classic "tip of the iceberg" sign may be produced by extensive shadowing. Other echogenic structures including hair, teeth, and bone may be seen.

On CT, the presence of low-attenuation (–20 to –120 HU) adipose tissue within a lesion, with or without calcification, is diagnostic. Fluid–fluid levels may also be present.

On MR, they are oval or round, well-marginated, and hyperintense on T1-WI. They classically demonstrate loss of signal on fat-saturated gradient echo T1 sequences. On T2-WI, they are variable in signal intensity, usually similar to subcutaneous fat. Calcifications are typically hypointense; a fluid–fluid level may be seen.

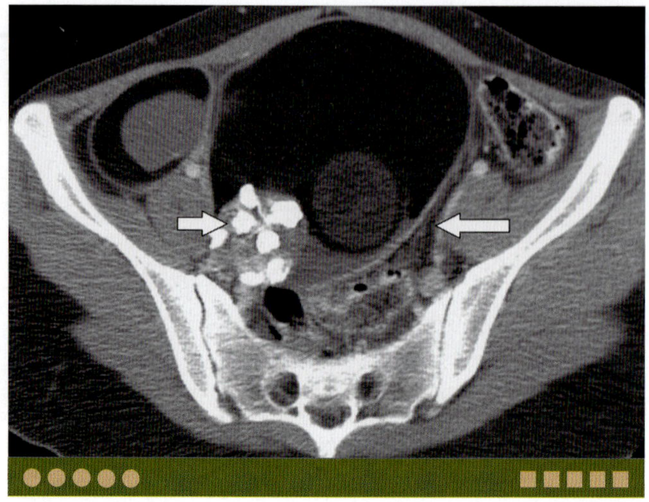

A. Axial CECT shows a large pelvic lesion, the majority of which is composed of fat. In addition, there are solid areas with coarse calcifications including teeth (short arrow), and a fluid–fluid level (long arrow).

Extracapsular growth of the tumor is very rare but important to appreciate on imaging because this may signify malignant transformation. Rupture and ovarian torsion are the most important complications. They are usually removed laparoscopically.

PEARLS

- **Dermoids are common ovarian lesions found in women in their 20's and 30's.**
- **On sonography, they typically have one or more echogenic, shadowing regions.**
- **On MR, they follow the signal intensity of fat and loss of signal on fat-saturated sequences should be seen.**
- **Rupture and torsion are the most important potential complications.**

ADDITIONAL IMAGES (B-D)

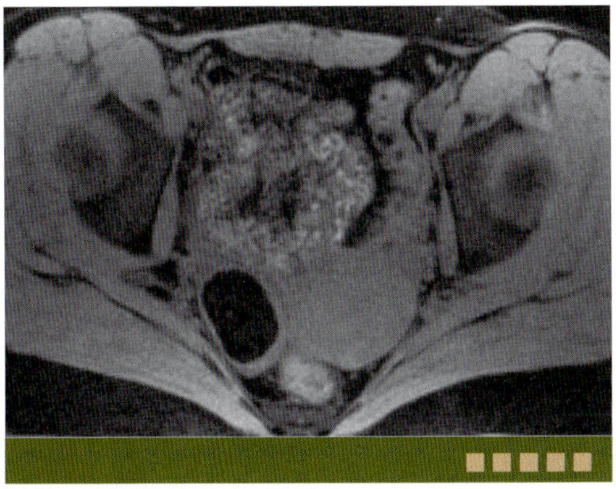

B. Axial noncontrast fat-suppressed T1-WI shows an oval hypointense lesion in the right posterior pelvis, adjacent to the uterus. Its signal is identical to the signal of the subcutaneous fat. Features are classic for a dermoid.

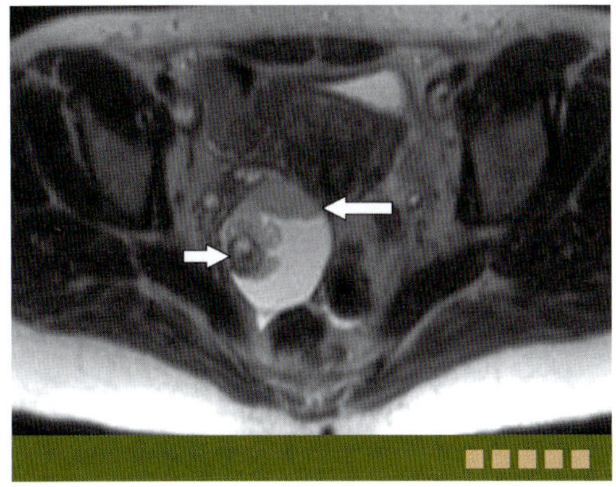

C. Axial T2-WI on another patient shows a complex lesion in the posterior pelvis. Note the presence of a fluid–fluid level (long arrow) and hypointense foci representing calcifications (short arrow).

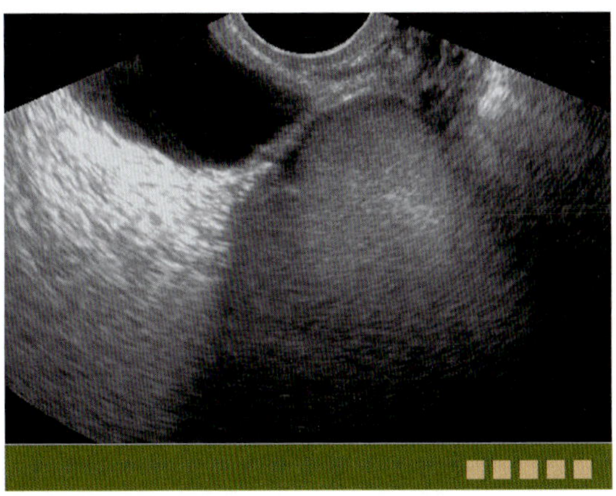

D. Transvaginal sonogram on another patient shows a large hyperechoic left ovarian lesion with extensive shadowing. This appearance is classic for a dermoid.

DIFFERENTIAL DIAGNOSES IMAGES (E-G)

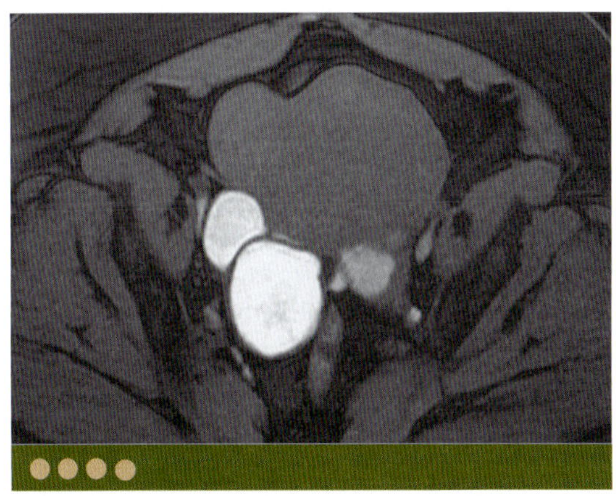

E. Endometrioma: Axial noncontrast fat suppressed T1-WI shows bilateral hyperintense adnexal lesions. This appearance is pathognomic for endometriomas. Dermoids would have shown fat suppression.

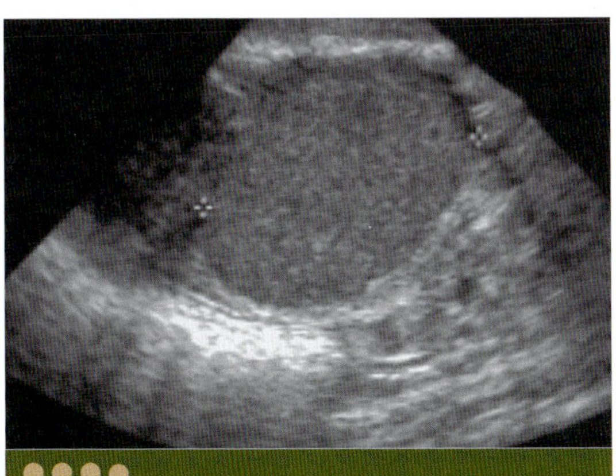

F. Endometrioma: Transvaginal sonogram in a different patient shows a right ovarian lesion with uniform low-level echoes. This persisted on a follow-up study 9 weeks later and was shown to represent an endometrioma on laparoscopy.

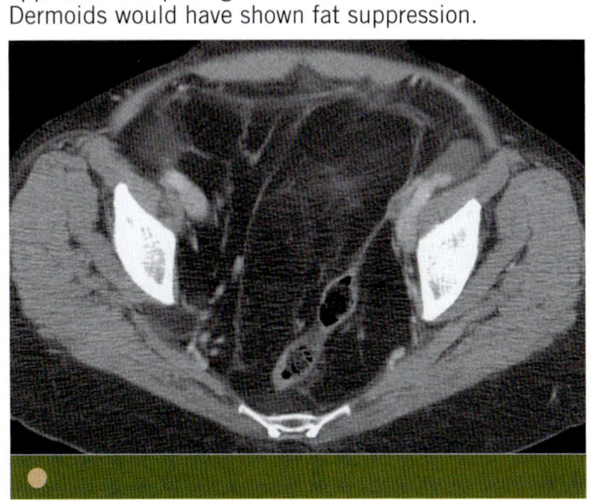

G. Liposarcoma: Axial CECT shows a large fatty lesion occupying a significant portion of the pelvis. It surrounds the sigmoid colon. It shows linear septations, a few areas of increased attenuation, and some nodular foci. This represented a large pelvic liposarcoma.

IMAGE KEY

Common

Rare

Typical

Unusual

16–33 Hemorrhagic Ovarian Cyst

Paul Nikolaidis

PRESENTATION

Unilateral pelvic or lower abdominal pain, often asymptomatic.

FINDINGS

Pelvic sonography shows an ovarian lesion with an internal reticular, lace-like appearance and increased posterior through transmission.

DIFFERENTIAL DIAGNOSES

- *Endometrioma*: Diffuse homogeneous low-level internal echoes are typically seen as opposed to the more reticular, lace-like appearance of a hemorrhagic cyst.
- *Cystic ovarian neoplasm*: Retracting thrombus within a hemorrhagic cyst may be confused for a mural nodule of a cystic neoplasm; however, mural nodules have convex margins. Also, color flow should be present in a mural nodule.

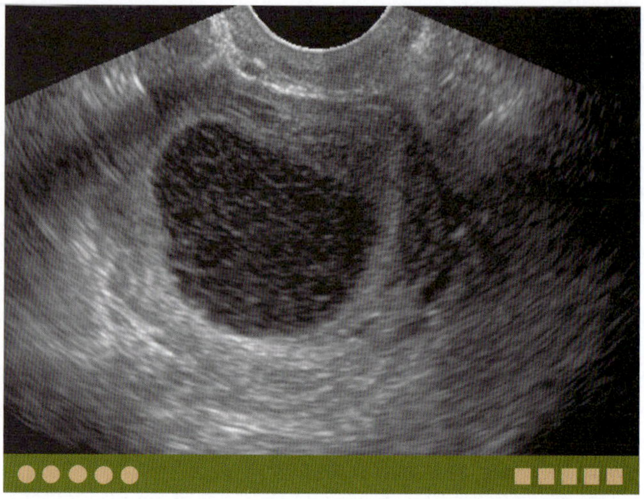

A. Sagittal transvaginal sonogram shows a 3.5-cm right adnexal lesion with smooth walls and an internal reticular appearance and some increased posterior through transmission. The lesion resolved on a follow-up ultrasound obtained 7 weeks later.

COMMENTS

Hemorrhagic ovarian cysts are common benign lesions. At mid-cycle, luteinizing hormone is released from the pituitary and a corpus luteum cyst is formed. Blood vessels within the wall of the cyst are very fragile and may rupture, giving rise to a hemorrhagic cyst. Hemorrhage into a cyst is often acutely painful.

The sonographic appearance of a hemorrhagic ovarian cyst is typically very specific (in more than 90% of cases). Size is variable, ranging from 2.5 to 10 cm. The wall of the cyst should be smooth and is usually quite thin, but may range from 2 mm to 2.2 cm. Internal flow is absent on color Doppler ultrasound. Increased posterior through transmission should be seen. The two most important gray-scale sonographic features are the presence of fibrin strands or a retracting clot. These fibrin strands give the classic lace-like, fishnet, or fine reticular pattern. Portions of a hemorrhagic ovarian cyst may appear more solid and may mimic a mural nodule of a cystic ovarian neoplasm, but blood flow should be absent.

CT may be obtained in cases of nonspecific pelvic pain, primarily to exclude other lower abdominal or pelvic pathology. A relatively hyperdense (more than 20 HU), nonenhancing adnexal cyst should be seen. Occasionally, hemorrhagic cysts will rupture, with blood entering the abdominal cavity.

The MR appearance of a hemorrhagic cyst is variable and depends on technical parameters, the quantity of blood or serous fluid, and age of the hemorrhage. Approximately two-thirds are low-signal on T1-WI. Most will show heterogenous signal intensity on T2-WI, but approximately 20% are hyperintense, mimicking simple cysts.

Correct diagnosis is imperative to avoid unnecessary surgery. Short-interval follow-up sonography of equivocal cases will nearly always show resolution. If a hemorrhagic ovarian cyst does not have a classic appearance, or is larger than 3 cm, follow-up ultrasound is generally recommended in 6 to 10 weeks.

PEARLS

- **One of the most frequently encountered ovarian lesions.**
- **Most important gray-scale ultrasound features are the presence of fibrin strands or a retracting clot.**
- **Flow within the lesion is entirely absent on color Doppler imaging.**
- **In some instances, hemorrhagic cysts will rupture, and patients may have an associated hemoperitoneum.**

ADDITIONAL IMAGES (B-D)

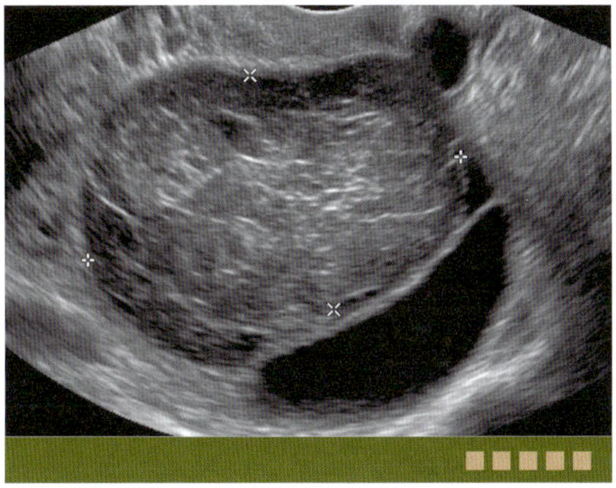

B. Sagittal transvaginal sonogram in another patient shows a 6-cm ovarian lesion (outlined by calipers) with a complex internal reticular appearance.

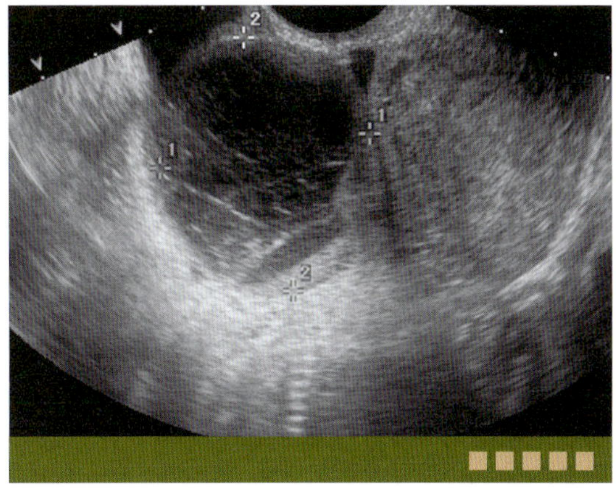

C. Sagittal transvaginal sonogram in another patient shows a 4.5-cm left ovarian hemorrhagic cyst (outlined by calipers).

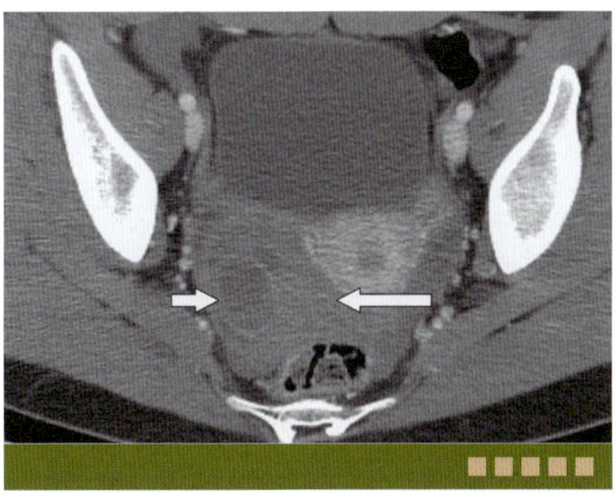

D. Axial CECT on a different patient shows a round right adnexal lesion (short arrow) with surrounding hemorrhage (long arrow).

DIFFERENTIAL DIAGNOSES IMAGES (E-G)

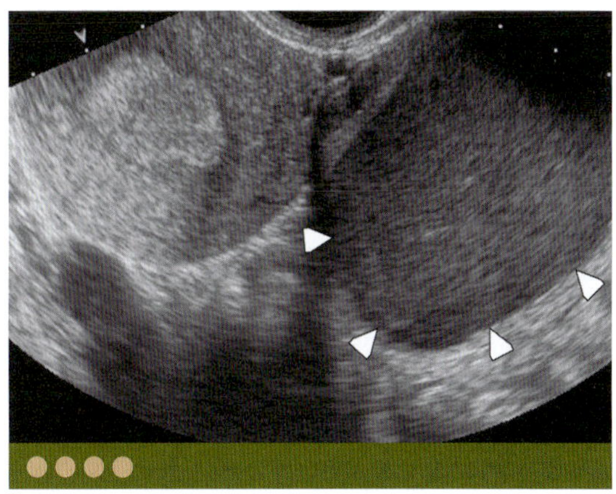

E. Endometrioma: Transverse transvaginal sonogram in a different patient shows a left ovarian lesion with diffuse uniformly low-level echoes (arrowheads).

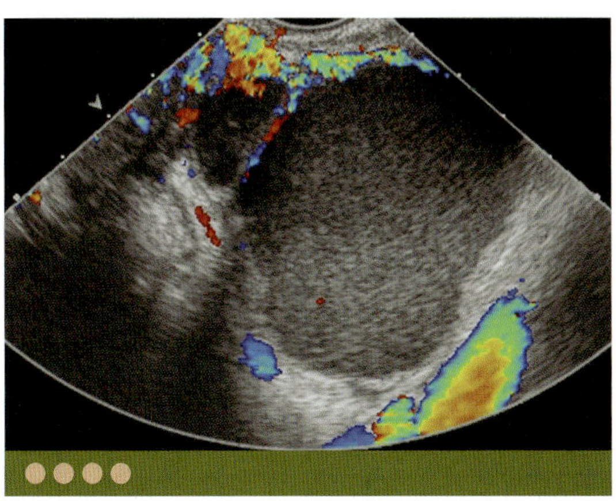

F. Endometrioma: Corresponding transverse transvaginal color Doppler sonogram shows that lesion is completely avascular.

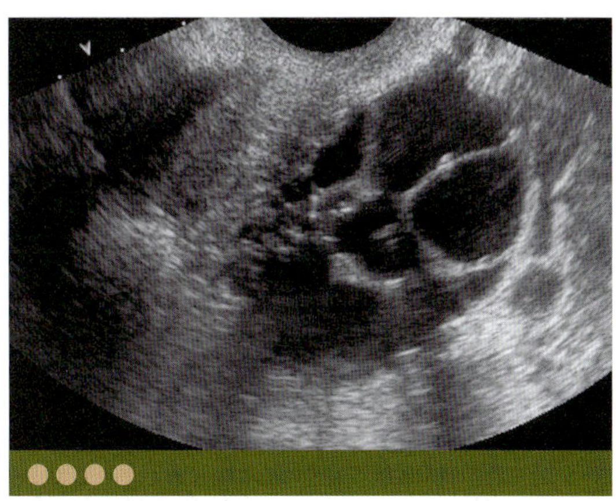

G. Ovarian cystadenoma: Transverse transvaginal sonogram shows a complex left ovarian lesion with multiple septa, some of which are thickened and nodular.

IMAGE KEY

Common

Rare

Typical

Unusual

16–34 Ovarian Fibroma

Paul Nikolaidis

PRESENTATION

Mostly asymptomatic, may rarely present with ascites and a pleural effusion.

FINDINGS

A well-marginated round homogenous adnexal mass with low-signal intensity on both T1-WI and T2-WI.

DIFFERENTIAL DIAGNOSIS

- *Subserosal uterine fibroid*: These should be shown to be separate from the ovary and connected to the uterus by a pedicle or more broad-based attachment.

COMMENTS

Ovarian fibromas are the most common sex-cord stromal tumors. Most are considered benign. They present as solid, unilateral, hormonally inactive masses, and most typically occur in postmenopausal women. Approximately 10% of patients have multiple lesions. They are sometimes associated with the presence of ascites and a pleural effusion that will resolve following resection (Meigs syndrome). In less than 1% of the cases, they may progress to fibrosarcomas.

The typical sonographic appearance is of a solid, hypoechoic ovarian mass that attenuates the ultrasound beam. This appearance along with the patient's age and lack of symptoms should suggest the diagnosis of a fibroma.

On CT, these lesions have a nonspecific appearance, although they are typically well-marginated, solid, homogenous (or somewhat heterogeneous) masses with delayed contrast enhancement.

MR characteristics of an ovarian fibroma include a well-marginated round or oval homogenous mass that may have a lobulated outline depending on its size. Fibromas are of low-signal intensity on both T1-WI and T2-WI because of their histologic composition (hyalinized fibrous tissue, collagen, and dense spindle cells). Uncommonly, in larger fibromas, there may be ill-defined surrounding increased signal as a result of edema, or high signal within the lesion resulting from cystic degeneration.

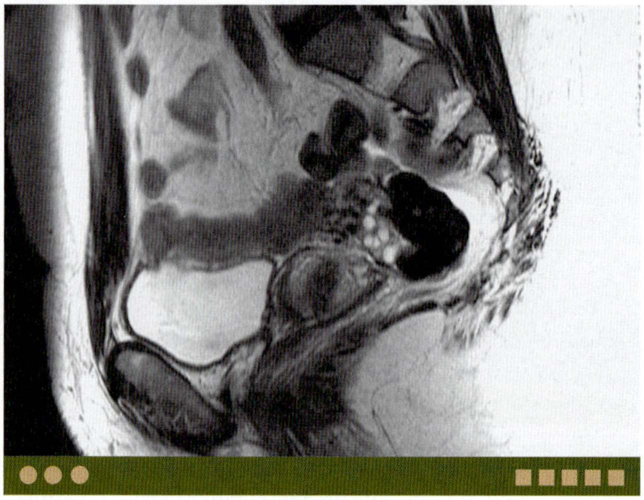

A. Sagittal T2-WI shows a hypointense mass immediately posterior to the right ovary. Note the multiple round hyperintense follicles in the normal portion of the ovary, anterior to the fibroma.

It is important to differentiate an ovarian fibroma from a subserosal or pedunculated uterine leiomyoma, which may have similar imaging characteristics because of its tissue composition. Ovarian fibromas should be surgically resected; most of them are benign.

PEARLS

- **Most common sex-cord stromal tumors; the majority are benign.**
- **Meigs syndrome: Ascites and a pleural effusion in a patient with a fibroma.**
- **Fibromas have similar sonographic and MR features with uterine fibroids.**
- **Fibromas display low-signal intensity on both T1-WI and T2-WI because of their histologic composition.**

ADDITIONAL IMAGES (B-D)

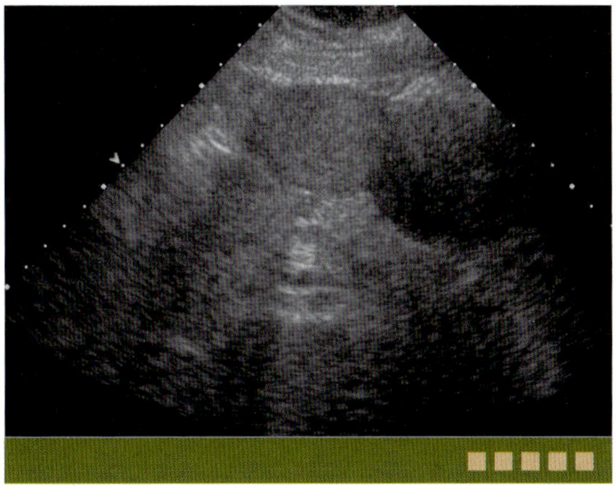

B. Transverse transvaginal sonogram shows a homogeneous solid lesion corresponding to an ovarian fibroma. It may be difficult to distinguish from a fibroid or even endometrioma on gray-scale sonography.

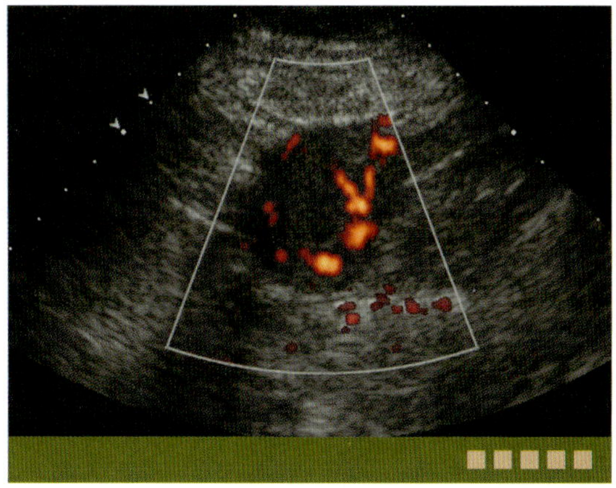

C. Transverse transvaginal sonogram with power Doppler shows this mass to be vascular, excluding the possibility of an endometrioma. It was also shown to be separate from the uterus, excluding a uterine fibroid.

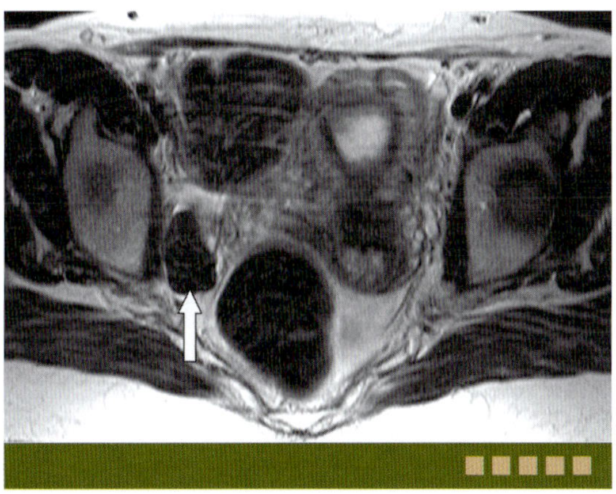

D. Axial T2-WI on another patient shows a homogeneously hypointense right adnexal mass (arrow), shown on surgical pathology to represent an ovarian fibroma.

DIFFERENTIAL DIAGNOSIS IMAGES (E-G)

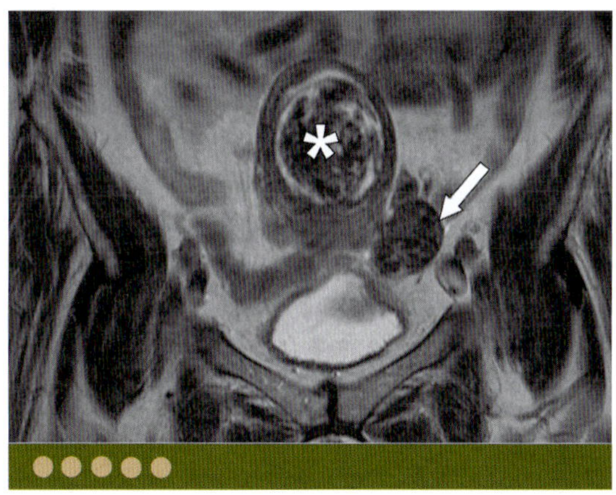

E. Subserosal uterine fibroid: Coronal T2-WI shows an oval hypointense mass immediately adjacent to the uterus (arrow). Note the presence of an additional submucosal fibroid (asterisk).

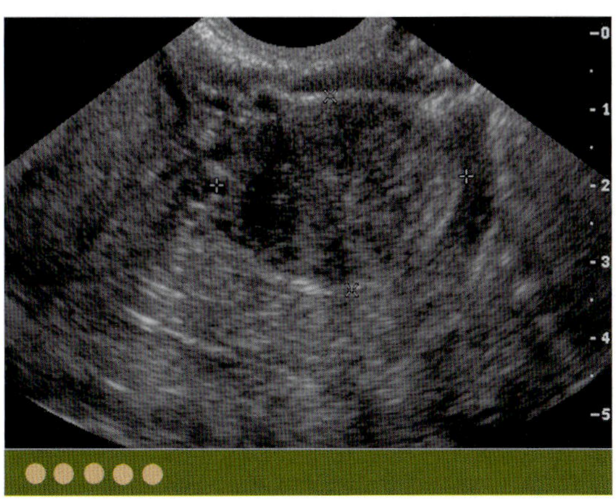

F. Subserosal uterine fibroid: Coronal transvaginal sonogram shows a 3-cm mildly heterogeneous solid pelvic mass (outlined by calipers) immediately adjacent to the uterus.

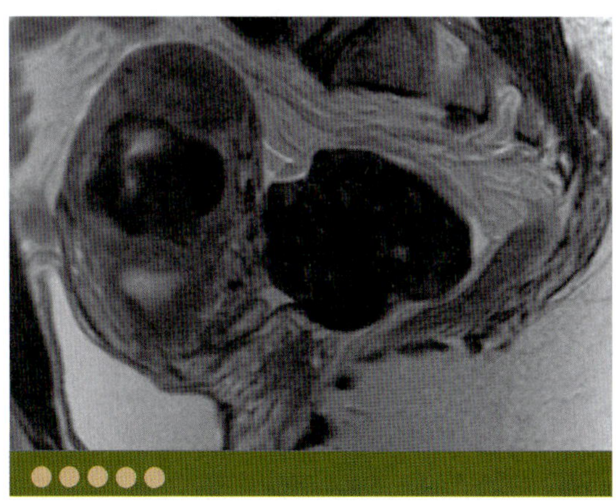

G. Subserosal uterine fibroid: Sagittal T2-WI on another patient shows a large hypointense mass, with a broad-based attachment to the uterus, representing a subserosal fibroid.

IMAGE KEY

Common

Rare

Typical

Unusual

16–35 Granulosa Cell Tumor of the Ovary

Paul Nikolaidis

PRESENTATION

Menometrorrhagia, postmenopausal bleeding, adnexal mass.

FINDINGS

MR shows a left adnexal mass anterior to the uterus with hyperintense cystic components on T2-WI and hyperintense hemorrhagic elements on T1-WI.

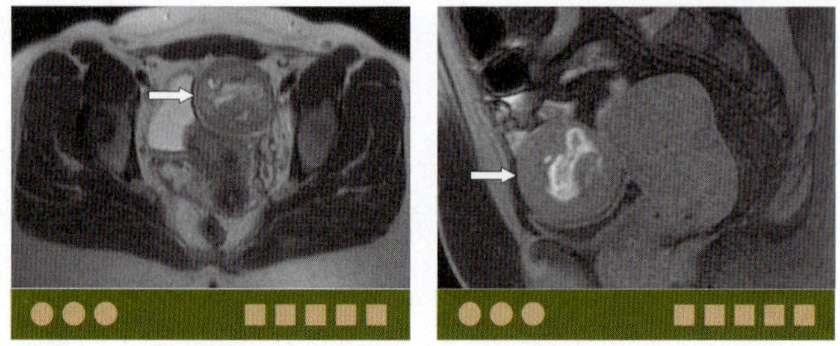

A. Axial T2-WI shows a large left adnexal mass anterior to the uterus with few internal cystic components (arrow).
B. Sagittal nonenhanced fat saturated T1-WI on the same patient shows internal areas of high signal in the mass (arrow). Intratumoral hemorrhage, a classic finding in granulosa cell tumors, is best seen as hyperintense foci on T1-WI.

DIFFERENTIAL DIAGNOSIS

- *Ovarian neoplasms*: The differential diagnosis of a hemorrhagic solid ovarian mass includes endometrioid carcinoma, malignant germ cell tumors (ie, yolk sac tumor), and serous carcinomas. These patients will not have symptoms relating to excess estrogen levels.

COMMENTS

Granulosa cell tumors of the ovary are a subtype of sex-cord stromal tumors. They arise from the germinal cells of ovarian follicles. They are the most common estrogen producing ovarian tumor but account for fewer than 2% of all ovarian neoplasms. They have low malignant potential. Their clinical presentation depends on the hormonal activity of the tumor, age of the patient, and size of the tumor. Most patients present with symptoms relating to excess estrogen levels. Less hormonally active tumors will present with an enlarging adnexal mass.

There are two types: adult and juvenile. The adult form is more prevalent and occurs in peri- and postmenopausal women (median age is 52 years). Patients present with menometrorrhagia or postmenopausal bleeding secondary to elevated estrogen levels. Affected women may also have endometrial abnormalities including hyperplasia, polyps, and carcinoma. The median age of patients with the juvenile form is 13. Excessive estrogen levels may lead to precocious puberty or menstrual abnormalities, including amenorrhea.

Granulosa cell tumors can range from solid to cystic; they typically have internal areas of hemorrhage. On ultrasound, smaller tumors are well-defined, solid, often with echogenicity similar to a uterine leiomyoma or ovarian fibroma. Larger masses are more commonly multilocular complex cystic lesions.

Areas of bleeding within the tumor are hyperdense on NECT but are difficult to discern on CECT.

MR typically shows a solid or complex adnexal mass with variable cystic components and hemorrhage. Intratumoral hemorrhage is best seen as areas of high signal on T1-WI. On T2-WI, these tumors have a characteristic "sponge-like" appearance, in which numerous hyperintense cysts are seen along with solid areas of lower signal intensity. The solid components typically enhance following contrast administration. Associated uterine and endometrial changes may be seen.

Medical management is different from other epithelial ovarian neoplasms. Patients with localized disease do not undergo chemotherapy. In young patients, the preferred initial treatment is unilateral salpingo-oophorectomy with preservation of the uterus.

PEARLS

- **Most common estrogen producing ovarian tumor.**
- **Clinical presentation depends on hormonal activity of the tumor, age, and tumor size.**
- **Granulosa cell tumors have nonspecific sonographic and CT features.**
- **On MR hyperintense hemorrhagic foci on T1-WI are typically seen.**

ADDITIONAL IMAGES (C-E)

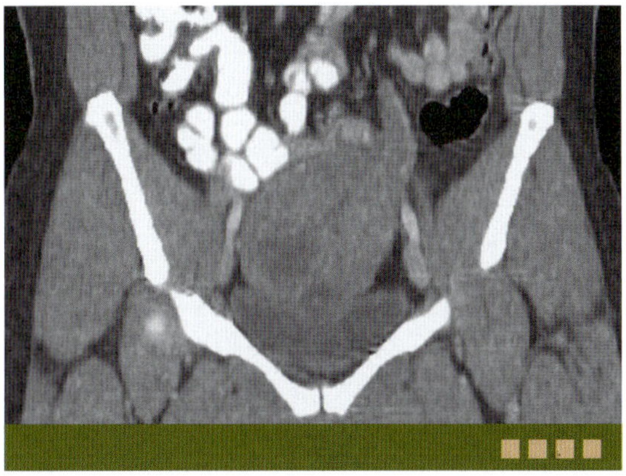

C. Coronal CECT reformation on the same patient shows a predominantly solid lesion with few hypodense cystic spaces.

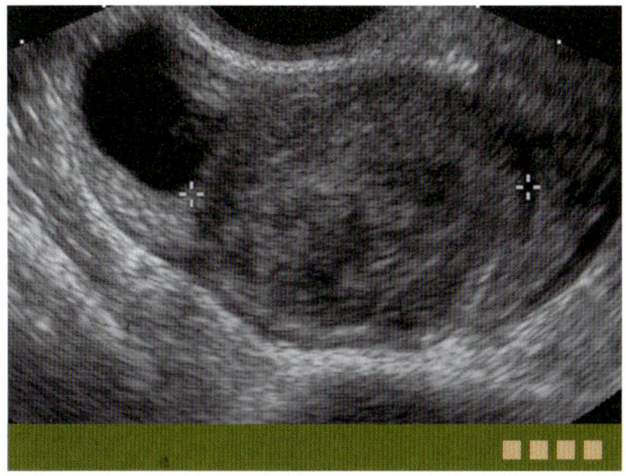

D. Transverse transvaginal sonogram on another patient shows a 4-cm right adnexal mass. There are some internal areas of heterogeneity along with areas of reticulation that may be caused by hemorrhage.

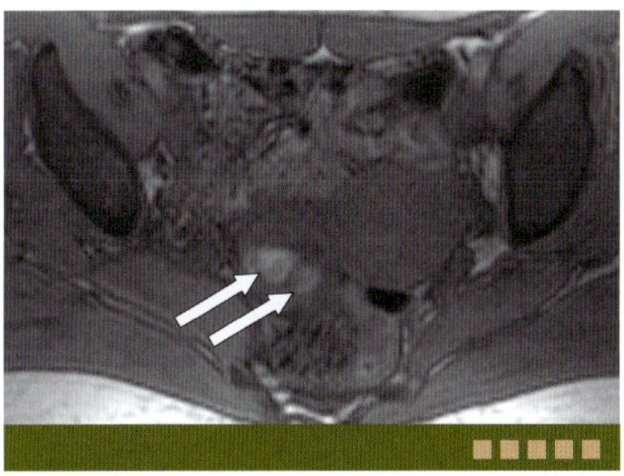

E. Corresponding nonenhanced T1-WI on the same patient shows a right adnexal mass with internal hyperintense areas representing intratumoral hemorrhage, a finding suggestive of a granulosa cell tumor.

DIFFERENTIAL DIAGNOSIS IMAGES (F-H)

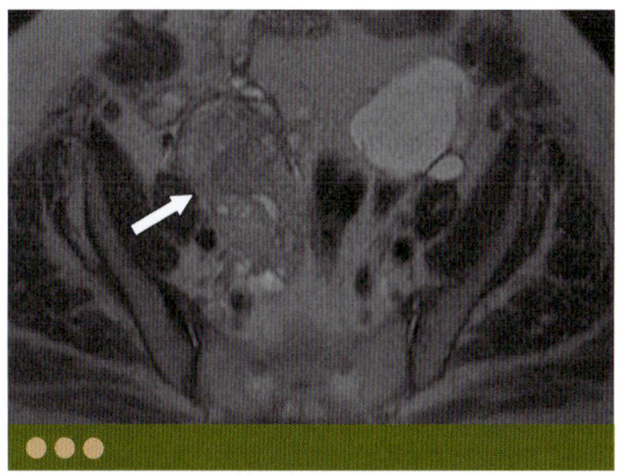

F. Sex cord stromal tumor: Axial T2-WI shows a nonspecific complex right adnexal mass (arrow). Imaging findings are nonspecific but highly suspicious for a neoplasm.

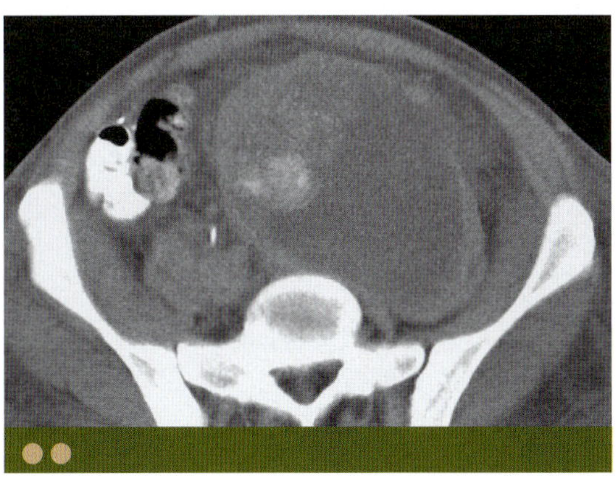

G. Yolk sac tumor: Axial CECT shows a large complex left ovarian lesion with large hypodense cystic spaces. Imaging findings in this case are also nonspecific.

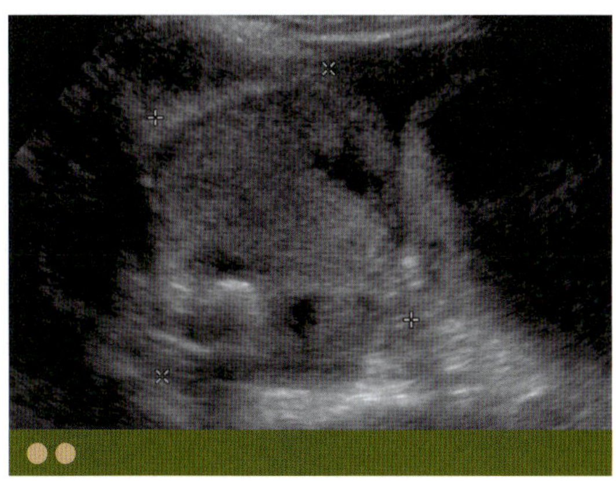

H. Endometrioid carcinoma of the ovary: Transverse transvaginal sonogram shows a large predominantly solid right adnexal mass (outlined by calipers).

IMAGE KEY

Common

Rare

Typical

Unusual

16–36 Brenner Tumor of the Ovary

Paul Nikolaidis

PRESENTATION

Mostly asymptomatic, sometimes in association with a cystic ovarian neoplasm.

FINDINGS

CT shows a round solid adnexal mass with numerous faint central calcifications.

DIFFERENTIAL DIAGNOSES

- *Ovarian fibroma*: Similarly T2-hypointense on MR; however Brenner tumors contain calcifications that are best seen on CT.
- *Subserosal uterine fibroid*: Similarly T2-hypointense on MR; degenerated fibroids may also have calcifications on CT that are often more chunky. Fibroids will be connected to the uterus and are separate from the ovary.

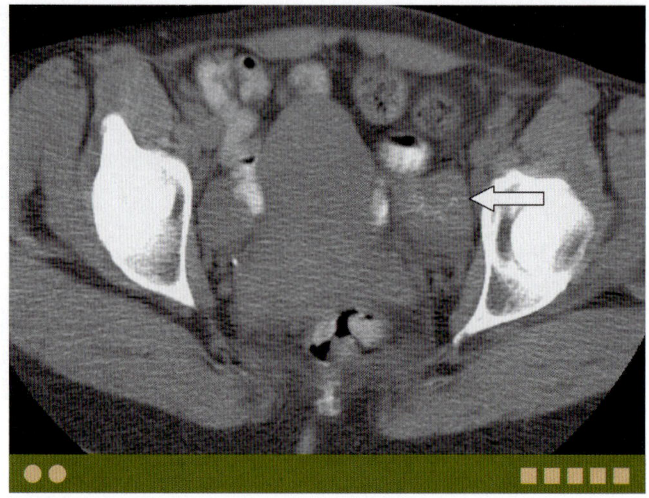

A. Axial NECT shows a solid left adnexal mass which is isodense to the myometrium (arrow). Note the multiple amorphous small calcifications within the lesion.

COMMENTS

Brenner tumors are uncommon epithelial neoplasms that account for 1% to 2% of all ovarian tumors. They are almost always benign. In 30%, they are discovered in conjunction with cystic neoplasms, usually mucinous or serous cystadenomas. However, they usually present as solid, unilateral, hormonally inactive masses, with a peak incidence between 40 and 50 years. Tumors are bilateral in approximately 6% to 7%.

They are also known as transitional cell tumors of the ovary, as they are composed of ovarian epithelial cells that undergo metaplasia to transitional cells with a histologic similarity to urothelial epithelium. These transitional cells are embedded in an extensive fibrous stroma.

The typical sonographic appearance of a Brenner tumor is a solid, hypoechoic mass that may resemble a fibroma, thecoma, or leiomyoma. Calcifications are seen in 50%. Some lesions may be partially cystic. A thorough search for concomitant cystic lesions is important.

On CT, they are typically well-marginated solid or partially solid masses. Calcifications may be present in the wall, and extensive amorphous calcifications within the solid component of the tumor are characteristic. The solid portion of the tumor shows mild-to-moderate enhancement on CECT.

The MR appearance is not as specific and includes a homogeneous, well-marginated, round or oval mass. Brenner tumors are isointense to myometrium on T1-WI and hypointense on T2-WI because of their high fibrous tissue component. They may be difficult to differentiate from a fibroma, or a subserosal uterine leiomyoma, which may have similar signal characteristics.

Ovarian Brenner tumors are surgically resected and almost all are benign. Rarely proliferative and malignant forms are encountered.

PEARLS

- **Mostly solid ovarian lesions, typically occuring in women aged 40 to 50 years.**
- **In 30%, they are found in conjunction with other cystic ovarian neoplasms.**
- **Calcifications are typically seen on ultrasound and particularly on CT.**
- **Brenner tumors have similar MR features with ovarian fibromas and uterine fibroids.**

ADDITIONAL IMAGES (B-D)

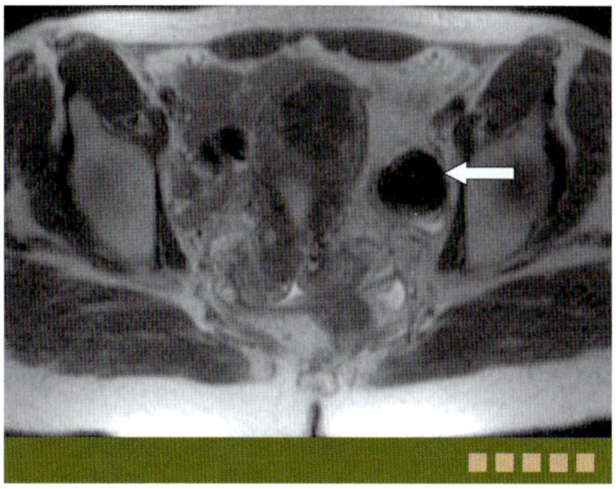

B. Axial T2-WI on the same patient shows a homogeneously hypointense left adnexal mass (arrow). It has signal characteristics identical to an ovarian fibroma.

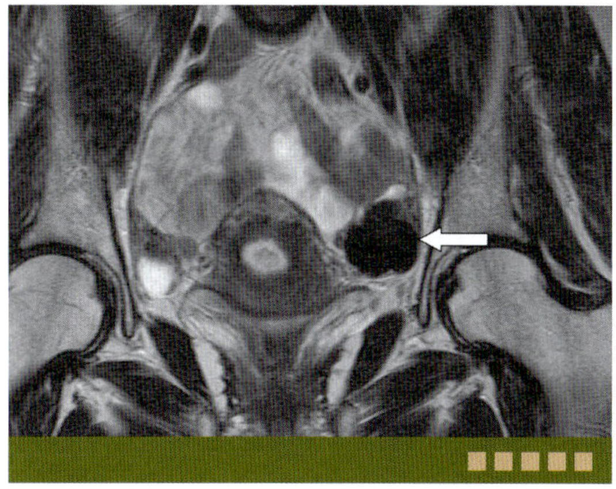

C. Coronal T2-WI on the same patient shows the hypointense left ovarian Brenner tumor (arrow).

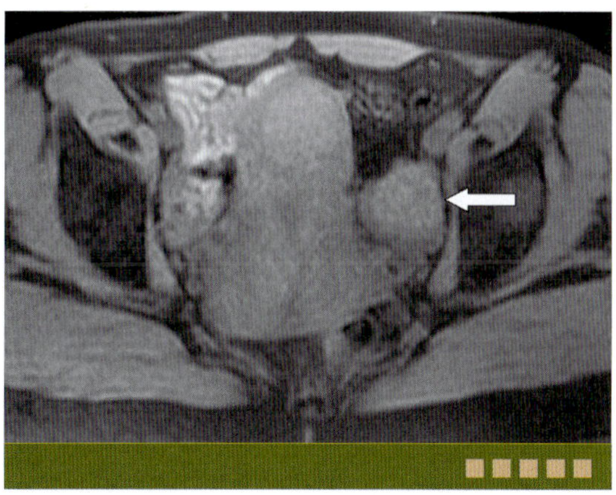

D. Axial noncontrast T1-WI shows the mass to be isointense to myometrium (arrow).

DIFFERENTIAL DIAGNOSES IMAGES (E-G)

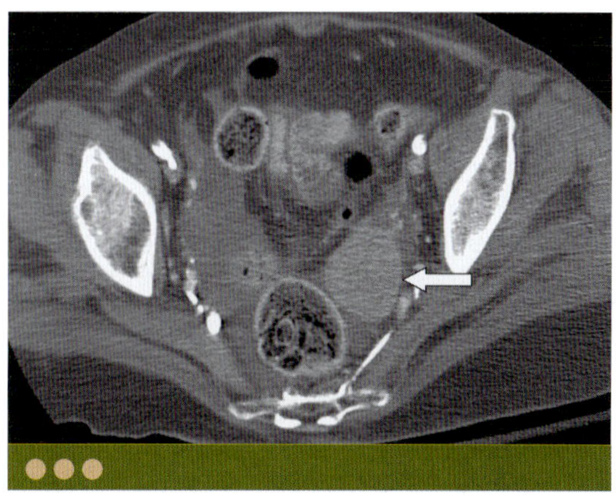

E. Ovarian fibroma: Axial CECT shows a nonspecific solid left adnexal mass (arrow). Note the absence of calcifications. Ascites in the pelvis was secondary to cirrhosis.

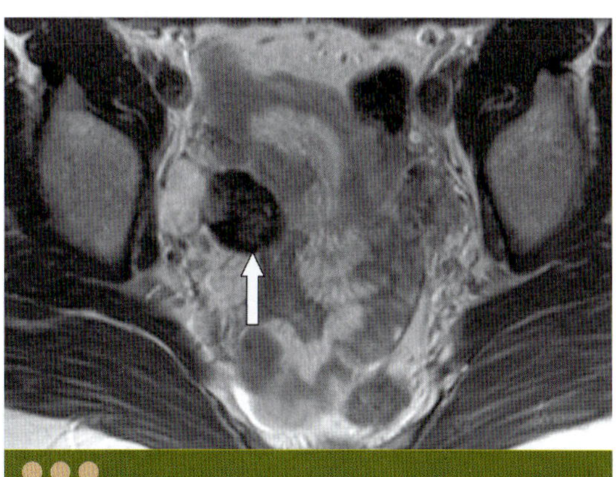

F. Ovarian fibroma: Axial T2-WI in another patient shows a uniformly hypointense solid mass attached to the right ovary (arrow). This was shown to represent an ovarian fibroma.

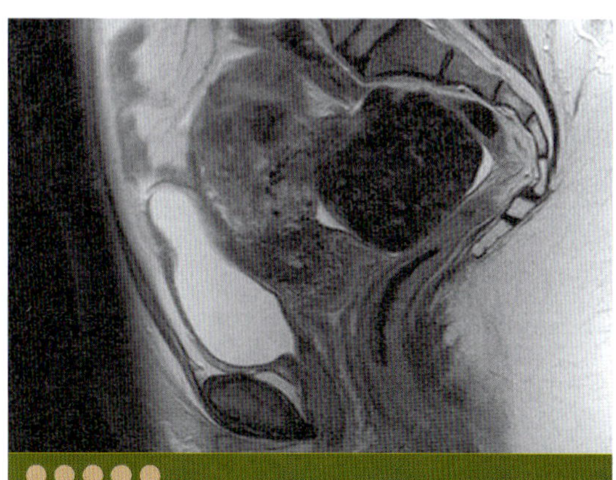

G. Subserosal uterine fibroid: Sagittal T2-WI on another patient shows a large posteriorly located hypointense mass, which is attached to the body of the uterus. Additional smaller intramural fibroids were also present.

IMAGE KEY

Common

Rare

Typical

Unusual

16–37 Ovarian Cystadenofibroma

Paul Nikolaidis

PRESENTATION

Pelvic/adnexal mass, asymptomatic.

FINDINGS

CT shows a large complex cystic pelvic mass with some solid components.

DIFFERENTIAL DIAGNOSIS

- *Primary ovarian neoplasms*: Usually impossible to distinguish on CT and ultrasound. On MR, a hypointense solid component with internal hyperintense cystic foci may be seen in cystadenofibromas.

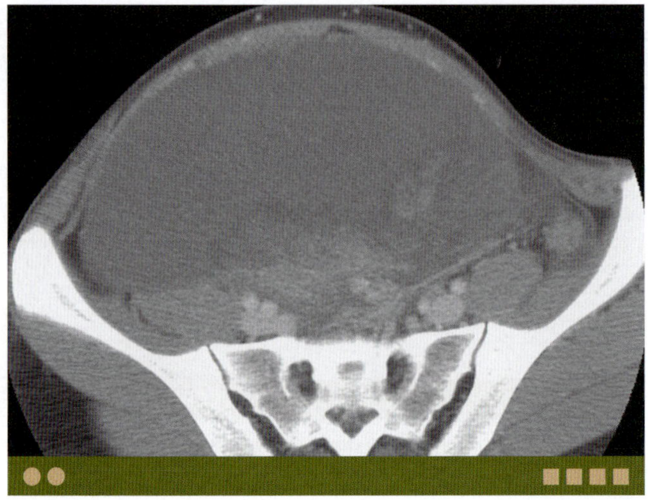

A. Axial CECT shows a large predominantly cystic pelvic mass with a large solid component posteriorly.

COMMENTS

Ovarian cystadenofibroma is an ovarian tumor composed of both benign epithelial and stromal components. It is rarely malignant, but it mimics ovarian cancer as lesions can get quite large and often display suspicious imaging features including thickened septations and solid nodules. Cystadenofibromas are believed to represent approximately 1.7% of all cystic ovarian neoplasms.

Ovarian cystadenofibromas are sub-classified according to their epithelial types as either serous, endometrioid, mucinous, clear cell, or mixed. In addition cystadenofibromas are divided into benign, borderline, and malignant. Almost all cystadenofibromas are benign.

On imaging, ovarian cystadenofibromas are usually nonspecific in appearance. They are more typically cystic, and mixed cystic and solid. The most frequent reported imaging finding is the presence of solid nodules, with a reported rate ranging between 33% and 80%. On ultrasound and CT, there are usually no specific features to differentiate ovarian cystadenofibromas from other primary ovarian neoplasms. In purely cystic lesions, findings on CT and ultrasound are similar to ovarian cystadenomas.

On MR, a more specific finding for cystadenofibromas on T2-WI that has been reported is the presence of a hypointense solid component. This is thought to be because of the presence of fibrous tissue.

Ovarian cystadenofibromas are surgically resected and almost all are benign. Rarely borderline and malignant forms are encountered. Cystadenocarcinofibroma is the malignant counterpart of cystadenofibroma. It is exceedingly rare.

PEARLS

- **Composed of both epithelial and stromal components.**
- **On imaging solid components may be seen in up to 80%.**
- **On ultrasound and CT, there are no specific features to differentiate cystadenofibromas from other ovarian neoplasms.**
- **On MR, a hypointense solid component may be seen.**

ADDITIONAL IMAGES (B-D)

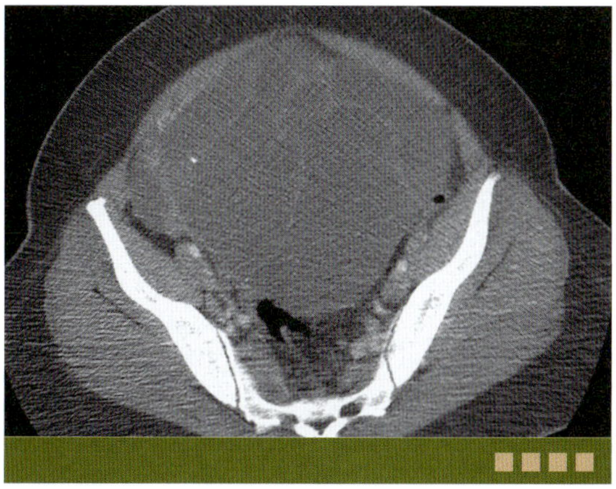

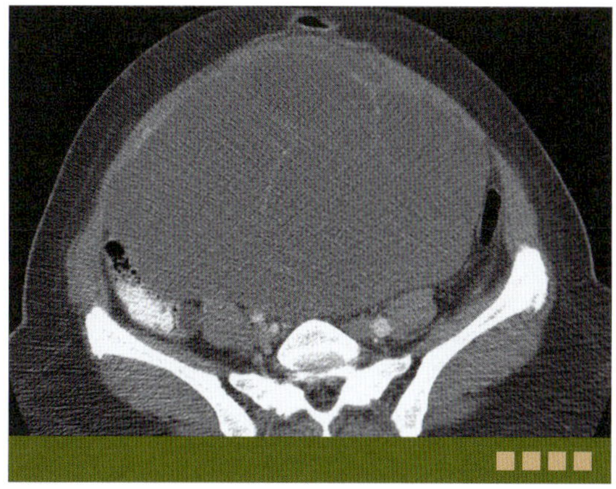

B. and **C.** Axial CECT on another patient shows a large cystic pelvic mass with numerous septations, some of which are more thickened and nodular anteriorly.

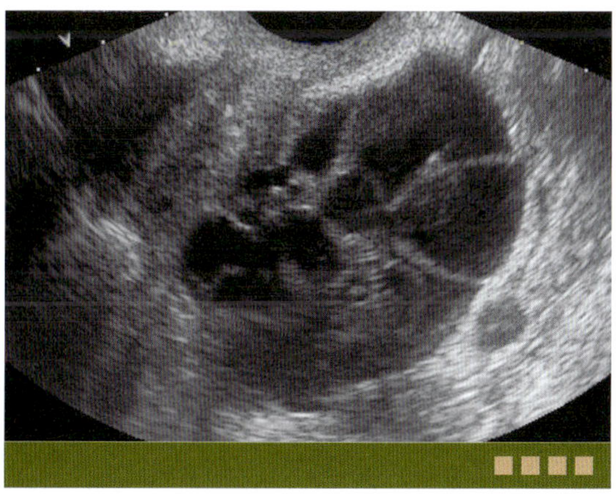

D. Transverse transvaginal sonogram on another patient with an ovarian cystadenofibroma shows a complex cystic adnexal mass with numerous thickened septations, and areas of nodularity and solid portions.

DIFFERENTIAL DIAGNOSIS IMAGES (E-G)

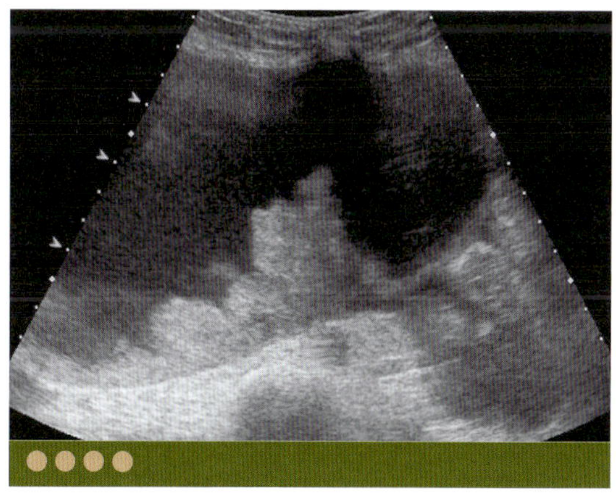

E. Serous cystadenocarcinoma of the ovary: Sagittal transabdominal sonogram shows a large mixed cystic and solid right ovarian mass. The lesion had a large solid component. It was a serous cystadenocarcinoma on pathology, but a cystadenofibroma might have an identical appearance.

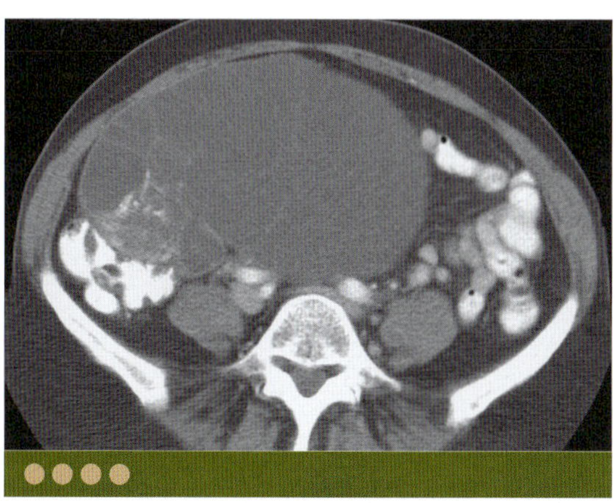

F. Mucinous cystadenocarcinoma of the ovary: Axial CECT on a different patient shows a predominantly cystic mass with septations, areas of soft-tissue nodularity and calcification in its right lateral aspect.

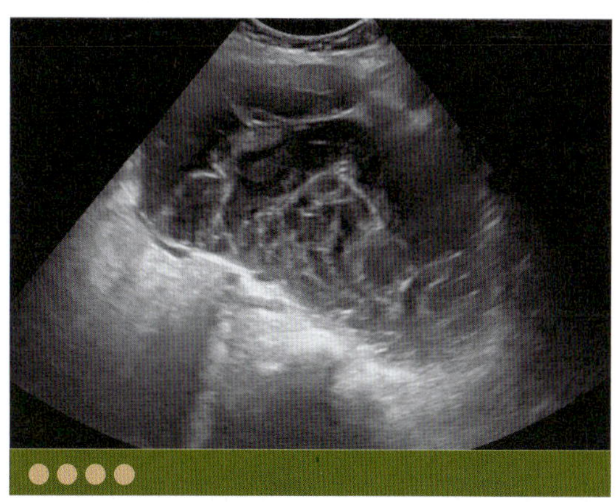

G. Mucinous cystadenocarcinoma of the ovary: Sagittal transabdominal sonogram on the same patient shows the septations and areas of nodularity within the mass.

IMAGE KEY

Common

Rare

Typical

Unusual

16–38 Ovarian Lymphoma

Paul Nikolaidis

PRESENTATION

Fatigue, fever, bilateral adnexal masses.

FINDINGS

CT shows bilateral solid enhancing adnexal masses in a patient with a history of non-Hodgkin lymphoma.

DIFFERENTIAL DIAGNOSES

- *Ovarian metastases*: Metastases are unilateral or bilateral masses with cystic and mixed cystic or solid components. Lymphoma is more typically bilateral and solid.
- *Ovarian cancer*: Especially if predominantly solid and/or with metastasis to the contralateral ovary. Unilateral solid lesions are more likely to be primary neoplasms.

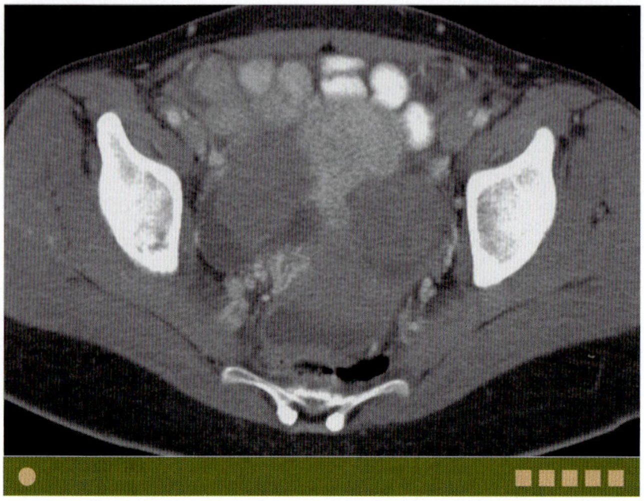

A. Axial CECT on a patient with Hodgkin lymphoma shows bilateral solid adnexal lesions. Both adnexal lesions were new since a prior study conducted 3 months ago.

COMMENTS

Lymphomas are a malignancy of lymphoid cell origin. Their presentation, manifestations, and prognosis largely depend on histologic subtype and stage. Staging of lymphoma depends on the extent of disease and nodal involvement.

Primary ovarian lymphoma is exceedingly rare. Involvement of the ovary is usually part of a more widespread disease process. Although tumor sizes may vary, lesions can get quite large, often exceeding 15 cm. In most patients, these tumors are solid and bilateral. At histologic examination, lymphoma involving the ovary is more typically non-Hodgkins and large cell type in older adults, and small non-cleaved cell type in children and young adults.

CT and MR are often vital in evaluating all ovarian neoplasms, and in cases of lymphoma, they are important for surveying the remainder of the chest, abdomen, and pelvis for additional sites of involvement. CT is excellent for diagnosing and staging lymphoma. On CT, ovarian lymphomas are homogeneously enhancing bilateral solid masses with well-defined margins.

On MR, ovarian lymphomas are well-circumscribed solid ovarian masses. The signal intensity of the mass is usually uniformly low on T1-WI and mildly hyperintense on T2-WI. Lesions show mild-to-moderate contrast enhancement following intravenous gadolinium administration.

PEARLS

- **Primary ovarian lymphoma is exceedingly rare.**
- **Typically bilateral well-circumscribed solid lesions.**
- **On CT and MR, they show mild-to-moderate contrast enhancement.**
- **On MR, lesions are usually uniformly low signal on T1-WI and mildly hyperintense on T2-WI.**

ADDITIONAL IMAGES (B-D)

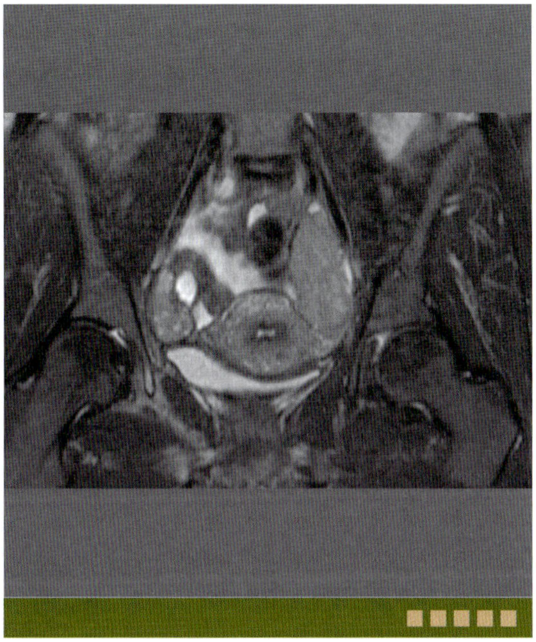

B. Coronal T2-WI on the same patient shows bilateral solid adnexal lesions. A small ovarian follicle is also seen on the right.

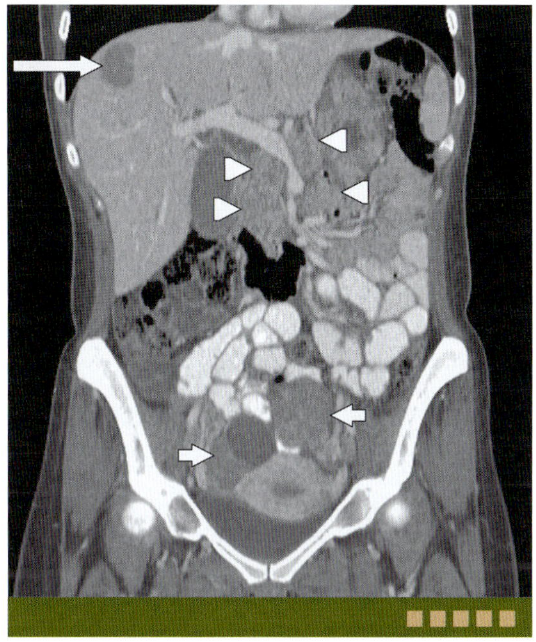

C. Coronal CECT reformation on the same patient nicely depicts both solid adnexal lesions (arrows). It also shows additional sites of involvement by lymphoma. There is extensive mesenteric and periportal lymphadenopathy (arrowheads), along with a solid liver lesion (long arrow) also representing lymphoma.

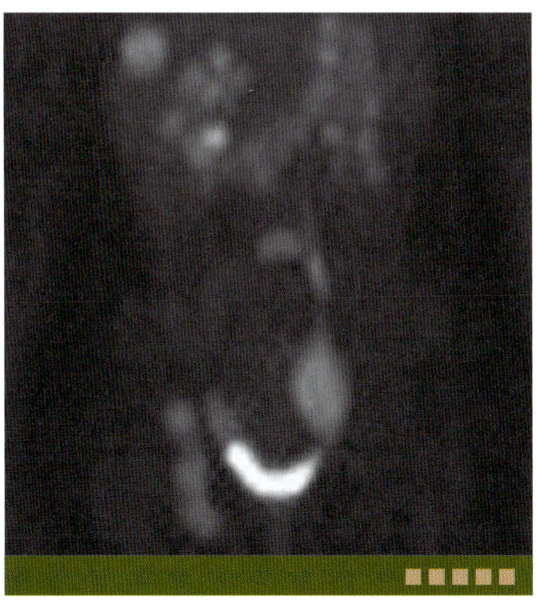

D. PET scan on the same patient shows multiple areas of increased metabolic activity in the abdomen and pelvis, including bilateral adnexal, hepatic, and renal lesions along with abdominal lymphadenopathy.

DIFFERENTIAL DIAGNOSES IMAGE

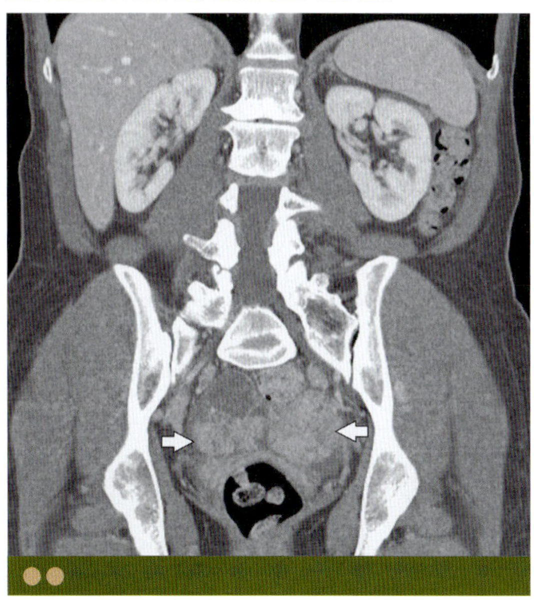

E. Ovarian metastases: Coronal CECT reformation on a patient with history of primary gastric adenocarcinoma shows bilateral predominantly solid adnexal lesions representing metastases (arrows).

IMAGE KEY

Common

Rare

Typical

Unusual

16–39 Ovarian Metastasis

Paul Nikolaidis

PRESENTATION

Pelvic/adnexal mass; asymptomatic.

FINDINGS

Sonography shows bilateral adnexal masses in a patient with a known primary malignancy.

DIFFERENTIAL DIAGNOSES

- *Primary ovarian cancer with contralateral metastasis*: Often difficult to distinguish, although in some cases the primary lesion may be larger.
- *Ovarian lymphoma*: Often difficult to distinguish without the clinical history. Bilateral solid ovarian masses with well-defined margins that show mild-to-moderate contrast enhancement are typically seen.

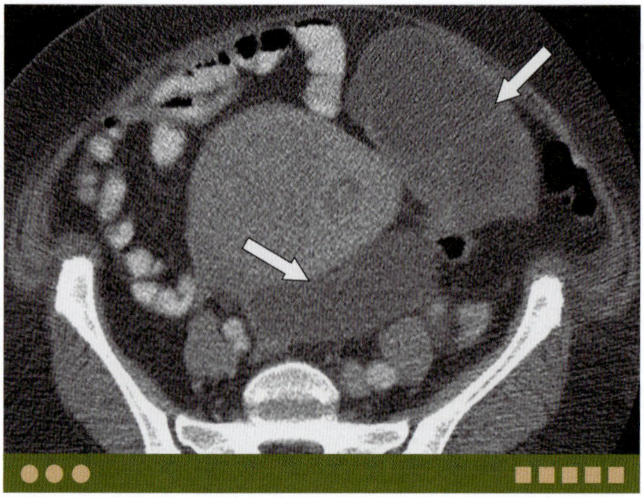

A. Axial CECT on a patient with history of primary colonic adenocarcinoma shows bilateral complex cystic adnexal lesions representing metastases (arrows). Metastases from colon cancer are typically cystic.

COMMENTS

Approximately 5% to 15% of malignant ovarian tumors are metastases. The most common primary malignancies to metastasize to the ovary are: colon and stomach (most common), pancreas, breast, lung, endometrial cancer, and carcinoma of the contralateral ovary. Although metastases may be unilateral (endometrial cancer in particular), metastatic ovarian lesions are typically bilateral (75%).

Ovarian metastases in premenopausal women may be more common secondary to the higher vascularity of the ovaries in younger females. It is important to differentiate primary ovarian cancer from a metastasis, in terms of prognosis and treatment. Imaging studies are important for surveying the remainder of the chest, abdomen, and pelvis for additional sites of involvement.

On imaging, metastatic ovarian lesions are usually nonspecific unilateral or bilateral masses. They are more typically cystic or mixed cystic and solid. There are no specific features to differentiate ovarian metastases from most primary ovarian neoplasms. Krukenberg tumors (signet ring cell metastases from the GI tract) may have a more specific appearance. They are typically bilateral oval masses that are predominantly solid, but may have large cystic or necrotic areas; colon cancer metastases are typically cystic.

On MR, a specific finding for Krukenberg tumors on T2-WI is peripheral or randomly distributed low-signal intensity, which corresponds histopathologically to dense collagenous stroma. Other findings on imaging may include areas of T2-hyperintensity (given the presence of mucin or central necrosis). Iso- or hypointense solid elements may be seen on T1-WI, likely related to dense stromal tissue.

PEARLS

- **Between 5% to 15% of ovarian malignancies are metastatic lesions.**
- **Most metastases are bilateral cystic and mixed cystic and solid lesions.**
- **Metastases from the GI tract are known as Krukenberg tumors.**

ADDITIONAL IMAGES (B-D)

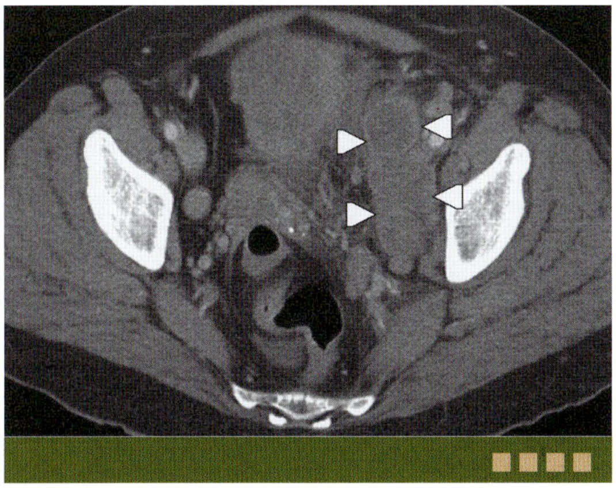

B. Axial CECT on a patient with a large uterine mass representing endometrial stromal sarcoma shows a large complex left adnexal lesion representing metastasis to the ovary (arrowheads).

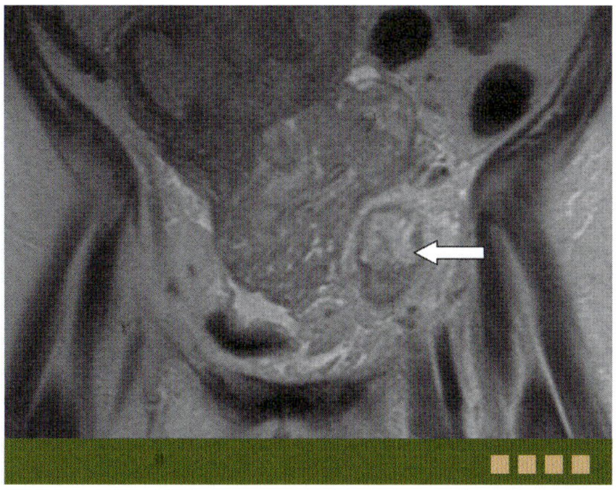

C. Coronal T2-WI on the same patient shows portion of the large uterine mass and the left ovarian metastasis (arrow).

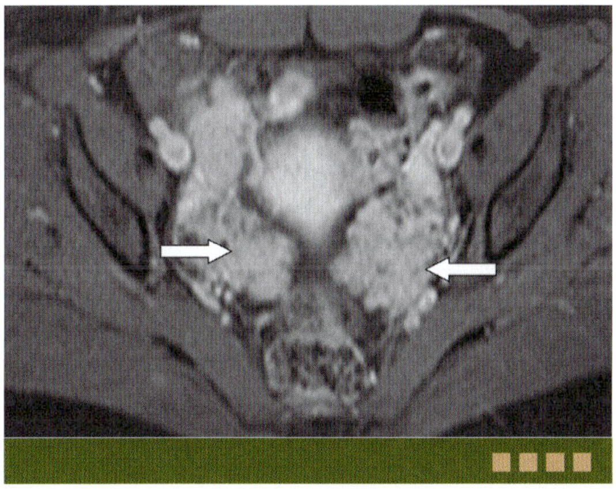

D. Axial postcontrast T1-WI on a patient with breast carcinoma shows bilateral solid adnexal lesions representing metastases (arrows). In some instances, ovarian metastases may be predominantly (or entirely) solid.

DIFFERENTIAL DIAGNOSES IMAGES (E-G)

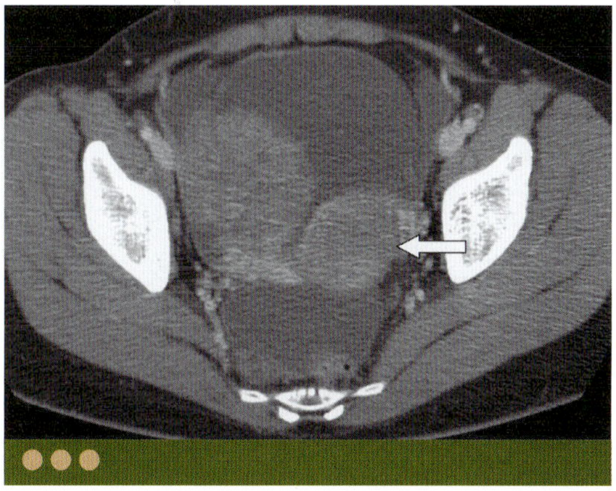

E. Primary ovarian carcinoma with contralateral metastasis: Axial CECT on a patient with a large right primary carcinoma of the ovary shows a solid left ovarian lesion representing a metastasis (arrow).

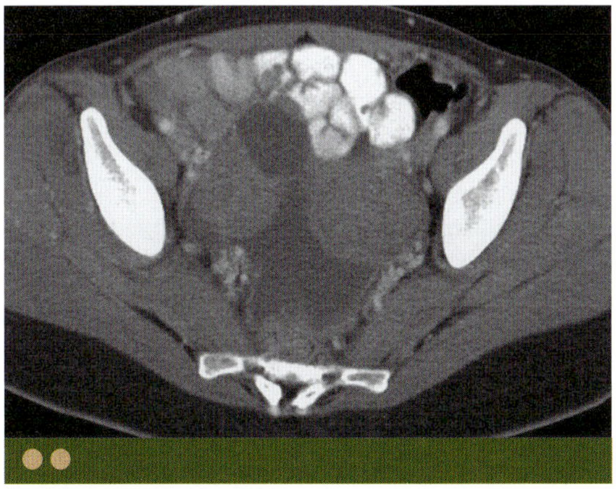

F. Ovarian lymphoma: Axial CECT on a patient with Hodgkin lymphoma shows bilateral solid adnexal lesions. The left ovarian lesion is larger. A small cystic lesion also arises from the right adnexa.

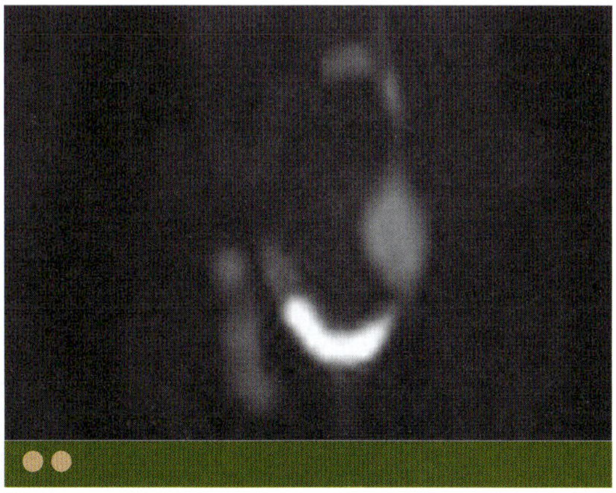

G. Ovarian lymphoma: Coronal PET scan on the same patient shows areas of increased metabolic activity corresponding to both solid ovarian lesions.

IMAGE KEY

Common

●●●●●
●●●●
●●●
●●
●

Rare

Typical

■■■■■
■■■■
■■■
■■
■

Unusual

16–40 Polycystic Ovarian Syndrome

Nancy A. Hammond

PRESENTATION

Amenorrhea.

FINDINGS

Enlarged ovaries with multiple, peripheral, small cysts.

DIFFERENTIAL DIAGNOSES

- *Ovarian torsion*: Enlarged ovary with multiple cortical follicles, usually unilateral, intraovarian flow may or may not be present, typically patient presents with acute abdomen.
- *Multifollicular ovaries*: Seen in mid to late normal puberty, demonstrates fewer cysts that are typically larger than Polycystic ovaries (PCO) and distributed diffusely throughout the ovary, no stromal hypertrophy.

COMMENTS

Polycystic ovarian syndrome (PCOS) is a complex endocrinologic disorder resulting in chronic anovulation. It was originally described in 1935 by Stein and Leventhal with the classic presentation including amenorrhea, infertility, hirsutism, and enlarged polycystic ovaries. It is now known that multiple clinical presentations exist for PCOS. Clinically, features of hyperandrogenism are the most consistent finding but manifestations of unopposed estrogen stimulation can also be present. The pathophysiology of PCOS is complex but includes failure of the normal cyclical changes in follicle-stimulating hormone (FSH) and luteinizing hormone (LH). The LH/FSH level is persistently elevated resulting in chronically stimulated and unruptured follicles. PCOS is most commonly diagnosed with laboratory studies with the initial evaluation including serum values of TSH, FSH, LH, and prolactin.

Polycystic ovaries is seen in approximately 3% to 7% of women worldwide and has been reported in up to 50% of women presenting to infertility clinics. Women present with infertility, amenorrhea, or irregular menses in their 20s or 30s. Alternatively, women present with signs of hyperandrogenism including hirsutism, acne, or male-pattern baldness.

Radiographic studies are used in patients with equivocal laboratory findings. Pelvic ultrasound is the imaging study of choice. The initial criteria for ultrasound diagnosis utilized a transabdominal approach. PCO was characterized as the presence of 10 or more cysts measuring 2 to 18 mm in diameter arranged peripherally around an increased amount of central ovarian stroma creating the "pearl necklace" appearance. Less commonly, multiple small cysts 2 to 4 mm in diameter distributed throughout abundant stroma may be present. PCO findings were later modified based on the advent of TVUS and the ability to image at a higher resolution. PCO based on TVUS is characterized as at least 15 cysts of 2 to 10 mm in diameter arranged around echogenic prominent stroma. Increased ovarian volume as a criterion has lessened in importance because several groups have demonstrated normal ovarian volumes in a larger percentage of patients presenting with PCOS. On MRI, multiple peripheral cysts are seen in both ovaries. The cysts are hypointense on T1-weighted sequences and hyperintense on T2-weighted sequences. The central ovarian tissue is low signal on both T1- and T2-weighted sequences and can enhance with contrast administration. The uterus can be hypoplastic but normal zonal anatomy is typically preserved. Additional features of PCO that have been described include increased ovarian volume, increased roundness index (ovarian width/ovarian length ratio) and decreased uterine width to ovarian length ratio. While the above radiographic findings in the ovaries are seen in 90% of women with PCOS, it should be noted that they are also seen in 25% of women without PCOS.

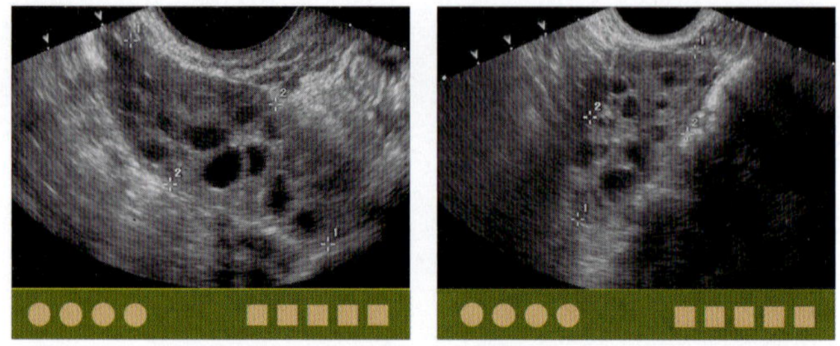

A. and **B.** Longitudinal TVUS shows bilateral ovarian enlargement. Both ovaries show multiple small cysts that are predominantly peripheral in location. This patient had laboratory proven diagnosis of PCOS.

PEARLS

- **PCOS is common in women of reproductive age presenting most commonly with infertility, menstrual irregularity, and/or signs of androgen excess.**
- **The radiographic findings of polycystic ovaries are not diagnostic of PCOS. Findings should be correlated with clinical and laboratory data.**
- **Multiple peripherally located cysts are present radiographically with central echogenic stroma on ultrasound and central low signal stroma on both T1-WI and T2-WI sequences.**

ADDITIONAL IMAGES (C-D)

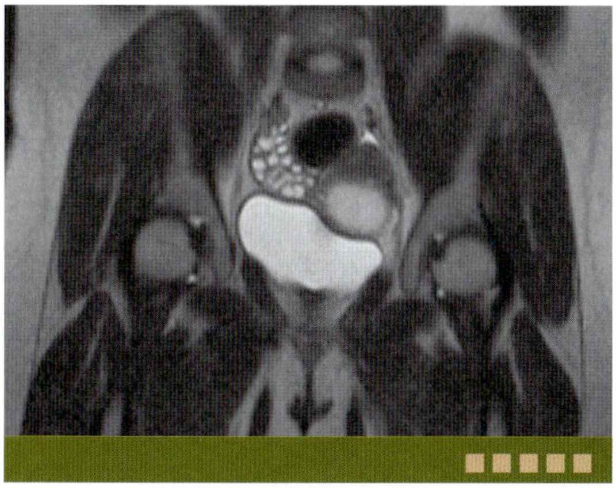

C. Coronal T2-WI shows a prominent right ovary with multiple, small peripheral cysts.

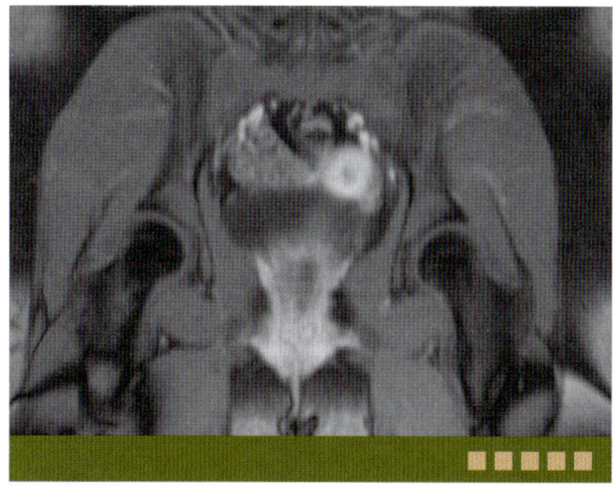

D. Coronal contrast-enhanced T1-WI in the same patient as Figure C further shows the enlarged right ovary with multiple small peripheral cysts.

DIFFERENTIAL DIAGNOSIS IMAGES (E-F)

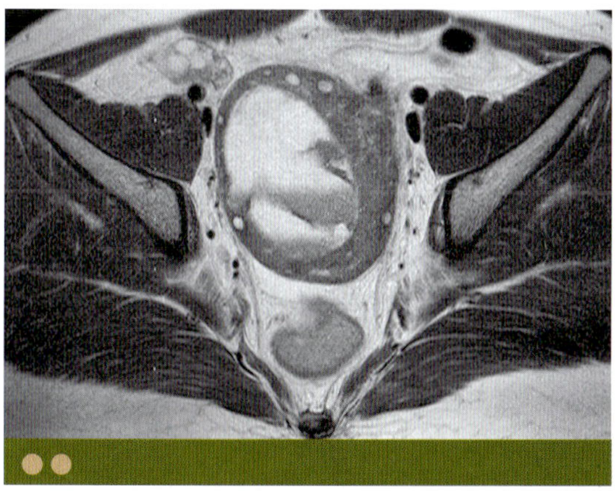

E. Ovarian torsion: Axial T2-WI in a patient presenting with right lower quadrant pain shows an enlarged left ovary with a complex cystic mass located centrally. Smaller cystic foci are present at the peripheral aspect of the ovary. Note the normal appearing right ovary located more anteriorly.

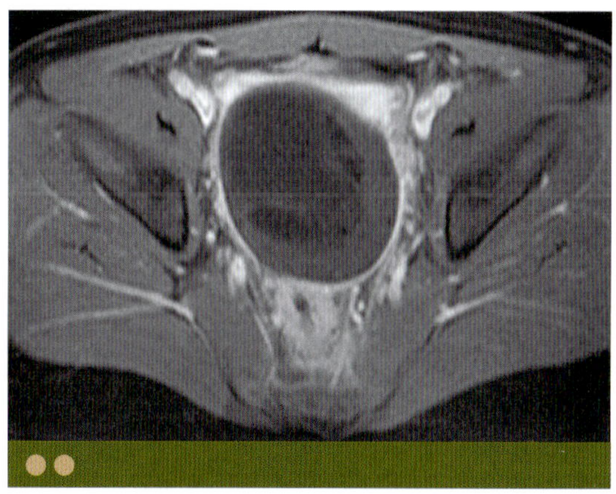

F. Ovarian torsion: Axial contrast-enhanced T1-WI in the same patient as Figure E shows the complex mass involving the left ovary with lack of enhancement of the ovarian parenchyma.

IMAGE KEY

Common

Rare

Typical

Unusual

16–41 Paraovarian Cyst

Nancy A. Hammond

PRESENTATION

Palpable pelvic mass on routine physical examination.

FINDINGS

Large cystic mass separate from the ovary.

DIFFERENTIAL DIAGNOSES

- *Ovarian cyst*: Cystic mass associated with the ovary.
- *Ovarian cystic neoplasm*: Complex cystic mass associated with the ovary.

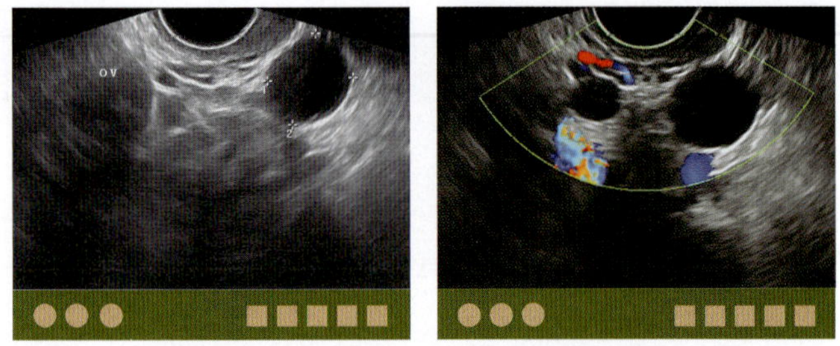

A. Longitudinal transvaginal sonogram shows a 2.0-cm cystic mass in the right adnexal region that appears to be separate from the right ovary
B. Longitudinal transvaginal Doppler image shows lack of flow to this cystic mass. A separate smaller cyst is seen associated with the right ovary and most consistent with a functional cyst in this premenopausal woman.

COMMENTS

Paraovarian or paratubal cysts are not ovarian masses but arise from mesothelial, paramesonephric (müllerian), or mesonephric (wolffian) structures and are located adjacent to the ovaries. They account for approximately 10% to 20% of adnexal masses and are typically seen in women aged 30 to 40 years. They most commonly originate from the hydatid of Morgagni which is a derivative of the paramesonephric ducts located in the broad ligament adjacent to the fimbrial end of the fallopian tube. As such, they usually occur in the mesosalpinx between the ovary and fallopian tube. Grossly, the cyst is thin walled and contains serous fluid. Clinically, most paraovarian cysts are small and asymptomatic. Complications may occur with larger cysts including torsion or internal hemorrhage. The rate of malignant degeneration is estimated to be approximately 2%.

Sonographically, paraovarian cysts appear as thin-walled, unilocular, anechoic masses. If complicated by hemorrhage, the fluid may appear complex. A separate normal ovary should be identified. On CT, simple paraovarian cysts are thin-walled hypodense masses demonstrating attenuation values compatible with simple fluid. MRI demonstrates a T1-hypointense, T2-hyperintense, nonenhancing mass located adjacent to the ovary within the broad ligament. If complicated by hemorrhage, the mass appears as T1 hyperintense. On all imaging modalities, a separate normal ovary should be identified to exclude an ovarian cystic neoplasm. Although uncommon, the presence of mural proliferation or papillary projections suggests malignant or borderline malignant tumors.

Treatment ranges from conservative to surgical management depending on the clinical presentation and imaging features of the cyst.

PEARLS

- **Account for 10% to 20% of all adnexal masses and are usually seen in women between 30 to 40 years of age.**
- **Typically asymptomatic but can hemorrhage or undergo torsion when large.**
- **Appear as simple, unilocular cystic masses that are clearly distinguishable from the adjacent ovary.**

ADDITIONAL IMAGES (C-E)

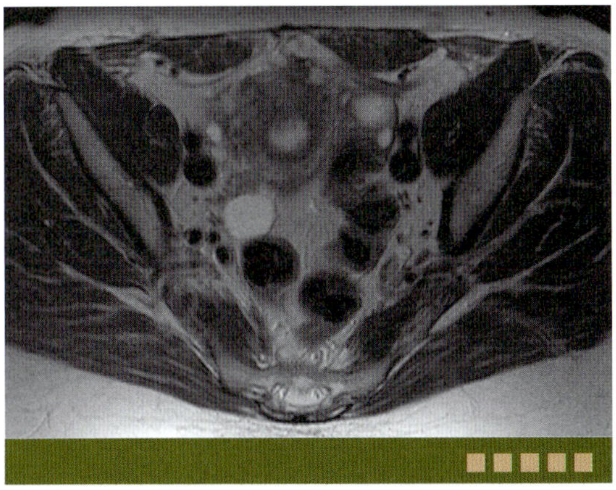

C. Axial T2-WI in the same patient as Figure A and B confirms the cystic nature of the mass in the right hemipelvis. No enhancement was seen on contrast-enhanced sequences (not shown).

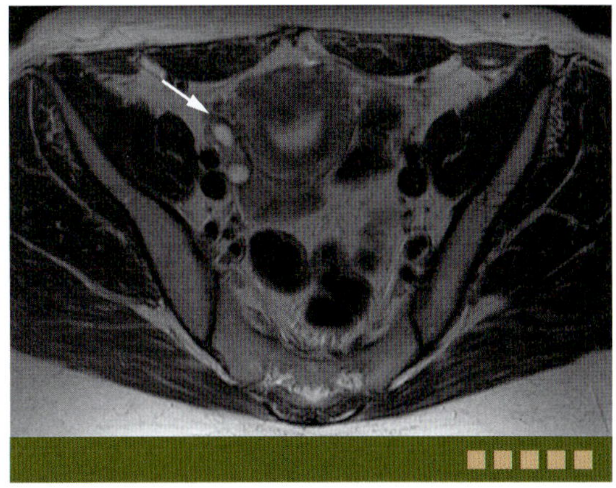

D. Axial T2-WI in the same patient confirms the presence of the right ovary more anteriorly in the pelvis (arrow).

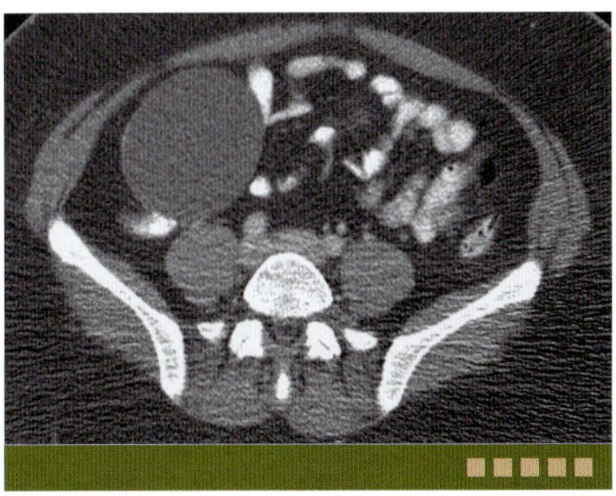

E. Axial CECT shows a hypodense mass in the right hemipelvis that was separate from the more inferiorly located right ovary.

DIFFERENTIAL DIAGNOSES IMAGES (F-G)

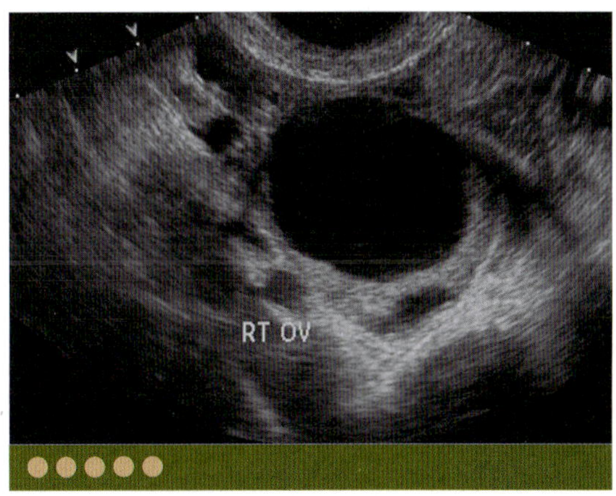

F. Functional ovarian cyst: Longitudinal transvaginal sonogram shows a simple appearing cyst clearly arising from the right ovary.

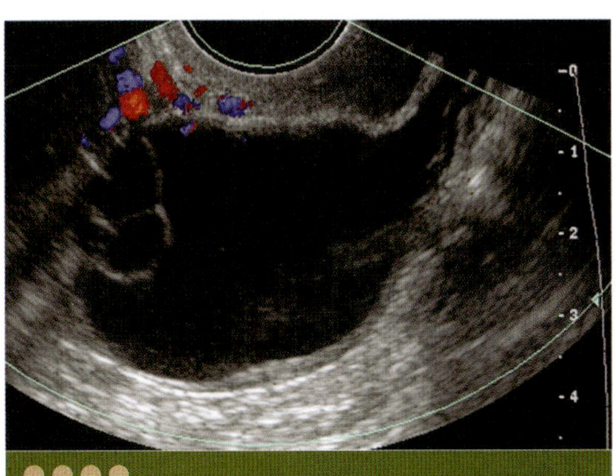

G. Cystic ovarian neoplasm: Longitudinal transvaginal sonogram shows a complex cystic adnexal mass with internal septations and mild mural nodularity. This was pathologically proven to represent a mucinous cystadenoma.

IMAGE KEY

Common

Rare

Typical

Unusual

16–42 Peritoneal Inclusion Cyst

Paul Nikolaidis

PRESENTATION

Cystic adnexal mass, pelvic mass/fullness if large, often asymptomatic.

FINDINGS

T2-WI MR shows a large multiloculated cystic lesion in the pelvis, surrounding the uterus and left ovary.

DIFFERENTIAL DIAGNOSES

- *Ovarian cystadenoma/cystadenocarcinoma*: Unlike peritoneal inclusion cysts, cystic ovarian neoplasms should not loculate or conform to their surrounding structures; they usually displace them.
- *Hydrosalpinx*: Usually have a characteristic folded tubular appearance with incomplete septations and plicae that appear as a mural nodule in one plane and a ridge in the perpendicular plane.
- *Lymphocele*: These also occur in patients with a history of pelvic surgery and may be difficult to distinguish; peritoneal inclusion cysts are usually larger and more likely to extend medially or surround the ovary.
- *Pelvic ascites*: Usually accumulates in the cul de sac; typically will not have a loculated appearance.

COMMENTS

Peritoneal inclusion cysts are also referred to in the medical literature as benign cystic mesothelioma, peritoneal pseudocysts, inflammatory cysts of the peritoneum, and multilocular peritoneal inclusion cysts.

They are collections of physiologic ovarian fluid that accumulate between peritoneal adhesions that may form caused by surgery, trauma, and inflammatory gynecological conditions, including endometriosis and pelvic inflammatory disease. Normally physiologic fluid from the ovary is resorbed by the peritoneum. In the setting of adhesions and peritoneal inflammation, this resorption is impaired, leading to the accumulation of fluid in potential spaces created by adhesions.

On transvaginal sonography, the most common finding is an ovary surrounded by septations and fluid. In cases of severe peritoneal adhesive disease, more irregular and thickened septations may be seen, making differentiation from cystic ovarian masses and tubo-ovarian abscess more difficult.

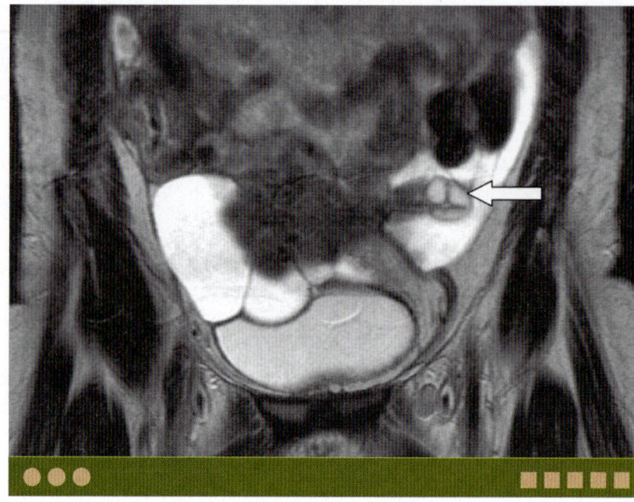

A. Coronal T2-WI shows a large multiloculated fluid intensity lesion occupying a significant portion of the pelvis. It surrounds the uterus and left ovary (arrow).

In many instances, MR is helpful, given its larger field-of-view and improved resolution. Peritoneal inclusion cysts are generally low signal on T1-WI and high on T2-WI. The signal intensity of fluid may vary depending on exact fluid composition; hemorrhagic or proteinaceous fluid may show higher signal intensity on T1-WI. Septations of varying thickness, usually thin, are present. A unique characteristic of peritoneal inclusion cysts is their tendency to loculate and conform to surrounding structures, rather than displace them. Larger lesions may exert mild mass effect.

Peritoneal inclusion cysts are unlikely to cause significant symptoms and therefore surgical management is usually not necessary.

PEARLS

- **Peritoneal inclusion cysts are collections of physiologic ovarian fluid that accumulate between peritoneal adhesions.**
- **Fluid tends to loculate and should conform to surrounding structures, rather than displace them.**
- **On MR, they typically are low signal on T1-WI and high signal on T2-WI.**
- **High signal on T1-WI may result from hemorrhagic or proteinaceous contents.**

ADDITIONAL IMAGES (B-D)

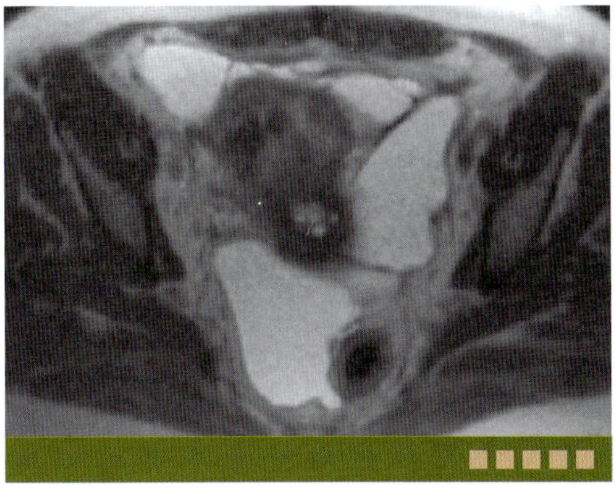

B. Axial T2-WI on the same patient shows the large peritoneal inclusion cyst. Note the numerous septations and how the locules of fluid seem to conform around the surrounding structures.

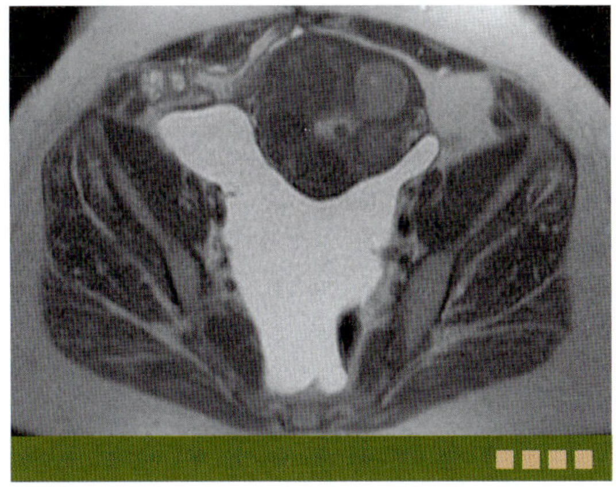

C. Axial T2-WI on another patient with a history of prior gynecologic surgeries shows a large anechoic fluid signal intensity structure with only few incomplete septations.

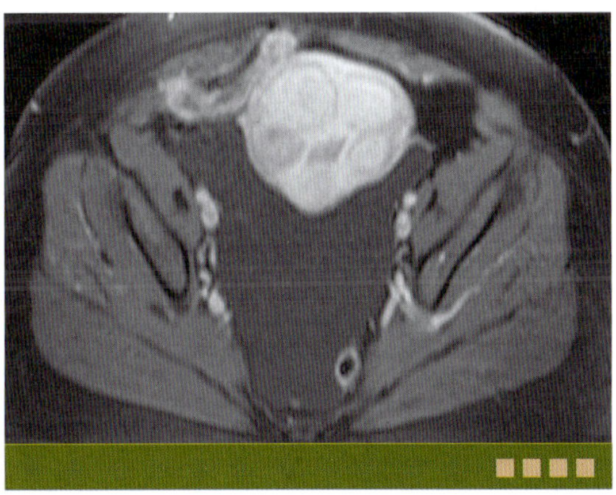

D. Axial contrast-enhanced T1-WI on the same patient shows that there are no enhancing components.

DIFFERENTIAL DIAGNOSES IMAGES (E-G)

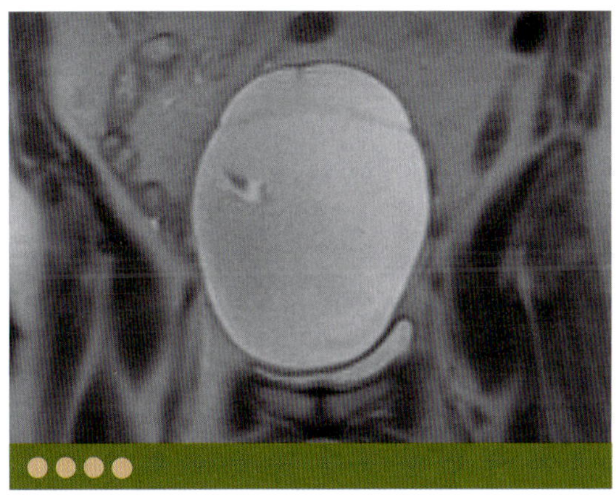

E. Ovarian cystadenocarcinoma: Coronal T2-WI shows a large, round hyperintense ovarian lesion with a few septations. This lesion exerted mass effect on surrounding structures, rather than conforming to them.

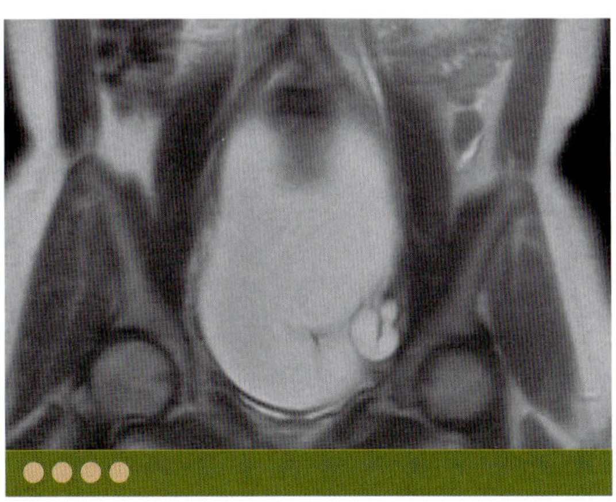

F. Hydrosalpinx: Coronal T2-WI shows a large cystic structure with a characteristic folded tubular appearance.

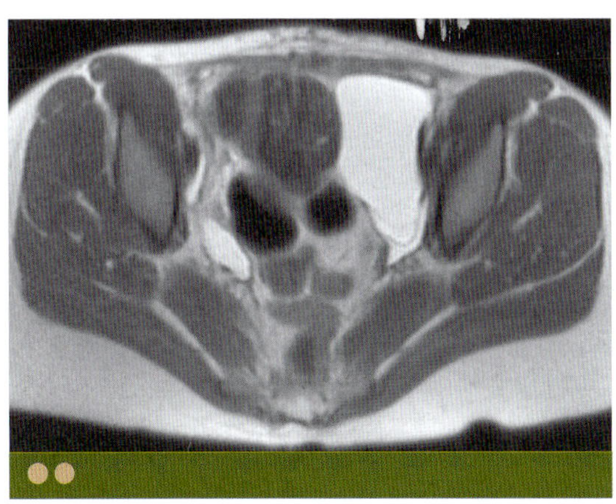

G. Lymphoceles: Axial T2-WI shows bilateral pelvic fluid intensity structures in a patient with prior external iliac lymph node dissection. Aspiration revealed lymphatic fluid.

IMAGE KEY

Common

Rare

Typical

Unusual

16–43 Ovarian Torsion

Paul Nikolaidis

PRESENTATION

Sudden onset of severe pain, pelvic mass.

FINDINGS

Pelvic sonography shows unilateral ovarian enlargement. Intraovarian vascular flow was absent.

DIFFERENTIAL DIAGNOSES

- *Ovarian neoplasm without torsion*: Most cases of torsion in adults occur in patients with ovarian masses. Ovarian masses without associated torsion should be differentiated by the preserved (and often increased) vascular flow and the lack of acute symptoms.
- *Polycystic Ovarian Syndrome*: Ovarian enlargement along with numerous peripherally displaced follicles is seen in PCOS. Color flow is preserved and the clinical presentation allows for differentiation from torsion.

COMMENTS

Ovarian torsion occurs when the ovary rotates around its axis on the structures that support it (the ovarian vessels and ligaments) resulting in arterial, venous and lymphatic obstruction. Patients typically present with acute lower abdominal pain or a unilateral abdominal/pelvic mass. Causes include the presence of a lead mass such as an ovarian tumor or cyst, but it may occur in a normal ovary especially in the pediatric population.

Ultrasound findings in ovarian torsion include unilateral ovarian enlargement. The affected ovary usually contains several uniform sized (8-12 mm) small immature follicles along its periphery. Free pelvic fluid is often present.

Findings on color Doppler ultrasound may vary. Initially, intra-ovarian venous flow may be absent, followed by arterial flow. Residual arterial and venous flow has been present in surgically proven cases of torsion. Flow within the adnexal vessels may be preserved. In few cases, the twisted pedicle of the torsed ovary may be recognized, a specific sign for ovarian torsion. In chronic torsion, arterial waveforms can mimic venous waveforms. When torsion is complete, no arterial waveforms should be detected.

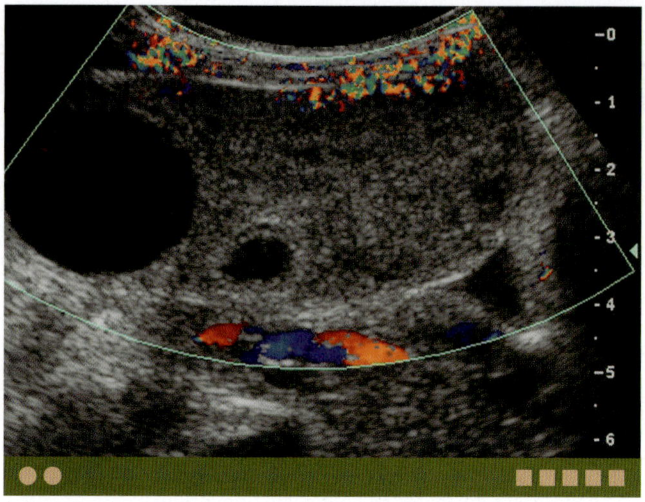

A. Longitudinal sonogram shows an enlarged ovary measuring approximately 7 cm with a dominant cyst/follicle and a few smaller peripherally located follicles. There was no internal flow on color Doppler examination.

CT and MR imaging findings include: unilateral ovarian enlargement, fallopian tube thickening, ascites, uterine deviation toward the involved side, engorgement of the vessels on the affected side, and hemorrhage. Tubal thickening may be present (>10 mm); this is a specific finding in torsion. Smooth thickening of the wall of the adnexal mass is thought to be secondary to edema and congestion. It is generally eccentric with a diameter greater than 10 mm, when associated with hemorrhagic infarction. Hemorrhage into the adnexal mass, fallopian tube, or peritoneum can also occur.

Early diagnosis is imperative, as it may result in vascular compromise of the ovary. Surgery is often required.

PEARLS

- **An ipsilateral lead mass is present in 50% to 80% of cases of adult patients.**
- **Pediatric patients usually do not have a lead mass.**
- **Sonographic features include ovarian enlargement with several prominent peripheral immature follicles.**
- **On Doppler, venous flow is initially absent, followed by arterial flow.**

ADDITIONAL IMAGES (B-E)

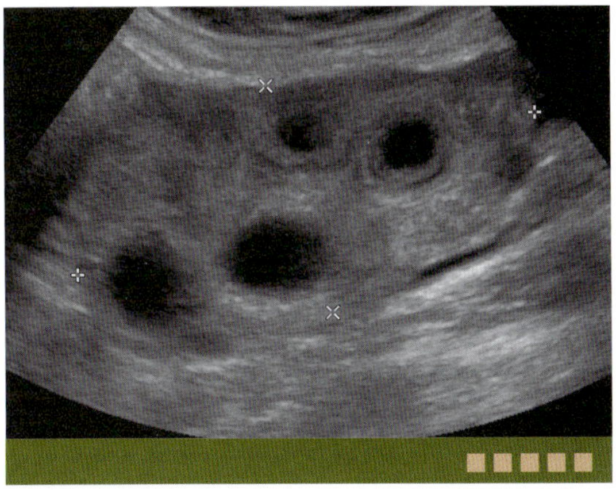

B. Longitudinal sonogram in another patient shows an enlarged right ovary, measuring 9 cm, with numerous prominent follicles/cysts.

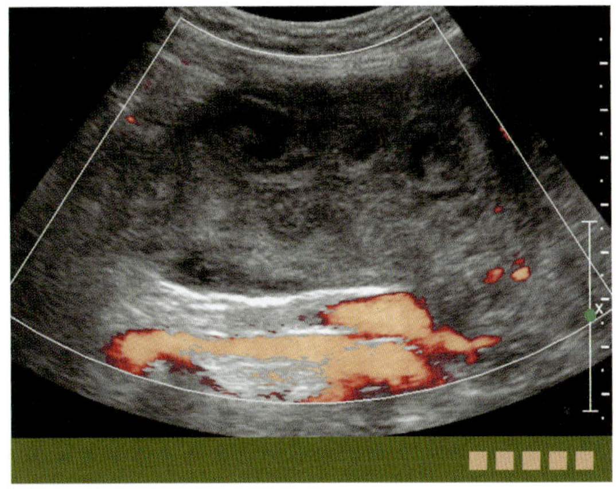

C. Sagittal power Doppler sonogram on the same patient shows no evidence of flow within the abnormally enlarged ovary.

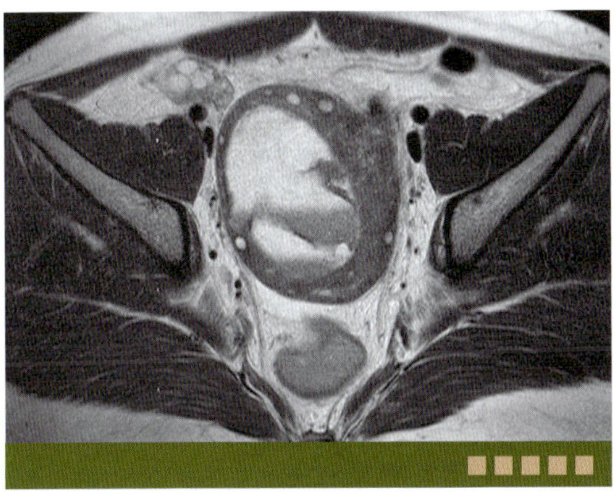

D. Axial T2-WI on a 16-year-old patient with a 3-day history of sharp pelvic pain shows an enlarged left ovary containing multiple small peripherally located follicles and a large central complex cystic lesion.

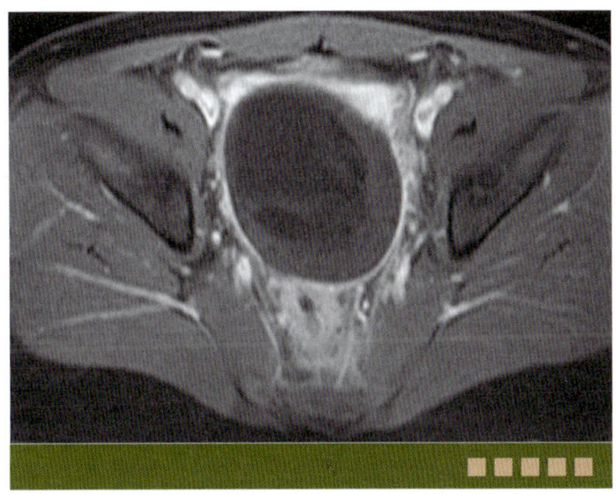

E. Axial contrast-enhanced fat-suppressed T1-WI shows complete lack of enhancement of the left ovarian mass.

DIFFERENTIAL DIAGNOSES IMAGES (F-G)

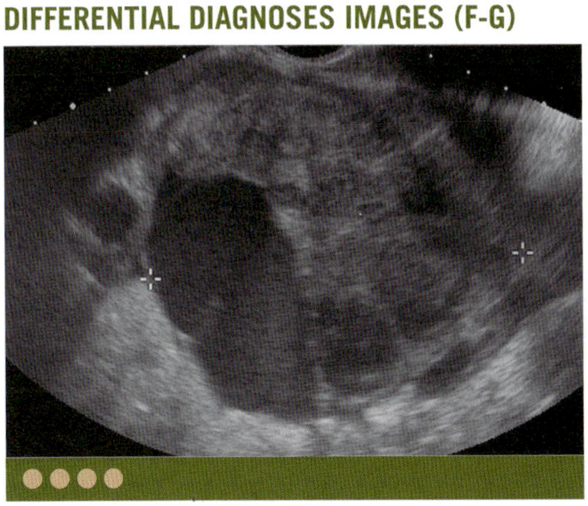

F. Ovarian carcinoma (without torsion): Transvaginal sonogram shows a 9-cm heterogeneous mass replacing the left ovary. There are large solid components. Note the absence of architectural features of a normal ovary, and the lack of any peripherally displaced prominent cysts/follicles, as can be seen in torsion.

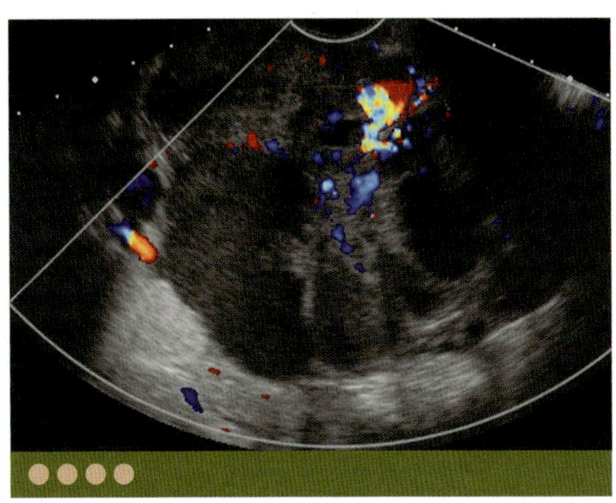

G. Ovarian carcinoma (without torsion): Corresponding color Doppler sonogram shows significant vascularity within the solid portions of this mass. The cystic components are avascular.

IMAGE KEY

Common

Rare

Typical

Unusual

16–44 Ovarian Vein Thrombosis

Nancy A. Hammond

PRESENTATION

Postpartum patient with pelvic pain and fever.

FINDINGS

Low-density tubular structure with rim enhancement in the expected location of the ovarian vein.

DIFFERENTIAL DIAGNOSIS

None

COMMENTS

Ovarian vein thrombosis (thrombophlebitis) is an uncommon disorder that is associated with a variety of conditions. Most commonly it is seen in the postpartum female but occurs in less than 1% of all pregnancies. Ovarian vein thrombosis occurs secondary to venous stasis and a hypercoagulable state and, therefore, is also associated with other hypercoaguable states including malignancy, Crohn disease, and the early postsurgical state. In the postpartum patient, it is commonly seen in patients with endometritis.

It affects the right ovarian vein 80% to 90% of the time but can be bilateral about 14% of the time. Clinically, it is usually seen on the second or third postpartum day with patients presenting with abdominal pain, fever, and an abdominal mass. Complications of ovarian vein thrombosis include sepsis, IVC thrombosis, pulmonary embolism (25%), and death (5%).

Ultrasound, CT, and MRI may be used for diagnosis. Ultrasound is often limited by poor visualization of the ovarian vein because of overlying bowel gas and its operator dependency. CT demonstrates a low-density, rim-enhancing tubular structure in the expected location of the ovarian vein. MRI demonstrates similar findings on gadolinium-enhanced T1 FS GRE sequences. T2-weighted sequences demonstrate loss of the normal signal void in the ovarian vein. There may be enlargement of the vein as a result of the acute thrombosis. It should be noted that ovarian vein thrombus can also be seen in patients who have undergone total abdominal hysterectomy with bilateral oopherectomy as an incidental finding.

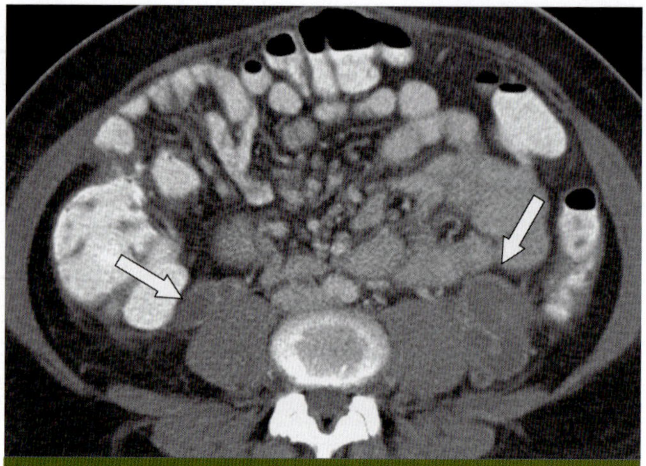

A. Axial CECT shows bilateral low-density, rim-enhancing structures adjacent to the psoas muscles (arrows) in this postpartum patient with fever.

Initial therapy for ovarian vein thrombosis consists of intravenous antibiotics and heparin. If resolution is not achieved, IVC filter or ligation of the involved vessel at the most proximal point of thrombosis should be considered.

PEARLS

- **Ovarian thrombosis is most commonly seen in the postpartum patient but be seen in other hypercoaguable states.**
- **Most commonly affects the right ovarian vein and is commonly associated with endometritis.**
- **CT demonstrates a rim-enhancing tubular structure along the course of the ovarian vein.**
- **Ultrasound diagnosis is frequently limited by overlying bowel gas.**

ADDITIONAL IMAGES (B-E)

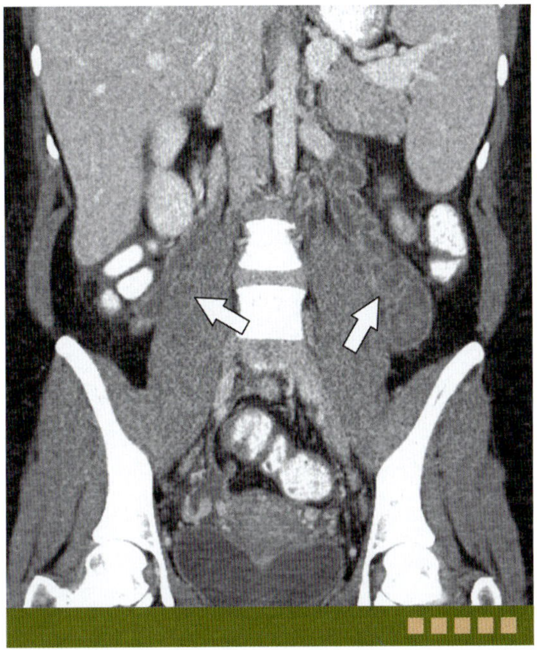

B. Coronal CECT in the same patient as Figure A shows elongation of these structures as they follow the expected course of the ovarian veins (arrows). The thrombosed, tortuous left ovarian vein is shown at its insertion into the left renal vein.

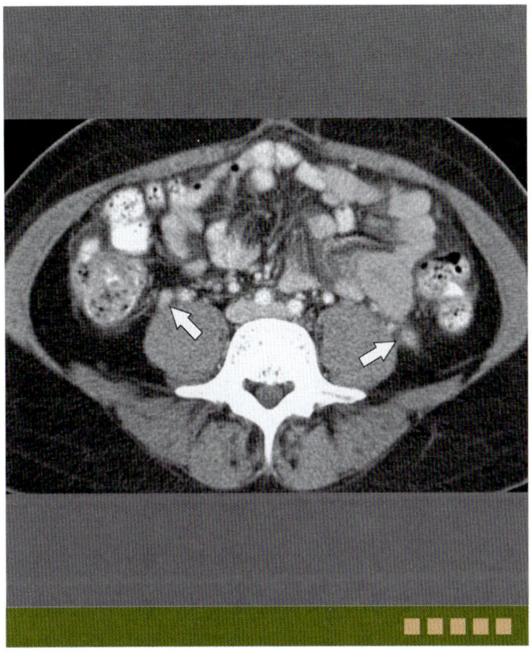

C. Axial CECT in the same patient performed three months after the initial study shows recanalization of both ovarian veins (arrows).

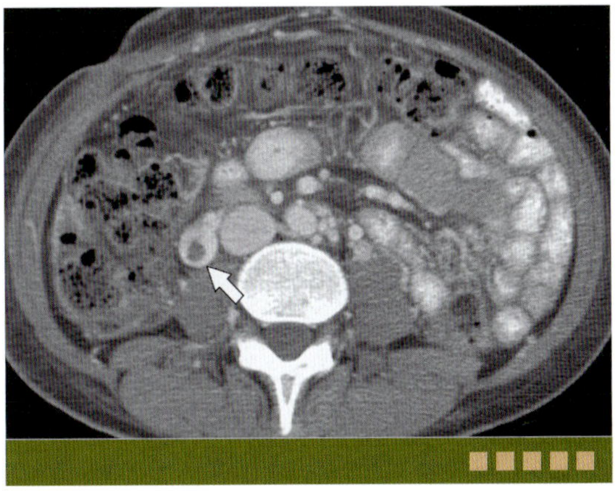

D. Axial CECT in a patient with a history of malignancy shows central low attenuation within the dilated right ovarian vein (arrow).

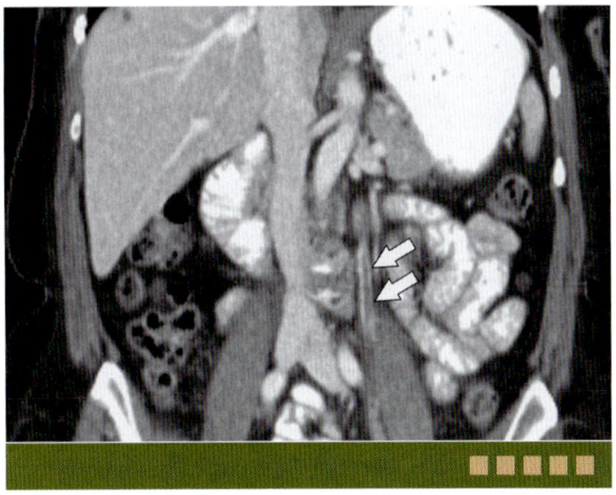

E. Coronal CECT shows thrombus in the left ovarian vein.

IMAGE KEY

Common

Rare

Typical

Unusual

Part 5

Fallopian Tube

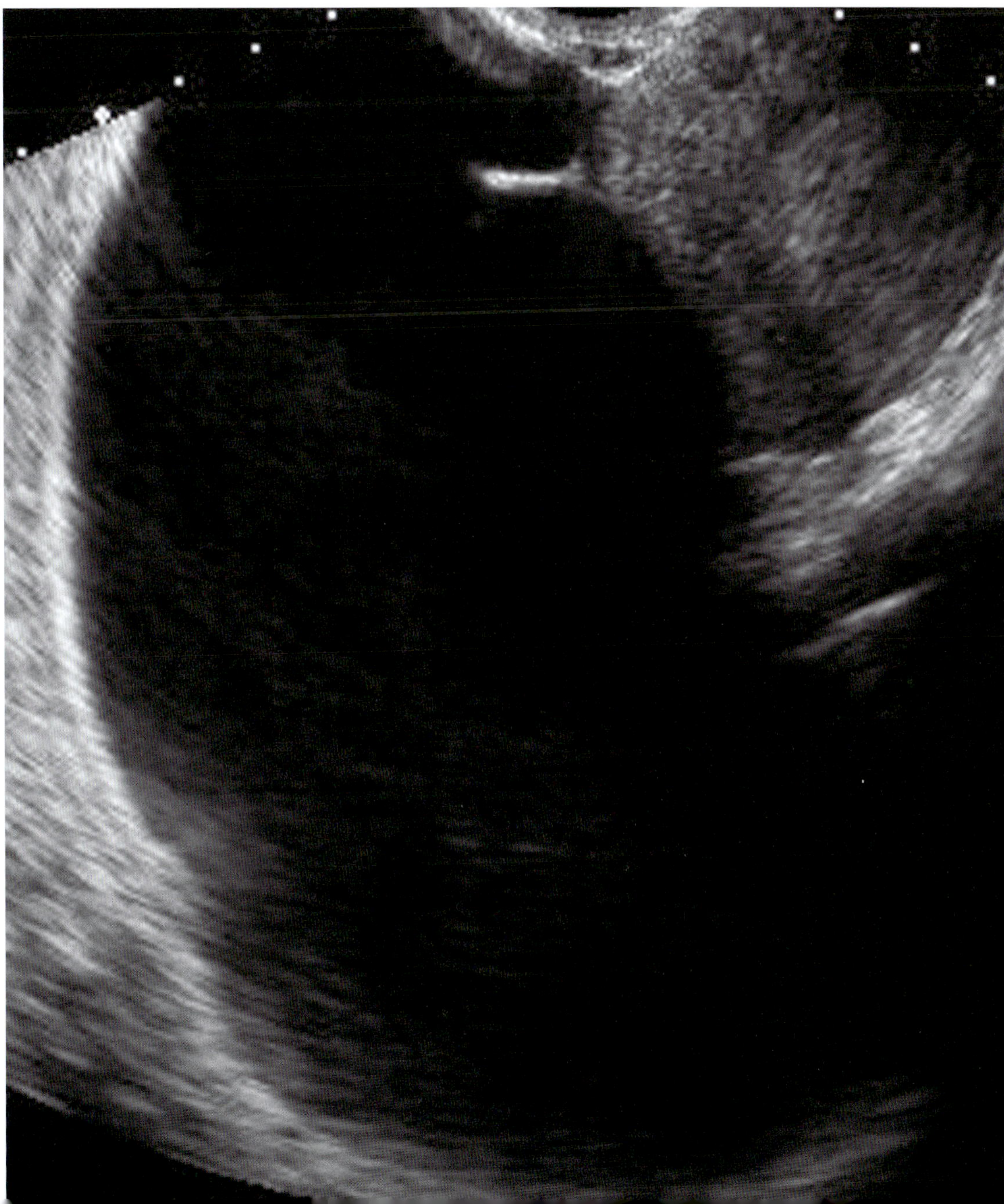

16–45 Fallopian Tube Carcinoma

Paul Nikolaidis

PRESENTATION

Vaginal bleeding, watery vaginal discharge, and pelvic mass.

FINDINGS

CT shows a complex left adnexal mass with a somewhat tubular appearance that contains both cystic and enhancing solid components.

DIFFERENTIAL DIAGNOSES

- *Tubo-ovarian abscess*: Appropriate clinical history and a thorough gynecologic examination are essential; patients with a fallopian tube neoplasm are also typically older. They may have vaginal bleeding, a watery vaginal discharge, or in cases of metastatic disease, a primary malignancy of the ovary or endometrium.
- *Hydrosalpinx*: There should be no nodular, enhancing, or soft-tissue components with a simple hydrosalpinx.

COMMENTS

The majority of malignancies involving the fallopian tube are metastatic, almost always originating from the ovary or endometrium. Approximately 80% of fallopian tube metastases are bilateral.

Primary carcinoma of the fallopian tube is a rare entity, comprising less than 1% of all gynecologic malignancies. The most common histologic type is adenocarcinoma. Other histologic subtypes include clear cell and MMMT. Patients classically present with vaginal bleeding, watery vaginal discharge, and a pelvic mass or lower abdominal pain. Hydrops tubae profluens is a pathognomonic finding in primary fallopian tube carcinoma consisting of the intermittent passage of vaginal fluid or blood, followed by shrinkage of the adnexal mass.

On CT, a complex adnexal mass is usually seen. There may be dilatation of the fallopian tube with associated solid and nodular components. On MR, these tumors are typically hypointense on T1-WI, whereas on T2-WI, they are homogenously or heterogeneously hyperintense. Other typical findings on MR or CT are peritumoral ascites, intrauterine fluid, and a hydrosalpinx. In cases of fallopian tube metastases, an ovarian or endometrial neoplasm should be readily identified on cross-sectional imaging.

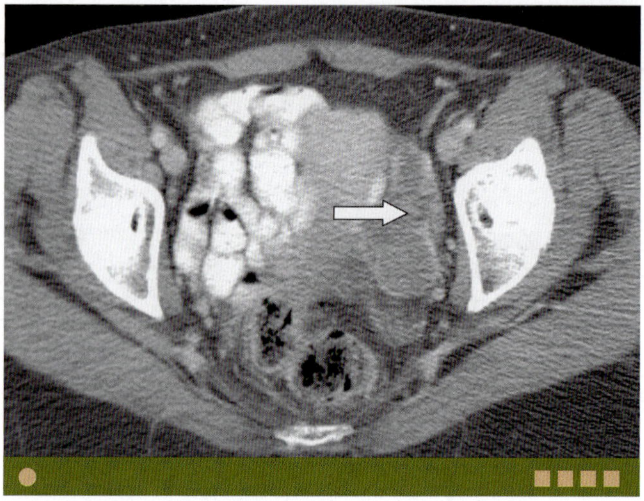

A. Axial CECT shows a tubular structure in the left adnexa with some nodular components (arrow).

The diagnosis is only definitively made with surgical resection. Accurate staging is vital as stage is the primary determinant of prognosis.

PEARLS

- **The large majority of fallopian tube neoplasms are metastatic.**
- **The most common primary fallopian tube malignancy is adenocarcinoma.**
- **A complex enhancing mass in the expected region of the fallopian tube is usually seen on CT or MR.**
- **Peritumoral ascites, intrauterine fluid and a hydrosalpinx may also be present.**

ADDITIONAL IMAGES (B-D)

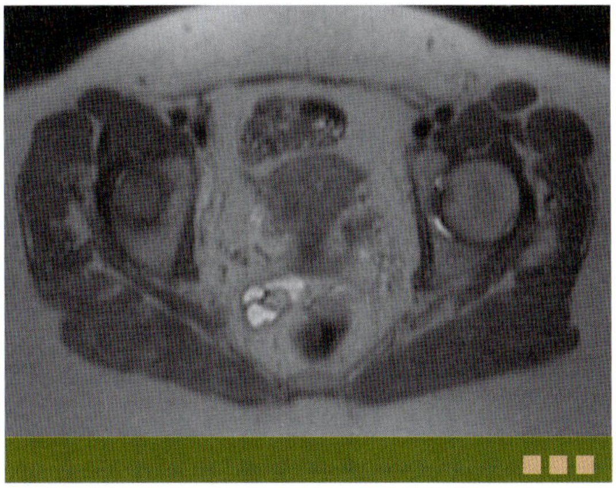

B. Axial T2-WI on another patient shows a small tubular structure posterior to the uterus with a mildly thickened wall and hyperintense components. Surgical pathology revealed early stage primary adenocarcinoma of the fallopian tube.

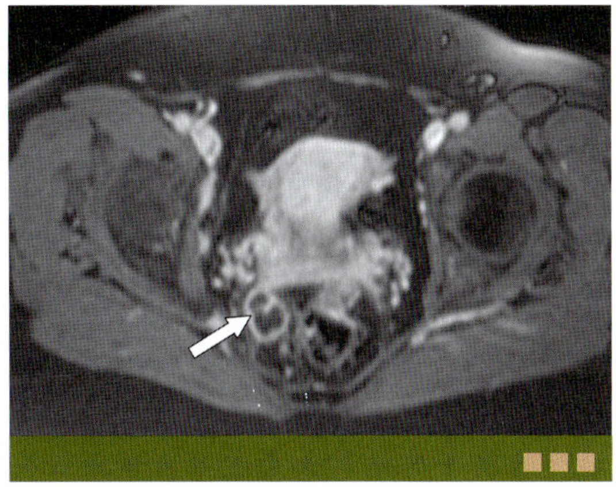

C. Axial contrast-enhanced T1-WI on the same patient shows that the wall of the fallopian tube enhances avidly (arrow).

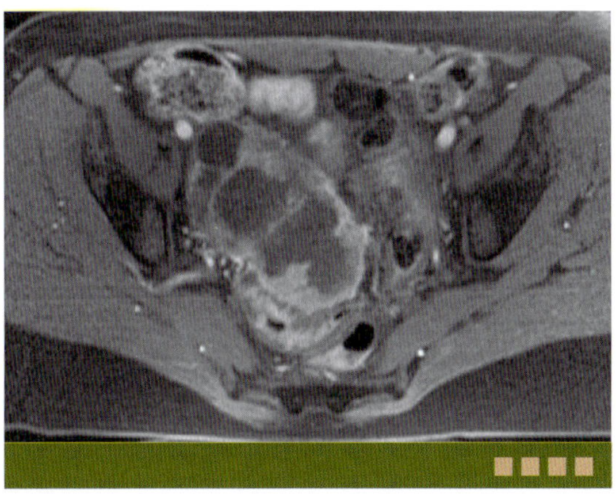

D. Axial contrast-enhanced T1-WI on a patient with known endometrial carcinoma shows a large right-sided cystic and solid lesion representing metastatic disease to the fallopian tube.

DIFFERENTIAL DIAGNOSES IMAGES (E-G)

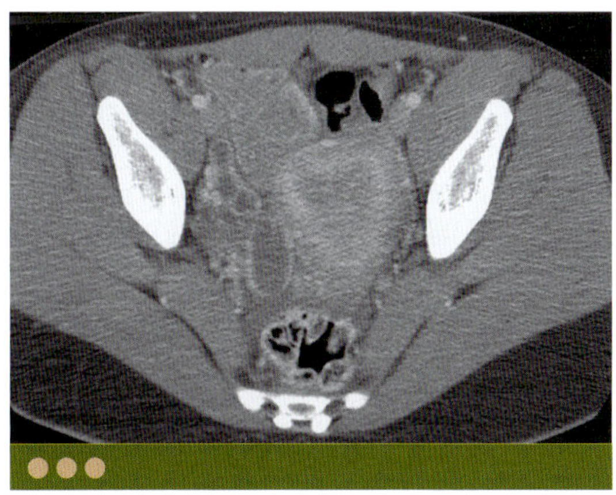

E. Tubo-ovarian abscess: Axial CECT in a young patient with clinical suspicion of pelvic inflammatory disease shows a complex tubular structure in the right adnexa with a thick wall and surrounding fluid.

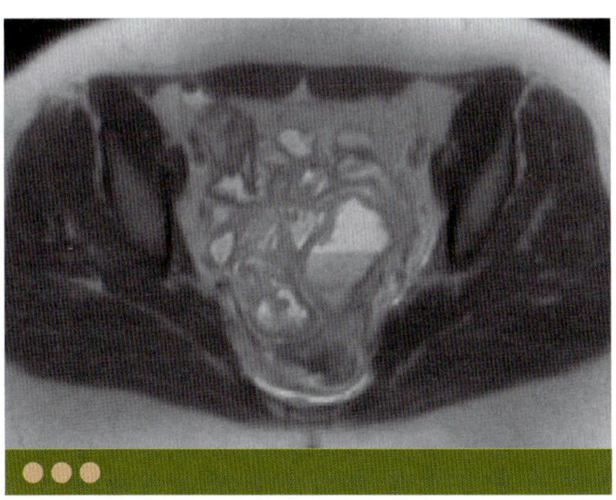

F. Tubo-ovarian abscess: Axial T2-WI on another patient shows large complex left adnexal mass with fluid–fluid levels. This patient also had signs and symptoms of severe pelvic inflammatory disease.

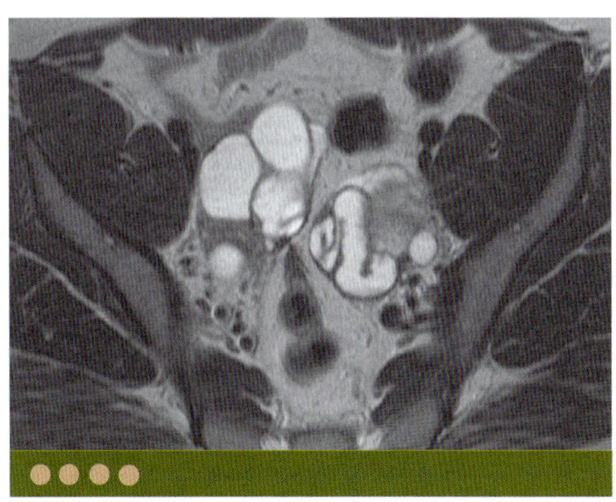

G. Hydrosalpinx: Axial T2-WI shows bilateral hyperintense tubular structures, representing dilated fallopian tubes. There are no suspicious solid or nodular components.

IMAGE KEY

Common

Rare

Typical

Unusual

16–46 Hydrosalpinx

Paul Nikolaidis

PRESENTATION

Infertility, endometriosis, history of pelvic inflammatory disease.

FINDINGS

Axial T2-WI MR shows bilateral tubular structures that connect to the ovaries and have a folded appearance. HSG shows dilated, obstructed fallopian tubes.

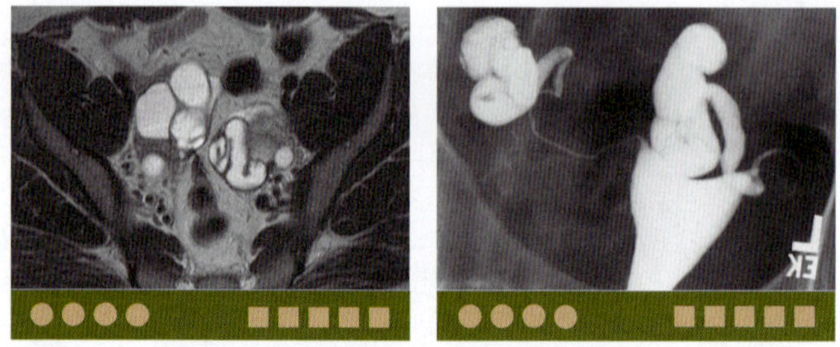

A. and B. Axial T2-WI MR (A) shows bilateral hyperintense tubular structures which connect to the ovaries. HSG (B) on the same patient performed 6 months later shows dilated fallopian tubes with no evidence of contrast spillage into the peritoneal cavity, indicating obstruction.

DIFFERENTIAL DIAGNOSES

- *Peritoneal inclusion cysts*: Septated and multiloculated rather than tubular in configuration; tend to loculate and conform to surrounding structures, rather than displace them.
- *Cystic ovarian lesions (cystadenoma or cystadenocarcinoma)*: Should not have a folded, tubular appearance; are usually rounder.

COMMENTS

A hydrosalpinx refers to a dilated, obstructed fallopian tube. A hydrosalpinx may be secondary to chronic or acute infection (salpingitis), endometriosis, or following pelvic surgery as a result of formation of adhesions. Patients are usually asymptomatic, although they may present with infertility or an adnexal mass.

A hydrosalpinx is easily detected sonographically, as a dilated tubular structure between the uterus and ovaries. If the fluid within the hydrosalpinx is simple, it should appear anechoic. It should not be mistaken for adnexal or bowel pathology. It must also be differentiated from fluid-filled bowel loops by watching for peristalsis.

A hydrosalpinx will be very well visualized on MR. The normal fallopian tubes are usually not identified on MR. A dilated tube should appear as a fluid-filled tubular structure that folds on itself to form a C or S shape. Attention to the coronal and sagittal planes is often useful in demonstrating its classic folded tubular structure. Incomplete septations within a cystic mass may be an indication of a tube folding on itself. Plicae are a feature specific to dilated tubes. Plicae typically appear as a mural nodule in one plane and a ridge in the perpendicular plane. Although the finding of plicae is specific for dilated tubes, they are frequently absent in hydrosalpinx secondary to salpingitis.

Specific signal characteristics on MR may help identify the cause of a hydrosalpinx. High-signal intensity of tubal fluid on T1-WI (especially with fat saturation) suggests a hemorrhagic component, likely from endometriosis of the pelvis and tubes. Low-signal intensity of tubal fluid is frequently seen on T2-WI in patients with acute salpingitis in addition to thickening, or a double-layered appearance of the fallopian tube wall.

PEARLS

- **Main causes of a hydrosalpinx include chronic or acute infection, endometriosis and adhesions from pelvic surgery.**
- **On ultrasound, should be differentiated from adnexal or bowel pathology, fluid-filled bowel loops, and prominent parametrial veins.**
- **High signal on T1-WI, especially on fat-saturated sequences is indicative of endometriosis.**
- **Lower signal tubal fluid on T2-WI suggests infection.**

ADDITIONAL IMAGES (C-D)

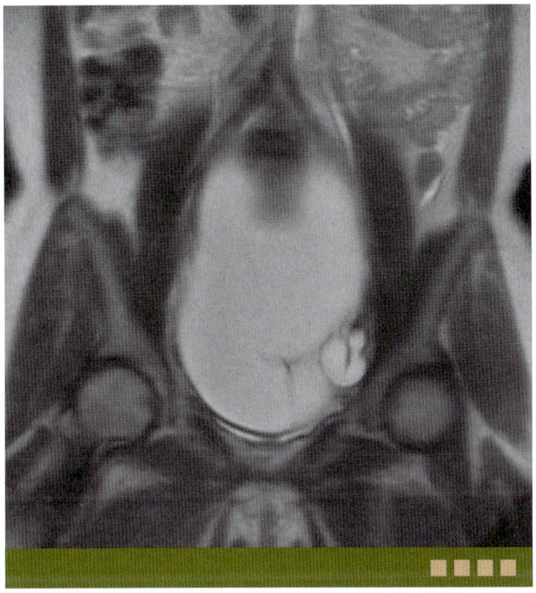

C. Coronal T2-WI MR on another patient shows a markedly dilated tubular structure representing a large hydrosalpinx.

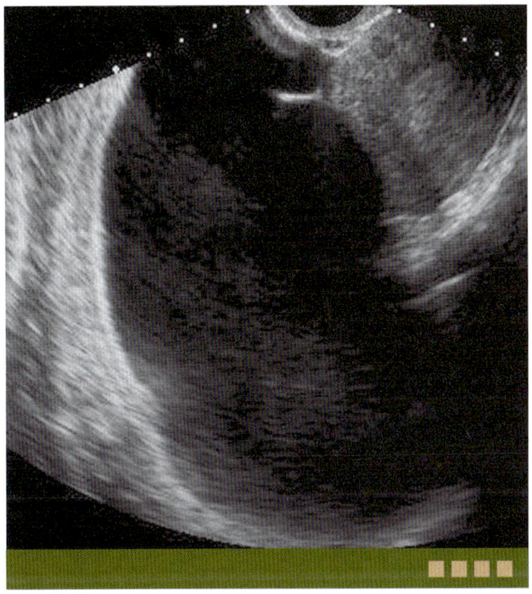

D. Coronal transvaginal sonogram on the same patient shows a large anechoic tubular structure representing the markedly dilated fallopian tube.

DIFFERENTIAL DIAGNOSES IMAGES (E-F)

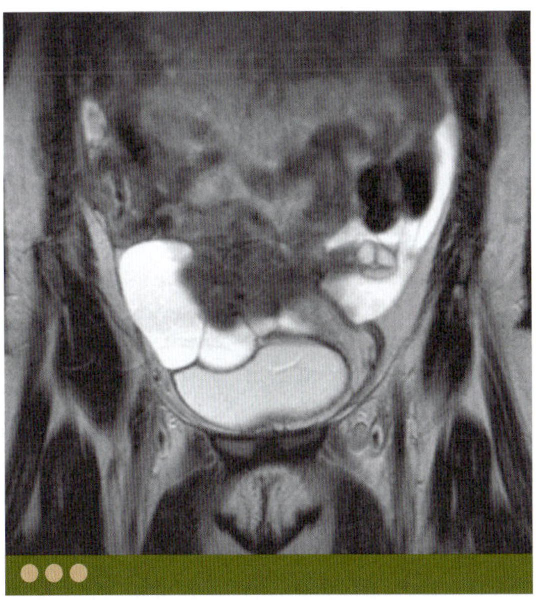

E. Peritoneal inclusion cyst: Axial T2-WI MR in a patient with a history of gynecologic surgery shows a large multiloculated fluid intensity lesion, with several septations. The fluid conforms to the surrounding structures, a feature classic of this entity.

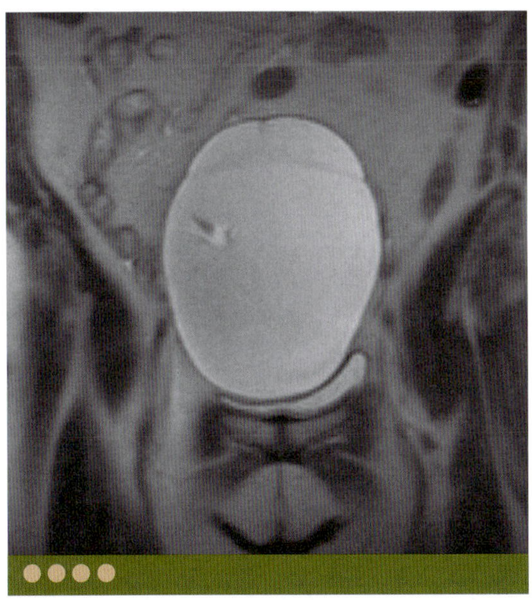

F. Ovarian cystadenocarcinoma: Coronal T2-WI MR shows a large round ovarian mass with few septations compressing the bladder. Surgical pathology revealed cystadenocarcinoma.

IMAGE KEY

Common

Rare

Typical

Unusual

16–47 Tubo-Ovarian Abscess

Paul Nikolaidis

PRESENTATION

High fever, cervical motion tenderness, adnexal tenderness and pain.

FINDINGS

MR of the pelvis shows a complex left-sided pelvic mass encompassing the left ovary, fallopian tube, and surrounding structures.

DIFFERENTIAL DIAGNOSES

- *Hydrosalpinx*: There should be no nodular, enhancing, or soft-tissue components in association with a simple hydrosalpinx.
- *Fallopian tube neoplasm*: Patients are typically older. They may have vaginal bleeding, a watery vaginal discharge, or in cases of metastatic disease, a primary malignancy of the ovary or endometrium.

COMMENTS

A tubo-ovarian abscess (TOA) is a serious complication of longstanding pelvic inflammatory disease (PID), an infection of the upper genital tract. TOA results from ascent of the infection into the fallopian tube and extension into the surrounding tissues, including the ovary. It occurs when a true abscess or an inflammatory mass results from the breakdown of the normal adnexal structures from severe inflammation. A TOA is typically caused by a polymicrobial infection with a mixture of aerobic, anerobic, and facultative organisms. The diagnosis of TOA is usually made with a combination of clinical, laboratory, and imaging findings.

TVUS should show a cystic or complex adnexal mass with internal echoes, representing debris. The abnormal, enlarged fallopian tube is often identified.

On CT, an inflammatory mass with accompanying soft tissue thickening and internal debris that is contiguous with the ovary may be seen. A thick-walled, enhancing, dilated fallopian tube is often identified. The finding of gas bubbles is a highly specific, but uncommon finding.

MR is typically reserved for cases in which the clinical or ultrasound findings are inconclusive. On MR, TOA will appear as a thick-walled, fluid-filled mass. On T2-WI, a hyperintense pus-filled cavity may be seen, surrounded by an area of hypointense fluid. The surrounding tissues are often inflamed and appear as low-signal intensity on T1-WI and intermediate- or high-signal intensity on T2-WI. Avid enhancement of its wall and surrounding tissues is commonly present after gadolinium administration.

Aggressive medical intervention with IV antibiotics for an extended period and surgical drainage when nonresponsive to antimicrobial therapy are the main treatment options.

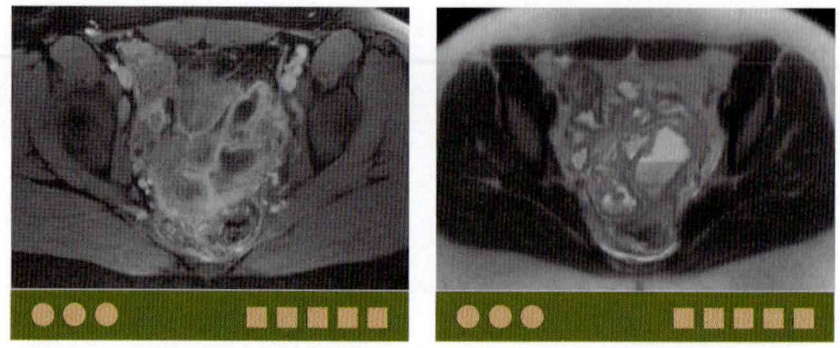

A. and **B.** Axial contrast-enhanced T1-WI (A) and T2-WI (B) of the pelvis show an enhancing large complex left-sided pelvic mass involving the left ovary, fallopian tube, and surrounding structures. Note the fluid–fluid level on T2-WI.

PEARLS

- **TOA results from spread of infection through the fallopian tube with extension into the surrounding tissues, including the ovary.**
- **It is usually a polymicrobial infection requiring aggressive medical treatment and often surgical intervention.**
- **TVUS shows a cystic or complex adnexal mass with internal echoes.**
- **CT and MR show a thick-walled enhancing adnexal mass, severe inflammatory changes and involvement of the ovary and surrounding structures.**

ADDITIONAL IMAGES (C-F)

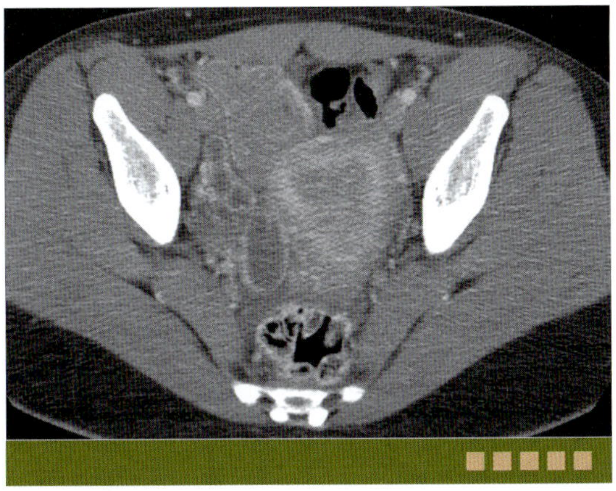

C. Axial CECT on a different patient shows a complex tubular right adnexal lesion in a patient with high-clinical suspicion of PID. The wall of the fallopian tube is thickened and enhancing.

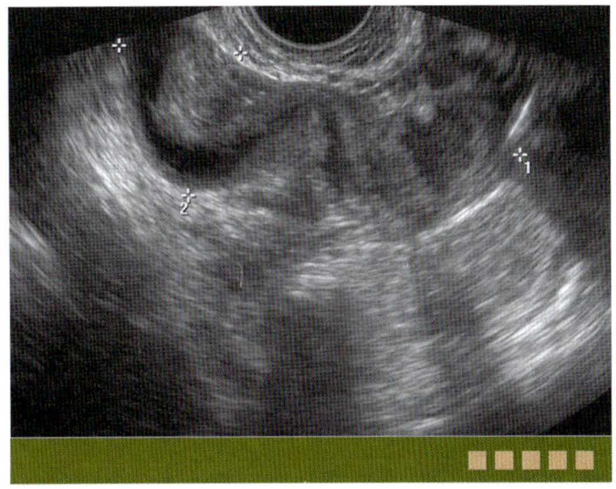

D. Sagittal sonogram on the same patient shows a complex tubular mass involving the right fallopian tube and ovary outlined by the calipers.

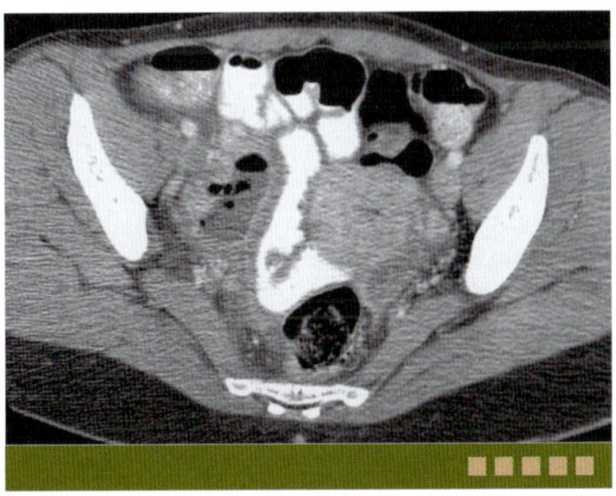

E. Axial CECT on a different patient shows a few foci of gas within the tubo-ovarian abscess. The finding of gas bubbles is a highly specific, but uncommon finding in TOA.

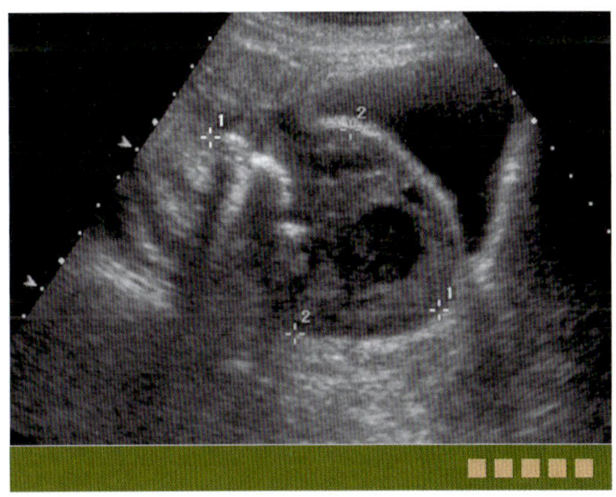

F. Corresponding sagittal sonogram on the same patient shows a complex right ovarian mass with linear echogenic foci (corresponding to the gas within the abscess).

DIFFERENTIAL DIAGNOSES IMAGES (G-H)

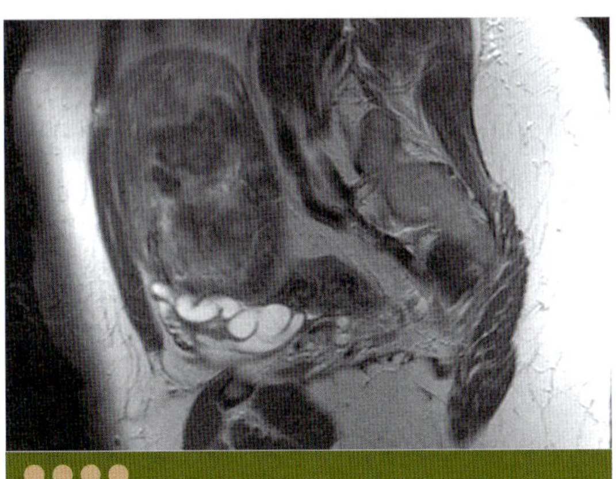

G. Hydrosalpinx: Sagittal T2-WI shows a tubular hyper-intense structure representing a simple hydrosalpinx.

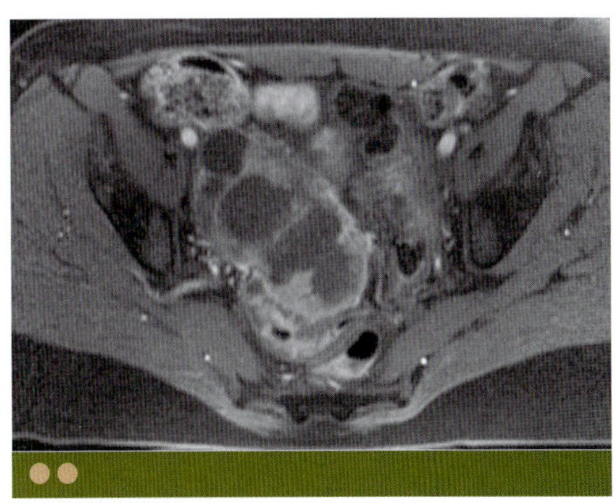

H. Fallopian tube metastasis: Axial contrast-enhanced T1-WI on an elderly female patient with history endometrial carcinoma shows a large complex mass involving the right fallopian tube and ovary.

IMAGE KEY

Common

Rare

Typical

Unusual

16–48 Salpingitis Isthmica Nodosa

Paul Nikolaidis

PRESENTATION

Infertility, history of PID or ectopic pregnancy.

FINDINGS

HSG shows multiple small diverticula extending outward from the lumen of the fallopian tubes.

DIFFERENTIAL DIAGNOSIS

- *Uterine adenomyosis*: Multiple small diverticular outpouchings extend from the endometrial cavity into the uterine wall, not from the fallopian tubes.

COMMENTS

Salpingitis isthmica nodosa (SIN) refers to the microscopic presence of tubal epithelium in the muscular portion of the fallopian tube, or beneath the tubal serosa. These pockets of epithelium protrude through the tube, similar to small diverticula. Salpingitis isthmica nodosa affects the isthmic, and occasionally, the ampullary segments of the fallopian tube. On histopathology, almost half the patients treated with salpingectomy for ectopic pregnancy had evidence of SIN.

The etiology of salpingitis isthmica nodosa is unclear. It was initially thought to represent a congenital abnormality. However, currently most authors believe that it represents an acquired condition. A pathogenesis similar to that of colonic diverticulosis has been proposed. Commonly accepted etiological theories are that SIN represents either an infectious entity, or an inflammatory entity related to endometriosis. A precise cause and effect relationship has not yet been established. Its incidence in healthy, fertile women ranges from 0.6% to 11%, but it occurs more often in the settings of ectopic pregnancy and infertility.

Diagnosis is usually made by either HSG or gynecologic surgery. Its appearance on HSG is pathognomonic. Multiple small diverticula are seen extending outward from the lumen of the isthmus or ampullary segment of the fallopian tube. There has been no established role for MR or sonography in the diagnosis of this entity.

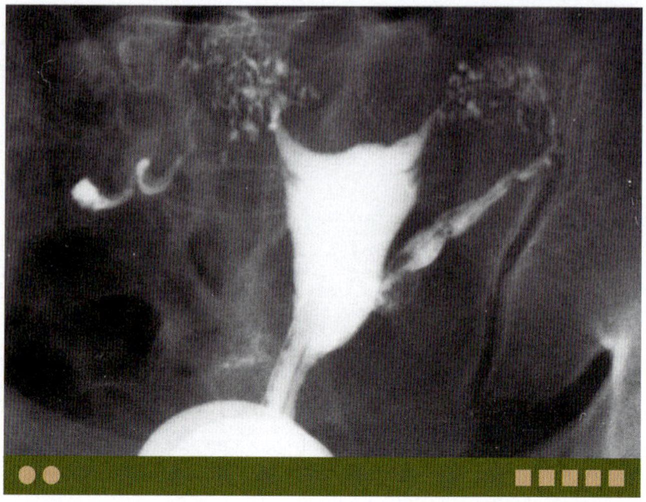

A. HSG shows multiple small diverticular outpouchings arising from the isthmic portions of both fallopian tubes. Note that neither tube is patent.

Salpingitis isthmica nodosa is often associated with tubal obstruction. A fairly high technical success rate has been reported with fluoroscopic transcervical fallopian tube recanalization.

PEARLS

- **Salpingitis isthmica nodosa refers to the presence of tubal epithelium in the muscular portion of the fallopian tube wall, or beneath the tubal serosa.**
- **These pockets of epithelium protrude through the tube, similar to small diverticula.**
- **Most likely a postinfectious or inflammatory process.**
- **On HSG, multiple small diverticula are seen protruding from the lumen of the fallopian tube.**

ADDITIONAL IMAGES (B-C)

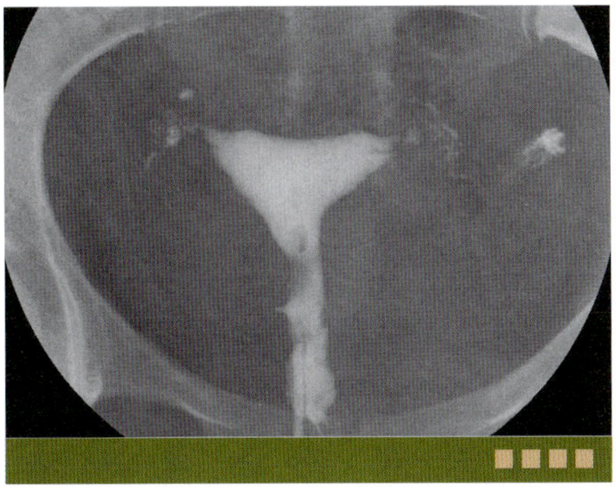

B. HSG on a different patient shows subtle, smaller diverticular outpouchings arising from the isthmic portions of both fallopian tubes.

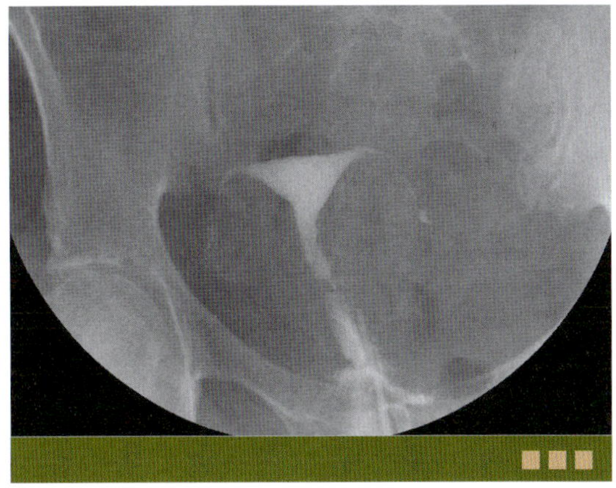

C. HSG on a different patient shows unilateral involvement of the ampullary portion of the right fallopian tube with SIN.

DIFFERENTIAL DIAGNOSIS IMAGES (D-E)

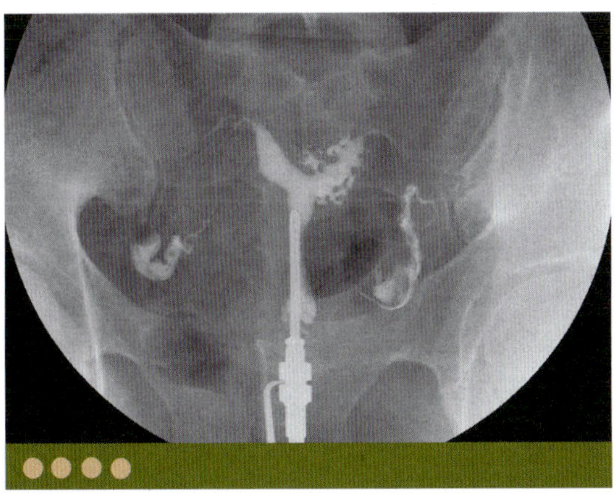

D. Adenomyosis on HSG: HSG shows normal, patent fallopian tubes and numerous small diverticular outpouchings into the left side of uterine wall, representing filling of endometrial glands extending into the myometrium.

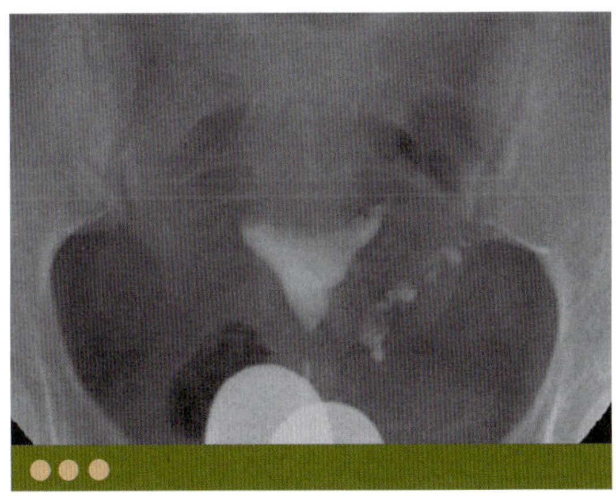

E. Irregularity of the left fallopian tube: HSG shows opacification of only the left fallopian tube that has a somewhat nodular appearance. This should not be confused with the diverticular outpouchings seen in SIN.

IMAGE KEY

Common

Rare

Typical

Unusual

INDEX

Page numbers followed by *f* indicate figures. Page numbers in **boldface** indicate major discussions.

S